Nelson
Essentials
of Pediatrics

EXCEL IN YOUR PE
rotation, residency or practice!

Nelson Textbook of Pediatrics, 19th Edition

Expert Consult — Online and Print

By Robert M. Kliegman, MD et al.

This streamlined edition covers the latest on **genetics, neurology, infectious disease, melamine poisoning, sexual identity and adolescent homosexuality, psychosis associated with epilepsy,** and more.

The Harriet Lane Handbook, 20th Edition

Expert Consult — Online and Print

By Johns Hopkins Hospital, Jamie Laubisch, MD and Branden Engorn, MD

Trusted by generations of **residents and practitioners**, this title remains your first choice for **fast, accurate information** on pediatric diagnosis and treatment.

Fetal & Neonatal Secrets, 3rd Edition

By Richard A. Polin, MD and Alan R. Spitzer, MD

With its user-friendly Q&A format, practical tips from neonatologists and fetal medicine experts, and "Key Points" boxes, this portable and easy-to-read reference provides **rapid access to the practical knowledge you need** to succeed both in practice and on exams.

Fetal and Neonatal Physiology, 4th Edition

Expert Consult — Online and Print

By Richard A. Polin, MD, William W. Fox, MD and Steven H. Abman, MD

latest information on genetic therapy, roimaging, and much more.

d Companion

. Stryjewski, MD, MPH
Competencies developed by rates the **thought processes** on pediatric presentations.

ide to Pediatrics

r workup plans for the with **quick, focused** ie patient.

tion

Dlitt(Hon)
is the **nuances of the child/family** ucial interpersonal skills, and important ons, and athletic participation.

today's child.

Order today! Ca   w.elsevierhealth.com!

Nelson
Essentials
of Pediatrics

7th Edition

Karen J. Marcdante, MD
Professor
Department of Pediatrics
Medical College of Wisconsin
Children's Hospital of Wisconsin
Milwaukee, Wisconsin

Robert M. Kliegman, MD
Professor and Chairman Emeritus
Department of Pediatrics
Medical College of Wisconsin
Children's Hospital of Wisconsin
Milwaukee, Wisconsin

ELSEVIER
SAUNDERS

1600 John F. Kennedy Blvd.
Ste 1800
Philadelphia, PA 19103-2899

NELSON ESSENTIALS OF PEDIATRICS, SEVENTH EDITION   ISBN: 978-1-4557-5980-4
INTERNATIONAL EDITION   ISBN: 978-0-323-22700-1
Copyright © 2015, 2011, 2006, 2002, 1998, 1994, 1990 by Saunders, an imprint of Elsevier Inc.

Notices

Knowledge and best practice in this field are constantly changing. As new research and experience broaden our understanding, changes in research methods, professional practices, or medical treatment may become necessary.

Practitioners and researchers must always rely on their own experience and knowledge in evaluating and using any information, methods, compounds, or experiments described herein. In using such information or methods they should be mindful of their own safety and the safety of others, including parties for whom they have a professional responsibility.

With respect to any drug or pharmaceutical products identified, readers are advised to check the most current information provided (i) on procedures featured or (ii) by the manufacturer of each product to be administered, to verify the recommended dose or formula, the method and duration of administration, and contraindications. It is the responsibility of practitioners, relying on their own experience and knowledge of their patients, to make diagnoses, to determine dosages and the best treatment for each individual patient, and to take all appropriate safety precautions.

To the fullest extent of the law, neither the Publisher nor the authors, contributors, or editors, assume any liability for any injury and/or damage to persons or property as a matter of products liability, negligence or otherwise, or from any use or operation of any methods, products, instructions, or ideas contained in the material herein.

Library of Congress Cataloging-in-Publication Data

Nelson essentials of pediatrics / [edited by] Karen J. Marcdante, Robert M. Kliegman.-- Seventh edition.
    p. ; cm.
  Essentials of pediatrics
  Includes bibliographical references and index.
  ISBN 978-1-4557-5980-4 (paperback : alk. paper)
  I. Marcdante, Karen J., editor of compilation. II. Kliegman, Robert, editor of compilation. III. Title:
Essentials of pediatrics.
  [DNLM: 1. Pediatrics. WS 100]
  RJ45
  618.92--dc23
                                                    2013044668

Senior Content Strategist: James Merritt
Senior Content Development Specialist: Jennifer Shreiner
Publishing Services Manager: Patricia Tannian
Project Manager: Amanda Mincher
Manager, Art and Design: Steven Stave

Printed in Canada

Last digit is the print number: 9 8 7 6 5 4 3 2 1

This book is dedicated to all of our colleagues (faculty, residents, and medical students) who demonstrate a passion for learning, a curiosity that drives advancement in the care of children, and an amazing dedication to the patients and families we are honored to serve.

Contributors

Lisa M. Allen, MD
Associate Professor
Department of Obstetrics and Gynecology
University of Toronto
The Hospital for Sick Children
Mount Sinai Hospital
Toronto, Ontario
Canada
Adolescent Medicine

Warren P. Bishop, MD
Professor
Department of Pediatrics
University of Iowa Carver College of Medicine
Director, Division of Gastroenterology
University of Iowa Children's Hospital
Iowa City, Iowa
The Digestive System

Kim Blake, MD, MRCP, FRCPC
Professor of General Pediatrics
IWK Health Centre
Division of Medical Education
Dalhousie University
Halifax, Nova Scotia
Canada
Adolescent Medicine

Nathan J. Blum, MD
Professor
Department of Pediatrics
The Perelman School of Medicine at the University
    of Pennsylvania
Director, Leadership Education in Neurodevelopmental
    Disabilities
Program Director, Developmental-Behavioral Pediatrics
    Fellowship Program
Division of Child Development and Metabolic Disease
The Children's Hospital of Philadelphia
Philadelphia, Pennsylvania
Psychosocial Issues

Raed Bou-Matar, MD
Associate Staff
Center for Pediatric Nephrology
Cleveland Clinic Foundation
Cleveland, Ohio
Fluids and Electrolytes

Scott J. Brown, MD
Developmental-Behavioral Pediatric Fellow
Department of Pediatrics
University of California, San Diego
La Jolla, California
Behavioral Disorders

April O. Buchanan, MD
Associate Professor
Department of Pediatrics
Academic Director, Years 3 and 4
University of South Carolina School of Medicine Greenville
Pediatric Hospitalist
Children's Hospital, Greenville Health System
Greenville, South Carolina
Pediatric Nutrition and Nutritional Disorders

Asriani M. Chiu, MD
Associate Professor of Pediatrics
Division of Pediatric Allergy and Immunology
Director, Asthma and Allergy
Director, Allergy and Immunology Fellowship Program
Medical College of Wisconsin
Milwaukee, Wisconsin
Allergy

Yvonne E. Chiu, MD
Assistant Professor
Department of Dermatology
Medical College of Wisconsin
Milwaukee, Wisconsin
Dermatology

Cindy W. Christian, MD
Professor
Department of Pediatrics
The Perelman School of Medicine at the University
    of Pennsylvania
Director, Safe Place
The Children's Hospital of Philadelphia
Philadelphia, Pennsylvania
Psychosocial Issues

David Dimmock, MD
Assistant Professor
Department of Pediatrics
Division of Pediatric Genetics
Medical College of Wisconsin
Milwaukee, Wisconsin
Metabolic Disorders

Dawn R. Ebach, MD
Clinical Associate Professor
Department of Pediatrics
University of Iowa Carver College of Medicine
Iowa City, Iowa
The Digestive System

Sheila Gahagan, MD, MPH
Professor and Chief
Academic General Pediatrics, Child Development and
    Community Health
Martin Stein Endowed Chair, Developmental-Behavioral
    Pediatrics
University of California, San Diego
La Jolla, California
Behavioral Disorders

Clarence W. Gowen, Jr., MD, FAAP
Associate Professor and Interim Chair
Department of Pediatrics
Eastern Virginia Medical School
Interim Senior Vice President for Academic Affairs
Director of Medical Education
Director of Pediatric Residency Program
Children's Hospital of The King's Daughters
Norfolk, Virginia
Fetal and Neonatal Medicine

Larry A. Greenbaum, MD, PhD
Marcus Professor of Pediatrics
Director, Division of Pediatric Nephrology
Emory University School of Medicine
Chief, Pediatric Nephrology
Emory-Children's Center
Atlanta, Georgia
Fluids and Electrolytes

Hilary M. Haftel, MD, MHPE
Clinical Associate Professor
Departments of Pediatrics and Communicable Diseases
    and Internal Medicine
Director of Pediatric Education
Pediatric Residency Director
University of Michigan Medical School
Ann Arbor, Michigan
Rheumatic Diseases of Childhood

MaryKathleen Heneghan, MD
Attending Physician
Division of Pediatric Endocrinology
Advocate Lutheran General Children's Hospital
Park Ridge, Illinois
Endocrinology

Matthew P. Kronman, MD, MSCE
Assistant Professor of Pediatrics
University of Washington School of Medicine
Division of Pediatric Infectious Diseases
Seattle Children's Hospital
Seattle, Washington
Infectious Diseases

K. Jane Lee, MD
Assistant Professor of Pediatrics, Bioethics, and Medical
    Humanities
Program Director, Pediatric Critical Care Fellowship
Medical College of Wisconsin
Institute for Health and Society
Milwaukee, Wisconsin
The Acutely Ill or Injured Child

David A. Levine, MD
Professor
Department of Pediatrics
Chief, Division of Pre-doctoral Education
Morehouse School of Medicine
Atlanta, Georgia
Growth and Development

Paul A. Levy, MD, FACMG
Assistant Professor
Departments of Pediatrics and Pathology
Albert Einstein College of Medicine of Yeshiva University
Attending Geneticist
Children's Hospital at Montefiore
Bronx, New York
Human Genetics and Dysmorphology

Yi Hui Liu, MD, MPH
Assistant Professor
Department of Pediatrics
University of California, San Diego
La Jolla, California
Behavioral Disorders

John D. Mahan, MD
Professor, Department of Pediatrics
Program Director, Pediatric Residency Program
Program Director, Pediatric Nephrology Fellowship Program
Vice-Chair for Education
The Ohio State University College of Medicine
Nationwide Children's Hospital
Columbus, Ohio
Nephrology and Urology

Robert W. Marion, MD
Professor
Department of Pediatrics
Department of Obstetrics and Gynecology and Women's
    Health
Ruth L. Gottesman Chair in Developmental Pediatrics
Chief, Section of Child Development
Chief, Section of Genetics
Department of Pediatrics
Albert Einstein College of Medicine of Yeshiva University
Bronx, New York
Human Genetics and Dysmorphology

Maria L. Marquez, MD
Associate Professor
Department of Pediatrics
Georgetown University School of Medicine
Director, Medical Student Education
Georgetown University Hospital
Washington, DC
Pediatric Nutrition and Nutritional Disorders

Susan G. Marshall, MD
Professor
Department of Pediatrics
University of Washington School of Medicine
Attending Physician
Pulmonary Division
Seattle Children's Hospital
Seattle, Washington
The Respiratory System

Thomas W. McLean, MD
Associate Professor
Department of Pediatrics
Wake Forest University Baptist Medical Center
Winston-Salem, North Carolina
Oncology

Thida Ong, MD
Assistant Professor
Department of Pediatrics
University of Washington School of Medicine
Attending Physician
Pulmonary Division
Seattle Children's Hospital
Seattle, Washington
The Respiratory System

Julie A. Panepinto, MD, MSPH
Professor
Department of Pediatrics
Medical College of Wisconsin
Division of Pediatric Hematology
The Children's Research Institute of the Children's Hospital
    of Wisconsin
Milwaukee, Wisconsin
Hematology

Hiren P. Patel, MD
Clinical Associate Professor
Department of Pediatrics
The Ohio State University College of Medicine
Chief, Section of Nephrology
Medical Director, Renal Dialysis Unit
Nationwide Children's Hospital
Columbus, Ohio
Nephrology and Urology

Rowena C. Punzalan, MD
Assistant Professor
Department of Pediatrics
Medical College of Wisconsin
Division of Pediatric Hematology
The Children's Research Institute of the Children's Hospital
    of Wisconsin
Milwaukee, Wisconsin
Hematology

Russell Scheffer, MD
Chair and Professor
Department of Psychiatry and Behavioral Sciences
Professor
Department of Pediatrics
University of Kansas School of Medicine–Wichita
Wichita, Kansas
Psychiatric Disorders

Jocelyn Huang Schiller, MD
Clinical Assistant Professor
Department of Pediatrics
University of Michigan Medical School
Division of Pediatric Neurology
C.S. Mott Children's Hospital
Ann Arbor, Michigan
Neurology

Daniel S. Schneider, MD
Associate Professor
Department of Pediatrics
University of Virginia School of Medicine
Charlottesville, Virginia
The Cardiovascular System

J. Paul Scott, MD
Professor
Department of Pediatrics
Medical College of Wisconsin
Medical Director, Wisconsin Sickle Cell Center
The Children's Research Institute of the Children's Hospital
    of Wisconsin
Milwaukee, Wisconsin
Hematology

Renée A. Shellhaas, MD, MS
Clinical Assistant Professor
Department of Pediatrics
University of Michigan Medical School
Division of Pediatric Neurology
C.S. Mott Children's Hospital
Ann Arbor, Michigan
Neurology

Benjamin S. Siegel, MD
Director, Medical Student Education in Pediatrics
Professor
Department of Pediatrics
Boston University School of Medicine
Boston, Massachusetts
The Profession of Pediatrics

Paola A. Palma Sisto, MD
Associate Professor
Department of Pediatrics
University of Connecticut School of Medicine
Director, Endocrinology Program
Division of Pediatric Endocrinology
Connecticut Children's Medical Center
Hartford, Connecticut
Endocrinology

Sherilyn Smith, MD
Professor of Pediatrics
Fellowship Director, Pediatric Infectious Disease
University of Washington School of Medicine
Associate Clerkship Director
Seattle Children's Hospital
Seattle, Washington
Infectious Diseases

Amanda Striegl, MD, MS
Assistant Professor
Department of Pediatrics
University of Washington School of Medicine
Attending Physician
Pulmonary Division
Seattle Children's Hospital
Seattle, Washington
The Respiratory System

J. Channing Tassone, MD
Associate Professor
Departments of Orthopedic Surgery and Pediatrics
Medical College of Wisconsin
Division of Pediatric Orthopedic Surgery
Children's Hospital of Wisconsin
Milwaukee, Wisconsin
Orthopedics

Aveekshit Tripathi, MD
Senior Psychiatry Resident
Department of Psychiatry and Behavioral Sciences
University of Kansas School of Medicine–Wichita
Wichita, Kansas
Psychiatric Disorders

James W. Verbsky, MD, PhD
Assistant Professor
Department of Pediatrics
Department of Microbiology and Molecular Genetics
Division of Pediatric Rheumatology
Medical College of Wisconsin
Children's Hospital of Wisconsin
Milwaukee, Wisconsin
Immunology

Kevin D. Walter, MD, FAAP
Assistant Professor
Departments of Orthopedic Surgery and Pediatrics
Medical College of Wisconsin
Program Director, Primary Care Sports Medicine
Children's Hospital of Wisconsin
Milwaukee, Wisconsin
Orthopedics

Marcia M. Wofford, MD
Associate Professor
Department of Pediatrics
Wake Forest University Baptist Medical Center
Winston-Salem, North Carolina
Oncology

Preface

Medicine and technology just don't stop! The amazing advancements we hear about as our scientist colleagues further delineate the pathophysiology and mechanisms of diseases must eventually be translated to our daily care of patients. Our goal, as the editors and authors of this textbook, is not only to provide the classic, foundational knowledge we use every day but to include these advances in a readable and concise text for medical students and residents.

This new edition has been updated with the advances that have occurred since the last edition. We have also incorporated technology by linking this book to the second edition of *Pediatric Decision Making Strategies* by Pomeranz, Busey, Sabnis, and Kliegman. This will allow you to read about the medical issues and then follow a link to an algorithm to facilitate efficient and effective evaluations.

We believe this integration will help you investigate the common and classic pediatric disorders in a time-honored, logical format to both acquire knowledge and apply knowledge to your patients. We have also once again asked our colleagues who serve as clerkship directors to write many of the sections so that you can gain the knowledge and skills necessary to succeed both in caring for patients and in preparing for clerkship or in-service examinations.

We are honored to be part of the journey of thousands of learners who rotate through pediatrics as well as those who will become new providers of pediatric care in the years to come.

Karen J. Marcdante, MD
Robert M. Kliegman, MD

Acknowledgments

The editors could never have published this edition without the assistance and attention to detail of James Merritt and Jennifer Shreiner. We also couldn't have accomplished this without Carolyn Redman, whose prompting, organizing, and overseeing of the process helped us create this new edition.

Contents

SECTION
1

The Profession of Pediatrics   1
Karen J. Marcdante and Benjamin S. Siegel

Chapter 1   POPULATION AND CULTURE: THE CARE OF CHILDREN IN SOCIETY   1

Chapter 2   PROFESSIONALISM   4

Chapter 3   ETHICS AND LEGAL ISSUES   5

Chapter 4   PALLIATIVE CARE AND END-OF-LIFE ISSUES   7

SECTION
2

Growth and Development   10
David A. Levine

Chapter 5   NORMAL GROWTH   10

Chapter 6   DISORDERS OF GROWTH   12

Chapter 7   NORMAL DEVELOPMENT   13

Chapter 8   DISORDERS OF DEVELOPMENT   15

Chapter 9   EVALUATION OF THE WELL CHILD   20

Chapter 10   EVALUATION OF THE CHILD WITH SPECIAL NEEDS   26

SECTION
3

Behavioral Disorders   37
Sheila Gahagan, Yi Hui Liu, and Scott J. Brown

Chapter 11   CRYING AND COLIC   37

Chapter 12   TEMPER TANTRUMS   39

Chapter 13   ATTENTION-DEFICIT/HYPERACTIVITY DISORDER   41

Chapter 14   CONTROL OF ELIMINATION   43

Chapter 15   NORMAL SLEEP AND PEDIATRIC SLEEP DISORDERS   47

SECTION
4

Psychiatric Disorders   51
Russell Scheffer and Aveekshit Tripathi

Chapter 16   SOMATOFORM DISORDERS, FACTITIOUS DISORDERS, AND MALINGERING   51

Chapter 17   ANXIETY AND PHOBIAS   55

Chapter 18   DEPRESSION AND BIPOLAR DISORDERS   59

Chapter 19   OBSESSIVE-COMPULSIVE DISORDER   62

Chapter 20   PERVASIVE DEVELOPMENTAL DISORDERS AND PSYCHOSES   63

SECTION
5

Psychosocial Issues   67
Cindy W. Christian and Nathan J. Blum

Chapter 21   FAILURE TO THRIVE   67

Chapter 22   CHILD ABUSE AND NEGLECT   70

Chapter 23   HOMOSEXUALITY AND GENDER IDENTITY   75

Chapter 24   FAMILY STRUCTURE AND FUNCTION   76

Chapter **25**   VIOLENCE   79

Chapter **26**   DIVORCE, SEPARATION, AND BEREAVEMENT   82

SECTION 6

Pediatric Nutrition and Nutritional Disorders   86

April O. Buchanan and Maria L. Marquez

Chapter **27**   DIET OF THE NORMAL INFANT   86

Chapter **28**   DIET OF THE NORMAL CHILD AND ADOLESCENT   89

Chapter **29**   OBESITY   90

Chapter **30**   PEDIATRIC UNDERNUTRITION   93

Chapter **31**   VITAMIN AND MINERAL DEFICIENCIES   96

SECTION 7

Fluids and Electrolytes   106

Larry A. Greenbaum and Raed Bou-Matar

Chapter **32**   MAINTENANCE FLUID THERAPY   106

Chapter **33**   DEHYDRATION AND REPLACEMENT THERAPY   107

Chapter **34**   PARENTERAL NUTRITION   111

Chapter **35**   SODIUM DISORDERS   112

Chapter **36**   POTASSIUM DISORDERS   116

Chapter **37**   ACID-BASE DISORDERS   119

SECTION 8

The Acutely Ill or Injured Child   124

K. Jane Lee

Chapter **38**   ASSESSMENT AND RESUSCITATION   124

Chapter **39**   RESPIRATORY FAILURE   128

Chapter **40**   SHOCK   129

Chapter **41**   INJURY PREVENTION   133

Chapter **42**   MAJOR TRAUMA   133

Chapter **43**   DROWNING   136

Chapter **44**   BURNS   137

Chapter **45**   POISONING   139

Chapter **46**   SEDATION AND ANALGESIA   144

SECTION 9

Human Genetics and Dysmorphology   146

Paul A. Levy and Robert W. Marion

Chapter **47**   PATTERNS OF INHERITANCE   146

Chapter **48**   GENETIC ASSESSMENT   154

Chapter **49**   CHROMOSOMAL DISORDERS   156

Chapter **50**   THE APPROACH TO THE DYSMORPHIC CHILD   160

SECTION 10

Metabolic Disorders   164

David Dimmock

Chapter **51**   METABOLIC ASSESSMENT   164

Chapter **52**   CARBOHYDRATE DISORDERS   172

Chapter **53**   AMINO ACID DISORDERS   174

Chapter **54**   ORGANIC ACID DISORDERS   177

Chapter **55**   FAT METABOLIC DISORDERS   179

Chapter **56**   LYSOSOMAL AND PEROXISOMAL DISORDERS   180

Chapter **57**   MITOCHONDRIAL DISORDERS   183

SECTION 11

Fetal and Neonatal Medicine 186
Clarence W. Gowen, Jr.

Chapter 58 ASSESSMENT OF THE MOTHER, FETUS, AND NEWBORN 186

Chapter 59 MATERNAL DISEASES AFFECTING THE NEWBORN 204

Chapter 60 DISEASES OF THE FETUS 208

Chapter 61 RESPIRATORY DISEASES OF THE NEWBORN 209

Chapter 62 ANEMIA AND HYPERBILIRUBINEMIA 216

Chapter 63 NECROTIZING ENTEROCOLITIS 223

Chapter 64 HYPOXIC-ISCHEMIC ENCEPHALOPATHY, INTRACRANIAL HEMORRHAGE, AND SEIZURES 224

Chapter 65 SEPSIS AND MENINGITIS 227

Chapter 66 CONGENITAL INFECTIONS 229

SECTION 12

Adolescent Medicine 234
Kim Blake and Lisa M. Allen

Chapter 67 OVERVIEW AND ASSESSMENT OF ADOLESCENTS 234

Chapter 68 WELL-ADOLESCENT CARE 240

Chapter 69 ADOLESCENT GYNECOLOGY 242

Chapter 70 EATING DISORDERS 248

Chapter 71 SUBSTANCE ABUSE 250

SECTION 13

Immunology 252
James W. Verbsky

Chapter 72 ASSESSMENT 252

Chapter 73 LYMPHOCYTE DISORDERS 256

Chapter 74 NEUTROPHIL DISORDERS 263

Chapter 75 COMPLEMENT SYSTEM 266

Chapter 76 HEMATOPOIETIC STEM CELL TRANSPLANTATION 269

SECTION 14

Allergy 271
Asriani M. Chiu

Chapter 77 ASSESSMENT 271

Chapter 78 ASTHMA 273

Chapter 79 ALLERGIC RHINITIS 282

Chapter 80 ATOPIC DERMATITIS 285

Chapter 81 URTICARIA, ANGIOEDEMA, AND ANAPHYLAXIS 288

Chapter 82 SERUM SICKNESS 292

Chapter 83 INSECT ALLERGIES 293

Chapter 84 ADVERSE REACTIONS TO FOODS 294

Chapter 85 ADVERSE REACTIONS TO DRUGS 296

SECTION 15

Rheumatic Diseases of Childhood 299
Hilary M. Haftel

Chapter 86 ASSESSMENT 299

Chapter 87 HENOCH-SCHÖNLEIN PURPURA 301

Chapter 88 KAWASAKI DISEASE 303

Chapter 89 JUVENILE IDIOPATHIC ARTHRITIS 305

Chapter 90 SYSTEMIC LUPUS ERYTHEMATOSUS 309

Chapter 91 JUVENILE DERMATOMYOSITIS 311

Chapter 92 MUSCULOSKELETAL PAIN SYNDROMES 312

SECTION 16

Infectious Diseases 315
Matthew P. Kronman and Sherilyn Smith

Chapter 93   ASSESSMENT 315

Chapter 94   IMMUNIZATION AND PROPHYLAXIS 317

Chapter 95   ANTI-INFECTIVE THERAPY 323

Chapter 96   FEVER WITHOUT A FOCUS 324

Chapter 97   INFECTIONS CHARACTERIZED BY FEVER AND RASH 329

Chapter 98   CUTANEOUS INFECTIONS 335

Chapter 99   LYMPHADENOPATHY 338

Chapter 100   MENINGITIS 342

Chapter 101   ENCEPHALITIS 344

Chapter 102   THE COMMON COLD 346

Chapter 103   PHARYNGITIS 347

Chapter 104   SINUSITIS 350

Chapter 105   OTITIS MEDIA 351

Chapter 106   OTITIS EXTERNA 353

Chapter 107   CROUP (LARYNGOTRACHEOBRONCHITIS) 354

Chapter 108   PERTUSSIS 356

Chapter 109   BRONCHIOLITIS 357

Chapter 110   PNEUMONIA 358

Chapter 111   INFECTIVE ENDOCARDITIS 364

Chapter 112   ACUTE GASTROENTERITIS 366

Chapter 113   VIRAL HEPATITIS 369

Chapter 114   URINARY TRACT INFECTION 372

Chapter 115   VULVOVAGINITIS 374

Chapter 116   SEXUALLY TRANSMITTED INFECTIONS 376

Chapter 117   OSTEOMYELITIS 381

Chapter 118   INFECTIOUS ARTHRITIS 384

Chapter 119   OCULAR INFECTIONS 386

Chapter 120   INFECTION IN THE IMMUNOCOMPROMISED PERSON 390

Chapter 121   INFECTIONS ASSOCIATED WITH MEDICAL DEVICES 394

Chapter 122   ZOONOSES 396

Chapter 123   PARASITIC DISEASES 402

Chapter 124   TUBERCULOSIS 407

Chapter 125   HIV AND AIDS 412

SECTION 17

The Digestive System 417
Warren P. Bishop and Dawn R. Ebach

Chapter 126   ASSESSMENT 417

Chapter 127   ORAL CAVITY 429

Chapter 128   ESOPHAGUS AND STOMACH 430

Chapter 129   INTESTINAL TRACT 437

Chapter 130   LIVER DISEASE 444

Chapter 131   PANCREATIC DISEASE 450

Chapter 132   PERITONITIS 453

SECTION 18

The Respiratory System 455
Thida Ong, Amanda Striegl, and Susan G. Marshall

Chapter 133   RESPIRATORY SYSTEM ASSESSMENT 455

Chapter 134   CONTROL OF BREATHING 461

Chapter 135   UPPER AIRWAY OBSTRUCTION 464

Chapter 136   LOWER AIRWAY, PARENCHYMAL, AND PULMONARY VASCULAR DISEASES 469

Chapter 137   CYSTIC FIBROSIS 475

Chapter 138   CHEST WALL AND PLEURA 478

SECTION 19

The Cardiovascular System   481
Daniel S. Schneider

Chapter 139   CARDIOVASCULAR SYSTEM ASSESSMENT   481

Chapter 140   SYNCOPE   486

Chapter 141   CHEST PAIN   487

Chapter 142   DYSRHYTHMIAS   488

Chapter 143   ACYANOTIC CONGENITAL HEART DISEASE   491

Chapter 144   CYANOTIC CONGENITAL HEART DISEASE   495

Chapter 145   HEART FAILURE   499

Chapter 146   RHEUMATIC FEVER   501

Chapter 147   CARDIOMYOPATHIES   502

Chapter 148   PERICARDITIS   504

SECTION 20

Hematology   506
Julie A. Panepinto, Rowena C. Punzalan, and J. Paul Scott

Chapter 149   HEMATOLOGY ASSESSMENT   506

Chapter 150   ANEMIA   509

Chapter 151   HEMOSTATIC DISORDERS   523

Chapter 152   BLOOD COMPONENT THERAPY   532

SECTION 21

Oncology   534
Thomas W. McLean and Marcia M. Wofford

Chapter 153   ONCOLOGY ASSESSMENT   534

Chapter 154   PRINCIPLES OF CANCER TREATMENT   538

Chapter 155   LEUKEMIA   542

Chapter 156   LYMPHOMA   544

Chapter 157   CENTRAL NERVOUS SYSTEM TUMORS   546

Chapter 158   NEUROBLASTOMA   548

Chapter 159   WILMS TUMOR   550

Chapter 160   SARCOMAS   551

SECTION 22

Nephrology and Urology   553
John D. Mahan and Hiren P. Patel

Chapter 161   NEPHROLOGY AND UROLOGY ASSESSMENT   553

Chapter 162   NEPHROTIC SYNDROME AND PROTEINURIA   556

Chapter 163   GLOMERULONEPHRITIS AND HEMATURIA   558

Chapter 164   HEMOLYTIC UREMIC SYNDROME   560

Chapter 165   ACUTE AND CHRONIC RENAL FAILURE   561

Chapter 166   HYPERTENSION   563

Chapter 167   VESICOURETERAL REFLUX   564

Chapter 168   CONGENITAL AND DEVELOPMENTAL ABNORMALITIES OF THE URINARY TRACT   565

Chapter 169   OTHER URINARY TRACT AND GENITAL DISORDERS   567

SECTION 23

Endocrinology   570
Paola A. Palma Sisto and MaryKathleen Heneghan

Chapter 170   ENDOCRINOLOGY ASSESSMENT   570

Chapter 171   DIABETES MELLITUS   572

Chapter 172   HYPOGLYCEMIA   579

Chapter **173**   SHORT STATURE   583

Chapter **174**   DISORDERS OF PUBERTY   589

Chapter **175**   THYROID DISEASE   596

Chapter **176**   DISORDERS OF PARATHYROID BONE AND MINERAL ENDOCRINOLOGY   602

Chapter **177**   DISORDERS OF SEXUAL DEVELOPMENT   604

Chapter **178**   ADRENAL GLAND DYSFUNCTION   607

SECTION 24

Neurology   612
Jocelyn Huang Schiller and Renée A. Shellhaas

Chapter **179**   NEUROLOGY ASSESSMENT   612

Chapter **180**   HEADACHE AND MIGRAINE   616

Chapter **181**   SEIZURES (PAROXYSMAL DISORDERS)   618

Chapter **182**   WEAKNESS AND HYPOTONIA   623

Chapter **183**   ATAXIA AND MOVEMENT DISORDERS   631

Chapter **184**   ALTERED MENTAL STATUS   634

Chapter **185**   NEURODEGENERATIVE DISORDERS   642

Chapter **186**   NEUROCUTANEOUS DISORDERS   645

Chapter **187**   CONGENITAL MALFORMATIONS OF THE CENTRAL NERVOUS SYSTEM   647

SECTION 25

Dermatology   650
Yvonne E. Chiu

Chapter **188**   ASSESSMENT   650

Chapter **189**   ACNE   652

Chapter **190**   ATOPIC DERMATITIS   653

Chapter **191**   CONTACT DERMATITIS   656

Chapter **192**   SEBORRHEIC DERMATITIS   657

Chapter **193**   PIGMENTED LESIONS   659

Chapter **194**   VASCULAR ANOMALIES   661

Chapter **195**   ERYTHEMA MULTIFORME, STEVENS-JOHNSON SYNDROME, AND TOXIC EPIDERMAL NECROLYSIS   662

Chapter **196**   CUTANEOUS INFESTATIONS   664

SECTION 26

Orthopedics   667
Kevin D. Walter and J. Channing Tassone

Chapter **197**   ORTHOPEDICS ASSESSMENT   667

Chapter **198**   FRACTURES   670

Chapter **199**   HIP   672

Chapter **200**   LOWER EXTREMITY AND KNEE   676

Chapter **201**   FOOT   681

Chapter **202**   SPINE   684

Chapter **203**   UPPER EXTREMITY   691

Chapter **204**   BENIGN BONE TUMORS AND CYSTIC LESIONS   693

The Profession of Pediatrics

Karen J. Marcdante and Benjamin S. Siegel

Chapter 1

POPULATION AND CULTURE: THE CARE OF CHILDREN IN SOCIETY

Health care professionals need to appreciate the interactions between medical conditions and social, economic, and environmental influences associated with the provision of pediatric care. New technologies and treatments help improve morbidity, mortality, and the quality of life for children and their families, but the costs may exacerbate disparities in medical care. The challenge for pediatricians is to deliver care that is socially equitable; integrates psychosocial, cultural, and ethical issues into practice; and ensures that health care is available to all children.

CURRENT CHALLENGES

Many challenges affect children's health outcomes. These include access to health care; health disparities; supporting their social, cognitive, and emotional lives in the context of families and communities; and addressing environmental factors, especially poverty. Early experiences and environmental stresses interact with the genetic predisposition of every child and, ultimately, may lead to the development of diseases seen in adulthood. Thus, pediatricians have the unique opportunity to address not only acute and chronic illnesses but also the aforementioned issues and toxic stressors to promote wellness and health maintenance in children.

Many scientific advances have an impact on the growing role of pediatricians. Incorporating the use of newer genetic technologies allows the diagnosis of diseases at the molecular level, aids in the selection of medications and therapies, and provides information on the prognosis of some diseases. Prenatal diagnosis and newborn screening improve the accuracy of early diagnosis of a variety of conditions, allowing for earlier treatment even when a cure is impossible. Functional magnetic resonance imaging allows a greater understanding of psychiatric and neurologic problems, such as dyslexia and attention-deficit/hyperactivity disorder.

Challenges persist with the incidence and prevalence of chronic illness having increased in recent decades. Chronic illness is now the most common reason for hospital admissions among children (excluding trauma and newborn admissions). From middle school and beyond, mental illness is the main non–childbirth-related reason for hospitalization among children. Pediatricians must also address the increasing concern about environmental toxins and the prevalence of physical, emotional, and sexual abuse, as well as violence. Since the September 11, 2001, destruction of the World Trade Center in New York City, fear of terrorism in the United States has increased the level of anxiety for many families and children.

To address these ongoing challenges, pediatricians must practice as part of a health care team. Many pediatricians already practice collaboratively with psychiatrists, psychologists, nurses, and social workers. Team composition can change, depending on location and patient needs. Although school health and school-based health clinics have improved access and outcomes for many common childhood and adolescent conditions, the shortage of available general pediatricians and family physicians has led to the development of retail medical facilities in pharmacies and retail stores.

Childhood antecedents of adult health conditions, such as alcoholism, depression, obesity, hypertension, and hyperlipidemias, are increasingly being recognized. Maternal health status can affect the fetus. Infants who are a smaller size and relatively underweight at birth because of maternal malnutrition have increased rates of coronary heart disease, stroke, type 2 diabetes mellitus, obesity, metabolic syndrome, and osteoporosis in later life. Because of improved neonatal care, a greater percentage of preterm, low birth weight, or very low birth weight newborns survive, increasing the number of children with chronic medical conditions and developmental delays with lifelong implications.

LANDSCAPE OF HEALTH CARE FOR CHILDREN IN THE UNITED STATES

Complex health, economic, and psychosocial challenges greatly influence the well-being and health outcomes of children. National reports from the Centers for Disease Control and Prevention (CDC) (e.g., http://www.cdc.gov/nchs/data/hus/hus11.pdf#102) provide information about many of these issues. Some of the key issues include the following:

- **Health insurance coverage.** In 2010 over eight million children in the United States had no health insurance coverage. In addition, 10 to 20 million were underinsured. Many children, despite public sector insurance, do not receive recommended immunizations. Although

Medicaid and the State Children's Health Insurance Program covered more than 42 million children in 2010 who otherwise would not have health care access, over a million U.S. children are unable to get needed medical care because their families cannot afford it.

- **Prenatal and perinatal care.** Ten to 25% of women do not receive prenatal care during the first trimester. In addition, a significant percentage of women continue to smoke, use illicit drugs, and consume alcohol during pregnancy.
- **Preterm births.** The incidence of preterm births (<37 weeks) peaked in 2006 and has been slowly declining (11.99% in 2010). However, the 2010 rates of low birth weight infants (≤2500 g [8.15% of all births]) and very low birth weight infants (≤1500 g [1.45% of all births]) are essentially unchanged since 2006.
- **Birth rate in adolescents.** The national birth rate among adolescents has been steadily dropping since 1990, reaching its lowest rate (34.2 per 1000) for 15- to 19-year-old adolescents in 2010.
- **Adolescent abortions.** In 2009 nearly 800,000 abortions were reported to the CDC, a continued decline over the last decade. Adolescents from 15 to 19 years of age accounted for 15.5% of abortions. Approximately 60% of sexually active adolescents report using effective contraception.
- **Infant mortality.** Although infant mortality rates have declined since 1960, the disparity among the ethnic groups persists. In 2011 the overall infant mortality rate was 6.05 per 1000 live births with a rate per 1000 live births of 5.05 for non-Hispanic whites, 5.27 for Hispanic infants, and 11.42 for black infants. In 2008 the United States ranked thirty-first in infant mortality. Marked variations in infant mortality exist by state with highest mortality rates in the South and Midwest.
- **Initiation and maintenance of breastfeeding.** Seventy-seven percent of women initiate breastfeeding following the birth of their infants. Breastfeeding rates vary by ethnicity (higher rates in non-Hispanic whites and Hispanic mothers) and education (highest in women with a bachelor's degree or higher). Only 47% of women continue breastfeeding for 6 months, with about 25% continuing at 12 months.
- **Cause of death in U.S. children.** The overall causes of death in all children (1 to 24 years of age) in the United States in 2010, in order of frequency, were accidents (unintentional injuries), assaults (homicide), suicide, malignant neoplasms, and congenital malformations (Table 1-1). There was a slight improvement in the rate of death from all causes.
- **Hospital admissions for children and adolescents.** In 2010 2.4% of children were admitted to a hospital at least once. Respiratory illnesses (asthma, pneumonia, and bronchitis/bronchiolitis) and injury are the causes of over 28% of hospitalization in children under 18 years of age. Mental illness is the most common cause of admissions for children 13 to 17 years of age.
- **Significant adolescent health challenges: substance use and abuse.** There is considerable substance use and abuse in U.S. high school students. Forty-six percent of high school students reported having tried cigarettes in 2009. In 2011 nearly 71% of high school students reported having had at least one drink; 21.9% admitted to more

Table 1-1	Causes of Death by Age in the United States, 2005
AGE GROUP (YR)	**CAUSES OF DEATH IN ORDER OF FREQUENCY**
1–4	Unintentional injuries (accidents) Congenital malformations, deformations, and chromosomal abnormalities Homicide Malignant neoplasms Diseases of the heart
5–14	Unintentional injuries (accidents) Malignant neoplasms Congenital malformations, deformations, and chromosomal abnormalities Homicide Diseases of the heart
15–24	Unintentional injuries (accidents) Homicide Suicide Malignant neoplasms Diseases of the heart

From Centers for Disease Control and Prevention: Health, United States, 2011: With special feature on socioeconomic status and health (website). http://www.cdc.gov/nchs/data/hus/hus11.pdf#102.

than five drinks on one day in the previous month, and 8.2% admitted to driving after drinking. Nearly 40% of high school students have tried marijuana; 11.4%, inhalants; 6.8%, cocaine; 3.8 %, methamphetamine; 2.9%, heroin; and 2%, injectables.
- **Children in foster care.** Currently there are about 400,000 children in the foster care system. Approximately 25,000 of these children must leave the child welfare system each year. Of those who leave, 25% to 50% experience homelessness and/or joblessness and will not graduate from high school. These children have a high incidence of mental health problems, substance abuse, and early pregnancy for females with an increased likelihood of having a low birth weight baby.

OTHER HEALTH ISSUES THAT AFFECT CHILDREN IN THE UNITED STATES

- **Obesity.** The prevalence of obesity continues to increase. The prevalence of **overweight** children 6 to 19 years of age has increased more than fourfold from 4% in 1965 to over 18% in 2010. Currently it is estimated that 32% of children 2 to 19 years of age are overweight or obese. An estimated 300,000 deaths a year and at least $147 billion in health care costs are associated with the 68% of Americans who are overweight or obese.
- **Sedentary lifestyle.** Among 6 to 11 year olds, 62% do not engage in recommended amounts of moderate or vigorous physical activity. Nearly 40% spend more than 2 hours of screen time (television/videos) per school day.
- **Motor vehicle accidents and injuries.** In 2009, 1314 children 14 years of age or younger died in motor vehicle crashes, and 179,000 were injured. Other causes of childhood injury included drowning, child abuse, and poisonings. The estimated cost of all unintentional childhood injuries is nearly $300 billion per year in the United States.

- **Child maltreatment.** Although there has been a slow decline in the prevalence of child maltreatment, there were over 760,000 reported cases of abuse in 2009. The majority (71%) of children were neglected; 16% suffered physical abuse, and nearly 9% were victims of sexual abuse.
- **Current social and economic stress on the U.S. population.** There are considerable societal stresses affecting the physical and mental health of children, including rising unemployment associated with the economic slowdown, financial turmoil, and political unrest. Millions of families have lost their homes or are at risk for losing their homes after defaulting on mortgage payments.
- **Toxic stress in childhood leading to adult health challenges.** The growing understanding of the interrelationship between biologic and developmental stresses, environmental exposure, and the genetic potential of patients is helping us recognize the adverse impact of toxic stressors on health and well-being. Pediatricians must screen for and act upon factors that promote or hinder early development to provide the best opportunity for long-term health.
- **Military deployment and children.** Current armed conflicts and political unrest have affected millions of adults and their children. There are an estimated 1.5 million active duty and National Guard/Reserve servicemen and women, parents to over a million children. An estimated 31% of troops returning from armed conflicts have a mental health condition (alcoholism, depression, and posttraumatic stress disorder) or report having experienced a traumatic brain injury. Their children are affected by these morbidities as well as by the psychological impact of deployment on children of all ages. Child maltreatment is more prevalent in families of U.S.-enlisted soldiers during combat deployment than in nondeployed soldiers.

HEALTH DISPARITIES IN HEALTH CARE FOR CHILDREN

Health disparities are the differences that remain after taking into account patients' needs, preferences, and the availability of health care. Social conditions, social inequity, discrimination, social stress, language barriers, and poverty are antecedents to and associated causes of health disparities. The disparities in infant mortality relate to poor access to prenatal care during pregnancy and the lack of access and appropriate heath services for women, such as preventive services, family planning, and appropriate nutrition and health care, throughout their life span.

- Infant mortality increases as the mother's level of education decreases.
- Children from poor families are less likely to be immunized at 4 years of age and less likely to receive dental care.
- Rates of hospital admission are higher for people who live in low-income areas.
- Children of ethnic minorities and children from poor families are less likely to have physician office or hospital outpatient visits and more likely to have hospital emergency department visits.

- Children with Medicaid/public coverage are less likely to be in excellent health than children with private health insurance.
- Access to care for children is easier for whites and for children of higher income families than for minority and low-income families.

CHANGING MORBIDITY: THE SOCIAL/ EMOTIONAL ASPECTS OF PEDIATRIC PRACTICE

- **Changing morbidity** reflects the relationship among environmental, social, emotional, and developmental issues; child health status; and outcome. These observations are based on significant interactions of **biopsychosocial** influences on health and illness, such as school problems, learning disabilities, and attention problems; child and adolescent mood and anxiety disorders; adolescent suicide and homicide; firearms in the home; school violence; effects of media violence, obesity, and sexual activity; and substance use and abuse by adolescents.
- Currently 20% to 25% of children are estimated to have some mental health problems; 5% to 6% of these problems are severe. Unfortunately it is estimated that pediatricians identify only 50% of mental health problems. The overall prevalence of psychosocial dysfunction of preschool and school-age children is 10% and 13%, respectively. Children from poor families are twice as likely to have psychosocial problems than children from higher income families. Nationwide, there is a lack of adequate mental health services for children.

Important influences on children's health, in addition to poverty, include homelessness, single-parent families, parental divorce, domestic violence, both parents working, and inadequate child care. Related pediatric challenges include improving the quality of health care, social justice, equality in health care access, and improving the public health system. For adolescents, there are special concerns about sexuality, sexual orientation, pregnancy, substance use and abuse, violence, depression, and suicide.

CULTURE

Culture is an active, dynamic, and complex process of the way people interact and behave in the world. Culture encompasses the concepts, beliefs, values (including nurturing of children), and standards of behavior, language, and dress attributable to people that give order to their experiences in the world, offer sense and purpose to their interactions with others, and provide meaning for their lives. The growing diversity of the United States requires that health care workers make an attempt to understand the impact of health, illness, and treatment on the patient and family from their perspective. This requires open-ended questions, such as: "What *worries* (concerns) you the most about your child's illness?" and "What do you *think* has caused your child's illness?" These can facilitate a discussion of parents' thoughts and feelings about the illness and its causes. Addressing concepts and beliefs about how one interacts with health professionals as well as the family's spiritual and religious approach to health and health care from a cultural perspective allows the pediatrician, patient, and family to incorporate differences in perspectives, values, or beliefs into the care plan. Significant conflicts may arise because religious or cultural practices may lead to the possibility of child abuse and neglect. In this circumstance, the pediatrician is required by law to report the suspected child abuse and neglect to the appropriate social service authorities (see Chapter 22).

Complementary and alternative medicine (CAM) practices constitute a part of the broad cultural perspective. Therapeutic modalities for CAM include biochemical, lifestyle, biomechanical, and bioenergetic treatments, as well as homeopathy. It is estimated that 20% to 30% of all children and 50% to 75% of adolescents use CAM. Of children with chronic illness, 30% to 70% use CAM therapies, especially for asthma and cystic fibrosis. Only 30% to 60% of children and families tell their physicians about their use of CAM. Some modalities may be effective, whereas others may be ineffective or even dangerous.

Chapter 2

PROFESSIONALISM

CONCEPT OF PROFESSIONALISM

Society provides a profession with economic, political, and social rewards. Professions have specialized knowledge and the potential to maintain a monopoly on power and control, remaining relatively autonomous. The profession's autonomy can be limited by societal needs. A profession exists as long as it fulfills its responsibilities for the social good.

Today the activities of medical professionals are subject to explicit public rules of accountability. Governmental and other authorities grant limited autonomy to the professional organizations and their membership. City and municipal government departments of public health establish and implement health standards and regulations. At the state level, boards of registration in medicine establish the criteria for obtaining and revoking medical licenses. The federal government regulates the standards of services, including Medicare, Medicaid, and the Food and Drug Administration. The Department of Health and Human Services regulates physician behavior in conducting research with the goal of protecting human subjects. The Health Care Quality Improvement Act of 1986 authorized the federal government to establish the National Practitioner Data Bank, which contains information about physicians (and other health care practitioners) who have been disciplined by a state licensing board, professional society, hospital, or health plan or named in medical malpractice judgments or settlements. Hospitals are required to review information in this data bank every 2 years as part of clinician recredentialing. There are accrediting agencies for medical schools, such as the Liaison Committee on Medical Education (LCME), and postgraduate training, such as the Accreditation Council for Graduate Medical Education (ACGME). The ACGME includes committees that review subspecialty training programs.

Historically the most privileged professions have depended on their legitimacy for serving the public interest. The public trust of physicians is based on the physician's commitment to altruism. Many medical schools include variations on the traditional Hippocratic Oath as part of the commencement ceremonies as a recognition of a physician's responsibility to put the interest of others ahead of self-interest.

The core of professionalism is embedded in the daily healing work of the physician and encompassed in the patient-physician relationship. Professionalism includes an appreciation for the cultural and religious/spiritual health beliefs of the patient, incorporating the ethical and moral values of the profession and the moral values of the patient. Unfortunately, the inappropriate actions of a few practicing physicians, physician investigators, and physicians in positions of power in the corporate world have created a societal demand to punish those involved and have led to the erosion of respect for the medical profession.

The American Academy of Pediatrics (AAP), the American Board of Pediatrics (ABP), the American Board of Internal Medicine, the LCME, the Medical School Objectives Project of the Association of American Medical Colleges, and the ACGME Outcome Project have called for increasing attention to professionalism in the practice of medicine and in the education of physicians.

PROFESSIONALISM FOR PEDIATRICIANS

The ABP adopted professional standards in 2000, and the AAP updated the policy statement and technical report on Professionalism in 2007, as follows:

- **Honesty/integrity** is the consistent regard for the highest standards of behavior and the refusal to violate one's personal and professional codes. Maintaining integrity requires awareness of situations that may result in conflict of interest or that may result in personal gain at the expense of the best interest of the patient.
- **Reliability/responsibility** includes accountability to one's patients and their families, to society to ensure that the public's needs are addressed, and to the profession to ensure that the ethical precepts of practice are upheld. Inherent in this responsibility is reliability in completing assigned duties or fulfilling commitments. There also must be a willingness to accept responsibility for errors.
- **Respect for others** is the essence of humanism. The pediatrician must treat all persons with respect and regard for their individual worth and dignity; be aware of emotional, personal, family, and cultural influences on a patient's well being, rights, and choices of medical care; and respect appropriate patient confidentiality.
- **Compassion/empathy** is a crucial component of medical practice. The pediatrician must listen attentively, respond humanely to the concerns of patients and family members, and provide appropriate empathy for and relief of pain, discomfort, and anxiety as part of daily practice.
- **Self-improvement** is the pursuit of and commitment to providing the highest quality of health care through lifelong learning and education. The pediatrician must seek to learn from errors and aspire to excellence through self-evaluation and acceptance of the critiques of others.
- **Self-awareness/knowledge of limits** includes recognition of the need for guidance and supervision when faced with new or complex responsibilities. The pediatrician

also must be insightful regarding the impact of his or her behavior on others and cognizant of appropriate professional boundaries.

- **Communication/collaboration** is crucial to providing the best care for patients. Pediatricians must work cooperatively and communicate effectively with patients and their families and with all health care providers involved in the care of their patients.
- **Altruism/advocacy** refers to unselfish regard for and devotion to the welfare of others. It is a key element of professionalism. Self-interest or the interests of other parties should not interfere with the care of one's patients and their families.

Chapter 3

ETHICS AND LEGAL ISSUES

ETHICS IN HEALTH CARE

The ethics of health care and medical decision making relies on **values** to determine what kinds of decisions are best or appropriate for all. Sometimes ethical decision making in medical care is a matter of choosing the least harmful option among many adverse alternatives. In the day-to-day practice of medicine, although all clinical encounters may have an ethical component, major ethical challenges are infrequent.

The legal system defines the minimal standards of behavior required of physicians and the rest of society through the legislative, regulatory, and judicial systems. Laws exist to provide for social order and adjudicate disputes, not to address ethical concerns. The laws support the principle of **confidentiality** for teenagers who are competent to decide about such issues. Using the concept of **limited confidentiality**, parents, teenagers, and the pediatrician may all agree to openly discuss serious health challenges, such as suicidal ideation and pregnancy. This reinforces the long-term goal of supporting the autonomy and identity of the teenager while encouraging appropriate conversations with parents.

Ethical problems derive from **value differences** among patients, families, and clinicians about choices and options in the provision of health care. Resolving these value differences involves several important ethical principles. **Autonomy**, which is based on the principle of **respect for persons**, means that competent adult patients can make choices about health care that they perceive to be in their best interests, after being appropriately informed about their particular health condition and the risks and benefits of alternatives of diagnostic tests and treatments. **Paternalism** challenges the principle of autonomy and involves the clinician deciding what is best for the patient, based on how much information is provided. Paternalism, under certain circumstances (e.g., when a patient has a life-threatening medical condition or a significant psychiatric disorder and is threatening self or others), may be more appropriate than autonomy. Weighing the values of autonomy and paternalism can challenge the clinician.

Other important ethical principles are those of **beneficence** (doing good), **nonmaleficence** (doing no harm or as little harm as possible), and **justice** (the values involved in the equality of the distribution of goods, services, benefits, and burdens to the individual, family, or society). End-of-life decision making must address quality of life and suffering in the provision of palliative and hospice care (see Chapter 4).

ETHICAL PRINCIPLES RELATED TO INFANTS, CHILDREN, AND ADOLESCENTS

Children vary from being totally dependent on parents or guardians to meet their health care needs to being more independent. Infants and young children do not have the capacity for making medical decisions. Paternalism by parents and pediatricians in these circumstances is appropriate. Adolescents (<18 years of age), if competent, have the legal right to make medical decisions for themselves. Children 8 to 9 years old can understand how the body works and the meaning of certain procedures; by age 14 to 15, young adolescents may be considered autonomous through the process of being designated a mature or emancipated minor or by having certain medical conditions. It is ethical for pediatricians to involve children in the decision-making process with information appropriate to their capacity to understand. The process of obtaining the **assent** of a child is consistent with this goal.

The principle of shared decision making is appropriate, but the process may be limited because of issues of confidentiality in the provision of medical care. A parent's concern about the side effects of immunization raises a conflict between the need to protect and support the health of the individual and the public with the rights of the individual and involves ethical issues of distributive justice in regard to the costs and distribution of the vaccinations and responsibility for side effects.

LEGAL ISSUES

All competent patients of an age defined legally by each state (usually ≥18 years of age) are considered autonomous with regard to their health decisions. To have the capacity to decide, patients must meet the following requirements:

- Understand the nature of the medical interventions and procedures, understand the risks and benefits of these interventions, and be able to communicate their decision.
- Reason, deliberate, and weigh the risks and benefits using their understanding about the implications of the decision on their own welfare.
- Apply a set of personal values to the decision-making process and show an awareness of the possible conflicts or differences in values as applied to the decisions to be made.

These requirements need to be placed within the context of medical care and applied to each case with its unique characteristics. Most young children are not able to meet the requirements for competency and need others, usually the parent, to make decisions for them. Legally parents are given great discretion in making decisions for their children. This discretion is legally limited when there is child abuse and neglect, which triggers a further legal process in determining the best interests of the child.

It is important to become familiar with state law because state law, not federal law, determines when an adolescent can consent to medical care and when parents may access confidential adolescent medical information. The Health Insurance Portability and Accountability Act (HIPAA) of 1996, which became effective in 2003, requires a minimal standard of confidentiality protection. The law confers less confidentiality protection to minors than to adults. It is the pediatrician's responsibility to inform minors of their confidentiality rights and help them exercise these rights under the HIPAA regulations.

Under special circumstances, nonautonomous adolescents are granted the legal right to consent under state law when they are considered mature or emancipated minors or because of certain public health considerations, as follows:

- **Mature minors.** Some states have legally recognized that many adolescents age 14 and older can meet the cognitive criteria and emotional maturity for competence and may decide independently. The Supreme Court has decided that pregnant, mature minors have the constitutional right to make decisions about abortion without parental consent. Although many state legislatures require parental notification, pregnant adolescents wishing to have an abortion do not have to seek parental consent. The state must provide a judicial procedure to facilitate this decision making for adolescents.
- **Emancipated minors.** Children who are legally emancipated from parental control may seek medical treatment without parental consent. The definition varies from state to state but generally includes children who have graduated from high school, are members of the armed forces, married, pregnant, runaways, are parents, live apart from their parents, and are financially independent or declared emancipated by a court.
- **Interests of the state (public health).** State legislatures have concluded that minors with certain medical conditions, such as sexually transmitted infections and other contagious diseases, pregnancy (including prevention with the use of birth control), certain mental illnesses, and drug and alcohol abuse, may seek treatment for these conditions autonomously. States have an interest in limiting the spread of disease that may endanger the public health and in eliminating barriers to access for the treatment of certain conditions.

ETHICAL ISSUES IN PRACTICE

From an ethical perspective, clinicians should engage children and adolescents, based on their developmental capacity, in discussions about medical plans so that they have a good understanding of the nature of the treatments and alternatives, the side effects, and expected outcomes. There should be an assessment of the patient's understanding of the clinical situation, how the patient is responding, and the factors that may influence the patient's decisions. Pediatricians should always listen to and appreciate patients' requests for confidentiality and their hopes and wishes. The ultimate goal is to help nourish children's capacity to become as autonomous as is appropriate to their developmental stage.

Confidentiality

Confidentiality is crucial to the provision of medical care and is an important part of the basis for a trusting patient-family-physician relationship. Confidentiality means that information about a patient should not be shared without consent. If confidentiality is broken, patients may experience great harm and may not seek needed medical care. See Chapter 67 for a discussion of confidentiality in the care of adolescents.

Ethical Issues in Genetic Testing and Screening in Children

The goal of **screening** is to identify diseases when there is no clinically identifiable risk factor for disease. Screening should take place only when there is a treatment available or when a diagnosis would benefit the child. **Testing** usually is performed when there is some clinically identifiable risk factor. Genetic testing and screening present special problems because test results have important implications. Some genetic screening (sickle cell anemia or cystic fibrosis) may reveal a carrier state, which may lead to choices about reproduction or create financial, psychosocial, and interpersonal problems (e.g., guilt, shame, social stigma, and discrimination in insurance and jobs). Collaboration with, or referral to, a clinical geneticist is appropriate in helping the family with the complex issues of genetic counseling when a genetic disorder is detected or likely to be detected.

Newborn screening should not be used as a surrogate for parental testing. Examples of diseases that can be diagnosed by genetic screening, even though the manifestations of the disease process do not appear until later in life, are polycystic kidney disease; Huntington disease; certain cancers, such as breast cancer in some ethnic populations; and hemochromatosis. Parents may pressure the pediatrician to order genetic tests when the child is still young, for the parents' purposes. Testing for these disorders should be delayed until the child has the capacity for informed consent or assent and is competent to make decisions, unless there is a direct benefit to the child at the time of testing.

Religious Issues and Ethics

The pediatrician is required to act in the best interests of the child, even when religious tenets may interfere with the health and well-being of the child. When an infant or child whose parents have a religious prohibition against a blood transfusion needs a transfusion to save his or her life, the courts always have intervened to allow a transfusion. In contrast, parents with strong religious beliefs under some state laws may refuse immunizations for their children. However, state governments can mandate immunizations for all children during disease outbreaks or epidemics. By requiring immunization of all, including individuals who object on religious grounds, the state government is using the principle of **distributive justice,** which states that all members of society must share in the burdens and the benefits to have a just society.

Children as Human Subjects in Research

The goal of research is to develop new and generalized knowledge. Parents may give informed permission for children to participate in research under certain conditions. Children cannot give consent but may assent or dissent to research protocols. Special federal regulations have been developed to protect child and adolescent participants in human investigation.

These regulations provide additional safeguards beyond the safeguards provided for adult participants in research, while still providing the opportunity for children to benefit from the scientific advances of research.

Many parents with seriously ill children hope that the research protocol will have a direct benefit for their particular child. The greatest challenge for researchers is to be clear with parents that research is not treatment. This fact should be addressed as sensitively and compassionately as possible.

Chapter **4**

PALLIATIVE CARE AND END-OF-LIFE ISSUES

The death of a child is one of life's most difficult experiences. The **palliative care** approach to a child's medical care should be instituted when medical diagnosis, intervention, and treatment cannot reasonably be expected to affect the imminence of death. In these circumstances, the goals of care focus on improving the quality of life, maintaining dignity, and ameliorating the suffering of the seriously ill child. Central to this approach is the willingness of clinicians to look beyond the traditional medical goals of curing disease and preserving life. They need to look toward enhancing the life of the child and working with family members and close friends when the child's needs are no longer met by curative goals. High-quality palliative care is an expected standard at the end of life.

Palliative care in pediatrics is not simply end-of-life care. There are conditions where death is not predictably imminent, and a child's needs are best met by the palliative care approach. Children needing palliative care have been described as having conditions that fall into four basic groups, based on the goal of treatment. These include conditions of the following scenarios:

- A cure is possible, but failure is not uncommon (e.g., cancer with a poor prognosis).
- Long-term treatment is provided with a goal of maintaining quality of life (e.g., cystic fibrosis).
- Treatment that is exclusively palliative after the diagnosis of a progressive condition is made (e.g., trisomy 13 syndrome).
- Treatments are available for severe, nonprogressive disability in patients who are vulnerable to health complications (e.g., severe spastic quadriparesis with difficulty in controlling symptoms).

These conditions present different timelines and different models of medical intervention. Yet they all share the need to attend to concrete elements, which affect the quality of a child's death, mediated by medical, psychosocial, cultural, and spiritual concerns.

The sudden death of a child also requires elements of the palliative care approach, although conditions do not allow for the full spectrum of involvement. Many of these deaths involve emergency medicine caregivers and first responders in the field, and they may involve dramatic situations where no relationship may exist between caregivers and the bereaved family. Families who have not had time to prepare for the tragedy of an unexpected death require considerable support. Palliative care can make important contributions to the end-of-life and bereavement issues that families face in these circumstances. This may become complicated in circumstances where the cause of the death must be fully explored. The need to investigate the possibility of child abuse or neglect subjects the family to intense scrutiny and may create guilt and anger directed at the medical team.

PALLIATIVE AND END-OF-LIFE CARE

Palliative treatment is directed toward the relief of symptoms as well as assistance with anticipated adaptations that may cause distress and diminish the quality of life of the dying child. Elements of palliative care include pain management; expertise with feeding and nutritional issues at the end of life; and management of symptoms, such as minimizing nausea and vomiting, bowel obstruction, labored breathing, and fatigue. Psychological elements of palliative care have a profound importance and include sensitivity to bereavement, a developmental perspective of a child's understanding of death, clarification of the goals of care, and ethical issues. Curative care and palliative care can coexist; aggressive pain medication may be provided while curative treatment is continued in the hopes of a remission or improved health status. Palliative care is delivered with a multidisciplinary approach, giving a broad range of expertise to patients and families as well as providing a supportive network for the caregivers. Caregivers involved may be pediatricians, nurses, mental health professionals, social workers, and pastors.

A model of integrated palliative care rests on the following principles:

- Article I. **Respect for the dignity of patients and families.** The clinician should respect and listen to patient and family goals, preferences, and choices. School-age children can articulate preferences about how they wish to be treated. Adolescents, by the age of 14, can engage in decision making (see Section 12). The pediatrician should assist the patient and the family in understanding the diagnosis, treatment options, and prognosis; help clarify the goals of care; promote informed choices; allow for the free flow of information; and listen to and discuss the social-emotional concerns. **Advanced care** (advance directives) should be instituted with the child and parents, allowing discussions about what they would like as treatment options as the end of life nears. Differences of opinion between the family and the pediatrician should be addressed by identifying the multiple perspectives, reflecting on possible conflicts, and altruistically coming to agreements that validate the patient and family perspectives, yet reflect sound practice. **Hospital ethics committees** and consultation services are important resources for the pediatrician and family members.
- Article II. **Access to comprehensive and compassionate palliative care.** The clinician should address the physical symptoms, comfort, and functional capacity, with special attention to pain and other symptoms associated with the dying process, and respond empathically to the psychological distress and human suffering, providing treatment options. Respite should be available at any time during the illness to allow the family caregivers to rest and renew.

- Article III. **Use of interdisciplinary resources.** Because of the complexity of care, no one clinician can provide all of the needed services. The team members may include primary and subspecialty physicians, nurses in the hospital/facility or for home visits, the pain management team, psychologists, social workers, pastoral ministers, schoolteachers, friends of the family, and peers of the child. The child and family should be in a position to decide who should know what during all phases of the illness process.
- Article IV. **Acknowledgment and support provisions for caregivers.** The death of a child is difficult to accept and understand. The primary caregivers of the child, family, and friends need opportunities to address their own emotional concerns. Siblings of the child who is dying react emotionally and cognitively, based on their developmental level. Team meetings to address thoughts and feelings of team members are crucial. Soon after the death of the child, the care team should review the experience with the parents and family and share their reactions and feelings. Institutional support may include time to attend funerals, counseling for the staff, opportunities for families to return to the hospital, and scheduled ceremonies to commemorate the death of the child.
- Article V. **Commitment to quality improvement of palliative care through research and education.** Hospitals should develop support systems and staff to monitor the quality of care continually, assess the need for appropriate resources, and evaluate the responses of the patient and family members to the treatment program. Issues often arise over less than completely successful attempts to control the dying child's symptoms or differences between physicians and family members in the timing of the realization that death is imminent. Consensus results in better palliative care from the medical and psychosocial perspective.

Hospice care is a treatment program for the end of life, providing the range of palliative care services by an interdisciplinary team, including specialists in the bereavement and end-of-life process. Typically, the hospice program uses the adult Medicare model, requiring a prognosis of death within 6 months and the cessation of curative efforts for children to receive hospice services. Recently some states have developed alternative pediatric models where curative efforts may continue while the higher level of coordinated end-of-life services may be applied.

BEREAVEMENT

Bereavement refers to the process of psychological and spiritual accommodation to death on the part of the child and the child's family. **Grief** has been defined as the emotional response caused by a loss, including pain, distress, and physical and emotional suffering. It is a normal adaptive human response to death. Palliative care attends to the grief reaction. Assessing the coping resources and vulnerabilities of the affected family before death takes place is central to the palliative care approach.

Parental grief is recognized as being more intense and sustained than other types of grief. Most parents work through their grief. Complicated grief, a pathologic manifestation of continued and disabling grief, is rare. Parents who share their problems with others during the child's illness, who have had access to psychological support during the last month of their child's life, and who have had closure sessions with the attending staff, are more likely to resolve their grief.

A particularly difficult issue for parents is whether to talk with their child about the child's imminent death. Although evidence suggests that sharing accurate and truthful information with a dying child is beneficial, each individual case presents its own complexities, based on the child's age, cognitive development, disease, timeline of disease, and parental psychological state. Parents are more likely to regret not talking with their child about death than having done so. Among those who did not talk with their child about death, parents who sensed their child was aware of imminent death, parents of older children, and mothers more than fathers were more likely to feel regretful.

COGNITIVE ISSUES IN CHILDREN AND ADOLESCENTS: UNDERSTANDING DEATH AND DYING

The pediatrician should communicate with children about what is happening to them, while respecting the cultural and personal preferences of the family. A developmental understanding of children's concepts of health and illness helps frame the discussion with children and can help parents understand how their child is grappling with the situation. Piaget's theories of cognitive development, which help illustrate children's concepts of death and disease, are categorized as sensorimotor, preoperational, concrete operations, and formal operations.

For very young children, up to 2 years of age (sensorimotor), death is seen as a separation, and there is probably no concept of death. The associated behaviors in grieving children of this age usually include protesting and difficulty of attachment to other adults. The degree of difficulty depends on the availability of other nurturing people with whom the child has had a good previous attachment.

Children from 3 to 5 years of age (preoperational) (sometimes called the *magic years*) have trouble grasping the meaning of the illness and the permanence of the death. Their language skills at this age make understanding their moods and behavior difficult. Because of a developing sense of guilt, death may be viewed as punishment. If a child previously wished a younger sibling to have died, the death may be seen psychologically as being caused by the child's wishful thinking. They can feel overwhelmed when confronted with the strong emotional reactions of their parents.

In children ages 6 to 11 years of age (late preoperational to concrete operational), the finality of death gradually comes to be understood. Magical thinking gives way to a need for detailed information to gain a sense of control. Older children in this range have a strong need to control their emotions by compartmentalizing and intellectualizing.

In adolescents (≥12 years of age) (formal operations), death is a reality and is seen as universal and irreversible. Adolescents handle death issues at the abstract or philosophical level and can be realistic. They may also avoid emotional expression and information, instead relying on anger or disdain. Adolescents can discuss withholding treatments. Their wishes, hopes, and fears should be attended to and respected.

CULTURAL, RELIGIOUS, AND SPIRITUAL CONCERNS ABOUT PALLIATIVE CARE AND END-OF-LIFE DECISIONS

Understanding the family's religious/spiritual or cultural beliefs and values about death and dying can help the pediatrician work with the family to integrate these beliefs, values, and practices into the palliative care plan. Cultures vary regarding the roles family members have, the site of treatment for dying people, and the preparation of the body. Some ethnic groups expect the clinical team to speak with the oldest family member or to only the head of the family outside of the patient's presence. Some families involve the entire extended family in decision making. For some families, dying at home can bring the family bad luck, whereas others believe that the patient's spirit will become lost if the death occurs in the hospital. In some traditions, the health care team cleans and prepares the body, whereas, in others, family members prefer to complete this ritual. Religious/spiritual or cultural practices may include prayer, anointing, laying on of the hands, an exorcism ceremony to undo a curse, amulets, and other religious objects placed on the child or at the bedside. Families differ in the idea of organ donation and the acceptance of autopsy. Decisions, rituals, and withholding of palliative or lifesaving procedures that could harm the child or are not in the best interests of the child should be addressed. Quality palliative care attends to this complexity and helps parents and families through the death of a child while honoring the familial, cultural, and spiritual values.

ETHICAL ISSUES IN END-OF-LIFE DECISION MAKING

Before speaking with a child about death, the caregiver should assess the child's age, experience, and level of development; the child's understanding and involvement in end-of-life decision making; the parents' emotional acceptance of death; their coping strategies; and their philosophical, spiritual, and cultural views of death. These may change over time, and the use of open-ended questions to repeatedly assess these areas contributes to the end-of-life process. The care of a dying child can create **ethical dilemmas** involving **autonomy, beneficence** (doing good), **nonmaleficence** (doing no harm), truth telling, confidentiality, or the physician's duty. It is extremely difficult for parents to know when the burdens of continued medical care are no longer appropriate for their child. The beliefs and values of what constitutes quality of life, when life ceases to be worth living, and religious/spiritual, cultural, and philosophical beliefs may differ between families and health care workers. The most important ethical principle is what is in the **best interest** of the child as determined through the process of **shared decision making**, **informed permission/consent** from the parents, and **assent** from the child. Sensitive and meaningful communication with the family, in their own terms, is essential. The physician, patient, and family must **negotiate** the goals of continued medical treatment while recognizing the burdens and benefits of the medical intervention plan. There is no ethical or legal difference between withholding treatment and withdrawing treatment, although many parents and physicians see the latter as more challenging. Family members and the patient should agree about what are appropriate **do not resuscitate** (also called **DNR**) orders. Foregoing some measures does not preclude other measures being implemented, based on the needs and wishes of the patient and family. When there are serious differences among parents, children, and physicians on these matters, the physician may consult with the **hospital ethics committee** or, as a last resort, turn to the legal system by filing a report about potential abuse or neglect.

Suggested Reading

American Academy of Pediatrics: Committee on Bioethics Fallat ME, Glover J: Professionalism in pediatrics: statement of principles, *Pediatrics* 120(4):895–897, 2007.

American Academy of Pediatrics: Committee on Psychosocial Aspects of Child and Family Health: The new morbidity revisited: a renewed commitment to the psychosocial aspects of pediatric care, *Pediatrics* 108(5):1227–1230, 2001.

Bloom B, Cohen RA: Summary health statistics for U.S. children: National health interview survey, 2006, National Center for Health Statistics, *Vital Health Stat* 10(234):1–79, 2007.

Flores G, Tomany-Korman SC: Racial and ethnic disparities in medical and dental health, access to care, and use of health services in US children, *Pediatrics* 121(2):e286–e298, 2008.

Gluckman PD, Hanson MA, Cooper C, et al.: Effect of in utero and early-life considerations on adult health and disease, *N Engl J Med* 359(1):61–73, 2008.

Hamilton BE, Martin JA, Ventura SJ: Births: preliminary data for 2006, *Natl Vital Stat Rep* 56(7):1–18, 2007.

National Center for Health Statistics: *Health, United States, 2007: with chartbook on trends in the health of Americans*, Hyattsville, MD, 2007.

Growth and Development

David A. Levine

THE HEALTH MAINTENANCE VISIT

The frequent office visits for health maintenance in the first 2 years of life are more than *physicals*. Although a somatic history and physical examination are important parts of each visit, many other issues are discussed, including nutrition, behavior, development, safety, and **anticipatory guidance**.

Disorders of growth and development are often associated with chronic or severe illness or may be the only symptom of parental neglect or abuse. Although normal growth and development does not eliminate a serious or chronic illness, in general, it supports a judgment that a child is healthy except for acute, often benign, illnesses that do not affect growth and development.

The processes of growth and development are intertwined. However, it is convenient to refer to **growth** as the increase in size and **development** as an increase in function of processes related to body and mind. Being familiar with normal patterns of growth and development allows those practitioners who care for children to recognize and manage abnormal variations.

The genetic makeup and the physical, emotional, and social environment of the individual determine how a child grows and develops throughout childhood. One goal of pediatrics is to help each child achieve his or her individual potential through periodically monitoring and screening for the normal progression or abnormalities of growth and development. The American Academy of Pediatrics recommends routine office visits in the first week of life (depending on timing of nursery discharge) at 2 weeks; at 1, 2, 4, 6, 9, 12, 15, and 18 months; at 2, 2½, and 3 years; then annually through adolescence/young adulthood (Fig. 9-1).

Chapter 5

NORMAL GROWTH

Deviations in growth patterns may be nonspecific or may be important indicators of serious and chronic medical disorders. An accurate measurement of length/height, weight, and head circumference should be obtained at every health supervision visit and compared with statistical norms on growth charts. Table 5-1 summarizes several convenient benchmarks to evaluate normal growth. Serial measurements are much more useful than single measurements to detect deviations from a particular growth pattern, even if the value remains within statistically defined normal limits (percentiles). Following the trend helps define whether growth is within acceptable limits or warrants further evaluation.

Growth is assessed by plotting accurate measurements on growth charts and comparing each set of measurements with previous measurements obtained at health visits. Please see examples in Figures 5-1 to 5-4. Complete charts can be found at www.cdc.gov/growthcharts/who_charts.htm for birth to 2 years and www.cdc.gov/growthcharts for 2 to 20 years. The body mass index is defined as body weight in kilograms divided by height in meters squared; it is used to classify adiposity and is recommended as a screening tool for children and adolescents to identify those overweight or at risk for being overweight (see Chapter 29).

Normal growth patterns have spurts and plateaus, so some shifting on percentile graphs can be expected. Large shifts in percentiles warrant attention, as do large discrepancies in height, weight, and head circumference percentiles. When caloric intake is inadequate, the weight percentile falls first, then the height, and the head circumference is last. Caloric intake may be poor as a result of inadequate feeding or because the child is not receiving adequate attention and stimulation (*nonorganic* failure to thrive [see Chapter 21]).

Caloric intake also may be inadequate because of increased caloric needs. Children with chronic illnesses, such as heart failure or cystic fibrosis, may require a significantly higher caloric intake to sustain growth. An increasing weight percentile in the face of a falling height percentile suggests hypothyroidism. Head circumference may be disproportionately

Table 5-1	Rules of Thumb for Growth
WEIGHT	
Weight loss in first few days: 5%–10% of birth weight	
Return to birth weight: 7–10 days of age	
Double birth weight: 4–5 months	
Triple birth weight: 1 year	
Daily weight gain:	
20–30 g for first 3–4 months	
15–20 g for rest of the first year	
HEIGHT	
Average length: 20 in. at birth, 30 in. at 1 year	
At age 4 years, the average child is double birth length or 40 in.	
HEAD CIRCUMFERENCE (HC)	
Average HC: 35 cm at birth (13.5 in.)	
HC increases: 1 cm per month for first year (2 cm per month for first 3 months, then slower)	

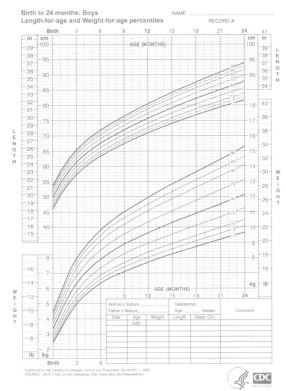

Figure 5-1 Length-by-age and weight-by-age percentiles for boys, birth to 2 years of age. Developed by the National Center for Health Statistics in collaboration with the National Center for Chronic Disease Prevention and Health Promotion. *(From Centers for Disease Control and Prevention:* WHO Child Growth Standards, *Atlanta, Ga, 2009. Available at* http://www.cdc.gov/growthcharts/who_charts.htm.)

Figure 5-3 Stature-for-age and weight-for-age percentiles for girls, 2 to 20 years of age. Developed by the National Center for Health Statistics in collaboration with the National Center for Chronic Disease Prevention and Health Promotion. *(From Centers for Disease Control and Prevention, Atlanta, Ga, 2001. Available at* http://www.cdc.gov/growthcharts.)

Figure 5-2 Head circumference and weight-by-length percentiles for boys, birth to 2 years of age. Developed by the National Center for Health Statistics in collaboration with the National Center for Chronic Disease Prevention and Health Promotion. *(From Centers for Disease Control and Prevention:* WHO Child Growth Standards, *Atlanta, Ga, 2009. Available at* http://www.cdc.gov/growthcharts/who_charts.htm.)

Figure 5-4 Body mass index–for-age percentiles for girls, 2 to 20 years of age. Developed by the National Center for Health Statistics in collaboration with the National Center for Chronic Disease Prevention and Health Promotion. *(From Centers for Disease Control and Prevention Atlanta, Ga, 2001. Available at* http://www.cdc.gov/growthcharts.)

large when there is familial megalocephaly, hydrocephalus, or merely *catch-up* growth in a neurologically normal premature infant. A child is considered microcephalic if the head circumference is less than the third percentile, even if length and weight measurements also are proportionately low. Serial measurements of head circumference are crucial during infancy, a period of rapid brain development, and should be plotted regularly until the child is 2 years of age. Any suspicion of abnormal growth warrants at least a close follow-up, further evaluation, or both.

Chapter 6

DISORDERS OF GROWTH

Decision-Making Algorithm
Available @ StudentConsult.com

Short stature

The most common reasons for deviant measurements are technical (i.e., faulty equipment and human errors). Repeating a deviant measurement is the first step. Separate growth charts are available and should be used for very low birth weight infants (weight <1500 g) and for those with Turner syndrome, Down syndrome, achondroplasia, and various other dysmorphology syndromes.

Variability in body proportions occurs from fetal to adult life. Newborns' heads are significantly larger in proportion to the rest of their body. This difference gradually disappears. Certain growth disturbances result in characteristic changes in the proportional sizes of the trunk, extremities, and head. Patterns requiring further assessment are summarized in Table 6-1.

Evaluating a child over time, coupled with a careful history and physical examination, helps determine whether the growth pattern is normal or abnormal. Parental heights may be useful when deciding whether to proceed with a further evaluation. Children, in general, follow their parents' growth pattern, although there are many exceptions.

For a girl, midparental height is calculated as follows:

$$\frac{Paternal\ height\ (inches)\ +\ Maternal\ heigh\ (inches)}{2} - 2.5$$

For a boy, midparental height is calculated as follows:

$$\frac{Paternal\ height\ (inches)\ +\ Maternal\ heigh\ (inches)}{2} + 2.5$$

Actual growth depends on too many variables to make an accurate prediction from midparental height determination for every child. The growth pattern of a child with low weight, length, and head circumference is commonly associated with **familial short stature** (see Chapter 173). These children are genetically normal but are smaller than most

PATTERN	REPRESENTATIVE DIAGNOSES TO CONSIDER	FURTHER EVALUATION
Weight, length, head circumference all <5th percentile	Familial short stature Constitutional short stature Intrauterine insult Genetic abnormality	Midparental heights Evaluation of pubertal development Examination of prenatal records Chromosome analysis
Discrepant percentiles (e.g., weight 5th, length 5th, head circumference 50th, or other discrepancies)	Normal variant (familial or constitutional) Endocrine growth failure Caloric insufficiency	Midparental heights Thyroid hormone Growth factors, growth hormone testing Evaluation of pubertal development
Declining percentiles	*Catch-down growth* Caloric insufficiency Endocrine growth failure	Complete history and physical examination Dietary and social history Growth factors, growth hormone testing

Table 6-1 Specific Growth Patterns Requiring Further Evaluation

children. A child who, by age, is preadolescent or adolescent and who starts puberty later than others may have the normal variant called **constitutional short stature** (see Chapter 173); careful examination for abnormalities of pubertal development should be done, although most are normal. An evaluation for primary amenorrhea should be considered for any female adolescent who has not reached menarche by 15 years or has not done so within 3 years of thelarche. Lack of breast development by age 13 years also should be evaluated (see Chapter 174).

Starting out in high growth percentiles, many children assume a lower percentile between 6 and 18 months until they match their genetic programming, then grow along new, lower percentiles. They usually do not decrease more than two major percentiles and have normal developmental, behavioral, and physical examinations. These children with *catch-down growth* should be followed closely, but no further evaluation is warranted.

Infants born small for gestational age, or prematurely, ingest more breast milk or formula and, unless there are complications that require extra calories, usually exhibit *catch-up growth* in the first 6 months. These infants should be fed on demand and provided as much as they want unless they are vomiting (not just spitting up [see Chapter 128]). Some may benefit from a higher caloric content formula. Many psychosocial risk factors that may have led to being born small or early may contribute to nonorganic failure to thrive (see Chapter 21). Conversely infants who recover from being low birth weight or premature have an increased risk of developing childhood obesity.

Growth of the nervous system is most rapid in the first 2 years, correlating with increasing physical, emotional, behavioral, and cognitive development. There is again rapid change during adolescence. Osseous maturation (bone age) is determined from radiographs on the basis of the number and size of calcified epiphyseal centers; the size, shape, density, and sharpness of outline of the ends of bones; and the distance separating the epiphyseal center from the zone of provisional calcification.

NORMAL DEVELOPMENT

PHYSICAL DEVELOPMENT
Parallel to the changes in the developing brain (i.e., cognition, language, behavior) are changes in the physical development of the body.

NEWBORN PERIOD
Observation of any asymmetric movement or altered muscle tone and function may indicate a significant central nervous system abnormality or a nerve palsy resulting from the delivery and requires further evaluation. Primitive neonatal reflexes are unique in the newborn period and can further elucidate or eliminate concerns over asymmetric function. The most important reflexes to assess during the newborn period are as follows:

The **Moro reflex** is elicited by allowing the infant's head to gently move back suddenly (from a few inches off of the mattress onto the examiner's hand), resulting in a startle, then abduction and upward movement of the arms followed by adduction and flexion. The legs respond with flexion.

The **rooting reflex** is elicited by touching the corner of the infant's mouth, resulting in lowering of the lower lip on the same side with tongue movement toward the stimulus. The face also turns toward the stimulus.

The **sucking reflex** occurs with almost any object placed in the newborn's mouth. The infant responds with vigorous sucking. The sucking reflex is replaced later by voluntary sucking.

The **grasp reflex** occurs when placing an object, such as a finger, onto the infant's palm (palmar grasp) or sole (plantar grasp). The infant responds by flexing fingers or curling the toes.

The **asymmetric tonic neck reflex** is elicited by placing the infant supine and turning the head to the side. This placement results in ipsilateral extension of the arm and the leg into a "fencing" position. The contralateral side flexes as well.

A delay in the expected disappearance of the reflexes may also warrant an evaluation of the central nervous system.

See Sections 11 and 26 for additional information on the newborn period.

LATER INFANCY
With the development of gross motor skills, the infant is first able to control his or her posture, then proximal musculature, and, last, distal musculature. As the infant progresses through these stages, the parents may notice orthopedic deformities (see Chapters 202 and 203). The infant also may have deformities that are related to intrauterine positioning. Physical examination should indicate whether the deformity is fixed or can be moved passively into the proper position. When a joint held in an abnormal fashion can be moved passively into the proper position, there is a high likelihood of resolving with the progression of gross motor development. Fixed deformities warrant immediate pediatric orthopedic consultation (see Section 26).

Evaluation of vision and ocular movements is important to prevent the serious outcome of strabismus. The cover test and light reflex should be performed at early health maintenance visits; interventions after age 2 decrease the chance of preserving binocular vision or normal visual acuity (see Chapter 179).

SCHOOL AGE/PREADOLESCENT
Older school-age children who begin to participate in competitive sports should have a comprehensive sports history and physical examination, including a careful evaluation of the cardiovascular system. The American Academy of Pediatrics 4th edition sports preparticipation form is excellent for documenting cardiovascular and other risks. The patient and parent should complete the history form and be interviewed to assess cardiovascular risk. Any history of heart disease or a murmur must be referred for evaluation by a pediatric cardiologist. A child with a history of dyspnea or chest pain on exertion, irregular heart rate (i.e., skipped beats, palpitations), or syncope should also be referred to a pediatric cardiologist. A family history of a primary (immediate family) or secondary (immediate family's immediate family) atherosclerotic disease (myocardial infarction or cerebrovascular disease) before 50 years of age or sudden unexplained death at any age requires additional assessment.

Children interested in contact sports should be assessed for special vulnerabilities. Similarly vision should be assessed as a crucial part of the evaluation before participation in sports.

ADOLESCENCE
Adolescents need annual comprehensive health assessments to ensure progression through puberty without major problems (see Chapters 67 and 68). Sexual maturity is an important issue in adolescents. All adolescents should be assessed to monitor progression through sexual maturity rating stages (see Chapter 67). Other issues in physical development include scoliosis, obesity, and trauma (see Chapters 29 and 203). Most scoliosis is mild and requires only observation for progression. Obesity may first manifest during childhood and is an issue for many adolescents.

DEVELOPMENTAL MILESTONES
The use of milestones to assess development focuses on discrete behaviors that the clinician can observe or accept as present by parental report. This approach is based on comparing the patient's behavior with that of many normal children whose behaviors evolve in a uniform sequence within specific age ranges (see Chapter 8). The development of the neuromuscular system, similar to that of other organ systems, is determined first by genetic endowment and then molded by environmental influences.

Although a sequence of specific, easily measured behaviors can adequately represent some areas of development (**gross motor, fine motor**, and **language**), other areas, particularly social and emotional development, are not as easy to assess. Easily measured developmental milestones are well established through age 6 years only. Other types of assessment (e.g., intelligence tests, school performance, and personality profiles) that expand the developmental milestone approach are available for older children but generally require time and expertise in administration and interpretation.

PSYCHOSOCIAL ASSESSMENT
Bonding and Attachment in Infancy

The terms *bonding* and *attachment* describe the affective relationships between parents and infants. **Bonding** occurs shortly after birth and reflects the feelings of the parents toward the newborn (unidirectional). **Attachment** involves reciprocal feelings between parent and infant and develops gradually over the first year.

Attachment of infants outside of the newborn period is crucial for optimal development. Infants who receive extra attention, such as parents responding immediately to any crying or fussiness, show less crying and fussiness at the end of the first year. **Stranger anxiety** develops between 9 and 18 months of age, when infants normally become insecure about separation from the primary caregiver. The infant's new motor skills and attraction to novelty may lead to headlong plunges into new adventures that result in fright or pain followed by frantic efforts to find and cling to the primary caregiver. The result is dramatic swings from stubborn independence to clinging dependence that can be frustrating and confusing to parents. With secure attachment, this period of ambivalence may be shorter and less tumultuous.

Developing Autonomy in Early Childhood

Toddlers build on attachment and begin developing autonomy that allows separation from parents. In times of stress, toddlers often cling to their parents, but in their usual activities they may be actively separated. Ages 2 to 3 years are a time of major accomplishments in fine motor skills, social skills, cognitive skills, and language skills. The dependency of infancy yields to developing independence and the "I can do it myself" age. Limit setting is essential to a balance of the child's emerging independence.

Early Childhood Education

There is a growing body of evidence that notes that children who are in high quality early learning environments are more prepared to succeed in school. Every dollar invested in early childhood education may save taxpayers up to 13 dollars in future costs. These children commit fewer crimes and are better prepared to enter the workforce after school. Early Head Start (less than 3 years), Head Start (3 to 4 years), and prekindergarten programs (4 to 5 years) all demonstrate better educational attainment, although the earlier the start, the better the results.

School Readiness

Readiness for preschool depends on the development of autonomy and the ability of the parent and the child to separate for hours at a time. Preschool experiences help children develop socialization skills; improve language; increase skill building in areas such as colors, numbers, and letters; and increase problem solving (puzzles).

Readiness for school (kindergarten) requires emotional maturity, peer group and individual social skills, cognitive abilities, and fine and gross motor skills (Table 7-1). Other issues include chronologic age and gender. Children tend to do better in kindergarten if their fifth birthday is at least 4 to 6 months before the beginning of school. Girls usually are ready earlier than boys. If the child is in less than the average developmental range, he or she should not be forced into early kindergarten. Holding a child back for reasons of developmental delay, in the false hope that the child will catch up, can also lead to difficulties. The child should enroll on schedule, and educational planning should be initiated to address any deficiencies.

Physicians should be able to identify children at risk for school difficulties, such as those who have developmental delays or physical disabilities. These children may require specialized school services.

Adolescence

Some define adolescence as 10 to 25 years of age but adolescence is perhaps better characterized by the developmental stages (*early, middle,* and *late* adolescence) that all teens must negotiate to develop into healthy, functional adults. Different behavioral and developmental issues characterize each stage. The age at which each issue manifests and the importance of these issues vary widely among individuals, as do the rates of cognitive, psychosexual, psychosocial, and physical development.

During **early adolescence**, attention is focused on the present and on the peer group. Concerns are primarily related

Table 7-1	Evaluating School Readiness
PHYSICIAN OBSERVATIONS (BEHAVIORS OBSERVED IN THE OFFICE)	
Ease of separation of the child from the parent	
Speech development and articulation	
Understanding of and ability to follow complex directions	
Specific pre-academic skills	
Knowledge of colors	
Counts to 10	
Knows age, first and last names, address, and phone number	
Ability to copy shapes	
Motor skills	
Stand on one foot, skip, and catch a bounced ball	
Dresses and undresses without assistance	
PARENT OBSERVATIONS (QUESTIONS ANSWERED BY HISTORY)	
Does the child play well with other children?	
Does the child separate well, such as a child playing in the backyard alone with occasional monitoring by the parent?	
Does the child show interest in books, letters, and numbers?	
Can the child sustain attention to quiet activities?	
How frequent are toilet-training *accidents*?	

to the body's physical changes and normality. Strivings for independence are ambivalent. These young adolescents are difficult to interview because they often respond with short, clipped conversation and may have little insight. They are just becoming accustomed to abstract thinking.

Middle adolescence can be a difficult time for adolescents and the adults who have contact with them. Cognitive processes are more sophisticated. Through abstract thinking, middle adolescents can experiment with ideas, consider things as they might be, develop insight, and reflect on their own feelings and the feelings of others. As they mature, these adolescents focus on issues of identity not limited solely to the physical aspects of their body. They explore their parents' and culture's values, sometimes by expressing the contrary side of the dominant value. Many middle adolescents explore these values in their minds only; others do so by challenging their parents' authority. Many engage in high-risk behaviors, including unprotected sexual intercourse, substance abuse, or dangerous driving. The strivings of middle adolescents for independence, limit testing, and need for autonomy often distress their families, teachers, or other authority figures. These adolescents are at higher risk for morbidity and mortality from accidents, homicide, or suicide.

Late adolescence usually is marked by formal operational thinking, including thoughts about the future (e.g., educational, vocational, and sexual). Late adolescents are usually more committed to their sexual partners than are middle adolescents. Unresolved separation anxiety from previous developmental stages may emerge, at this time, as the young person begins to move physically away from the family of origin to college or vocational school, a job, or military service.

MODIFYING PSYCHOSOCIAL BEHAVIORS

Child behavior is determined by heredity and by the environment. Behavioral theory postulates that behavior is primarily a product of external environmental determinants and that manipulation of the environmental antecedents and consequences of behavior can be used to modify maladaptive behavior and to increase desirable behavior (operant conditioning). The four major methods of operant conditioning are positive reinforcement, negative reinforcement, extinction, and punishment. Many common behavioral problems of children can be ameliorated by these methods.

Positive reinforcement increases the frequency of a behavior by following the behavior with a favorable event (e.g., praising a child for excellent school performance). **Negative reinforcement** usually decreases the frequency of a behavior by removal, cessation, or avoidance of an unpleasant event. Conversely sometimes this reinforcement may occur unintentionally, increasing the frequency of an undesirable behavior. For example, a toddler may purposely try to stick a pencil in a light socket to obtain attention, whether it be positive or negative. **Extinction** occurs when there is a decrease in the frequency of a previously reinforced behavior because the reinforcement is withheld. Extinction is the principle behind the common advice to ignore behavior such as crying at bedtime or temper tantrums, which parents may unwittingly reinforce through attention and comforting. **Punishment** decreases the frequency of a behavior through unpleasant consequences.

Positive reinforcement is more effective than punishment. Punishment is more effective when combined with positive reinforcement. A toddler who draws on the wall with a crayon may be punished, but he or she learns much quicker when positive reinforcement is given for the proper use of the crayon—on paper, not the wall. Interrupting and modifying behaviors are discussed in detail in Section 3.

TEMPERAMENT

Significant individual differences exist within the normal development of temperament (behavioral style). Temperament must be appreciated because, if an expected pattern of behavior is too narrowly defined, normal behavior may be inappropriately labeled as abnormal or pathologic. Three common constellations of temperamental characteristics are as follows:

1. The **easy child** (about 40% of children) is characterized by regularity of biologic functions (consistent, predictable times for eating, sleeping, and elimination), a positive approach to new stimuli, high adaptability to change, mild or moderate intensity in responses, and a positive mood.
2. The **difficult child** (about 10%) is characterized by irregularity of biologic functions, negative withdrawal from new stimuli, poor adaptability, intense responses, and a negative mood.
3. The **slow to warm up child** (about 15%) is characterized by a low activity level, withdrawal from new stimuli, slow adaptability, mild intensity in responses, and a somewhat negative mood.

The remaining children have more mixed temperaments. The individual temperament of a child has important implications for parenting and for the advice a pediatrician may give in anticipatory guidance or behavioral problem counseling.

Although, to some degree, temperament may be hardwired (*nature*) in each child, the environment (*nurture*) in which the child grows has a strong effect on the child's adjustment. Social and cultural factors can have marked effects on the child through differences in parenting style, educational approaches, and behavioral expectations.

Chapter **8**

DISORDERS OF DEVELOPMENT

DEVELOPMENTAL SURVEILLANCE AND SCREENING

Developmental and behavioral problems are more common than any category of problems in pediatrics, except acute infections and trauma. In 2008 15% of children ages 3 to 7 had a developmental disability, and others had behavioral disabilities. As many as 25% of children have serious psychosocial problems. Parents often neglect to mention these problems because they think the physician is uninterested or cannot help. It is necessary to monitor development and screen for the presence of these problems at health supervision visits, particularly in the years before preschool or early childhood learning center enrollment.

Development surveillance, done at every office visit, is an informal process comparing skill levels to lists of milestones. If suspicion of developmental or behavioral issues recurs, further evaluation is warranted (Table 8-1). Surveillance does not have a standard, and screening tests are necessary.

Developmental screening involves the use of standardized screening tests to identify children who require further diagnostic assessment. The American Academy of Pediatrics recommends the use of validated standardized screening tools at three of the health maintenance visits: 9 months, 18 months, and 30 months. Clinics and offices that serve a higher risk patient population (children living in poverty) often perform a screening test at *every* health maintenance visit. A child who fails to pass a developmental screening test requires more comprehensive evaluation but does not necessarily have a delay; definitive testing must confirm. Developmental evaluations for children with suspected delays and intervention services for children with diagnosed disabilities are available free to families. A combination of U.S. state and federal funds provides these services.

Screening tests can be categorized as general screening tests that cover all behavioral domains or as targeted screens that focus on one area of development. Some may be administered in the office by professionals, and others may be completed at home (or in a waiting room) by parents. Good developmental/behavioral screening instruments have a sensitivity of 70% to 80% in detecting suspected problems and a specificity of 70% to 80% in detecting normal development. Although 30% of children screened may be *over-referred* for definitive developmental testing, this group also includes children whose skills are below average and who may benefit from testing that may help address relative developmental deficits. The 20% to 30% of children who have disabilities that are not detected by the single administration of a screening instrument are likely to be identified on repeat screening at subsequent health maintenance visits.

Table 8-1	Developmental Milestones				
AGE	**GROSS MOTOR**	**FINE MOTOR–ADAPTIVE**	**PERSONAL-SOCIAL**	**LANGUAGE**	**OTHER COGNITIVE**
2 wk	Moves head side to side		Regards face	Alerts to bell	
2 mo	Lifts shoulder while prone	Tracks past midline	Smiles responsively	Cooing Searches for sound with eyes	
4 mo	Lifts up on hands Rolls front to back If pulled to sit from supine, no head lag	Reaches for object Raking grasp	Looks at hand Begins to work toward toy	Laughs and squeals	
6 mo	Sits alone	Transfers object hand to hand	Feeds self Holds bottle	Babbles	
9 mo	Pulls to stand Gets into sitting position	Starting to pincer grasp Bangs two blocks together	Waves bye-bye Plays pat-a-cake	Says *Dada* and *Mama*, but nonspecific Two-syllable sounds	
12 mo	Walks Stoops and stands	Puts block in cup	Drinks from a cup Imitates others	Says *Mama* and *Dada*, specific Says one to two other words	
15 mo	Walks backward	Scribbles Stacks two blocks	Uses spoon and fork Helps in housework	Says three to six words Follows commands	
18 mo	Runs	Stacks four blocks Kicks a ball	Removes garment "Feeds" doll	Says at least six words	
2 yr	Walks up and down stairs Throws overhand	Stacks six blocks Copies line	Washes and dries hands Brushes teeth Puts on clothes	Puts two words together Points to pictures Knows body parts	Understands concept of *today*
3 yr	Walks steps alternating feet Broad jump	Stacks eight blocks Wiggles thumb	Uses spoon well, spilling little Puts on T-shirt	Names pictures Speech understandable to stranger 75% Says three-word sentences	Understands concepts of *tomorrow* and *yesterday*
4 yr	Balances well on each foot Hops on one foot	Copies O, maybe + Draws person with three parts	Brushes teeth without help Dresses without help	Names colors Understands adjectives	
5 yr	Skips Heel-to-toe walks	Copies □		Counts Understands opposites	
6 yr	Balances on each foot 6 sec	Copies ▵ Draws person with six parts		Defines words	Begins to understand *right* and *left*

Mo, Month; *sec,* second; *wk,* week; *yr,* year.

The **Denver Developmental Screening Test II** was the classic test used by general pediatricians (Figs. 8-1 and 8-2). The Denver II assesses the development of children from birth to 6 years of age in the following four domains:

1. Personal-social
2. Fine motor–adaptive
3. Language
4. Gross motor

The advantage of this test is that it teaches developmental milestones when administered. Items on the Denver II are carefully selected for their reliability and consistency of norms across subgroups and cultures. The Denver II is a useful screening instrument, but it cannot assess adequately the complexities of socioemotional development. Children with *suspect* or *untestable* scores must be followed carefully.

The pediatrician asks questions (items labeled with an "R" may be asked of parents to document the task "by report") or directly observes behaviors. On the scoring sheet, a line is drawn at the child's chronologic age. Tasks that are entirely to the left of the line that the child has not accomplished are considered delayed. If the test instructions are not followed accurately or if items are omitted, the validity of the test becomes

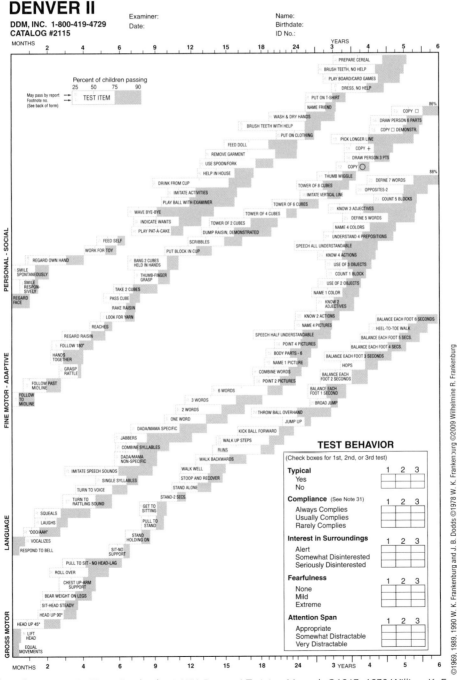

Figure 8-1 Scoring form for Denver II. *(From Frankenburg WK: Denver I Training Manual. ©1967, 1970 William K. Frankenburg and Josiah B. Dodds; 1975, 1976, 1978 William K. Frankenburg; 1990, 1992 William K. Frankenburg and Josiah B. Dodds; © 2009 Wilhelmine R. Frankenburg - Contact DDM, Inc. 1-800-419-4729 or Info@denverii.com.)*

DIRECTIONS FOR ADMINISTRATION

1. Try to get child to smile by smiling, talking or waving. Do not touch him/her.
2. Child must stare at hand several seconds.
3. Parent may help guide toothbrush and put toothpaste on brush.
4. Child does not have to be able to tie shoes or button/zip in the back.
5. Move yarn slowly in an arc from one side to the other, about 8" above child's face.
6. Pass if child grasps rattle when it is touched to the backs or tips of fingers.
7. Pass if child tries to see where yarn went. Yarn should be dropped quickly from sight from tester's hand without arm movement.
8. Child must transfer cube from hand to hand without help of body, mouth, or table.
9. Pass if child picks up raisin with any part of thumb and finger.
10. Line can vary only 30 degrees or less from tester's line.
11. Make a fist with thumb pointing upward and wiggle only the thumb. Pass if child imitates and does not move any fingers other than the thumb.

12. Pass any enclosed form. Fail continuous round motions.
13. Which line is longer? (Not bigger.) Turn paper upside down and repeat. (pass 3 of 3 or 5 of 6)
14. Pass any lines crossing near midpoint.
15. Have child copy first. If failed, demonstrate.

When giving items 12, 14, and 15, do not name the forms. Do not demonstrate 12 and 14.

16. When scoring, each pair (2 arms, 2 legs, etc.) counts as one part.
17. Place one cube in cup and shake gently near child's ear, but out of sight. Repeat for other ear.
18. Point to picture and have child name it. (No credit is given for sounds only.)
    If less than 4 pictures are named correctly, have child point to picture as each is named by tester.

19. Using doll, tell child: Show me the nose, eyes, ears, mouth, hands, feet, tummy, hair. Pass 6 of 8.
20. Using pictures, ask child: Which one flies?...says meow?...talks?...barks?...gallops? Pass 2 of 5, 4 of 5.
21. Ask child: What do you do when you are cold?...tired?...hungry? Pass 2 of 3, 3 of 3.
22. Ask child: What do you do with a cup? What is a chair used for? What is a pencil used for? Action words must be included in answers.
23. Pass if child correctly places <u>and</u> says how many blocks are on paper. (1,5).
24. Tell child: Put block **on** table; **under** table; **in front of** me, **behind** me. Pass 4 of 4. (Do not help child by pointing, moving head or eyes.)
25. Ask child: What is a ball?...lake?...desk?...house?...banana?...curtain?...fence?...ceiling? Pass if defined in terms of use, shape, what it is made of, or general category (such as banana is fruit, not just yellow). Pass 5 of 8, 7 of 8.
26. Ask child: If a horse is big, a mouse is ___? If fire is hot, ice is ___? If the sun shines during the day, the moon shines during the ___? Pass 2 of 3.
27. Child may use wall or rail only, not person. May not crawl.
28. Child must throw ball overhand 3 feet to within arm's reach of tester.
29. Child must perform standing broad jump over width of test sheet (8 1/2 inches).
30. Tell child to walk forward, ⊂⊃⊂⊃⊂⊃⊂⊃➤ heel within 1 inch of toe. Tester may demonstrate. Child must walk 4 consecutive steps.
31. In the second year, half of normal children are non-compliant.

OBSERVATIONS:

Denver Developmental Materials, Inc.
P.O. Box 371075
Denver, Colorado 80237-5075
Tele. #: (303) 355-4729
(800) 419-4729

Catalog #2115   **TO REORDER CALL: (800) 419-4729**

Figure 8-2 Instructions for the Denver II. Numbers are coded to a scoring form (see Fig. 8-1). "Abnormal" is defined as two or more delays (failure of an item passed by 90% at that age) in two or more categories or two or more delays in one category with one other category having one delay and an age line that does not intersect one item that is passed. *(From Frankenburg WK: Denver I Training Manual. ©1967, 1970 William K. Frankenburg and Josiah B. Dodds; 1975, 1976, 1978 William K. Frankenburg; 1990, 1992 William K. Frankenburg and Josiah B. Dodds; © 2009 Wilhelmine R. Frankenburg - Contact DDM, Inc. 1-800-419-4729 or Info@denverii.com.)*

worse. To assist physicians in using the Denver II, the scoring sheet also features a table to document confounding behaviors, such as interest, fearfulness, or an apparent short attention span. Repeat screening at subsequent health maintenance visits often detects abnormalities that a single screen was unable to detect.

Other developmental screening tools include parent-completed Ages and Stages Questionnaires (also milestone driven), and Parents' Evaluation of Developmental Status. The latter is a simple, 10-item questionnaire that parents complete at office visits based on concerns with function and progression of development. Parent-reported screens have good validity compared to office-based screening measures.

Autism screening is recommended for all children at 18 to 24 months of age. Although there are several tools, many pediatricians use the Modified Checklist for Autism in Toddlers (M-CHAT). M-CHAT is an office-based questionnaire that asks parents about 23 typical behaviors, some of which are more predictive than others for autism or other pervasive developmental disorders. If the child demonstrates more than two predictive or three total behaviors, further assessment

Table 8-2	Rules of Thumb for Speech Screening		
AGE (YR)	SPEECH PRODUCTION	ARTICULATION (AMOUNT OF SPEECH UNDERSTOOD BY A STRANGER)	FOLLOWING COMMANDS
1	One to three words		One-step commands
2	Two- to three-word phrases	One half	Two-step commands
3	Routine use of sentences	Three fourths	
4	Routine use of sentence sequences; conversational give-and-take	Almost all	
5	Complex sentences; extensive use of modifiers, pronouns, and prepositions	Almost all	

Table 8-3	Conditions Considered High Risk for Associated Hearing Deficit

Congenital hearing loss in first cousin or closer relative

Bilirubin level of ≥20 mg/dL

Congenital rubella or other nonbacterial intrauterine infection

Defects in the ear, nose, or throat

Birth weight of ≤1500 g

Multiple apneic episodes

Exchange transfusion

Meningitis

Five-minute Apgar score of ≤5

Persistent fetal circulation (primary pulmonary hypertension)

Treatment with ototoxic drugs (e.g., aminoglycosides and loop diuretics)

Table 8-4	Context of Behavioral Problems

CHILD FACTORS

Health (past and current)

Developmental status

Temperament (e.g., difficult, slow to warm up)

Coping mechanisms

PARENTAL FACTORS

Misinterpretations of stage-related behaviors

Mismatch of parental expectations and characteristics of child

Mismatch of personality style between parent and child

Parental characteristics (e.g., depression, lack of interest, rejection, overprotective)

Coping mechanisms

ENVIRONMENTAL FACTORS

Stress (e.g., marital discord, unemployment, personal loss)

Support (e.g., emotional, material, informational, child care)

Poverty

Racism

with an interview algorithm is indicated to distinguish normal variant behaviors from those children needing a referral for definitive testing. The test is freely distributed on the Internet (see Chapter 20).

Language screening correlates best with cognitive development in the early years. Table 8-2 provides some rules of thumb for language development that focus on speech production (expressive language). Although expressive language is the most obvious language element, the most dramatic changes in language development in the first years involve recognition and understanding (receptive language).

Whenever there is a speech and/or language delay, a **hearing deficit** must be considered. The implementation of universal newborn hearing screening detects many, if not most, of these children in the newborn period, and appropriate early intervention services may be provided. Conditions that present a high risk of an associated hearing deficit are listed in Table 8-3. Dysfluency (*stuttering*) is common in a 3- and 4-year-old child. Unless the dysfluency is severe, is accompanied by tics or unusual posturing, or occurs after 4 years of age, parents should be counseled that it is normal and transient and to accept it calmly and patiently.

After the child's sixth birthday and until adolescence, developmental assessment is initially done by inquiring about school performance (academic achievement and behavior). Inquiring about concerns raised by teachers or other adults who care for the child (after-school program counselor, coach, religious leader) is prudent. Formal developmental testing of these older children is beyond the scope of the primary care pediatrician. Nonetheless the health care provider should be the coordinator of the testing and evaluation performed by other specialists (e.g., psychologists, psychiatrists, developmental pediatricians, and educational professionals).

OTHER ISSUES IN ASSESSING DEVELOPMENT AND BEHAVIOR

Ignorance of the environmental influences on child behavior may result in ineffective or inappropriate management

(or both). Table 8-4 lists some contextual factors that should be considered in the etiology of a child's behavioral or developmental problem.

Building rapport with the parents and the child is a prerequisite for obtaining the often sensitive information that is essential for understanding a behavioral or developmental issue. Rapport usually can be established quickly if the parents sense that the clinician respects them and is genuinely interested in listening to their concerns. The clinician develops rapport with the child by engaging the child in developmentally appropriate conversation or play, perhaps providing toys while interviewing the parents, and being sensitive to the fears the child may have. Too often the child is ignored until it is time for the physical examination. Similar to their parents, children feel more comfortable if they are greeted by name and involved in pleasant interactions before they are asked sensitive questions or threatened with examinations. Young children can be engaged in conversation on the parent's lap, which provides security and places the child at the eye level of the examiner.

With adolescents emphasis should be placed on building a physician-patient relationship that is distinct from the relationship with the parents. The parents should not be excluded; however the adolescent should have the opportunity to express concerns to and ask questions of the physician in confidence. Two intertwined issues must be taken into consideration—consent and confidentiality. Although laws vary from state to state, in general, adolescents who are able to give informed consent (i.e., mature minors) may consent to visits and care related to high-risk behaviors (i.e., substance abuse; sexual health, including prevention, detection, and treatment of sexually transmitted infections; and pregnancy). Most states support the physician who wishes the visit to be confidential. Physicians should become familiar with the governing law in the state where they practice (see www.guttmacher.org/statecenter/updates/index.html). Providing confidentiality is crucial, allowing for optimal care (especially for obtaining a history of risk behaviors). When assessing development and behavior, confidentiality can be achieved by meeting with the adolescent alone for at least part of each visit. However parents must be informed when the clinician has significant and immediate concerns about the health and safety of the child. Often the clinician can convince the adolescent to inform the parents directly about a problem or can reach an agreement with the adolescent about how the parents will be informed by the physician (see Chapter 67).

EVALUATING DEVELOPMENTAL AND BEHAVIORAL ISSUES

Responses to open-ended questions often provide clues to underlying, unstated problems and identify the appropriate direction for further, more directed questions. Histories about developmental and behavioral problems are often vague and confusing; to reconcile apparent contradictions, the interviewer frequently must request clarification, more detail, or mere repetition. By summarizing an understanding of the information at frequent intervals and by recapitulating at the close of the visit, the interviewer and patient and family can ensure that they understand each other.

If the clinician's impression of the child differs markedly from the parent's description, there may be a crucial parental concern or issue that has not yet been expressed, either because it may be difficult to talk about (e.g., marital problems), because it is unconscious, or because the parent overlooks its relevance to the child's behavior. Alternatively the physician's observations may be atypical, even with multiple visits. The observations of teachers, relatives, and other regular caregivers may be crucial in sorting out this possibility. The parent also may have a distorted image of the child, rooted in parental psychopathology. A sensitive, supportive, and noncritical approach to the parent is crucial to appropriate intervention. More information about referral and intervention for behavioral and developmental issues is covered in Chapter 10.

Chapter 9

EVALUATION OF THE WELL CHILD

Health maintenance or supervision visits should consist of a comprehensive assessment of the child's health and of the parent's/guardian's role in providing an environment for optimal growth, development, and health. Bright Futures standardizes each of the health maintenance visits and provides resources for working with the children and families of different ages (see www.brightfutures.aap.org). Elements of each visit include evaluation and management of parental concerns; inquiry about any interval illness since the last physical, growth, development, and nutrition; anticipatory guidance (including safety information and counseling); physical examination; screening tests; and immunizations (Table 9-1). The *Bright Futures'* "Recommendations for Preventive Pediatric Health Care," found at http://brightfutures.aap.org/clinical_practice.html, summarizes requirements and indicates the ages that specific prevention measures should be undertaken, including risk screening and performance items for specific measurements. Bright Futures is now the enforced standard for the Medicaid

Table 9-1	Topics for Health Supervision Visits
FOCUS ON THE CHILD	
Concerns (parent's or child's)	
Past problem follow-up	
Immunization and screening test update	
Routine care (e.g., eating, sleeping, elimination, and health habits)	
Developmental progress	
Behavioral style and problems	
FOCUS ON THE CHILD'S ENVIRONMENT	
Family	
Caregiving schedule for caregiver who lives at home	
Parent-child and sibling-child interactions	
Extended family role	
Family stresses (e.g., work, move, finances, illness, death, marital and other interpersonal relationships)	
Family supports (relatives, friends, groups)	
Community	
Caregivers outside of the family	
Peer interaction	
School and work	
Recreational activities	
Physical environment	
Appropriate stimulation	
Safety	

and the Children's Health Insurance Program, along with many insurers. Health maintenance and immunizations now are covered without co-pays for insured patients as part of the Patient Protection and Affordable Care Act.

SCREENING TESTS

Children usually are quite healthy and only the following screening tests are recommended: newborn metabolic screening with hemoglobin electrophoresis, hearing and vision evaluation, anemia and lead screening, and tuberculosis testing. Children born to families with dyslipidemias or early heart disease should also be screened for lipid disorders. (Items marked by a *star* in *Bright Futures'* recommendations should be performed if a risk factor is found.) Sexually experienced adolescents should be screened for sexually transmissible infections. When an infant or child begins care after the newborn period, the pediatrician should perform any missing screening tests and immunizations.

Newborn Screening
Metabolic Screening

Every state in the United States mandates newborn metabolic screening. Each state determines its own priorities and procedures, but the following diseases are usually included in metabolic screening: phenylketonuria, galactosemia, congenital hypothyroidism, maple sugar urine disease, and organic aciduria (see Section 10). Many states now screen for cystic fibrosis, testing for immunoreactive trypsinogen. If that test is positive, then a deoxyribonucleic acid (commonly referred to as *DNA*) analysis for cystic fibrosis mutations is performed.

Hemoglobin Electrophoresis

Children with hemoglobinopathies are at higher risk for infection and complications from anemia, which early detection may prevent or ameliorate. Infants with sickle cell disease are begun on oral penicillin prophylaxis to prevent sepsis, the major cause of mortality in these infants (see Chapter 150).

Hearing Evaluation

Because speech and language are central to a child's cognitive development, the hearing screening is performed before discharge from the newborn nursery. An infant's hearing is tested by placing headphones over the infant's ears and electrodes on the head. Standard sounds are played, and the transmission of the impulse to the brain is documented. If abnormal, a further evaluation is indicated, using evoked response technology of sound transmission.

Hearing and Vision Screening of Older Children
Infants and Toddlers

Inferences about hearing are drawn from asking parents about responses to sound and speech and by examining speech and language development closely. Inferences about vision may be made by examining gross motor milestones (children with vision problems may have a delay) and by physical examination of the eye. Parental concerns about vision should be sought until the child is 3 years of age and about hearing until the child is 4 years of age. If there are concerns, definitive testing should be arranged. Hearing can be screened by auditory evoked responses, as mentioned for newborns. For toddlers and older children who cannot cooperate with formal audiologic testing with headphones, behavioral audiology may be used. Sounds of a specific frequency or intensity are provided in a standard environment within a soundproof room, and responses are assessed by a trained audiologist. Vision may be assessed by referral to a pediatric ophthalmologist and by visual evoked responses.

Children 3 Years of Age and Older

At various ages, hearing and vision should be screened objectively using standard techniques as specified in the *Bright Futures'* recommendations. Asking the family and child about any concerns or consequences of poor hearing or vision accomplishes subjective evaluation. At 3 years of age, children are screened for vision for the first time if they are developmentally able to be tested. Many children at this age do not have the interactive language or interpersonal skills to perform a vision screen; these children should be re-examined at a 3- to 6-month interval to ensure that their vision is normal. Because most of these children do not yet identify letters, using a Snellen eye chart with standard shapes is recommended. When a child is able to identify letters, the more accurate letter-based chart should be used. Audiologic testing of sounds with headphones should be begun on the fourth birthday (although Head Start requires that pediatricians attempt the hearing screening at 3 years of age). Any suspected audiologic problem should be evaluated by a careful history and physical examination, with referral for comprehensive testing. Children who have a documented vision problem, failed screening, or parental concern should be referred, preferably to a pediatric ophthalmologist.

Anemia Screening

Children are screened for anemia at ages when there is a higher incidence of iron deficiency anemia. Infants are screened at birth and again at 4 months if there is a documented risk, such as low birth weight or prematurity. Healthy term infants usually are screened at 12 months of age because this is when a high incidence of iron deficiency is noted. Children are assessed at other visits for risks or concerns related to anemia (denoted by a ★ in the Bright Futures' recommendations at http://brightfutures.aap.org/clinical_practice.html). Any abnormalities detected should be evaluated for etiology. Anemic infants do not perform as well on standard developmental testing. When iron deficiency is strongly suspected, a therapeutic trial of iron may be used (see Chapter 150).

Lead Screening

Lead intoxication may cause developmental and behavioral abnormalities that are not reversible, even if the hematologic and other metabolic complications are treated. Although the Centers for Disease Control and Prevention (CDC) recommends environmental investigation at blood lead levels of 20 µg/dL on a single visit or persistent 15 µg/dL over a 3-month period, levels of 5 to 10 µg/dL may cause learning problems. Risk factors for lead intoxication include living in older homes with cracked or peeling lead-based paint, industrial exposure, use of foreign remedies (e.g., a diarrhea remedy from Central or South America), and use of pottery with lead paint glaze. Because of the significant association of lead intoxication with poverty, the CDC recommends blood lead screening at 12 and 24 months. In addition, standardized screening questions for risk of lead intoxication should be asked for all children between 6 months and 6 years of age (Table 9-2). Any positive or suspect response is an indication for obtaining a blood lead level. Capillary blood sampling may produce false-positive results, thus, a venous blood sample should be obtained. County health departments, community organizations, and private companies provide lead inspection and detection services to determine the source of the lead. Standard decontamination techniques should be used to remove the lead while avoiding aerosolizing the toxic metal that a child might breathe or creating dust that a child might ingest (see Chapters 149 and 150).

Tuberculosis Testing

The prevalence of tuberculosis is increasing, largely as a result of the adult human immunodeficiency virus (HIV) epidemic. Children often present with serious and multisystem disease (miliary tuberculosis). All children should be assessed for risk of tuberculosis at health maintenance visits, especially after 1 year of age. The high-risk groups, as defined by the CDC, are listed in Table 9-3. In general the standardized purified protein derivative intradermal test is used with evaluation by a health care provider 48 to 72 hours after injection. The size of induration, not the color of any mark, denotes a positive test. For most patients, 10 mm of induration is a positive test. For HIV-positive patients, those with recent tuberculosis contacts, patients with evidence of old healed tuberculosis on chest film, or immunosuppressed patients, 5 mm is a positive test (see Chapter 124). The CDC has approved (in adults) the QuantiFERON-TB Gold Test, which has the advantage of needing one office visit only.

Cholesterol

Children and adolescents who have a family history of cardiovascular disease or have at least one parent with a high blood cholesterol level are at increased risk of having high blood cholesterol levels as adults and increased risk of coronary heart disease. The American Academy of Pediatrics (AAP) recommends dyslipidemia screening in the context of regular health care for at-risk populations (Table 9-4) by obtaining a fasting lipid profile. The recommended screening levels are the same for all children 2 to 18 years. Total cholesterol of less than 170 mg/dL is normal, 170 to 199 mg/dL is borderline, and greater than 200 mg/dL is elevated. In addition, in 2011, the AAP endorsed the National Heart, Lung, and Blood Institute of the National Institutes of Health recommendation to test all children between ages 9 and 11.

Sexually Transmitted Infection Testing

Annual office visits are recommended for adolescents. A full adolescent psychosocial history should be obtained in confidential fashion (see Section 12). Part of this evaluation is a comprehensive sexual history that often requires creative questioning. Not all adolescents identify oral sex as sex, and some adolescents misinterpret the term *sexually active* to mean that one has many sexual partners or is very vigorous during intercourse. The questions, "Are you having sex?" and "Have you ever had sex?" should be asked. In the Bright Futures guidelines, any child or adolescent who has had any form of sexual intercourse should have at least an annual evaluation (more often if there is a history of high-risk sex) for sexually transmitted diseases by physical examination (genital warts, genital herpes, and pediculosis) and laboratory testing (chlamydia, gonorrhea, syphilis, and HIV) (see Chapter 116). Young women should be assessed for human papillomavirus and precancerous lesions by Papanicolaou smear at 21 years of age.

IMMUNIZATIONS

Immunization records should be checked at each office visit, regardless of the reason. Appropriate vaccinations should be administered (see Chapter 94).

Table 9-2	Lead Poisoning Risk Assessment Questions to be Asked between 6 Months and 6 Years
Does the child spend any time in a building built before 1960 (e.g., home, school, barn) that has cracked or peeling paint?	
Is there a brother, sister, housemate, playmate, or community member being followed or treated (or even rumored to be) for lead poisoning?	
Does the child live with an adult whose job or hobby involves exposure to lead (e.g., lead smelting and automotive radiator repair)?	
Does the child live near an active lead smelter, battery recycling plant, or other industry likely to release lead?	
Does the family use home remedies or pottery from another country?	

Table 9-3	Groups at High Risk for Tuberculosis
Close contact with persons known to have tuberculosis (TB), positive TB test, or suspected to have TB	
Foreign-born persons from areas with high TB rates (Asia, Africa, Latin America, Eastern Europe, Russia)	
Health care workers	
High-risk racial or ethnic minorities or other populations at higher risk (Asian, Pacific Islander, Hispanic, African American, Native American, groups living in poverty [e.g., Medicaid recipients], migrant farm workers, homeless persons, substance abusers)	
Infants, children, and adolescents exposed to adults in high-risk categories	

Table 9-4	Cholesterol Risk Screening Recommendations
Risk screening at ages 2, 4, 6, 8, 10 and annually in adolescence:	
1. Children and adolescents who have a family history of high cholesterol or heart disease	
2. Children whose family history is unknown	
3. Children who have other personal risk factors: obesity, high blood pressure, or diabetes	
Universal screening at ages 9–11 and ages 18–20	

DENTAL CARE

Many families in the United States, particularly poor families and ethnic minorities, underuse dental health care. Pediatricians may identify gross abnormalities, such as large caries, gingival inflammation, or significant malocclusion. All children should have a dental examination by a dentist at least annually and a dental cleaning by a dentist or hygienist every 6 months. Dental health care visits should include instruction about preventive care practiced at home (brushing and flossing). Other prophylactic methods shown to be effective at preventing caries are concentrated fluoride topical treatments (dental varnish) and acrylic sealants on the molars. Pediatric dentists recommend beginning visits at age 1 year to educate families and to screen for milk bottle caries. Some recommend that pediatricians apply dental varnish to the children's teeth, especially in communities that do not have pediatric dentists. Fluoridation of water or fluoride supplements in communities that do not have fluoridation are important in the prevention of cavities (see Chapter 127).

NUTRITIONAL ASSESSMENT

Plotting a child's growth on the standard charts is a vital component of the nutritional assessment. A dietary history should be obtained because the content of the diet may suggest a risk of nutritional deficiency (see Chapters 27 and 28).

ANTICIPATORY GUIDANCE

Anticipatory guidance is information conveyed to parents verbally, in written materials, or even directing parents to certain Internet websites to assist them in facilitating optimal growth and development for their children. Anticipatory guidance that is age relevant is another part of the Bright Futures guidelines. Bright Futures has a "toolkit" that includes the topics and one-page handouts for families (and for older children) about the highest yield issues for the specific age. Table 9-5 summarizes representative issues that might be discussed. It is important to review briefly the safety topics previously discussed at other visits for reinforcement. Age-appropriate discussions should occur at each visit.

Safety Issues

The most common cause of death for infants 1 month to 1 year of age is **motor vehicle crashes**. No newborn should be discharged from a nursery unless the parents have a functioning and properly installed car seat. Many automobile dealerships offer services to parents to ensure that safety seats are installed properly in their specific model. Most states have laws that mandate use of safety seats until the child reaches 4 years of age or at least 40 pounds in weight. The following are age-appropriate recommendations for car safety:

- Infants and toddlers should ride in a **rear-facing safety seat** until they are 2 years of age, or until they reach the highest weight or height allowed by the safety seat manufacturer.
- Toddlers and preschoolers over age 2 or who have outgrown the rear-facing car seat should use a **forward-facing car seat** with harness for as long as possible, up to the highest weight or height recommended by the manufacturer.
- School-age children, whose weight or height is above the forward-facing limit for their car seat, should use a **belt-positioning booster seat** until the vehicle seat belt fits properly, typically when they have reached 4 ft 9 in. in height and are between 8 and 12 years of age.
- Older children should always use **lap and shoulder seat belts** for optimal protection. All children younger than 13 years should be restrained in the rear seats of vehicles for optimal protection. This is specifically to protect them from airbags, which may cause more injury than the crash in young children.

The **_Back to Sleep_ initiative** has reduced the incidence of sudden infant death syndrome (SIDS). Before the initiative, infants routinely were placed prone to sleep. Since 1992 when the AAP recommended this program, the annual SIDS rate has decreased by more than 50%. Another initiative is aimed at day care providers, because 20% of SIDS deaths occur in day care settings.

Fostering Optimal Development

See Table 9-5 as well as the Bright Futures' recommendations (found at http://brightfutures.aap.org/clinical_practice.html) for presentation of age-appropriate activities that the pediatrician may advocate for families.

Discipline means to teach, not merely to punish. The ultimate goal is the child's self-control. Overbearing punishment to control a child's behavior interferes with the learning process and focuses on external control at the expense of the development of self-control. Parents who set too few reasonable limits may be frustrated by children who cannot control their own behavior. Discipline should teach a child exactly what is expected by supporting and reinforcing positive behaviors and responding appropriately to negative behaviors with proper limits. It is more important and effective to reinforce good behavior than to punish bad behavior.

Commonly used techniques to control undesirable behaviors in children include scolding, physical punishment, and threats. These techniques have potential adverse effects on children's sense of security and self-esteem. The effectiveness of scolding diminishes the more it is used. Scolding should not be allowed to expand from an expression of displeasure about a specific event to derogatory statements about the child. Scolding also may escalate to the level of psychological abuse. It is important to educate parents that they have a _good child who does bad things from time to time_, so parents do not think and tell the child that he or she is "bad."

Frequent mild physical punishment (corporal punishment) may become less effective over time and tempt the parent to escalate the physical punishment, increasing the risk of child abuse. Corporal punishment teaches a child that in certain situations it is proper to strike another person. Commonly in households that use spanking, older children who have been raised with this technique are seen responding to younger sibling behavioral problems by hitting their siblings.

Threats by parents to leave or to give up the child are perhaps the most psychologically damaging ways to control a child's behavior. Children of any age may remain fearful and anxious about loss of the parent long after the threat is made; however many children are able to see through empty threats. Threatening a mild loss of privileges (no video games for 1 week or grounding a teenager) may be appropriate, but the consequence must be enforced if there is a violation.

Table 9-5	Anticipatory Guidance Topics Suggested by Age				
AGES	**INJURY PREVENTION**	**VIOLENCE PREVENTION**	**SLEEP POSITION**	**NUTRITIONAL COUNSELING**	**FOSTERING OPTIMAL DEVELOPMENT**
Birth and/ or 3–5 days	Crib safety Hot water heaters <120° F Car safety seats Smoke detectors	Assess bonding and attachment Identify family strife, lack of support, pathology Educate parents on nurturing	Back to sleep Crib safety	Exclusive breastfeeding encouraged Formula as a second-best option	Discuss parenting skills Refer for parenting education
2 weeks or 1 month	Falls	Reassess* Discuss sibling rivalry Assess if guns in the home	Back to sleep	Assess breastfeeding and offer encouragement, problem solving	Recognize and manage postpartum blues Child care options
2 months	Burns/hot liquids	Reassess firearm safety	Back to sleep		Parent getting enough rest and managing returning to work
4 months	Infant walkers Choking/ suffocation	Reassess	Back to sleep	Introduction of solid foods	Discuss central to peripheral motor development Praise good behavior
6 months	Burns/hot surfaces	Reassess		Assess status	Consistent limit-setting versus "spoiling" an infant Praise good behavior
9 months	Water safety Home safety review Ingestions/ poisoning	Assess parents' ideas on discipline and "spoiling"		Avoiding juice Begin to encourage practice with cup drinking	Assisting infants to sleep through the night if not accomplished Praise good behavior
12 months	Firearm hazards Auto-pedestrian safety	Discuss timeout versus corporal punishment Avoiding media violence Review firearm safety		Introduction of whole cow's milk (and constipation with change discussed) Assess anemia, discuss iron-rich foods	Safe exploration Proper shoes Praise good behavior
15 months	Review and reassess topics	Encourage nonviolent punishments (timeout or natural consequences)		Discuss decline in eating with slower growth Assess food choices and variety	Fostering independence Reinforce good behavior Ignore annoying but not unsafe behaviors
18 months	Review and reassess topics	Limit punishment to high yield (not spilled milk!) Parents consistent in discipline		Discuss food choices, portions, "finicky" feeders	Preparation for toilet training Reinforce good behavior
2 years	Falls—play equipment	Assess and discuss any aggressive behaviors in the child		Assess body proportions and recommend low-fat milk Assess family cholesterol and atherosclerosis risk	Toilet training and resistance
3 years	Review and reassess topics	Review, especially avoiding media violence		Discuss optimal eating and the food pyramid Healthy snacks	Read to child Socializing with other children Head Start if possible
4 years	Booster seat versus seat belts			Healthy snacks	Read to child Head Start or pre-K options
5 years	Bicycle safety Water/pool safety	Developing consistent, clearly defined family rules and consequences Avoiding media violence		Assess for anemia Discuss iron-rich foods	Reinforcing school topics Read to child Library card Chores begun at home
6 years	Fire safety	Reinforce consistent discipline Encourage nonviolent strategies Assess domestic violence Avoiding media violence		Assess content, offer specific suggestions	Reinforcing school topics After-school programs Responsibility given for chores (and enforced)
7–10 years	Sports safety Firearm hazard	Reinforcement Assess domestic violence Assess discipline techniques Avoiding media violence Walking away from fights (either victim or spectator)		Assess content, offer specific suggestions	Reviewing homework and reinforcing school topics After-school programs Introduce smoking and substance abuse prevention (concrete)

	INJURY PREVENTION	**VIOLENCE PREVENTION**	**SLEEP POSITION**	**NUTRITIONAL COUNSELING**	**FOSTERING OPTIMAL DEVELOPMENT**
AGES					
11–13 years	Review and reassess	Discuss strategies to avoid interpersonal conflicts Avoiding media violence Avoiding fights and walking away Discuss conflict resolution techniques		Junk food versus healthy eating	Reviewing homework and reinforcing school topics Smoking and substance abuse prevention (begin abstraction) Discuss and encourage abstinence; possibly discuss condoms and contraceptive options Avoiding violence Offer availability
14–16 years	Motor vehicle safety Avoiding riding with substance abuser	Establish new family rules related to curfews, school, and household responsibilities		Junk food versus healthy eating	Review school work Begin career discussions and college preparation (PSAT) Review substance abuse, sexuality, and violence regularly Discuss condoms, contraception options, including emergency contraception Discuss sexually transmitted diseases, HIV Providing no questions–asked ride home from at-risk situations
17–21 years	Review and reassess	Establish new rules related to driving, dating, and substance abuse		Heart healthy diet for life	Continuation of above topics Off to college or employment New roles within the family

Table 9-5 | Anticipatory Guidance Topics Suggested by Age—cont'd

HIV, Human immunodeficiency virus; PSAT, Preliminary Scholastic Aptitude Test.
*Reassess means to review the issues discussed at the prior health maintenance visit.

Parenting involves a dynamic balance between **setting limits** on the one hand and allowing and encouraging freedom of expression and exploration on the other. A child whose behavior is out of control improves when clear limits on their behavior are set and enforced. However parents must agree on where the limit will be set and how it will be enforced. The limit and the consequence of breaking the limit must be clearly presented to the child. Enforcement of the limit should be consistent and firm. Too many limits are difficult to learn and may thwart the normal development of autonomy. The limit must be reasonable in terms of the child's age, temperament, and developmental level. To be effective, both parents (and other adults in the home) must enforce limits. Otherwise, children may effectively *split* the parents and seek to test the limits with the more indulgent parent. In all situations, to be effective, punishment must be brief and linked directly to a behavior. More effective behavioral change occurs when punishment also is linked to praise of the intended behavior.

Extinction is an effective and systematic way to eliminate a frequent, annoying, and relatively harmless behavior by ignoring it. First parents should note the frequency of the behavior to appreciate realistically the magnitude of the problem and to evaluate progress. Parents must determine what reinforces the child's behavior and what needs to be consistently eliminated. An appropriate behavior is identified to give the child a positive alternative that the parents can reinforce. Parents should be warned that the annoying behavior usually increases in frequency and intensity (and may last for weeks) before it decreases when the parent ignores it (removes the reinforcement). A child who has an attention-seeking temper tantrum should be ignored or placed in a secure environment. This action may anger the child more, and the behavior may get louder and angrier. Eventually with no audience for the tantrum, the tantrums decrease in intensity and frequency. In each specific instance, when the child's behavior has become appropriate, he or she should be praised, and extra attention should be given. This is an effective technique for early toddlers, before their capacity to understand and adhere to a timeout.

The **timeout** consists of a short period of isolation *immediately* after a problem behavior is observed. Timeout interrupts the behavior and immediately links it to an unpleasant consequence. This method requires considerable effort by the parents because the child does not wish to be isolated. A parent may need to hold the child physically in timeout. In this situation, the parent should become *part of the furniture* and should not respond to the child until the timeout period is over. When established, a simple isolation technique, such as making a child stand in the corner or sending a child to his or her room, may be effective. If such a technique is not helpful, a more systematic procedure may be needed. One effective protocol for the timeout procedure involves interrupting the child's play when the behavior occurs and having the child sit in a dull, isolated place for a brief period, measured by a portable kitchen timer (the clicking noises document that time is passing and the bell alarm at the end signals the end of the punishment). Timeout is simply punishment and is not a time for a young child to *think* about the behavior (these children do not possess the capacity for abstract thinking) or a time to de-escalate the behavior. The amount of timeout should be appropriate to the child's short attention span. One minute per year of a child's age is recommended. This inescapable and unpleasant consequence of the undesired behavior motivates the child to learn to avoid the behavior.

Chapter **10**

EVALUATION OF THE CHILD WITH SPECIAL NEEDS

Children with disabilities, severe chronic illnesses, congenital defects, and health-related educational and behavioral problems are **children with special health care needs (SHCN).** Many of these children share a broad group of experiences and encounter similar problems, such as school difficulties and family stress. The term *children with special health care needs* defines these children noncategorically, without regard to specific diagnoses, in terms of increased service needs. Approximately 19% of children in the United States younger than 18 years of age have a physical, developmental, behavioral, or emotional condition requiring services of a type or amount beyond those required by children, generally.

The goal in managing a child with SHCN is to maximize the child's potential for productive adult functioning by treating the primary diagnosis and by helping the patient and family deal with the stresses and secondary impairments incurred because of the disease or disability. Whenever a chronic disease is diagnosed, family members typically grieve, show anger, denial, negotiation (in an attempt to forestall the inevitable), and depression. Because the child with SHCN is a constant reminder of the object of this grief, it may take family members a long time to accept the condition. A supportive physician can facilitate the process of acceptance by education and by allaying guilty feelings and fear. To minimize denial, it is helpful to confirm the family's observations about the child. The family may not be able to absorb any additional information initially, so written material and the option for further discussion at a later date should be offered.

The primary physician should provide a **medical home** to maintain close oversight of treatments and subspecialty services, provide preventive care, and facilitate interactions with school and community agencies. A major goal of *family-centered care* is for the family and child to feel in control. Although the medical management team usually directs treatment in the acute health care setting, the locus of control should shift to the family as the child moves into a more routine, home-based life. Treatment plans should allow the greatest degree of normalization of the child's life. As the child matures, self-management programs that provide health education, self-efficacy skills, and techniques such as symptom monitoring help promote good long-term health habits. These programs should be introduced at 6 or 7 years of age or when a child is at a developmental level to take on chores and benefit from being given responsibility. Self-management minimizes *learned helplessness* and the *vulnerable child syndrome*, both of which occur commonly in families with chronically ill or disabled children.

MULTIFACETED TEAM ASSESSMENT OF COMPLEX PROBLEMS

When developmental screening and surveillance suggest the presence of significant developmental lags, the physician should take responsibility for coordinating the further assessment of the child by the team of professionals and provide continuity of care. The physician should become aware of local facilities and programs for assessment and treatment. If the child is at high risk for delay (e.g., prematurity), a structured follow-up program to monitor the child's progress may already exist. Under federal law, all children are entitled to assessments if there is a suspected developmental delay or a risk factor for delay (e.g., prematurity, failure to thrive, and parental mental retardation [MR]). Special programs for children up to 3 years of age are developed by states to implement this policy. Developmental interventions are arranged in conjunction with third-party payers with local programs funding the cost only when there is no insurance coverage. After 3 years of age, development programs usually are administered by school districts. Federal laws mandate that special education programs be provided for all children with developmental disabilities from birth through 21 years of age.

Children with special needs may be enrolled in pre-K programs with a therapeutic core, including visits to the program by therapists, to work on challenges. Children who are of traditional school age (kindergarten through secondary school) should be evaluated by the school district and provided an **individualized educational plan (IEP)** to address any deficiencies. An IEP may feature individual tutoring time (resource time), placement in a special education program, placement in classes with children with severe behavioral problems, or other strategies to address deficiencies. As part of the comprehensive evaluation of developmental/behavioral issues, all children should receive a thorough medical assessment. A variety of other specialists may assist in the assessment and intervention, including subspecialist pediatricians (e.g., neurology, orthopedics, psychiatry, developmental/behavioral), therapists (e.g., occupational, physical, oral-motor), and others (e.g., psychologists, early childhood development specialists).

Medical Assessment

The physician's main goals in team assessment are to identify the cause of the developmental dysfunction, if possible (often a specific cause is not found), and identify and interpret other medical conditions that have a developmental impact. The comprehensive history (Table 10-1) and physical examination (Table 10-2) include a careful graphing of growth parameters and an accurate description of dysmorphic features. Many of the diagnoses are rare or unusual diseases or syndromes. Many of these diseases and syndromes are discussed further in Sections 9 and 24.

Motor Assessment

The comprehensive neurologic examination is an excellent basis for evaluating motor function, but it should be supplemented by an adaptive functional evaluation (see Chapter 179). Observing the child at play aids assessment of function. Specialists in early childhood development and therapists (especially occupational and physical therapists who have experience with children) can provide excellent input into the evaluation of age-appropriate adaptive function.

| Table 10-1 | Information to Be Sought during the History Taking of a Child with Suspected Developmental Disabilities |

ITEM	POSSIBLE SIGNIFICANCE	ITEM	POSSIBLE SIGNIFICANCE
Parental concerns	Parents are quite accurate in identifying development problems in their children.	Mental functioning	Increased hereditary and environmental risks
Current levels of developmental functioning	Should be used to monitor child's progress	Illnesses (e.g., metabolic diseases)	Hereditary illness associated with developmental delay
Temperament	May interact with disability or may be confused with developmental delay	Family member died young or unexpectedly	May suggest inborn error of metabolism or storage disease
PRENATAL HISTORY		Family member requires special education	Hereditary causes of developmental delay
Alcohol ingestion	Fetal alcohol syndrome; index of caregiving risk	**SOCIAL HISTORY**	
Exposure to medication, illegal drug, or toxin	Development toxin (e.g., phenytoin); may be an index of caregiving risk	Resources available (e.g., financial, social support)	Necessary to maximize child's potential
Radiation exposure	Damage to CNS	Educational level of parents	Family may need help to provide stimulation.
Nutrition	Inadequate fetal nutrition	Mental health problems	May exacerbate child's conditions
Prenatal care	Index of social situation	High-risk behaviors (e.g., illicit drugs, sex)	Increased risk for HIV infection; index of caregiving risk
Injuries, hyperthermia	Damage to CNS	Other stressors (e.g., marital discord)	May exacerbate child's conditions or compromise care
Smoking	Possible CNS damage	**OTHER HISTORY**	
HIV exposure	Congenital HIV infection	Gender of child	Important for X-linked conditions
Maternal illness (so-called "TORCH" infections)	**T**oxoplasmosis, Syphilis (**O**ther in the mnemonic), **R**ubella, **C**ytomegalovirus, **H**erpes simplex virus infections	Developmental milestones	Index of developmental delay; regression may indicate progressive condition.
PERINATAL HISTORY		Head injury	Even moderate trauma may be associated with developmental delay or learning disabilities.
Gestational age, birth weight	Biologic risk from prematurity and small for gestational age	Serious infections (e.g., meningitis)	May be associated with developmental delay
Labor and delivery	Hypoxia or index of abnormal prenatal development	Toxic exposure (e.g., lead)	May be associated with developmental delay
APGAR scores	Hypoxia, cardiovascular impairment	Physical growth	May indicate malnutrition; obesity, short stature, genetic syndrome
Specific perinatal adverse events	Increased risk of CNS damage	Recurrent otitis media	Associated with hearing loss and abnormal speech development
NEONATAL HISTORY		Visual and auditory functioning	Sensitive index of impaired vision and hearing
Illness—seizures, respiratory distress, hyperbilirubinemia, metabolic disorder	Increased risk of CNS damage	Nutrition	Malnutrition during infancy may lead to delayed development.
Malformations	May represent genetic syndrome or new mutation associated with developmental delay	Chronic conditions such as renal disease	May be associated with delayed development or anemia
FAMILY HISTORY			
Consanguinity	Autosomal recessive condition more likely		

Adapted and updated from Liptak G: Mental retardation and developmental disability. In Kliegman RM, editor: *Practical Strategies in Pediatric Diagnosis and Therapy*, Philadelphia, 1996, WB Saunders.
CNS, Central nervous system; *HIV*, human immunodeficiency virus.

Psychological Assessment

Psychological assessment includes the testing of cognitive ability (Table 10-3) and the evaluation of personality and emotional well-being. The IQ and mental age scores, taken in isolation, are only partially descriptive of a person's functional abilities, which are a combination of cognitive, adaptive, and social skills. Tests of achievement are subject to variability based on culture, educational exposures, and experience and must be standardized for social factors. Projective and non-projective tests are useful in understanding the child's emotional status.

Although a child should not be labeled as having a problem solely on the basis of a standardized test, these tests provide important and reasonably objective data for evaluating a child's progress within a particular educational program.

Educational Assessment

Educational assessment involves the evaluation of areas of specific strengths and weaknesses in reading, spelling, written expression, and mathematical skills. Schools routinely screen

Table 10-2	Information to Be Sought during the Physical Examination of a Child with Suspected Developmental Disabilities

ITEM	POSSIBLE SIGNIFICANCE	ITEM	POSSIBLE SIGNIFICANCE
General appearance	May indicate significant delay in development or obvious syndrome	**LIVER**	
STATURE		Hepatomegaly	Fructose intolerance, galactosemia, glycogenosis types I to IV, mucopolysaccharidosis I and II, Niemann-Pick disease, Tay-Sachs disease, Zellweger syndrome, Gaucher disease, ceroid lipofuscinosis, gangliosidosis
Short stature	Williams syndrome, malnutrition, Turner syndrome; many children with severe retardation have associated short stature.		
Obesity	Prader-Willi syndrome	**GENITALIA**	
Large stature	Sotos syndrome	Macro-orchidism (usually not noted until puberty)	Fragile X syndrome
HEAD			
Macrocephaly	Alexander syndrome, Sotos syndrome, gangliosidosis, hydrocephalus, mucopolysaccharidosis, subdural effusion	Hypogenitalism	Prader-Willi syndrome, Klinefelter syndrome, CHARGE association
		EXTREMITIES	
Microcephaly	Virtually any condition that can retard brain growth (e.g., malnutrition, Angelman syndrome, de Lange syndrome, fetal alcohol effects)	Hands, feet, dermatoglyphics, and creases	May indicate specific entity such as Rubinstein-Taybi syndrome or be associated with chromosomal anomaly
FACE		Joint contractures	Sign of muscle imbalance around joints (e.g., with meningomyelocele, cerebral palsy, arthrogryposis, muscular dystrophy; also occurs with cartilaginous problems such as mucopolysaccharidosis)
Coarse, triangular, round, or flat face; hypotelorism or hypertelorism, slanted or short palpebral fissure; unusual nose, maxilla, and mandible	Specific measurements may provide clues to inherited, metabolic, or other diseases such as fetal alcohol syndrome, cri du chat syndrome (5p- syndrome), or Williams syndrome.		
		SKIN	
EYES		Café au lait spots	Neurofibromatosis, tuberous sclerosis, Bloom syndrome
Prominent	Crouzon syndrome, Seckel syndrome, fragile X syndrome	Eczema	Phenylketonuria, histiocytosis
Cataract	Galactosemia, Lowe syndrome, prenatal rubella, hypothyroidism	Hemangiomas and telangiectasia	Sturge-Weber syndrome, Bloom syndrome, ataxia-telangiectasia
Cherry-red spot in macula	Gangliosidosis (GM_1), metachromatic leukodystrophy, mucolipidosis, Tay-Sachs disease, Niemann-Pick disease, Farber lipogranulomatosis, sialidosis III	Hypopigmented macules, streaks, adenoma sebaceum	Tuberous sclerosis, hypomelanosis of Ito
		HAIR	
Chorioretinitis	Congenital infection with cytomegalovirus, toxoplasmosis, or rubella	Hirsutism	de Lange syndrome, mucopolysaccharidosis, fetal phenytoin effects, cerebro-oculo-facio-skeletal syndrome, trisomy 18 syndrome
Corneal cloudiness	Mucopolysaccharidosis I and II, Lowe syndrome, congenital syphilis		
EARS		**NEUROLOGIC**	
Pinnae, low set or malformed	Trisomies such as 18, Rubinstein-Taybi syndrome, Down syndrome, CHARGE association, cerebro-oculo-facio-skeletal syndrome, fetal phenytoin effects	Asymmetry of strength and tone	Focal lesion, cerebral palsy
		Hypotonia	Prader-Willi syndrome, Down syndrome, Angelman syndrome, gangliosidosis, early cerebral palsy
Hearing	Loss of acuity in mucopolysaccharidosis; hyperacusis in many encephalopathies		
HEART		Hypertonia	Neurodegenerative conditions involving white matter, cerebral palsy, trisomy 18 syndrome
Structural anomaly or hypertrophy	CHARGE association, CATCH-22, velocardiofacial syndrome, glycogenosis II, fetal alcohol effects, mucopolysaccharidosis I; chromosomal anomalies such as Down syndrome; maternal phenylketonuria; chronic cyanosis may impair cognitive development.	Ataxia	Ataxia-telangiectasia, metachromatic leukodystrophy, Angelman syndrome

Adapted and updated from Liptak G: Mental retardation and developmental disability. In Kliegman RM, Greenbaum LA, Lye PS, editors: Practical Strategies in Pediatric Diagnosis and Therapy, ed 2, Philadelphia, 2004, Saunders, p 540.
*CATCH-22, **C**ardiac defects, **a**bnormal face, **t**hymic hypoplasia, **c**left palate, **h**ypocalcemia, defects on chromosome **22**; CHARGE, **c**oloboma, **h**eart defects, **a**tresia choanae, **r**etarded growth, **g**enital anomalies, **e**ar anomalies (deafness).*

Table 10-3	Tests of Cognition		
TEST		**AGE RANGE**	**SPECIAL FEATURES**
INFANT SCALES			
Bayley Scales of Infant Development (3rd ed)		1–42 mo	Mental, psychomotor scales, behavior record; weak intelligence predictor
Cattell Infant Intelligence Scale		2–30 mo	Used to extend Stanford-Binet downward
Gesell Developmental Observation-Revised (GDO-R)		Birth–3 yr	Used by many pediatricians
Ordinal Scales of Infant Psychological Development		Birth–24 mo	Six subscales; based on Piaget's stages; weak in predicting later intelligence
PRESCHOOL SCALES			
Stanford-Binet Intelligence Scale (4th ed)		2 yr–adult	Four area scores, with subtests and composite IQ score
McCarthy Scales of Children's Abilities		2½–8½ yr	6–18 subtests; good at defining learning disabilities; strengths/weaknesses approach
Wechsler Primary and Preschool Test of Intelligence–Revised (WPPSI-R)		2 ½–7¼ yr	11 subtests; verbal, performance IQs; long administration time; good at defining learning disabilities
Merrill-Palmer Scale of Mental Tests		18 mo–4 yr	19 subtests cover language skills, motor skills, manual dexterity, and matching ability
Differential Abilities Scale – II (2nd ed)		2½–18 yr	Special nonverbal composite; short administration time
SCHOOL-AGE SCALES			
Stanford-Binet Intelligence Scale (4th ed)		2 yr–adult	Four area scores, with subtests and composite IQ score
Wechsler Intelligence Scale for Children (4th ed) (WISC IV)		6–16 yr	See comments on WPPSI-R
Leiter International Performance Scale, Revised		2–20 yr	Nonverbal measure of intelligence ideal for use with those who are cognitively delayed, non-English speaking, hearing impaired, speech impaired, or autistic
Wechsler Adult Intelligence Scale–Revised (WAIS-III)		16 yr–adult	See comments on WPPSI-R
Differential Abilities Scale – II (2nd ed)		2½ yr–adult	Special nonverbal composite; short administration time
ADAPTIVE BEHAVIOR SCALES			
Vineland Adaptive Behavior Scale – II (2nd ed)		Birth–90 yr	Interview/questionnaire; typical persons and blind, deaf, developmentally delayed, and retarded
American Association on Mental Retardation (AAMR) Adaptive Behavioral Scale		4–21 yr	Useful in mental retardation, other disabilities

children with grouped tests to aid in problem identification and program evaluation. For the child with special needs, this screening ultimately should lead to individualized testing and the development of an IEP that would enable the child to progress comfortably in school. Diagnostic teaching, in which the child's response to various teaching techniques is assessed, also may be helpful.

Social Environment Assessment

Assessments of the environment in which the child is living, working, playing, and growing are important in understanding the child's development. A home visit by a social worker, community health nurse, and/or home-based intervention specialist can provide valuable information about the child's social milieu. Often the home visitor can suggest additional adaptive equipment or renovations if there are challenges at home. If there is a suspicion of inadequate parenting, and, especially, if there is a suspicion of neglect or abuse (including emotional abuse), the child and family must be referred to the local child protection agency. Information about reporting hotlines and local child protection agencies usually is found inside the front cover of local telephone directories (see Chapter 22).

MANAGEMENT OF DEVELOPMENTAL PROBLEMS

Intervention in the Primary Care Setting

The clinician must decide whether a problem requires referral for further diagnostic workup and management or whether management in the primary care setting is appropriate. Counseling roles required in caring for these children are listed in Table 10-4. When a child is young, much of the counseling interaction takes place between the parents and the clinician, and, as the child matures, direct counseling shifts increasingly toward the child.

The assessment process may be therapeutic in itself. By assuming the role of a nonjudgmental, supportive listener, the clinician creates a climate of trust, allowing the family to express difficult or painful thoughts and feelings. Expressing emotions may allow the parent or caregiver to move on to the work of understanding and resolving the problem.

Table 10-4	Primary Care Counseling Roles
Allow ventilation	
Facilitate clarification	
Support patient problem solving	
Provide specific reassurance	
Provide education	
Provide specific parenting advice	
Suggest environmental interventions	
Provide follow-up	
Facilitate appropriate referrals	
Coordinate care and interpret reports after referrals	

Interview techniques may facilitate clarification of the problem for the family and for the clinician. The family's ideas about the causes of the problem and attempts at coping can provide a basis for developing strategies for problem management that are much more likely to be implemented successfully because they emanate, in part, from the family. The clinician shows respect by endorsing the parent's ideas when appropriate; this can increase self-esteem and sense of competency.

Educating parents about normal and aberrant development and behavior may prevent problems through early detection and anticipatory guidance and communicates the physician's interest in hearing parental concerns. Early detection allows intervention before the problem becomes entrenched and associated problems develop.

The severity of developmental and behavioral problems ranges from variations of normal to problematic responses to stressful situations to frank disorders. The clinician must try to establish the severity and scope of the patient's symptoms so that appropriate intervention can be planned.

Counseling Principles

For the child, behavioral change must be learned, not simply imposed. It is easiest to learn when the lesson is simple, clear, and consistent and presented in an atmosphere free of fear or intimidation. Parents often try to impose behavioral change in an emotionally charged atmosphere, most often at the time of a behavioral *violation*. Similarly clinicians may try to *teach* parents with hastily presented advice when the parents are distracted by other concerns or not engaged in the suggested behavioral change.

Apart from management strategies directed specifically at the problem behavior, regular times for positive parent-child interaction should be instituted. Frequent, brief, affectionate physical contact over the day provides opportunities for positive reinforcement of desirable child behaviors and for building a sense of competence in the child and the parent.

Most parents feel guilty when their children have a developmental/behavioral problem. Guilt may be caused by the fear that the problem was caused by inadequate parenting or by previous angry responses to the child's behavior. If possible and appropriate, the clinician should find ways to alleviate guilt, which may be a serious impediment to problem solving.

Interdisciplinary Team Intervention

In many cases, a team of professionals is required to provide the breadth and quality of services needed to appropriately serve the child who has SHCN. The primary care physician should monitor the progress of the child and continually reassess that the requisite therapy is being accomplished.

Educational intervention for a young child begins as home-based infant stimulation, often with an early childhood specialist (e.g., nurse/therapist), providing direct stimulation for the child and training the family to provide the stimulation. As the child matures, a center-based nursery program may be indicated. For the school-age child, special services may range from extra attention in the classroom to a self-contained special education classroom.

Psychological intervention may be directed to the parent or family or, with an older child, primarily child-directed. Examples of therapeutic approaches are guidance therapies, such as directive advice giving, counseling to create their own solutions to problems, psychotherapy, behavioral management techniques, psychopharmacologic methods (from a psychiatrist), and cognitive therapy.

Motor intervention may be performed by a physical or occupational therapist. *Neurodevelopmental therapy* (NDT), the most commonly used method, is based on the concept that nervous system development is hierarchical and subject to some plasticity. The focus of NDT is on gait training and motor development, including daily living skills; perceptual abilities, such as eye-hand coordination; and spatial relationships. *Sensory integration therapy* is also used by occupational therapists to structure sensory experience from the tactile, proprioceptive, and vestibular systems to allow for adaptive motor responses.

Speech-language intervention by a speech and language therapist/pathologist (oral-motor therapist) is usually part of the overall educational program and is based on the tested language strengths and weaknesses of the child. Children needing this type of intervention may show difficulties in reading and other academic areas and develop social and behavioral problems because of their difficulties in being understood and in understanding others. **Hearing intervention**, performed by an audiologist (or an otolaryngologist), includes monitoring hearing acuity and providing amplification when necessary via hearing aids.

Social and environmental intervention generally includes nursing or social work involvement with the family. Frequently the task of coordinating services falls to these specialists. Case managers may be in the private sector, from the child's insurance or Medicaid plan, or part of a child protection agency.

Medical intervention for a child with a developmental disability involves providing primary care as well as specific treatment of conditions associated with the disability. Although curative treatment often is not possible, functional impairment can be minimized through thoughtful medical management. Certain general medical problems are found more frequently in delayed and developmentally disabled people (Table 10-5), especially if the delay is part of a known syndrome. Some children may have a limited life expectancy. Supporting the family through palliative care, hospice, and bereavement is another important role of the primary care pediatrician.

Table 10-5	Recurring Medical Issues in Children with Developmental Disabilities
PROBLEM	**ASK ABOUT OR CHECK**
Motor	Range of motion examination; scoliosis check; assessment of mobility; interaction with orthopedist, physical medicine and rehabilitation (PM&R), and physical therapist/occupational therapist as needed
Diet	Dietary history, feeding observation, growth parameter measurement and charting, supplementation as indicated by observations, oro-motor therapist as needed
Sensory impairments	Functional vision and hearing screening; interaction as needed with ophthalmologist, audiologist
Dermatologic	Examination of *all* skin areas for decubitus ulcers or infection
Dentistry	Examination of teeth and gums; confirmation of access to dental care (preferably with ability to use sedation)
Behavioral problems	Aggression, self-injury, pica; sleep problems; psychotropic drug levels and side effects
Seizures	Major motor, absence, other suspicious symptoms; monitoring of anticonvulsant levels and side effects
Infectious diseases	Ear infections, diarrhea, respiratory symptoms, aspiration pneumonia, immunizations (especially hepatitis B and influenza)
Gastrointestinal problems	Constipation, gastroesophageal reflux, gastrointestinal bleeding (stool for occult blood)
Sexuality	Sexuality education, preventing abuse, hygiene, contraception, menstrual suppression, genetic counseling
Other syndrome-specific problems	Ongoing evaluation of other "physical" problems as indicated by known mental retardation/developmental disability etiology
Advocacy for services and enhancing access to care	Educational program, family supports, financial supports, legislative advocacy to support programs

SELECTED CLINICAL PROBLEMS: THE SPECIAL NEEDS CHILD
Mental Retardation
MR is defined as significantly subnormal intellectual functioning for a child's developmental stage, existing concurrently with deficits in adaptive behaviors (self-care, home living, communication, and social interactions). MR is defined statistically as cognitive performance that is two standard deviations below the mean (roughly below the 3rd percentile) of the general population as measured on standardized intelligence testing. The last known estimate of the prevalence of MR is that about 2% of the U.S. population is affected. Levels of MR from IQ scores derived from two typical tests are shown in Table 10-6. Caution must be exercised in interpretation because these categories do not reflect actual functional level of the tested individual.

The etiology of the central nervous system insult resulting in MR may involve genetic disorders, teratogenic influences,

Table 10-6	Levels of Mental Retardation		
LEVEL OF RETARDATION	**ICD-10 IQ SCORE**	**WISC-IV IQ SCORE**	**EDUCATIONAL LABEL**
Mild	50–69	50–55 to 70	Educable mentally retarded (EMR)
Moderate	35–49	35–40 to 50–55	Trainable mentally retarded (TMR)
Severe	20–34	20–25 to 35–50	
Profound	<20	<20–25	

ICD-10, International Classification of Diseases (WHO), ed 10; *WISC-IV*, Wechsler Intelligence Scale for children, ed 4.

perinatal insults, acquired childhood disease, and environmental and social factors (Table 10-7). Mild MR correlates with socioeconomic status, although profound MR does not. Although a single organic cause may be found, each individual's performance should be considered a function of the interaction of environmental influences with the individual's organic substrate. Behavioral difficulties resulting from the MR itself and from the family's reaction to the child and the condition are common. More severe forms of MR can be traced to biologic factors. The earlier the cognitive slowing is recognized, the more severe the deviation from normal is likely to be.

The first step in the diagnosis and management of a child with MR is to identify functional strengths and weaknesses for purposes of medical and habilitative therapies. A history and physical examination may suggest a diagnostic approach that, then, may be confirmed by laboratory testing and/or imaging. Frequently used laboratory tests include chromosomal analysis and magnetic resonance imaging of the brain. Almost one third of individuals with MR do not have readily identifiable reasons for their disability.

Vision Impairment
Significant visual impairment is a problem in many children. **Partial vision** (defined as visual acuity between 20/70 and 20/200) occurs in 1 in 500 school-age children in the United States. **Legal blindness** is defined as distant visual acuity of 20/200 or worse and affects about 35,000 children in the United States. Such impairment can be a major barrier to optimal development.

The most common cause of **severe visual impairment** in children is retinopathy of prematurity (see Chapter 61). Congenital cataracts may lead to significant amblyopia. Cataracts also are associated with other ocular abnormalities and developmental disabilities. **Amblyopia** is a pathologic alteration of the visual system characterized by a reduction in visual acuity in one or both eyes with no clinically apparent organic abnormality that completely accounts for the visual loss. Amblyopia is due to a distortion of the normal clearly formed retinal image (from congenital cataracts or severe refractive errors); abnormal binocular interaction between the eyes as one eye competitively inhibits the other (strabismus); or a combination of both mechanisms. Albinism, hydrocephalus, congenital cytomegalovirus infection, and birth asphyxia are other significant contributors to blindness in children.

Table 10-7	Differential Diagnosis of Mental Retardation*

EARLY ALTERATIONS OF EMBRYONIC DEVELOPMENT

Sporadic events affecting embryogenesis, usually a stable developmental challenge

Chromosomal changes (e.g., trisomy 21 syndrome)

Prenatal influences (e.g., substance abuse, teratogenic medications, intrauterine TORCH infections) †

UNKNOWN CAUSES

No definite issue is identified, or multiple elements present, none of which is diagnostic (may be multifactorial)

ENVIRONMENTAL AND SOCIAL PROBLEMS

Dynamic influences, commonly associated with other challenges

Deprivation (neglect)

Parental mental illness

Environmental intoxications (e.g., significant lead intoxication)*

PREGNANCY PROBLEMS AND PERINATAL MORBIDITY

Impingement on normal intrauterine development or delivery; neurologic abnormalities frequent, challenges are stable or occasionally worsening

Fetal malnutrition and placental insufficiency

Perinatal complications (e.g., prematurity, birth asphyxia, birth trauma)

HEREDITARY DISORDERS

Preconceptual origin, variable expression in the individual infant, multiple somatic effects, frequently a progressive or degenerative course

Inborn errors of metabolism (e.g., Tay-Sachs disease, Hunter disease, phenylketonuria)

Single-gene abnormalities (e.g., neurofibromatosis or tuberous sclerosis)

Other chromosomal aberrations (e.g., fragile X syndrome, deletion mutations such as Prader-Willi syndrome)

Polygenic familial syndromes (pervasive developmental disorders)

ACQUIRED CHILDHOOD ILLNESS

Acute modification of developmental status, variable potential for functional recovery

Infections (all can ultimately lead to brain damage, but most significant are encephalitis and meningitis)

Cranial trauma (accidental and child abuse)

Accidents (e.g., near-drowning, electrocution)

Environmental intoxications (prototype is lead poisoning)

TORCH, Toxoplasmosis, other (congenital syphilis), rubella, cytomegalovirus, and herpes simplex virus.
*Some health problems fit in several categories (e.g., lead intoxication may be involved in several areas).
†This also may be considered as an acquired childhood disease.

Children with **mild to moderate visual impairment** usually have an uncorrected refractive error. The most common presentation is myopia or nearsightedness. Other causes are hyperopia (farsightedness) and astigmatism (alteration in the shape of the cornea leading to visual distortion). In children younger than 6 years, high refractive errors in one or both eyes also may cause amblyopia, aggravating visual impairment.

The diagnosis of severe visual impairment commonly is made when an infant is 4 to 8 months of age. Clinical suspicion is based on parental concerns aroused by unusual behavior, such as lack of smiling in response to appropriate stimuli, the presence of nystagmus, other wandering eye movements, or motor delays in beginning to reach for objects. Fixation and visual tracking behavior can be seen in most infants by 6 weeks of age. This behavior can be assessed by moving a brightly colored object (or the examiner's face) across the visual field of a quiet but alert infant at a distance of 1 ft. The eyes also should be examined for red reflexes and pupillary reactions to light. Optical alignment (binocular vision with both eyes consistently focusing on the same spot) should not be expected until the infant is beyond the newborn period. Persistent nystagmus is abnormal at any age. If ocular abnormalities are identified, referral to a pediatric ophthalmologist is indicated.

During the newborn period, vision may be assessed by physical examination and by **visual evoked response**. This test evaluates the conduction of electrical impulses from the optic nerve to the occipital cortex of the brain. The eye is stimulated by a bright flash of light or with an alternating checkerboard of black-and-white squares, and the resulting electrical response is recorded from electrodes strategically placed on the scalp, similar to an electroencephalogram.

There are many developmental implications of visual impairment. Perception of body image is abnormal, and imitative behavior, such as smiling, is delayed. Delays in mobility may occur in children who are visually impaired from birth, although their postural milestones (ability to sit) usually are achieved appropriately. Social bonding with the parents also is often affected.

Visually impaired children can be helped in various ways. Classroom settings may be augmented with resource-room assistance to present material in a nonvisual format. Fine motor activity development, listening skills, and Braille reading and writing are intrinsic to successful educational intervention for a child with severe visual impairment.

Hearing Impairment

Decision-Making Algorithm
Available @ StudentConsult.com

Hearing Loss

The clinical significance of hearing loss varies with its type (conductive versus sensorineural), its frequency, and its severity as measured in the number of decibels heard or the number of decibels of hearing lost. The most common cause of mild to moderate hearing loss in children is a conduction abnormality caused by acquired middle ear disease (acute and chronic otitis media). This abnormality may have a significant effect on the development of speech and language development, particularly if there is chronic fluctuating middle ear fluid. If hearing impairment is more severe, sensorineural hearing loss is more common. Causes of sensorineural deafness include congenital infections (e.g., rubella and cytomegalovirus), meningitis, birth asphyxia, kernicterus, ototoxic drugs (especially aminoglycoside antibiotics), and tumors and their treatments. Genetic deafness may be either dominant or recessive in inheritance; this is the main cause of hearing impairment in schools for the deaf. In Down syndrome, there is a predisposition to conductive loss caused by middle ear infection

Table 10-8	Neurodevelopmental-Behavioral Complications of Hearing Loss				
		COMPLICATIONS			
SEVERITY OF HEARING LOSS	**POSSIBLE ETIOLOGIC ORIGINS**	**SPEECH-LANGUAGE**	**EDUCATIONAL**	**BEHAVIORAL**	**TYPES OF THERAPY**
Slight 15–25 dB (ASA)	Chronic otitis media/ middle ear effusions	Difficulty with hearing distant or faint speech	Possible auditory learning dysfunction	Usually none	May require favorable class setting, speech therapy, or auditory training
	Perforation of tympanic membrane		May reveal a slight verbal deficit		Possible value in hearing aid, surgery
	Sensorineural loss				Favorable class setting
	Tympanosclerosis				
Mild 25–40 dB (ASA)	Chronic otitis media/ middle ear effusions	Difficulty with conversational speech over 3–5 ft	May miss 50% of class discussions	Psychological problems	Special education resource help, surgery
	Perforation of tympanic membrane	May have limited vocabulary and speech disorders	Auditory learning dysfunction	May act inappropriately if directions are not heard well	Hearing aid, surgery
	Sensorineural loss			Acting out behavior	Favorable class setting
	Tympanosclerosis			Poor self-concept	Lip reading instruction Speech therapy
Moderate 40–65 dB (ASA)	Chronic otitis media/ middle ear effusions	Conversation must be loud to be understood.	Learning disability	Emotional and social problems	Special education resource or special class, surgery
	Middle ear anomaly	Defective speech	Difficulty with group learning or discussion	Behavioral reactions of childhood	Special help in speech-language development
	Sensorineural loss	Deficient language use and comprehension	Auditory processing dysfunction	Acting out	Hearing aid and lip reading
			Limited vocabulary	Poor self-concept	Speech therapy
Severe 65–95 dB (ASA)	Sensorineural loss	Loud voices may be heard 2 ft from ear.	Marked educational retardation	Emotional and social problems that are associated with handicap	Full-time special education for deaf children, cochlear implant
	Severe middle ear disease	Defective speech and language No spontaneous speech development if loss present before 1 yr	Marked learning disability, limited vocabulary	Poor self-concept	Full-time special education for deaf children, hearing aid, lip reading, speech therapy, surgery, cochlear implant
Profound ≥95 dB (ASA)	Sensorineural or mixed loss	Relies on vision rather than hearing Defective speech and language Speech and language will not develop spontaneously if loss present before 1 yr.	Marked learning disability because of lack of understanding of speech	Congenital and prelingually deaf may show severe emotional problems.	Full-time special education for deaf children, hearing aid, lip reading, speech therapy, surgery, cochlear implant

Adapted and updated from Gottlieb MI: Otitis media. In Levine MD, Carey WB, Crocker AC, et al, editors: Developmental-Behavioral Pediatrics, Philadelphia, 1983, WB Saunders.
ASA, Acoustical Society of America.

and sensorineural loss caused by cochlear disease. Any hearing loss may have a significant effect on the child's developing communication skills. These skills then affect all areas of the child's cognitive and skills development (Table 10-8).

It is sometimes quite difficult to accurately determine the presence of hearing in infants and young children. Inquiring about a newborn's or infant's response to sounds or even observing the response to sounds in the office is unreliable for identifying hearing-impaired children. Universal screening of newborns is required prior to nursery discharge and includes the following:

- **Auditory brainstem response (ABR)** measures how the brain responds to sound. Clicks or tones are played through soft earphones into the infant's ears. Three electrodes placed on the infant's head measure the brain's response.

- **Otoacoustic emissions** measure sound waves produced in the inner ear. A tiny probe is placed just inside the infant's ear canal. It measures the response (echo) when clicks or tones are played into the infant's ears.

Both of these tests are quick (5 to 10 minutes), painless, and may be performed while the infant is sleeping or lying still. The tests are sensitive but not as specific as more definitive tests. Infants who do not pass these tests are referred for more comprehensive testing. Many of these infants have normal hearing on definitive testing. Infants who do not have normal hearing should be immediately evaluated or referred for etiologic diagnosis and early intervention.

For children not screened at birth (such as children of immigrant parents) or children with suspected acquired hearing loss, later testing may allow early appropriate intervention. Hearing can be screened by means of an office audiogram, but other techniques are needed (ABR, behavior audiology) for young, neurologically immature or impaired, and behaviorally difficult children. The typical audiologic assessment includes pure-tone audiometry over a variety of sound frequencies (pitches), especially over the range of frequencies in which most speech occurs. **Pneumatic otoscopic** examination and **tympanometry** are used to assess middle ear function and the tympanic membrane compliance for pathology in the middle ear, such as fluid, ossicular dysfunction, and eustachian tube dysfunction (see Chapter 9).

The treatment of conductive hearing loss (largely due to otitis media and middle ear effusions) is discussed in Chapter 105. Treatment of sensorineural hearing impairment may be medical or surgical. If amplification is indicated, hearing aids can be tuned preferentially to amplify the frequency ranges in which the patient has decreased acuity. Educational intervention typically includes speech-language therapy and teaching American Sign Language. Even with amplification, many hearing-impaired children show deficits in processing auditory information, requiring special educational services for helping to read and for other academic skills. **Cochlear implants** are surgically implantable devices that provide hearing sensation to individuals with severe to profound hearing loss. The implants are designed to substitute for the function of the middle ear, cochlear mechanical motion, and sensory cells, transforming sound energy into electrical energy that initiates impulses in the auditory nerve. Cochlear implants are indicated for children older than 12 months with profound bilateral sensorineural hearing loss who have limited benefit from hearing aids, have failed to progress in auditory skill development, and have no radiologic or medical contraindications. Implantation in children as young as possible gives them the most advantageous auditory environment for speech-language learning.

Speech-Language Impairment

Parents often bring the concern of speech delay to the physician's attention when they compare their young child with others of the same age (Table 10-9). The most common causes of the speech delay are MR, hearing impairment, social deprivation, autism, and oral-motor abnormalities. If a problem is suspected based on screening with tests such as Ages and Stages Questionnaires or the Parents' Evaluation of Developmental Status test (see Chapter 8) or other standard screening test (Early Language Milestone Scale), a referral to a specialized hearing and speech center is indicated. While awaiting

Table 10-9	Clues to When a Child with a Communication Disorder Needs Help

0–11 MONTHS

Before 6 months, the child does not startle, blink, or change immediate activity in response to sudden, loud sounds.

Before 6 months, the child does not attend to the human voice and is not soothed by his or her mother's voice.

By 6 months, the child does not babble strings of consonant and vowel syllables or imitate gurgling or cooing sounds.

By 10 months, the child does not respond to his or her name.

At 10 months, the child's sound-making is limited to shrieks, grunts, or sustained vowel production.

12–23 MONTHS

At 12 months, the child's babbling or speech is limited to vowel sounds.

By 15 months, the child does not respond to "no," "bye-bye," or "bottle."

By 15 months, the child does not imitate sounds or words.

By 18 months, the child is not consistently using at least six words with appropriate meaning.

By 21 months, the child does not respond correctly to "Give me . . . ," "Sit down," or "Come here" when spoken without gestural cues.

By 23 months, two-word phrases that are spoken as single units (e.g., "whatszit," "thankyou," "allgone") have not emerged.

24–36 MONTHS

By 24 months, at least 50% of the child's speech is not understood by familiar listeners.

By 24 months, the child does not point to body parts without gestural cues.

By 24 months, the child is not combining words into phrases (e.g., "go bye-bye," "go car," "want cookie").

By 30 months, the child does not show understanding of spatial concepts: on, in, under, front, and back.

By 30 months, the child is not using short sentences (e.g., "Daddy went bye-bye").

By 30 months, the child has not begun to ask questions (using *where, what, why*).

By 36 months, the child's speech is not understood by unfamiliar listeners.

ALL AGES

At any age, the child is consistently dysfluent with repetitions, hesitations; blocks or struggles to say words. Struggle may be accompanied by grimaces, eye blinks, or hand gestures.

Adapted and updated from Weiss CE, Lillywhite HE: Communication Disorders: a handbook for prevention and early detection, *St Louis, 1976, Mosby.*

the results of testing or initiation of speech-language therapy, parents should be advised to speak slowly and clearly to the child (and avoid *baby talk*). Parents and older siblings should read frequently to the speech-delayed child.

Speech disorders include **articulation, fluency,** and **resonance disorders.** Articulation disorders include difficulties producing sounds in syllables or saying words incorrectly to the point that other people cannot understand what is being said. Fluency disorders include problems such as **stuttering,** the condition in which the flow of speech is interrupted by abnormal stoppages, repetitions (*st-st-stuttering*), or prolonging sounds and syllables (*ssssstuttering*). Resonance or voice disorders include problems with the pitch, volume, or quality of a child's voice that distract listeners from what is being said.

Language disorders can be either receptive or expressive. Receptive disorders refer to difficulties understanding or processing language. Expressive disorders include difficulty putting words together, limited vocabulary, or inability to use language in a socially appropriate way.

Speech-language pathologists (speech or oral-motor therapists) assess the speech, language, cognitive communication, and swallowing skills of children; determine what types of communication problems exist; and identify the best way to treat these challenges. Speech-language pathologists skilled at working with infants and young children are also vital in training parents and infants in other oral-motor skills, such as how to feed an infant born with a cleft lip and palate.

Speech-language therapy involves having a speech-language specialist work with a child on a one-on-one basis, in a small group, or directly in a classroom to overcome a specific disorder using a variety of therapeutic strategies. Language intervention activities involve having a speech-language specialist interact with a child by playing and talking to him or her, using pictures, books, objects, or ongoing events to stimulate language development. Articulation therapy involves having the therapist model correct sounds and syllables for a child, often during play activities.

Children enrolled in therapy early (<3 years of age) tend to have better outcomes than children who begin therapy later. Older children can make progress in therapy, but progress may occur more slowly because these children often have learned patterns that need to be modified or changed. Parental involvement is crucial to the success of a child's progress in speech-language therapy.

Cerebral Palsy

Decision-Making Algorithms
Available @ StudentConsult.com

Limp
In-Toeing, Out-Toeing, and Toe-Walking
Bowlegs and Knock-Knees
Hypotonia and Weakness

Cerebral palsy (CP) refers to a group of nonprogressive, but often changing, motor impairment syndromes secondary to anomalies or lesions of the brain arising before or after birth. The prevalence of CP at age 8 in the United States is 3.6 per 1000; prevalence is much higher in premature and twin births. Prematurity and low birth weight infants (leading to perinatal asphyxia), congenital malformations, and kernicterus are causes of CP noted at birth. Ten percent of children with CP have acquired CP, developing at later ages. Meningitis and head injury (accidental and nonaccidental) are the most common causes of acquired CP (Table 10-10). Nearly 50% of children with CP have no identifiable risk factors. As genomic medicine advances, many of these causes of idiopathic CP may be identified.

Most children with CP, except in its mildest forms, are diagnosed in the first 18 months of life when they fail to attain motor milestones or show abnormalities such as asymmetric

Table 10-10	Risk Factors for Cerebral Palsy

PREGNANCY AND BIRTH

Low socioeconomic status

Prematurity

Low birth weight/fetal growth retardation (<1500 g at birth)

Maternal seizures/seizure disorder

Treatment with thyroid hormone, estrogen, or progesterone

Pregnancy complications

  Polyhydramnios

  Eclampsia

  Third-trimester bleeding (including threatened abortion and placenta previa)

    Multiple births

    Abnormal fetal presentation

    Maternal fever

Congenital malformations/syndromes

Newborn hypoxic-ischemic encephalopathy

Bilirubin (kernicterus)

ACQUIRED AFTER THE NEWBORN PERIOD

Meningitis

Head injury

  Car crashes

  Child abuse

Near-drowning

Stroke

Table 10-11	Descriptions of Cerebral Palsy by Site of Involvement

Hemiparesis (hemiplegia)—predominantly unilateral impairment of the arm and leg on the same (e.g., right or left) side

Diplegia—motor impairment primarily of the legs (often with some limited involvement of the arms; some authors challenge this specific type as not being different from quadriplegia)

Quadriplegia—all four limbs (whole body) are functionally compromised.

gross motor function, hypertonia, or hypotonia. CP can be characterized further by the affected parts of the body (Table 10-11) and descriptions of the predominant type of motor disorder (Table 10-12). Comorbidities in these children often include epilepsy, learning difficulties, behavioral challenges, and sensory impairments. Many of these children have an isolated motor defect. Some affected children may be intellectually gifted.

Treatment depends on the pattern of dysfunction. Physical and occupational therapy can facilitate optimal positioning and movement patterns, increasing function of the affected parts. Spasticity management also may include oral medications (dantrolene, benzodiazepines, and baclofen), botulinum toxin injections, and implantation of intrathecal baclofen pumps. Management of seizures, spasticity, orthopedic impairments, and sensory impairments may help improve

Table 10-12	Classification of Cerebral Palsy by Type of Motor Disorder

Spastic cerebral palsy: the most common form of cerebral palsy, it accounts for 70%–80% of cases. It results from injury to the upper motor neurons of the pyramidal tract. It may occasionally be bilateral. It is characterized by at least two of the following: abnormal movement pattern, increased tone, or pathologic reflexes (e.g., Babinski response, hyperreflexia).

Dyskinetic cerebral palsy: occurs in 10%–15% of cases. It is dominated by abnormal patterns of movement and involuntary, uncontrolled, recurring movements.

Ataxic cerebral palsy: accounts for <5% of cases. This form results from cerebellar injury and features abnormal posture or movement and loss of orderly muscle coordination or both.

Dystonic cerebral palsy: also uncommon. It is characterized by reduced activity and stiff movement (hypokinesia) and hypotonia.

Choreoathetotic cerebral palsy: rare now that excessive hyperbilirubinemia is aggressively prevented and treated. This form is dominated by increased and stormy movements (hyperkinesia) and hypotonia.

Mixed cerebral palsy: accounts for 10%–15% of cases. This term is used when more than one type of motor pattern is present and when one pattern does not clearly dominate another. It typically is associated with more complications, including sensory deficits, seizures, and cognitive-perceptual impairments.

educational attainment. CP cannot be cured, but a host of interventions can improve functional abilities, participation in society, and quality of life. Like all children, an assessment and reinforcement of strengths are important, especially for intellectually intact or gifted children who have simple motor deficits.

Suggested Reading

Brosco J, Mattingly M, Sanders L: Impact of specific medical interventions on reducing the prevalence of mental retardation, *Arch Pediatr Adolesc Med* 160:302–309, 2006.

Council on Children With Disabilities; Section on Developmental Behavioral Pediatrics; Bright Futures Steering Committee; Medical Home Initiatives for Children With Special Needs Project Advisory Committee: Identifying infants and young children with developmental disorders in the medical home: an algorithm for developmental surveillance and screening. *Pediatrics* 118(1):405–420, 2006.

Daniels S, Greer F: Committee on Nutrition: Lipid screening and cardiovascular health in childhood, *Pediatrics* 122:198–208, 2008.

Gardner HG: American Academy of Pediatrics Committee on Injury, Violence, and Poison Prevention. Office-based counseling for unintentional injury prevention, *Pediatrics* 119(1):202–206, 2007.

Hagan J, Shaw J, Duncan P: *Bright Futures: guidelines for health supervision of infants, children, and adolescents*, ed 3, Elk Grove Village IL, 2008, American Academy of Pediatrics.

Kliegman R, Behrman R, Jenson H, et al: *Nelson Textbook of Pediatrics*, ed 18, Philadelphia, 2007, Elsevier.

Behavioral Disorders
Sheila Gahagan, Yi Hui Liu, and Scott J. Brown

Chapter 11

CRYING AND COLIC

Infant crying, a sign of pain, distress, hunger, or fatigue, is interpreted by caregivers according to the context of the crying. The cry just after birth heralds the infant's health and vigor. The screams of the same infant, 6 weeks later, may be interpreted as a sign of illness, difficult temperament, or poor parenting. Crying is a manifestation of infant arousal influenced by the environment and interpreted through the lens of the family, social, and cultural context.

NORMAL DEVELOPMENT

Crying is best understood by the characteristics of timing, duration, frequency, intensity, and modifiability of the cry (Fig. 11-1). Most infants cry little during the first 2 weeks of life, gradually increasing to 3 hours per day by 6 weeks and decreasing to 1 hour per day by 12 weeks.

Cry **duration** differs by culture and infant care practices. For example, !Kung San hunter–gatherer infants, who are continuously carried and fed four times per hour, cry 50% less than infants in the United States. Crying may also relate to health status. Premature infants cry little before 40 weeks gestational age but tend to cry more than term infants at 6 weeks' corrected age. Crying behavior in former premature infants also may be influenced by ongoing medical conditions, such as bronchopulmonary dysplasia, visual impairments, and feeding disorders. The duration of crying is often modifiable by caregiving strategies.

Frequency of crying is less variable than duration of crying. At 6 weeks of age, the mean frequency of combined crying and fussing is 10 episodes in 24 hours. Diurnal variation in crying is the norm, with crying concentrated in the late afternoon and evening.

The **intensity** of infant crying varies, with descriptions ranging from fussing to screaming. An intense infant cry (pitch and loudness) is more likely to elicit concern or even alarm from parents and caregivers than an infant who frets more quietly. Pain cries of newborns are remarkably loud: 80 dB at a distance of 30.5 cm from the infant's mouth. Although pain cries have a higher frequency than hunger cries, when not attended to for a protracted period, hunger cries become acoustically similar to pain cries. Fortunately most infant crying is of a lesser intensity, consistent with fussing.

COLIC

Colic often is diagnosed using **Wessel's rule of threes**—crying for more than 3 hours per day, at least 3 days per week, for more than 3 weeks. The limitations of this definition include the lack of specificity of the word *crying* (e.g., does this include fussing?) and the necessity to wait 3 weeks to make a diagnosis in an infant who has excessive crying. Colicky crying is often described as paroxysmal and may be characterized by facial grimacing, leg flexion, and passing flatus.

Etiology

Fewer than 5% of infants evaluated for excessive crying have an organic etiology. Because the etiology of colic is unknown, this syndrome may represent the extreme of the normal phenomenon of infant crying. Nonetheless evaluation of infants with excessive crying is warranted.

Epidemiology

Cumulative incidence rates of colic vary from 5% to 19% in different studies. Girls and boys are affected equally. Studies vary by how colic is defined and by data collection methodology, such as maintaining a cry diary or actual recording of infant vocalizations. Concern about infant crying also varies by culture, and this may influence what is recorded as crying or fussing.

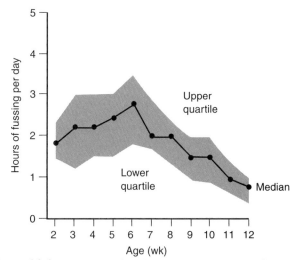

Figure 11-1 Distribution of total crying time among 80 infants studied from 2 to 12 weeks of age. Data derived from daily crying diaries recorded by mothers. *(From Brazelton TB: Crying in infancy. Pediatrics 29:582, 1962.)*

Clinical Manifestations

Decision-Making Algorithm
Available @ StudentConsult.com

Irritable Infant

The clinician who evaluates a crying infant must differentiate serious disease from colic, which has no identifiable etiology. The history includes a description of the crying, including duration, frequency, intensity, and modifiability. Associated symptoms, such as leg flexion, facial grimacing, vomiting, or back arching, should be identified. Other important historical clues include the onset, diurnal pattern, any changes in quality, and triggers or activities that relieve crying. A review of systems can identify or eliminate other serious illnesses. Medical history also is important because infants with perinatal problems are at increased risk for neurologic causes of crying. Attention to the feeding history can reveal feeding-related problems, including hunger, air swallowing (worsened by crying), gastroesophageal reflux, and food intolerance. Questions concerning the family's ability to handle the stress of the infant's crying and their knowledge of infant soothing strategies assist the clinician in assessing risk for parental mental health comorbidities and developing an intervention plan suitable for the family.

The diagnosis of colic is made only when the **physical examination** reveals no organic cause for the infant's excessive crying. The examination begins with vital signs, weight, length, and head circumference, looking for effects of systemic illness on growth. A thorough inspection of the infant is important to identify possible sources of pain, including skin lesions, **corneal abrasions, hair tourniquets, skeletal infections,** or signs of child abuse such as **fractures** (see Chapters 22 and 199). Infants with common conditions such as otitis media, urinary tract infections, mouth ulcerations, and insect bites may present with crying. A neurologic examination may reveal previously undiagnosed neurologic conditions, such as perinatal brain injuries, as the cause of irritability and crying. Observation of the infant during a crying episode is invaluable to assess the infant's potential for calming and the parents' skills in soothing the infant.

Laboratory and imaging studies are reserved for infants in whom there are history or physical examination findings suggesting an organic cause for excessive crying. An algorithm for the medical evaluation of an infant with excessive crying inconsistent with colic is presented in Figure 11-2.

Differential Diagnosis

The differential diagnosis for colic is broad and includes any condition that can cause pain or discomfort in the infant and conditions associated with *nonpainful* distress, such as fatigue or sensory overload. Cow's milk protein intolerance, maternal drug effects (including fluoxetine hydrochloride via breastfeeding), and anomalous left coronary artery all have been reported as causes of persistent crying. In addition, situations associated with poor infant regulation, including fatigue, hunger, parental anxiety, and chaotic environmental conditions, may increase the risk of excessive crying. In most cases, the

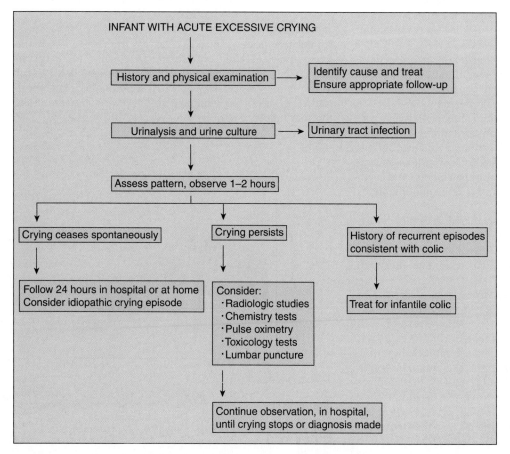

Figure 11-2 Algorithm for medical evaluation of infants with acute excessive crying. *(From Barr RG, Hopkins B, Green JA, editors: Crying complaints in the emergency department. In Crying as a Sign, a Symptom, and a Signal, London, 2000, MacKeith Press, p. 99.)*

cause of crying in infants is unexplained. If the condition began before 3 weeks' corrected age, the crying has a diurnal pattern consistent with colic (afternoon and evening clustering), the infant is otherwise developing and thriving, and no organic cause is found, a diagnosis of colic is indicated.

Treatment

The management of colic begins with education and demystification. When the family and the physician are reassured that the infant is healthy, without infection, trauma, or underlying disease, education about the normal pattern of infant crying is appropriate. Learning about the temporal pattern of colic can be reassuring; the mean crying duration begins to decrease at 6 weeks of age and decreases by half by 12 weeks of age. Colic does not always resolve by 3 months of age. Approximately 15% of infants with colic continue to have excessive crying after 3 months of age.

Helping families develop caregiving schedules for the infant's fussy period is useful. Techniques for calming infants include soothing vocalizations or singing, swaddling, slow rhythmic rocking, walking, white noise, and gentle vibration (e.g., a ride in a car). Giving caregivers permission to allow the infant to rest when soothing strategies are not working may alleviate overstimulation in some infants; this also relieves families of guilt and allows them a wider range of responses to infant crying. **Avoidance** of dangerous soothing techniques, such as **shaking the infant** or placing the infant on a vibrating clothes dryer (which has resulted in injury from falls), should be stressed.

Medications, including phenobarbital, diphenhydramine, alcohol, simethicone, dicyclomine, and lactase, are of no benefit in reducing colic and should be avoided. Parents, especially from Mexico and Eastern Europe, often use chamomile, fennel, vervain, licorice, and balm-mint teas. These teas have not been studied scientifically as remedies for colic. Families should be counseled to limit the volume of tea given because it displaces milk from the infant's diet and may limit caloric intake.

In most circumstances, **dietary changes** are not effective in reducing colic but should be considered in certain specific circumstances. There is rationale for change to a non-cow's milk formula if the infant has signs of cow's milk protein colitis. If the infant is breastfeeding, the mother can eliminate dairy products from her diet.

Prognosis

There is no evidence that infants with colic have adverse long-term outcomes in health or temperament after the neonatal period. Similarly infantile colic does not have untoward long-term effects on maternal mental health. When colic subsides, the maternal distress resolves. Rarely cases of child abuse have been associated with inconsolable infant crying.

Prevention

Much can be done to prevent colic, beginning with education of prospective parents about the normal pattern of infant crying. Prospective parents often imagine that their infant will cry only briefly for hunger. Increased contact and carrying of the infant in the weeks before the onset of colic may decrease the duration of crying episodes. Similarly other soothing strategies may

be more effective if the infant has experienced them before the onset of excessive crying. Infants who have been tightly swaddled for sleep and rest during the first weeks of life often calm to swaddling during a crying episode; this is not true for infants who have not experienced swaddling before a crying episode. Parents also can be coached to learn to read their infant's cues of hunger, discomfort, boredom, or overstimulation. It is important to understand that there are times when the infant's cry is not interpretable, and caregivers can do only their best.

Chapter **12**

TEMPER TANTRUMS

A temper tantrum, defined as out-of-control behavior, including screaming, stomping, hitting, head banging, falling down, and other violent displays of frustration, can include breath-holding, vomiting, and serious aggression, including biting. Tantrums are seen most often when the young child experiences frustration, anger, or simple inability to cope with a situation. Temper tantrums can be considered normal behavior in 1- to 3-year-old children, when the temper tantrum period is of short duration and the tantrums are not manipulative in nature.

ETIOLOGY

Temper tantrums are believed to be a normal human developmental stage. Child temperament may be a determinant of tantrum behavior.

EPIDEMIOLOGY

This behavior is common in children 18 months to 4 years of age. In U.S. studies, 50% to 80% of 2- to 3-year-old children have had regular tantrums, and 20% are reported to have daily tantrums. The behavior appears to peak late in the third year of life. Approximately 20% of 4-year-olds are still having regular temper tantrums, and explosive temper occurs in approximately 5% of school-age children. Tantrums occur equally in boys and girls during the preschool period.

CLINICAL MANIFESTATIONS

Temper tantrums are the most commonly reported behavioral problem in 2- and 3-year-old children. The typical frequency of tantrums is approximately one per week, with a great deal of variability (Fig. 12-1). The duration of each tantrum is 2 to 5 minutes, and duration increases with age (Fig. 12-2). Helping the family identify the typical antecedents of the child's tantrums is essential to evaluation and intervention. A child who has tantrums only when he or she misses a routine nap can be treated differently than a child who has frequent tantrums related to minor difficulties or disappointments.

The **evaluation** of a child who is having temper tantrums requires a complete history, including perinatal and developmental information. Careful attention to the child's daily routines may reveal problems associated with hunger, fatigue, inadequate physical activity, or overstimulation. A social

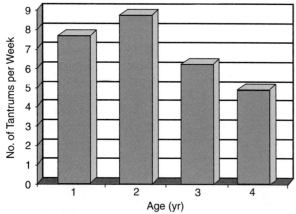

Figure 12-1 Mean tantrum frequency per week. Children 1 to 4 years of age who have tantrums typically have four to nine tantrums per week.

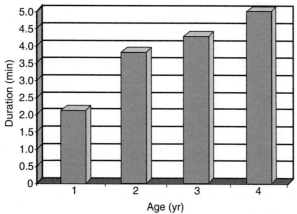

Figure 12-2 Mean duration of tantrums. The typical duration of a tantrum increases with the age of the child.

history is important, because family stress can exacerbate or prolong what begins as a normal developmental phase. The coexistence of other behavioral problems, such as sleep problems, learning problems, and social problems, suggests the possibility of a more serious mental health disorder.

The physical examination focuses on discovering an underlying illness that could decrease the child's ability to self-regulate. A thorough examination of the skin to identify child abuse is recommended (see Chapter 22). The neurologic examination identifies underlying brain disorders. Dysmorphic features may reveal a genetic syndrome. Behavioral observations reveal a child's ability to follow instructions, play with age-appropriate toys, and interact with parents and the clinician.

Laboratory studies screening for iron deficiency anemia and lead exposure are important. Other laboratory and imaging studies are performed only when the history and physical examination suggest a possible underlying etiology. Some children with excessive tantrums should have a formal developmental evaluation.

DIFFERENTIAL DIAGNOSIS

Most children who have temper tantrums have no underlying medical problem. Hearing loss and language delay may be associated with temper tantrums. Children with brain injury and other brain disorders are at increased risk for prolonged temper

tantrum behavior (in terms of actual tantrum duration and continued manifestation after the normal tantrum age). These children include former premature infants and children with autism, traumatic brain injury, cognitive impairment, and Prader-Willi and Smith-Magenis syndromes. Children with rare conditions, such as congenital adrenal hyperplasia and precocious puberty, also may present with severe and persistent tantrums. Children with intellectual disability may exhibit tantrums when their developmental age is comparable to 3 to 4 years.

TREATMENT

Intervention begins with parental education about temper tantrums, stressing that tantrums are a normal developmental phase. Parents may have unwarranted concerns about their child's mental health. The clinician can help parents understand their role in helping the child move toward self-regulation of frustration and anger. The environment can be structured to limit toddler frustration; age-inappropriate demands on the child; and hunger, fatigue, loneliness, or hyperstimulation. It is important to review the child's daily routine to understand whether the child's tantrums are communicating essential unmet needs. Children who behave well all day at day care and exhibit temper tantrums at home in the evening may be signaling fatigue or need for parental attention. Identification of underlying stress is the cornerstone of treatment because many stressors can be eliminated. Parents may consider some changes in the home environment so that they do not have to say "No" to the child as frequently.

In some cases, parents inadvertently reinforce tantrum behavior by complying with the child's demands. The child's behavior can be seen as manipulative or simply as learned behavior from a prior successful experience. Parental ambivalence about acceptable toddler behavior also may lead to inconsistent expectations and restrictions. Helping parents clarify what behavior is allowed and what is off limits can avert the temptation to give in when the child screams loudly or publicly.

Distraction is an effective means of short-circuiting impending tantrums. Physically removing the child from an environment that is associated with the child's difficulty is sometimes helpful. Further behavioral interventions are recommended only after engaging in strategies to help the child gain control by meeting basic needs, altering the environment, and anticipating meltdowns. Recommended behavioral strategies include behavior modification with positive and negative reinforcement or extinction. During the first week of any behavioral intervention, tantrum behavior may increase. Parents must be warned that it will probably get worse before it gets better. At the same time that parents are working to extinguish or decrease the tantrums, it is important that they provide positive reinforcement for good behavior.

PREVENTION

Providing parents with knowledge about the temper tantrum stage and strategies for assisting the child with emotional regulation is recommended at a health care maintenance visit between 12 and 18 months of age. Regular routines for sleeping, eating, and physical activity in a childproofed home (or day care center) provided by well-rested and psychologically healthy parents (or caregivers) usually result in a quick transition through this challenging period.

Chapter 13

ATTENTION-DEFICIT/ HYPERACTIVITY DISORDER

Attention deficit/hyperactivity disorder (ADHD) is a neurobehavioral disorder defined by symptoms of inattention, hyperactivity, and impulsivity. Clinical guidelines emphasize the use of the *Diagnostic and Statistical Manual of Mental Health Disorders, Fifth Edition,* criteria (available at http://www.cdc.gov/ncbddd/adhd/diagnosis.html) to diagnose ADHD. Diagnosis of children up to the age of 16 years requires the presence of at least 6 symptoms of inattention or 6 symptoms of hyperactivity-impulsivity for at least 6 months in two or more environments. Children 17 years of age and older must exhibit at least 5 symptoms of inattention or at least 5 symptoms of hyperactivity-impulsivity. Symptoms of inattention include: failing to pay close attention to details, appearing to not listen when spoken to directly, failing to follow through on instructions or finish assigned work, having difficulty sustaining attention during tasks or play, having difficulty organizing tasks or activities, avoiding or disliking activities that require sustained mental effort (e.g., schoolwork), frequently losing things required for tasks and activities, becoming easily distracted, and experiencing frequent forgetfulness in daily activities. Symptoms of hyperactivity include: being fidgety or restless, leaving a seat when expected to remain seated, running or climbing excessively in inappropriate situations, having difficulty in playing quietly, acting as if "driven by a motor," and talking excessively. Symptoms of impulsivity include: blurting out answers before a question has been completed, having difficulty awaiting his or her turn, and causing frequent interruptions or intrusions. In addition, several symptoms must have been present prior to 12 years of age; evidence of significant impairment in social, academic, or work settings must occur; and other mental disorders must be excluded.

ETIOLOGY

ADHD is multifactorial in origin, with genetic, neural, and environmental contributions. Twin studies and family studies demonstrate high heritability (0.8) and greater risk of developing ADHD in first-degree relatives. Candidate genes include those involving the dopaminergic and noradrenergic neurotransmitter systems. Neuroimaging studies (functional magnetic resonance imaging and positron emission tomography, commonly recognized as fMRI and PET, respectively) have shown structural and functional differences, particularly of the frontal lobes, inferior parietal cortex, basal ganglia, corpus callus, and cerebellar vermis. Prenatal exposure to substances (e.g., nicotine, alcohol) and damage to the central nervous system from trauma or infection increase the risk of ADHD.

EPIDEMIOLOGY

U.S. prevalence rates for ADHD vary, depending on criteria used and population studied, with rates typically in the 5% to 10% range. The male to female ratio is 2 to 6:1, with greater male predominance for the hyperactive/impulsive and combined types. Girls often present with inattentive symptoms and are more likely to be underdiagnosed or to receive later diagnoses. Symptoms of ADHD, particularly impulsivity and inattention, persist into adolescence and adulthood in 60% to 80% of patients.

CLINICAL MANIFESTATIONS

ADHD is diagnosed clinically by **history.** Open-ended questions should focus on specific behaviors and their impact on academic performance, family and peer relationships, safety, self-esteem, and daily activities. Information should be gathered from the family and the school via ADHD-specific rating scales such as the Conners' Rating Scales or the Vanderbilt Rating Scales.

A **physical examination** is essential to identify medical (e.g., neurologic, genetic) or developmental problems (e.g., cognitive impairment, language disorder, learning disability, autism spectrum disorder) that may underlie, coexist, or provide an alternative explanation for the child's behaviors. Observation of the child, the parents, and their interactions is part of the evaluation. Keep in mind that children with ADHD can typically focus without hyperactivity in environments with low stimulation and little distraction (e.g., clinician's office).

Laboratory and imaging studies are not routinely recommended but may help exclude other conditions. Consider thyroid function studies, blood lead levels, genetic studies, and brain imaging studies if indicated by medical history, environmental history, or physical examination.

DIFFERENTIAL DIAGNOSIS

The clinician should first consider the child's developmental level to determine whether the behaviors are within the range of normal. Medical conditions, such as sleep disordered breathing, seizure disorders, substance use, hyperthyroidism, lead intoxication, and sensory deficits, should be considered as possible causes for a child's hyperactivity and distractibility. Inattention and hyperactivity may be present as features of genetic disorders such as fragile X, 22q11.2 deletion syndrome, and neurofibromatosis 1. Chaotic living situations or psychological stress (e.g., bullying, abuse) can also lead to symptoms of hyperactivity, impulsivity, and inattention. Children who have symptoms of ADHD in only one setting may be having problems due to cognitive level, level of emotional maturity, or feelings of well-being in that setting.

More important, coexisting conditions are present in up to 60% of children with ADHD. These include psychiatric conditions, particularly oppositional defiant disorder, conduct disorder, anxiety disorder, and depression; learning disabilities; language disorders; and tic disorders. These conditions are also part of the differential diagnosis of ADHD.

TREATMENT

Management begins with recognizing ADHD as a chronic condition and educating affected children and their parents about the diagnosis, treatment options, and prognosis.

Table 13-1	**FDA-Approved Medications for Attention-Deficit/Hyperactivity Disorder**		
GENERIC MEDICATION	**BRAND NAME**	**INITIAL-MAXIMUM DOSE**	**DURATION (h)**
STIMULANTS			
Mixed amphetamine salts	Adderall*	2.5 mg–40 mg	6
	Adderall XR*	5 mg–40 mg	10
Lisdexamfetamine	Vyvanse	20 mg–70 mg	10–12
Methylphenidate	Concerta	18–54 mg (<13 years)	12
	Daytrana	18–72 mg (≥13 years)	12
	Metadate CD	10 mg†–30 mg†	Apply for 9 h
	Methyl ER	20 mg–60 mg	6–8
	Methylin	10 mg–60 mg	8
	Ritalin*	5 mg–60 mg	3–5
	Ritalin LA	5 mg–60 mg	3–5
	Ritalin SR*	20 mg–60 mg	6–8
		20 mg–60 mg	2–6
ᴅexmethylphenidate	Focalin*	2.5 mg–20 mg	3–5
	Focalin XR	5 mg–30 mg	8–12
NOREPINEPHRINE-REUPTAKE INHIBITOR			
Atomoxetine	Strattera	0.5 mg/kg/d then increase to 1.2 mg/kg with max 1.4 mg/kg 40 mg/d for adults and children weighing >154 lb titrate up to 100 mg/d	At least 10–12
ALPHA AGONISTS			
Clonidine	Kapvay	0.1 mg/d–0.4 mg/d	At least 10–12
Guanfacine	Intuniv	1 mg/d–4 mg/d	At least 10–12

Adapted from AAP: Implementing the key action statements: an algorithm and explanation for process of care for the evaluation, diagnosis, treatment, and monitoring of ADHD in children and adolescents. Pediatrics SI1–SI21, 2011.
*Available in generic form.
†Dosages for the dermal patch are not equivalent to those of the oral preparations.

Anticipatory guidance includes providing proactive strategies to mediate adverse effects on learning, school functioning, social relationships, family life, and self-esteem. Children with ADHD respond to **behavioral management,** including structure, routine, consistency in adult responses to their behaviors, and appropriate behavioral goals. Children also benefit when parents and clinicians work with teachers to address the child's needs. Daily behavior report cards and accommodations may be helpful. Social skills training or additional mental health treatments may assist some children with behavior change or preservation of self-esteem, particularly when they have coexisting developmental or mental health conditions also requiring treatment.

Stimulant medications (methylphenidate or amphetamine compounds) are the first-line agents for treatment of ADHD due to extensive evidence of effectiveness and safety. Stimulant medications are available in short-acting, intermediate-acting, and long-acting forms. Preparations include liquid, tablets, capsules, and a transdermal patch. These options allow the clinician to tailor the choice of medication to the child's needs. Nonstimulant medications, including atomoxetine (norepinephrine-reuptake inhibitor), guanfacine, or clonidine (alpha agonists), may be helpful in situations such as nonresponse to stimulant medication, family preference, concerns about medication abuse or diversion, and coexisting tic or sleep problems. ADHD medication options are listed in Table 13-1. Common side effects include appetite suppression and sleep disturbance with stimulant medications, gastrointestinal tract symptoms with atomoxetine, and sedation with alpha agonists. These side effects usually can be managed by careful adjustment of medication dosage and timing. Screening (by history and exam) for cardiac disease and monitoring of cardiac status is prudent given concerns raised by a retrospective study suggesting extremely rare but slightly increased odds of sudden cardiac death in those taking stimulant medication.

COMPLICATIONS
ADHD may be associated with academic underachievement, difficulties in interpersonal relationships, and poor self-esteem. These can have long-reaching effects (e.g., lower levels of educational, employment attainment). Adolescents with ADHD, particularly those who are untreated, are at increased risk for high-risk behaviors such as drug use, early sexual activity, and automobile accidents. Despite parental concerns of illicit drug use and addiction from stimulant medication, there is actually decreased risk of drug abuse in children and adolescents with ADHD who are appropriately medically managed.

PREVENTION
Child-rearing practices including promoting calm environments and opportunities for age-appropriate activities that require increasing levels of focus may be helpful. Limiting time spent watching television and playing rapid-response video games also may be prudent because these activities reinforce short attention span. Early implementation of behavior management techniques may assist in curtailing problematic behaviors before they result in significant impairment. Secondary disabilities can be prevented by educating medical professionals and teachers about the signs and symptoms of ADHD and the most appropriate behavioral and pharmaceutical interventions. Collaboration between health care providers, educational professionals, and mental health clinicians will enhance the early identification of and provision of services to children at risk for ADHD.

CONTROL OF ELIMINATION

NORMAL DEVELOPMENT OF ELIMINATION

Development of control of urination and defecation involves physical and cognitive maturation and is strongly influenced by cultural norms, socioeconomic status, and practices within the United States and throughout the world. In the first half of the twentieth century, toilet mastery by 18 months of age was the norm in the United States. Concern about harsh toilet training and possible later psychological distress led to professional endorsement of later toilet training. In 1962 Brazelton introduced the *child-centered approach,* which respects the child's autonomy and pride in mastery. The invention of disposable diapers also facilitated later toilet training. Social changes, including increased maternal work outside of the home and group child care, also have influenced this trend. Some families choose to wait until the child is older because the duration of the training period may be shorter. Toilet training usually begins after the second birthday and is achieved at about 3 years of age in middle-class white U.S. populations. Toilet training between 12 and 18 months of age continues to be accepted in lower-income families.

Prerequisites for achieving elimination in the toilet include the child's ability to recognize the urge for urination and defecation, to get to the toilet, to understand the sequence of tasks required, to avoid oppositional behavior, and to take pride in achievement. The entire process of toilet training can take 6 months and need not be hurried. Successful parent-child interaction around the goal of toilet mastery can set the stage for future active parental teaching and training (e.g., manners, kindness, rules and laws, and limit setting).

ENURESIS

Enuresis is urinary incontinence in a child who is adequately mature to have achieved continence. Enuresis is classified as diurnal (daytime) or nocturnal (nighttime). In the United States, daytime and nighttime dryness are expected by 4 and 6 years of age, respectively. Another useful classification of enuresis is **primary** (incontinence in a child who has never achieved dryness) and **secondary** (incontinence in a child who has been dry for at least 6 months).

Etiology

Enuresis is a symptom with multiple possible etiologic factors, including developmental difference, organic illness, or psychological distress. Primary enuresis often is associated with a family history of delayed acquisition of bladder control. A genetic etiology has been hypothesized, and familial groups with autosomal dominant phenotypic patterns for nocturnal enuresis have been identified. Although most children with enuresis do not have a psychiatric disorder, stressful life events can trigger loss of bladder control. Sleep physiology

may play a role in the etiology of nocturnal enuresis, with a high arousal threshold commonly noted. In a subgroup of enuretic children, nocturnal polyuria relates to a lack of a nocturnal vasopressin peak. Another possible etiology is malfunction of the detrusor muscle with a tendency for involuntary contractions even when the bladder contains small amounts of urine. Reduced bladder capacity can be associated with enuresis and is commonly seen in children who have chronic constipation with a large dilated distal colon, which impinges on the bladder.

Epidemiology

Enuresis is the most common urologic condition in children. Nocturnal enuresis has a reported prevalence of 15% in 5-year-olds, 7% in 8-year-olds, and 1% in 15-year-olds. The spontaneous remission rate is reported to be 15% per year. The odds ratio of nocturnal enuresis in boys compared with girls is 1.4:1. The prevalence of daytime enuresis is lower than nocturnal enuresis but has a female predominance, 1.5:1 at 7 years of age. Of children with enuresis, 22% wet during the day only, 17% wet during the day and at night, and 61% wet at night only.

Clinical Manifestations

Decision-Making Algorithm
Available @ StudentConsult.com

Enuresis

The history focuses on elucidating the pattern of voiding: How often does wetting occur? Does it occur during the day, night, or both? Are there any associated conditions with wetting episodes (e.g., bad dreams, consumption of caffeinated beverages, or exhausting days)? Has the child had a period of dryness in the past? Did a stressful event precede the change in wetting pattern? A review of systems should include a developmental history and detailed information about the neurologic, urinary, and gastrointestinal systems (including patterns of defecation). A history of sleep patterns also is important, including snoring, parasomnias, and timing of nighttime urination. A family history often reveals that one or both parents had enuresis as children. Although enuresis is rarely associated with child abuse, physical and sexual abuse history should be included as part of the psychosocial history. Many families have tried numerous interventions before seeking a physician's help. Identifying these interventions and how they were carried out aids the understanding of the child's condition and its role within the family.

The **physical examination** begins with observation of the child and the parent for clues about child developmental and parent-child interaction patterns. Special attention is paid to the abdominal, neurologic, and genital examination. A rectal examination is recommended if the child has constipation. Observation of voiding is recommended if a history of voiding problems, such as hesitancy or dribbling, is elicited. The lumbosacral spine should be examined for signs of spinal dysraphism or a tethered cord.

For most children with enuresis, the only laboratory test recommended is a clean catch urinalysis to look for chronic urinary tract infection (UTI), renal disease, and diabetes mellitus. Further testing, such as a urine culture, is based on the urinalysis. Children with complicated enuresis, including children with previous or current UTI, severe voiding dysfunction, or a neurologic finding, are evaluated with a renal sonogram and a voiding cystourethrogram. If vesicoureteral reflux, hydronephrosis, or posterior urethral valves are found, the child is referred to a urologist for further evaluation and treatment.

Differential Diagnosis

Commonly there is no identified cause of enuresis and, in most cases, enuresis resolves by adolescence without treatment. Children with primary nocturnal enuresis are most likely to have a family history and are least likely to have an identified etiology. Children with secondary diurnal and nocturnal enuresis are more likely to have an organic etiology, such as UTI, diabetes mellitus, or diabetes insipidus, to explain their symptoms. Children with primary diurnal and nocturnal enuresis may have a neurodevelopmental condition or a problem with bladder function. Children with secondary nocturnal enuresis may have a psychosocial stressor or a sleep disturbance as a predisposing condition for enuresis.

Treatment

Treatment begins with treating any diagnosed underlying organic causes of enuresis. Elimination of underlying chronic constipation is often curative. For a child whose enuresis is not associated with an identifiable disorder, all therapies must be considered in terms of cost in time, money, disruption to the family, the treatment's known success rate, and the child's likelihood to recover from the condition without treatment. The most commonly used treatment options are **conditioning therapy and pharmacotherapy.** The clinician can also assist the family in making a plan to help the child cope with this problem until it is resolved. Many children have to live with enuresis for months to years before a cure is achieved; a few children have symptoms into adulthood. A plan for handling wet garments and linens in a nonhumiliating and hygienic manner preserves the child's self-esteem. The child should take as much responsibility as he or she is able, depending on age, development, and family culture.

The most widely used **conditioning therapy** for nocturnal enuresis is the **enuresis alarm.** Enuresis alarms have an initial success rate of 70% with a relapse rate of 10%. The alarm is worn on the wrist or clipped onto the pajama and has a probe that is placed in the underpants or pajamas in front of the urethra. The alarm sounds when the first drop of urine contacts the probe. The child is instructed to get up and finish voiding in the bathroom when the alarm sounds. After 3 to 5 months, 70% of children are dry through the night.

Pharmacotherapy for nighttime enuresis includes desmopressin acetate and, rarely, tricyclic antidepressants. **Desmopressin** decreases urine production and has proved to be safe in the treatment of enuresis. The oral medication is started at 0.2 mg per dose (one dose at bedtime) and on subsequent nights is increased to 0.4 mg and then to 0.6 mg if needed. This treatment must be considered symptomatic, not curative, and has a relapse rate of 90% when the medication is discontinued. **Imipramine,** now rarely used for enuresis, reduces the frequency of nighttime wetting. The initial success rate is 50%. Imipramine is effective during treatment only, with a relapse

rate of 90% on discontinuation of the medication. The most important contraindication is risk of overdose (associated with fatal cardiac arrhythmia).

Complications

The psychological consequences can be severe. Families can minimize the impact on the child's self-esteem by avoiding punitive approaches and ensuring that the child is competent to handle issues of their own comfort, hygiene, and aesthetics.

Prevention

Appropriate anticipatory guidance to educate parents that bed-wetting is common in early childhood helps alleviate considerable anxiety.

FUNCTIONAL CONSTIPATION AND SOILING

Constipation is decreased frequency of bowel movements usually associated with a hard stool consistency. The occurrence of pain at defecation frequently accompanies constipation. Although underlying gastrointestinal, endocrinologic, or neurologic disorders can cause constipation, *functional constipation* implies that there is no identifiable causative organic condition. **Encopresis** is the regular, voluntary or involuntary passage of feces into a place other than the toilet after 4 years of age. Encopresis without constipation is uncommon and may be a symptom of oppositional defiant disorder or other psychiatric illness. *Soiling* is the involuntary passage of stool and often is associated with fecal impaction. The normal frequency of bowel movements declines between birth and 4 years of age, beginning with greater than four stools per day to approximately one per day.

Etiology

The etiology of functional constipation and soiling includes a low-fiber diet, slow gastrointestinal transit time for neurologic or genetic reasons, and chronic withholding of bowel movements, usually because of past painful defecation experiences. Approximately 95% of children referred to a subspecialist for encopresis have no other underlying pathologic condition.

Epidemiology

In U.S. studies, 16% to 37% of children experience constipation between 5 and 12 years of age. Constipation with overflow soiling occurs in 1% to 2% of preschool children and 4% of school-age children. The incidence of constipation and soiling is equal in preschool girls and boys, whereas there is a male predominance during school age.

Clinical Manifestations

Decision-Making Algorithms
Available @ StudentConsult.com

Constipation
Irritable Infant

The presenting complaint for constipation with soiling is typically a complaint of uncontrolled defecation in the underwear. Parents may report that the child has diarrhea because of soiling of liquid stool. Soiling may be frequent or continuous. On further questioning, the clinician learns that the child is passing large-caliber bowel movements that may occasionally block the toilet. Children younger than 3 years of age often present with painful defecation, impaction, and withholding. The history should include a complete review of systems for gastrointestinal, endocrine, and neurologic disorders and a developmental and psychosocial history.

Stool impaction can be felt on abdominal examination in about 50% of patients at presentation. Firm packed stool in the rectum is highly predictive of fecal impaction. A rectal examination allows assessment of sphincter tone and size of the rectal vault. Evaluation of anal placement and existence of anal fissures also is helpful in considering etiology and severity. A neurologic examination, including lower extremity reflexes, anal wink, and cremasteric reflexes, may reveal underlying spinal cord abnormalities.

Abdominal x-ray is not required. It can be helpful to show to the family the degree of colonic distention and fecal impaction. In general further studies, such as barium enema and rectal biopsy, are indicated only if an organic cause for the constipation is indicated by history or physical examination (see Chapter 129). Similarly although endocrinologic conditions such as hypothyroidism can cause chronic constipation, laboratory studies are not indicated without history or physical examination suggesting such a disorder.

Differential Diagnosis

The differential diagnosis for functional constipation and soiling includes organic causes of constipation (e.g., neurogenic, anatomic, endocrinologic, gastrointestinal, and pharmacologic). A child with chronic constipation and soiling who had delayed passage of meconium and has an empty rectum and tight sphincter may have Hirschsprung disease (see Chapter 129). Chronic constipation may be a presenting sign of spinal cord abnormalities, such as a spinal cord tumor or a tethered cord. Physical examination findings of altered lower extremity reflexes, absent anal wink, or a sacral hairy tuft or sacral sinus may be a clue to these anomalies. Hypothyroidism can present with chronic constipation and typically is accompanied by poor linear growth and bradycardia. Anal stenosis may lead to chronic constipation. The use of opiates, phenothiazine, antidepressants, and anticholinergics also may lead to chronic constipation. Developmental problems, including mental retardation and autism, may be associated with chronic constipation.

Treatment

Treatment begins with education and demystification for the child and family about chronic constipation and soiling, emphasizing the chronic nature of this condition and the good prognosis with optimal management. Explaining the physiologic basis of constipation and soiling to the child and the family alleviates blame and enlists cooperation. Education may improve adherence to the long-term treatment plan (Table 14-1). One half to two thirds of children with functional constipation recover completely and no longer require medication.

Table 14-1	Education about Chronic Constipation and Soiling

Constipation affects 16% to 37% of children.

1% to 4% of children have functional constipation and soiling.

Functional constipation with/without soiling begins early in life due to a combination of factors:

    Uncomfortable/painful stool passage

    Withholding of stool to avoid discomfort

    Diets higher in constipating foods and lower in fiber and fluid intake*

    Use of medications that are constipating

    Developmental features—increasing autonomy; perhaps toilet avoidance

    Possible family genetic factors—slower colonic transit

When chronic impaction, physiologic changes at the rectum reduce a child's bowel control.

Dilated rectal vault results in reduced sensation to standard fecal volume.

Rehabilitation of rectal musculature and strength requires several months.
    Until then, dilated rectal musculature may be less able to expel stool effectively.

Paradoxical anal sphincter contraction may occur when the urge to defecate is felt; it can lead to incomplete emptying of stool at defecation attempt.

Many children do not recognize their soiling accidents owing to olfactory accommodation.

Low self-esteem or other behavioral concerns are common on presentation.
    Improve for most with education and management for the constipation and soiling.

Effective management of functional constipation requires a substantial commitment of the child/family, usually for 6–24 mo.

Degree of child and family adherence is likely a predictor of the child's success.

*The common features of the transition to the toddler diet (decreased fluid intake, continued high dairy intake, and *finicky* eating patterns) make this a high-risk time during development for constipation problems.

The younger the child is when diagnosis and treatment begin, the higher the success rate. Treatment involves a combination of behavioral training and laxative therapy. Successful treatment requires 6 to 24 months. The next step is adequate colonic cleanout or disimpaction. Clean-out methods include enemas alone or combinations of enema, suppository, and oral laxatives. High-dose oral mineral oil is a slower approach to clean-out. Choice of disimpaction method depends on the age of the child, family choice, and the clinician's experience with a particular method. Methods and side effects are summarized in Table 14-2. The child and family should be included in the process of choosing the clean-out method. Because enemas may be invasive and oral medication may be unpleasant, allowing points of choice and control for the child and praising all signs of cooperation are important.

Behavioral training is essential to the treatment of chronic constipation and soiling. The child and family are asked to monitor and document stool output. Routine toilet sitting is instituted for 5 to 10 minutes three to four times per day. The child is asked to demonstrate proper toilet sitting position with the upper body flexed forward slightly and feet on the floor

Table 14-2	Clean-Out Disimpaction

MEDICATION	SIDE EFFECTS/COMMENTS
INFANTS	
Glycerin suppositories	No side effects
Enema—6 mL/kg up to 4.5 oz (135 mL)	If enemas are considered, administer first in physician's office.
CHILDREN	
Rapid Cleanout	
Enema—6 mL/kg up to 4.5 oz (135 mL) every 12–24 h × 1–3	Invasive; risk of mechanical trauma Large impaction: mineral oil enema followed 1–3 h later by normal saline or phosphate enema Small impaction: normal saline or phosphate enema
Mineral oil	Lubricates hard impaction; may not see return after administration
Normal saline	Abdominal cramping; may not be as effective as hypertonic phosphate
Hypertonic phosphate	Abdominal cramping; risk of hyperphosphatemia, hypokalemia, and hypocalcemia, especially with Hirschsprung or renal insufficiency or if retained. Some experts do not recommend phosphate enema for children <4 yr, others for children <2yr.
Milk of molasses: 1:1 milk:molasses	For difficult to clear impaction
Combination: enema, suppository, oral laxative	
Day 1: Enema q12–24 h	See enemas above
Day 2: Bisacodyl suppository (10 mg) q12–24 h	Abdominal cramping, diarrhea, hypokalemia
Day 3: Bisacodyl tablet (5 mg) q12–24 h	Abdominal cramping, diarrhea, hypokalemia
Repeat 3-day cycle if needed × 1–2	
Oral/nasogastric tube: Polyethylene glycol electrolyte solution (GoLYTELY or NuLYTELY)—25 mL/kg/h up to 1000 mL/h × 4 h/day	Nausea, cramping, vomiting, bloating, aspiration. Large volume. Usually requires nasogastric tube and hospitalization to administer
Slower Cleanout	
Oral high-dose mineral oil—15–30 mL per year of age per day up to 8 oz × 3–4 days	Aspiration—lipoid pneumonia. Give chilled.
X-Prep (senna): 15 mL q12h × 3	Abdominal cramping. May not see output until dose 2 or 3
Magnesium citrate: 1 oz/yr of age to maximum of 10 oz per day for 2–3 days	Hypermagnesemia
Maintenance medications—also may be used for cleanout	

or foot support. The child should be praised for all components of cooperation with this program, and punishment and embarrassment should be avoided. As symptoms resolve, toilet sitting is decreased to twice daily and finally to once a day.

When disimpaction is achieved, the child begins the maintenance phase of treatment. This phase promotes regular stool production and prevents reimpaction. It involves attention to diet, medications to promote stool regularity, and behavioral training. Increasing dietary fiber and fluid are recommended. For children with chronic constipation, the recommended daily dose of fiber is calculated as 10 grams plus the child's age in years (e.g., a 10-year-old should take 20 grams of fiber per day). At least 2 oz of nondairy fluid intake per gram of fiber intake is recommended. Sorbitol-based juices, including prune, pear, and apple juice, increase the water content of bowel movements. Lubricants or osmotic laxatives are used to promote regular soft bowel movements. Maintenance medications, including side effects, are listed in Table 14-3. Polyethylene glycol powder is well tolerated because the taste and texture are palatable. Some children may require the use of a lubricant in addition to an osmotic laxative; children with severe constipation may require a stimulant laxative.

Treatment failure occurs in approximately one in five children secondary to problems with adherence or poor recognition of inadequate treatment resulting in reimpaction.

Complications

Chronic constipation and soiling interfere with social functioning and self-esteem. Discomfort and fear of accidents may distract children from their schoolwork and other important tasks. Children also may develop unusual eating habits in response to chronic constipation and their beliefs about this condition. Case reports of child abuse related to soiling have been published.

Prevention

The primary care physician can recommend adequate fiber intake in all children and encourage families to help their children institute regular toileting habits at an early age as preventive measures. Earlier diagnosis of chronic constipation can prevent much secondary disability and shorten the length of treatment required.

Table 14-3	Maintenance Medications*	
MEDICATION		**SIDE EFFECTS/COMMENTS**
INFANTS		
Oral Medications/Other		
Juices containing sorbitol		Pear, prune, apple
Lactulose or sorbitol: 1–3 mL/kg/day ÷ doses bid		See below
Corn syrup (light or dark): 1–3 mL/kg/day ÷ doses bid *Per Rectum*		Not considered risk for *Clostridium botulinum* spores
Glycerin suppository		No side effects
CHILDREN		
Oral Medications		
Lubricant		Softens stool and eases passage
Mineral oil: 1–3 mL/kg day as one dose or ÷ bid		Aspiration—lipoid pneumonia
		Chill or give with juice
		Adherence problems
		Leakage: dose too high or impaction
Osmotics		Retain water in stool, aiding bulk and softness
Lactulose: 10 g/15 mL, 1–3 cc/kg/day ÷ doses bid		Synthetic disaccharide: abdominal cramping, flatus
Magnesium hydroxide (milk of magnesia): 400 mg/5 mL, 1–3 mL/kg/day ÷ bid 800 mg/5 mL, 0.5 mL/kg ÷ bid		Risk of hypermagnesemia, hypophosphatemia, secondary hypocalcemia with overdose or renal insufficiency
MiraLAX (polyethylene glycol powder): 17 g/240 cc water or juice stock, 1.0 g/kg/day ÷ doses bid (approximately 15 cc/kg/day)		Titrate dose at 3-day intervals to achieve mushy stool consistency May make stock solutions to administer over 1–2 days
		Excellent adherence
Sorbitol: 1–3 mL/kg/day ÷ doses bid		Less costly than lactulose
Stimulants†		Improve effectiveness of colonic and rectal muscle contractions
Senna: syrup—8.8 g sennoside/5 mL		Idiosyncratic hepatitis, melanosis coli, hypertrophic osteoarthropathy, analgesic nephropathy; abdominal cramping
2–6 yr: 2.5–7.5 cc/day ÷ doses bid		
6–12 yr: 5–15 cc/day ÷ doses bid (Tablets and granules available)		Improvement of melanosis coli after medication stopped
Bisacodyl: 5-mg tablets, 1–3 tablets/dose 1–2 × daily		Abdominal cramping, diarrhea, hypokalemia
Per Rectum		
Glycerin suppository		No side effects
Bisacodyl: 10-mg suppositories, 0.5–1 suppository, 1–2 × daily		Abdominal cramping, diarrhea, hypokalemia

*Single agent may suffice to achieve daily, comfortable stools.
†Stimulants should be reserved for short-term use.

Chapter **15**

NORMAL SLEEP AND PEDIATRIC SLEEP DISORDERS

Sleep is a universal phenomenon that is critical to child health, development, and daily functioning. This complex behavioral and physiologic process is characterized by a reversible state of partial unresponsiveness and disengagement from the environment. Sleep is broadly categorized by polysomnographic patterns into rapid eye movement (REM) sleep and non-REM (NREM) sleep. REM sleep is characterized by an active, awake-like electroencephalography (EEG) pattern and muscle atonia. NREM sleep is further divided into three stages—from stage 1 (N1), which is the lightest sleep stage and consists of low-amplitude, high-frequency EEG activity, to stage 3 (N3), also known as *deep* or *slow-wave* sleep, characterized by low-frequency, high-amplitude delta waves. REM and NREM sleep alternate in cycles throughout the night.

Sleep architecture changes from fetal life through infancy and childhood. Sleep cycles last approximately 60 minutes in newborns and gradually lengthen to 90 minutes in children and adults. Neonates typically begin their sleep cycle in REM sleep, whereas older children and adults begin sleep in NREM sleep. REM sleep in neonates is termed *active sleep,* and frequent muscle twitches and facial grimaces are common. REM sleep comprises up to 50% of total sleep time in newborns and gradually decreases to 25% to 30% by adolescence. Slow-wave sleep is not seen before 3 to 6 months of age. Beginning from 6 to 12 months and continuing through adulthood, the amount of REM sleep shifts toward the last third of the night, while NREM sleep predominates during the first third of the night.

The timing and duration of sleep also change with age. Sleep patterns become more diurnal and total daily sleep time gradually decreases. Full-term infants sleep on average 16 to 18 hours per day in fragmented intervals throughout the day and night. One-year-old children sleep on average 10 to 11 hours per night and nap for 2 to 3 hours during the day. Naps decrease from two naps to one during the second year of life. In the United States, over 80% of 2-year-olds nap, decreasing to 50% by age 3. By 12 years old, the average child sleeps 9 to 10 hours per day. By adolescence, the average sleep duration has dropped to 7½ hours per day, even though adolescents need an average of 9 hours per day. Adolescents also develop a physiologically based shift toward later sleep-onset and wake times relative to those in middle childhood.

Cultural factors strongly influence multiple sleep practices, including whether children sleep independently (the norm in the United States) or with parents, other siblings, or grandparents (the norm in many other cultures). Awareness of the varying cultural practices regarding sleep is essential to respectful and effective intervention.

SLEEP DISORDERS

Sleep problems are one of the most frequent complaints in pediatric practice. Numerous sleep disorders exist, including behavioral insomnias (bedtime refusal, delayed sleep onset, nighttime awakenings), parasomnias, and circadian rhythm disorders (Table 15-1). Obstructive sleep apnea (OSA) and sleep disorders associated with mental and physical illness should also be considered.

Epidemiology

Sleep problems occur in 20% to 30% of children at some point during childhood. Behavioral sleep disorders are common and found across all age groups but are most prevalent from infancy through preschool age. Bedtime resistance occurs in 10% to 15% of toddlers, and 15% to 30% of preschool-aged children have difficulties achieving and/or maintaining sleep. Although generally benign, parasomnias occur commonly in young children, including sleep walking (15% to 40%) and sleep terrors (1% to 6%). OSA is reported in 1% to 4% of children. Circadian rhythm disorders occur in 7% to 16% of adolescents.

Clinical Manifestations and Evaluation

Decision-Making Algorithms
Available @ StudentConsult.com

Seizures and Other Paroxysmal Disorders
Sleep Disturbances

Sleep disorders may manifest in a variety of ways and often go unrecognized. Some children present with daytime behavioral problems, including inattentiveness, hyperactivity, or irritability rather than overt sleepiness. Screening for sleep disorders is recommended as part of primary care. Clinicians should inquire about bedtime problems, excessive daytime sleepiness, wakenings during the night, regularity and duration of sleep, and presence of snoring and sleep-disordered breathing.

The assessment of sleep complaints begins with a detailed **history** of sleep habits, including bedtime, sleep-onset, and wake times. A detailed description of the sleep environment can result in a dynamic understanding of the challenges to and resources for achieving normal sleep. The recommended history includes the type of bed, who shares it, the ambient light, noise, temperature, and the bedtime routine. Household structure, routines, and cultural practices may be important and influence the timing and ease of sleep (e.g., parental work patterns, evening activities, number of household members). Dietary practices influence sleep, including timing of meals and caffeine intake. A detailed history assessing for symptoms of OSA (gasps, snorting noises, breathing pauses, and so on) should be obtained in all children who snore regularly. New-onset sleep disorders may be associated with a psychological trauma. When the history does not reveal the cause of the sleep disorder, a sleep diary can be helpful.

A complete **physical examination** is important to rule out medical causes of sleep disturbance, such as conditions that cause pain, neurologic conditions that could be associated with seizure disorder, and other central nervous system disorders. Children with genetic syndromes associated with developmental delay may have sleep disorders. Similarly children with attention-deficit/hyperactivity disorder and fetal alcohol syndrome are at higher risk for sleep disorders than other children. Careful attention to the upper airway and pulmonary examination may reveal enlarged tonsils or adenoids or other signs of obstruction.

A **polysomnogram** is used to detect OSA, excessive limb movements, and seizure disorder. This consists of an all-night observation and recording performed in a sleep laboratory. Polysomnography is not indicated in children with primary insomnia (difficulty initiating or maintaining sleep), circadian rhythm disorders, uncomplicated parasomnias, or behaviorally based sleep problems.

Differential Diagnosis

Behavioral insomnia of childhood is divided into two subtypes: *Sleep-onset association subtype* manifests as frequent or prolonged nighttime wakenings that occur in infants or young children. During periods of normal brief arousal with each sleep cycle, the child awakens under conditions different from those experienced as they fell asleep. Thus they are unable to return to sleep independently. *Limit-setting subtype* is most common in preschool-aged and older children and is characterized by bedtime resistance or refusal that stems from a caregiver's unwillingness or inability to enforce bedtime rules and expectations. Nighttime fears are also common causes of bedtime refusal.

Parasomnias include sleepwalking, sleep terrors, and confusional arousals. These occur during NREM sleep and are more likely during the first third of the night. They are most common in preschool children and are likely to resolve with time and developmental maturation. Sleepwalking is common and often benign but is sometimes associated with agitation or dangerous behaviors. Sleep terrors consist of an abrupt awakening with a loud scream, agitation, and unresponsiveness to caregivers' attempts to console. Sleep terrors are differentiated

Table 15-1	Childhood Sleep Disruption Disorders		
TYPE	**CAUSE**	**SYMPTOMS**	**TREATMENT**
BEHAVIORAL AND ENVIRONMENTAL			
Behavioral insomnia of childhood Sleep-onset association subtype	Child falls asleep in conditions different from those of the rest of the night	Frequent or prolonged night wakenings requiring intervention	Put child to bed drowsy but awake; allow to fall asleep independently Minimize nocturnal parental response
Behavioral insomnia of childhood Limit-setting subtype	Parental anxiety, unwillingness/ inability to enforce bedtime rules and limits	Bedtime resistance/refusal Excessive expression of "needs" by child	Modify parental behavior to improve limit-setting (provide rewards/positive reinforcement, appropriate consequences).
Nighttime fears	Anxiety, stress, traumatic events	Bedtime resistance Crying, clinging, seeking parental reassurance	Reassurance of safety Teach coping skills Nightlights, security objects
Social disruptions	Family stressors	Night waking Refusal to sleep	Regularize routines Family counseling
PARASOMNIAS			
Sleepwalking Sleep terrors Confusional arousals	Stage N3 (deep) sleep instability Genetic predisposition	Awakening 1–3 h after falling asleep with characteristic behaviors (see text)	Reassurance Protective environment Scheduled awakenings
Sleep enuresis	? Stage N3 instability Metabolic disease (e.g., diabetes) Urinary tract infection Urinary anatomic anomaly	Bed-wetting	Rule out medical conditions Fluid limitation, pre-bed voiding Behavioral approaches (bell and pad) Emotional support Medication (e.g., imipramine, DDAVP) Reassurance
CIRCADIAN RHYTHM DISORDERS			
Irregular sleep-wake pattern	No defined sleep schedule	Variable waking and sleeping	Regularize schedule
Delayed sleep phase	Shift in sleep-wake schedule with resetting of circadian _ _ _	Not sleepy at bedtime Sleep onset at a consistently late time _ _ _ _ _me sleepiness	Enforce wake-up time Gradually move bedtime earlier or keep awake overnight to create drowsy state Melatonin
ORGANIC			
Obstructive apnea		_ _ing, gasps/snorts, _ _ _nea, labored _ _ _ing sleep, _ _ _iness, attention _ _ _g problems	Polysomnography (for diagnosis) Adenotonsillectomy Weight loss Nasal steroids Continuous positive airway pressure (CPAP)
Illness		_ _ out	Treat disease symptomatically
Neurodevel_ _ and central _ _ system disc_		_ disruptions	Evaluate environment Sleep hygiene Sedatives as last resort

DDAVP, 1-des_

from night_
from arous_
remember_
terrors. Co_
to be less d_

Circadi_ _websi_
adolescenc_
gerated delayed sleep phase, leading to the inability to _
in the mornings and failure to meet sleep requirements. Many adolescents attempt to recoup lost sleep on the weekends. The resulting sleep deprivation leads to problems with cognition and emotional regulation.

Obstructive sleep apnea in childhood is not always obvious or easy to diagnose. OSA is commonly caused by tonsillar or adenoidal hypertrophy. A history of snoring is typical; some children may have excessive daytime sleepiness. Obese

children are at increased risk for OSA. In toddlers OSA often is associated with poor growth, which improves when the obstruction is relieved by a tonsillectomy or adenoidectomy. Many children with OSA experience cognitive difficulties and school problems. Hyperactivity is also more common in these children than in age-matched controls.

Primary sleep disorders must be differentiated from sleep disorders associated with psychiatric and medical disorders. Psychoses, anxiety disorders, and substance abuse can present with disordered sleep. The clinician should also consider sleep-related epilepsy and developmental disorders.

Prevention and Treatment

Establishing a baseline of healthy sleep habits is essential to both prevention and treatment of sleep disorders at all ages.

Table 15-2	Prevention of Pediatric Behavioral Sleep Disorders

Consistent and appropriate bedtime and wake-up time

Consistent bedtime routine (~30 min) to cue sleep
Consistent ambient noise, light, temperature in bedroom
Adequate food, hydration, socialization, and physical activity during the day

No television or other electronics in bedroom
Avoidance of naps (unless developmentally appropriate)

Caffeine avoidance
Child feels safe and protected

Child allowed to develop self-soothing strategies

Parents are comfortable setting limits/boundaries

These include having a consistent and appropriate bedtime and bedtime routine, and close attention to sleep hygiene (see Table 15-2). A bedtime routine should consist of three or four soothing activities that help calm the child and signal that it is time for sleep. It should last no more than 30 minutes. Activities may include bathing, brushing teeth, reading a story, or singing a song. Even older children and adolescents require a consistent pre-bed routine. A transitional object such as a blanket or stuffed animal can be used to promote positive sleep associations and encourage self-soothing. The bedtime should be set early enough to allow for sufficient nighttime sleep, and both bedtime and morning wake time should be consistent, including on weekends. Televisions and other electronic devices should be removed from the bedroom because these can lead to delayed sleep onset and maladaptive sleep associations.

Sleep-onset association disorder in infancy usually can be prevented by parental understanding of infant sleep physiology, developmentally appropriate expectations, and planning the infant sleep environment to coincide with family needs. It is recommended that infants be put in bed drowsy, but still awake, after they have had a diaper change, food, and comfort. Some toleration of infant crying is required for the infant to achieve self-regulation of sleep. A safe sleep environment is essential. It is important for parents to understand that it is normal for their infant to wake frequently for the first 6 weeks before settling into a routine of waking every 3 to 4 hours for feeding. Infants typically do not sleep through the night before 6 months of age, and some do not sleep through the night before 12 to 18 months of age. Even though co-sleeping (mother and infant sleeping together) is common, it is not recommended because of increased risk of SIDS. Proactively considering the desirability of bed sharing allows parents to be in control rather than ceding control to the young child.

Behavioral interventions comprise the mainstay of treatment for behavioral sleep disorders. In addition to meticulous attention to sleep hygiene and bedtime practices, difficulty falling asleep and bedtime resistance in young children are treated by specific behavioral strategies. *Systematic ignoring* consists of not responding to a child's demands for parental attention at bedtime. *Unmodified extinction* ("cry it out") involves putting the child to bed and then ignoring the child's demands until the next morning. *Graduated extinction* involves waiting successively longer periods of time before briefly checking on the child. Both methods are effective in decreasing bedtime resistance and enabling young children to fall asleep independently. Positive reinforcement strategies can also be used in preschool-aged and older children. These include rewards (e.g., stickers) for meeting a bedtime goal (e.g., staying in bed). Rewards should be provided immediately (first thing in the morning) to increase effectiveness and better link the reward with the positive behavior. Children with nighttime fears can benefit from behavioral therapy aimed at reinforcing feelings of safety.

Infrequent or nonintrusive parasomnias do not need treatment beyond education and reassurance. Ensuring a safe environment is important. Sleep terrors are best managed by minimal intervention, because conversation with the child is impossible during the episode. Anticipatory brief awakening of the child shortly before the typical occurrence of a parasomnia may be effective in aborting the event. Children with frequent or prolonged parasomnias may need a sleep study to evaluate for possible coexisting sleep disorders or nocturnal seizures. Medications that suppress slow-wave sleep may be indicated in severe cases.

Circadian rhythm disorders are also treated by ensuring sleep hygiene practices and gradual resetting of the biologic clock. Bedtime fading involves allowing the child to go to bed at the time he or she naturally feels tired, then gradually advancing the bedtime forward over the course of several weeks.

Rarely children with insomnia are treated pharmacologically. Melatonin (dose, 2.5 to 10 mg) has soporific properties useful in treating delayed sleep phase syndrome. It has been used successfully in both children with normal development and those with developmental delays. Melatonin is available without prescription in stores that sell dietary supplements. The α-agonist clonidine acts preferentially on presynaptic α_2 neurons to inhibit noradrenergic activity. Somnolence is a side effect of clonidine, which can be put to use in cases of refractory sleep difficulties; this is an *off-label* use in children. Clonidine is usually started with a dose of 0.05 mg at bedtime and increased to 0.1 mg if needed. There are data on treating children as young as 4 years old with clonidine. Weaning off clonidine is recommended at the end of treatment.

Complications

The most obvious and serious complication associated with childhood sleep disorders is impairment of cognitive ability and emotional regulation. This impairment puts children at risk for school failure, family difficulties, and social problems. It is likely that sleep-deprived children are at increased risk for acute illness and psychiatric disorders.

Suggested Reading

Blass EM, Camp CA: Changing determinants of crying termination in 6- to 12-week-old human infants, *Dev Psychobiol* 42:312–316, 2003.

Glazener CM, Evans JH, Peto RE: Alarm interventions for nocturnal enuresis in children, *Cochrane Database of Syst Rev*(2): CD002911, 2005.

Mindell JA, Owens JA: *A Clinical Guide to Pediatric sleep: Diagnosis and Management of Sleep Problems*, ed 2, Philadelphia, 2010, Lippincott Williams and Wilkins.

Potegal M, Davidson RJ: Temper tantrums in young children: 1. Behavioral composition. 2. Tantrum duration and temporal organization, *J Dev Behav Pediatr* 24:140–154, 2003.

Rubin G, Dale A: Chronic constipation in children, *BMJ* 333:1051–1055, 2006.

Subcommittee on Attention-Deficit/Hyperactivity Disorder. Steering Committee on Quality Improvement and Management Wolraich M, Brown L, Brown RT, et al: ADHD: clinical practice guideline for the diagnosis, evaluation, and treatment of attention-deficit/hyperactivity disorder in children and adolescents, *Pediatrics* 128(5):1007–1022, 2011.

Psychiatric Disorders

Russell Scheffer and Aveekshit Tripathi

Chapter 16

SOMATOFORM DISORDERS, FACTITIOUS DISORDERS, AND MALINGERING

The somatoform disorders are groups of disorders in which physical symptoms (pain or loss of function) are inconsistent and cannot be explained by a medical condition (Table 16-1). While transient symptoms, as "signals of distress," are responsible for up to 50% of outpatient visits in the pediatric age group, somatoform disorders represent only the severe end of this continuum. Somatization that occurs in the context of a physical illness is identified by symptoms that go beyond the expected pathophysiology, affecting the child's school, home life, and peer relationships and becoming the focus of the patient and the family's life. Somatization is often associated with psychosocial stress and often persists beyond the acute stressor, leading to the belief by the child and the family that the correct medical diagnosis has not yet been found.

A somatization disorder occurs in as many as 10% to 20% of first-degree relatives and has a higher concordance rate in monozygotic twin studies. Lifetime prevalence of somatoform disorders is 3%, and that of subclinical somatoform illness is as high as 10%. Adolescent girls tend to report nearly twice as many functional somatic symptoms as adolescent boys, whereas prior to puberty the ratio is equal.

Affected children are more likely to have difficulty expressing emotional distress, come from families with a history of marital conflict, child maltreatment (including emotional, sexual, physical abuse), or history of physical illness. In early childhood, symptoms often include recurrent abdominal pain (RAP). Later headaches, neurologic symptoms, insomnia, and fatigue are more common.

Explainable medical conditions and a somatoform disorder (e.g., seizures and pseudoseizures) can coexist in up to 50% of patients and present difficult diagnostic dilemmas. The list of systemic medical disorders that could present with unexplained physical symptoms includes chronic fatigue syndrome (CFS), multiple sclerosis, myasthenia gravis, endocrine disorders, chronic systemic infections, vocal cord dysfunction, periodic paralysis, acute intermittent porphyria, fibromyalgia, polymyositis, and other myopathies.

Depression is a common comorbid condition and frequently precedes the somatic symptoms. Anxiety disorders can present with somatic complaints.

DSM-IV classifies somatoform disorders as somatization disorder, undifferentiated somatoform disorder, somatoform disorder not otherwise specified, conversion disorder, pain disorder, body dysmorphic disorder (BDD), and hypochondriasis. The diagnostic criteria for somatoform disorders are established for adults and need additional study in pediatric populations.

Somatization disorder involves multiple unexplained physical complaints, including pain, gastrointestinal, sexual, and pseudoneurologic symptoms not caused by known mechanisms. The criteria used to diagnose this disorder are listed in Table 16-2. Given the requirement for at least one sexual or reproductive symptom, the diagnosis is unusual in children and the onset is common during adolescence. Prevalence estimates range from 0.2% to 2% in females and less than 0.2% in males. Early onset of somatization disorder is associated with poor prognosis.

Undifferentiated somatoform disorder (Table 16-3) includes one or more unexplained physical complaints accompanied by functional impairment that last for at least 6 months. Children and adolescents are more likely to meet *DSM-IV* criteria for an undifferentiated somatoform disorder than for a somatization disorder, and no evidence exists to predict which patients will go on to develop the full symptom criteria for somatization disorder.

Conversion disorder involves symptoms affecting voluntary motor or sensory function and is suggestive of a neurologic illness in the absence of a disease process (Table 16-4). Adjustment difficulties, recent family stress, unresolved grief reactions, and family psychopathology occur at a high frequency in conversion symptoms. A physical condition and a conversion disorder (e.g., epileptic and nonepileptic seizures) may coexist in the same patient. There are four subtypes of conversion disorder based on whether the symptoms presented are primarily motor, sensory, nonepileptic (seizures), or mixed.

Presenting symptoms follow the psychological stressor by hours to weeks and may cause more distress for others than for the patient. This seeming lack of concern regarding potentially serious symptoms is referred to as *la belle indifference.*

Table 16-1	Features of Somatoform Disorders of Children and Adolescents

PSYCHOPHYSIOLOGIC DISORDER

Presenting complaint is a physical symptom.

Physical symptom is caused by a known physiologic mechanism.

Physical symptom is stress induced.

Patient may recognize association between symptom and stress.

Symptom frequently responds to medication, biofeedback, and stress reduction.

CONVERSION REACTION

Presenting complaint is physical (loss of function, pain, or both).

Physical symptom is not caused by a known physiologic mechanism.

Physical symptom is related to unconscious idea, fantasy, or conflict.

Patient does not recognize association between symptom and the unconscious.

Symptom responds slowly to resolution of unconscious factors.

SOMATIZATION DISORDER

Requires more than 13 physical symptoms in girls, more than 11 in boys (see Table 16-2)

Physical symptoms are not caused by a known physiologic or pathologic mechanism.

Physical symptoms are related to need to maintain the sick role.

Patient convinced that symptoms are unrelated to psychological factors.

Symptoms tend to persist or change character despite treatment.

HYPOCHONDRIASIS

Presenting complaint is a physical sign or symptom.

Patient interprets physical symptom to indicate disease.

Conviction regarding illness may be related to depression or anxiety.

Symptom does not respond to reassurance.

Medication directed at underlying psychological problems often helps.

MALINGERING

Presenting complaint is a physical symptom.

Physical symptom is under voluntary control.

Physical symptom is used to gain reward (e.g., money, avoidance of military service).

Patient consciously recognizes symptom as factitious.

Symptom may not lessen when reward is attained (need to retain reward).

FACTITIOUS DISORDER (AS IN MUNCHAUSEN SYNDROME)

Presenting complaint is symptom complex mimicking known syndrome.

Symptom complex is under voluntary control.

Symptom complex is used to attain medical treatment (including surgery).

Patient consciously recognizes symptom complex as factitious but is often psychologically disturbed so that unconscious factors also are operating.

Symptom complex often results in multiple diagnoses and multiple operations.

Table 16-2	Criteria for Diagnosis of Somatization Disorder

Each of the following criteria must be met. Individual symptoms may occur at any time during the course of disturbance.

1. **Four pain symptoms:** pain related to at least four different sites or functions (e.g., head, abdomen, back, joints, extremities, chest, rectum; during menstruation, sexual intercourse, or urination)

2. **Two gastrointestinal symptoms:** at least two gastrointestinal symptoms other than pain (e.g., nausea, bloating, vomiting, diarrhea, or intolerance of several foods)

3. **One sexual symptom:** at least one sexual or reproductive symptom other than pain (e.g., sexual indifference, erectile or ejaculatory dysfunction, irregular menses, excessive menstrual bleeding, vomiting throughout pregnancy)

4. **One pseudoneurologic symptom:** at least one symptom or deficit suggesting a neurologic condition not limited to pain (conversion symptoms such as impaired coordination or balance, paralysis or localized weakness, difficulty swallowing or lump in throat, aphonia, urinary retention, hallucinations, loss of touch or pain sensation, double vision, blindness, deafness, seizures; dissociative symptoms such as amnesia; or loss of consciousness other than fainting)

Either (1) or (2)

1. After appropriate investigation, each of the symptoms is not fully explained by a known general medical condition or the direct effects of a substance (e.g., drug, medication).

2. When there is a related general medical condition, the physical complaints, social or occupational impairment are in excess of what is expected from the history, physical examination, or laboratory findings.

Table 16-3	Criteria for Diagnosis of Undifferentiated Somatoform Disorder

A. One or more physical complaints (e.g., fatigue, loss of appetite, gastrointestinal complaints)

B. Either (1) or (2)

1. After appropriate investigation, the symptoms cannot be fully explained by a known general medical condition or the direct effects of a substance (e.g., drug or medication).

2. When there is a related general medical condition, the physical complaints, social, or occupational impairment is in excess of what is expected from the history, physical examination, or laboratory findings.

C. The symptoms cause clinically significant distress or impairment in social, occupational, or other important areas of functioning.

D. At least 6 months of disturbance

E. The disturbance is not better accounted for by another mental disorder (e.g., another somatoform disorder, sexual dysfunction, mood disorder, anxiety disorder, sleep disorder, or psychotic disorder).

F. The symptom is not intentionally produced or feigned (factitious disorder, malingering).

Symptoms are often self-limited but may be associated with chronic sequelae, such as contractures or iatrogenic injury.

Falling out syndrome (falling down with altered consciousness) is common in several cultures throughout the world, including the United States. **Stocking glove** (nonanatomic) **anesthesia** is another common finding. Symptoms are

Table 16-4	Criteria for Diagnosis of Conversion Disorder

A. One or more symptoms affect voluntary motor or sensory function, suggesting a neurologic or other general medical condition.

B. Psychological factors are judged to be associated with the symptom or deficit because the initiation or exacerbation is preceded by conflicts or other stressors.

C. The symptom is not intentionally produced or feigned (factitious disorder, malingering).

D. After appropriate investigation, the symptom cannot be fully explained by a general medical condition, by the direct effects of a substance, or as a culturally sanctioned behavior or experience.

E. The symptom causes clinically significant distress or impairment in social, occupational, or other function or warrants medical evaluation.

F. The symptom is not limited to pain or sexual dysfunction, does not occur exclusively during the course of somatization disorder, and is not better accounted for by another mental disorder.

Table 16-5	Criteria for Diagnosis of Pain Disorder

A. Pain in one or more anatomic sites is the predominant focus and is of sufficient severity to warrant clinical attention.

B. The pain causes clinically significant distress or impairment in social, occupational, or other important functions.

C. Psychological factors have an important role in the onset, severity, exacerbation, or maintenance of the pain.

D. The symptom or deficit is not intentionally produced or feigned (factitious disorder, malingering).

E. The pain is not better accounted for by a mood, anxiety, or psychotic disorder and does not meet criteria for dyspareunia.

Specify the following:

• Acute: duration <6 months

• Chronic: duration ≥6 months

often inconsistent; patients may move a *paralyzed* extremity when they think that no one is watching.

Nonepileptic seizures, sometimes described as *pseudoseizures,* resemble epileptic seizures but are not associated with the electroencephalographic abnormalities or a clinical course characteristic of true epilepsy. Most cases resolve within 3 months of diagnosis. Referring to nonclassic presentations for seizures as *spells* can help avoid medicalization of these symptoms.

The course of the condition is often benign, although 20% to 25% of patients experience a recurrence. Good prognostic characteristics include symptoms of paralysis, aphonia, blindness; acute onset; above-average intelligence; presence of an identifiable stressor; and early diagnosis and psychiatric treatment. Poor prognostic characteristics include tremor and pseudoseizures. The rate of misdiagnosis of conversion symptoms averages 4%. Myasthenia gravis, multiple sclerosis, dystonias, and dyskinesias (abnormal movements) are conditions commonly mistaken for conversion disorder.

Pain disorder is diagnosed instead of a conversion disorder if pain is the predominant physical symptom. The *DSM-IV* divides pain disorders into those associated with psychological factors, those with both psychological and medical factors, and those in which the medical condition is the major factor in the pain symptom (Table 16-5). The diagnosis is considered acute if the condition lasts less than 6 months and chronic when it lasts 6 months or more.

RAP is the most common recurrent pain complaint of childhood and accounts for 2% to 4% of pediatric office visits. It is defined by intermittent pain with full recovery between episodes lasting more than 3 months. There is a strong relation between RAP and anxiety in children. Approximately 90% of pediatric patients have no clinical findings to account for their abdominal pain.

Common types of headaches are migraine and tension-type headache. Migraine may be associated with dizziness, gastrointestinal symptoms, and cyclic vomiting syndrome, characterized by recurrent and stereotypic episodes of intense, unexplained vomiting. Psychological factors frequently play a significant role in the complaint of a headache.

Functional chest pain can be seen in 10% of school-aged children and adolescents. Other common pain disorders are musculoskeletal pains (limb pain and back pain), fibromyalgia, and complex regional pain syndrome type I (previously known as *reflex sympathetic dystrophy*).

Reassurance is the primary treatment of pain disorder. Symptom diaries, including the events that precede and follow the pain episode, aid in initial assessment and ongoing management of the problem. Minimizing secondary psychological consequences of recurrent pain syndromes is important.

Hypochondriasis is the preoccupation with the fear of having a serious disease based on misinterpretation of bodily symptoms and functions. This fear should be present for 6 months. The presenting complaint is a physical sign or symptom, which is normal but is interpreted by the patient to indicate disease despite reassurance of a physician (e.g., a tension headache perceived as a brain tumor). This diagnosis is more commonly seen in late adolescence and adulthood. An underlying depression or anxiety disorder may be related to the symptoms. Prevalence of obsessive-compulsive disorder (OCD) is four times greater than in the general population. When the belief or preoccupation is limited to an imagined defect in appearance, the diagnosis is body dysmorphic disorder (BDD), not hypochondriasis.

Body dysmorphic disorder is a preoccupation with an imagined or slight defect in physical appearance that causes clinically significant distress or impairment in functioning. It is usually seen in adolescents (the male-to-female ratio being almost equal) and is distinguished from common developmental preoccupations with appearance by the presence of clinically significant distress and/or impairment in functioning. Any bodily area can be a focus, but excessive concerns about the skin (scars and acne) and body shape are common. Because BDD can be associated with shame and the need for secrecy, the diagnosis may be missed unless clinicians ask directly about symptoms. Parents of children with BDD report excessive mirror checking, grooming, attempts to *camouflage* a particular body area, and reassurance-seeking. Patients may cause self-injury as a consequence of attempts to fix the perceived flaw.

Many of these patients have had consultations with surgeons and dermatologists and often seek interventions but are unlikely to be satisfied with the results.

BDD is considered to be related to OCD. The prevalence of BDD has been reported to be 0.7% in children, 2% in adolescents, and up to 5% in patients seeking cosmetic surgery. Many individuals with BDD report a history of childhood maltreatment; comorbid psychiatric disorders, including depression, OCD, social phobia, and anorexia nervosa; gender identity disorder; delusional disorder; and narcissistic personality disorder. BDD is also associated with high rates of suicidal ideation and attempts, with 28% of sufferers having attempted suicide.

Fatigue is a common physical complaint, affecting up to 50% of adolescents. CFS specifically refers to a condition characterized by at least 6 months of severe, disabling fatigue associated with self-reported limitations in concentration and short-term memory, sleep disturbance, and musculoskeletal aches and pains, where alternative medical and psychiatric explanations have been excluded. CFS is often associated with depression and can be incapacitating. CFS is rare in childhood and uncommon in adolescence, with prevalence below 1%. Onset typically follows an acute post-viral illness in approximately two thirds of pediatric cases. Treatment is nonspecific, unless a psychological or general medical cause is uncovered.

Screening tools for somatoform disorders include the Children's Somatization Inventory (child and parent versions) and the Illness Attitude Scales and Soma Assessment Interview (parental interview questionnaires). The Functional Disability Inventory assesses the severity of symptoms.

Treatment for somatoform disorders should use an integrated medical and psychiatric approach. The goals are to identify concurrent psychiatric disorders, rule out concurrent physical disorders, improve overall functioning, and minimize unnecessary invasive tests and doctor shopping. This works when mental health consultation is presented as part of a comprehensive evaluation, thereby minimizing stigma and distrust.

Antidepressant medications (fluoxetine, sertraline, citalopram, and clomipramine) may be of benefit in the treatment of unexplained headaches, fibromyalgia, BDD, somatoform pain, irritable bowel syndrome, and functional gastrointestinal disorders. Tricyclic antidepressants (clomipramine and others) should be avoided in youth with **functional abdominal pain (FAP)** because they have no proven efficacy in either pain management or mood disorders and are very dangerous in overdose. In **chronic fatigue syndrome** with comorbid depression and anxiety, a more activating antidepressant, like bupropion, can be useful. Stimulants may also be helpful in CFS.

Cognitive-behavioral methods, which reward health-promoting behaviors and discourage disability and illness behaviors, help in the treatment of recurrent pain, CFS, fibromyalgia, and FAP. Interpersonal and expressive psychotherapies in the presence of psychological trauma are particularly useful. Self-management strategies, such as self-monitoring, relaxation, hypnosis, and biofeedback, provide some symptomatic relief and encourage more active coping strategies. Family therapy and family-based interventions can be very useful. Home schooling should be avoided, and school attendance and performance should be emphasized as important

indicators of appropriate functioning. In dealing with pain symptoms (e.g., headaches, stomachaches) parents should remove or limit attention for pain behavior; strongly encourage sticking to schedule (e.g., going to school); help the child identify stress at home and school; provide attention and special activities on days when child does not have symptoms; and limit activities and interactions on sick days. Discussions about excessive discomfort or illness should be replaced with having the child practice relaxation techniques and educating personnel working with their child about these approaches.

FACTITIOUS DISORDERS AND MALINGERING

In contrast to somatoform disorders, patients intentionally simulate or create their problems in factitious disorders and malingering.

Factitious disorder is a condition in which physical or psychological symptoms are produced intentionally but for unconscious reasons to assume a sick role. This diagnosis is made either by direct observation or by eliminating other possible causes. Most patients are immature, passive, and hypochondriacal. They show improvement when confronted with their behavior or acknowledge the factitious nature of their symptoms. It has been associated with borderline personality traits and substance abuse disorders. Approximate answers (e.g., 20−3=13) reported during a mental status examination are most commonly found in factitious disorders.

Munchausen syndrome by proxy (MBP) is a form of factitious disorder by proxy, where a parent (usually mother) mimics symptoms in his or her child. The motivation is believed to be a psychological need to assume a sick role through the child. Of these mothers, more than 72% have a history of factitious disorder or a somatoform disorder, and up to 80% of involved parents have some health care background. MBP is a type of child abuse. Boys are more commonly abused in this way, and neonates and preschoolers are the most common victims. Both *factitious disorder by proxy* (diagnosis of the abuser) and *pediatric condition falsification* (diagnosis of the child) are needed for diagnosis.

Common presenting symptoms include vomiting, diarrhea, respiratory arrest, asthma, seizures, incoordination, fever, bleeding, failure to thrive, rash, hypoglycemia, and loss of consciousness. Simulation of psychiatric disorders is rare. Nearly 75% of the morbidity to the child occurs in hospitals from invasive procedures. Once confronted with negative test results or discharge planning, the perpetrators may become intensely enraged and acutely suicidal or may initiate legal action so the treatment team should take appropriate precautions. Mortality in MBP may be as high as 33%, and siblings of these children are also at risk. Virtually all children suffer serious psychological sequelae from this form of abuse. Treatment involves protecting the child from further abuse and reporting to child protective services.

Malingering is a condition in which a physical symptom that is under voluntary control is used to gain reward (e.g., money or avoidance of school, jail, or obtaining drugs). The patient has conscious intent in production of symptoms. Symptoms may not lessen when the reward is attained. Malingering is difficult to prove unless the patient is directly observed or confesses.

Chapter 17

ANXIETY AND PHOBIAS

ANXIETY DISORDERS

Anxiety disorders are characterized by uneasiness, excessive rumination, and apprehension about the future. The conditions tend to be chronic, recurring, and vary in intensity over time. They affect 5% to 10% of children and adolescents (Table 17-1). Some common anxiety disorders are discussed in the following sections.

Panic disorder is the presence of recurrent, unexpected panic attacks. A **panic attack** is a sudden unexpected onset of intense fear associated with a feeling of impending doom in the absence of real danger. At least 1 month of persistent worrying about having another panic attack is required to make the diagnosis (Table 17-2). Panic disorder most often begins in adolescence or early adulthood. Symptom severity waxes and wanes. Characteristic symptoms include shortness of breath, palpitations, chest pain, a choking or smothering sensation, and a fear of losing control or going "crazy" (Table 17-3). Symptoms generally last approximately 15 minutes and are generally time-limited. It is common for patients to think that they are about to die of a heart attack. Panic attacks are classified as (1) spontaneous, (2) bound to situations (occur immediately on exposure), and (3) predisposed to situations (attacks occur while at school, but not every time). **Agoraphobia** is a condition describing fear of situations where escape is difficult or would draw unwanted attention to the person. Agoraphobia is often persistent and can leave people homebound. Panic disorder is seen in 95% of patients with agoraphobia. The condition is more common in females. Consider the diagnosis of a specific phobia (as opposed to agoraphobia) if the avoidance is limited to one or a few specific situations or social phobia if avoidance is limited to social situations in general.

Generalized anxiety disorder (GAD) is characterized by 6 or more months of persistent, out of proportion worry and anxiety that includes a historical diagnosis of overanxious disorder of childhood. The worries should be multiple, not paroxysmal, and not focused on a single theme and should cause significant impairment (Table 17-4). The anxiety must be accompanied by at least three of the following symptoms: restlessness, easy fatigability, difficulty concentrating, irritability, muscle tension, and disturbed sleep. Physical signs of anxiety are often present,

		GENERALIZED		**SEPARATION**	**SPECIFIC**
FEATURE	**PANIC DISORDER**	**ANXIETY DISORDER**	**PTSD**	**ANXIETY DISORDER**	**PHOBIAS**
Epidemiology	Prevalence is 0.2%–10%; rates are similar in all racial groups. Half have agoraphobia. Eight times more common and of early onset in family members of affected individuals than general population.	Prevalence is 5%. The sex ratio is equal. Genetic factors play only a modest role in the etiology.	Prevalence is around 8%. Twin studies suggest some genetic role.	Prevalence is 2%–4% of children and adolescents. The sex ratio is almost equal. Heritability of SAD is greater for girls than for boys.	Prevalence is 2%. Sex ratio is 2:1 females:males. Increased risk of specific phobias in first-degree relatives of patients with specific phobias.
Onset	Average age at onset is 15–19 years; earlier in 25%.	The average age at onset is 10 years.		The average age at onset is 8–9 years.	
Differential diagnosis	Anxiety disorder due to a general medical condition. Substance-induced anxiety disorder due to caffeine or other stimulants.	Other anxiety disorders, anorexia nervosa, somatoform disorders, and major depression. Substance-induced (caffeine and sedative-hypnotic withdrawal).	Other anxiety disorders, adjustment disorders, psychotic disorders, and substance-induced disorders. If financial compensation is at issue, malingering should be ruled out.	Other anxiety disorders.	-
Comorbidities	Separation anxiety disorder (common). Substance abuse, major depression, obsessive-compulsive disorder (OCD), and other anxiety disorders. Asthma patients have a high incidence of panic attacks.	Depression, other anxiety disorders, ADHD.	Depression, other anxiety disorders, ADHD.	Depression, Social phobia, other anxiety disorders, ADHD.	Depression and other anxiety symptoms.
Prognosis	Frequently chronic with a relative high rate of suicide attempts and completions.	One study showed that 65% of children cease to have the diagnosis in 2 years.	Variable. Time may diminish symptoms. Substance abuse and suicidality increased over time in this group.	Variable. Affected children are likely to develop panic disorder, agoraphobia, or depressive disorders later in life.	Social phobia in childhood may become associated with alcohol abuse in adolescence.

ADHD, Attention-deficit/hyperactivity disorder; *PTSD,* posttraumatic stress disorder.

Table 17-2	Criteria for Diagnosis of a Panic Disorder

A. Both (1) and (2)

1. Recurrent unexpected panic attacks

2. At least one attack is followed by ≥1 month of one or more of the following:

   a. Persistent concern about having additional attacks

   b. Worry about the implications of the attack or its consequences (e.g., losing control, having a heart attack, "going crazy")

   c. A significant change in behavior related to the attacks

B. The presence of agoraphobia

C. The panic attacks are not due to direct physiologic effects of drugs or abuse or medication or a general medical condition (e.g., hyperthyroidism).

D. The panic attacks are not better accounted for by another mental disorder, such as social phobia, specific phobia, obsessive-compulsive disorder, posttraumatic stress disorder, or separation anxiety disorder.

Table 17-3	Criteria for Diagnosis of a Panic Attack

A discrete period of intense fear or discomfort, in which four or more of the following symptoms developed abruptly and reached a peak within 10 minutes:

Palpitations, pounding heart, or accelerated heart rate

Sweating

Trembling or shaking

Sensations of shortness of breath or smothering

Feeling of choking

Chest pain or discomfort

Nausea or abdominal distress

Feeling dizzy, unsteady, lightheaded, or faint

Derealization (feelings of unreality) or depersonalization (being detached from oneself)

Fear of losing control or going crazy

Paresthesias (numbness or tingling sensations)

Chills or hot flashes

Table 17-4	Criteria for Diagnosis of Generalized Anxiety Disorder

A. Excessive anxiety and worry (apprehensive expectation), occurring more days than not for at least 6 months, about numerous events or activities

B. The person finds it difficult to control the worry.

C. The anxiety and worry are associated with three or more of the following six symptoms (with at least some symptoms present for more days than not for the past 6 months). Note: Only one symptom is required in children.

   1. Restlessness or feeling keyed up or on edge

   2. Being easily fatigued

   3. Difficulty concentrating or mind going blank

   4. Irritability

   5. Muscle tension

   6. Sleep disturbance (difficulty falling or staying asleep or restless, unsatisfying sleep)

D. The focus of the anxiety and worry is not confined to features of a disorder (e.g., panic disorder, social phobia, obsessive-compulsive disorder, separation anxiety disorder, anorexia nervosa, somatization disorder, hypochondriasis), and the anxiety and worry do not occur exclusively during posttraumatic stress disorder.

E. The anxiety, worry, or physical symptoms cause clinically significant distress or impairment in social, occupational, or other important areas of functioning.

F. The disturbance is not due to the direct physiologic effects of a drug or a general medical condition (e.g., hyperthyroidism) and does not occur exclusively during a mood disorder, a psychotic disorder, or a pervasive developmental disorder.

including shakiness, trembling, and myalgias. Gastrointestinal symptoms (nausea, vomiting, diarrhea) and autonomic symptoms (tachycardia, shortness of breath) commonly coexist. In children and adolescents, the specific symptoms of autonomic arousal are less prominent, and symptoms are often related to school performance or sports. Children with GAD are often exceedingly self-conscious, exhibit behavioral inhibition, have low self-esteem, and have more sleep disturbance than patients with other kinds of anxiety disorder. Care must be taken to elicit internalizing symptoms of negative cognitions about the self (hopelessness, helplessness, worthlessness, suicidal ideation), as well as those concerning relationships (embarrassment, self-consciousness) and associated with anxieties. Inquiry about eating, weight, energy, and interests should also be carried out to eliminate a mood disorder.

Posttraumatic stress disorder (PTSD) is characterized by re-experiencing a traumatic event in which actual or threatened death or serious injury was possible. The reexperiencing

is accompanied by avoidance of stimuli that remind the person of the trauma and by autonomic hyperarousal (Table 17-5). Type, severity, duration, and proximity of the traumatic event are the most likely predictors of PTSD. Presentation often depends on the age group of the child. In preverbal children, there are changes in behavior: regressed clingy behavior, increased aggression, unwillingness to explore the environment, alterations in feeding, sleeping behaviors, and difficulty soothing child. Preschool children may display rapidly changing emotional states like anger, sadness, and excitement and play may have compulsive reenactments linked to the traumatic event. Later symptomatology is more typical of adult PTSD, except that flashbacks are more daydream quality than the sudden intrusive events seen in adults, and complaint of restriction of effect and numbing are less frequent.

Dissociative states lasting a few seconds to many hours, in which the person relives the traumatic event, are referred to as *flashbacks.* Reexperiencing trauma in children may be nonspecific to the trauma (e.g., dreams of monsters). In adolescents anticipation of unwanted visual imagery increases the risk of irritable mood, anger, and voluntary sleep deprivation. When faced with reminders of the original trauma, physical signs of anxiety or increased arousal occur, including difficulty falling or staying asleep, hypervigilance, exaggerated startle response, irritability, angry outbursts, and difficulty concentrating.

Typically an acute stress disorder is present immediately after the trauma. The risk of chronic PTSD increases when symptoms are unresolved by 6 weeks and there are higher premorbid levels of anxiety or depression. PTSD usually begins

Table 17-5	Criteria for Diagnosis of Posttraumatic Stress Disorder

A. The person has been exposed to a traumatic event in which both of the following were present:

1. The person experienced, witnessed, or was confronted with an event or events that involved actual or threatened death or serious injury or a threat to the physical integrity of self or others.

2. The person's response involved intense fear, helplessness, or horror. Note: In children, this may be expressed instead by disorganized or agitated behavior.

B. The traumatic event is persistently reexperienced in one or more of the following ways:

1. Recurrent and intrusive distressing recollections of the event, including images, thoughts, or perceptions. Note: In young children, repetitive play may occur in which themes or aspects of the trauma are expressed.

2. Recurrent distressing dreams of the event. Note: In children, there may be frightening dreams without recognizable content.

3. Acting or feeling as if the traumatic event were recurring (includes a sense of reliving the experience, illusions, hallucinations, and dissociative flashback episodes, including flashbacks that occur on awakening or when intoxicated). Note: In young children, trauma-specific re-enactment may occur.

4. Intense psychological distress at exposure to internal or external cues that symbolize or resemble an aspect of the traumatic event.

5. Physiologic reactivity on exposure to internal or external cues that symbolize or resemble an aspect of the traumatic event.

C. Persistent avoidance of stimuli associated with the trauma and numbing of general responsiveness (not present before the trauma), as indicated by three or more of the following:

1. Efforts to avoid thoughts, feelings, or conversations associated with the trauma

2. Efforts to avoid activities, places, or people that arouse recollections of the trauma

3. Inability to recall an important aspect of the trauma

4. Markedly diminished interest or participation in significant activities

5. Feeling of detachment or estrangement from others

6. Restricted range of affect (e.g., unable to have loving feelings)

7. Sense of a foreshortened future (e.g., does not expect to have a career, marriage, children, or a normal life span)

D. Persistent symptoms of increased arousal (not present before the trauma), as indicated by two or more of the following:

1. Difficulty falling or staying asleep

2. Irritability or outbursts of anger

3. Difficulty concentrating

4. Hypervigilance

5. Exaggerated startle response

E. Duration of the disturbance (symptoms in criteria B, C, and D) is >1 month

F. The disturbance causes clinically significant distress or impairment in social, occupational, or other important areas of functioning

Specify the following:

• Acute: if duration of symptoms is <3 months

• Chronic: if duration of symptoms is ≥3 months

• With delayed onset: if onset of symptoms is at least 6 mo after the stressor

within 3 months of the trauma, although delay in symptom expression can occur. Rates of suicide attempts are threefold higher than unaffected controls.

Acute stress disorder is characterized by the same signs and symptoms as PTSD but occurs immediately after a traumatic event. If impaired function persists after 1 month, the diagnosis is PTSD.

Anxiety disorder not otherwise specified is a common condition in clinical practice. This diagnosis is used when there is impairing anxiety or phobic symptoms that do not meet full criteria for another anxiety disorder.

Separation anxiety disorder (SAD) is seen in children and adolescents who express vague somatic symptoms (e.g., headaches, abdominal pain, fatigue) to avoid or refuse to go to school. Patients may have a valid or an irrational concern about a parent or have had an unpleasant experience in school. They often have been seen by numerous specialists and have undergone elaborate medical evaluations. Their absence from school often is mistakenly seen as a consequence of their symptoms. The prospect of returning to school provokes extreme anxiety and escalating symptoms. True phobia related to schoolwork is rare. SAD is a strong (78%) risk factor for developing problems in adulthood, such as panic disorder, agoraphobia, and depression. School phobia that first presents during adolescence may be an expression of a severe underlying psychopathologic condition. Psychiatric consultation is needed.

Specific phobias are marked persistent fears of things or situations, which often lead to avoidance behaviors (Table 17-6). The associated anxiety is almost always felt immediately when the person is confronted with the feared object or situation. The greater the proximity or the more difficult it is to escape, the higher the anxiety. Many patients have had actual fearful experiences with the object or situation (traumatic event). The response to the fear can range from limited symptoms of anxiety to full panic attacks. Children may not recognize that their fears are out of proportion to the circumstances, unlike adolescents and adults, and express their anxiety as crying, tantrums, freezing, or clinging.

School phobia is one of a range of reasons for school nonattendance. In severely worried children, defensive aggression may be used to prevent attendance. Otherwise these patients do not have antisocial tendencies. Boys and girls are equally affected and there is no association with social class, intelligence, or academic ability. The youngest in a family of several children is more likely to be affected as well as children of older parents. Truancy is generally associated with older adolescents with lower levels of fear. Unlike anxious school refusers, truants hide their school nonattendance from their parents.

Social phobia is a common (3% to 13% prevalence; girls predominate over boys) type of phobia characterized by a marked and persistent fear of social or performance situations in which embarrassment might occur (Table 17-7).

There is a wariness of strangers and social apprehension or anxiety when encountering new, strange, or socially threatening situations. Children appear to have a lower rate of negative cognitions (e.g., embarrassment, overconcern, self-consciousness) than adults. Children with simple avoidant disorders are younger than those with more socialized phobic conditions. Left untreated or poorly treated, phobias can become immobilizing and result in significant morbidity and restriction of their lives.

Table 17-6	Criteria for Diagnosis of Specific Phobia

A. Marked and persistent fear that is excessive or unreasonable, cued by the presence or anticipation of a specific object or situation (e.g., flying, heights, animals, receiving an injection, seeing blood)

B. Exposure to the phobic stimulus almost invariably provokes an immediate anxiety response, which may take the form of a situationally bound or situationally predisposed panic attack. Note: In children, the anxiety may be expressed by crying, tantrums, freezing, or clinging.

C. The person recognizes that the fear is excessive or unreasonable. Note: In children, this feature may be absent.

D. The phobic situation is avoided or else is endured with intense anxiety or distress.

E. The avoidance, anxious anticipation, or distress in the feared situation interferes significantly with the person's normal routine, occupational (or academic) functioning, or social activities or relationships, or there is marked distress about having the phobia.

F. In children <18 years, the duration is at least 6 months.

G. The anxiety, panic attacks, or phobic avoidance associated with the specific object or situation are not better accounted for by another mental disorder, such as obsessive-compulsive disorder, posttraumatic stress disorder, separation anxiety disorder, social phobia, panic disorder with agoraphobia, or agoraphobia without history of panic disorder.

Specify type:

• Animal type is fear elicited by animals or insects.

• Natural environment type (e.g., heights, storms, water).

• Blood/injection/injury type is fear related to seeing blood, injuries, injections, or having an invasive medical procedure.

• Situational type is fear caused by specific situations (e.g., airplanes, elevators, enclosed places).

• Other type (e.g., fear of choking, vomiting, or contracting an illness; in children, fear of loud sounds or costumed characters)

Table 17-7	Criteria for Diagnosis of Social Phobia

A. A marked and persistent fear of one or more social or performance situations in which the person is exposed to unfamiliar people or to possible scrutiny by others. The individual fears that he or she will act in a way (or show anxiety symptoms) that will be humiliating or embarrassing. Note: In children, there must be evidence of the capacity for age-appropriate social relationships with familiar people, and the anxiety must occur in peer settings, not just in interactions with adults.

B. Exposure to the feared social situation almost invariably provokes anxiety, which may take the form of a situationally bound or situationally predisposed panic attack. Note: In children, the anxiety may be expressed by crying, tantrums, freezing, or shrinking from social situations or unfamiliar people.

C. The person recognizes that the fear is excessive or unreasonable. Note: In children, this feature may be absent.

D. The feared social or performance situations are avoided or else are endured with intense anxiety or distress.

E. The avoidance, anxious anticipation, or distress in the feared social or performance situation interferes significantly with the person's normal routine, occupational (academic) functioning, or social activities or relationships, or there is marked distress about having the phobia.

F. In children <18 years, the duration is at least 6 months.

G. The fear or avoidance is not due to the direct physiologic effects of a drug of abuse, a medication, or a general medical condition and is not better accounted for by another mental disorder (e.g., panic disorder with or without agoraphobia, separation anxiety disorder, body dysmorphic disorder, pervasive developmental disorder, or schizoid personality disorder).

H. If a general medical condition or another mental disorder is present, the fear in criterion A is unrelated to it (e.g., the fear is not of stuttering or exhibiting abnormal eating behavior in anorexia nervosa or bulimia nervosa).

Specify the following:

Generalized: if the fears include most social situations (e.g., initiating or maintaining conversations, participating in small groups, dating, speaking to authority figures, attending parties). Note: Also consider the additional diagnosis of avoidant personality disorder.

In the **management of anxiety disorders,** likely medical conditions, including hyperthyroidism, medication side effects, substance abuse, or other medical conditions, should be ruled out. The patient should be screened for comorbid psychiatric disorders, such as mood disorders, psychosis, eating disorders, tic disorders, and disruptive behavior disorders. A history from multiple sources is important because the child may be unable to effectively communicate symptoms. A detailed history that includes the nature of the anxiety triggers; psychosocial history; and family history of tics, anxiety disorders, depression, and other mood disorders should be taken. The younger child may better communicate his or her anxieties through drawings or play.

Treatment consists of psychotherapy and psychopharmacology. For mild to moderate anxiety, evidence-based psychotherapies and psychoeducation should be used first. Combined therapy usually has better efficacy than psychotherapy and psychopharmacology alone. Cognitive and behavioral therapy (including systematic desensitization, exposure, operant conditioning, modeling, and cognitive restructuring) can be beneficial in a variety of anxiety disorders. Patients with anxiety disorders are often less tolerant of medication side effects, and supportive therapy helps them maintain treatment regimens.

Family and individual psychotherapy and care coordination with a patient's school is helpful. Reassurance that the patient does not have a life-threatening illness is important. Other psychosocial treatments include stress management, supportive therapies, and biofeedback. Emphasis is placed on decreasing morbidity through proper treatment. Panic disorder tends to be chronic but usually is responsive to treatment. In PTSD trauma-focused cognitive behavioral therapy has shown efficacy. Critical-incident stress debriefing and "psychological first aid," soon after the event, greatly reduce distress and involve discussing the nature and impact of the trauma event in a group format.

Selective serotonin reuptake inhibitors (SSRIs) are the medication of choice. The SSRIs approved for children by the U.S. Food and Drug Administration (FDA) are fluoxetine, sertraline, and fluvoxamine. They can initially exacerbate anxiety or even panic symptoms. Clomipramine requires electrocardiographic and blood level monitoring but may be effective and is approved by the FDA for obsessive-compulsive disorder. Tricyclic antidepressants have also shown efficacy. Benzodiazepines (alprazolam and clonazepam) include a risk of causing disinhibition in children. Alpha-2a-agonists (guanfacine and clonidine) may be useful if autonomic symptoms are present. Anticonvulsant agents (gabapentin, topiramate, and oxcarbazepine) are used when other agents are ineffective. β-Blockers help with performance anxiety.

Co-occurrence of the inattentive type of attention-deficit/hyperactivity disorder (ADHD) and an anxiety disorder is common. When using a stimulant, it is advisable to start at a low dose, increasing slowly to minimize the risk of increasing anxiety.

For PTSD, antidepressants may be augmented by clonidine (also useful in hyperarousal and impulsivity) in the presence of severe affective dyscontrol. Atypical antipsychotics are used if self-injurious behavior, dissociation, psychosis, and aggression are present. Atomoxetine is useful in PTSD with concurrent ADHD.

Chapter 18

DEPRESSION AND BIPOLAR DISORDERS

DEPRESSION

Major depressive disorder (MDD) requires a minimum of 2 weeks of symptoms, including either depressed mood or loss of interest or pleasure in nearly all activities. Four additional symptoms must also be present (Table 18-1). In children and adolescents, a new onset of irritability, restlessness, or boredom may be seen instead of depressed mood. A sudden drop in grades is often present. A change in appetite (usually decreased but can be increased) with carbohydrate craving with or without accompanying weight changes and sleep disturbance along with somatic complaints (fatigue, vague aches and pains) may also be present. Psychotic symptoms, seen in severe cases of major depression, are generally mood-congruent (e.g., derogatory auditory hallucinations, guilt associated delusional thinking). Suicidal thoughts and attempts are common and should be evaluated.

The prevalence of MDD in prepubertal children is 2% with 1:1 female-to-male ratio; in adolescents the prevalence is 6% to 8%, with a female-to-male ratio of 2:1 (similar to adults). If untreated, major depression can become chronic in 10% of patients.

Depression has a clear genetic predisposition, with family history as the strongest single factor for developing MDD. Twin studies show 40% to 65% heritability for depression. Family studies show a twofold to fourfold increased risk for depression in offspring of depressed parents. Other potential responsible factors for depression include dysregulation of central serotonergic and/or noradrenergic systems, hypothalamic-pituitary-adrenal axis dysfunction, and the influence of pubertal sex hormones. The stress-diathesis model relates to the interaction of genes and environment; for example, a less functional genetic variant of the serotonin receptor in presence of stressful life events could contribute to depression.

Table 18-1	Criteria for Diagnosis of a Major Depressive Episode

A. Five or more of the following symptoms present during the same 2-week period and represent a change from previous functioning; at least one of the symptoms is either (1) depressed mood or (2) loss of interest or pleasure. Note: Do not include symptoms that are clearly due to a general medical condition or mood-incongruent delusions or hallucinations

1. Depressed mood most of the day, nearly every day, as indicated by either subjective report (e.g., feels sad or empty) or observation made by others (e.g., appears tearful). Note: In children and adolescents, mood can be irritable.

2. Markedly diminished interest or pleasure in all, or almost all, activities most of the day, nearly every day (as indicated by subjective account or observation by others)

3. Significant weight loss when not dieting or weight gain or decrease or increase in appetite nearly every day. Note: In children, consider failure to make expected weight gains

4. Insomnia or hypersomnia nearly every day

5. Psychomotor agitation or retardation nearly every day (observable by others)

6. Fatigue or loss of energy nearly every day

7. Feelings of worthlessness or excessive or inappropriate guilt (which may be delusional) nearly every day (not self-reproach or guilt about being sick)

8. Diminished ability to think, concentrate, or be decisive nearly every day (subjective account or as observed by others)

9. Recurrent thoughts of death (not just fear of dying), recurrent suicidal ideation without a specific plan, a suicide attempt or a specific plan for committing suicide

B. The symptoms do not meet criteria for a mixed manic episode.

C. The symptoms cause clinically significant distress or impairment in social, occupational, or other important areas of functioning.

D. The symptoms are not due to the direct physiologic effects of a drug or abuse, a medication, or a general medical condition (e.g., hypothyroidism).

E. The symptoms are not better accounted for by bereavement, and the symptoms persist >2 mo or are characterized by marked functional impairment, morbid preoccupation with worthlessness, suicidal ideation, psychotic symptoms, or psychomotor retardation.

Dysthymic disorder and anxiety disorders (prevalence 30% and 80%, respectively), substance abuse (20% to 30%), and disruptive behavior disorders (10% to 20%) are frequent comorbid disorders in depressed children and adolescents. Twenty percent of patients diagnosed with depression develop bipolar disorder (BD); this is more common in cases with a family history of mania or concurrent psychotic features.

The differential diagnoses for MDD are diverse and many. It is always prudent to rule out mood disorder due to a general medical condition or substance-induced mood disorders before considering MDD. Schizophrenia in its initial stages and the dysphoria related to untreated attention-deficit/hyperactivity disorder (ADHD) may also be mistakenly diagnosed as depression. Hypothyroidism, anemia, diabetes, and folate and B_{12} vitamin deficiencies need to be ruled out.

Dysthymic disorder (prevalence rate 0.6% to 1.7%) is a chronic, milder form of depression characterized by a depressed or irritable mood (subjectively or described by others) present for at least 1 year. Two of the following symptoms are also required: changes in appetite; sleep difficulty, fatigue; low self-esteem; poor concentration or difficulty with making decisions; and feelings of hopelessness. About 70% of children and adolescents with dysthymic disorder eventually develop major depression. The development of MDD after dysthymia is often referred to as *double depression.*

Atypical depression is MDD characterized by hypersomnia, increased appetite with carbohydrate craving, weight gain, interpersonal rejection sensitivity, and mood reactivity.

Adjustment disorder with depressed mood is the most common depressive disorder in children and adolescents. Symptoms start within 3 months of an identifiable stressor (e.g., loss of a relationship), with distress in excess of what would be expected and interference with social, occupational, or school functioning. Symptoms should not meet criteria for another psychiatric disorder, should not be caused by bereavement, and should not last longer than 6 months after the stressor has stopped.

Seasonal affective disorder is a condition common in northern or extreme southern latitudes, in which depressive symptoms occur in the late fall and early winter when the hours of daylight are shortening.

Depressive disorder not otherwise specified is a diagnosis used when patients have functionally impairing depressive symptoms that do not meet criteria for another condition.

Treatment of depression involves psychopharmacy and psychotherapy. First line antidepressant selective serotonin reuptake inhibitors (SSRIs) have response rates of 50% to 70% despite high-placebo response rate. Fluoxetine is the only agent approved by the U.S. Food and Drug Administration (FDA) for treatment of youth. Citalopram, escitalopram, paroxetine, and venlafaxine have positive clinical trial results as well. An antidepressant should be given an adequate trial (6 weeks at therapeutic doses) before switching or discontinuing unless there are serious side effects. For a first episode of depression in children and adolescents, treatment for 6 to 9 months after remission of symptoms is recommended. Patients with recurrent or chronic depression may need to take antidepressants for extended periods (years or even a lifetime). If a patient does not respond to adequate trials of two or more antidepressants, a child psychiatrist should be consulted. The psychiatrist's evaluation should focus on diagnostic clarity and psychosocial issues that might be preventing a full response. The psychiatrist may use augmentation strategies that may include lithium, thyroid hormone, lamotrigine, or bupropion.

For acute depression, more frequent visits are indicated, and the risks of medication (including suicidal and self-destructive behavior) should be discussed with parents, guardians, and patients. Higher frequency of monitoring can include phone calls or collaborative care with a psychotherapist. Parents and patients should also be educated about warning signs and to call immediately if these new symptoms occur. Notable side effects are thoughts of suicide, increased agitation, or restlessness. Other side effects include headache, dizziness, gastrointestinal symptoms, sleep cycle disturbance, sexual dysfunction, akathisia, serotonin syndrome, and risk of increased bruising (due to platelet inhibition.) There is also a risk of SSRI-induced mania.

In 2004 the FDA issued warnings for all antidepressants regarding suicidal thinking or behavior. The data suggest that antidepressants pose a 4% risk, versus a 2% risk in placebo. An increase in suicides in children and adolescents since that

year has many experts believing that it might be related to low prescription of antidepressants and resultant untreated depression. Substance use, concomitant conduct problems, and impulsivity increase the risk of suicide.

Psychotherapy appears to have good efficacy in mild to moderate depression. In moderate to severe depression, combined treatment with psychotherapy and medication has the greatest rate of response, although in severe cases the efficacy was equivalent to medication alone. Cognitive-behavioral therapy and interpersonal therapies are the empirically supported psychotherapies. Cognitive behavioral therapy and its derivative, dialectic behavioral therapy (for borderline personality disorder), involve techniques and skills-building to mitigate cognitive distortions and maladaptive processing; whereas interpersonal therapy focuses on collaborative decisions between the therapist and patient and is based on the exploration and recognition of precipitants of depression. Family therapy is often used as an adjunct to other treatments for depression.

Light therapy has been shown to be beneficial for seasonal affective disorder and in MDD with a seasonal component. Electroconvulsive therapy is used in refractory and life-threatening depression.

Depression is a chronic and debilitating illness that often starts in childhood or adolescence. It increases risk for future suicide, substance use, and other psychiatric sequelae. Adolescent depressive disorders are more likely to be recurrent into adulthood than childhood onset depression.

Suicide is a fatal complication of MDD and surpasses motor vehicle accidents as a **cause of death in adolescents**. It has high prevalence among high school students with 20% having contemplated suicide and 8% having attempted each year. While the risk of suicide during an MDD episode is high, it can be paradoxically higher during start of treatment as energy and motivation improve with cognitive recovery from depression.

Treatment is targeted toward decreasing morbidity and suicide. Along with treatments mentioned previously, modalities such as hospitalization, partial hospital, therapeutic after-school programs, or psychoeducation may be needed.

BIPOLAR DISORDERS

Bipolar disorder consists of distinct periods of mania (elevated, expansive, or irritable moods and distractibility) that may alternate with periods of severe depression (Table 18-2).

To diagnose mania associated with BD, euphoria (elevated or expansive mood) and three additional symptoms; or irritability and four additional manic symptoms are required. Children and adolescents with euphoric mood are bubbly, giggly, and "over-the-top" happy, to a degree that is socially unacceptable to others. Grandiosity in children is often dramatic. Children act as if they are superior even when it is obvious that it is not true, and they behave as if the laws of nature do not apply to them. Racing thoughts are common in BD. Periods of extreme rage also are common. Children with BD often present with rapid or ultra-rapid cycling with multiple shifts between euthymia, mania, and depression.

A decreased need for sleep is a hallmark of mania. There are no other diagnoses where a child has a greatly decreased amount of total sleep (compared with age-appropriate norms) and is not fatigued. Sleep deprivation, substance abuse, and antidepressants may trigger mania. BD onset often begins with an episode of depression. It is estimated that 33% of youth will develop BD

Table 18-2	Mania Symptoms

A. A distinct period of abnormally and persistently elevated, expansive, or irritable mood, lasting at least 1 week (or any duration if hospitalization is necessary)

B. During the period of mood disturbance, three or more of the following symptoms have persisted (four if the mood is only irritability) and are present to a significant degree:

1. Inflated self-esteem or grandiosity

2. Decreased need for sleep (e.g., feels rested after only 3 hours of sleep)

3. More talkative than usual or pressure to keep talking

4. Flight of ideas or subjective experience that thoughts are racing

5. Distractibility (i.e., easily drawn to unimportant or irrelevant external stimuli)

6. Increased goal-directed activity (socially, at work or school, or sexually) or psychomotor agitation

C. Excessive involvement in pleasurable activities that have a high potential for painful consequences (e.g., unrestrained buying sprees, sexual indiscretions, or foolish investments)

D. The symptoms do not meet criteria for a mixed episode.

E. The mood disturbance is sufficiently severe to cause marked impairment in occupational functioning, usual social activities or relationships with others or to necessitate hospitalization to prevent harm to self or others, or with psychotic features.

F. The symptoms are not due to the direct physiologic effects of a substance or a general medical condition. Note: Manic-like episodes that are clearly caused by somatic antidepressant treatment (e.g., medication, electroconvulsive therapy) should not count toward a diagnosis of bipolar I disorder.

within 5 years of a depressive episode. Features associated with switching include early-onset depression, psychomotor retardation, psychosis, mood lability, seasonal pattern, family history of BD or mood disorders, and antidepressant-induced hypomania. A *mixed episode* requires 1 week of symptoms of both a manic and major depressive episode. *Dysphoric mania* is another term used to describe periods of mania that are accompanied by "bad feelings." *Hypomania* is used to describe a period of more than 4 but fewer than 7 days of manic symptoms. It also is used less specifically to describe less intense mania. The prevalence of psychosis in adolescence (often auditory hallucinations) is 16% to 60%. Although high, it is still less than its prevalence in adult BD.

Bipolar II disorder includes at least one full major depressive episode and at least one period of hypomania. **Bipolar disorder not otherwise specified** is used to describe prominent symptoms of BD that do not meet full diagnostic criteria or when historical information is unclear.

Cyclothymic disorder is characterized by 2 years or more (1 year in children) of numerous periods of hypomania and depression that do not meet full criteria for either a manic or a major depressive episode.

BD occurs in up to 4% of the general population. It is estimated that 1% of children and adolescents meet diagnostic criteria for BD. According to retrospective studies, 60% of BD onset occurs before 20 years of age. Although BD in adults tends to be gender neutral, it is estimated that prepubertal BD is almost four times more frequently diagnosed in boys. This may be because aggression is the main reason for referral for psychiatric services.

The etiology of BD is multifactorial. Studies in BD point to a highly familial etiology with family history of mental illness, including major depression, BD, schizophrenia, or ADHD. A first-degree relative with BD leads to a 10-fold increase in a child's chance of developing BD. An earlier onset of BD in a parent increases the risk of early onset BD in offspring with a more chronic and debilitating course that may be less responsive to treatment.

The differential diagnosis for BD includes ADHD, major depression, conduct disorder (CD), mood disorder due to a general medical condition, substance-induced mood disorder, pervasive developmental disorder, and schizophrenia.

Patients with BD often have concurrent conditions that warrant treatment. ADHD occurs in approximately 60% to 90% of children with BD. Anxiety disorders also commonly occur with BD and do not respond to antimanic agents. Substance abuse can precipitate and perpetuate mania and depression. The alteration between highs and lows related to some types of substance abuse often mimics BD. Patients with BD may also self-medicate in attempts to alleviate symptoms. Many patients with BD may commit crimes and meet criteria for CD due to aggression and impulsivity. Prominent symptoms of mania assist in differentiating between CD and BD. Patients with BD generally exhibit reactive aggression, whereas those with CD are more likely to preplan and develop a typical pattern of crimes.

No laboratory or imaging studies can diagnose BD. Physical examination, careful history, review of systems, and laboratory testing are done to rule out suspected medical etiologies, including neurologic and substance-induced disorders.

Treatment of BD includes decreasing acute symptoms. The FDA has approved lithium, divalproex sodium, carbamazepine, olanzapine, risperidone, quetiapine, ziprasidone, and aripiprazole for adults with BD. Lithium is the oldest proven treatment for mania in adults and has been used effectively in children and adolescents for years. Common side effects of lithium include hypothyroidism, polyuria, and acne. Divalproex is also a first-line agent (preferable for mixed or rapid cycling cases) for adults. It has been used effectively for decades in youth, but it is not FDA-approved. Periodic monitoring of blood levels for select medications (lithium and divalproex sodium) can help ensure both treatment safety and the receipt of therapeutic amounts of the medication. Antipsychotics (risperidone, olanzapine, quetiapine, aripiprazole, and ziprasidone) have had positive results in youth with BD. It is likely that newer antipsychotics will also be effective in BD.

Treating comorbid psychiatric disorders must be done carefully. Stimulants may be used to treat ADHD once the patient has been stabilized on a mood stabilizer. Antidepressants should be avoided; if the youth is depressed or has significant anxiety and is not responsive to other pharmacotherapy, cautious use of antidepressants may be necessary. Careful monitoring for manic reactivation, cycling, and suicidality is needed.

Cognitive and behavioral therapies are aimed at improving adherence to medication treatments and ameliorating anxiety and depressive symptoms. Psychoeducation and family therapy are needed to stabilize the patient's environment and improve prognosis. There should be continuous ongoing safety assessment. Because developmental delays are also common in young children with BD due to poor learning while symptomatic, collaboration with school regarding behavioral management, special educational needs, and an appropriate individualized educational plan is also needed.

BD is an even higher risk factor for suicide than depression. Forty percent of children and 50% of adolescents with BD attempt suicide. High levels of irritability, impulsivity, and poor ability to consider consequences (substance abuse, and so on) increase the risk of completed suicide. Attempters are usually older, more likely to have mixed episodes and psychotic features, comorbid substance use, panic disorder, nonsuicidal self-injurious behaviors, a family history of suicide attempts, history of hospitalizations, and history of physical or sexual abuse. Ensuring safety is the first consideration. Hospitalization, partial hospitalization, intensive outpatient treatment, and intensive in-home services are used as needed for stabilization and safety.

Chapter 19

OBSESSIVE-COMPULSIVE DISORDER

Obsessive-compulsive disorder (OCD) is characterized by obsessions, compulsions, or both in the absence of another psychiatric disorder that better explains the symptoms (Table 19-1). Obsessions are persistent intrusive thoughts, images, or impulses. Compulsions are non-gratifying repeated behaviors aimed at reducing or preventing distress or anxiety. Usually the compulsions are performed to offset anxiety created by the obsessions. In children, due to low level of insight, rituals or compulsive symptoms may predominate over worries or obsessions. Symptoms are usually recognized as being excessive or unreasonable. Common examples of obsessions in children are fears of contamination, repeated doubts, need for orderliness, and aggressive or horrific impulses. Common compulsions are hand washing, ordering, checking, requesting or demanding reassurance, praying, counting, repeating words silently, and hoarding.

Prevalence of OCD in children and adolescents ranges from 1% to 4%, increasing with age. It is more common in boys at a younger age and in girls during adolescence.

At least 50% of youth with OCD have at least one other psychiatric illness. Psychiatric comorbidities include tics (20% to 30%), mood and anxiety disorders (up to 75%), disruptive behavior disorders (attention-deficit/hyperactivity disorder [ADHD] and oppositional defiant disorder), developmental disorders, body dysmorphic disorder, hypochondriasis, and obsessive-compulsive personality disorder.

Twin studies suggest that obsessive-compulsive symptoms are moderately heritable, with genetic factors accounting for 45% to 65% of variance.

Streptococcal infection causing inflammation in the basal ganglia may account for 10% of childhood-onset OCD and is a part of a condition referred to as *pediatric autoimmune neuropsychiatric disorders associated with streptococcal* (also known as *PANDAS*) infection. Antistreptolysin O, antistreptococcal DNAase B titers, and a throat culture assist in diagnosing a

group A beta-hemolytic streptococcal infection. Early antibiotic therapy may help treat these cases.

OCD has been linked to a disruption in the brain's serotonin, glutamate, and dopamine systems. Overactivity in neural pathways involving orbital frontal cortex and the caudate nucleus has been implicated in OCD.

Physical examination may reveal rough, cracked skin as evidence of excessive hand washing. The Yale-Brown Obsessive-Compulsive Scale (also known as *Y-BOCS*) is regarded as the gold standard measure of obsessive-compulsive symptom severity. Although somewhat lengthy, it can be helpful in the clinical setting.

Cognitive-behavioral therapy (CBT) involving exposure and response prevention is considered the **treatment** of choice in milder cases. CBT provides durability of symptom relief and avoidance of potential pharmacotherapy-associated side effects. As with other anxiety disorders, CBT is at least

Table 19-1	Criteria for Diagnosis of Obsessive-Compulsive Disorder

A. Either obsessions or compulsions

Obsessions are defined by (1), (2), (3), and (4).

1. Recurrent and persistent thoughts, impulses, or images experienced at some time during the disturbance as intrusive and inappropriate and causing marked anxiety or distress

2. Thoughts, impulses, or images are not simply excessive worries about real-life problems.

3. The person attempts to ignore or suppress such thoughts, impulses, or images or to neutralize them with some other thought or action.

4. The person recognizes that the obsessional thoughts, impulses, or images are a product of his or her own mind (not imposed from without as in thought insertion).

Compulsions are defined by (1) and (2).

1. Repetitive behaviors (e.g., hand washing, ordering, checking) or mental acts (e.g., praying, counting, repeating words silently) that the person feels driven to perform in response to an obsession or according to rigidly applied rules.

2. The behaviors or mental acts are aimed at preventing or reducing distress or preventing some dreaded event or situation; however, these behaviors or mental acts are not realistically connected with what they are designed to neutralize/prevent or are clearly excessive.

B. At some point, the person recognizes that the obsessions or compulsions are excessive or unreasonable. Note: This is not required for children.

C. The obsessions or compulsions cause marked distress; are time-consuming (taking >1 hour a day); or significantly interfere with a normal routine, occupational (or academic) functioning, or usual social activities or relationships.

D. If another Axis I disorder is present, the content of the obsessions or compulsions is not restricted to it (e.g., preoccupation with food in the presence of an eating disorder).

E. The disturbance is not due to the direct physiologic effects of a drug of abuse, a medication, or a general medical condition.

Specify the following:

With poor insight: if, for most of the time during the current episode, the person does not recognize that the obsessions and compulsions are excessive or unreasonable as good, if not better, than medications. The combination of medications and CBT has shown the best response.

Selective serotonin reuptake inhibitors (SSRI) are useful for higher severity of symptoms and complications with comorbidities or when cognitive or emotional ability are insufficient to cooperate in CBT. If quality CBT is not available, treatment with medications alone while psychotherapy referral is pursued is a reasonable choice.

SSRI (paroxetine, fluoxetine, fluvoxamine, sertraline, citalopram and escitalopram) treatment is generally thought to show a favorable risk-to-benefit ratio in OCD. Side effects such as activation, akathisia, disinhibition, impulsivity, and hyperactivity may be seen. Monitoring of height may be advisable due to possible growth suppression associated with the SSRIs.

If an SSRI trial is unsuccessful, clomipramine can be tried next. Combination therapy using an SSRI with an antipsychotic medication (risperidone or another atypical antipsychotic) is also considered especially with specific comorbidities, for example, in tic disorders. Antipsychotics are also useful when the intrusive thoughts associated with OCD become nearly delusional in nature. Psychostimulants are used with comorbid ADHD, even though there is a risk that stimulants may increase obsessional symptoms and tics.

Most *responders* exhibit partial response only, and as many as one third of young people with OCD are refractory to treatment. Poor prognostic factors include comorbid psychiatric illness and a poor initial treatment response.

Deep brain stimulation of the basal ganglia, through surgically implanted electrodes and surgical interventions (anterior capsulotomy, anterior cingulotomy, subcaudate tractotomy, and limbic leucotomy), are reserved for very severe cases or highly refractory cases.

The differential diagnosis for OCD includes psychotic disorders, complex tics, other anxiety disorders, and obsessive-compulsive personality disorder. Often a patient with OCD recognizes that the intrusive thoughts are created by their own brain, whereas psychotic patients feel they are not created by them. This may be less clear in youth. A delusional fixation on appearance in **body dysmorphic disorder** and impulsive hair pulling to relieve anxiety or tension in **trichotillomania** can be confused with OCD. **Obsessive-compulsive personality disorder** is a character style involving preoccupation with orderliness, perfectionism, and control. No true obsessions or compulsions are present.

Chapter 20

PERVASIVE DEVELOPMENTAL DISORDERS AND PSYCHOSES

Pervasive developmental disorders, also known as **autism spectrum disorders** (ASDs), consist of five disorders: autism, Asperger syndrome, childhood disintegrative disorder, Rett syndrome, and pervasive developmental disorder not otherwise specified.

Onset of these disorders is in infancy and preschool years. Hallmarks of these disorders include impaired communication and impaired social interaction as well as stereotypic behaviors, interests, and activities. Mental retardation is common, with a few children showing remarkable isolated abilities (savant or splinter skills).

ASDs are seen in less than 1% of the population with equal prevalence among all racial and ethnic groups. The prevalence is greater in boys (except for Rett syndrome), but girls with the disorders tend to be more severely affected.

Differentiating features of the pervasive developmental disorders are listed in Table 20-1.

Treatment of ASD is symptomatic and multimodal. At present there are no treatments for the core symptoms of ASDs. Antipsychotics (risperidone, olanzapine, quetiapine, aripiprazole, ziprasidone, paliperidone, haloperidol, thioridazine) are used for aggression, agitation, irritability, hyperactivity, and self-injurious behavior. Anticonvulsants and lithium can be used for aggression. Naltrexone has been used to decrease self-injurious behavior, presumably by blocking endogenous opioids. Selective serotonin reuptake inhibitors are given for anxiety, perseveration, compulsions, depression, and social isolation. Stimulants are useful for hyperactivity and inattention (better response with Asperger syndrome). There are reports of significant worsening of irritability and aggression in some patients treated with stimulants. Alpha-2 agonists (guanfacine, clonidine) are used for hyperactivity, aggression, and sleep dysregulation, although melatonin is first-line medication for sleep dysregulation. Behavioral management training for parents is useful in teaching protocols to help their child learn appropriate behavior. Special educational services should be individualized for the child. Occupational, speech, and physical therapy are often required. Referral for disability services and support is often warranted. Potentially useful therapies tailored to the individual include applied behavioral analysis, discrete trial training, and structured teaching. There is a need for family support groups and individual supportive counseling for parents. The prognosis for autism is guarded. There are no known methods of primary prevention. Treatment and educational interventions are aimed at decreasing morbidity and maximizing function.

AUTISM

Autism, the prototypic pervasive developmental disorder, is characterized by lifelong marked impairment in reciprocal social interaction, communication, and a restricted range of activities and interests (Table 20-2). Approximately 20% of parents report relatively normal development until 1 or 2 years of age, followed by a steady or sudden decline. If no clinical manifestations of the disorder are present by 3 years of age, Rett syndrome or childhood disintegrative disorder need to be considered. As an infant, there is delayed or absent social smiling. The young child may spend hours in solitary play and be socially withdrawn with indifference to attempts at communication. Patients with autism often are not able to understand nonverbal communication (eye contact, facial expressions) and do not interact with people as significantly different from objects. Speech often is delayed and, when present, it is frequently dominated by echolalia (sometimes mistaken as a sign of obsessive-compulsive disorder [OCD]), perseveration (confused with psychosis or

Table 20-1	Pervasive Developmental Disorder: Characteristics				
FEATURE	**AUTISM**	**ASPERGER**	**RETT**	**CDD**	**PDD-NOS**
Epidemiology	10 cases per 10,000; 5:1 male-to-female ratio	2.5 per 10,000; 5:1 male-to-female ratio	0.44 to 2.1 per 10,000; diagnosed only in girls; associated with *MECP2* gene mutation	0.11 per 10,000	2 to 16 per 10,000
Onset	Before age 3 yr	Usually first recognized in preschool age; Motor delays seen	Before age 5 yr; Head circumference growth dramatically decelerates and child begins losing skills.	Child appears normal until age 2 yr, then dramatic autistic-like picture	Variable; Child does not meet full criteria for other PDD
Language/communication impairment	Marked	Good verbal ability but poor communication	Very marked	Marked (normal previously)	Variable
Motor issues	Poor; May be preserved previously	Fine and gross motor difficulties	Significant loss of motor abilities, hand-washing stereotypes; A characteristic hand-wringing movement exists.	Often preserved but child may lose some skills	Variable
Restricted interests	Marked, mannerisms, trouble with change, occasionally savant ability	Highly circumscribed interests that may interfere with functioning	Significant psychomotor retardation	Marked, as in autism	Variable; mannerisms may be less prominent, but child is often troubled by change.

CDD, Childhood disintegrative disorder; *PDD-NOS*, pervasive developmental disorder-not otherwise specified.

OCD), pronoun reversal, nonsense rhyming, and other abnormalities. Intense absorbing interests, ritualistic behavior, and compulsive routines are characteristic, and their disruption often invokes tantrum or rage reactions. Head banging, teeth grinding, rocking, diminished responsiveness to pain and external stimuli, and self-mutilation may be noted.

Although the etiology of autistic disorder is unknown, there is an increased risk of autistic disorder in siblings compared to the general population. Twin studies have revealed high levels of concordance for monozygotic twins. Family studies reveal prevalence rates of between 2% and 10% in siblings, and, when absent, there may be increased risk for language, learning, and social development problems.

It is proposed that the brain connectivity is adversely affected. Abnormalities in the limbic system, temporal, and frontal lobes have been suggested. Some postmortem studies reveal abnormalities in the brain microarchitecture, size, and neuronal packing. Functional magnetic resonance imaging (MRI) studies show hypoactivity of the fusiform gyrus of the amygdala, a location involved in face processing tasks and facial expression recognition involved in social and affective judgments.

The American Academy of Pediatrics recommends screening for autism at 18 and 24 months of age. Comprehensive testing should be done if there is an affected sibling or parental, other caregiver, or pediatric concern.

There are no definitive laboratory studies for autistic disorder, but they can help rule out other diagnoses. A hearing test (may account for the language deficits), chromosomal testing (to identify fragile X syndrome, tubular sclerosis, and genetic polymorphisms), congenital viral infections, and metabolic disorders (phenylketonuria) should be performed. Electroencephalography abnormalities may be seen in 20% to 25% of children with autism but are not diagnostic. Psychological tests in children with autism often show strengths in nonverbal tasks (e.g., puzzles) and marked deficiency in verbal cognitive abilities. IQ is usually low, though savant skills and hyperlexia (a precocious interest in letters and numbers) are sometimes

observed. Speech pathology consultation can be helpful in evaluating the communication difficulties.

Common comorbidities are mental retardation (in up to 80%), seizure disorder (in 25%), anxiety disorders, OCD, and attention-deficit/hyperactivity disorder. Seizures often start around the onset of puberty. Higher IQ and better language skills are related to improved prognosis. Good communication by the age of 6 years and average nonverbal cognitive skills predict the likelihood of living independently or in a less structured group living situation.

The earliest studies of autism suggested a relatively poor prognosis, with only a small number of individuals (1% to 2%) being able to function independently as adults. Recent research reveals major gains, but not a cure, with early diagnosis and treatment.

SCHIZOPHRENIA

Schizophrenia generally presents in adolescence or early adulthood. The same diagnostic criteria are applied as in adults but must be interpreted in terms of the developmental stage of the child (Table 20-3).

Childhood-onset schizophrenia is a rare disorder (<1 in 10,000 children) and usually indicates a more severe form of schizophrenia. The frequency increases between 13 and 18 years of age. Boys tend to be affected about twice as often as girls, regardless of ethnic or other cultural factors. The etiology of schizophrenia is unknown. Numerous studies have shown genetic predisposition and linkages for the disorder. In addition, family studies consistently show a higher risk in monozygotic twins compared with dizygotic twins and siblings. First-degree relatives of patients with schizophrenia have a 10-fold higher risk.

The symptoms of schizophrenia typically fall into four broad categories:

• **Positive symptoms** include hallucinations and delusions. Hallucinations are auditory or visual misperceptions that occur without external stimuli. Delusions are fixed false

Table 20-2	Criteria for Diagnosis of Autistic Disorder

A. Six or more items from (1), (2), and (3), with at least two from (1) and one each from (2) and (3)

1. Qualitative impairment in social interaction, as manifested by at least two of the following:

   a. Marked impairment in the use of multiple nonverbal behaviors, such as eye-to-eye gaze, facial expression, body postures, and gestures to regulate social interaction

   b. Failure to develop peer relationships appropriate to developmental level

   c. A lack of spontaneously seeking to share enjoyment, interests, or achievements with other people (e.g., by a lack of showing, bringing, or pointing out objects of interest)

   d. Lack of social or emotional reciprocity

2. Qualitative impairments in communication as manifested by at least one of the following:

   a. Delay in, or total lack of, the development of spoken language (not accompanied by attempts to compensate through alternative modes of communication, such as gesture or mime)

   b. In individuals with adequate speech, marked impairment in the ability to initiate or sustain a conversation with others

   c. Stereotyped and repetitive use of language or idiosyncratic language

   d. Lack of varied, spontaneous make-believe play or social imitative play appropriate to developmental level

3. Restricted repetitive and stereotyped patterns of behavior, interests, and activities, as manifested by at least one of the following:

   a. Encompassing preoccupation with stereotyped and restricted patterns of interest that is abnormal either in intensity or focus

   b. Apparently inflexible adherence to specific, nonfunctional routines or rituals

   c. Stereotyped and repetitive motor mannerisms (e.g., hand- or finger-flapping or twisting or complex whole body movements)

   d. Persistent preoccupation with parts of objects

B. Delays or abnormal functioning in at least one of the following areas, with onset before age 3 yr

   1. Social interaction

   2. Language as used in social communication

   3. Symbolic or imaginative play

C. The disturbance is not better accounted for by Rett syndrome or childhood disintegrative disorder.

Table 20-3	Criteria for Diagnosis of Schizophrenia

A. Characteristic symptoms: two of the following, each present for a significant portion of time during a 1-month period (or less if successfully treated)

   1. Delusions

   2. Hallucinations

   3. Disorganized speech (e.g., frequent derailment or incoherence)

   4. Grossly disorganized or catatonic behavior

   5. Negative symptoms (i.e., affective flattening, alogia, or avolition)

Note: Only one criterion A symptom is required if delusions are bizarre or hallucinations consist of a voice keeping up a running commentary on the person's behavior or thoughts or two or more voices conversing with each other.

B. Social/occupational dysfunction: for a significant portion of the time since the onset of the disturbance, major areas of functioning, such as work, interpersonal relations, or self-care, are markedly below the level achieved before the onset (or when the onset is in childhood or adolescence, failure to achieve expected level of interpersonal, academic, or occupational achievement).

C. Duration: continuous signs of the disturbance persist for at least 6 months with at least 1 month of symptoms (or less if successfully treated) that meet criterion A (i.e., active-phase symptoms) and may include periods of prodromal or residual symptoms. During prodromal or residual periods, signs of disturbance may be manifested by only negative symptoms or symptoms listed in criterion A present in an attenuated form (e.g., odd beliefs, unusual perceptual experiences).

D. Schizoaffective and mood disorder exclusion: schizoaffective disorder and mood disorder with psychotic features have been ruled out because either (1) no major depressive, manic, or mixed episodes have occurred concurrently with the active-phase symptoms or (2) if mood episodes have occurred during active-phase symptoms, their total duration has been brief relative to the duration of the active and residual periods.

E. The disturbance is not due to the direct physiologic effects of a drug abuse, a medication, or a general medical condition.

F. If there is a history of autistic disorder or another pervasive developmental disorder, the additional diagnosis of schizophrenia is made only if prominent delusions or hallucinations also are present for at least 1 month (or less if successfully treated).

Classification of longitudinal course (can be applied only after at least 1 year has elapsed since the initial onset of active-phase symptoms):

Episodic with inter-episode residual symptoms (episodes are defined by the reemergence of prominent psychotic symptoms); also specify if: with prominent negative symptoms.

Episodic with no inter-episode residual symptoms

Continuous (prominent psychotic symptoms are present throughout the period of observation); also specify if: with prominent negative symptoms.

---

beliefs and can be bizarre or non-bizarre, depending on cultural norms.

- **Negative symptoms** include a lack of motivation and social interactions and flat effect. Negative symptoms are most frequent in early childhood and later adolescence. Children with high IQs often show more positive and fewer negative symptoms than children with low IQs.
- **Disorganization of thoughts and behavior** can cause significant impairment.
- **Cognitive impairment** is common and is perhaps the most disabling feature of schizophrenia, causing marked social and functional impairment.

There are five subtypes of schizophrenia: paranoid, disorganized, catatonic, undifferentiated, and residual.

- **Paranoid type:** prominent hallucinations and delusions with relatively normal cognition. The delusions are often persecutory, but other types of delusions also may occur.
- **Disorganized type:** disorganized speech, disorganized behavior, and flat or inappropriate affect.

- **Catatonic type:** prominent psychomotor abnormalities that may include extreme inactivity or excessive motor activity. **Cataplexy** (waxy flexibility) is rare in children and adolescents.
- **Undifferentiated type:** case in which a patient meets the diagnostic criteria for schizophrenia but not paranoid, disorganized, or catatonic type.
- **Residual type:** clinical situation in which full diagnostic criteria have been met previously but no current, prominent, positive symptoms.

To meet criteria for diagnosing schizophrenia, clinical symptoms should be present for at least 6 months. If symptoms are present for less than 1 month, the condition is called a **brief psychotic disorder.** If symptoms are present for more than 1 month but less than 6 months, a diagnosis of **schizophreniform disorder** is made. Psychotic symptoms that do not meet full diagnostic criteria for schizophrenia but are clinically significant are diagnosed as **psychotic disorder not otherwise specified.**

There are several disorders that have to be distinguished from schizophrenia. These include the following:

Schizoaffective disorder is diagnosed when a person has clear symptoms of schizophrenia for at least 2 weeks without active symptoms of depression or mania. These affective syndromes occur at other times, even when psychotic symptoms are present.

Major depression with psychotic features and **bipolar disorder with psychotic features** are diagnoses made when psychotic symptoms occur during the course of depression or mania only. Psychotic disorder due to a general medical condition describes psychotic symptoms that are judged to be the direct result of a general medical condition.

Substance-induced psychotic disorders have psychotic symptoms related to drug or alcohol ingestion.

Shared psychotic disorder, folie à deux, occurs when delusional symptoms from one person influence delusions, with similar content, in another person.

Other disorders in the differential diagnoses are autism, childhood disintegrative disorder (Heller syndrome), Asperger syndrome, drug-induced psychosis, and organic brain disorders.

No diagnostic tests or imaging studies are specific for schizophrenia. It is a clinical diagnosis of exclusion. Obtaining a family history with attention to mental illness is critical. The workup of schizophrenia includes physical and neurologic examinations, MRI, electroencephalography (to rule out epilepsy, especially temporal lobe epilepsy), drug screening, and metabolic screening for endocrinopathies. Evaluation to rule out Wilson disease and delirium is also indicated. Psychotic symptoms in younger children must be differentiated from manifestations of normal vivid fantasy life or abuse-related symptoms. Youth with posttraumatic stress disorder often have vivid recollections and nightmares related to abuse but sometimes are less specific and can include nightmares with other negative topics. Psychological testing can be helpful in identifying psychotic thought processes.

Treatment is based on a multimodal approach, including use of antipsychotic medications. First-line drugs are atypical antipsychotics (e.g., risperidone, olanzapine, quetiapine, aripiprazole, ziprasidone, and paliperidone). Second-line medications are typical antipsychotics (e.g., haloperidol, thiothixene, chlorpromazine, trifluoperazine, loxapine, and molindone). It is likely that the newer antipsychotics approved for adults will also work in youth. However, these are not yet approved in youth by the U.S. Food and Drug Administration. Antipsychotics can be augmented with lithium or another mood stabilizer. Clozapine or electroconvulsive therapy is generally reserved for resistant cases.

Psychosocial treatments, including skills training, supportive psychotherapy, behavior modification, and cognitive-behavioral therapy, are all appropriate and should be considered as needed for individual patients. Attention should be paid to psychoeducation for parents and the child about the disease and its treatments. School interventions are needed to ensure that any special learning needs are addressed.

The course of illness for schizophrenia varies in exacerbations and remissions of psychotic symptoms. The poorest prognosis is seen if the onset is at an age younger than 13 years, with poor premorbid function, when marked negative symptoms are present, and when a family history of schizophrenia exists.

Suggested Reading

American Psychiatric Association (APA): *Practice guideline for the treatment of patients with panic disorder,* ed 2, Washington (DC), 2009 Jan, American Psychiatric Association (APA). Available from the PsychiatryOnline website. Available at http://psychiatryonline.org/content.aspx?bookid=28§ionid=1680635.

Hagerman RJ, Berry-Kravis E, Kaufmann WE, et al: Advances in the treatment of fragile X syndrome, *Pediatrics* 123(1):378–390, 2009.

Huyser C, Veltman DJ, de Haan E, et al: Paediatric obsessive-compulsive disorder, a neurodevelopmental disorder? Evidence from neuroimaging, *Neurosci Biobehav Rev.* 33(6):818–830, 2009.

Ibeziako PI, Shaw J, DeMaso DR: Psychosomatic illness. In Kliegman RM, Stanton BF, St. Geme J, et al: *Nelson Textbook of Pediatrics,* 20, ed 19, Philadelphia, 2011, Elsevier, pp 67–69.

Ponniah K, Hollon SD: Empirically supported psychological treatments for adult acute stress disorder and posttraumatic stress disorder: a review, *Depress Anxiety* 26(12):1086–1109, 2009.

Shattuck PT, Durkin M, Maenner M, et al: Timing of identification among children with an autism spectrum disorder: findings from a population-based surveillance study, *J Am Acad Child Adolesc Psychiatry* 48(5):474–483, 2009.

Silber TJ: Somatization disorders: diagnosis, treatment, and prognosis, *Pediatr Rev* 32(2):56–63, 2011 quiz 63–64.

Psychosocial Issues

Cindy W. Christian and Nathan J. Blum

Chapter 21

FAILURE TO THRIVE

Failure to thrive (FTT) is a descriptive term given to malnourished infants and young children who fail to meet expected standards of growth. FTT is most often used to describe malnutrition related to environmental or psychosocial causes. In many children with inadequate growth, however, organic and environmental contributors coexist, underscoring the importance of assessing potential medical, nutritional, developmental, psychosocial, and environmental contributors in all cases.

FTT is often diagnosed by weight that falls or remains below the 3rd percentile for age; decreases, crossing two major percentile lines on the growth chart over time; or is less than 80% of the median weight for the height of the child. Caveats to these definitions exist. According to growth chart standards, 3% of the population naturally falls below the 3rd percentile. These children, who typically have short stature or constitutional delay of growth, usually are proportional (normal weight for height). Additionally in the first few years of life, large fluctuations in percentile position can occur in normal children. Changes in weight should be assessed in relation to height (length) and head circumference.

Weight that decreases from a disproportionately high percentile to one that is proportional causes no concern, but weight that decreases to a disproportionately low percentile is of concern. Allowances must be made for prematurity; weight corrections are needed until 24 months of age, height corrections until 40 months of age, and head circumference corrections until 18 months of age. Although some growth variants can be difficult to distinguish from FTT, growth velocity and height-for-weight determinations can be useful in distinguishing the cause. In children with FTT, malnutrition initially results in wasting (deficiency in weight gain). Stunting (deficiency in linear growth) generally occurs after months of malnutrition, and head circumference is spared except with chronic, severe malnutrition. FTT that is *symmetric* (proportional weight, height/length, and head circumference) suggests long-standing malnutrition, chromosomal abnormalities, congenital infection, or teratogenic exposures. FTT is a common problem in pediatrics, affecting 5% to 10% of young children, 3% to 5% of children admitted to hospitals, and 15% of children living in poverty and foster care.

ETIOLOGY

Because possible causes of growth failure are diverse and often multifactorial, the management of FTT begins with a careful search for its etiology (Table 21-1). The common causes of FTT vary by age, which should be reflected in the evaluation (Table 21-2). In most cases, a comprehensive history and physical examination are sufficient to suggest or eliminate medical disease as the primary cause of FTT. Medical diseases are diagnosed in fewer than 50% of children hospitalized for growth failure and even less frequently in children managed in the outpatient setting. Growth failure is often a manifestation of more extensive family problems. It is clinically useful to categorize the causes of malnutrition into inadequate nutritional intake, inadequate nutrient absorption, or increased metabolic demand.

DIAGNOSIS AND CLINICAL MANIFESTATIONS

Decision-Making Algorithm
Available @ StudentConsult.com

Failure to Thrive

A medical history should include prenatal history prematurity, birth size (weight, length, and head circumference), as well as family and travel history. Indicators of medical diseases, such as vomiting, diarrhea, fever, respiratory symptoms, and fatigue, should be noted. A careful diet history is essential. Lactation problems in breastfed infants and improper formula preparation are frequent causes of growth failure early in infancy. It is crucial to evaluate intake of solid foods and liquids for older infants and children. Due to parental dietary beliefs, some children have inappropriately restricted diets; others drink excessive amounts of fruit juice, leading to malabsorption or anorexia. The child's daily meal schedule (timing, frequency, location) should also be noted. Mealtime practices, especially distractions that interfere with completing meals, can influence growth. A complete psychosocial assessment of the child and family is required. Child factors (temperament, development), parental factors (depression, domestic violence, social isolation, mental retardation, substance abuse), and environmental and societal factors (poverty, unemployment, illiteracy, lead toxicity) all may contribute to growth failure.

A complete physical examination and developmental screening should assess signs of inflicted injury; oral or dental problems; indicators of pulmonary, cardiac, or gastrointestinal

Table 21-1	Causes of Failure to Thrive

ENVIRONMENTAL (COMMON)

Emotional deprivation

Rumination

Child maltreatment

Maternal depression

Poverty

Poor feeding techniques

Improper formula preparation

Improper mealtime environment

Unusual parental nutritional beliefs

GASTROINTESTINAL

Cystic fibrosis and other causes of pancreatic insufficiency

Celiac disease

Other malabsorption syndromes

Gastrointestinal reflux

CONGENITAL/ANATOMIC

Chromosomal abnormalities, genetic syndromes

Congenital heart disease

Gastrointestinal abnormalities (e.g., pyloric stenosis, malrotation)

Vascular rings

Upper airway obstruction

Dental caries

Congenital immunodeficiency syndromes

INFECTIONS

Human immunodeficiency virus

Tuberculosis

Hepatitis

Urinary tract infection, chronic sinusitis, parasitic infection

METABOLIC

Thyroid disease

Adrenal or pituitary disease

Aminoaciduria, organic aciduria

Galactosemia

NEUROLOGIC

Cerebral palsy

Hypothalamic and other central nervous system tumors

Hypotonia syndromes

Neuromuscular diseases

Degenerative and storage diseases

RENAL

Chronic renal failure

Renal tubular acidosis

Urinary tract infection

HEMATOLOGIC

Sickle cell disease

Iron deficiency anemia

Table 21-2	Common Causes of Malnutrition in Early Life

NEONATE

Failed breastfeeding

Improper formula preparation

Congenital syndromes

Prenatal infections

Teratogenic exposures

EARLY INFANCY

Maternal depression

Improper formula preparation

Gastroesophageal reflux

Poverty

Congenital heart disease

Cystic fibrosis

Neurologic abnormalities

Child neglect

LATER INFANCY

Celiac disease

Food intolerance

Child neglect

Delayed introduction of age-appropriate foods

Juice consumption

AFTER INFANCY

Acquired diseases

Highly distractible child

Juice consumption

Autonomy struggles

Inappropriate mealtime environment

Inappropriate diet

disease; and dysmorphic features that may suggest a genetic or teratogenic cause for growth failure. A complete neurologic examination may reveal spasticity or hypotonia, which can have untoward effects on feeding and growth. Physical findings related to malnutrition include decreased subcutaneous fat, decreased muscle mass, dermatitis, hepatomegaly, cheilosis, or edema (see Chapter 30). Additionally children with FTT have more otitis media, respiratory, and gastrointestinal infections than age-matched controls; severely malnourished children are at risk for a variety of serious infections.

The history and physical examination findings should guide the laboratory evaluation. Simple screening tests are recommended to identify common illnesses that cause growth failure and to search for medical problems resulting from malnutrition. Initial tests may include a complete blood count; screening for iron deficiency anemia and lead toxicity; urinalysis, urine culture, and serum electrolytes to assess renal infection or dysfunction; thyroid stimulating hormone; liver function tests; and a protein purified derivative test to screen for tuberculosis. Human immunodeficiency virus testing may also be indicated. For children with diarrhea, abdominal pain, or malodorous stools, a stool sample for culture and ova and parasites may be indicated. A review of the child's newborn screen may also be warranted. Observation during feeding and home visitation, if possible, is of great diagnostic value in assessing feeding problems, food preferences, mealtime distractions, unusual or disruptive parent-child interactions, and the home environment.

TREATMENT

Treatment must address the child's nutritional requirements and the social issues of the family. Initial treatment should focus on the nutritional and medical management of the child while engaging the family in the treatment plan. Parents of malnourished children may feel personally responsible and threatened by the diagnosis of FTT. Parents may be so depressed or dysfunctional they cannot focus on their child's needs; they may not recognize the psychosocial and family contributors to the malnutrition. These issues can have a profound effect on the success of treatment, and they need to be addressed.

Children with mild malnutrition whose cause is easily identified can be managed by the primary care physician and family. In more challenging cases, a multidisciplinary team, including pediatricians, nutritionists, developmental specialists, nurses, and social workers, improves nutritional outcome in children with FTT. Most children with FTT can be treated in the outpatient setting. Children with severe malnutrition, underlying diagnoses that require hospitalization for evaluation or treatment, or whose safety is in jeopardy because of maltreatment require hospitalization. Admitting children to the hospital to induce and document weight gain is not recommended unless intensive outpatient evaluation and intervention has failed or the social circumstances are a contraindication for attempting outpatient management.

Nutritional management is the cornerstone of treatment, regardless of the etiology. Children with FTT may require more than 1.5 times the expected calorie and protein intake for their age for catch-up growth. Children with FTT who are anorexic and picky eaters may not be able to consume this amount in volume and require calorically dense foods. For formula-fed infants, the concentration of formula can be adjusted appropriately (Table 21-3). For toddlers dietary changes should include increasing the caloric density of favorite foods by adding butter, oil, sour cream, peanut butter, or other high-calorie foods. High-calorie oral supplements (30 cal/oz) are often well tolerated by toddlers. In some cases, specific carbohydrate, fat, or protein additives are used to boost calories by increasing calories without increasing volume requirements. Additionally vitamin and mineral supplementation is needed, especially during catch-up growth. In general the simplest and least costly approach to dietary change is warranted.

Depending on the severity of the malnutrition, initiation of catch-up growth may take 2 weeks. Initial weight gain two to three times normal growth can be seen. Weight improvement precedes improvement in stature. For children with chronic, severe malnutrition, many months are needed to reverse all trends in growth. Although many children with FTT eventually reach normal size, they remain at risk for developmental, learning, and behavioral problems.

COMPLICATIONS

Malnutrition causes defects in host defenses. Children with FTT may suffer from a **malnutrition-infection cycle,** in which

Table 21-3	Infant Formula Preparation*	
AMOUNT OF POWDER/ LIQUID	AMOUNT OF WATER (OZ)	FINAL CONCENTRATION
1 cup powdered formula	29	20 kcal/oz
4 scoops powdered formula	8	20 kcal/oz
13 oz liquid concentrate	13	20 kcal/oz
1 cup powdered formula	24	24 kcal/oz
5 scoops powdered formula	8	24 kcal/oz
13 oz liquid concentrate	9	24 kcal/oz
1 cup powdered formula	21	27 kcal/oz
5.5 scoops powdered formula	8	27 kcal/oz
13 oz liquid concentrate	6	27 kcal/oz

From Jew R, editor: Department of Pharmacy Services Pharmacy Handbook and Formulary, 2000–2001. Hudson, Ohio, 2000, Department of Pharmacy Services, p 422.
*Final concentrations are reached by adding formula to water. One scoop of powdered formula = one measuring tablespoon. For healthy infants, formulas are prepared to provide 20 kcal/oz.

recurrent infections exacerbate malnutrition, leading to greater susceptibility to infection. Children with FTT must be evaluated and treated promptly for infection and followed closely.

During starvation, the body slows metabolic processes and growth to minimize the need for nutrients and uses its stores of glycogen, fat, and protein to maintain normal metabolic requirements. The body also generally maintains homeostasis and normal serum concentrations of electrolytes. With the rapid reinstitution of feeding after starvation, fluid and electrolyte homeostasis may be lost. Changes in serum electrolyte concentrations and the associated complications are collectively termed the **refeeding syndrome.** These changes typically affect phosphorus, potassium, calcium, and magnesium and can result in life-threatening cardiac, pulmonary, or neurologic problems. Infants and children with marasmus, kwashiorkor, and anorexia nervosa and those who have had prolonged fasting are at risk for refeeding syndrome. Refeeding syndrome can be avoided by slow institution of nutrition, close monitoring of serum electrolytes during the initial days of feeding, and prompt replacement of depleted electrolytes.

Occasionally children who live in psychological deprivation develop short stature with or without concomitant FTT or delayed puberty, a syndrome called **psychosocial short stature.** The signs and symptoms include polyphagia, polydipsia, hoarding and stealing of food, gorging and vomiting, drinking from toilet bowls, and other notable behaviors. Affected children are often shy and passive and are typically depressed and socially withdrawn. Endocrine dysfunction is often identified in affected children, who may have decreased growth hormone secretion and a muted response to exogenous growth hormone. Removal of the child from the adverse environment typically results in rapid improvement in endocrine function and subsequent rapid somatic and pubertal growth of the child. The prognosis for children with psychosocial short stature depends on the age at diagnosis and the degree of psychological trauma. Early identification and removal from the environment portends a healthy prognosis. Those diagnosed in later childhood or adolescence may not reach their genetic potential for growth and have a poorer psychosocial prognosis.

Chapter 22

CHILD ABUSE AND NEGLECT

Few social problems have as profound an impact on the well-being of children as child abuse and neglect. Each year in the United States, 3 million reports of suspected maltreatment are made to child welfare agencies. Approximately 1 million of these reports are substantiated after investigation by Child Protective Services (CPS). These reports represent only a small portion of the children who suffer from maltreatment. Parental surveys indicate that several million adults admit to physical violence against their children each year, and many more adults report abusive experiences as children. Federal and state laws define child abuse and neglect. Each state determines the process of investigating abuse, protecting children, and holding perpetrators accountable for their actions or inactions. Adverse childhood events, such as child abuse and neglect, increase the risk of the individual's developing behaviors in adolescence and adulthood that predict adult morbidity and early mortality. The ability to recognize child maltreatment and effectively advocate for the protection and safety of a child is a great challenge in pediatric practice that can have a profound influence on the health and future well-being of a child.

Child abuse is parental behavior destructive to the normal physical or emotional development of a child. Because personal definitions of abuse vary according to religious and cultural beliefs, individual experiences, and family upbringing, various physicians have different thresholds for reporting suspected abuse to CPS. In every state, physicians are mandated by law to identify and report all cases of *suspected* child abuse and neglect. It is the responsibility of CPS to investigate reports of suspected abuse to ensure the ongoing safety of the child. State laws also define intentional or reckless acts that cause harm to a child as crimes. Law enforcement investigates crimes such as sexual abuse and serious physical abuse or neglect for possible criminal charges against a perpetrator.

Child abuse and neglect are often considered in broad categories that include physical abuse, sexual abuse, emotional abuse, and neglect. Neglect is the most common, accounting for approximately half of the reports made to child welfare agencies. **Child neglect** is defined by omissions that prevent a child's basic needs from being met. These needs include adequate food, clothing, supervision, housing, health care, education, and nurturance. Child abuse and neglect result from a complex interaction of individual, family, and societal risk factors. Although some risk factors, such as parental substance abuse, maternal depression, and domestic violence, are strong risk factors for maltreatment, they are better considered as broadly defined markers to alert a physician to a potential risk, rather than determinants of specific abuse and neglect.

The ability to identify victims of child abuse varies by the age of the patient and the type of maltreatment sustained. Children who are victims of sexual abuse are often brought for medical care after the child makes a disclosure, and the diagnosis is straightforward. Physically abused infants may be brought for medical evaluation of irritability or lethargy, without a disclosure of trauma. If the infant's injuries are not severe or visible, the diagnosis may be missed. Approximately one third of infants with abusive head trauma initially are misdiagnosed by unsuspecting physicians, only to be identified after sustaining further injury. Although physicians are inherently trusting of parents, a constant awareness of the possibility of abuse is needed.

PHYSICAL ABUSE

Decision-Making Algorithms
Available @ StudentConsult.com

Extremity Pain
Altered Mental Status
Alopecia

The physical abuse of children by parents affects children of all ages. It is estimated that 1% to 2% of children are physically abused during childhood and that approximately 1500 children are fatally injured each year. Although mothers are most frequently reported as the perpetrators of physical abuse, serious injuries, such as head or abdominal trauma, are more likely to be inflicted by fathers or maternal boyfriends. The diagnosis of physical abuse can be made easily if the child is battered, has obvious external injuries, or is capable of providing a history of the abuse. In many cases, the diagnosis is not obvious. The history provided by the parent is often inaccurate because the parent is unwilling to provide the correct history or is a nonoffending parent who is unaware of the abuse. The child may be too young or ill to provide a history of the assault. An older child may be too scared to do so or may have a strong sense of loyalty to the perpetrator.

A **diagnosis** of physical abuse initially is suggested by a history that seems incongruent with the clinical presentation of the child (Table 22-1). Although injury to any organ system can occur from physical abuse, some injuries are more common. Bruises are universal findings in healthy ambulatory children but also are among the most common injury identified in abused children. Bruises suggestive of abuse include those that are patterned, such as a slap mark on the face or looped extension cord marks on the body (Fig. 22-1). Bruises

Table 22-1	Clues to the Diagnosis of Physical Abuse

A child presents for medical care with significant injuries, and a history of trauma is denied, especially if the child is an infant or toddler.

The history provided by the caregiver does not explain the injuries identified.

The history of the injury changes significantly over time.

A history of self-inflicted trauma does not correlate with the child's developmental abilities.

There is an unexpected or unexplained delay in seeking medical care.

Multiple organ systems are injured, including injuries of various ages.

The injuries are pathognomonic for child abuse.

in healthy children generally are distributed over bony prominences; bruises that occur in an unusual distribution, such as isolated to the torso, ears or neck, should raise concern. Bruises in nonambulatory infants are unusual, occurring in less than 2% of healthy infants seen for routine medical care. Occasionally a subtle bruise may be the only external clue to abuse and can be associated with significant internal injury.

Burns are common pediatric injuries and usually represent preventable unintentional trauma (see Chapter 44). Approximately 10% of children hospitalized with burns are victims of abuse. Inflicted burns can be the result of contact with hot objects (irons, radiators, or cigarettes) but more commonly the result of scalding injuries (Fig. 22-2). Hot tap water burns in infants and toddlers are sometimes the result of intentional immersion injuries, which often occur around toilet training issues. These burns have clear lines of demarcation, uniformity of burn depth, and characteristic pattern.

Inflicted fractures occur more commonly in infants and young children. Although diaphyseal fractures are most common in abuse, they are nonspecific for inflicted injury. Fractures that should raise suspicion for abuse include fractures that are unexplained; occur in young, nonambulatory children; or involve multiple bones. Certain fractures have a high specificity for abuse, such as rib, metaphyseal, scapular, vertebral, or other unusual fractures (Fig. 22-3). Some metabolic diseases can be confused with abuse and should be considered in the differential diagnosis when appropriate.

Abdominal injury is an uncommon but serious form of physical abuse. Blunt trauma to the abdomen is the primary mechanism of injury, and infants and toddlers are the most common victims. Injuries to solid organs, such as the liver or pancreas, predominate and hollow viscus injury occurs more commonly with inflicted trauma than accidental. Even

Figure 22-1 Multiple looped cord marks on a 2-year-old abused child who presented to the hospital with multiple untreated burns to the back, arms, and feet.

Figure 22-2 A 1-year-old child brought to the hospital with a history that she sat on a hot radiator. Suspicious injuries such as this require a full medical and social investigation, including a skeletal survey to look for occult skeletal injuries and a child welfare evaluation.

Figure 22-3 A, Metaphyseal fracture of the distal tibia in a 3-month-old infant admitted to the hospital with severe head injury. There also is periosteal new bone formation of that tibia, perhaps from a previous injury. **B,** Bone scan of same infant. Initial chest x-ray showed a single fracture of the right posterior fourth rib. A radionuclide bone scan performed 2 days later revealed multiple previously unrecognized fractures of the posterior and lateral ribs. **C,** Follow-up radiographs 2 weeks later showed multiple healing rib fractures. This pattern of fracture is highly specific for child abuse. The mechanism of these injuries is usually violent squeezing of the chest.

Figure 22-4 Acute subdural hemorrhage in the posterior interhemispheric fissure in an abused infant.

in severe cases of trauma, there may be no bruising to the abdominal wall. The lack of external trauma, along with the usual inaccurate history, can cause delay in diagnosis. A careful evaluation often reveals additional injuries. Abdominal trauma is the second leading cause of mortality from physical abuse, although the prognosis is generally good for children who survive the acute assault.

Abusive head trauma is the leading cause of mortality and morbidity from physical abuse. Most victims are young; infants predominate. Shaking and blunt impact trauma cause injuries. The perpetrators are most commonly fathers and boyfriends, and the trauma typically is precipitated by the perpetrator's intolerance to a crying, fussy infant. Victims present with neurologic symptoms ranging from lethargy and irritability to seizures, apnea, and coma. Unsuspecting physicians misdiagnose approximately one third of infants, and of these, more than 25% are reinjured before diagnosis. A common finding on presentation is subdural hemorrhage, often associated with progressive cerebral edema (Fig. 22-4). Hypoxic-ischemic injury is a significant contributor to the pathophysiology of the brain injury. Associated findings include retinal hemorrhages (seen in many, but not all, victims) and skeletal trauma, including rib and classic metaphyseal fractures. At the time of diagnosis, many head-injured infants have evidence of previous injury. Survivors are at high risk for permanent neurologic sequelae.

The extensive **differential diagnosis** of physical abuse depends on the type of injury (Table 22-2). For children who present with pathognomonic injuries to multiple organ systems, an exhaustive search for medical diagnoses is unwarranted. Children with unusual medical diseases have been incorrectly diagnosed as victims of abuse, emphasizing the need for careful, objective assessments of all children. All infants and young toddlers who present with suspicious

Table 22-2	Differential Diagnosis of Physical Abuse*

BRUISES

Accidental injury (common)

Dermatologic disorders

   Mongolian spots

   Erythema multiforme

   Phytophotodermatitis

Hematologic disorders

   Idiopathic thrombocytopenic purpura

   Leukemia

   Hemophilia

   Vitamin K deficiency

   Disseminated intravascular coagulopathy

Cultural practices

   Cao gio (coining)

   Quat sha (spoon rubbing)

Infection

   Sepsis

   Purpura fulminans (meningococcemia)

Genetic diseases

   Ehlers-Danlos syndrome

   Familial dysautonomia (with congenital indifference to pain)

   Vasculitis

   Henoch-Schönlein purpura

BURNS

Accidental burns (common)

Infection

   Staphylococcal scalded skin syndrome

   Impetigo

Dermatologic

   Phytophotodermatitis

   Stevens-Johnson syndrome

   Fixed drug eruption

   Epidermolysis bullosa

   Severe diaper dermatitis, including Ex-Lax ingestion

Cultural practices

   Cupping

   Moxibustion

FRACTURES

Accidental injury

Birth trauma

Metabolic bone disease

   Osteogenesis imperfecta

   Copper deficiency

Rickets

Infection

   Congenital syphilis

   Osteomyelitis

Table 22-2	Differential Diagnosis of Physical Abuse*—cont'd

HEAD TRAUMA

Accidental head injury

Hematologic disorders

    Vitamin K deficiency (hemorrhagic disease of the newborn)

    Hemophilia

Intracranial vascular abnormalities

Infection

Metabolic diseases

    Glutaric aciduria type I, Menkes kinky hair syndrome

From Christian CW: Child abuse physical. In Schwartz MW, editor: The 5-minute Pediatric Consult, ed 3, Philadelphia, 2003, Lippincott Williams & Wilkins.

*The differential diagnosis of physical abuse varies by the type of injury and organ system involved.

injuries should undergo a skeletal survey looking for occult or healing fractures. One third of young infants with multiple fractures, facial injuries, or rib fractures may have occult head trauma. Brain imaging may be indicated for these infants.

SEXUAL ABUSE

Child sexual abuse is the involvement of children in sexual activities that they cannot understand, for which they are developmentally unprepared and cannot give consent to, and that violates societal taboos. Sexual abuse can be a single event, but more commonly it is chronic. Most perpetrators are adults or adolescents who are known to the child and who have real or perceived power over the child. Most sexual abuse involves manipulation and coercion and does not involve physical violence. Although assaults by strangers occur, they are infrequent. Perpetrators are more often male than female and include parents, relatives, teachers, family friends, members of the clergy, and other individuals who have access to children. All perpetrators strive to keep the child from disclosing the abuse and often do so with coercion or threats.

Approximately 80% of victims are girls, although the sexual abuse of boys is underrecognized and underreported. Children generally come to attention after they have made a disclosure of their abuse. They may disclose to a nonoffending parent, sibling, relative, friend, or teacher. Children commonly delay disclosure for many weeks, months, or years after their abuse, especially if the perpetrator has ongoing access to the child. Sexual abuse also should be considered in children who have behavioral problems, although no behavior is pathognomonic. Hypersexual behaviors should raise the possibility of abuse, although some children with these behaviors are exposed to inappropriate sexual behaviors on television or videos or by witnessing adult sexual activity. Sexual abuse occasionally is recognized by the discovery of an unexplained vaginal, penile, or anal injury or by the discovery of a sexually transmitted infection.

In most cases, the diagnosis of sexual abuse is made by the history obtained from the child. In cases in which the sexual abuse has been reported to CPS or the police (or both), and the child has been interviewed before the medical visit,

a complete, forensic interview at the physician's office is not needed. Many communities have systems in place to ensure quality investigative interviews of sexually abused children. However if no other professional has spoken to the child about the abuse, or the child makes a spontaneous disclosure to the physician, the child should be interviewed with questions that are open-ended and non-leading. In all cases, the child should be questioned about medical issues related to the abuse, such as timing of the assault and symptoms (bleeding, discharge, or genital pain).

The **physical examination** should be complete, with careful inspection of the genitals and anus. Most sexually abused children have a normal genital examination at the time of the medical evaluation. Genital injuries are seen more commonly in children who present for medical care within 72 hours of their most recent assault and in children who report genital bleeding, but they are diagnosed in only 5% to 10% of sexually abused children. Many types of sexual abuse (fondling, vulvar coitus, oral genital contact) do not injure genital tissue, and genital mucosa heals so rapidly and completely that injuries often heal by the time of the medical examination. For children who present within 72 hours of the most recent assault, special attention should be given to identifying acute injury and the presence of blood or semen on the child. Injuries to the oral mucosa, breasts, or thighs should not be overlooked. Forensic evidence collection is needed in a few cases and has the greatest yield when collected in the first 24 hours after an acute assault. Few findings are diagnostic of sexual assault, but findings with the most specificity include acute, unexplained lacerations or ecchymoses of the hymen, posterior fourchette or anus, complete transection of the hymen, unexplained anogenital scarring, or pregnancy in an adolescent with no other history of sexual activity.

The **laboratory evaluation** of a sexually abused child is dictated by the child's age, history, and symptoms. Universal screening for sexually transmitted infections for prepubertal children is unnecessary because the risk of infection is low in asymptomatic young children. The type of assault, identity and known medical history of the perpetrator, and the epidemiology of sexually transmitted infections in the community also are considered. Many clinicians use nucleic acid amplification testing to screen for sexually transmitted infections in sexually abused children because these tests have excellent sensitivity while maintaining good specificity for STIs in children and adolescents. The diagnosis of most sexually transmitted infections in young children requires an investigation for sexual abuse (see Chapter 116).

MANAGEMENT

The management of child abuse includes medical treatment for injuries and infections, careful medical documentation of verbal statements and findings, and ongoing advocacy for the safety and health of the child (Fig. 22-5). Parents always should be informed of the suspicion of abuse and the need to report to CPS, focusing on the need to ensure the safety and well-being of the child. Crimes that are committed against children also are investigated by law enforcement, so the police become involved in some, but not all, cases of suspected abuse. Physicians occasionally are called to testify in court hearings regarding civil issues, such as dependency and custody, or criminal issues. Careful review of the medical records and preparation for court are needed to provide an educated, unbiased account of the child's medical condition and diagnoses.

The prevention of child maltreatment is a great challenge. There are a few partially successful primary prevention programs. Visiting home nursing programs that begin during pregnancy and continue through early childhood may reduce the risk of abuse and neglect. Physician training in screening for risk factors in parents has shown to be supportive of families and reduce child maltreatment in some populations. Ultimately physicians always need to remain cognizant of the diagnosis, aware of their professional mandates, and willing to advocate on behalf of these vulnerable patients.

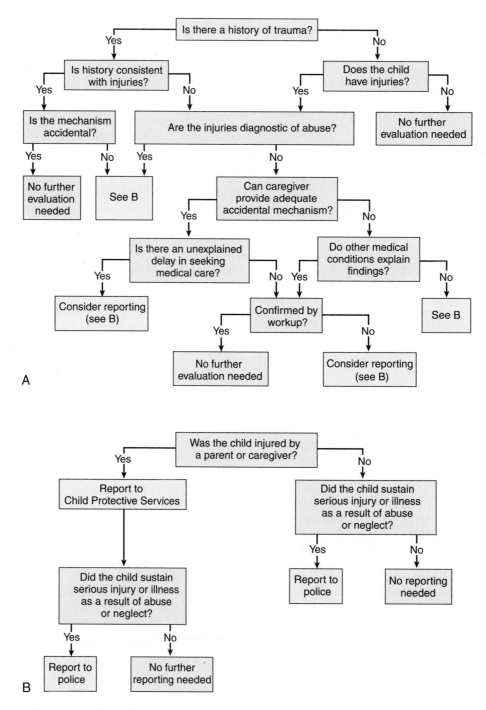

Figure 22-5 A, Approach to initiating the civil and criminal investigation of suspected abuse. **B,** Reporting to Child Protective Services (CPS) or law enforcement or both in child abuse cases. CPS reports are required when a child is injured by a parent, by an adult acting as a parent, or by a caregiver of the child. The police investigate crimes against children committed by any person, including parents or other caregivers. *(From Christian CW: Child abuse. In Schwartz MW, editor: Clinical Handbook of Pediatrics, ed 3, Baltimore, 2003, Lippincott Williams & Wilkins, pp 192–193.)*

Chapter 23

HOMOSEXUALITY AND GENDER IDENTITY

The development of sexuality occurs throughout a child's life. Sexuality includes gender roles, gender identity, sexual orientation, and sexual behaviors. It is influenced by biologic and social factors and individual experience. Pediatricians are likely to be consulted if parents have a concern about their child's sexual development. A pediatrician who provides an open and nonjudgmental environment may be a valuable resource for an adolescent with questions about heterosexual behaviors, homosexuality, or gender identity (Table 23-1).

DEVELOPMENT OF SEXUAL IDENTITY

Sexual behaviors occur throughout childhood. Early in life, male infants can have erections and female infants are capable of vaginal lubrication. During the preschool period, masturbation occurs in both sexes. Between 2 and 3 years of age, children identify themselves as a boy or a girl, but the understanding that one is always a male or always a female may not develop until 4 to 5 years of age. Stating that one wants to be a member of the opposite sex and pretending to be a member of the opposite sex are not unusual behaviors in this age group. Preschool children need to begin to learn that genitals and sexual behaviors are private; it is common for preschool children to touch their genitals in public, show their genitals to others, or undress in public. It would be highly unusual for a preschool child to imitate intercourse or other adult sexual behaviors. If this behavior is occurring, the child should be evaluated for exposure to inappropriate sexual material and possible sexual abuse (see Chapter 22).

Most elementary school–age children show a strong and consistent **gender identity,** and their behaviors (**gender roles**) reflect this. If a child this age is engaging in cross sex gender role behaviors, parents may be concerned about teasing and the possibility of their child having a homosexual sexual orientation. This concern is particularly likely if a boy is engaged in effeminate behaviors that are generally viewed as less socially acceptable than a

girl acting as a "tomboy." By this age, dressing as a member of the opposite sex and, particularly, stating a desire to be the opposite sex are uncommon, but playing with toys designed for the opposite sex remains common. In assessing parental concerns about atypical gender role behaviors, the type of behavior exhibited and its consistency should be considered. Reassurance that the behavior is consistent with typical development is appropriate when these behaviors are part of a flexible repertoire of male and female gender role behaviors. Reassurance is appropriate if the behaviors occur in response to a stress, such as the birth of an infant of the opposite sex or divorce of the parents. In contrast if these behaviors occur as a consistent and persistent pattern of nearly exclusive interest in behaviors typical of the gender role opposite that of the child's anatomic sex, referral for evaluation for **gender identity disorder** (GID) would be appropriate.

The biologic, social, and cognitive changes during adolescence place a focus on sexuality. Becoming comfortable with one's sexuality is one of the principal developmental tasks of this period and is likely to include questioning and experimentation. Almost half of high school students report that they have had sexual intercourse. Ten to 25% have at least one homosexual experience, with this behavior being reported more commonly by boys than girls. Although many adolescents have sexual experiences with a same-sex partner, only a few have a homosexual sexual orientation by late adolescence. When adolescents develop a consistent sexual orientation is probably affected by many different factors (societal, family, individual). Some adolescents report that they are certain of their sexual orientation in the early teenage years, whereas for others this does not develop until later. By 18 years of age, only a small proportion of individuals report being uncertain of their sexual orientation.

GENDER IDENTITY DISORDER

GID is characterized by intense and persistent cross-gender identification and discomfort with one's own sex. In children these feelings may be manifested by behaviors such as cross-dressing, stating that one wants to be or is the opposite sex, and a strong and almost exclusive preference for cross-sex roles, games, and playmates. The onset of these behaviors often can be traced back to the preschool period. However referral for evaluation typically occurs at school age or later, when it becomes clear that the behaviors do not represent a transient phase, and the behaviors may begin to interfere with social relationships. Forty to 80% of children with GID will have a bisexual or homosexual sexual orientation as adults. However there is no reliable way to predict adult sexual orientation, and there is no evidence that parental behavior would alter the developmental pathway toward homosexual or heterosexual behavior.

In adults GID may be characterized by a belief that one was born the wrong sex and by a persistent desire to live and be treated as the opposite sex. Adults may request hormones or surgical procedures to alter sexual characteristics to simulate the other sex, but, when these procedures are done in individuals who have completed puberty, they often fail to fully achieve the appearance of the desired gender. Long-term follow-up studies of children with GID suggest that only 2% to 20% have GID as adults, but gender dysphoria that intensifies with the onset of puberty is likely to persist. In 2009 the Endocrine Society published guidelines that recommended

Table 23-1	Terminology
Gender identity	
Perception of oneself as male or female	
Gender role	
Behaviors and appearance that signal to others of being male or female	
Heterosexual	
Sexual attraction to members of the opposite sex with weak attraction to members of the same sex	
Homosexual	
Sexual attraction to members of the same sex with weak attraction to members of the opposite sex	

considering reversible suppression of puberty using gonado-tropin releasing hormone analogs at Tanner stages 2 through 3 for individuals with GID because this allows the adolescent more time to decide whether to begin cross-sex hormone treatment.

HOMOSEXUALITY

Identical twins (even twins raised in separate families) show a higher concordance rate for sexual orientation than would be expected by chance alone, but nowhere near 100%, as would be expected if genetics alone determined sexual orientation. Some studies have found differences in the size of certain brain regions in homosexual individuals, but the findings are inconsistent. The levels of androgens and estrogens have not been found to differ in homosexual and heterosexual adults. Although it is well documented that parents tend to treat boys and girls differently, if, or how, these interactions affect sexual orientation is unknown.

It is currently estimated that about 1% to 4% of adults identify themselves as homosexual. Given the prevalent negative societal attitudes toward homosexuality, these children are at high risk for having a negative self-esteem, being isolated, being verbally harassed, and often being physically assaulted. Although sexual behaviors, not sexual orientation, determine risk of sexually transmitted infections, homosexual male adolescents engage in high-risk behaviors despite the threat of infection from the human immunodeficiency virus (HIV). For medical and psychosocial reasons, health care providers need to provide an environment in which adolescents feel comfortable discussing their sexual orientation (Table 23-2).

Acknowledging that one is homosexual and disclosing it to one's parents is often extremely stressful. Although many parents come to accept their child's homosexuality, some parents, particularly those who view this behavior as immoral, may reject their child. Homosexual youth are at a high risk for homelessness. Adolescents need to be made aware that even parents who eventually come to accept their child's homosexuality initially may be shocked, fearful about their child's well-being, or upset about the loss of the adulthood they had expected for their child. Parents may need to be reassured that they did not cause their child to have a homosexual orientation. Likewise they may need to be informed that therapies designed to change sexual orientation not only are

unsuccessful, but also often lead to the child having more feelings of guilt and a lower self-esteem. The health care provider should have knowledge of support groups and counselors who can discuss these issues with the adolescent or his or her parents when the information the health care provider offers is not sufficient.

The homosexual youth is affected by how homosexuality is addressed in schools, by peers, and by other community groups. Unbiased information about homosexuality is often not available in these settings, and homophobic jokes, teasing, and violence are common. It is not surprising that homosexual youth and adults have higher rates of anxiety and mood disorders than are found in the general population. Increased rates of substance abuse and suicide are reported. Health care providers have an important role in detecting these problems.

Although education about safe sexual practices should be part of all adolescent well-child visits, health care providers should be aware that certain sexual behaviors of homosexual males increase the risk of certain types of sexually transmitted infections. Anal intercourse is an efficient route for infection by hepatitis B virus, cytomegalovirus, and HIV. Proctitis caused by gonorrhea, chlamydia, herpes simplex virus, syphilis, or human papillomavirus may occur (see Chapter 116).

Chapter **24**

FAMILY STRUCTURE AND FUNCTION

A family is a dynamic system of interactions among biologically, socially, or legally related individuals; families have a unique power to promote or interfere with health and development. When a family functions well, interactions support the physical and emotional needs of all family members, and the family serves as a resource for an individual member who is having difficulty. Alternatively the problems of an individual member or the interactions among members may prevent the family from meeting the physical or emotional needs of one or more family members or, in the worst-case scenario, may cause physical or emotional harm to a member of the family. These situations are often referred to as **family dysfunction.**

FAMILY FUNCTIONS

The functions that families carry out in support of their children can be categorized broadly as providing for physical needs, emotional support, education, and socialization (Table 24-1). Within these categories, all families have strengths and weaknesses. The amount of support that an individual child needs in these categories varies with the child's development, personality, temperament, health status, experiences, and stressors. Too much and too little support can interfere with optimal child health and development. Most cases of child abuse involve the failure of the family to provide a safe environment for the child and, in cases of neglect, inappropriate

Table 23-2	Providing Supportive Health Care Environments for Homosexual Youth

Ensure confidentiality

Implement policies against homophobic jokes and remarks

Ensure that information-gathering forms use gender-neutral language (e.g., *partner* as opposed to *husband/wife*)

Ensure that one uses gender-neutral questions when asking about dating or sexual behaviors

Display posters, brochures, and information that show concern for issues important to homosexual youth and their families

Provide information about support groups and other resources for homosexual youth and their families

Adapted from Perrin EC: Sexual Orientation in Child and Adolescent Health Care, New York, 2002, Kluwer Academic/Plenum Publishers.

support for the child's physical, emotional, or social development. At the other extreme, overprotective parents may limit friendships and other growth-promoting experiences or seek excessive health care, as may occur in the vulnerable child syndrome. Parental perfectionism may create intense pressure on children related to achievement that may contribute to problems such as anxiety disorders.

FAMILY STRUCTURE

The traditional family consists of a married mother and father and their biologic children. The diversity in the structure of the family in the United States has increased dramatically; less than half of children now live in the traditional nuclear family. Today children may live with unmarried parents, single parents of either gender, a parent and a stepparent, grandparents, parents living as a same-sex couple, or foster care families. There is little evidence that family structure alone is a significant predictor of child health or development. Regardless of family structure, the presence of a loving adult or adults serving as a parent or parents committed to fulfilling a child's physical, emotional, and socialization needs is the best predictor of good health and development. Different family structures create different types of family stresses.

Single-Parent Families

At any one point in time, approximately 30% of children are living in single parent families, and more than 40% of children are born to unmarried mothers. In some cases this is the mother's choice, but often times this results from a young woman's unplanned pregnancy. Children may also live in single-parent families because of divorce or the death of a parent (see Chapter 26). Although most single parent families are still headed by mothers, single-father families are increasing and in 2009 nearly 5% of children lived in single-father families.

Single parents often have limited financial resources and social supports. For households headed by single mothers,

Table 24-1	Important Roles Families Play in Supporting Children

PHYSICAL NEEDS

Safety

Food

Shelter

Health and health care

EMOTIONAL SUPPORT

Affection

Stimulation

Communication

Guidance/discipline

EDUCATION AND SOCIALIZATION

Values

Relationships

Community

Formal schooling

the median income is only 40% of the income of two-parent families and for single fathers it is only 60% of the income of two parent families. Thus the frequency of children living in poverty is three to five times higher in single-parent families. These parents must also rely to a greater extent on other adults for child care. Although these adults may be sources of support for the single parent, they also may criticize the parent, decreasing confidence in parenting skills. Fatigue associated with working and raising a child may also make consistent parenting difficult. Single parents are likely to have less time for a social life or other activities, which may increase their isolation. When the increased burdens of being a single parent are associated with exhaustion, isolation, and depression, developmental and behavioral problems in the child are more likely.

When the parent is a teenage mother, problems of parenting may be exacerbated further (see Section 12). Being a teenage parent is associated with lower educational attainment, lower paying jobs without much opportunity for autonomy or advancement, and lower self-esteem. They are even less likely than other single mothers to have any support from the child's father. Children of adolescent mothers are at high risk for cognitive delays, behavioral problems, and difficulties in school. Referral to early intervention services or Head Start programs is important in these situations.

When a single parent has good social supports, is able to collaborate well with other care providers, and has sufficient financial resources, he or she is likely to be successful in raising a child. Pediatricians can improve parental confidence through education about child development and behavior and validation of parenting behaviors. Empathetic understanding of the difficulties of being a single parent can have a healing effect or help a parent discuss difficulties that may suggest the need for a referral to other professionals.

Children Living with Homosexual Parents

Many children with a gay or lesbian parent were conceived in the context of a heterosexual relationship. Some parents were unaware of their homosexuality at the time that they married, whereas others may view themselves as bisexual or marry despite the recognition that they are homosexual. Gay men and lesbian women also become parents on their own or in the context of an already established relationship with a same-sex partner through adoption, insemination, or surrogacy. Children living with homosexual parents may encompass many possible family structures.

Parents in these families are likely to have concerns about how disclosure of the homosexuality and the associated social stigma will affect the child. In general earlier disclosure of a parent's homosexuality to children, especially before adolescence, is associated with better acceptance. Most children of homosexual parents experience some social stigma associated with having a gay or lesbian parent; this may occur in the form of teasing by peers, disapproval from adults, and stress or isolation related to keeping the parent's homosexuality a secret.

Evidence suggests that having a homosexual parent does not cause increased problems in the parent-child relationship or the child's social-emotional development. Gender and gender role behaviors are typical for the child's age. Nonetheless distress related to teasing or maintaining the parent's secret may be great for some children, especially in early adolescence when issues of peer acceptance, sexual identity, and separation from one's parents are especially strong.

Adoption

Adoption is a legal and social process that provides full family membership to a child not born to the adoptive parents. Approximately 2% of children in the United States are adopted. A significant proportion of legal and informal adoptions are by stepparents or relatives of the child. Most adoptions in the United States involve U.S. parents adopting U.S. children, but shifting cultural trends have increased the diversity in the ways in which adoptions occur (e.g., international adoptions, single-parent adoptions, privately arranged adoptions, and the use of a surrogate parent). These types of adoption each raise unique issues for families and health care providers. *Open adoptions* in which the biologic parents and birth parents agree to interact are occurring with increased frequency and create new issues for the adoption triad (biologic parent, adoptive parent, and child).

Pediatricians are in an ideal position to help adoptive parents obtain and evaluate medical information, consider the unique medical needs of the adopted child, and provide a source of advice and counseling from the preadoption period through the issues that may arise when the child is an adolescent. A *preadoption visit* may allow discussion of medical information that the prospective parents have received about the child and identify important missing information such as the medical history of the biologic family and the educational and social history of the biologic parents. The preadoption period is the time that families are most likely to be able to obtain this information. Depending on the preadoption history, there may be risks of infections, in utero substance exposure, poor nutrition, or inadequate infant care that should be discussed with adoptive parents.

When the adopted child is first seen, screening for medical disorders beyond the typical age-appropriate screening tests should be considered. If the child has not had the standard newborn screening tests, the pediatrician may need to obtain these tests. Documented immunizations should be reviewed and, if needed, a plan developed to complete the needed immunizations (see Chapter 94). Children may be at high risk for infection based on the biologic mother's social history or the country from which the child was adopted, including infection with human immunodeficiency virus, hepatitis B, cytomegalovirus, tuberculosis, syphilis, and parasites. A complete blood count may be needed to screen for iron deficiency.

A knowledgeable pediatrician also can be a valuable source of support and advice about psychosocial issues. The pediatrician should help the adoptive parents think about how they will raise the child while helping the child to understand the fact that he or she is adopted. Neither denial of nor intense focus on the adoption is healthy. Parents should use the term *adoption* around their children during the toddler years and explain the simplest facts first. Children's questions should be answered honestly. Parents should expect the same or similar questions repeatedly, and that during the preschool period the child's cognitive limitations make it likely the child will not fully understand the meaning of adoption. As children get older, they may have fantasies of being reunited with their biologic parents, and there may be new challenges as the child begins to interact more with individuals outside of the family. Families may want advice about difficulties created by school assignments such as creating a genealogic chart or teasing by peers. During the teenage years, the child may have questions about his or her identity and a desire to find his or her biologic parents. Adoptive parents may need reassurance that these desires do not represent rejection of the adoptive family but the child's desire to understand more about his or her life. In general adopted adolescents should be supported in efforts to learn about their past, but most experts recommend encouraging children to wait until late adolescence before deciding to search actively for the biologic parents.

Although adopted children have a higher rate of school, learning, and behavioral problems, much of this increase is likely to be related to biologic and social influences before the adoption. The pediatrician can play an important role in helping families distinguish developmental and behavioral variations from problems that may require recommendations for early intervention, counseling, or other services.

Foster Care

Foster care is a means of providing protection for children who require out-of-home placement, most commonly because of homelessness, parental inability to care for the child, parental substance abuse, or child neglect or abuse. From the late 1990s through 2005, over half a million children were in foster care, but between 2005 and 2010, the number of children living in foster care decreased by about 20%. These decreases were associated with changes in federal and state policies that have emphasized shortened stays in foster care, promoted more rapid adoptions, and expanded efforts to support troubled families.

The 400,000 children in foster care are at extremely high risk for medical, nutritional, developmental, behavioral, and mental health problems. At the time of placement in foster care, most of these children have received incomplete medical care and have had multiple detrimental life experiences. Comprehensive assessments at the time of placement reveal many untreated acute medical problems, and nearly half of the children have a chronic illness. Developmental delays and serious behavioral or emotional disorders are common.

Ideally foster care provides a healing service for these children and families, leading to reunification or adoption. Too often children experience multiple changes in placement within the foster care system, further exacerbating the problems foster children may have in forming a secure relationship with adult caregivers. Children may manifest this difficulty by resisting foster parents' attempts to develop a close relationship. This detachment from the foster parent may be difficult for the foster parent to endure, which may perpetuate a cycle of placement failures. The trauma or neglect experienced that led to the need for foster care in combination with instability of placements causes enduring long-term difficulties. Foster care alumni report rates of anxiety disorders, depression, substance abuse, and posttraumatic stress disorder that are two to six times higher than in the general population. Furthermore although the *protections* of the foster care system often end at 18 years of age, these adolescents rarely have the skills and maturity needed to allow them to be successful living independently. Thus the Fostering Connections to Success and Increasing Adoptions Act of 2008 mandates that effective transition to adulthood planning be done with youth in foster care.

The challenges for the foster care system are great. However when children are placed with competent and nurturing foster parents and provided coordinated care from skilled professionals, significant improvements in a child's health status, development, and academic achievement usually occur.

FAMILY DYSFUNCTION
Physical Needs
Failure to meet a child's physical needs for protection or nutrition results in some of the most severe forms of family dysfunction (see Chapters 21 and 22). There are many other ways in which parental behaviors can interfere with a child having a healthy and safe environment, such as prenatal and postnatal substance abuse. Prenatal use of alcohol can damage the fetus resulting in spectrum disorders known as **fetal alcohol spectrum disorders (FASD).** At the most severe end of the spectrum, this teratogen causes **fetal alcohol syndrome (FAS)** characterized by in utero and postnatal growth retardation, microcephaly, intellectual disability, and a characteristic dysmorphic facial appearance. Other manifestations of FASD include birth defects and problems with coordination, attention, hyperactivity, impulsivity, learning, or behavior. Children with these difficulties may be diagnosed with *alcohol-related neurodevelopmental disorder, alcohol-related birth defects,* or *partial FAS.*

Other substances also may affect the fetus, but investigation of these effects is complicated by the fact that often more than one substance is used, and nutrition and prenatal care are not optimal. Cigarette smoking during pregnancy is associated with lower birth weight and increased child behavioral problems. Use of cocaine in the perinatal period has been associated with prematurity, intracranial hemorrhages, and abruptio placentae. Exposure to opiates in utero can result in prematurity and a neonatal withdrawal syndrome. Investigations of the effects of cocaine and opiates on cognitive development have produced mixed results.

Parental substance abuse after the child's birth is associated with increased family conflict, decreased organization, increased isolation, and increased family stress related to marital and work problems. Family violence may be more frequent. Despite the fact that these parents often have difficulty providing discipline and structure, they may expect their children to be competent at a variety of tasks at a younger age than non-substance–abusing parents. This sets the children up for failure and contributes to increased rates of depression, anxiety, and low self-esteem. The parents' more accepting attitude toward alcohol and drugs seems to increase the chance that their children will use substances during adolescence.

Parents also may expose children directly to the harmful effects of other substances, such as exposure to *second hand cigarette smoke,* which is consistently associated with increased rates of childhood respiratory illnesses, otitis media, and sudden infant death syndrome. Despite these effects, only a few parents restrict smoking in their homes. There are many other ways in which parents may not physically protect their children. Failing to immunize children, to childproof the home adequately, and to provide adequate supervision are other examples.

Parents' attempts to provide too much protection for their child also can cause problems. One example of this is the **vulnerable child syndrome** in which a child who is ill early in life continues to be viewed as vulnerable by the parents despite that the child has fully recovered. Behavioral difficulties may result if parents are overindulgent and fail to set limits. Parental reluctance to leave the child may contribute to the child having separation anxiety. Parents may be particularly attentive to minor variations in bodily functions, leading them to seek excess medical care. If the physician does not recognize this situation, the child may be exposed to unnecessary medical procedures.

Emotional Support, Education, and Socialization
Failure to meet a child's emotional or educational needs can have a severe and enduring negative impact on child development and behavior. Infants need a consistent adult who learns to understand their signals and meets the infant's needs for attention as well as food. As the adult caregiver learns these signals, he or she responds more rapidly and appropriately to the infant's attempts at communication. Through this process, often referred to as **attachment,** the special relationship between parent and child develops. When affectionate and responsive adults are not consistently available, infants often are less willing to explore the environment and may become unusually clingy, angry, or difficult to comfort.

Appropriate stimulation also is vital for a child's cognitive development. Children whose parents do not read to them and do not play developmentally appropriate games with them have lower scores on intelligence tests and more school problems. In these situations, early intervention has been shown to be particularly effective in improving skill development and subsequent school performance. At the other extreme, there are increasing concerns that some parents may provide too much stimulation and scheduling of the child's day. There may be such emphasis on achievement that children come to feel that parental love is contingent on achievement. There are concerns that this narrow definition of success may contribute to problems with anxiety and self-esteem for some children.

Chapter 25

VIOLENCE

INTIMATE PARTNER VIOLENCE AND CHILDREN
Intimate partner violence (IPV) is a pattern of purposeful coercive behaviors aimed at establishing control of one partner over the other that may include inflicted physical injury, psychological abuse, sexual assault, progressive social isolation, stalking, deprivation, intimidation, and threats. Such violence between adults affects the lives of millions of children each year. Children experience IPV by seeing or hearing the violence and its aftermath. Children who live in households with

IPV often develop psychological and behavioral problems that interfere with their ability to function normally in school, at home, and with peers. They may be injured during violent outbursts, sometimes while attempting to intervene on behalf of a parent. Many children are victims of abuse themselves. It is estimated that there is at least a 50% concurrence rate between IPV and child abuse. Children who grow up in violent households learn that violence is appropriate in intimate relationships. A history of having witnessed IPV as a child is a strong predictor for becoming a batterer in adulthood. In addition to sporadic outbursts of violence, children who live in households with IPV experience disruptive events that can overtly or subtly affect the child's development. Although partner violence often occurs between male perpetrators and female victims, it may also occur bi-directionally and may be better conceptualized as family or interpersonal-violence. Violence may escalate during the peri-natal period.

There is no particular behavioral consequence or disturbance that is specific to children who witness IPV. Some children are traumatized by fear for their caregiver's safety and feel helpless. Others may blame themselves for the violence. Children may have symptoms of **posttraumatic stress disorder,** depression, anxiety, aggression, or hypervigilance. Older children may have conduct disorders, poor school performance, low self-esteem, or other nonspecific behaviors. Infants and young toddlers are at risk for disrupted attachment and routines around eating and sleeping. Preschoolers may show signs of regression, irritable behavior, or temper tantrums. During school-age years, children may show both externalizing (aggressive or disruptive) and internalizing (withdrawn and passive) behaviors. Because of family isolation, some children have no opportunity to participate in extracurricular activities at school and do not form friendships. Adolescents in homes where IPV is present have higher rates of school failure, substance abuse, and risky sexual behaviors. These adolescents are more likely than their peers to enter into a violent dating relationship.

Because of the high concurrence of IPV and child abuse, asking about IPV is part of the screening for violence against children. Recognizing the importance of IPV screening in pediatric practice, the American Academy of Pediatrics has endorsed universal screening in this setting and suggests that intervening on behalf of battered women may be one of the most effective means of preventing child abuse. Without standardized screening, pediatricians may underestimate the IPV prevalence in their practices. Parents should not be screened together. Questions about family violence should be direct, nonjudgmental, and done in the context of child safety and anticipatory guidance (Table 25-1).

Intervention is needed for caregivers who disclose IPV. It is appropriate to show concern and to provide available community resources. It is important to assess for the safety of the victim and the children. In some states, physicians are mandated to report IPV. Information for families that provides details about community resources and state laws is helpful.

YOUTH VIOLENCE

Youth violence is a leading cause of pediatric mortality in the United States. Homicide is the second leading cause of death for all children 1 to 19 years of age. Each year nearly 6000 children, primarily adolescents, are victims of homicide, and 4000

Table 25-1	Questions for Adults and Children Related to Family Violence

FOR THE CHILD

How are things at home and at school?

Who lives with you?

How do you get along with your family members?

What do you like to do with them?

What do you do if something is bothering you?

Do you feel safe at home?

Do people fight at home? What do they fight about? How do they fight?

ADDITIONAL QUESTIONS FOR THE ADOLESCENT

Do your friends get into fights often? How about you?

When was your last physical fight?

Have you ever been injured during a fight?

Has anyone you know been injured or killed?

Have you ever been forced to have sex against your will?

Have you ever been threatened with a gun or a knife?

How do you avoid getting in fights?

Do you carry a weapon for self-defense?

FOR THE PARENT

Do you have any concerns about your child?

Who helps with your children?

How do you feel about your neighborhood?

Do you feel safe at home?

Is there any fighting or violence at home?

Does anyone at home use drugs?

Have you been frightened by your partner?

Does your partner ever threaten you or hurt you?

more commit suicide. Youth violence is a problem in urban, suburban, and rural communities and affects children across race and gender. Surveys of adolescents show that 30% to 40% of boys and 15% to 30% of girls report having committed a serious violent offense during childhood, including robbery, rape, aggravated assault, or homicide. Most of these crimes are not reported to the police, and the perpetrator is arrested in a few cases only. Although boys commit more crimes than girls, this gap has narrowed. Boys are much more likely to be arrested for their crimes. Self-reported violent events do not differ much between white and minority adolescents; the latter are more likely to be arrested for their crimes.

Most violent youth begin to exhibit their violent behaviors during early adolescence. **Bullying,** which peaks in middle school, is a form of aggression in which a child repeatedly and intentionally intimidates, harasses, or physically harms another child. Technology-assisted bullying behavior or cyber-bullying has become a major concern. Psychosocial consequences of being bullied include depression and suicidal ideation. Children who bully others are more likely to be involved with other problem behaviors, such as smoking and alcohol use. Bullying and being bullied are both associated with higher rates of weapon carriage and fighting. Although most bullies

Table 25-2	Risk and Protective Factors for Serious Youth Violence by Age of Onset		
FACTORS	**EARLY ONSET (<12 yr)**	**LATER ONSET (>12 yr)**	**PROTECTIVE FACTORS**
Individual	**Substance use***	General offenses	Intolerance toward deviance
	General offenses	Aggression†	High IQ
	Being male	Being male	Being female
	Antisocial behavior	Physical violence	Positive social orientation
	Aggression**	Antisocial attitudes	Perceived sanctions for transgressions
	Hyperactivity	Crimes against persons	
	Exposure to TV violence	Low IQ	
	Low IQ	Substance abuse	
	Antisocial attitudes	Risk-taking behaviors	
	Dishonesty**		
Family	Low SES/poverty	Poor parent-child relations	Supportive parents or other adults
	Antisocial parents	Low parent involvement	Parental monitoring
	Poor parent-child relations	Antisocial parents	Parents' positive evaluation of peers
	Broken home	Broken home	
	Abusive, neglectful	Low SES/poverty	
	parents	Abusive parents	
School	Poor attitude	Poor attitude	Commitment to school
	Poor performance	Poor performance; academic failure	Recognition for involvement in school activities
Peer	Weak social ties	**Weak social ties**	Friends who engage in conventional behavior
	Antisocial peers	**Antisocial delinquent peers**	
Community		**Gang membership**	
		Neighborhood crime	
		Neighborhood drugs	
		Neighborhood disorganization	

From National Center for Injury Prevention and Control, Substance Abuse and Mental Health Services Administration: Youth violence: a report of the surgeon general. *Rockville, MD, 2001, U.S. Department of Health and Human Services.*
SES, Socioeconomic status.
***Bold** = factors with strongest effect.
†Males only.

do not progress into serious violent offenders, violent behavior that continues into high school years indicates the potential for severe violent behavior in adulthood. Another subset of violent youth begins at a very young age. These children tend to be more serious offenders, perpetrate more crimes, and more often continue their violence into adulthood. Most adolescent violence ends by young adulthood. Most violent youth are only intermittently violent. Frequent acts of violence are committed more commonly by youth who start their violence before the onset of puberty. These violent youth need to be evaluated for cognitive impairments or mental illness.

Serious youth violence is not an isolated problem but usually coexists with other adolescent risk-taking behaviors, such as drug use, truancy and school dropout, early sexual activity, and gun ownership. Risk factors for youth violence are slightly different for children who begin their violence early in life compared with youth who begin during adolescence. Often these risk factors exist in clusters, and they tend to be additive. Although understanding risk factors for violence is crucial for developing prevention strategies, the risk factors do not predict whether a particular individual will become violent. For children who begin their violence early in life, the strongest risk factors are early substance abuse (<12 years of age)

and perpetration of nonviolent, serious crimes during childhood. Additional risk factors include poverty, male gender, and antisocial behavior. For children who begin their violence during adolescence, individual risk factors are less important, whereas factors related to peer groups are most important. Gang membership, associating with antisocial or delinquent friends, being unpopular in school, and having weak ties to conventional peer groups are important risk factors for adolescent-onset violence (Table 25-2). The strength of the listed risk factors is not uniform, and some factors show a small effect only. Table 25-2 also lists protective factors that seem to buffer the effects of risk factors. One important protective factor is the child's level of school connectedness, such as involvement in class and extracurricular activities, and how positively the child regards the school's personnel. Another protective factor is the support of nonviolent family members and close friends.

Violence prevention efforts that target risk and protective factors need to be developmentally appropriate. Education about the dangers of substance abuse should begin before the onset of puberty, whereas adolescent programs must consider the importance of peer group identification. Many violence prevention programs fail to show long-term effects. Effective violence prevention programs must address simultaneously individual, family, and environmental (school, peer group, social) risk factors; capitalize on the child's strengths; involve family and other supports; and be implemented over an extended period.

DATING VIOLENCE AND DATE RAPE

Dating violence and date rape are common. It is estimated that 15% to 40% of adolescents have experienced violence in a dating relationship. Adolescent women experience higher rates of sexual assault than any other age group. An acquaintance or partner of the victim perpetrates most adolescent sexual assaults. Risk factors for date rape include initiating dating at a young age, initiating early sexual activity, and having a history of past sexual abuse or victimization. A history of child abuse by parents or siblings increases the risk of dating violence. Adolescent boys who believe that it is appropriate to strike a girl if she insults or embarrasses him or intentionally tries to make him jealous are at risk for becoming perpetrators. Date-specific factors put some teens at risk for date rape, including who initiated the date, the date activities, which person drove, and who paid.

Alcohol use is common in episodes of adolescent sexual assault, occurring in approximately 50% of cases. Drugs such as benzodiazepines, cocaine, and marijuana may also contribute. Flunitrazepam (Rohypnol) and gamma hydroxybutyrate are two commonly implicated drugs that cause sedation and amnesia, especially when used in conjunction with alcohol.

Relatively few victims of date rape report the assault to law enforcement. Reporting rates are even lower when the victim knows the perpetrator. Women who report assaults to the police are more likely to receive timely medical care; it is likely that many sexually assaulted adolescents do not receive medical attention, putting them at risk for physical and mental health consequences. Routine adolescent health care should screen for adolescent dating violence, provide routine sexually transmitted infection evaluation, and be able to identify counseling resources for teens who are victims or perpetrators of dating violence (see Chapter 116).

Chapter 26

DIVORCE, SEPARATION, AND BEREAVEMENT

The family is the child's principal resource for meeting needs for protection, emotional support, education, and socialization. A variety of different disruptions may cause the child to be separated from his or her parents. At times these separations may be relatively brief but unexpected (e.g., a parent's acute illness or injury). The separation may occur in the context of significant parental discord, as often occurs with a divorce. The death of a parent results in a permanent separation that may be anticipated or unanticipated. All of these disruptions cause significant stress for the child, with the potential for long-term adverse consequences. The child's adaptation to these stresses is affected by the reasons for the separation and the child's age, temperament, and available support systems.

DIVORCE

Approximately 40% to 50% of first marriages end in divorce. About half of these divorces occur in the first 10 years of marriage, so there are often young children in the family when the parents divorce. At least 25% of children experience the divorce or separation of their parents. Few events in childhood are as dramatic and challenging for the child as divorce.

Divorce is likely to be accompanied by changes in behavioral and emotional adjustment. In the immediate post-divorce period, many children exhibit anger, noncompliance, anxiety, and depression. Children from divorced families require psychological help two to three times more frequently than children with married parents. Long-term studies suggest that in the absence of ongoing stressors, most children demonstrate good adjustment a few years after the divorce, but some have enduring difficulties.

Divorce is not a single event, but a process that occurs over time. In most cases, marital conflict begins long before the physical or legal separation, and the divorce brings about permanent changes in the family structure. Multiple potential stressors for the child are associated with divorce, including parental discord before and after the divorce, changes in living arrangements and sometimes location, and changes in the child's relationship with both parents.

The child's relationship with each parent is changed by the divorce. In the short-term, the parent is likely to experience new burdens and feelings of guilt, anger, or sadness that may disrupt parenting skills and family routines. Contact with the noncustodial parent may decline greatly. Parents may be perceived by their children as being unaware of the child's distress around the time of the divorce. Pediatricians can help parents understand things they can do that will be reassuring to the child. Maintaining contact with both parents, seeing where the noncustodial parent is living, and, in particular, maintaining familiar routines are comforting to the child in the midst of the turmoil of a separation and divorce. The child should attend school and continue to have opportunities to interact with friends. Given the parents' distress, assistance from the extended family can be helpful, but these family members may not offer to help for fear of "interfering." It may be helpful for pediatricians to encourage parents to ask for this assistance. Pediatricians should look for maladaptive coping responses. Some parents may respond to their increased burdens and distress by treating their children as friends with whom they share their distress. Alternatively they may place excessive responsibilities on the child or leave the child unsupervised for longer periods of time. Responses such as these increase the chance that the child will develop behavioral or emotional problems.

Reaction to Divorce at Different Ages

The child's reaction to the divorce is influenced by the child's age and developmental level. Although infants do not react directly to the divorce, they require special considerations in relation to custody and visitation because infants need a stable daily routine and regular contact with a primary caregiver to develop secure attachment. Separations from a primary caregiver should be brief. Increased infant irritability or listlessness and withdrawal may be signs of distress for an infant. **Preschool children** are characterized by having magical beliefs about cause and effects and an egocentric view of the world. They may believe that something they did caused the divorce, leading them to be particularly upset. They may engage in unusual behaviors that they believe will bring the parents back together again. At this age, parents need to deliver a clear message that the divorce was related to disagreements between the parents, that nothing the child did caused the divorce, and that nothing the child could do would bring the parents back together again. Preschool children may reason that if the parents left each other they also might leave the child. To counteract this fear of abandonment, children may need to be reassured that although parents separated, they will not abandon the child and that the child's relationship with both parents will endure.

School-age children have a concrete understanding of cause and effect; if something bad happened, they understand that something caused it to happen. However they are not likely to understand fully the subtleties of parental conflict or the idea that multiple factors contribute to a conflict. Children at this age may still worry that something they did caused the divorce. They may express more anger than younger children and often feel rejected. Many young school-age children worry about what will happen to one or both parents. School performance often deteriorates. Older elementary school–age children may believe that one parent was wronged by the other. This belief, in conjunction with their concrete understanding of cause and effect, allows children to be easily co-opted by one parent to take sides against the other. Parents need to understand this vulnerability and resist the temptation to support their child in taking sides.

Adolescents may respond to the divorce by acting out, becoming depressed, or experiencing somatic symptoms. Adolescents are developing a sense of autonomy, a sense of morality, and the capacity for intimacy, and divorce may lead them to question previously held beliefs. They may be concerned about what the divorce means for their future and whether they too will experience marital failure. Questioning of previous beliefs in conjunction with decreased supervision may set the stage for risk-taking behaviors, such as truancy, sexual behaviors, and alcohol or drug use.

Outcome of Divorce

One of the best predictors of children's adaptation to divorce is whether the physical separation is associated with a decrease in the child's exposure to parental discord. In most cases, divorced parents still must interact with each other around the child's schedule, child custody and support, and other parenting issues. These types of issues create the potential for the child to have ongoing exposure to significant discord between the parents. For example if one parent tends to keep the child up much later than the bedtime at the other parent's house, sleep problems may develop. When children feel caught in the middle of ongoing conflicts between their divorced parents, behavior or emotional problems are much more likely. Regardless of how angry parents are with each other, the parents should be counseled that they must shield their child from this animosity. Clear rules about schedules, discipline, and other parenting roles is ideal, but in cases of conflict it can also be helpful for the pediatrician to help a parent accept that he or she can only control his or her actions and decisions related to the child. When parents have trouble resolving these issues, mediation may be helpful. Pediatricians need to be wary of parents' attempts to recruit them into custody battles to substantiate claims of poor parenting, unless the pediatrician has first-hand knowledge that the concerns are valid.

Although the primary physical residence for most children is still with the mother, the court's bias toward preferring mothers in custody decisions has decreased, and there is more emphasis on including both parents in the child's life. In the early 1980s, 50% of children had no contact with their fathers 2 or 3 years after a divorce, whereas today only 20% to 25% of children have no contact with their father. Most states now allow joint physical or legal custody. In joint physical custody, the child spends a significant amount of time with each parent, and in joint legal custody, parents share authority in decision making. Although joint custody arrangements may promote the involvement of both parents in the child's life, they also can be a vehicle through which parents continue to express their anger at each other. When parents have severe difficulty working together, joint custody is an inappropriate arrangement and has been associated with deterioration in the child's psychological and social adjustment.

Divorce often creates financial difficulties. Family income usually declines in the first year after the divorce. Only about half of mothers who have child support awards receive the full amount, and one fourth receive no money at all. These financial changes may have multiple adverse affects on the child. A move to a new house may require the child to attend a new school disrupting peer relationships and other potential supports. The child may spend more time in child care if one or both parents have to increase work hours.

Role of the Pediatrician

Pediatricians may be confronted with issues related to marital discord before the divorce, may be consulted around the time of the divorce, or may be involved in helping the family to manage issues in the years after the divorce. The pediatrician can be an important voice in helping the parents understand and meet the child's needs (Table 26-1). Before the divorce, parents may wonder what they should tell their children. Children should be told of the parents' decision before the physical separation. The separation should be presented as a rational step in managing marital conflict and should prepare the child for the changes that will occur. Parents should be prepared to answer children's questions, and they should expect that the questions will be repeated over the next months. Once parents have told children of the separation, it may be confusing to the child if the parents continue to appear to live together and may raise false hopes that the parents will not divorce.

Many parents report not feeling like their life had stabilized until 2 to 3 years or more after the divorce, and for some the divorce remains a painful issue 10 years later. The child's emotional adjustment to divorce is closely predicted by the parents' adjustment so parents should be encouraged to get help for themselves if they are struggling emotionally after a divorce.

Table 26-1	General Recommendations for Pediatricians to Help Children During Separation, Divorce, or Death of a Close Relative

Acknowledge and provide support for grief that the parent/caregiver is experiencing.

Help parent/caregiver consider child's needs.

Encourage parent/caregiver to maintain routines familiar to the child.

Encourage continued contact between child and his or her friends.

If primary residence changes, the child should take transitional objects, familiar toys, and other important objects to the new residence.

Minimize frequent changes in caregivers, and for infants keep brief the times spent away from primary caregiver.

Have parent/caregiver reassure the child that he or she will continue to be cared for.

Have parent/caregiver reassure the child that he or she did not cause the separation, divorce, or death (especially important in preschool children).

Encourage parent/caregiver to create times or rituals that allow the child to discuss questions and feelings if the child wishes.

Although most children ultimately show good adjustment to the divorce, some have significant acting-out behaviors or depression that requires referral to a mental health professional. Some parents need the assistance of a mediator or family therapist to help them stay focused on their child's needs. In the most contentious situations, a guardian ad litem may need to be appointed by the court. This individual is usually a lawyer or mental health professional with the power to investigate the child and family's background and relationships to make a recommendation to the court as to what would be in the best interests of the child.

SEPARATIONS FROM PARENTS

Children experience separations from their primary caregiver for a variety of reasons. Brief separations, such as those to attend school, camp, or other activities, are nearly a universal experience. Many children experience longer separations for a variety of reasons, including parental business trips, military service, or hospitalization. Child adjustment to separation is affected by child factors, such as the age of the child and the child's temperament; factors related to the separation, such as the length of and reason for the separation, whether the separation was planned or unplanned; and factors related to the caregiving environment during the separation, such as how familiar the child is with the caregiver and whether the child has access to friends and familiar toys and routines.

Children between 6 months and 3 to 4 years of age often have the most difficulty adjusting to a separation from their primary caregiver. Older children have cognitive and emotional skills that help them adjust. They may be better able to understand the reason for the separation, communicate their feelings, and comprehend the passage of time, allowing them to anticipate the parent's return. For older children, the period immediately before a planned separation may be particularly difficult if the reason for the separation causes significant family tension, as it may in the case of hospitalization or military service.

If parents anticipate a separation, they should explain the reason for the separation and, to the extent possible, give concrete information about when they will be in contact with the child and when they will return home. If the child can remain at home with a familiar and responsive caregiver, this is likely to help adjustment. If children cannot remain at home, they should be encouraged to take with them transitional objects, such as a favorite blanket or stuffed animal, familiar toys, and important objects such as a picture of the parent. Maintenance of familiar family routines and relationships with friends should be encouraged.

DEATH OF A PARENT OR FAMILY MEMBER AND BEREAVEMENT

Death of a close family member is a sad and difficult experience. When a child loses a parent, it is a devastating experience. This experience is not rare. By 15 years of age, 4% of children in the United States experience the death of a parent. This experience is likely to alter forever the child's view of the world as a secure and safe place. Similar to the other separations, a child's cognitive development and temperament along with the available support systems affect the child's adjustment after the death of a parent. Many of the recommendations in Table 26-1 are helpful. The death of a parent or close family member also brings up some unique issues.

Explaining Death to a Child

Children's understanding of death changes with their cognitive development and experiences (see Chapter 4). Preschool children often do not view death as permanent and may have magical beliefs about what caused death. As children become older, they understand death as permanent and inevitable, but the concept that death represents the cessation of all bodily functions and has a biologic cause may not be fully appreciated until adolescence.

Death should not be hidden from the child. It should be explained in simple and honest terms that are consistent with the family's beliefs. The explanation should help the child to understand that the dead person's body stopped functioning and that the dead person will not return. Preschool children should be reassured that nothing they did caused the individual to die. One should be prepared to answer questions about where the body is and let the child's questions help determine what information the child is prepared to hear. False or misleading information should be avoided. Comparisons of death to sleep may contribute to sleep problems in the child.

There are many possible reactions of children to the death of a parent or close relative. Sadness and a yearning to be with the dead relative are common. Sometimes a child might express a wish to die so that he or she can visit the dead relative, but a plan or desire to commit suicide is uncommon and would need immediate evaluation. A decrease in academic functioning, lack of enjoyment with activities, and changes in appetite and sleep can occur. About half of children have their most severe symptoms about 1 month after the death, but for many the most severe symptoms in reaction to the death do not occur until 6 to 12 months after the death.

Should the Child Attend the Funeral?

Children often find it helpful to attend the funeral. It may help the child to understand that the death occurred and provide an opportunity to say good-bye. Seeing others express their grief and sadness may help the child to express these feelings. Going to the funeral helps prevent the child from having fears or fantasies about what happened at the funeral. If the child is going to attend the funeral, he or she should be informed of what will happen. If a preschool-age child expresses a desire not to attend the funeral, he or she should not be encouraged to attend. For older children, it may be appropriate to encourage attendance, but a child who feels strongly about not wanting to go to the funeral should not be required to attend.

Suggested Readings

Bair-Merritt M: Intimate partner violence, *Pediatr Rev* 31:145–150, 2001.

Cole S, Lanham J: Failure to thrive: an update, *Am Fam Physician* 83(7): 829–834, 2011.

Dubowitz H, Feigelman S, Lane W, et al: Pediatric primary care to help prevent child maltreatment: the Safe Environment for Every Kid (SIIK) Model, *Pediatrics* 123:858–864, 2009.

Kellogg: ND and the Committee on Child Abuse and Neglect. The evaluation of sexual behaviors in children, *Pediatrics* 124:992–998, 2009.

Kleinsorge C, Civitz LM: Impact of divorce on children: developmental considerations, *Pediatr Rev* 33:147–155, 2012.

Minnes S, Lang A, Singer L: Prenatal tobacco, marijuana, stimulant, and opiate exposure: outcomes and practical implications, *Addict Sci Clin Pract* 6:57–70, 2011.

Reece RM, Christian CW, editors: *Child abuse: medical diagnosis and management*, ed 3, Elk Grove Village, Ill, 2009, American Academy of Pediatrics. (Role of the pediatrician in youth violence prevention. *Pediatrics* 124:393–402, 2009.

Sedlak AJ, Mettenburg J, Basena M, et al: *Fourth national incidence study of child abuse and neglect (NIS-4): report to Congress.* U.S. Department of Health and Human Services, Administration for Children and Families. Washington, DC, 2010, (website). www.acf.hhs.gov/sites/default/files/opre/nis4_report_congress_full_pdf_jan2010.pdf. Accessed October 8, 2012.

Shonkoff JP, Thomas Boyce W, McEwen BS: Neuroscience, molecular biology, and the childhood roots of health disparities: building a new framework for health promotion and disease prevention, *JAMA* 301:2252–2259, 2009.

Smith GA and the Committee on Injury, Violence, and Poison Prevention. Policy Statement. Role of the pediatrician in youth violence prevention. *Pediatrics* 124(1):393–402, 2009.

Spack NP, Edwards-Leeper L, Feldman HA, et al: Children and adolescents with gender identity disorder referred to a pediatric medical center, *Pediatrics* 129:418–425, 2012.

Pediatric Nutrition and Nutritional Disorders

April O. Buchanan and Maria L. Marquez

Chapter 27

DIET OF THE NORMAL INFANT

Proper nutrition in infancy is essential for normal growth, resistance to infections, long-term adult health, and optimal neurologic and cognitive development. Healthy nutrition is especially important during the first 6 months, a period of exceptionally accelerated growth and high nutrient requirements relative to body weight (see Chapter 5). Breastfeeding is associated with a reduced risk of many diseases in infants, children, and mothers (for more details visit http://www.nutrition.gov/).

BREASTFEEDING

Human milk and breastfeeding are the ideal and normative standards for infant feeding and nutrition. The American Academy of Pediatrics (AAP) recommends human milk as the sole source of nutrition for the first 6 months of life, with continued intake for the first year, and as long as desired thereafter. Breastfeeding has short- and long-term advantages for infant neurodevelopment. Pediatric health care providers should approach breastfeeding at multiple levels (individual, community, social, and political) to reach the goals of "Healthy People in 2020"; its targets include 82% of infants with any breastfeeding, 23.7% of infants with exclusive breastfeeding for the first 6 months of life, and lactation support at work of 38%. In collaboration with national and global organizations, including the AAP, World Health Organization (WHO), UNICEF, the Centers for Disease Control and Prevention (CDC), and the Joint Commission, hospitals are asked to promote and facilitate breastfeeding.

The first 2 days of breastfeeding, and perhaps the first hour of life, may determine the success of breastfeeding. The current rate of breastfeeding initiation for the total U.S. population is 75% (Figure 27-1). There is greater emphasis to improve and standardize hospital practices with "Baby Friendly" programs for breastfeeding support.

The Department of Health and Human Services and the CDC recognize that breastfeeding offers infants, mothers, and society compelling advantages in industrialized *and* developing countries. Human milk feeding decreases the incidence and severity of diarrhea, respiratory illnesses, otitis media, bacteremia, bacterial meningitis, and necrotizing enterocolitis.

There are beneficial effects of feeding *preterm* infants with human milk on long-term neurodevelopment (IQ) in preterm infants. Preterm breastfed infants also have a lower readmission rate in the first year of life.

Mothers who breastfeed experience both short- and long-term health benefits. Decreased risk of postpartum hemorrhages, more rapid uterine involution, longer period of amenorrhea, and decreased postpartum depression have been observed. Similarly, there is an association between a long lactation of 12 to 23 months (cumulative lactation of all pregnancies) and a significant reduction of hypertension, hyperlipidemia, cardiovascular disease, and diabetes in the mother. Cumulative lactation of more than 12 months also correlates with reduced risk of ovarian and breast cancer.

Adequacy of milk intake can be assessed by voiding and stooling patterns of the infant. A well-hydrated infant voids six to eight times a day. Each voiding should soak, not merely moisten, a diaper, and urine should be colorless. By 5 to 7 days, loose yellow stools should be passed at least four times a day. Rate of weight gain provides the most objective indicator of adequate milk intake. Total weight loss after birth should not exceed 7%, and birth weight should be regained by 10 days. The mean feeding frequency during the early weeks postpartum is 8 to 12 times per day. An infant may be adequately hydrated while not receiving enough milk to achieve adequate energy and nutrient intake. Telephone follow-up is valuable during the interim between discharge and the first doctor visit to monitor the progress of lactation. A follow-up visit should be scheduled by 3 to 5 days of age, and again by 2 weeks of age.

In the newborn period, elevated concentrations of serum bilirubin are present more often in breastfed infants than in formula-fed infants (Chapter 62). Feeding frequency during the first 3 days of life of breastfed infants is inversely related to the level of bilirubin; frequent feedings stimulate meconium passage and excretion of bilirubin in the stool. Infants who have insufficient milk intake and poor weight gain in the first week of life may have an increase in unconjugated bilirubin secondary to an exaggerated enterohepatic circulation of bilirubin. This is known as **breastfeeding jaundice**. Attention should be directed toward improved milk production and intake. The use of water supplements in breastfed infants has no effect on bilirubin levels and is not recommended.

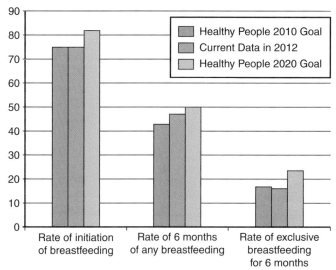

Figure 27-1 The 2010 and 2020 Healthy People Targets and the current 2012 rates of breastfeeding initiation, 6 months of any breastfeeding, and 6 months of exclusive breastfeeding in the United States.

After the first week of life in a breastfed infant, prolonged elevated serum bilirubin may be due to presence of an unknown factor in milk that enhances intestinal absorption of bilirubin. This is termed **breast milk jaundice**, which is a diagnosis of exclusion and should be made only if an infant is otherwise thriving, with normal growth and no evidence of hemolysis, infection, biliary atresia, or metabolic disease (Chapter 62). Breast milk jaundice usually lasts no more than 1 to 2 weeks. The American Academy of Pediatrics recommends vitamin D supplementation (400 IU/day starting soon after birth), and, when needed, fluoride after 6 months for breastfed infants.

Common Breastfeeding Problems

Breast tenderness, engorgement, and cracked nipples are the most common problems encountered by breastfeeding mothers. Engorgement, one of the most common causes of lactation failure, should receive prompt attention because milk supply can decrease quickly if the breasts are not adequately emptied. Applying warm or cold compresses to the breasts before nursing and hand expression or pumping of some milk can provide relief to the mother and make the areola easier to grasp by the infant. Nipple tenderness requires attention to proper latch-on and positioning of the infant. Supportive measures include nursing for shorter periods, beginning feedings on the less sore side, air drying the nipples well after nursing, and applying lanolin cream after each nursing session. Severe nipple pain and cracking usually indicate improper latch-on. Temporary pumping, which is well tolerated, may be needed. Meeting with a lactation consultant may help minimize these problems and allow the successful continuation of breastfeeding.

If a lactating woman reports fever, chills, and malaise, **mastitis** should be considered. Treatment includes frequent and complete emptying of the breast and antibiotics. Breastfeeding usually should not be stopped because the mother's mastitis commonly has no adverse effects on the breastfed infant.

Table 27-1	Maternal Contraindications and Recommendations for Breastfeeding
MATERNAL CONTRAINDICATIONS	**RECOMMENDATIONS FOR MOTHER**
Tuberculosis (active)	Should not breastfeed; expressed milk may be provided to child.
Varicella	Should not breastfeed; expressed milk may be provided to child.
H1N1 influenza	Should not breastfeed; expressed milk may be provided to child.
Herpes simplex infection of the breast	Should not breastfeed; expressed milk may be provided to child.
Human immunodeficiency virus (HIV)	In industrialized countries mothers are not recommended to breastfeed. In developing countries women are recommended to combine breastfeeding with antiretroviral therapy (ART) for 6 months.
Use of phencyclidine (PCP), cocaine, or amphetamines	Recommended to stop use of drugs as it can affect infant neurobehavioral development. Mothers enrolled in supervised methadone programs are encouraged to breastfeed.
Alcohol	Limit ingestion to less than 0.5 mg of alcohol per kg of body weight due to association with motor development.
Radiopharmaceutical agents	Express milk before exposure to feed infant. Express milk and discard during therapies. Radioactivity may be present in milk from 2 to 14 days, depending on agent. Consult with nuclear medicine expert.
Antineoplastic and immunosuppressive agents	Substitute formula.

Modified from Eidelman AI, Schanler RJ: American Academy of Pediatrics Section on Breastfeeding. Breastfeeding and the use of human milk, Pediatrics 129(3):827–841, 2012.

Untreated mastitis may also progress to a **breast abscess**. If an abscess is diagnosed, treatment includes incision and drainage, antibiotics, and regular emptying of the breast. Nursing from the contralateral breast can be continued with a healthy infant. If maternal comfort allows, nursing can continue on the affected side.

Maternal infection with human immunodeficiency virus (HIV) is considered a contraindication for breastfeeding in developed countries. When the mother has active tuberculosis, syphilis, or varicella, restarting breastfeeding may be considered after therapy is initiated. If a woman has herpetic lesions on her breast, nursing and contact with the infant on that breast should be avoided. Women with genital herpes can breastfeed. Proper hand-washing procedures should be stressed.

There are limited numbers of medical contraindications for breastfeeding, including pediatric metabolic disorders such as galactosemia, and infants with phenylketonuria, although infants with the latter may alternate breastfeeding with special protein-free or modified formulas. Maternal contraindications are shown in Table 27-1.

Maternal Drug Use

Any drug prescribed therapeutically to newborns usually can be consumed via breast milk without ill effect. The factors that determine the effects of maternal drug therapy on the nursing infant include the route of administration, dosage, molecular weight, pH, and protein binding. Few therapeutic drugs are absolutely contraindicated; these include radioactive compounds, antimetabolites, lithium, and certain antithyroid drugs. The mother should be advised against the use of unprescribed drugs, including alcohol, nicotine, caffeine, or "street drugs."

Maternal use of illicit or recreational drugs is a contraindication to breastfeeding. If a woman is unable to discontinue drug use, she should not breastfeed. Expression of milk for a feeding or two after use of a drug is not acceptable. Breastfed infants of mothers taking methadone (but no alcohol or other drugs) as part of a treatment program generally have not experienced ill effects.

FORMULA FEEDING

Cow's milk–based formulas are the vast majority of commercial formulas. Most milk-based formulas have added iron, which the AAP recommends, and parents should use only iron-fortified formula unless advised otherwise by the primary health care provider. Infant formula manufacturers have begun to examine the benefits of adding a variety of nutrients and biological factors to infant formula to mimic the composition and quality of breast milk. These include long-chain polyunsaturated fatty acids, nucleotides, prebiotics, and probiotics. Soy-based formulas, which sometimes have added iron, may be used for newborns who may be allergic to cow's milk. However, some newborns allergic to cow's milk are also allergic to the protein in soy formulas. There are hypoallergenic formulas for infants who can't tolerate the basic formulas, such as those with allergies to milk or soy proteins. The proteins in these hypoallergenic formulas are broken down to their basic components and are therefore easier to digest (Table 27-2). Specialized formulas are designed for premature, low birth weight babies. The carbohydrate is generally lactose, although lactose-free cow's milk–based formulas are available. The caloric density of formulas is 20 kcal/oz (0.67 kcal/mL), similar to that of human milk. A relatively high-fat and calorically dense diet (human milk or formula) is needed to deliver adequate

| Table 27-2 | Composition of Breast Milk, Breast Milk after Freezing and Pasteurization, and Representative Infant Formulas |

COMPONENT	BREAST MILK	BREAST MILK AFTER FREEZING AND PASTEURIZING	STANDARD FORMULA	SOY FORMULA	HYPOALLERGENIC FORMULA
Protein	1.1 per dL	Reduced	1.5 per dL	1.7 per dL	1.9 per d/L
Fat	4.0 per dL	4.0 per dL	3.6 per dL	3.6 per dL	3.8–3.3 per d/L
Carbohydrate	7.2 per dL	7.2 per dL	6.9–7.2 per dL	6.8 per dL	6.9–7.3 per d/L
Calcium	290 mg/L	290 mg/L	420–550 mg/L	700 mg/L	635–777 mg/L
Phosphorus	140 mg/L	140 mg/L	280–390 mg/L	500 mg/L	420–500 mg/L
Sodium	8.0 mg/L	8.0 mg/L	6.5–8.3 mg/L	13 mg/L	14 mg/L
Vitamin D	Variable	Variable	400 per dL	400 per dL	400 per d/L
Vitamin A	100%	100%			
Osmolality	253 mOsm/L	253 mOsm/L	230 mOsm/L	200–220 mOsm/L	290 mOSm/L
Renal solute load	75 mOsm/L	75 mOsm/L	100–126 mOsm/L	126–150 mOsm/L	125–175 mOSm/L
IgA and SIgA	Present	Reduced 30%	0	0	0
IgM	Present	Present	0	0	0
IgG	Present	Reduced 30%	0	0	0
Lactoferrin	Present	Reduced 30%	0	0	0
Lysozyme	Present	Reduced 25%	0	0	0
Lipases	Present	0	0	0	0
Monoglycerides	Present	Present	Added to some formulas	Added to some formulas	Added to some formulas
Free fatty acids	Present	Present	Added to some formulas	Added to some formulas	Added to some formulas
Linoleic acid	Present	Present	Added to some formulas	Added to some formulas	Added to some formulas
Alpha-linoleic acid	Present	Present	Added to some formulas	Added to some formulas	Added to some formulas
Bifidus factor	Present	Present			
Oligosaccharides	Present	Present			

calories (around 18 to 30 oz per day). Formula-fed infants are at higher risk for obesity later in childhood; this may be related to self regulation of volumes ingested by the newborns and infants.

COMPLEMENTARY FOODS

By approximately 6 months, complementary feeding of semisolid foods is suggested. By this age, an exclusively breastfed infant requires additional sources of several nutrients, including protein, iron, and zinc. Cereals commonly are mixed with breast milk, formula, or water and later with fruits. To help identify possible allergies or food intolerances that may arise when new foods are added to the diet, single-grain cereals (rice, oatmeal, barley) are recommended as starting cereals. If juice is given, it should be started only after 6 months of age, be given in a cup (as opposed to a bottle), and limited to 4 oz daily of 100% natural unsweetened juice. An infant should never be put to sleep with a bottle or cup filled with milk, formula, or juice because this can result in Early Childhood Caries (ECC) (see Chapter 127).

Green vegetables bring nutrients, vitamin, minerals, and micronutrients. Children should get two to three servings of vegetables. For infants with a strong family history of food allergy, foods with high allergic potential, such as fish, peanuts, tree nuts, dairy products, and eggs, should probably be avoided. All foods with the potential to obstruct the young infant's main airway should be avoided in general until 4 years of age or older. Because of the risk of infant botulism, honey should not be given before 1 year of age.

Commercially prepared or homemade foods help meet the nutritional needs of the infant. If the introduction of solid foods is delayed, nutritional deficiencies can develop, and oral sensory issues (texture and oral aversion) may occur. General signs of readiness include the ability to hold the head up, maturity (around double the birth weight), opening their mouths wide, showing eager anticipation of eating food and interest in foods, sitting unassisted, bringing objects to the mouth, and the ability to track a spoon. The choice of foods to meet micronutrient needs is less critical for formula.

Caries are tooth infections that start as early as when the deciduous teeth (baby teeth) have erupted. A tooth cavity is caused by a combination of sugar and bacteria in the mouth. Eating a healthy diet and brushing regularly will control sugar and bacteria. Rubbing infant gums with a wet washcloth can be the first step in oral hygiene. There are also ergonomically designed tooth brushes, comfortable and safe for infants, used to rub their gums and create the habit of oral hygiene. A variety of feeding habits beyond nursing and bottle feeding are implicated as causes of dental caries in childhood that can lead to problems with adult teeth and health. This infection can be prevented by healthy food choices and habits starting in infancy. Exposure to different textures and the process of self-feeding are important neurodevelopmental experiences for infants. A healthy diet is recommended to take full advantage of the child's developmental milestones and for the child's well-being. For the first 2 months it is important to set the stage by making distinctions between sleeping and feeding time. At 4 to 6 months of age, beginning to actively separate mealtime from bedtime is recommended.

DIET OF THE NORMAL CHILD AND ADOLESCENT

NUTRITION ISSUES FOR TODDLERS AND OLDER CHILDREN

Learning healthy eating behaviors at an early age is an important preventive measure because of the association of diet with several chronic and noncommunicable diseases (NCDs), such as obesity, diabetes, and cardiovascular disease, which may account for approximately 60% of all deaths worldwide. These diseases share risk factors that can be modified by lifestyle changes such as eating less processed food and increasing physical activity. Diets high in fruits and vegetables together with increased physical activity improve metabolic risk factors. The first 1000 days of life are an important time to engage in healthy nutrition behaviors that will promote well-being. Accelerated postnatal growth in infants and young children is an important risk factor for obesity; interventions should be aimed at identifying underlying causes for early prevention. For a discussion of nutrient needs for children and adolescents, see http://www.health.gov/dietaryguidelines.

MILK

The consumption of cow's milk is ideally not introduced until approximately 1 year of age when it is better tolerated. Low-fat (2%) or whole milk is recommended until 2 years or age, after which fat-free or 1% milk is recommended. Excessive milk intake (more than 24 oz/day) should be avoided in toddlers because larger intakes may reduce the intake of a good variety of nutritionally important solid foods and also result in iron deficiency anemia; large intakes also may contribute to excessive caloric intake.

JUICES

Juice intake for toddlers and young children should be limited to 4 oz, and juice intake for children 7 to 18 years of age should be limited to 8 oz/day. Water and milk are the recommended drinks during the day.

GENERAL RECOMMENDATIONS

"ChooseMyPlate" by the U.S. Department of Agriculture can provide parents with a general guideline for the types of foods to be offered on a regular basis. A child should eat three meals a day and two healthy snacks. A general rule for the quantity of food to offer to a child is one tablespoon per age of each food provided per meal, with more given if the child requests. As a rule of thumb, children should not be eating more than an adult palm per serving. By 1 year of age, infants should be eating meals with the family, have a regular schedule of meals and snacks, and be encouraged to self-feed with appropriate finger foods.

The "plate" image is divided into five sections: Fruits, Grains, Vegetables, Protein, and Dairy (Figure 28-1; Table 28-1). Half of the "plate" should be vegetables and fruits, and the other half grains and proteins, with dairy on the side. The "plate" is simple, organized, and serves as a guide for healthy eating. A weekly recommendation for vegetable intake is also provided (Table 28-1). Other suggestions include the following: switch to fat free or low-fat (1%) milk; make at least half of the grains whole instead of refined grains; avoid oversize proportions; compare sodium (salt) in foods such as soup, bread, and frozen meals; choose foods with lower sodium content; and drink water instead of sugary drinks. After 2 years, it is recommended that the fat intake gradually be reduced to approximately 30% and not less than 20% of calories. Replace proteins from red meat with a mix of fish, chicken, nuts, and legumes. Power struggles over eating are common between parents and toddlers. The parent's role is to decide the what, when, and where of the meals. The child's role is to decide if, what, and how much to eat.

IRON INTAKE

Iron intake may be inadequate in some children between 1 and 3 years of age in the United States. Significant iron deficiency anemia exists in some high-risk minority or low-income populations of young children. Toddlers with excessive milk intakes (>32 oz/day) and/or those who consume little meat, green leaves rich in iron, or grains are at risk for iron deficiency.

NUTRITION ISSUES FOR ADOLESCENTS

Teen nutrition can be a challenge. Ads for junk food and images of incredibly thin adolescents provide conflicting and unhealthy ideas about what they should eat. Girls ages 14 to 18 need anywhere from 1800 to 2400 calories per day, depending on their activity level and stage of development. Boys of the same age group need 2000 to 3200 calories daily. Poor eating habits may develop during adolescence. Skipped meals (especially breakfast), binge eating with friends or alone, dieting, and consumption of nutrient-poor, calorically dense foods are common problems. Excessive consumption of sugar from soda, fruit drinks, and specialty coffee and tea drinks may contribute to excess weight gain as well as tooth decay and may displace other needed nutrients. Poor calcium intake during adolescence may predispose the adult to future osteoporotic hip fracture. Osteoporosis (osteopenia) during adolescence caused by poor dietary calcium or vitamin D intake or poor absorption of ingested calcium in children and adolescents is a potential problem. Only 1 of 10 teenage girls and 1 of 4 teenage boys get enough calcium every day. Adolescents ages 9 to 18 need 1300 milligrams of calcium daily. Good sources include milk, yogurt, fortified orange juice, cheese, soybeans, and tofu.

Inadequate iron intake may results in symptoms of fatigue and iron deficiency anemia. Iron needs increase during growth spurts, which is why teens are more likely to suffer from iron deficiency anemia. Teenage girls are especially prone to anemia. Student athletes are also vulnerable to inadequate iron intakes, severely restrictive eating patterns, and use of inappropriate nutritional and vitamin supplements. Adolescents should be counseled on specific and healthy dietary choices (see Chapter 70).

Table 28-1	Recommended Weekly Vegetable Intake (in cups)				
AGE (YEARS)	GREEN	ORANGE	STARCH	DRY BEANS/ PEAS	OTHER*
2-3	1	½	1½	½	4
4-8	1½	1	2½	5½	4½
>9 Girls	2	1½	2½	2½	5½
>9 Boys	3	2	3	3	6½

From www.ChooseMyPlate.gov
*Including cabbage, cauliflower, green beans, lettuce, zucchini.

Figure 28-1 "ChooseMyPlate" guidelines developed by the U.S. Department of Agriculture. (From www.ChooseMyPlate.gov)

OBESITY

EPIDEMIOLOGY

Childhood obesity is an epidemic in the United States. Data indicate that approximately 17% of children in the United States ages 2 to 20 are obese (body mass index of ≥95th percentile) and more than 30% of U.S. adults are obese. Many obese children become obese adults, and the risk of remaining obese increases with age and degree of obesity. Obesity runs in families and is rarely related to genetic influences. The largest increases in the prevalence of obesity are seen in the most severely overweight classifications and in certain ethnic groups, such as African-American and Mexican-American children. In 2008, obesity cost the nation $147 billion in medical costs. The associations between obesity and television watching and excessive dietary intake as well as the different rates of obesity observed in urban versus rural areas support the important influence of environment. One important risk factor is maternal obesity during pregnancy. Children born to obese mothers are three to five times more likely to be obese in childhood. Women who gain much more weight than recommended during pregnancy have children who have a higher BMI than normal in adolescence. Also, some small for gestational age (SGA) newborns have higher risks for abnormal postnatal weight gain and diabetes.

CLINICAL MANIFESTATIONS

Decision-Making Algorithm
Available @ StudentConsult.com

Obesity

Complications of obesity in children and adolescents can affect virtually every major organ system. High BMI increases the risk of metabolic and cardiovascular diseases and some cancers; it is also the most important modifiable risk factor for glycemia and diabetes. The history and physical examination should screen for many potential complications noted among obese patients (Table 29-1), in addition to specific syndromes associated with obesity (Table 29-2). Medical complications are often related to the degree of obesity and usually decrease in severity or resolve with weight reduction. Obesity is associated with the presence of precursors of coronary heart disease that are already evident in 12- and 13-year-old children. Type 2 diabetes is also increasing in children.

ASSESSMENT

The **diagnosis** of obesity depends on the measurement of excess body fat. Actual measurement of body composition is not practical in most clinical situations.

BMI (body mass index; BMI = wt (kg) ÷ Ht^2 (m)) is a convenient screening tool that correlates fairly strongly with body fatness in children and adults. **BMI age-specific and gender-specific percentile curves** (for 2- to 20-year-olds) allow an assessment of BMI percentile (available online at http://www.cdc.gov/growthcharts). Table 29-3 provides BMI interpretation guidelines. For children younger than 2 years of age, weight-for-length measurements greater than 95th percentile may indicate overweight and warrant further assessment. A BMI for age and gender above the 95th percentile is strongly associated with excessive body fat and is associated with multiple cardiovascular disease risk factors.

Early recognition of excessive rates of weight gain, overweight, or obesity in children is essential because the earlier the interventions, the more likely they are to be successful.

Table 29–2	Diseases Associated with Childhood Obesity*	
SYNDROME	**MANIFESTATIONS**	
Alström syndrome	Hypogonadism, retinal degeneration, deafness, diabetes mellitus	
Carpenter syndrome	Polydactyly, syndactyly, cranial synostosis, mental retardation	
Cushing syndrome	Adrenal hyperplasia or pituitary tumor	
Fröhlich syndrome	Hypothalamic tumor	
Hyperinsulinism	Nesidioblastosis, pancreatic adenoma, hypoglycemia, Mauriac syndrome	
Laurence-Moon-Bardet-Biedl	Retinal degeneration, syndactyly, hypogonadism, mental retardation, autosomal recessive syndrome	
Muscular dystrophy	Late onset of obesity	
Myelodysplasia	Spina bifida	
Prader-Willi syndrome	Neonatal hypotonia, normal growth immediately after birth, small hands and feet, mental retardation, hypogonadism; some have partial deletion of chromosome 15	
Pseudohypoparathyroidism	Variable hypocalcemia, cutaneous calcifications	
Turner syndrome	Ovarian dysgenesis, lymphedema, web neck; XO chromosome	

*These diseases represent <5% of cases of childhood obesity.

Table 29-1	Complications of Obesity
COMPLICATION	**EFFECTS**
Psychosocial	Peer discrimination, teasing, reduced college acceptance, isolation, depression, eating disorders (binge-eating), reduced job promotion*
Growth	Advance bone age, increased height, early menarche
Central nervous system	Pseudotumor cerebri
Respiratory	Obstructive sleep apnea
Cardiovascular	Hypertension, cardiac hypertrophy, arrhythmias, ischemic heart disease,* sudden death*
Orthopedic	Slipped capital femoral epiphysis, Blount disease
Metabolic	Insulin resistance, type 2 diabetes mellitus, hypertriglyceridemia, hypercholesterolemia, gout,* hepatic steatosis, polycystic ovary disease, cholelithiasis

*Complications unusual until adulthood.

Table 29-3	Body Mass Index (BMI)* Interpretation
BMI/AGE PERCENTILE	**INTERPRETATION**
<5th	Underweight
5th–85th	Normal
85th–95th	Overweight
>95th	Obese

From www.cdc.gov/healthyweight.

*BMI = $\dfrac{\text{wt (kg)}}{\text{Ht}^2 \text{ (m)}}$

Routine evaluation at well-child visits should include the following:

1. **Anthropometric data**, including weight, height, and calculation of BMI. Data should be plotted on age-appropriate and gender-appropriate growth charts and assessed for BMI trends (see Table 29-3).
2. **Dietary and physical activity history** (Table 29-4). Assess patterns and potential targets for behavioral change.
3. **Physical examination.** Assess blood pressure, adiposity distribution (central versus generalized), markers of comorbidities (acanthosis nigricans, hirsutism, hepatomegaly, orthopedic abnormalities), and physical stigmata of a genetic syndrome (explains fewer than 5% of cases).
4. **Laboratory studies.** These are generally reserved for children who are obese (BMI > 95th percentile), who have evidence of comorbidities, or both. Other studies should be guided by findings in the history and physical examination. The American Academy of Pediatrics endorses the government guidelines from 2011, which recommend that all 9- to 11-year-olds be screened for cholesterol. Other useful laboratory tests may include hemoglobin A1c, fasting lipid profile, fasting glucose levels, liver function tests, and thyroid function tests (if there is a faster increase in weight than height).

PREVENTION

The approach to therapy and aggressiveness of treatment should be based on risk factors, including age, severity of overweight and obesity, and comorbidities, as well as family history and support. The primary goal for all children with uncomplicated obesity and fast-rising weight-for-height is to achieve **healthy eating and activity patterns.** For children with a secondary complication, specific treatment of the complication is an important goal. Childhood and adolescent obesity treatment programs can lead to sustained weight loss and decreases in BMI when treatment focuses on behavioral changes and is family centered. Concurrent changes in dietary and physical activity patterns are most likely to provide success (Table 29-5).

Goal setting needs to be specific and attainable. Instead of recommending that the child walk or bike to school, suggest walking or biking to school two or more days a week. Rather than recommending that a child watch less television, suggest watching no television on school days. It is important to keep it simple and set one or two short-term goals at a time. In addition, behavioral risk factors need to be identified, such as avoiding fast food when family life gets hectic. Helping the family think of healthy alternatives is important.

Families need to be counseled on age-appropriate and healthy eating patterns, beginning with the promotion of **breastfeeding.** For infants, transition to complementary and table foods and the importance of regularly scheduled meals and snacks, versus grazing behavior, should be emphasized. Age-appropriate **portion sizes** for meals and snacks should be encouraged. Children should be taught to recognize hunger and satiety cues, guided by reasonable portions and healthy food choices by parents. Smaller bowls should be used, and children should never eat directly from a bag or box. No juices or soda should be the rule. Children should never be forced

Table 29-4	Eating and Activity Habits for Overweight/ Obesity Prevention
	ACTIVITIES FOR OVERWEIGHT/OBESITY PREVENTION
INDIVIDUAL	■ Be physically active >1 hour per day ■ Limit screen time (television, computer games/Internet, video games) to <1–2 hours per day (no TV for child <2 yr of age) ■ Consume five or more servings of fruits and vegetables per day ■ Minimize consumption of sugar-sweetened beverages ■ Consume a healthy breakfast every day
FAMILY	■ Eat at table, as a family, at least five to six times per week ■ Prepare more meals at home rather than purchasing restaurant food ■ Allow child to self-regulate his or her meals and avoid overly restrictive feeding behaviors ■ Do not reward children with food or drinks ■ Have only healthy foods available for snacking ■ Encourage outdoor activity
COMMUNITY	Schools ■ Serve healthy foods ■ Limit what is available in vending machines ■ Have physical activity daily ■ Have outdoor recess daily ■ Teach healthy eating Health Care Providers ■ Take a nutrition history ■ Speak to patients about healthy weight and good nutrition ■ Advise exercise
GOVERNMENT	■ Increase access to healthy food and eliminate food deserts ■ Regulate food ads or serving sizes ■ Add more sidewalks and parks ■ Emphasize safety

to eat when they are not willing, and overemphasis on food as a reward should be avoided. "Choose My Plate" by the U.S. Department of Agriculture can provide parents with a general guideline for the types of foods to be offered on a regular basis, including fruits, vegetables, grains, protein, and dairy.

The importance of physical activity should be emphasized. For some children, organized sports and school-based activities provide opportunities for vigorous activity and fun, whereas for others a focus on activities of daily living, such as increased walking, using stairs, and more active play may be better received. Time spent in **sedentary behavior**, such as television viewing and video/computer games, should be limited. Television in children's rooms is associated with more television time and with higher rates of overweight, and the risks of this practice should be discussed with parents. Clinicians may need to help families identify alternatives to sedentary activities, especially for families with deterrents to activity, such as unsafe neighborhoods or lack of supervision after school.

TREATMENT

More aggressive therapies are considered only for those who have not responded to other interventions. Treatment includes

Table 29-5	Setting Explicit Goals to Prevent or Treat Obesity	
FIGHT OBESITY EFFECTIVELY	**AMBIGUOUS GOALS**	**SPECIFIC GOALS**
Keep it simple	Walk or bike more	Walk or bike to school 2 days a week
Countable goals/unambiguous	Watch less TV	Watch no TV on school days
2 short-term goals/time		
Be able to count	Decrease size of serving	Small bowls (parent palm)
Aim to change behaviors		Avoid eating from the box
Don't focus on consumption of carbohydrates, fat, protein	Decrease to 20 g of fat	Eat fish once a week
Focus on specific categories	Decrease sugars	Avoid sweetened foods
Focus on healthier preparation methods		Avoid frying
Focus on eating patterns		Avoid double dinner
Focus on portion size		Portion parent's palm size
Eating fast food	Eat less junk food	Limit trips to McDonalds to once a week
Sweetened beverages	Avoid soda/juices	No soda or juices
Healthy beverages		Drink only milk or water
Fruits	Buy fewer juices	Have no juices in the refrigerator
	Increase eating fruits	Keep a bowl of fruits in the kitchen
Vegetables	Increase eating veggies	Have a bowl of veggies in the refrigerator
		Cooperation, competition, and social interaction such as building a house of veggies
Physical activities	Walk more	Family hikes every Sunday
		Specific activity time for activities and sedentary behavior
	Increase walking from school	Parents picking up from school 2 days a week

a systematic approach that promotes multidisciplinary brief, office-based interventions for obese children as well as reducing weight. Before enrolling any patient in a weight-loss program, the clinician must have a clear idea of that individual's expectations. Patients with unrealistic expectations should not be enrolled until these are changed to realistic and attainable goals. Using the pneumonic described, the clinician should guide the patient who seeks weight reduction to create **SMART** goals: Specific, Measurable, Attainable, Realistic, and Timely.

Surgical treatment may be advocated as a preferred and cost-effective solution for certain children and adolescents. The role of bariatric surgery in the treatment of obese children or adolescents is controversial. The concerns about surgery to treat obesity in young populations include whether or not surgery is cost effective; how to ensure healthy growth through to adulthood; what support services are needed after surgery; compliance with the postoperative nutrition regimen; and attendance at appointments for long-term follow-up and care. There is very limited evidence available to adequately estimate long-term safety, effectiveness, cost effectiveness or durability of bariatric surgery in growing children. The existing evidence suggests that bariatric surgery in severely obese adolescent results in significant weight loss and improvements in comorbidities and quality of life. Postoperative complications (both physical and psychological), compliance, and follow-up may be more problematic in adolescents than adults, and long-term data on safety, effectiveness, and cost remain largely unavailable.

Chapter 30

PEDIATRIC UNDERNUTRITION

Pediatric undernutrition is usually the result of inadequate food supply, access, or utilization; poor access to health and sanitation; and/or inappropriate feeding or child care practices. The greatest risk of undernutrition is in utero through age 2. Various guidelines can be used to classify pediatric malnutrition (Table 30-1). International references are established that allow normalization of anthropometric measures in terms of z scores. Other measurements include height and weight for age, weight for height, BMI, and mid-upper arm circumference. The greatest consequence of undernutrition is death, but significant intellectual and physical disability exists in many who survive.

Protein-energy malnutrition (PEM) is a spectrum of conditions caused by varying levels of protein and calorie deficiencies. Primary PEM is caused by social or economic factors that result in a lack of food. Secondary PEM occurs in children with various conditions associated with increased caloric requirements (infection, trauma, cancer) (Fig. 30-1), increased caloric loss (malabsorption), reduced caloric intake (anorexia, cancer, oral intake restriction, social factors), or a combination of these three variables. Protein and calorie malnutrition may

Table 30-1	Definitions of Malnutrition		
CLASSIFICATION	**DEFINITION**	**GRADING**	
Gomez	Weight below % median WFA	Mild (grade 1)	75%–90% WFA
		Moderate (grade 2)	60%–74% WFA
		Severe (grade 3)	<60% WFA
Waterlow	z-scores (SD) below median WFH	Mild	80%–90% WFH
		Moderate	70%–80% WFH
		Severe	<70% WFH
WHO (wasting)	z-scores (SD) below median WFH	Moderate	$-3 \leq$ z-score <-2
		Severe	z-score <-3
WHO (stunting)	z-scores (SD) below median HFA	Moderate	$-3 \leq$ z-score <-2
		Severe	z-score <-3
Kanawati	MUAC divided by occipitofrontal head circumference	Mild	<0.31
		Moderate	<0.28
		Severe	<0.25
Cole	z-scores of BMI for age	Grade 1	BMI for age z-score <-1
		Grade 2	BMI for age z-score <-2
		Grade 3	BMI for age z-score <-3

From Grover Z, Ee LC: Protein energy malnutrition, Pediatr Clin North Am *56:1055–1068, 2009*
BMI, Body mass index; HFA, height for age; MUAC, mid-upper arm circumference; NCHS, U.S. National Center for Health Statistics; SD, standard deviation; WFA, weight for age; WFH, weight for height; WHO, World Health Organization.

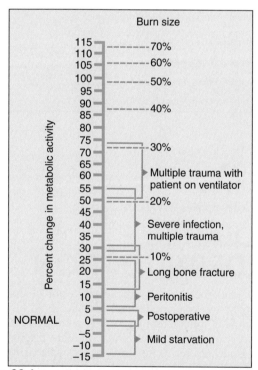

Figure 30-1 Increased energy needs with stress. *(Adapted from Wilmore D:* The Metabolic Management of the Critically Ill, *New York, 1977, Plenum Publishing. Revised in Walker W, Watkins J, editors:* Nutrition in Pediatrics: Basic Science and Clinical Application. *Boston, 1985, Little, Brown.)*

be associated with other nutrient deficiencies, which may be evident on physical examination (Table 30-2).

FAILURE TO THRIVE

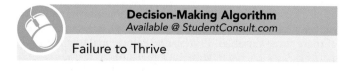

Decision-Making Algorithm
Available @ StudentConsult.com

Failure to Thrive

Pediatric **undernutrition** in the United States is often termed **failure to thrive** and describes circumstances in which a child fails to gain weight appropriately or, in more severe cases, experiences failure in linear growth or head circumference. The terms **organic** and **nonorganic** failure to thrive have lost favor in recognition of the frequent interplay between underlying medical conditions that may cause maladaptive behaviors. Similarly, social and behavioral factors that initially may have been associated with feeding problems (see Chapter 21), and poor growth also may be associated with medical problems, including frequent minor acute illnesses.

MARASMUS

Marasmus results from the body's physiologic response to inadequate calories and nutrients. Loss of muscle mass and subcutaneous fat stores can be confirmed by inspection or palpation and quantified by anthropometric measurements. The head may appear large but generally is proportional to the body length. Edema usually is absent. The skin is dry and thin, and the hair may be thin, sparse, and easily pulled out. Marasmic children may be apathetic, weak, and may be irritable when touched. Bradycardia and hypothermia signify severe and life-threatening malnutrition. Inappropriate or inadequate weaning practices and chronic diarrhea are common findings in developing countries. Stunting (impaired linear growth) results from a combination of malnutrition, especially micronutrients, and recurrent infections.

KWASHIORKOR

Kwashiorkor results from inadequate protein intake in the presence of fair to good caloric intake. The hypoalbuminemic state results in pitting edema that starts in the lower extremities and ascends with increasing severity. Other factors, such as acute infection, toxins, and possibly specific micronutrient or amino acid imbalances, are likely to contribute to the etiology. The major **clinical manifestation** of kwashiorkor is that the body weight is near normal for age; weight alone does not accurately reflect the nutritional status because of edema. **Physical**

Table 30-2 | Physical Signs of Nutritional Deficiency Disorders

SYSTEM	SIGN	DEFICIENCY	SYSTEM	SIGN	DEFICIENCY
General appearance	Reduced weight for height	Calories		Atrophic papillae	Riboflavin, iron, niacin, folate, vitamin B_{12}
Skin and hair	Pallor	Anemias (iron, vitamin B_{12}, vitamin E, folate, and copper)		Smooth tongue	Iron
				Red tongue (glossitis)	Vitamins B_6, B_{12}, niacin, riboflavin, folate
	Edema	Protein, thiamine		Parotid swelling	Protein
	Nasolabial seborrhea	Calories, protein, vitamin B_6, niacin, riboflavin		Caries	Fluoride
				Anosmia	Vitamins A, B_{12}, zinc
	Dermatitis	Riboflavin, essential fatty acids, biotin		Hypogeusia	Vitamin A, zinc
				Goiter	Iodine
	Photosensitivity dermatitis	Niacin	Cardiovascular	Heart failure	Thiamine, selenium, nutritional anemias
	Acrodermatitis	Zinc	Genital	Hypogonadism	Zinc
	Follicular hyperkeratosis (sandpaper-like)	Vitamin A	Skeletal	Costochondral beading	Vitamins D, C
	Depigmented skin	Calories, protein		Subperiosteal hemorrhage	Vitamin C, copper
	Purpura	Vitamins C, K		Cranial bossing	Vitamin D
	Scrotal, vulval dermatitis	Riboflavin		Wide fontanel	Vitamin D
	Alopecia	Zinc, biotin, protein		Epiphyseal enlargement	Vitamin D
	Depigmented, dull hair, easily pluckable	Protein, calories, copper		Craniotabes	Vitamin D, calcium
				Tender bones	Vitamin C
Subcutaneous tissue	Decreased	Calories		Tender calves	Thiamine, selenium, vitamin C
Eye (vision)	Adaptation to dark	Vitamins A, E, zinc		Spoon-shaped nails (koilonychia)	Iron
	Color discrimination	Vitamin A		Transverse nail line	Protein
	Bitot spots, xerophthalmia, keratomalacia	Vitamin A	Neurologic	Sensory, motor neuropathy	Thiamine, vitamins E, B_6, B_{12}
	Conjunctival pallor	Nutritional anemias		Ataxia, areflexia	Vitamin E
	Fundal capillary microaneurysms	Vitamin C		Ophthalmoplegia	Vitamin E, thiamine
Face, mouth, and neck	Moon facies	Kwashiorkor		Tetany	Vitamin D, Ca^{2+}, Mg^{2+}
				Retardation	Iodine, niacin
	Simian facies	Marasmus		Dementia, delirium	Vitamin E, niacin, thiamine
	Angular stomatitis	Riboflavin, iron		Poor position sense, ataxia	Thiamine, vitamin B_{12}
	Cheilosis	Vitamins B_6, niacin, riboflavin			
	Bleeding gums	Vitamins C, K			

examination reveals a relative maintenance of subcutaneous adipose tissue and a marked atrophy of muscle mass. Edema varies from a minor pitting of the dorsum of the foot to generalized edema with involvement of the eyelids and scrotum. The hair is sparse; is easily plucked; and appears dull brown, red, or yellow-white. Nutritional repletion restores hair color, leaving a band of hair with altered pigmentation followed by a band with normal pigmentation (flag sign). Skin changes are common and range from hyperpigmented hyperkeratosis to an erythematous macular rash (pellagroid) on the trunk and extremities. In the most severe form of kwashiorkor, a superficial desquamation occurs over pressure surfaces ("flaky paint" rash). Angular cheilosis, atrophy of the filiform papillae of the tongue, and monilial stomatitis are common. Enlarged parotid glands and facial edema result in moon facies; apathy and disinterest in eating are typical of kwashiorkor. Examination of the abdomen may reveal an enlarged, soft liver with an indefinite edge. Lymph node and tonsils are commonly atrophic. Chest examination may reveal basilar rales. The abdomen is distended, and bowel sounds tend to be hypoactive.

MIXED MARASMUS-KWASHIORKOR
These children often have concurrent wasting and edema in addition to stunting. These children exhibit features of dermatitis, neurologic abnormalities, and fatty liver.

TREATMENT OF MALNUTRITION
The basal metabolic rate and immediate nutrient needs decrease in cases of malnutrition. When nutrients are provided, the metabolic rate increases, stimulating anabolism and increasing

nutrient requirements. The body of the malnourished child may have compensated for micronutrient deficiencies with lower metabolic and growth rates, and refeeding may unmask these deficiencies. Nutritional rehabilitation should be initiated and advanced *slowly* to minimize these complications. The initial approach involves correction of dehydration and anti-infective (bacteria, parasites) therapy if indicated. Oral rehydration is recommended over intravenous fluid to avoid excessive fluid and solute load and resultant heart or renal failure.

When nutritional rehabilitation is initiated, calories can be safely started at 20% above the child's recent intake. If no estimate of the caloric intake is available, 50% to 75% of the normal energy requirement is safe. High-calorie oral solutions or ready-to-use therapeutic foods (a mixture of powdered milk, peanuts, sugar, vitamins, and minerals) are frequently used in developing countries. Nutritional rehabilitation can be complicated by **refeeding syndrome**, which is characterized by fluid retention, hypophosphatemia, hypomagnesemia, and hypokalemia. Careful monitoring of laboratory values and clinical status with severe malnutrition is essential.

When nutritional rehabilitation has begun, caloric intake can be increased 10% to 20% per day, monitoring for electrolyte imbalances, poor cardiac function, edema, or feeding intolerance. If any of these occurs, further caloric increases are not made until the child's status stabilizes. Caloric intake is increased until appropriate regrowth or catch-up growth is initiated. Catch-up growth refers to gaining weight at greater than 50th percentile for age and may require 150% or more of the recommended calories for an age-matched, well-nourished child. A general rule of thumb for infants and children up to 3 years of age is to provide 100 to 120 kcal/kg based on *ideal* weight for height. Protein needs also are increased as anabolism begins and are provided in proportion to the caloric intake. Vitamin and mineral intake in excess of the daily recommended intake is provided to account for the increased requirements; this is frequently accomplished by giving an age-appropriate daily multiple vitamin, with other individual micronutrient supplements as warranted by history, physical examination, or laboratory studies. Iron supplements are not recommended during the acute rehabilitation phase, especially for children with kwashiorkor, for whom ferritin levels are often high. Additional iron may pose an oxidative stress; iron supplementation is associated with higher morbidity and mortality.

In most cases, cow's milk–based formulas are tolerated and provide an appropriate mix of nutrients. Other easily digested foods, appropriate for the age, also may be introduced slowly. If feeding intolerance occurs, lactose-free or semielemental formulas should be considered.

COMPLICATIONS OF MALNUTRITION

Malnourished children are more susceptible to **infection,** especially sepsis, pneumonia, and gastroenteritis. Hypoglycemia is common after periods of severe fasting but may also be a sign of sepsis. Hypothermia may signify infection or, with bradycardia, may signify a decreased metabolic rate to conserve energy. Bradycardia and poor cardiac output predispose the malnourished child to heart failure, which is exacerbated by acute fluid or solute loads. **Micronutrient deficiencies** also can complicate malnutrition. Vitamin A and zinc deficiencies are common in the developing world and are an important cause of altered immune response and increased morbidity

and mortality. Depending on the age at onset and the duration of the malnutrition, malnourished children may have permanent growth stunting (from malnutrition in utero, infancy, or adolescence) and delayed development (from malnutrition in infancy or adolescence). Environmental (social) deprivation may interact with the effects of the malnutrition to impair further development and cognitive function.

Chapter **31**

VITAMIN AND MINERAL DEFICIENCIES

Micronutrients include vitamins and trace elements. In industrialized societies, frank clinical deficiencies are unusual in healthy children, but they can and do occur in certain high-risk circumstances. Risk factors include diets that are consistently limited in variety, especially with the exclusion of entire food groups, malabsorption syndromes, and conditions causing high physiologic requirements. Various common etiologies of vitamin and nutrient deficiency states are highlighted in Table 31-1, and characteristics of vitamin deficiencies are outlined in Table 31-2. Treatment is noted in Table 31-3.

WATER-SOLUBLE VITAMINS

Water-soluble vitamins are not *stored* in the body except for vitamin B_{12}; intake therefore alters tissue levels. Absorption from the diet is usually high, and the compounds exchange readily between intracellular and extracellular fluids; excretion is via the urine. Water-soluble vitamins typically function as coenzymes in energy, protein, amino acid, and nucleic acid metabolism; as cosubstrates in enzymatic reactions; and as structural components.

Ascorbic Acid

Decision-Making Algorithm
Available @ StudentConsult.com

Anemia

The principal forms of vitamin C are ascorbic acid and the oxidized form, dehydroascorbic acid. Ascorbic acid accelerates hydroxylation reactions in many biosynthetic reactions, including hydroxylation of proline in the formation of collagen. The needs of full-term infants for ascorbic acid and dehydroascorbic acid are calculated by estimating the availability in human milk.

A deficiency of ascorbic acid results in the clinical manifestations of **scurvy**. Infantile scurvy is manifested by irritability, bone tenderness with swelling, and pseudoparalysis of the legs. The disease may occur if infants are fed unsupplemented cow's milk in the first year of life or if the diet is devoid of fruits

Table 31-1	Etiology of Vitamin and Nutrient Deficiency States
ETIOLOGY	**DEFICIENCY**
DIET	
Vegans (strict)	Protein, vitamins B_{12}, D, riboflavin, iron
Breastfed infant	Vitamins K, D
Cow's milk–fed infant	Iron
Bulimia, anorexia nervosa	Electrolytes, other deficiencies
Parenteral alimentation	Essential fatty acids, trace elements
Alcoholism	Calories, vitamin B_1, B_6, folate
MEDICAL PROBLEMS	
Malabsorption syndromes	Vitamins A, D, E, K, zinc, essential fatty acids
Cholestasis	Vitamins E, D, K, A, zinc, essential fatty acids
MEDICATIONS	
Sulfonamides	Folate
Phenytoin, phenobarbital	Vitamins D, K, folate
Mineral oil	Vitamins A, D, E, K
Antibiotics	Vitamin K
Isoniazid	Vitamin B_6
Antacids	Iron, phosphate, calcium
Digitalis	Magnesium, calcium
Penicillamine	Vitamin B_6
SPECIFIC MECHANISMS	
Transcobalamin II or intrinsic factor deficiency	Vitamin B_{12}
Other digestive enzyme	Carbohydrate, fat, protein deficiencies
Menkes kinky hair syndrome	Copper
Acrodermatitis enteropathica	Zinc
Reduced exposure to direct sunlight	Vitamin D

and vegetables. Subperiosteal hemorrhage, bleeding gums and petechiae, hyperkeratosis of hair follicles, and a succession of mental changes characterize the progression of the illness. Anemia secondary to bleeding, decreased iron absorption, or abnormal folate metabolism is also seen in chronic scurvy. Treatment is noted in Table 31-3.

B Vitamins

Decision-Making Algorithms
Available @ StudentConsult.com

Anemia
Neutropenia

The B vitamins thiamine, riboflavin, and niacin are routinely added to enriched grain products; deficiencies in normal hosts

are rare in the United States. Levels from human milk reflect maternal intake, and deficiency can develop in breastfed infants of deficient mothers.

Thiamine
Vitamin B_1 functions as a coenzyme in biochemical reactions related to carbohydrate metabolism, decarboxylation of α-ketoacids and pyruvate, and transketolase reactions of the pentose pathway. Thiamine also is involved in the decarboxylation of branched-chain amino acids. Thiamine is lost during milk pasteurization and sterilization.

Thiamine deficiency occurs in alcoholics and has been reported in adolescents who have undergone bariatric surgery for severe obesity. **Infantile beriberi** occurs between 1 and 4 months of age in breastfed infants whose mothers have a thiamine deficiency (alcoholism), in infants with protein-calorie malnutrition, in infants receiving unsupplemented hyperalimentation fluid, and in infants receiving boiled milk. Acute **wet beriberi** with cardiac symptoms and signs predominates in infantile beriberi. Anorexia, apathy, vomiting, restlessness, and pallor progress to dyspnea, cyanosis, and death from heart failure. Infants with beriberi have a characteristic aphonic cry; they appear to be crying, but no sound is uttered. Other signs include peripheral neuropathy and paresthesias. For treatment see Table 31-3.

Riboflavin
Vitamin B_2 is a constituent of two coenzymes, riboflavin 5′-phosphate and flavin-adenine dinucleotide, essential components of glutathione reductase and xanthine oxidase, which are involved in electron transport. A deficiency of riboflavin affects glucose, fatty acid, and amino acid metabolism. Riboflavin and its phosphate are decomposed by exposure to light and by strong alkaline solutions.

Ariboflavinosis is characterized by an angular stomatitis; glossitis; cheilosis; seborrheic dermatitis around the nose and mouth; and eye changes that include reduced tearing, photophobia, corneal vascularization, and the formation of cataracts. Subclinical riboflavin deficiencies have been found in diabetic subjects, children in families with low socioeconomic status, children with chronic cardiac disease, and infants undergoing prolonged phototherapy for hyperbilirubinemia.

Niacin
Niacin consists of the compounds nicotinic acid and nicotinamide (niacinamide). Nicotinamide, the predominant form of the vitamin, functions as a component of the coenzymes nicotinamide adenine dinucleotide (NAD) and nicotinamide adenine dinucleotide phosphate (NADP). Niacin is involved in multiple metabolic processes, including fat synthesis, intracellular respiratory metabolism, and glycolysis.

In determining the needs for niacin, the content of tryptophan in the diet must be considered because tryptophan is converted to niacin. Niacin is stable in foods and withstands heating and prolonged storage. Approximately 70% of the total niacin equivalents in human milk are derived from tryptophan. **Pellagra,** or niacin deficiency disease, is characterized by weakness, lassitude, dermatitis, photosensitivity, inflammation of mucous membranes, diarrhea, vomiting, dysphagia, and, in severe cases, dementia.

Table 31-2	Characteristics of Vitamin Deficiencies			
VITAMIN	**PURPOSE**	**DEFICIENCY**	**COMMENTS**	**SOURCE**
WATER SOLUBLE				
Thiamine (B_1)	Coenzyme in ketoacid decarboxylation (e.g., pyruvate → acetyl-CoA transketolase reaction)	*Beriberi:* polyneuropathy, calf tenderness, heart failure, edema, ophthalmoplegia	Inborn errors of lactate metabolism; boiling milk destroys B_1	Liver, meat, milk, cereals, nuts, legumes
Riboflavin (B_2)	FAD coenzyme in oxidation-reduction reactions	Anorexia, mucositis, anemia, cheilosis, nasolabial seborrhea	Photosensitizer	Milk, cheese, liver, meat, eggs, whole grains, green leafy vegetables
Niacin (B_3)	NAD coenzyme in oxidation-reduction reactions	*Pellagra:* photosensitivity, dermatitis, dementia, diarrhea, death	Tryptophan is a precursor	Meat, fish, liver, whole grains, green leafy vegetables
Pyridoxine (B_6)	Cofactor in amino acid metabolism	Seizures, hyperacusis, microcytic anemia, nasolabial seborrhea, neuropathy	Dependency state: deficiency secondary to drugs	Meat, liver, whole grains, peanuts, soybeans
Pantothenic acid	CoA in Krebs cycle	None reported		Meat, vegetables
Biotin	Cofactor in carboxylase reactions of amino acids	Alopecia, dermatitis, hypotonia, death	Bowel resection, inborn error of metabolism,* and ingestion of raw eggs	Yeast, meats; made by intestinal flora
B_{12}	Coenzyme for 5-methyltetrahydrofolate formation; DNA synthesis	Megaloblastic anemia, peripheral neuropathy, posterior lateral spinal column disease, vitiligo	Vegans; fish tapeworm; short gut syndrome; transcobalamin or intrinsic factor deficiencies	Meat, fish, cheese, eggs
Folate	DNA synthesis	Megaloblastic anemia; neural tube defects	Goat milk deficient; drug antagonists; heat inactivates	Liver, greens, vegetables, cereals, cheese
Ascorbic acid (C)	Reducing agent; collagen metabolism	*Scurvy:* irritability, purpura, bleeding gums, periosteal hemorrhage, aching bones	May improve tyrosine metabolism in preterm infants	Citrus fruits, green vegetables; cooking destroys it
FAT SOLUBLE				
A	Epithelial cell integrity; vision	Night blindness, xerophthalmia, Bitot spots, follicular hyperkeratosis; immune defects	Common with protein-calorie malnutrition; malabsorption	Liver, milk, eggs, green and yellow vegetables, fruits
D	Maintain serum calcium, phosphorus levels	*Rickets:* reduced bone mineralization	Prohormone of 25- and 1,25-vitamin D	Fortified milk, cheese, liver; sunlight
E	Antioxidant	Hemolysis in preterm infants; areflexia, ataxia, ophthalmoplegia	May benefit patients with G6PD deficiency	Seeds, vegetables, germ oils, grains
K	Post-translation carboxylation of clotting factors II, VII, IX, X and proteins C, S	Prolonged prothrombin time; hemorrhage; elevated protein induced in vitamin K absence (PIVKA)	Malabsorption; breastfed infants	Liver, green vegetables; made by intestinal flora

CoA, Coenzyme A; *FAD,* flavin adenine dinucleotide; *G6PD,* glucose-6-phosphate dehydrogenase; *NAD,* nicotinamide adenine dinucleotide.
*Biotinidase deficiency.

Vitamin B6

Vitamin B_6 refers to three naturally occurring pyridines: pyridoxine (pyridoxol), pyridoxal, and pyridoxamine. The phosphates of the latter two pyridines are metabolically and functionally related and are converted in the liver to the coenzyme form, pyridoxal phosphate. The metabolic functions of vitamin B_6 include interconversion reactions of amino acids, conversion of tryptophan to niacin and serotonin, metabolic reactions in the brain, carbohydrate metabolism, immune development, and the biosynthesis of heme and prostaglandins. The pyridoxal and pyridoxamine forms of the vitamin are destroyed by heat; heat treatment was responsible for vitamin B_6 deficiency and seizures in infants fed improperly processed formulas. Goat's milk is deficient in vitamin B_6.

Dietary deprivation or malabsorption of vitamin B_6 in children results in hypochromic microcytic anemia, vomiting, diarrhea, failure to thrive, listlessness, hyperirritability, and seizures. Children receiving isoniazid or penicillamine may require additional vitamin B_6 because the drug binds to the vitamin. Vitamin B_6 is unusual as a water-soluble vitamin in that very large doses ($\geq$500 mg/day) have been associated with a sensory neuropathy.

Folate

Decision-Making Algorithms
Available @ StudentConsult.com

Anemia
Neutropenia

Table 31-3	Treatment of Vitamin Deficiencies	
	CLINICAL FEATURES	**SUGGESTED DOSES**
Vitamin A	Severe deficiency with xerophthalmia	Infants: 7,500–15,000 U/day IM, followed by oral 5000–10,000 U/day for 10 days. Children 1–8 yr of age: oral 5,000–10,000 U/kg/day for 5 days or until recovery. Children >8 yr of age and adults: oral 500,000 U/day for 3 days; then 50,000 U/day for 14 days; then 10,000–20,000 U/day for 2 mo.
	Deficiency without corneal changes	Infants <1 yr of age: 100,000 U/day orally, q4–6mo. Children 1–8 yr of age: 200,000 U/day orally, q4–6mo. Children >8 yr and adults: 100,000 U/day for 3 days, followed by 50,000 U/day for 10 days.
	Deficiency	IM given only to those patients with malabsorption in whom oral dosing is not possible. Infants: 7,500–15,000 U/day for 10 days. Children 1–8 yr of age: 17,500–35,000 U/day for 10 days. Children >8 yr of age and adults: 100,000 U/day for 3 days, then 50,000 U/day for 14 days. Give follow-up oral multivitamin that contains vitamin A: LBW infants: no dose established, children ≤8 years of age: 5,000–10,000 U/day, children >8 yr of age and adults: 10,000–20,000 U daily.
	Malabsorption syndrome (prophylaxis)	Children >8 yr of age and adults: oral 10,000–50,000 U/day of water-miscible product.
	Cystic fibrosis	1,500–10,000 U/day prophylaxis (CF Foundation).
	Measles	WHO recommendations: single dose, repeating the dose next day and at 4 wk for children with eye findings: 6 mo to 1 yr of age: 100,000 U; >1 yr of age: 200,000 U.
Vitamin D	Liver disease	4,000–8,000 U/day ergocalciferol.
	Malabsorption	1000 U/day ergocalciferol
	Nutritional rickets and osteomalacia	Ergocalciferol: children and adults with normal absorption: 1,000–5,000 U/day. Children with malabsorption: 10,000–25,000 U/day. Adults with malabsorption: 10,000–300,000 U/day.
	Renal disease and failure	Ergocalciferol: child: 4,000–40,000 U/day; adults: 20,000 U/day.
	Cystic fibrosis	Ergocalciferol: 400–800 U/day PO (CF Foundation).
	Hypoparathyroidism	Children: 50,000–200,000 U/day ergocalciferol and calcium supplements. Adults: 25,000–200,000 U/day ergocalciferol and calcium supplements.
	Vitamin D-dependent rickets	Children: 3000–5000 U/day ergocalciferol; max: 60,000 U/day. Adults: 10,000–60,000 U/day ergocalciferol.
	Vitamin D-resistant rickets	Children: initial 40,000–80,000 U/day with phosphate supplements, daily dosage is increased at 3- to 4-mo intervals in 10,000–20,000 U increments. Adults: 10,000–60,000 U/day with phosphate supplements.
Vitamin E	Premature infant, neonates, infants of low birth weight	D–α–tocopherol: 25–50 U/day for 1 wk orally.
	Fat malabsorption and liver disease	10–25 U/kg/day of water–miscible vitamin E preparation.
	Cystic fibrosis	<1 yr of age: 25–50 U/day; 1–2 years of age: 100 U/day; >2 yr of age: 100 U/day bid or 200 U daily orally (CF Foundation).
	Sickle cell disease	450 U/day orally.
	β-Thalassemia	750 U/day orally.
Vitamin K	Hemorrhagic disease of the newborn	Phytonadione: 0.5–1.0 mg SC or IM as prophylaxis within 1 hr of birth, may repeat 6–8 hours later; 1–2 mg/day as treatment.
	Deficiency	Infants and children: 2.5–5 mg/day orally, or 1–2 mg/dose SC, IM, IV as a single dose; adults: 5–25 mg/day or 10 mg IM, IV.
	Cystic fibrosis	2.5 mg, twice a week (CF Foundation).
Folate, folic acid, and folacin	Deficiency	Infants: 50 µg daily. Children 1–10 yr of age: 1 mg/day initially, then 0.1–0.4 mg/day as maintenance. Children >11 yr of age and adults: 1 mg/day initially, then 0.5 mg/day as maintenance.
	Hemolytic anemia	May require higher doses than those listed previously.
Niacin	Pellagra	Children: 50–100 mg tid. Adults: 50–100 mg/day, max 100 mg/day.

Continued

Table 31-3	Treatment of Vitamin Deficiencies—cont'd	
	CLINICAL FEATURES	**SUGGESTED DOSES**
Pyridoxine (B_6)	Seizures	Neonates and infants: initial 50–100 mg/day orally, IM, IV, SC.
	Drug-induced deficiencies	Children: 10–50 mg/day as treatment, 1–2 mg/kg/day as prophylaxis.
		Adults: 100–200 mg/day as treatment, 25–100 mg/day as prophylaxis.
	Dietary deficiency	Children: 5–25 mg/day for 3 wk, then 1.5–2.5 mg/day in a multivitamin product.
		Adults: 10–20 mg/day for 3 wk.
Riboflavin (B_2)		Children: 2.5–10 mg/day in divided doses.
		Adults: 5–30 mg/day in divided doses.
Thiamine (B_1)	Beriberi: critically ill	Children: 10–25 mg/day IM or IV.
		Adults: 5–30 mg/dose IM, IV tid, then 5–30 mg/day orally in a single or three divided doses for 1 mo.
	Beriberi: not critically ill	Children: 10–50 mg/day orally for 2 wk, then 5–10 mg/day for 1 mo.
	Metabolic disease	Adults: 10–20 mg/day orally.
	Wernicke encephalopathy	Adults: initially 100 mg IV, then 50–100 mg/day IM/IV until eating a balanced diet.
Cyanocobalamin (B_{12})	Nutritional deficiency	Intranasal gel: 500 µg once a wk.
		Orally: 25–250 µg/wk.
	Anemia	Give IM or deep SC; oral route not recommended because of poor absorption and IV route not recommended because of more rapid elimination.
	Pernicious anemia	If evidence of neurologic involvement in neonates and infants (congenital), 1,000 µg/day IM, SC, for at least 2 wk, and then maintenance, 50–100 µg/mo or 100 µg/day for 6–7 days. If clinical improvement, give 100 µg every other day for 7 doses, then every 3–4 days for 2–3 wk, followed by 100 µg/mo for life. Administer with folic acid if needed (1 mg/day for 1 mo concomitantly).
		Children: 30–50 µg/day for 2 or more wk (total dose of 1000 µg) IM, SC, then 100 µg/mo as maintenance.
		Adults: 100 µg/day for 6–7 days; if improvement, administer same dose on alternate days for 7 doses, then every 3–4 days for 2–3 wk. Once hematologic values are normal, give maintenance doses of 100 µg/mo parenterally.
	Hematologic remission	No evidence of neurologic involvement: use intranasal gel: 500 µg per wk.
	Vitamin B_{12} deficiency	Children with neurologic signs: 100 µg/day for 10–15 days (total dose of 1–1.5 mg), then 1–2/wk for several mo and taper to 60 µg/mo.
		Children with hematologic signs: 10–50 µg/day for 5–10 days, followed by 100–250 µg/day every 2–4 wk.
		Adults: 30 µg/day for 5–10 days, followed by maintenance doses of 100–200 µg/mo.
Ascorbic acid	Scurvy	Children: 100–300 mg/day in divided doses orally, IM, IV, or SC for several days.
		Adults: 100–250 mg/day one to two times/day.

Data from Lexi-Comp Inc., Hudson, Ohio, 2004; table from Kronel S, Mascarenhas: Vitamin deficiencies and excesses. In Burg FD, Ingelfinger JR, Polin RA, Gershon AA, editors: Current Pediatric Therapy, Philadelphia, 2006, Elsevier, Table 3, pp 104–105.
bid, Two times per day; CF, cystic fibrosis; IM, intramuscular; IV, intravenous; LBW, low birth weight; PO, by mouth; q, every; SC, subcutaneous; tid, three times per day; WHO, World Health Organization.

A variety of chemical forms of folate are nutritionally active. Folate functions in transport of single-carbon fragments in synthesis of nucleic acids and for normal metabolism of certain amino acids and in conversion of homocysteine to methionine. Food sources include green leafy vegetables, oranges, and whole grains; folate fortification of grains is now routine in the United States.

Folate deficiency, characterized by **hypersegmented neutrophils**, **macrocytic anemia**, and glossitis, may result from a low dietary intake, malabsorption, or vitamin-drug interactions. Deficiency can develop within a few weeks of birth because infants require 10 times as much folate as adults relative to body weight but have scant stores of folate in the newborn period. Folate is particularly heat labile. Heat-sterilizing home-prepared formula can decrease the folate content by half. Evaporated milk and goat's milk are low in folate. Patients with chronic hemolysis (sickle cell anemia, thalassemia) may require extra folate to avoid deficiency because of the relatively high requirement of the vitamin to support erythropoiesis. Other conditions with risk of deficiency include pregnancy, alcoholism, and treatment with anticonvulsants (phenytoin) or antimetabolites (methotrexate). First occurrence and recurrence of **neural tube defects** are reduced significantly by maternal supplementation during embryogenesis. Because closure of the neural tube occurs before usual recognition of pregnancy, all women of reproductive age are recommended to have a folate intake of at least 400 µg/day as prophylaxis.

Vitamin B_{12}

Decision-Making Algorithms
Available @ StudentConsult.com

Anemia
Neutropenia

Vitamin B_{12} is one of the most complex of the vitamin molecules, containing an atom of cobalt held in a *corrin ring* (similar to that of iron in hemoglobin). The cobalt ion is at the active center of the ring and serves as the site for attachment of alkyl groups during their transfer. The vitamin functions in single-carbon transfers and is intimately related to folate function and interconversions. Vitamin B_{12} is essential for normal lipid and carbohydrate metabolism in energy production and in protein biosynthesis and nucleic acid synthesis.

In contrast to other water-soluble vitamins, absorption of vitamin B_{12} is complex, involving cleavage of the vitamin from dietary protein and binding to a glycoprotein called *intrinsic factor*, which is secreted by the gastric mucosa (parietal cells). The cobalamin–intrinsic factor complex is efficiently absorbed from the distal ileum.

As vitamin B_{12} is absorbed into the portal circulation, it is transported bound to a specific protein, transcobalamin II. Its large stores in the liver also are unusual for a water-soluble vitamin. Efficient enterohepatic circulation normally protects from deficiency for months to years. Dietary sources of the vitamin are animal products only. Strict vegetarians should take a vitamin B_{12} supplement.

Vitamin B_{12} deficiency in children is rare. Early diagnosis and treatment of this disorder in childhood are important because of the danger of irreversible neurologic damage. Most cases in childhood result from a specific defect in absorption (see Table 31-2). Such defects include **congenital pernicious anemia** (absent intrinsic factor), **juvenile pernicious anemia** (autoimmune), and deficiency of transcobalamin II transport. Gastric or intestinal resection and small bowel bacterial overgrowth also cause vitamin B_{12} deficiency. Exclusively breastfed infants ingest adequate vitamin B_{12} unless the mother is a strict vegetarian without supplementation.

Depression of serum vitamin B_{12} and the appearance of hypersegmented neutrophils and macrocytosis (indistinguishable from folate deficiency) are early clinical manifestations of deficiency. Vitamin B_{12} deficiency also causes **neurologic manifestations**, including depression, peripheral neuropathy, posterior spinal column signs, dementia, and eventual coma. The neurologic signs do not occur in folate deficiency, but administration of folate may mask the hematologic signs of vitamin B_{12} deficiency, while the neurologic manifestations progress. Patients with vitamin B_{12} deficiency also have increased urine levels of methylmalonic acid. Most cases of vitamin B_{12} deficiency in infants and children are not of dietary origin and require treatment throughout life. Maintenance therapy consists of repeated monthly intramuscular injections, although a form of vitamin B_{12} is administered intranasally.

FAT-SOLUBLE VITAMINS

Fat-soluble vitamins generally have stores in the body, and dietary deficiencies generally develop more slowly than for water-soluble vitamins. Absorption of fat-soluble vitamins depends on normal fat intake, digestion, and absorption. The complexity of normal fat absorption and the potential for perturbation in many disease states explains the more common occurrence of deficiencies of these vitamins.

Vitamin A

Decision-Making Algorithms
Available @ StudentConsult.com

Hepatomegaly
Hypercalcemia

The basic constituent of the vitamin A group is retinol. Ingested plant carotene or animal tissue retinol esters release retinol after hydrolysis by pancreatic and intestinal enzymes. Chylomicron-transported retinol esters are stored in the liver as retinol palmitate. Retinol is transported from the liver to target tissues by retinol-binding protein, releasing free retinol to the target tissues. The kidney then excretes the retinol-binding protein. Diseases of the kidney diminish excretion of retinol-binding protein, whereas liver parenchymal disease or malnutrition lowers the synthesis of retinol-binding protein. Specific cellular binding proteins facilitate the uptake of retinol by target tissues. In the eye, retinol is metabolized to form **rhodopsin**; the action of light on rhodopsin is the first step of the visual process. Retinol also influences the growth and differentiation of epithelia. The clinical manifestations of vitamin A deficiency in humans appear as a group of ocular signs termed **xerophthalmia.** The earliest symptom is **night blindness**, which is followed by **xerosis** of the conjunctiva and cornea. Untreated, xerophthalmia can result in ulceration, necrosis, keratomalacia, and a permanent corneal scar. Clinical and subclinical vitamin A deficiencies are associated with **immunodeficiency**; increased risk of infection, especially measles; and increased risk of mortality, especially in developing nations. Xerophthalmia and vitamin A deficiency should be urgently treated. Hypervitaminosis A also has serious sequelae, including headaches, pseudotumor cerebri, hepatotoxicity, and teratogenicity.

Vitamin E

Eight naturally occurring compounds have vitamin E activity. The most active of these, α-tocopherol, accounts for 90% of the vitamin E present in human tissues and is commercially available as an acetate or succinate. Vitamin E acts as a biologic **antioxidant** by inhibiting the peroxidation of polyunsaturated fatty acids present in cell membranes. It scavenges free radicals generated by the reduction of molecular oxygen and by the action of oxidative enzymes.

Vitamin E deficiency occurs in children with fat malabsorption secondary to liver disease, untreated celiac disease, cystic fibrosis, and abetalipoproteinemia. In these children, without vitamin E supplementation, a syndrome of progressive **sensory and motor neuropathy** develops; the first sign of deficiency is loss of deep tendon reflexes. Deficient preterm infants at 1 to 2 months of age have hemolytic anemia characterized by an elevated reticulocyte count, an increased sensitivity of the erythrocytes to hemolysis in hydrogen peroxide, peripheral edema, and thrombocytosis. All the abnormalities are corrected after oral, lipid, or water-soluble vitamin E therapy.

Vitamin D

Decision-Making Algorithms
Available @ StudentConsult.com

Hypertension
Hypocalcemia

Cholecalciferol (vitamin D_3) is the mammalian form of vitamin D and is produced by ultraviolet irradiation of inactive precursors in the skin. Ergocalciferol (vitamin D_2) is derived from plants. Vitamin D_2 and vitamin D_3 require further metabolism to become active. They are of equivalent potency. Clothing, lack of sunlight exposure, and skin pigmentation decrease generation of vitamin D in the epidermis and dermis.

Vitamin D (D_2 and D_3) is metabolized in the liver to calcidiol, or 25-hydroxyvitamin D (25-[OH]-D); this metabolite, which has little intrinsic activity, is transported by a plasma-binding globulin to the kidney, where it is converted to the most active metabolite calcitriol, or 1,25-dihydroxyvitamin D (1,25-[OH]$_2$-D). The action of 1,25-(OH)$_2$-D results in a decrease in the concentration of messenger RNA (mRNA) for collagen in bone and an increase in the concentration of mRNA for vitamin D–dependent calcium-binding protein in the intestine (directly mediating increased intestinal calcium transport). The antirachitic action of vitamin D probably is mediated by provision of appropriate concentrations of calcium and phosphate in the extracellular space of bone and by enhanced intestinal absorption of these minerals. Vitamin D also may have a direct anabolic effect on bone. 1,25-(OH)$_2$-D has direct feedback to the parathyroid gland and inhibits secretion of parathyroid hormone.

Vitamin D deficiency appears as **rickets** in children and as **osteomalacia** in postpubertal adolescents. Inadequate direct sun exposure and vitamin D intake are sufficient causes, but other factors, such as various drugs (phenobarbital, phenytoin) and malabsorption, may increase the risk of development of vitamin-deficiency rickets. Breastfed infants, especially those with dark-pigmented skin, are at risk for vitamin D deficiency.

The pathophysiology of rickets results from defective bone growth, especially at the epiphyseal cartilage matrix, which fails to mineralize. The uncalcified osteoid results in a wide, irregular zone of poorly supported tissue, the rachitic metaphysis. This soft, rather than hardened, zone produces many of the skeletal deformities through compression and lateral bulging or flaring of the ends of bones.

The **clinical manifestations** of rickets are most common during the first 2 years of life and may become evident only after several months of a vitamin D–deficient diet. **Craniotabes** is caused by thinning of the outer table of the skull, which when compressed feels like a Ping-Pong ball to the touch. Enlargement of the costochondral junction (**rachitic rosary**) and thickening of the wrists and ankles may be palpated. The anterior fontanelle is enlarged, and its closure may be delayed. In advanced rickets, scoliosis and exaggerated lordosis may be present. Bowlegs or knock-knees may be evident in older infants, and greenstick fractures may be observed in long bones.

The **diagnosis** of rickets is based on a history of poor vitamin D intake and little exposure to direct ultraviolet sunlight. The serum calcium usually is normal but may be low; the serum phosphorus level usually is reduced, and serum alkaline phosphatase activity is elevated. When serum calcium levels decline to less than 7.5 mg/dL, tetany may occur. Levels of 24,25-(OH)$_2$-D are undetectable, and serum 1,25-(OH)2-D levels are commonly less than 7 ng/mL, although 1,25-(OH)$_2$-D levels also may be normal. The best measure of vitamin D status is the level of 25-(OH)-D. Characteristic **radiographic** changes of the distal ulna and radius include widening; concave cupping; and frayed, poorly demarcated ends. The increased space seen between the distal ends of the radius and ulna and the metacarpal bones is the enlarged, nonossified metaphysis.

Breastfed infants born of mothers with adequate vitamin D stores usually maintain adequate serum vitamin D levels for at least 2 months, but rickets may develop subsequently if these infants are not exposed to the sun or do not receive supplementary vitamin D. The American Academy of Pediatrics recommends vitamin D supplementation of all breastfed infants in the amount of 400 IU/day, started soon after birth and given until the infant is taking more than 1000 mL/day of formula or vitamin D–fortified milk (for age >1 year). Toxic effects of excessive chronic vitamin D may include hypercalcemia, muscle weakness, polyuria, and nephrocalcinosis.

Vitamin K

Decision-Making Algorithm
Available @ StudentConsult.com

Bleeding

The plant form of vitamin K is phylloquinone, or vitamin K_1. Another form is menaquinone, or vitamin K_2, one of a series of compounds with unsaturated side chains synthesized by intestinal bacteria. Plasma factors II (prothrombin), VII, IX, and X in the cascade of blood coagulation factors depend on vitamin K for synthesis and for post-translational conversion of their precursor proteins. The post-translational conversion of glutamyl residues to carboxyglutamic acid residues of a prothrombin molecule creates effective calcium-binding sites, making the protein active.

Other vitamin K–dependent proteins include proteins C, S, and Z in plasma and γ-carboxyglutamic acid–containing proteins in several tissues. Bone contains a major vitamin K–dependent protein, osteocalcin, and lesser amounts of other glutamic acid–containing proteins.

Phylloquinone is absorbed from the intestine and transported by chylomicrons. The rarity of dietary vitamin K deficiency in humans with normal intestinal function suggests that the absorption of menaquinones is possible. Vitamin K deficiency has been observed in subjects with impaired fat absorption caused by obstructive jaundice, pancreatic insufficiency, and celiac disease; often these problems are combined with the use of antibiotics that change intestinal flora.

Hemorrhagic disease of the newborn, a disease more common among breastfed infants, occurs in the first few weeks of life. It is rare in infants who receive prophylactic intramuscular vitamin K on the first day of life. Hemorrhagic disease of the newborn usually is marked by generalized ecchymoses, gastrointestinal hemorrhage, or bleeding from a circumcision or umbilical stump; intracranial hemorrhage can occur, but

Table 31-4	Characteristics of Trace Mineral Deficiencies			
MINERAL	**FUNCTION**	**MANIFESTATIONS OF DEFICIENCY**	**COMMENTS**	**SOURCES**
Iron	Heme-containing macromolecules (e.g., hemoglobin, cytochrome, and myoglobin)	Anemia, spoon nails, reduced muscle and mental performance	History of pica, cow's milk, gastrointestinal bleeding	Meat, liver, grains, legumes
Copper	Redox reactions (e.g., cytochrome oxidase)	Hypochromic anemia, neutropenia, osteoporosis, hypotonia, hypoproteinemia	Inborn error, Menkes kinky hair syndrome	Liver, nuts, grains, legumes, chocolate
Zinc	Metalloenzymes (e.g., alkaline phosphatase, carbonic anhydrase, DNA polymerase); wound healing	*Acrodermatitis enteropathica*: poor growth, acro-orificial rash, alopecia, delayed sexual development, hypogeusia, infection	Protein-calorie malnutrition; weaning; malabsorption syndromes	Meat, grains, legumes
Selenium	Antioxidant; glutathione peroxidase	Keshan cardiomyopathy in China	Endemic areas; long-term TPN without Se	Meat, vegetables
Chromium	Insulin cofactor	Poor weight gain, glucose intolerance, neuropathy	Protein-calorie malnutrition, long-term TPN without Cr	Yeast, breads
Fluoride	Strengthening of dental enamel	Caries	Supplementation during tooth growth, narrow therapeutic range, fluorosis may cause staining of the teeth	Seafood, fortified water
Iodine	Thyroxine, triiodothyronine production	Simple endemic goiter *Myxedematous cretinism*: congenital hypothyroidism *Neurologic cretinism*: mental retardation, deafness, spasticity, normal thyroxine level at birth	Endemic in New Guinea, the Congo; endemic in Great Lakes area before use of iodized salt	Seafood, iodized salt

TPN, Total parenteral nutrition.

is uncommon. The American Academy of Pediatrics recommends that parenteral vitamin K (0.5 to 1 mg) be given to all newborns shortly after birth.

MINERALS

The major minerals are those that require intakes of more than 100 mg/day and contribute at least 0.1% of total body weight. There are seven essential major minerals: calcium, phosphorus, magnesium, sodium, potassium, chloride, and sulfur. Ten trace minerals, which constitute less than 0.1% of body weight, have essential physiologic roles. Characteristics of trace mineral deficiencies are listed in Table 31-4.

Calcium

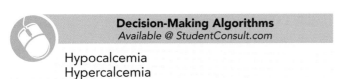

Decision-Making Algorithms
Available @ StudentConsult.com

Hypocalcemia
Hypercalcemia

Calcium is the most abundant major mineral. Ninety-nine percent of calcium is in the skeleton; the remaining 1% is in extracellular fluids, intracellular compartments, and cell membranes. The nonskeletal calcium has a role in nerve conduction, muscle contraction, blood clotting, and membrane permeability. There are two distinct bone calcium phosphate pools—a large, crystalline form and a smaller, amorphous phase. Bone calcium constantly turns over, with concurrent

bone reabsorption and formation. Approximately half of **bone mineral accretion** occurs during adolescence. Bone mineral density peaks in early adulthood and is influenced by prior and concurrent dietary calcium intake, exercise, and hormone status (testosterone, estrogen).

Calcium intake can come from a variety of sources, with dairy products providing the most common and concentrated source. The calcium equivalent of 1 cup of milk (about 300 mg of calcium) is ¾ cup of plain yogurt, 1.5 oz of cheddar cheese, 2 cups of ice cream, ⅕ cup of almonds, or 2.5 oz of sardines. Other sources of calcium include some leafy green vegetables (broccoli, kale, collards); lime-processed tortillas; calcium-precipitated tofu; and calcium-fortified juices, cereals, and breads.

There is no classic calcium deficiency syndrome because blood and cell levels are closely regulated. The body can mobilize skeletal calcium and increase the absorptive efficiency of dietary calcium. **Osteoporosis** that occurs in childhood is related to protein-calorie malnutrition, vitamin C deficiency, steroid therapy, endocrine disorders, immobilization and disuse, osteogenesis imperfecta, or calcium deficiency (in premature infants). It is believed that the primary method of prevention of **postmenopausal osteoporosis** is to ensure maximum peak bone mass by providing optimal calcium intake during childhood and adolescence. Bone mineral status can be monitored by dual-energy x-ray absorptiometry.

No adverse effects are observed in adults with dietary calcium intakes of 2.5 g/day. There is concern that higher intakes may increase the risk of urinary stone formation, constipation, and decreased renal function and may inhibit intestinal absorption of other minerals (iron, zinc).

Iron

Decision-Making Algorithms
Available @ StudentConsult.com

Gastrointestinal Bleeding
Anemia
Failure to Thrive

Iron, the most abundant trace mineral, is used in the synthesis of hemoglobin, myoglobin, and enzyme iron. Body iron content is regulated primarily through modulation of iron absorption, which depends on the state of body iron stores, the form and amount of iron in foods, and the mixture of foods in the diet. There are two categories of iron in food. The first is *heme iron,* present in hemoglobin and myoglobin, which is supplied by meat and rarely accounts for more than one fourth of the iron ingested by infants. The absorption of heme iron is relatively efficient and is not influenced by other constituents of the diet. The second category is **nonheme iron,** which represents the preponderance of iron intake consumed by infants and exists in the form of iron salts. The absorption of nonheme iron is influenced by the composition of consumed foods. Enhancers of nonheme iron absorption are ascorbic acid, meat, fish, and poultry. Inhibitors are bran, polyphenols (including the tannates in tea), and phytic acid, a compound found in legumes and whole grains. The percent intestinal absorption of the small amount of iron in human milk is 10%; 4% is absorbed from iron-fortified cow's milk formula and from iron-fortified infant dry cereals.

In a normal term infant, there is little change in total body iron and little need for exogenous iron before 4 months of age. Iron deficiency is rare in term infants during the first 4 months, unless there has been substantial blood loss (see Chapter 62). After about 4 months of age, iron reserves become marginal, and, unless exogenous sources of iron are provided, the infant becomes progressively at risk for anemia as the iron requirement to support erythropoiesis and growth increases (see Chapter 150). Premature or low birth weight infants have a lower amount of stored iron because significant amounts of iron are transferred from the mother in the third trimester. In addition, their postnatal iron needs are greater because of rapid rates of growth and when frequent phlebotomy occurs. Iron needs can be met by supplementation (ferrous sulfate) or by iron-containing complementary foods. Under normal circumstances, iron-fortified formula should be the only alternative to breast milk in infants younger than 1 year of age. Premature infants fed human milk may develop iron deficiency anemia earlier unless they receive iron supplements. Formula-fed preterm infants should receive iron-fortified formula.

In older children, iron deficiency may result from inadequate iron intake with excessive cow's milk intake or from intake of foods with poor iron bioavailability. Iron deficiency also can result from blood loss from such sources as menses or gastric ulceration. Iron deficiency affects many tissues (muscle and central nervous system) in addition to producing anemia. **Iron deficiency** and **anemia** have been associated with lethargy and decreased work capacity and **impaired neurocognitive development,** the deficits of which may be irreversible when onset is in the first 2 years of life.

The diagnosis of iron deficiency anemia is established by the presence of a microcytic hypochromic anemia, low serum ferritin levels, low serum iron levels, reduced transferrin saturation, normal to elevated red blood cell width distribution, and enhanced iron-binding capacity. The mean corpuscular volume and red blood cell indices are reduced, and the reticulocyte count is low. Iron deficiency may be present without anemia. Clinical manifestations are noted in Table 31-4.

Treatment of iron deficiency anemia includes changes in the diet to provide adequate iron and the administration of 2 to 6 mg iron/kg/24 hr (as ferrous sulfate) divided bid or tid. Reticulocytosis is noted within 3 to 7 days of starting treatment. Oral treatment should be continued for 5 months. Rarely, intramuscular or intravenous iron therapy is needed if oral iron cannot be given. Parenteral therapy carries the risk of anaphylaxis and should be administered according to a strict protocol, including a test dose.

Zinc

Decision-Making Algorithms
Available @ StudentConsult.com

Diarrhea
Vesicles and Bullae

Zinc is the second most abundant trace mineral and is important in protein metabolism and synthesis, in nucleic acid metabolism, and in stabilization of cell membranes. Zinc functions as a cofactor for more than 200 enzymes and is essential to numerous cellular metabolic functions. Adequate zinc status is especially crucial during periods of growth and for tissue proliferation (immune system, wound healing, skin and gastrointestinal tract integrity); physiologic functions for which zinc is essential include normal growth, sexual maturation, and immune function.

Dietary zinc is absorbed (20% to 40%) in the duodenum and proximal small intestine. The best dietary sources of zinc are animal products, including human milk, from which it is readily absorbed. Whole grains and legumes also contain moderate amounts of zinc, but phytic acid inhibits absorption from these sources. On a global basis, poor bioavailability secondary to phytic acid is thought to be a more important factor than low intake in the widespread occurrence of zinc deficiency. Excretion of zinc occurs from the gastrointestinal tract. In the presence of ongoing losses, such as in chronic diarrhea, requirements can drastically increase.

Zinc deficiency dwarfism syndrome was first described in a group of children in the Middle East with low levels of zinc in their hair, poor appetite, diminished taste acuity, hypogonadism, and short stature. Zinc supplementation reduces morbidity and mortality from **diarrhea** and **pneumonia** and enhances growth in developing countries. Mild to moderate zinc deficiency is considered to be highly prevalent in developing countries, particularly in populations with high rates of **stunting**. Mild zinc deficiency occurs in older breastfed infants without adequate zinc intake from complementary foods or in young children with poor total or bioavailable zinc intake in the general diet. A high infectious burden also may increase the risk of zinc deficiency in developing countries. Acute, acquired severe zinc deficiency occurs in patients receiving total parenteral nutrition without zinc supplementation and in premature infants fed human milk without fortification. **Clinical manifestations** of mild zinc deficiency include anorexia, growth faltering, and immune impairment. Moderately severe manifestations include delayed sexual maturation, rough skin, and hepatosplenomegaly. The signs of severe deficiency include acral and periorificial erythematous, scaling dermatitis; growth and immune impairment; diarrhea; mood changes; alopecia; night blindness; and photophobia.

Diagnosis of zinc deficiency is challenging. Plasma zinc concentration is most commonly used, but levels are frequently normal in conditions of mild deficiency; levels in moderate to severe deficiency are typically less than 60 μg/dL. Acute infection also can result in depression of circulating zinc levels. The standard for the diagnosis of deficiency is response to a trial of supplementation, with outcomes such as improved linear growth or weight gain, improved appetite, and improved immune function. Because there is no pharmacologic effect of zinc on these functions, a positive response to supplementation is considered evidence of a preexisting deficiency. Clinically an empirical trial of zinc supplementation (1 μg/kg/day) is a safe and reasonable approach in situations in which deficiency is considered possible.

Acrodermatitis enteropathica is an autosomal recessive disorder that begins within 2 to 4 weeks after infants have been weaned from breast milk. It is characterized by an acute perioral and perianal dermatitis, alopecia, and failure to thrive. The disease is caused by severe zinc deficiency from a specific defect of intestinal zinc absorption. Plasma zinc levels are markedly reduced, and serum alkaline phosphatase activity is low. **Treatment** is with high-dose oral zinc supplements. A relatively uncommon condition associated with presentation of severe zinc deficiency is due to a defect in the secretion of zinc from the mammary gland, resulting in abnormally low milk zinc concentrations. Breastfed infants, especially those born prematurely, present with classic signs of zinc deficiency: growth failure, diarrhea, and dermatitis. Because there is no defect in the infant's ability to absorb zinc, treatment consists of supplementing the infant with zinc for the duration of breastfeeding, which can be successfully continued. Subsequent infants born to the mother will also need zinc supplementation if breastfed. Zinc is relatively nontoxic. Excess intake produces nausea, emesis, abdominal pain, headache, vertigo, and seizures.

Fluoride

Dental enamel is strengthened when fluoride is substituted for hydroxyl ions in the hydroxyapatite crystalline mineral matrix of the enamel. The resulting fluoroapatite is more resistant to chemical and physical damage. Fluoride is incorporated into the enamel during the mineralization stages of tooth formation and by surface interaction after the tooth has erupted. Fluoride is similarly incorporated into bone mineral and may protect against osteoporosis later in life.

Because of concern about the risk of **fluorosis**, infants should not receive fluoride supplements before 6 months of age. Commercial formulas are made with defluoridated water and contain small amounts of fluoride. The fluoride content of human milk is low and is not influenced significantly by maternal intake. Practitioners should evaluate all potential fluoride sources and conduct a caries risk assessment before prescribing fluoride supplementation.

Suggested Readings

Kliegman RM, Stanton B, St. Geme J, et al: *Nelson textbook of pediatrics*, ed 19, Philadelphia, 2011, Saunders. Chap. 41–51.

Eidelman AI, Schanler RJ: American Academy of Pediatrics Section on Breastfeeding. Breastfeeding and the Use of Human Milk, *Pediatrics* 129(3):827–841, 2012.

Centers for Disease Control and Prevention: Racial and ethnic differences in breastfeeding initiation and duration, by state National Immunization Survey, United States, 2004–2008, *MMWR Morb Mortal Wkly Rep* 59(11):327–334, 2010.

http://www.nal.usda.gov

http://www.choosemyplate.gov

www.pediatrics.org/cgi/content/full/102/3/e38

Gribble JN, Murray NJ, Menotti EP: Reconsidering childhood undernutrition: can birth spacing make a difference? An analysis of the 2002–2003 El Salvador National Family Health Survey, *Matern Child Nutr* 5:49–63, 2009.

Boschert S, Robinson T: Fight obesity with specific, countable goals, *Pediatric News* 1, Oct 2012.

Grover Z, Ee LC: Protein energy malnutrition, *Pediatr Clin North Am* 56:1055–1068, 2009.

Krebs NF, Hambidge KM: Trace elements. In Duggan C, Watkins JB, Walker WA, editors: *Nutrition in pediatrics: basic science and clinical applications*, ed 4, Hamilton, Ontario, 2008, BC Decker, pp 67–82.

Penny ME: Protein-energy malnutrition: pathophysiology, clinical consequences, and treatment. In Duggan C, Watkins JB, Walker WA, editors: *Nutrition in pediatrics: basic science and clinical applications*, ed 4, Hamilton, Ontario, 2008, BC Decker, pp 127–142.

Wagner CL, Greer FR: Section on Breastfeeding and Committee on Nutrition, American Academy of Pediatrics: Prevention of rickets and vitamin D deficiency: new guidelines for vitamin D intake, *Pediatrics* 122:1142–1152, 2008.

Fluids and Electrolytes

Larry A. Greenbaum and Raed Bou-Matar

MAINTENANCE FLUID THERAPY

BODY COMPOSITION

Water is the most plentiful constituent of the human body. **Total body water** (TBW) as a percentage of body weight varies with age. The fetus has a high TBW, which gradually decreases to about 75% of birth weight for a term infant. Premature infants have a higher TBW content than term infants. During the first year of life, TBW decreases to about 60% of body weight and basically remains at this level until puberty. At puberty, the fat content of females increases more than that of males, who acquire more muscle mass than females. Because fat has low water content, and muscle has high water content, by the end of puberty TBW in males remains at 60%, but it decreases to 50% of body weight in females. During dehydration, TBW decreases and is a smaller percentage of body weight.

TBW has two main compartments: **intracellular fluid (ICF)** and **extracellular fluid (ECF)**. In the fetus and newborn, the ECF volume is larger than the ICF volume. The normal postnatal diuresis causes an immediate decrease in the ECF volume. This decrease in ECF volume is followed by continued expansion of the ICF volume because of cellular growth. By 1 year of age, the ratio of the ICF volume to the ECF volume approaches adult levels. The ECF volume is 20% to 25% of body weight, and the ICF volume is 30% to 40% of body weight (Fig. 32-1). With puberty, the increased muscle mass of males results in a higher ICF volume than in females.

The ECF is divided further into **plasma water** and **interstitial fluid** (see Fig. 32-1). Plasma water is about 5% of body weight. The blood volume, given a hematocrit of 40%, is usually 8% of body weight, although it is higher in newborns and young infants. The interstitial fluid, normally 15% of body weight, can increase dramatically in diseases associated with edema, such as heart failure, protein-losing enteropathy, liver failure, and nephrotic syndrome.

The composition of solutes in the ICF and ECF is different. Sodium and chloride are the dominant cation and anion in the ECF. Potassium is the most abundant cation in the ICF, and proteins, organic anions, and phosphate are the most plentiful anions in the ICF. The dissimilarity between the anions in the ICF and the ECF is determined largely by the presence of intracellular molecules that do not cross the cell membrane, the barrier separating the ECF and the ICF. In contrast, the difference in the distribution of cations—sodium and potassium—is due to the activity of the Na^+,K^+-ATPase pump, which extrudes sodium from cells in exchange for potassium.

REGULATION OF INTRAVASCULAR VOLUME AND OSMOLALITY

Proper cell functioning requires close regulation of plasma osmolality and intravascular volume; these are controlled by independent systems for water balance, which determines osmolality, and sodium balance, which determines volume status. Maintenance of a normal **osmolality** depends on control of water balance. Control of **volume status** depends on regulation of sodium balance.

The plasma osmolality is tightly controlled between 285 and 295 mOsm/kg through regulation of water intake and urinary water losses. A small increase in the plasma osmolality stimulates thirst. Urinary water losses are regulated by the secretion of **antidiuretic hormone** (ADH), which increases in response to an increasing plasma osmolality. ADH, by stimulating renal tubular reabsorption of water, decreases urinary water losses. Control of osmolality is subordinate to maintenance of an adequate intravascular volume. When significant volume depletion is present, ADH secretion and thirst are stimulated, regardless of the plasma osmolality.

Volume depletion and volume overload may cause significant morbidity and mortality. Because sodium is the principal extracellular cation and is restricted to the ECF, adequate body sodium is necessary for maintenance of intravascular volume. The kidney determines sodium balance because there is little homeostatic control of sodium intake, although salt craving occasionally occurs, typically in children with chronic renal salt loss. The kidney regulates sodium balance by altering the percentage of filtered sodium that is reabsorbed along the nephron. The **renin-angiotensin system** is an important regulator of renal sodium reabsorption and excretion. The juxtaglomerular apparatus produces renin in response to decreased *effective* intravascular volume. Renin cleaves angiotensinogen, producing angiotensin I, which angiotensin-converting enzyme converts into angiotensin II. The actions of angiotensin

Figure 32-1 Compartments of total body water, expressed as percentage of body weight, in an older child or adult. *(From Greenbaum LA: Pathophysiology of body fluids and fluid therapy. In Kliegman RM, Stanton, BF, St Geme JW, et al, editors: Nelson Textbook of Pediatrics, 19th ed. Philadelphia, 2011, Saunders, p 212.e1.)*

Table 32-1	Body Weight Method for Calculating Maintenance Fluid Volume and Rate	
BODY WEIGHT (KG)	**VOLUME PER DAY**	**HOURLY RATE**
0–10	100 mL/kg	4 mL/kg/h
11–20	1000 mL + 50 mL/kg for each 1 kg >10 kg	40 mL/h + 2 mL/kg/h × (wt − 10)
>20	1500 mL + 20 mL/kg for each 1 kg >20 kg*	60 mL/h + 1 mL/kg/h × (wt − 20)†

*The maximum total fluid per day is normally 2400 mL.
†The maximum fluid rate is normally 100 mL/hr.

maintenance therapy indefinitely; parenteral nutrition (see Chapter 34) should be used for children who cannot be fed enterally for more than a few days.

Daily water losses are measurable (urine and stool) and not measurable (*insensible losses* from the skin and lungs). Failure to replace these losses leads to a thirsty child and, ultimately, a dehydrated child. Table 32-1 provides a system for calculating **24-hour maintenance water** needs based on the patient's weight. Sodium and potassium are given in maintenance fluids to replace losses from urine and stool.

After calculation of water needs and electrolyte needs, children typically receive either 5% dextrose (D5) in ¼ normal saline (NS) plus 20 mEq/L of potassium chloride (KCl) or D5 in ½ NS plus 20 mEq/L of KCl. Children weighing less than 10 kg do best with the solution containing ¼ NS (38.5 mEq/L) because of their high water needs per kilogram. In contrast, larger children and adults may receive the solution with ½ NS (77 mEq/L). These guidelines assume that there is no disease process present that would require an adjustment in either the volume or the electrolyte composition of maintenance fluids. Children with renal insufficiency may be hyperkalemic or unable to excrete potassium and may not tolerate 20 mEq/L of KCl. In children with complicated pathophysiologic derangements, it may be necessary to adjust the electrolyte composition and rate of maintenance fluids empirically based on electrolyte measurements and assessment of fluid balance.

II include direct stimulation of the proximal tubule to increase sodium reabsorption and stimulation of the adrenal gland to increase aldosterone secretion, which increases sodium reabsorption in the distal nephron. In contrast, volume expansion stimulates the synthesis of **atrial natriuretic peptide**, which increases urinary sodium excretion.

MAINTENANCE FLUIDS

Maintenance intravenous (IV) fluids are used in children who cannot be fed enterally. Along with maintenance fluids, children may require concurrent **replacement fluids** if they have excessive **ongoing losses**, such as may occur with drainage from a nasogastric tube. In addition, if dehydration is present, the patient also needs to receive deficit replacement (see Chapter 33).

Maintenance fluids are composed of a solution of water, glucose, sodium, potassium, and chloride. This solution replaces electrolyte losses from the urine and stool, as well as water losses from the urine, stool, skin, and lungs. The glucose in maintenance fluids provides approximately 20% of the normal caloric needs of the patient. This percentage is enough to prevent the development of starvation ketoacidosis and diminishes the protein degradation that would occur if the patient received no calories.

Maintenance fluids do not provide adequate calories, protein, fat, minerals, or vitamins. Patients should not remain on

Chapter 33

DEHYDRATION AND REPLACEMENT THERAPY

REPLACEMENT THERAPY

There are three sources of normal water loss—the components of maintenance water (see Chapter 32): urine (60%), **insensible losses** from the skin and lungs (35%), and stool (5%) (Table 33-1). Sweating is not insensible and, in contrast to evaporative losses, sweat contains water and electrolytes.

Table 33-1	Components of Maintenance Water	
Urine		60%
Insensible losses (skin and lungs)		35%
Stool		5%

Table 33-2	Adjustments in Maintenance Water	
SOURCE	CAUSES OF INCREASED WATER NEEDS	CAUSES OF DECREASED WATER NEEDS
Skin	Radiant warmer Phototherapy Fever Sweat Burns	Mist tent Incubator (premature infants)
Lungs	Tachypnea Tracheostomy	Humidified ventilator Mist tent
Gastrointestinal	Diarrhea Emesis Nasogastric suction	
Renal	Polyuria	Oliguria/anuria
Miscellaneous	Surgical drain Third space losses	Hypothyroidism

A variety of clinical situations modify normal maintenance water balance (Table 33-2). Evaporative skin water losses can be higher in neonates, especially premature infants who are under radiant warmers or undergoing phototherapy. Burns can result in massive losses of water and electrolytes (see Chapter 44). Fever increases insensible losses. Tachypnea or a tracheostomy increases evaporative losses from the lungs.

The gastrointestinal tract is potentially a source of considerable water and electrolyte losses. A child who has large amounts of gastrointestinal losses should have these losses measured and replaced with an appropriate **replacement solution** (Table 33-3).

Urine output is normally the largest cause of *water* loss. Diseases such as renal failure and the syndrome of inappropriate antidiuretic hormone (SIADH) can lead to a decrease in urine volume. Maintenance fluids in a patient with oliguria or anuria produce fluid overload. In contrast, other conditions produce an increase in urine volume; these include the polyuric phase of acute tubular necrosis, diabetes mellitus, and diabetes insipidus. When the urine output is excessive, the patient must receive more than standard maintenance fluids to prevent dehydration.

The approach to decreased or increased urine output is similar (Table 33-4). Insensible losses are replaced by a solution that is administered at a rate one third of the normal maintenance rate. Placing the **anuric** child on "insensibles" theoretically maintains an even fluid balance, with the caveat that one third of maintenance fluid is only an *estimate* of insensible losses. This rate may need to be adjusted based on monitoring of the patient's weight and hydration status. An **oliguric** child needs to receive a urine replacement solution. Most children with **polyuria** (except for children with diabetes mellitus [see Chapter 171]) should be placed on insensible fluids plus urine replacement.

Table 33-3	Adjusting Fluid Therapy for Gastrointestinal Losses	
AVERAGE COMPOSITION	**APPROACH TO REPLACEMENT**	
DIARRHEA	REPLACEMENT OF ONGOING STOOL LOSSES	
Sodium: 55 mEq/L	Solution: 5% dextrose in ¼ normal saline + 20 mEq/L sodium bicarbonate + 20 mEq/L potassium chloride Replace stool mL/mL every 1–6 hr	
Potassium: 25 mEq/L		
Bicarbonate: 15 mEq/L		
GASTRIC FLUID	REPLACEMENT OF ONGOING GASTRIC LOSSES	
Sodium: 60 mEq/L	Solution: normal saline + 10 mEq/L potassium chloride Replace output mL/mL every 1–6 hr	
Potassium: 10 mEq/L		
Chloride: 90 mEq/L		

Table 33-4	Adjusting Fluid Therapy for Altered Renal Output	
OLIGURIA/ANURIA	**POLYURIA**	
Place the patient on insensible fluids (⅓ maintenance)	Place the patient on insensible fluids (⅓ maintenance)	
Replace urine output mL/mL with half normal saline	Measure urine electrolytes	
	Replace urine output mL/mL with a solution that is based on the measured urine electrolytes	

Output from surgical drains and chest tubes, when significant, should be measured and replaced. **Third space losses** manifest with edema and ascites and are due to a shift of fluid from the intravascular space into the interstitial space. Third space losses cannot be quantitated. Nonetheless, these losses can be large and lead to intravascular volume depletion, despite weight gain from edema or ascites. Replacement of third space fluid is empirical but should be anticipated in patients who are at risk, such as children who have burns or abdominal surgery. Third space losses and chest tube output are isotonic and usually require replacement with an **isotonic fluid,** such as normal saline or Ringer's lactate. Adjustments in the amount of replacement fluid for third space losses are based on continuing assessment of the patient's intravascular volume status.

DEHYDRATION

Dehydration, most often due to gastroenteritis, is common in children. The first step in caring for a dehydrated child is to assess the degree of dehydration. The degree of dehydration dictates the urgency of the situation and the volume of fluid needed for rehydration. Table 33-5 summarizes the clinical features that are present with varying degrees of dehydration.

A patient with **mild dehydration** has few clinical signs or symptoms. The history may describe decreased intake but

Table 33-5	Assessment of Degree of Dehydration		
	MILD	**MODERATE**	**SEVERE**
Infant	5%	10%	15%
Adolescent	3%	6%	9%
Infants and young children	Thirsty, alert; restless	Thirsty; restless or lethargic; irritable	Drowsy; limp, cold, sweaty, cyanotic extremities; may be comatose
Older children	Thirsty, alert	Thirsty, alert (usually)	Usually conscious (but at reduced level), apprehensive; cold, sweaty, cyanotic extremities; wrinkled skin on fingers and toes; muscle cramps
SIGNS AND SYMPTOMS			
Tachycardia	Absent	Present	Present
Palpable pulses	Present	Present (weak)	Decreased
Blood pressure	Normal	Orthostatic hypotension	Hypotension
Cutaneous perfusion	Normal	Normal	Reduced and mottled
Skin turgor	Normal	Slight reduction	Reduced
Fontanelle	Normal	Slightly depressed	Sunken
Mucous membrane	Moist	Dry	Very dry
Tears	Present	Present or absent	Absent
Respirations	Normal	Deep, may be rapid	Deep and rapid
Urine output	Normal	Oliguria	Anuria and severe oliguria

Data from World Health Organization.

more often increased fluid losses. An infant with **moderate dehydration** has demonstrable physical signs and symptoms. The patient needs fairly prompt intervention. A patient with **severe dehydration** is gravely ill. The decrease in blood pressure indicates that vital organs may be receiving inadequate perfusion (shock) (see Chapter 40). Such a patient should receive immediate and aggressive intravenous (IV) therapy. Clinical assessment of dehydration is only an estimate; the patient must be continually re-evaluated during therapy. The degree of dehydration is underestimated in hypernatremic dehydration because the osmotically driven shift of water from the intracellular space to the extracellular space helps to preserve the intravascular volume.

Laboratory Evaluation
Serum blood urea nitrogen (BUN) and creatinine concentrations are useful in assessing a child with dehydration. Volume depletion without renal insufficiency may cause a disproportionate increase in the BUN, with little or no change in the creatinine concentration. This is secondary to increased passive reabsorption of urea in the proximal tubule caused by appropriate renal conservation of sodium and water. This increase in the BUN may be absent or blunted in a child with poor protein intake because urea production depends on protein degradation. Conversely, the BUN may be disproportionately increased in a child with increased urea production, as occurs in a child with a gastrointestinal bleed or a child who is receiving glucocorticoids. A significant elevation of the creatinine concentration suggests renal injury.

The urine specific gravity is usually elevated (≥1.025) in cases of significant dehydration but decreases after rehydration.

With dehydration, a urinalysis may show hyaline and granular casts, a few white blood cells and red blood cells, and 30 to 100 mg/dL of proteinuria. These findings usually are not associated with significant renal pathology, and they remit with therapy. Hemoconcentration from dehydration causes an increase in the hematocrit and hemoglobin.

Calculation of Fluid Deficit
A child with dehydration has lost water; there is usually a concurrent loss of sodium and potassium. The fluid deficit is the percentage of dehydration multiplied by the patient's weight (for a 10-kg child, 10% of 10 kg =1 L deficit).

Approach to Dehydration
The child with dehydration requires acute intervention to ensure that there is adequate tissue perfusion (see Chapter 40). This resuscitation phase requires rapid restoration of the circulating intravascular volume, which should be done with an isotonic solution, such as normal saline (NS) or Ringer's lactate. Blood is an appropriate fluid choice for a child with acute blood loss. The child is given a fluid bolus, usually 20 mL/kg of the isotonic solution, over about 20 minutes. A child with severe dehydration may require multiple fluid boluses and may need to receive fluid at a faster rate. The initial resuscitation and rehydration is complete when signs of intravascular volume depletion resolve. The child typically becomes more alert and has a lower heart rate, normal blood pressure, and improved perfusion.

With adequate intravascular volume, it is now appropriate to plan the fluid therapy for the next 24 hours (Table 33-6). To

Table 33-6	Fluid Management of Dehydration

Restore intravascular volume

    Normal saline: 20 mL/kg over 20 minutes

    Repeat as needed

Rapid volume repletion: 20 mL/kg normal saline (maximum = 1 L) over 2 hours

Calculate 24-hour fluid needs: maintenance + deficit volume

Subtract isotonic fluid already administered from 24-hour fluid needs

Administer remaining volume over 24 hours using D5 ½ normal saline + 20 mEq/L KCl

Replace ongoing losses as they occur

Table 33-7	Monitoring Therapy

Vital signs

    Pulse

    Blood pressure

Intake and output

    Fluid balance

    Urine output and specific gravity

Physical examination

    Weight

    Clinical signs of depletion or overload

Electrolytes

ensure that the intravascular volume is restored, the patient receives an additional 20 mL/kg bolus of isotonic fluid over 2 hours. The child's total fluid needs are added together (maintenance + deficit). The volume of isotonic fluids the patient has received as acute resuscitation is subtracted from this total. The remaining fluid volume is then administered over 24 hours. Potassium usually is not included in the IV fluids until the patient voids, unless significant hypokalemia is present. *Children with significant ongoing losses need to receive an appropriate replacement solution.*

Monitoring and Adjusting Therapy

Decision-Making Algorithms
Available @ StudentConsult.com

Hypernatremia
Hyponatremia

All calculations in fluid therapy are only approximations. Thus, the patient needs to be monitored during treatment with therapy modifications based on the clinical situation (Table 33-7).

Hyponatremic dehydration occurs in children who have diarrhea and consume a hypotonic fluid (water or diluted formula). Volume depletion stimulates secretion of antidiuretic hormone, preventing the water excretion that should correct the hyponatremia. Some patients develop symptoms, predominantly neurologic, from the hyponatremia (see Chapter 35). Most patients with hyponatremic dehydration do well with the same general approach outlined in Table 33-6. Overly rapid correction of hyponatremia (>12 mEq/L/24 hr) should be avoided because of the remote risk of **central pontine myelinolysis.**

Hypernatremic dehydration is usually a consequence of an inability to take in fluid, because of a lack of access, a poor thirst mechanism (neurologic impairment), intractable emesis, or anorexia. The movement of water from the intracellular space to the extracellular space during hypernatremic dehydration partially protects the intravascular volume. Urine output may be preserved longer, and there may be less tachycardia. Children with hypernatremic dehydration are often lethargic and irritable. Hypernatremia may cause fever,

hypertonicity, hyperreflexia, and seizures. More severe neurologic symptoms may develop if cerebral bleeding or thrombosis occurs.

Overly rapid treatment of hypernatremic dehydration may cause significant morbidity and mortality. **Idiogenic osmoles** are generated within the brain during the development of hypernatremia. Idiogenic osmoles increase the osmolality within the cells of the brain, providing protection against brain cell shrinkage secondary to movement of water out of cells into the hypertonic extracellular fluid. These idiogenic osmoles dissipate slowly during correction of hypernatremia. With rapid lowering of the extracellular osmolality during correction of hypernatremia, a new gradient may be created that causes water movement from the extracellular space into the cells of the brain, producing **cerebral edema.** Possible manifestations of the resultant cerebral edema include altered mental status, seizures, and potentially lethal brain herniation.

To minimize the risk of cerebral edema during correction of hypernatremic dehydration, the serum sodium concentration should not decrease more than 12 mEq/L every 24 hours (Figure 33-1). The deficits in severe hypernatremic dehydration may need to be corrected over 2 to 4 days. The choice and rate of fluid are not nearly as important as vigilant monitoring of the serum sodium concentration and adjustment of the therapy based on the result (see Figure 33-1). Nonetheless, the initial resuscitation-rehydration phase of therapy remains the same as for other types of dehydration.

Oral Rehydration

Mild to moderate dehydration from diarrhea of any cause can be treated effectively using a simple, oral rehydration solution (ORS) containing glucose and electrolytes (see Chapter 112). The ORS relies on the coupled transport of sodium and glucose in the intestine. Oral rehydration therapy has significantly reduced the morbidity and mortality from acute diarrhea but is underused in developed countries. It should be attempted for most patients with mild to moderate diarrheal dehydration. Oral rehydration therapy is less expensive than IV therapy and has a lower complication rate. IV therapy may still be required for patients with severe dehydration; patients with uncontrollable vomiting; patients unable to drink because of extreme fatigue, stupor, or coma; or patients

Figure 33-1 Strategy for correcting hypernatremic dehydration.

with gastric or intestinal distention. Rapidly absorbed ondansetron may be used to treat vomiting, thus facilitating oral rehydration.

As a guideline for oral rehydration, 50 mL/kg of the ORS should be given within 4 hours to patients with mild dehydration, and 100 mL/kg should be given over 4 hours to patients with moderate dehydration. Supplementary ORS is given to replace ongoing losses from diarrhea or emesis. An additional 10 mL/kg of ORS is given for each stool. Fluid intake should be decreased if the patient appears fully hydrated earlier than expected or develops periorbital edema. After rehydration, patients should resume their usual diet (breast milk, formula).

When rehydration is complete, maintenance therapy should be started, using 100 mL of ORS/kg in 24 hours until the diarrhea stops. Breastfeeding or formula feeding should be maintained and not delayed for more than 24 hours. Patients with more severe diarrhea require continued supervision. The volume of ORS ingested should equal the volume of stool losses. If stool volume cannot be measured, an intake of 10 to 15 mL of ORS/kg/hr is appropriate.

Chapter 34

PARENTERAL NUTRITION

Parenteral nutrition (PN) is necessary when enteral feeding is inadequate to meet the nutritional needs of a patient. Enteral nutrition is always preferred because it is more physiologic, less expensive, and associated with fewer complications. Fewer complications are expected if at least some nutrition can be provided enterally.

INDICATIONS

A variety of clinical situations necessitate PN (Table 34-1). Acute PN is frequently given in an intensive care unit when there is poor tolerance of enteral feeds, potentially secondary to a transient ileus; concerns regarding bowel ischemia; or the

Table 34-1	Indications for Parenteral Nutrition
ACUTE	
Prematurity	
Trauma	
Burns	
Bowel surgery	
Multiorgan system failure	
Bone marrow transplantation	
Malignancy	
CHRONIC	
Short bowel	
Intractable diarrhea syndromes	
Intestinal pseudo-obstruction	
Inflammatory bowel disease	
Immunodeficiency	

risk of aspiration pneumonia. **Short bowel syndrome** is the most common indication for long-term PN; it may be caused by a congenital gastrointestinal anomaly or acquired after necrotizing enterocolitis (see Chapter 63). Some patients with a chronic indication for PN eventually may be transitioned to partial or full enteral feedings.

ACCESS FOR PARENTERAL NUTRITION

PN can be given via either a peripheral intravenous (IV) line or a central venous line. Long-term PN should be given via a central venous line (CVL). Acute PN may be given peripherally, although a temporary CVL often is used. Most children with cancer or receiving a bone marrow transplant have a CVL. A **peripherally inserted central catheter** is an excellent source of central access for acute PN because of the lower risk for complications than with a standard CVL.

A peripheral IV line has two major limitations. First, it frequently fails, necessitating interruption of PN and potentially painful placement of a new line. Second, high-osmolality solutions cause **phlebitis** of peripheral veins; this limits the dextrose and amino acid content of peripheral PN. The dextrose content of peripheral PN cannot be greater than 12%, with a lower limit if the amino acid concentration is high. Lipid emulsion has a low osmolality; therefore, it can be administered peripherally via the same IV line as the dextrose and amino acid solution. Patients can receive adequate nutrition via a peripheral IV line, but the volume of PN needs to be higher than is necessary when central access is available because of the limitations on dextrose and amino acid concentration. This situation may be problematic in patients who cannot tolerate larger fluid volumes.

COMPOSITION OF PARENTERAL NUTRITION

PN can provide calories, amino acids, electrolytes, minerals, essential fatty acids, vitamins, iron, and trace elements. The **calories** in PN are from dextrose and fat. The amino acids in PN are a potential source of calories, but they should be used predominantly for protein synthesis. PN is given as two separate solutions: a dextrose plus amino acid solution and a 20% lipid emulsion. The dextrose solution has all of the other components of PN except for fat.

The dextrose concentration of peripheral PN is typically 10% to 12%, whereas central PN has a concentration of about 20%, although it may be increased to 25% to 30% in patients who are fluid restricted. To avoid hyperglycemia, the dextrose delivery is increased gradually when starting PN. Protein delivery in PN is via amino acids in the dextrose solution. The goal is 0.8 to 2 g protein/kg/24 hr for older children, 1.5 to 3 g/kg/24 hr for full-term and older infants, and 2.5 to 3.5 g/kg/24 hr for preterm infants.

The electrolyte and mineral composition of PN depends on the age and the underlying illness. The 20% lipid emulsion provides essential fatty acids and calories. The lipid emulsion is started at a rate of 0.5 to 1 g/kg/24 hr, gradually increasing the rate so that the patient receives adequate calories; this typically requires 2.5 to 3.5 g/kg/24 hr. The lipid emulsion usually provides 30% to 40% of the required calories; it should not exceed 60%. The serum triglyceride concentration is monitored as the rate of lipid emulsion is increased, with reduction of the lipid emulsion rate if significant hypertriglyceridemia develops.

COMPLICATIONS

There are many potential complications of PN. CVLs are associated with complications during insertion (pneumothorax or bleeding) and long-term issues (thrombosis). **Catheter-related sepsis,** most commonly due to coagulase-negative staphylococci, is common and, on occasion, necessitates catheter removal. Other potential pathogens are *Staphylococcus aureus,* gram-negative bacilli, and fungi. Electrolyte abnormalities, nutritional deficiencies, hyperglycemia, and complications from excessive protein intake (azotemia or hyperammonemia) can be detected with careful monitoring.

The most concerning complication of long-term PN is **cholestatic liver disease,** which can lead to cirrhosis and liver failure. Current PN decreases the risk of liver disease by including reduced amounts of hepatotoxic amino acids. The best preventive strategy is early use of the gastrointestinal tract, even if only trophic feeds are tolerated.

Chapter **35**

SODIUM DISORDERS

The kidney regulates sodium balance and is the principal site of sodium excretion. Sodium is unique among electrolytes because **water balance,** not sodium balance, usually determines its concentration. When the sodium concentration increases, the resultant higher plasma osmolality causes increased thirst and increased secretion of antidiuretic hormone (ADH), which leads to renal conservation of water. Both of these mechanisms increase the water content of the body, and the sodium concentration returns to normal. During hyponatremia, the fall in plasma osmolality decreases ADH secretion, and consequent renal water excretion leads to an increase in the sodium concentration. Although water balance usually is regulated by osmolality, volume depletion stimulates thirst, ADH secretion, and renal conservation of water. In fact, volume depletion takes precedence over osmolality; volume depletion stimulates ADH secretion, even if a patient has hyponatremia.

The excretion of sodium by the kidney is not determined by the plasma osmolality. The patient's effective plasma volume regulates the amount of sodium in the urine through a variety of regulatory systems, including the renin-angiotensin-aldosterone system. In hyponatremia or hypernatremia, the underlying pathophysiology determines the urinary sodium concentration, not the serum sodium concentration.

HYPONATREMIA

Decision-Making Algorithm
Available @ StudentConsult.com

Hyponatremia

Etiology

Different mechanisms can cause hyponatremia (Fig. 35-1). **Pseudohyponatremia** is a laboratory artifact that is present when the plasma contains high concentrations of protein or lipid. It does not occur when a direct ion-selective electrode determines the sodium concentration, a technique that is increasingly used in clinical laboratories. In true hyponatremia, the *measured* osmolality is low, whereas it is normal in pseudohyponatremia. **Hyperosmolality**, resulting from mannitol infusion or hyperglycemia, causes a low serum sodium concentration because water moves down its osmotic gradient from the intracellular space into the extracellular space, diluting the sodium concentration. For every 100 mg/dL increment of the serum glucose, the serum sodium decreases by 1.6 mEq/L. Because the manifestations of hyponatremia are due to the low plasma osmolality, patients with hyponatremia caused by hyperosmolality do not have symptoms of hyponatremia and do not require correction of hyponatremia.

Classification of true hyponatremia is based on the patient's volume status (see Fig. 35-1). In **hypovolemic hyponatremia,** the child has lost sodium from the body. Water balance may be positive or negative, but there has been a higher net sodium loss than water loss; this is often due to oral or intravenous (IV) water intake, with water retention by the kidneys to compensate for the intravascular volume depletion. If the sodium loss is due to a nonrenal disease (e.g., diarrhea), the urine sodium concentration is very low, as the kidneys attempt to preserve the intravascular volume by conserving sodium. In renal diseases, the urine sodium is inappropriately elevated.

Patients with hyponatremia and no evidence of volume overload or volume depletion have **euvolemic hyponatremia.** These patients typically have an excess of total body water and a slight decrease in total body sodium. Some of these patients have an increase in weight, implying that they are volume overloaded. Nevertheless, they usually appear normal or have only subtle signs of fluid overload. In **syndrome of inappropriate ADH (SIADH),** there is secretion of ADH that is not inhibited by either low serum osmolality or expanded intravascular volume. Retention of water causes hyponatremia, and the expansion of the intravascular volume results in an increase in renal sodium excretion. Hyponatremia in hospitalized patients is often due to SIADH secondary to stress in the presence of hypotonic fluids.

Figure 35-1 Differential diagnosis of hyponatremia. Assessment of hyponatremia is a three-step process: (1) Determine if the osmolality is low; if yes, the patient has true hyponatremia. (2) Evaluate the patient's volume status. (3) Determine the urine sodium concentration to help narrow the differential diagnosis. *ATN,* Acute tubular necrosis; *SIADH,* syndrome of inappropriate secretion of antidiuretic hormone.

SIADH is also associated with pneumonia, mechanical ventilation, meningitis, and other central nervous system disorders (trauma). Ectopic (tumor) production of ADH is rare in children. Infants can develop euvolemic hyponatremia as a result of excessive water consumption or inappropriately diluted formula.

In **hypervolemic hyponatremia,** there is an excess of total body water and sodium, although the increase in water is greater than the increase in sodium. In renal failure, there is an inability to excrete sodium or water; the urine sodium may be low or high, depending on the cause of the renal insufficiency. In other causes of hypervolemic hyponatremia, there is a decrease in the effective blood volume because of either third space fluid loss or poor cardiac output (see Chapter 145). In response to the low effective blood volume, ADH causes renal water retention, and the kidneys also retain sodium, leading to a low urine sodium concentration. The patient's serum sodium concentration decreases when water intake exceeds sodium intake, and ADH prevents the normal loss of excess water.

Clinical Manifestations

Hyponatremia causes a fall in the osmolality of the extracellular space. Because the intracellular space then has a higher osmolality, water moves from the extracellular space to the intracellular space to maintain osmotic equilibrium. The increase in intracellular water may cause cells to swell. **Brain cell swelling** is responsible for most of the symptoms of hyponatremia. Neurologic symptoms of hyponatremia include anorexia, nausea, emesis, malaise, lethargy, confusion, agitation, headache, seizures, coma, and decreased reflexes. Patients may develop hypothermia and Cheyne-Stokes respirations. Hyponatremia can cause muscle cramps and weakness. Symptoms are more severe when hyponatremia develops rapidly; chronic hyponatremia can be asymptomatic because of a compensatory decrease in brain cell osmolality, which limits cerebral swelling.

Treatment

Rapid correction of hyponatremia can produce **central pontine myelinolysis.** Avoiding more than a 12-mEq/L increase in the serum sodium every 24 hours is prudent, especially in chronic hyponatremia. Treatment of hypovolemic hyponatremia requires administration of IV fluids with sodium to provide maintenance requirements and deficit correction, as well as to replace ongoing losses (see Chapter 33). For children with SIADH, water restriction is the cornerstone of therapy. Children with hyponatremia secondary to hypothyroidism or cortisol deficiency need specific hormone replacement. **Acute water intoxication** rapidly self-corrects with transient restriction of water intake, which is followed by introduction of a normal diet. Treatment of hypervolemic hyponatremia centers on restriction of water and sodium intake, but disease-specific measures, such as dialysis in renal failure, also may be necessary.

Emergency treatment of **symptomatic hyponatremia,** such as seizures, uses IV hypertonic saline to increase the serum sodium concentration rapidly, which leads to a decrease in brain edema. One milliliter per kilogram of 3% sodium chloride increases the serum sodium by approximately 1 mEq/L.

A child often improves after receiving 4 to 6 mL/kg of 3% sodium chloride.

HYPERNATREMIA

Decision-Making Algorithm
Available @ StudentConsult.com

Hypernatremia

Etiology

There are three basic mechanisms of hypernatremia (Fig. 35-2). **Sodium intoxication** is frequently iatrogenic in a hospital setting resulting from correction of metabolic acidosis with sodium bicarbonate. In hyperaldosteronism, there is renal retention of sodium and resultant hypertension; the hypernatremia is mild.

Hypernatremia resulting from water losses develops only if the patient does not have access to water or cannot drink adequately because of neurologic impairment, emesis, or anorexia. Infants are at high risk because of their inability to control their own water intake. Ineffective breastfeeding, often in a primiparous mother, can cause severe hypernatremic dehydration. High insensible losses of water are especially common in premature infants; the losses increase further as a result of radiant warmers or phototherapy for hyperbilirubinemia. Children with extrarenal causes of water loss have high levels of ADH and very concentrated urine.

Children with diabetes insipidus have inappropriately diluted urine. Hereditary **nephrogenic diabetes insipidus** causes massive urinary water losses. Because it is most commonly an X-linked disorder due to a mutation in the gene for the ADH receptor, it usually occurs in boys, who may have episodes of severe hypernatremic dehydration and failure to thrive. *Acquired nephrogenic diabetes insipidus* may be secondary to interstitial nephritis, sickle cell disease, hypercalcemia, hypokalemia, or medications (lithium or amphotericin). If the defect is due to **central diabetes insipidus,** urine output decreases and urine osmolality increases in response to administration of an ADH analog. Central causes of ADH deficiency include tumor, infarction, or trauma. There is no response to an ADH analog in a child with nephrogenic diabetes insipidus.

Diarrhea results in sodium and water depletion. Most children with gastroenteritis do not develop hypernatremia because they drink enough hypotonic fluid to compensate at least partially for stool water losses. Hypernatremia is most likely in a child with diarrhea who has inadequate intake because of emesis, lack of access to water, or anorexia. Some renal diseases, including obstructive uropathy, renal dysplasia, and juvenile nephronophthisis, can cause losses of sodium and water, potentially producing hypernatremia if the patient consumes insufficient water.

In situations with combined sodium and water deficits, analysis of the urine differentiates renal and nonrenal etiologies. When the losses are extrarenal, the kidney responds to volume depletion with low urine volume, a concentrated urine, and sodium retention (urine sodium <10 mEq/L). With renal causes, the urine volume is usually high, the urine is not maximally concentrated, and the urine sodium may be inappropriately elevated.

Figure 35-2 Differential diagnosis of hypernatremia by mechanism. *GI,* Gastrointestinal; *NG,* nasogastric.

Clinical Manifestations

Most children with hypernatremia are dehydrated and have the typical signs and symptoms of dehydration (see Chapter 33). Children with hypernatremic dehydration tend to have better preservation of intravascular volume owing to the shift of water from the intracellular space to the extracellular space. Hypernatremic infants potentially become more dehydrated before seeking medical attention. Probably because of intracellular water loss, the pinched abdominal skin of a dehydrated, hypernatremic infant has a *doughy* feel.

Hypernatremia, even without dehydration, causes central nervous system symptoms that tend to parallel the degree of sodium elevation and the acuity of the increase. Patients are irritable, restless, weak, and lethargic. Some infants have a high-pitched cry and hyperpnea. Alert patients are very thirsty, although nausea may be present. Hypernatremia causes fever, although many patients have an underlying process that contributes to the fever.

Brain hemorrhage is the most devastating consequence of hypernatremia. As the extracellular osmolality increases, water moves out of brain cells, resulting in a decrease in brain volume. This decrease in volume can result in tearing of intracerebral veins and bridging blood vessels as the brain moves away from the skull and the meninges. Patients may have subarachnoid, subdural, and parenchymal hemorrhage. Seizures and coma are possible sequelae of the hemorrhage.

Treatment

As hypernatremia develops, the brain generates idiogenic osmoles to increase the intracellular osmolality and prevent the loss of brain water. This mechanism is not instantaneous and is most prominent when hypernatremia has developed gradually. If the serum sodium concentration is lowered rapidly, there is movement of water from the serum into the brain cells to equalize the osmolality in the two compartments. The resultant brain swelling manifests as seizures or coma. Because of these dangers, corrected hypernatremia should be treated gradually. The goal is to decrease the serum sodium by less than 12 mEq/L every 24 hours (see Fig. 33-1). The most important component of correcting moderate or severe hypernatremia is frequent monitoring of the serum sodium to allow adjustment of fluid therapy and provide adequate correction that is neither too slow nor too fast.

In a child with hypernatremic dehydration, as in any child with dehydration, the first priority is restoration of intravascular volume with isotonic fluid. Figure 33-1 outlines a general approach for correcting hypernatremic dehydration secondary to gastroenteritis. If the hypernatremia and dehydration are secondary to water loss, as occurs with diabetes insipidus, a more hypotonic IV fluid is appropriate. A child with central diabetes insipidus should receive an ADH analog to prevent further excessive water loss. A child with nephrogenic diabetes insipidus requires a urine replacement solution to offset ongoing water losses. Chronically, reduced sodium intake, thiazide diuretics, and nonsteroidal anti-inflammatory drugs can decrease water losses in nephrogenic diabetes insipidus.

Acute, severe hypernatremia, usually secondary to sodium administration, can be corrected more rapidly because idiogenic osmoles have not had time to accumulate; this balances the high morbidity and mortality from severe, acute hypernatremia with the dangers of overly rapid correction. When hypernatremia is due to sodium intoxication, and the hypernatremia is severe, it may be impossible to administer enough water to correct the hypernatremia rapidly without worsening volume overload. Some patients require use of a loop diuretic or dialysis.

Chapter 36

POTASSIUM DISORDERS

The kidneys are the principal regulator of potassium balance, adjusting excretion based on intake. Factors affecting renal potassium excretion include aldosterone, acid-base status, serum potassium concentration, and renal function. The intracellular potassium concentration is approximately 30 times the extracellular potassium concentration. A variety of conditions alter the distribution of potassium between the intracellular and extracellular compartments, potentially causing either hypokalemia or hyperkalemia. The plasma concentration does not always reflect the total body potassium content.

HYPOKALEMIA

Decision-Making Algorithm
Available @ StudentConsult.com

Hypokalemia

Etiology

Hypokalemia is common in children, with most cases related to gastroenteritis. Spurious hypokalemia occurs in patients with leukemia and elevated white blood cell counts if plasma for analysis is left at room temperature, permitting the white blood cells to take up potassium from the plasma. There are four basic mechanisms of hypokalemia (Table 36-1). Low intake, nonrenal losses, and renal losses all are associated with total body potassium depletion. With a **transcellular shift**, total body potassium is normal unless there is concomitant potassium depletion secondary to other factors.

The transcellular shift of potassium after initiation of insulin therapy in children with diabetic ketoacidosis (see Chapter 171) can be dramatic. These patients have reduced total body potassium because of urinary losses, but they often have a normal serum potassium level before insulin therapy from a transcellular shift into the extracellular space secondary to insulin deficiency and metabolic acidosis. Children receiving aggressive doses of β-adrenergic agonists (albuterol) for asthma can have hypokalemia resulting from the intracellular movement of potassium. Poor intake is an unusual cause of hypokalemia, unless also associated with significant weight loss (anorexia nervosa).

Diarrhea has a high concentration of potassium, and the resulting hypokalemia usually is associated with a metabolic acidosis secondary to stool losses of bicarbonate. With emesis or nasogastric suction, there is gastric loss of potassium, but this is fairly minimal given the low potassium content of gastric fluid (approximately 10 mEq/L). More important is the gastric loss of hydrochloride, leading to a metabolic alkalosis and a state of volume depletion. Metabolic alkalosis and volume depletion increase urinary losses of potassium.

Urinary potassium wasting may be accompanied by a metabolic acidosis (proximal or distal renal tubular acidosis) (see Chapter 37). Loop and thiazide diuretics lead to hypokalemia

and a metabolic alkalosis. **Bartter syndrome** and **Gitelman syndrome** are autosomal recessive disorders resulting from defects in tubular transporters. Both disorders are associated with hypokalemia and a metabolic alkalosis. Bartter syndrome is usually associated with hypercalciuria, often with nephrocalcinosis; children with Gitelman syndrome have low urinary calcium losses, but hypomagnesemia secondary to urinary losses.

In the presence of a high aldosterone level, there is urinary loss of potassium, hypokalemia, and a metabolic alkalosis. There also is renal retention of sodium, leading to hypertension. A variety of genetic and acquired disorders can cause high aldosterone levels. **Liddle syndrome**, an autosomal dominant disorder caused by constitutively active sodium channels, has the same clinical features as hyperaldosteronism, but the serum aldosterone level is low.

Clinical Manifestations

The heart and skeletal muscle are especially vulnerable to hypokalemia. **Electrocardiographic (ECG) changes** include a flattened T wave, a depressed ST segment, and the appearance of a U wave, which is located between the T wave (if still visible) and P wave. Ventricular fibrillation and torsades de pointes may occur, although usually only in the context of underlying heart disease. Hypokalemia makes the heart especially susceptible to digitalis-induced arrhythmias.

The clinical consequences in skeletal muscle include muscle weakness and cramps. **Paralysis** is a possible complication (generally only at potassium levels <2.5 mEq/L). Paralysis usually starts with the legs, followed by the arms. Respiratory paralysis may require mechanical ventilation.

Some hypokalemic patients develop **rhabdomyolysis**, especially following exercise. Hypokalemia slows gastrointestinal motility; potassium levels less than 2.5 mEq/L may cause an ileus. Hypokalemia impairs bladder function, potentially leading to urinary retention. Hypokalemia causes polyuria by producing secondary nephrogenic diabetes insipidus. Chronic hypokalemia may cause kidney damage, including interstitial nephritis and renal cysts. In children, chronic hypokalemia, as in Bartter syndrome, leads to poor growth.

Diagnosis

It is important to review the child's diet, history of gastrointestinal losses, and medications. Emesis and diuretic use can be surreptitious. The presence of hypertension suggests excess mineralocorticoids. Concomitant electrolyte abnormalities are useful clues. The combination of hypokalemia and metabolic acidosis is characteristic of diarrhea, distal renal tubular acidosis, and proximal renal tubular acidosis. A concurrent metabolic alkalosis is characteristic of gastric losses, aldosterone excess, diuretics, Bartter syndrome, or Gitelman syndrome.

Treatment

Factors that influence the therapy of hypokalemia include the potassium level, clinical symptoms, renal function, presence of transcellular shifts of potassium, ongoing losses, and the patient's ability to tolerate oral potassium. Severe, symptomatic hypokalemia requires aggressive treatment. Supplementation

Table 36-1	Causes of Hypokalemia

Spurious	With metabolic alkalosis
High white blood cell count	Low urine chloride
Transcellular shifts	Emesis/nasogastric suction
Alkalemia	Pyloric stenosis
Insulin	Chloride-losing diarrhea
β-Adrenergic agonists	Cystic fibrosis
Drugs/toxins (theophylline, barium, toluene)	Low-chloride formula
Hypokalemic periodic paralysis	Posthypercapnia
Refeeding syndrome	Previous loop or thiazide diuretic use
Decreased intake	High urine chloride and normal blood pressure
Extrarenal losses	Gitelman syndrome
Diarrhea	Bartter syndrome
Laxative abuse	Loop and thiazide diuretics
Sweating	High urine chloride and high blood pressure
Renal losses	Adrenal adenoma or hyperplasia
With metabolic acidosis	Glucocorticoid-remediable aldosteronism
Distal RTA	Renovascular disease
Proximal RTA	Renin-secreting tumor
Ureterosigmoidostomy	17α-Hydroxylase deficiency
Diabetic ketoacidosis	11β-Hydroxylase deficiency
Without specific acid-base disturbance	Cushing syndrome
Tubular toxins (amphotericin, cisplatin, aminoglycosides)	11β-Hydroxysteroid dehydrogenase deficiency
Interstitial nephritis	Licorice ingestion
Diuretic phase of acute tubular necrosis	Liddle syndrome
Postobstructive diuresis	
Hypomagnesemia	
High urine anions (e.g., penicillin or penicillin derivatives)	

RTA, renal tubular acidosis.

is more cautious if renal function is decreased because of the kidney's limited ability to excrete excessive potassium. The plasma potassium level does not always provide an accurate estimation of the total body potassium deficit because there may be shifts of potassium from the intracellular space to the plasma. Clinically, this shift occurs most commonly with metabolic acidosis and as a result of the insulin deficiency of diabetic ketoacidosis; the plasma potassium underestimates the degree of total body potassium depletion. When these problems are corrected, potassium moves into the intracellular space, and these patients require more potassium supplementation to correct the hypokalemia. Patients who have ongoing losses of potassium need correction of the deficit and replacement of the ongoing losses.

Because of the risk of hyperkalemia, intravenous (IV) potassium should be used cautiously. Oral potassium is safer in nonurgent situations. The dose of IV potassium is 0.5 to 1 mEq/kg, usually given over 1 hour. The adult maximum dose is 40 mEq. Conservative dosing is generally preferred. For patients with excessive urinary losses, potassium-sparing diuretics are effective. When hypokalemia, metabolic alkalosis, and volume depletion are present, restoration of intravascular volume decreases urinary potassium losses.

HYPERKALEMIA

Decision-Making Algorithm
Available @ StudentConsult.com

Hyperkalemia

Etiology

Three basic mechanisms cause hyperkalemia (Table 36-2). In the individual patient, the etiology is sometimes multifactorial. **Factitious hyperkalemia** is usually due to hemolysis during phlebotomy, but it can be the result of prolonged tourniquet application or fist clenching, which causes local potassium release from muscle. Falsely elevated serum potassium levels can occur when serum levels are measured in patients with markedly elevated white blood cell or platelet counts; a promptly analyzed plasma sample usually provides an accurate result.

Because of the kidney's ability to excrete potassium, it is unusual for excessive intake, by itself, to cause hyperkalemia. This mechanism can occur in a patient who is receiving large quantities of IV or oral potassium for excessive losses that are no longer present. Frequent or rapid blood transfusions can increase the potassium level acutely secondary to the high

Table 36-2 | Causes of Hyperkalemia

Spurious laboratory value	Acquired Addison disease
Hemolysis	21-Hydroxylase deficiency
Tissue ischemia during blood drawing	3β-Hydroxysteroid-dehydrogenase deficiency
Thrombocytosis	Lipoid congenital adrenal hyperplasia
Leukocytosis	Adrenal hypoplasia congenita
Increased intake	Aldosterone synthase deficiency
IV or PO	Adrenoleukodystrophy
Blood transfusions	Hyporeninemic hypoaldosteronism
Transcellular shifts	Urinary tract obstruction
Acidemia	Sickle cell disease
Rhabdomyolysis	Kidney transplant
Tumor lysis syndrome	Lupus nephritis
Tissue necrosis	Renal tubular disease
Hemolysis/hematomas/gastrointestinal bleeding	Pseudohypoaldosteronism type 1
Succinylcholine	Pseudohypoaldosteronism type 2
Digitalis intoxication	Urinary tract obstruction
Fluoride intoxication	Sickle cell disease
β-Adrenergic blockers	Kidney transplant
Exercise	Medications
Hyperosmolality	ACE inhibitors
Insulin deficiency	Angiotensin II blockers
Malignant hyperthermia	Potassium-sparing diuretics
Hyperkalemic periodic paralysis	Cyclosporine
Decreased excretion	NSAIDs
Renal failure	Trimethoprim
Primary adrenal disease	

ACE, Angiotensin-converting enzyme; *IV,* intravenous; *NSAIDs,* nonsteroidal anti-inflammatory drugs; *PO,* oral.

potassium content of stored blood. Increased intake may precipitate hyperkalemia if there is an underlying defect in potassium excretion.

The intracellular space has a high potassium concentration, so a **shift of potassium from the intracellular space** to the extracellular space can have a significant impact on the plasma potassium. This shift occurs with acidosis, cell destruction (rhabdomyolysis or tumor lysis syndrome), insulin deficiency, medications (succinylcholine, β-blockers), malignant hyperthermia, and hyperkalemic periodic paralysis.

Hyperkalemia secondary to decreased excretion occurs with renal insufficiency. Aldosterone deficiency or unresponsiveness to aldosterone causes hyperkalemia, often with associated metabolic acidosis (see Chapter 37) and hyponatremia. A form of congenital adrenal hyperplasia, **21-hydroxylase deficiency,** is the most frequent cause of aldosterone deficiency in children. Male infants typically present with hyperkalemia, metabolic acidosis, hyponatremia, and volume depletion. Female infants with this disorder usually are diagnosed as newborns because of ambiguous genitalia.

Renin, via angiotensin II, stimulates aldosterone production. A deficiency in renin, resulting from kidney damage, can lead to decreased aldosterone production. These patients typically have hyperkalemia and a metabolic acidosis, without hyponatremia. Some patients have impaired renal function, partially accounting for the hyperkalemia, but the impairment in potassium excretion is more extreme than expected for the degree of renal insufficiency.

Children with **pseudohypoaldosteronism type 1** have hyperkalemia, metabolic acidosis, and salt wasting, leading to hyponatremia and volume depletion; aldosterone levels are elevated. In the autosomal recessive variant, there is a defect in the renal sodium channel that is normally activated by aldosterone. In the autosomal dominant form, patients have a defect in the aldosterone receptor, and the disease is milder, often remitting in adulthood. Pseudohypoaldosteronism type 2, also called **Gordon syndrome,** is an autosomal dominant disorder characterized by hypertension secondary to salt retention and impaired excretion of potassium and acid leading to hyperkalemia and metabolic acidosis. The risk of hyperkalemia secondary to medications that decrease renal potassium excretion is greatest in patients with underlying renal insufficiency.

Clinical Manifestations

The most import effects of hyperkalemia are due to the role of potassium in membrane polarization. The cardiac conduction system is usually the dominant concern. **ECG changes** begin with peaking of the T waves. As the potassium level increases, an increased P-R interval, flattening of the P wave, and widening of the QRS complex occur; this eventually can progress to ventricular fibrillation. Asystole also may occur. Some patients have paresthesias, weakness, and tingling, but cardiac toxicity usually precedes these clinical symptoms.

Diagnosis

The etiology of hyperkalemia is often readily apparent. Spurious hyperkalemia is common in children, so a repeat potassium level is often appropriate. If there is a significant elevation of the white blood cells or platelets, the repeat sample should be from plasma that is evaluated promptly. The history initially should focus on potassium intake, risk factors for transcellular shifts of potassium, medications that cause hyperkalemia, and the presence of signs of renal insufficiency, such as oliguria or an abnormal urinalysis. Initial laboratory evaluation should include serum creatinine and assessment of acid-base status. Many causes of hyperkalemia, such as renal insufficiency and aldosterone insufficiency or resistance, cause a metabolic acidosis. Cell destruction, as seen in rhabdomyolysis or tumor lysis syndrome, can cause concomitant hyperphosphatemia, hyperuricemia, and an elevated serum lactate dehydrogenase.

Treatment

The plasma potassium level, the ECG, and the risk of the problem worsening determine the aggressiveness of the therapeutic approach. A high serum potassium level with ECG changes requires more vigorous treatment. An additional source of concern is a patient with increasing plasma potassium despite minimal intake. This situation can occur if there is cellular release of potassium (tumor lysis syndrome), especially in the setting of diminished excretion (renal failure).

The first action in a child with a concerning elevation of plasma potassium is to stop all sources of additional potassium (oral and IV). If the potassium level is greater than 6.5 mEq/L, an ECG should be obtained to help assess the urgency of the situation. Therapy of hyperkalemia has two basic goals:
1. Prevent life-threatening arrhythmias.
2. Remove potassium from the body (Table 36-3)

Table 36-3	Treatment of Hyperkalemia
Rapidly decrease the risk of life-threatening arrhythmias	
Shift potassium intracellularly	
Sodium bicarbonate administration (IV)	
Insulin and glucose (IV)	
β-Agonist (albuterol via nebulizer)	
Cardiac membrane stabilization	
IV calcium	
Remove potassium from the body	
Loop diuretic (IV or PO)	
Sodium polystyrene (PO or rectal)	
Dialysis	

IV, Intravenous; *PO,* oral.

Treatments that acutely prevent arrhythmias all work quickly (within minutes), but do not remove potassium from the body.

Long-term management of hyperkalemia includes reducing intake via dietary changes and eliminating or reducing medications that cause hyperkalemia. Some patients require medications, such as sodium polystyrene sulfonate and loop or thiazide diuretics, to increase potassium losses. The disorders due to a deficiency in aldosterone respond to replacement therapy with fludrocortisone, a mineralocorticoid.

Chapter **37**

ACID-BASE DISORDERS

Close regulation of pH is necessary for cellular enzymes and other metabolic processes, which function optimally at a normal pH (7.35 to 7.45). Chronic, mild derangements in acid-base status may interfere with normal growth and development, whereas acute, severe changes in pH can be fatal. Control of acid-base balance depends on the kidneys, the lungs, and intracellular and extracellular buffers.

The lungs and the kidneys maintain a normal acid-base balance. Carbon dioxide (CO_2) generated during normal metabolism is a weak acid. The lungs prevent an increase in the partial pressure of CO_2 (PCO_2) in the blood by excreting the CO_2. Production of CO_2 varies depending on the body's metabolic needs. The rapid pulmonary response to changes in CO_2 concentration occurs via central sensing of the PCO_2 and a subsequent increase or decrease in ventilation to maintain a normal PCO_2 (35 to 45 mm Hg).

The kidneys excrete endogenous acids. An adult normally produces about 1 to 2 mEq/kg/day of hydrogen ions, whereas a child produces 2 to 3 mEq/kg/day. The hydrogen ions from endogenous acid production are neutralized by bicarbonate, potentially causing the bicarbonate concentration to fall. The kidneys regenerate this bicarbonate by secreting hydrogen ions, maintaining the serum bicarbonate concentration in the normal range (20 to 28 mEq/L).

CLINICAL ASSESSMENT OF ACID-BASE DISORDERS

Decision-Making Algorithms
Available @ StudentConsult.com

Acidemia
Alkalemia

Acidemia is a pH below normal (<7.35), and **alkalemia** is a pH above normal (>7.45). **Acidosis** is a pathologic process that causes an increase in the hydrogen ion concentration, and **alkalosis** is a pathologic process that causes a decrease in the hydrogen ion concentration. A **simple acid-base disorder** is a single primary disturbance. During a simple metabolic disorder, there is respiratory compensation; the P_{CO_2} decreases during a metabolic acidosis and increases during a metabolic alkalosis. With metabolic acidosis, the decrease in the pH increases the ventilatory drive, causing a decrease in the P_{CO_2}. The fall in the CO_2 concentration leads to an increase in the pH. This **appropriate respiratory compensation** for a metabolic process happens quickly and is complete within 12 to 24 hours.

During a primary respiratory process, there is metabolic compensation mediated by the kidneys. The kidneys respond to a respiratory acidosis by increasing hydrogen ion excretion, increasing bicarbonate generation, and raising the serum bicarbonate concentration. The kidneys increase bicarbonate excretion to compensate for a respiratory alkalosis; the serum bicarbonate concentration decreases. In contrast to a rapid respiratory compensation, it takes 3 to 4 days for the kidneys to complete **appropriate metabolic compensation.** However, there is a small and rapid compensatory change in the bicarbonate concentration during a primary respiratory process. The expected appropriate metabolic compensation for a respiratory disorder depends on whether the process is acute or chronic.

A **mixed acid-base disorder** is present when there is more than one primary acid-base disturbance. An infant with bronchopulmonary dysplasia may have a respiratory acidosis from chronic lung disease and a metabolic alkalosis from a diuretic used to treat the chronic lung disease. Formulas are available for calculating the appropriate metabolic or respiratory compensation for the six primary simple acid-base disorders (Table 37-1). Appropriate compensation is expected in a simple disorder; it is not optional. If a patient does not have appropriate compensation, a mixed acid-base disorder is present.

METABOLIC ACIDOSIS

Decision-Making Algorithm
Available @ StudentConsult.com

Acidemia

Metabolic acidosis occurs frequently in hospitalized children; diarrhea is the most common cause. For a patient with

an unknown medical problem, the presence of a metabolic acidosis is often helpful diagnostically because it suggests a relatively narrow differential diagnosis (Table 37-2).

Etiology

Diarrhea causes a loss of bicarbonate from the body. The amount of bicarbonate lost in the stool depends on the volume of diarrhea and the bicarbonate concentration of the stool, which tends to increase with more severe diarrhea. Diarrhea often causes volume depletion because of losses of sodium and water, potentially exacerbating the acidosis by causing hypoperfusion (shock) and a lactic acidosis. There are three forms of renal tubular acidosis (RTA):

- Distal (type I)
- Proximal (type II)
- Hyperkalemic (type IV)

In **distal RTA,** children may have accompanying hypokalemia, hypercalciuria, nephrolithiasis, and nephrocalcinosis; rickets is a less common finding. Failure to thrive, resulting from chronic metabolic acidosis, is the most common presenting complaint. Autosomal dominant and autosomal recessive forms of distal RTA exist. The autosomal dominant form is relatively mild. Autosomal recessive distal RTA is more severe and often associated with deafness secondary to a defect in the gene for a H^+-ATPase that is present in the kidney and the inner ear. Distal RTA also may be secondary to medications or congenital or acquired renal disease. Patients with distal RTA cannot acidify their urine and have a urine pH greater than 5.5, despite a metabolic acidosis.

Proximal RTA is rarely present in isolation. In most patients, proximal RTA is part of **Fanconi syndrome,** a generalized dysfunction of the proximal tubule. Along with renal wasting of bicarbonate, Fanconi syndrome causes glycosuria, aminoaciduria, and excessive urinary losses of phosphate and uric acid. The chronic hypophosphatemia is more clinically significant because it ultimately leads to rickets in children. Rickets or failure to thrive may be the presenting complaint. Fanconi syndrome is rarely an isolated genetic disorder, with pediatric cases usually secondary to an underlying genetic disorder, most commonly **cystinosis.** Medications, such as ifosfamide or valproate, may cause Fanconi syndrome. The ability to acidify the urine is intact in proximal RTA, and untreated patients have a urine pH less than 5.5. However, bicarbonate therapy increases bicarbonate losses in the urine, and the urine pH increases.

In **hyperkalemic RTA,** renal excretion of acid and potassium is impaired because of either an absence of aldosterone

Table 37-1	Appropriate Compensation During Simple Acid-Base Disorders
DISORDER	**EXPECTED COMPENSATION***
Metabolic acidosis	$P_{CO_2} = 1.5 \times [HCO_3^-] + 8 \pm 2$
Metabolic alkalosis	P_{CO_2} increases by 7 mm Hg for each 10-mEq/L increase in the serum $[HCO_3^-]$
Respiratory acidosis	
Acute	$[HCO_3^-]$ increases by 1 for each 10-mm Hg increase in the P_{CO_2}
Chronic	$[HCO_3^-]$ increases by 3.5 for each 10-mm Hg increase in the P_{CO_2}
Respiratory alkalosis	
Acute	$[HCO_3^-]$ falls by 2 for each 10-mm Hg decrease in the P_{CO_2}
Chronic	$[HCO_3^-]$ falls by 4 for each 10-mm Hg decrease in the P_{CO_2}

*$[HCO_3^-]$ is expressed in mEq/L.

Table 37-2	Causes of Metabolic Acidosis
NORMAL ANION GAP	
Diarrhea	
Renal tubular acidosis	
Urinary tract diversions	
Posthypocapnia	
Ammonium chloride intake	
INCREASED ANION GAP	
Lactic acidosis (shock)	
Ketoacidosis (diabetic, starvation, or alcoholic)	
Kidney failure	
Poisoning (e.g., ethylene glycol, methanol, or salicylates)	
Inborn errors of metabolism	

or an inability of the kidney to respond to aldosterone. In severe aldosterone deficiency, as occurs with congenital adrenal hyperplasia secondary to 21α-hydroxylase deficiency, the hyperkalemia and metabolic acidosis are accompanied by hyponatremia and volume depletion from renal salt wasting. Incomplete aldosterone deficiency causes less severe electrolyte disturbances; children may have isolated hyperkalemic RTA, hyperkalemia without acidosis, or isolated hyponatremia.

Lactic acidosis most commonly occurs when inadequate oxygen delivery to the tissues leads to anaerobic metabolism and excess production of lactic acid. Lactic acidosis may be secondary to shock, severe anemia, or hypoxemia. Inborn errors of carbohydrate metabolism produce a severe lactic acidosis (see Chapter 52). In diabetes mellitus, inadequate insulin leads to hyperglycemia and diabetic ketoacidosis (see Chapter 171). Renal failure (see Chapter 165) causes a metabolic acidosis because the kidneys are unable to excrete the acid produced by normal metabolism.

A variety of **toxic ingestions** cause a metabolic acidosis. Acute **salicylate** intoxication occurs after a large overdose. Chronic salicylate intoxication is possible because of the gradual buildup of the drug. In addition to a metabolic acidosis, some patients may have a respiratory alkalosis. Other symptoms of salicylate intoxication include fever, seizures, lethargy, and coma. Hyperventilation may be particularly marked. Tinnitus, vertigo, and hearing impairment are more likely with chronic salicylate intoxication. **Ethylene glycol**, a component of antifreeze, is converted in the liver to glyoxylic and oxalic acids, causing a severe metabolic acidosis. Excessive oxalate excretion causes calcium oxalate crystals to appear in the urine, and calcium oxalate precipitation in the kidney tubules can cause renal failure. The toxicity of **methanol** ingestion also depends on liver metabolism; formic acid is the toxic end product that causes the metabolic acidosis and other sequelae, which include damage to the optic nerve and central nervous system.

There are many **inborn errors of metabolism** that may cause a metabolic acidosis (see Section 10). The metabolic acidosis may be due to excessive production of ketoacids, lactic acid, or other organic anions. Some patients have accompanying hyperammonemia. In most patients, acidosis occurs only episodically during acute decompensations, which may be precipitated by ingestion of specific dietary substrates (proteins), the stress of a mild illness (fasting, catabolism), or poor compliance with dietary or medical therapy.

Clinical Manifestations

The underlying disorder usually produces most of the signs and symptoms in children with a mild or moderate metabolic acidosis. The clinical manifestations of the acidosis are related to the degree of acidemia; patients with appropriate respiratory compensation and less severe acidemia have fewer manifestations than patients with a concomitant respiratory acidosis. At a serum pH less than 7.20, there is impaired cardiac contractility and an increased risk of arrhythmias, especially if underlying heart disease or other predisposing electrolyte disorders are present. With acidemia, there is a decrease in the cardiovascular response to catecholamines, potentially exacerbating hypotension in children with volume depletion or shock. Acidemia causes vasoconstriction of the pulmonary vasculature, which is especially problematic in neonates with primary pulmonary hypertension of the newborn (see Chapter 61). The normal respiratory response to metabolic acidosis—compensatory hyperventilation—may be subtle with mild metabolic acidosis, but it causes discernible increased respiratory effort with worsening acidemia. Chronic metabolic acidosis causes failure to thrive.

Diagnosis

The plasma **anion gap** is useful for evaluating patients with a metabolic acidosis. It divides patients into two diagnostic groups: normal anion gap and increased anion gap. The following formula determines the anion gap:

$$\text{Anion gap} = [Na^+] - [Cl^-] - [HCO_3^-]$$

A normal anion gap is 3 to 11. A decrease in the albumin concentration of 1 g/dL decreases the anion gap by roughly 4 mEq/L. Similarly, albeit less commonly, an increase in unmeasured cations, such as calcium, potassium, or magnesium, decreases the anion gap. Conversely, a decrease in unmeasured cations is a rare cause of an increased anion gap. Because of these variables, the broad range of a normal anion gap, and other factors, the presence of a normal or increased anion gap is not always reliable in differentiating the causes of a metabolic acidosis, especially when the metabolic acidosis is mild. Some patients have more than one explanation for their metabolic acidosis, such as a child with diarrhea and lactic acidosis secondary to hypoperfusion. The anion gap should not be interpreted in dogmatic isolation; consideration of other laboratory abnormalities and the clinical history improves its diagnostic utility.

Treatment

The most effective therapeutic approach for patients with a metabolic acidosis is correction of the underlying disorder, if possible. The administration of insulin in diabetic ketoacidosis or restoration of adequate perfusion in lactic acidosis from shock eventually results in normalization of acid-base balance. The use of bicarbonate therapy is indicated when the underlying disorder is irreparable; examples include RTA and chronic renal failure. In salicylate poisoning, alkali administration increases renal clearance of salicylate and decreases the amount of salicylate in brain cells. Short-term base therapy is often necessary in other poisonings and inborn errors of metabolism.

METABOLIC ALKALOSIS
Etiology

The causes of a metabolic alkalosis are divided into two categories based on the urinary chloride (Table 37-3). The alkalosis in patients with a low urinary chloride is maintained by volume depletion. They are called **chloride responsive** because volume repletion with fluid containing sodium chloride and potassium chloride is necessary to correct the metabolic alkalosis. Emesis, which causes loss of hydrochloride and volume depletion, is the most common cause of a metabolic alkalosis. Diuretic use increases chloride excretion in the urine. Consequently, while a patient is receiving diuretics, the urinary chloride is typically high (>20 mEq/L). After the diuretic effect resolves, the urinary chloride is low (<15 mEq/L), because of appropriate renal chloride retention in response to volume depletion. Categorization of diuretics based on urinary chloride depends on the timing of the measurement. The metabolic alkalosis from diuretics is clearly chloride responsive; it corrects only after adequate volume repletion. This is the rationale for including it among the chloride-responsive causes of a metabolic alkalosis.

The **chloride-resistant** causes of metabolic alkalosis can be subdivided based on blood pressure. Patients with the rare disorders that cause a metabolic alkalosis and hypertension either have increased aldosterone or act as if they have increased aldosterone. Patients with Bartter syndrome or Gitelman syndrome (Chapter 36) have metabolic alkalosis, hypokalemia, and normal blood pressure secondary to renal tubular defects that cause continuous urinary losses of chloride.

Clinical Manifestations

The symptoms in patients with a metabolic alkalosis often are related to the underlying disease and associated electrolyte disturbances. Hypokalemia is often present, and occasionally severe, in the diseases that cause a metabolic alkalosis (see Chapter 36). Children with chloride-responsive causes of metabolic alkalosis often have symptoms related to volume depletion (see Chapter 33). In contrast, children with chloride-unresponsive causes may have symptoms related to hypertension. Severe alkalemia may cause arrhythmias, hypoxia secondary to hypoventilation, or decreased cardiac output.

Table 37-3 | Causes of Metabolic Alkalosis

CHLORIDE RESPONSIVE (URINARY CHLORIDE <15 Meq/L)

Gastric losses (emesis or nasogastric suction)

Pyloric stenosis

Diuretics (loop or thiazide)

Chloride-losing diarrhea

Chloride-deficient formula

Cystic fibrosis (sweat losses of chloride)

Posthypercapnia (chloride loss during respiratory acidosis)

CHLORIDE RESISTANT (URINARY CHLORIDE >20 Meq/L)

High Blood Pressure

Adrenal adenoma or hyperplasia

Glucocorticoid-remediable aldosteronism

Renovascular disease

Renin-secreting tumor

17α-Hydroxylase deficiency

11β-Hydroxylase deficiency

Cushing syndrome

11 β-Hydroxysteroid dehydrogenase deficiency

Licorice ingestion

Liddle syndrome

Normal Blood Pressure

Gitelman syndrome

Bartter syndrome

Base administration

Diagnosis

Measurement of the urinary chloride concentration is the most helpful test in differentiating among the causes of a metabolic alkalosis. The history usually suggests a diagnosis, although no obvious explanation may be present in the patient with bulimia, surreptitious diuretic use, or an undiagnosed genetic disorder, such as Bartter syndrome or Gitelman syndrome.

Treatment

The approach to therapy of metabolic alkalosis depends on the severity of the alkalosis and the underlying etiology. In children with a mild metabolic alkalosis ($[HCO_3^-] < 32$ mEq/L), intervention is often unnecessary. Patients with chloride-responsive metabolic alkalosis respond to correction of hypokalemia and volume repletion with sodium and potassium chloride, but aggressive volume repletion may be contraindicated if mild volume depletion is medically necessary in the child receiving diuretic therapy. In children with chloride-resistant causes of a metabolic alkalosis that are associated with hypertension, volume repletion is contraindicated because it exacerbates the hypertension and does not repair the metabolic alkalosis. Treatment focuses on eliminating or blocking the action of the excess mineralocorticoid. In children with Bartter syndrome or Gitelman syndrome, therapy includes oral potassium supplementation and potassium-sparing diuretics.

RESPIRATORY ACID-BASE DISTURBANCES

During a respiratory acidosis, there is a decrease in the effectiveness of CO_2 removal by the lungs. The causes of a respiratory acidosis are either pulmonary or nonpulmonary (Table 37-4). A respiratory alkalosis is an inappropriate reduction in the blood CO_2 concentration. A variety of stimuli can increase the ventilatory drive and cause a respiratory alkalosis (Table 37-5). Treatment of respiratory acid-base disorders focuses on correction of the underlying disorder. Mechanical ventilation may be necessary in a child with a refractory respiratory acidosis.

Table 37-4 | Causes of Respiratory Acidosis

Central nervous system depression (encephalitis or narcotic overdose)

Disorders of the spinal cord, peripheral nerves, or neuromuscular junction (botulism or Guillain-Barré syndrome)

Respiratory muscle weakness (muscular dystrophy)

Pulmonary disease (pneumonia or asthma)

Upper airway disease (laryngospasm)

Table 37-5 | Causes of Respiratory Alkalosis

Hypoxemia or tissue hypoxia (carbon monoxide poisoning or cyanotic heart disease)

Lung receptor stimulation (pneumonia or pulmonary embolism)

Central stimulation (anxiety or brain tumor)

Mechanical ventilation

Hyperammonemias

Suggested Reading

Colletti JE, Brown KM, Sharieff GQ, et al: The management of children with gastroenteritis and dehydration in the emergency department, *J Emerg Med* 38:686–698, 2010.

Friedman A: Fluid and electrolyte therapy: a primer, *Pediatr Nephrol* 25:843–846, 2010.

Gennari FJ: Pathophysiology of metabolic alkalosis: a new classification based on the centrality of stimulated collecting duct ion transport, *Am J Kidney Dis* 58:626–636, 2011.

Greenbaum LA: Pathophysiology of body fluids and fluid therapy. In Kliegman RM, Stanton BF, St. Geme JW, et al, editors: *Nelson textbook of pediatrics*, ed 19, Philadelphia, 2011, Elsevier Science, pp 212–249.

Kraut JA, Madias NE: Differential diagnosis of nongap metabolic acidosis: value of a systematic approach, *Clin J Am Soc Nephrol* 7:671–679, 2012.

Pepin J, Shields C: Advances in diagnosis and management of hypokalemic and hyperkalemic emergencies, *Emerg Med Pract* 14:1–17, 2012.

Simpson JN, Teach SJ: Pediatric rapid fluid resuscitation, *Curr Opin Pediatr* 23:286–292, 2011.

Unwin RJ, Luft FC, Shirley DG: Pathophysiology and management of hypokalemia: a clinical perspective, *Nat Rev Nephrol* 7:75–84, 2011.

The Acutely Ill or Injured Child

K. Jane Lee

Chapter **38**

ASSESSMENT AND RESUSCITATION

INITIAL ASSESSMENT

Initial assessment (the **ABCs—airway, breathing, and circulation**) of an acutely ill or injured child includes rapid identification of physiologic derangements in **tissue perfusion and oxygenation.** Once identified, immediate resuscitation must be implemented before pursuing the usual information needed to develop a differential diagnosis. Initial resuscitation measures are directed at achieving and maintaining adequate tissue perfusion and oxygenation. **Oxygen delivery** depends on cardiac output, hemoglobin concentration, and hemoglobin-oxygen saturation. The last mentioned depends on air movement, alveolar gas exchange, pulmonary blood flow, and oxygen-hemoglobin binding characteristics.

HISTORY

In the resuscitation phase, access to historical information may be limited. Characterization of the onset of symptoms, details of events, and a brief identification of underlying medical problems should be sought by members of the team not actively involved in the resuscitation. Attempts at identifying historical issues that affect the ABCs are useful but should not delay intervention if tissue oxygenation and perfusion are markedly impaired.

PHYSICAL EXAMINATION

Initial examination must focus rapidly on the **ABCs** (Table 38-1) to address the issues of oxygen delivery to tissues systematically. Airway patency is the first to be addressed, including assessment of the neurologically injured child's ability to protect the airway. Protection of the cervical spine also should be initiated at this step in any child with traumatic injury or who presents with altered mental status of uncertain etiology. Assessment of breathing includes auscultation of air movement and application of a pulse oximeter (when available) to identify current oxygenation status. Circulatory status is assessed by palpation for distal and central pulses, focusing on

the presence and quality of the pulses. Bounding pulses and a wide pulse pressure are often the first sign of the vasodilatory phase of shock and require immediate resuscitation measures. Weak, thready, or absent pulses are indicators for fluid resuscitation, initiation of chest compressions, or both. When assessment of the **ABCs** is complete and measures have been taken to achieve an acceptable level of tissue oxygenation, a more complete physical examination is performed. The sequence of this examination depends on whether the situation involves an acute medical illness or trauma. In trauma patients, the examination follows the **ABCDE pathway. D** stands for disability and prompts assessment of the neurologic system and evaluation for major traumatic injuries. **E** stands for exposure; the child is disrobed and examined for evidence of any life-threatening or limb-threatening problems. For the acutely ill and the injured child, the subsequent physical examination should identify evidence of organ dysfunction, starting with areas suggested in the chief complaint and progressing to a thorough and systematic investigation of the entire patient.

COMMON MANIFESTATIONS

The physiologic responses to acute illness and injury are mechanisms that attempt to correct inadequacies of tissue oxygenation and perfusion. When initial changes, such as increasing heart and respiratory rates, fail to meet the body's needs, other manifestations of impending cardiopulmonary failure occur (Table 38-2). **Respiratory failure,** the most common cause of acute deterioration in children, may result in inadequate tissue oxygenation and in respiratory acidosis. Signs and symptoms of respiratory failure (tachypnea, tachycardia, increased work of breathing, abnormal mentation) progress as tissue oxygenation becomes more inadequate. Inadequate perfusion (shock) leads to inadequate oxygen delivery and a resulting metabolic acidosis. **Shock** is characterized by signs of inadequate tissue perfusion (pallor, cool skin, poor pulses, delayed capillary refill, oliguria, and abnormal mentation). The presence of any of these symptoms demands careful assessment and intervention to correct the abnormality and to prevent further deterioration.

INITIAL DIAGNOSTIC EVALUATION
Screening Tests

During the initial phase of resuscitation, monitoring vital signs and physiologic status is the key screening activity. Continuous monitoring with attention to changes may indicate response to

Table 38-1	Rapid Cardiopulmonary Assessment

AIRWAY PATENCY

Able to be maintained independently

Maintainable with positioning, suctioning

Unmaintainable, requires assistance

BREATHING

Rate

Mechanics

- Retractions
- Grunting
- Use of accessory muscles
- Nasal flaring

Air movement

- Chest expansion
- Breath sounds
- Stridor
- Wheezing
- Paradoxical chest motion

Color

CIRCULATION

Heart rate

Peripheral and central pulses

- Present/absent
- Volume/strength

Skin perfusion

- Capillary refill time
- Skin temperature
- Color
- Mottling

Blood pressure

CENTRAL NERVOUS SYSTEM PERFUSION

Responsiveness (AVPU)

Recognition of parents or caregivers

Pupil size

Posturing

AVPU, Alert, responds to voice, responds to pain, unresponsive.

Table 38-2	Warning Signs and Symptoms Suggesting the Need for Resuscitation*

SYSTEM	SIGNS AND SYMPTOMS
Central nervous system	Lethargy, agitation, delirium, obtundation, confusion
Respiratory	Apnea, grunting, nasal flaring, dyspnea, retracting, tachypnea, poor air movement, stridor, wheezing
Cardiovascular	Arrhythmia, bradycardia, tachycardia, weak pulses, poor capillary refill, hypotension
Skin and mucous membranes	Mottling, pallor, cyanosis, diaphoresis, poor membrane turgor, dry mucous membranes

*Action would seldom be taken if only one or two of these signs and symptoms were present, but the occurrence of several in concert foreshadows grave consequences. Intervention should be directed at the primary disorder.

trauma patients is focused on identifying evidence of hemorrhage and organ and tissue injury. For an acutely ill child with respiratory distress, a chest x-ray is important. Appropriate cultures should be obtained when sepsis is suspected. Children with historical or physical evidence of inadequate intravascular volume should have serum electrolyte levels obtained, including bicarbonate, blood urea nitrogen, and creatinine.

RESUSCITATION

Resuscitation is focused on correcting identified abnormalities of oxygenation and perfusion and preventing further deterioration. **Oxygen supplementation** may improve oxygen saturation but may not completely correct tissue oxygenation. When oxygen supplementation is insufficient or air exchange is inadequate, assisted ventilation must be initiated. Inadequate perfusion is usually best managed initially by providing a fluid bolus. **Isotonic crystalloids** (normal saline, lactated Ringer solution) are the initial fluid of choice. A bolus of 10 to 20 mL/kg should be delivered in monitored conditions. Improvement, but not correction, after an initial bolus should prompt repeated boluses until circulation has been re-established. Because most children with shock have noncardiac causes, fluid administration of this magnitude is well tolerated. If hemorrhage is known or highly suspected, administration of packed red blood cells is appropriate. Monitoring for deteriorating physiologic status during fluid resuscitation (increase in heart rate, decrease in blood pressure) identifies children who may have decreased cardiac function. Fluid resuscitation increases preload, which may worsen pulmonary edema and cardiac function. If deterioration occurs, fluid administration should be interrupted, and resuscitation should be aimed at improving cardiac function.

When respiratory support and fluid resuscitation are insufficient, introduction of **vasoactive substances** is the next step. The choice of which agent to use depends on the type of shock present. Hypovolemic shock (when further volume is contraindicated) and distributive shock benefit from drugs that increase systemic vascular resistance (drugs with α-agonist activity, such as epinephrine or norepinephrine). The treatment of cardiogenic shock is more complex. To improve cardiac output by increasing the heart rate, drugs with positive chronotropy are used (epinephrine, norepinephrine, and dopamine). Afterload reduction, using drugs such as

therapy or further deterioration requiring additional intervention. During the initial rapid assessment, diagnostic evaluation often is limited to pulse oximetry and bedside measurement of glucose levels. The latter is important in any child with altered mental status or at risk for inadequate glycogen stores (infants, malnourished patients). After resuscitation measures, further diagnostic tests and imaging are often necessary.

Diagnostic Tests and Imaging

The choice of appropriate diagnostic tests and imaging is determined by the mechanism of disease and results of evaluation after initial resuscitation. The initial evaluation of major dobutamine, nitroprusside, or milrinone, also may be needed. Measuring mixed venous oxygen saturation, central venous pressure, and regional oxygen saturations helps guide therapy.

CARDIOPULMONARY ARREST

The outcome of cardiopulmonary arrest in children is poor; survival to hospital discharge is about 6% for out-of-hospital arrest and about 27% for in-hospital arrest, with most survivors having permanent neurologic disability. The ability to anticipate or recognize pre–cardiopulmonary arrest conditions and initiate prompt and appropriate therapy not only is lifesaving, but also preserves the quality of life (see Table 38-2).

Children who need cardiopulmonary resuscitation (CPR) usually have a primary respiratory arrest. Hypoxia usually initiates the cascade leading to arrest and also produces organ dysfunction or damage (Table 38-3). The approach to cardiopulmonary arrest extends beyond CPR and includes efforts to preserve vital organ function. The goal in resuscitating a pediatric patient following a cardiopulmonary arrest should be to optimize **cardiac output** and tissue oxygen delivery, which may be accomplished by using artificial ventilation and chest compression and by the judicious administration of pharmacologic agents.

Pediatric Advanced Life Support and CPR

In 2010 the American Heart Association revised the recommendations for resuscitation for adults, children, and infants. The biggest change is the recommendation to start chest compressions immediately, rather than beginning with airway and breathing.

Circulation

Chest compressions should be initiated if a pulse cannot be palpated or if the heart rate is less than 60 beats/min with signs of poor systemic perfusion. Chest compressions should be performed immediately by one person while a second person prepares to begin ventilation. **Ventilation** is extremely important in pediatric arrests because of the high likelihood of a primary respiratory cause; however, ventilation requires

Table 38-3	Target Organs for Hypoxic-Ischemic Damage
ORGAN	**EFFECT**
Brain	Seizures, cerebral edema, infarction, herniation, anoxic damage, SIADH, diabetes insipidus
Cardiovascular	Heart failure, myocardial infarct
Lung and pulmonary vasculature	Acute respiratory distress syndrome, pulmonary hypertension
Liver	Infarction, necrosis, cholestasis
Kidney	Acute tubular necrosis, acute cortical necrosis
Gastrointestinal tract	Gastric ulceration, mucosal damage
Hematologic	Disseminated intravascular coagulation

SIADH, Syndrome of inappropriate secretion of antidiuretic hormone.

equipment and is, therefore, sometimes delayed. For this reason the recommendation is to start chest compressions first while preparing for ventilation.

For optimal chest compressions, the child should be supine on a flat, hard surface. Effective CPR requires a compression depth of one third to one half of the anterior-posterior diameter of the chest with complete recoil after each compression. The compression rate should be at least 100/min with breaths delivered 8 to 10 times per minute. If an advanced airway is in place, compressions should not pause for ventilation; both should continue simultaneously.

Airway

Ventilation requires a **patent airway**. In children, airway patency often is compromised by a loss of muscle tone, allowing the mandibular block of tissue, including the tongue, bony mandible, and the soft surrounding tissues, to rest against the posterior pharyngeal wall. The head tilt–chin lift maneuver should be used to open the airway in children with no sign of head or neck trauma. In children with signs of head or neck trauma, the jaw thrust maneuver should be used.

Bag-mask ventilation can be as effective as, and possibly safer than, endotracheal intubation for short periods of time in an out-of-hospital setting. If skilled personnel and proper equipment are available, pediatric patients requiring resuscitation should be endotracheally intubated. Before intubation, the patient should be ventilated with 100% oxygen using a bag and mask. Cricoid pressure should be used to minimize inflation of the stomach. Many conscious patients may benefit from the use of induction medications (sedatives, analgesics, and paralytics) to assist intubation, but caution is necessary to prevent further cardiovascular compromise from vasodilating effects of many sedatives. The correct size of the tube may be estimated according to the size of the child's mid-fifth phalanx or the following formula: 4 + (patient age in years/4).

When the endotracheal tube is in place, the adequacy of ventilation and the position of the tube must be assessed. Use of both clinical assessment and confirmatory devices is recommended. Clinical assessment may include looking for adequate chest wall movement and auscultation of the chest to detect bilateral and symmetric breath sounds. Confirmatory devices such as end-tidal carbon dioxide (CO_2) monitoring devices are useful for validation of endotracheal placement, but low levels of detected CO_2 may be seen secondary to lack of pulmonary circulation. If the patient's condition fails to improve or deteriorates, consider the possibilities of tube **D**isplacement or **O**bstruction, **P**neumothorax, or **E**quipment failure (mnemonic DOPE).

Breathing

The major role of endotracheal intubation is to protect or maintain the airway and ensure the delivery of adequate oxygen to the patient. Because hypoxemia is the final common pathway in pediatric cardiopulmonary arrests, providing oxygen is more important than correcting the respiratory acidosis. The clinician should deliver 100% oxygen at a rate of 8 to 10 breaths/min during CPR, or 12 to 20 breaths/min for a patient who has a perfusing rhythm. Use only the tidal volume necessary to produce visible chest rise. Care should be taken not to hyperventilate the patient.

Drugs

When mechanical means fail to re-establish adequate circulation, pharmacologic intervention is essential (Table 38-4). If intravascular access is not present or rapidly established, administration through an intraosseous route is recommended. Some drugs can also be administered effectively through the endotracheal tube.

Epinephrine, a catecholamine with mixed α-agonist and β-agonist properties, constitutes the mainstay of drug therapy for CPR. The α-adrenergic effects are most important during acute phases of resuscitation, causing an increase in systemic vascular resistance that improves coronary blood flow. Standard dose therapy is recommended for the first and subsequent boluses. There is no benefit offered by high-dose epinephrine. Vasopressin, an endogenous hormone, causes constriction of capillaries and small arterioles and may be useful. Insufficient data support its routine use, but vasopressin may be considered in children failing standard medication administration.

The routine use of **sodium bicarbonate** is currently not recommended. Sodium bicarbonate may be judiciously used to treat toxidromes or hyperkalemic arrest; however, oxygen delivery and elimination of CO_2 must be established first. Side effects include hypernatremia, hyperosmolality, hypokalemia, metabolic alkalosis (shifting the oxyhemoglobin curve to the left and impairing tissue oxygen delivery), reduced ionized calcium level, and impaired cardiac function.

Routine administration of **calcium** is not recommended. It may be useful in cases of documented hypocalcemia, calcium channel blocker overdose, hypermagnesemia, or hypokalemia, but is otherwise not beneficial and potentially harmful.

Hypoglycemia is not uncommon in infants and children who sustain cardiac arrest. Blood glucose should be checked and hypoglycemia should be promptly treated with **glucose**.

Prompt electrical **defibrillation** is indicated when ventricular fibrillation or pulseless ventricular tachycardia is noted (Table 38-5). CPR should continue until immediately before defibrillation and resume immediately afterward, minimizing interruptions in compressions. If a second attempt at defibrillation is necessary, it should be followed by a dose of epinephrine. Children failing two episodes of defibrillation may benefit from administration of amiodarone. Defibrillation should be distinguished from **cardioversion** of supraventricular tachycardias, which also may compromise cardiac output. Cardioversion requires a lower starting dose and synchronization of the discharge to the electrocardiogram to prevent discharging during a susceptible period, which may convert supraventricular tachycardia to ventricular tachycardia or fibrillation.

Table 38-5	Recommendations for Defibrillation and Cardioversion in Children

DEFIBRILLATION

Place self-adhesive defibrillation pads or paddles with electrode gel at the apex of the heart and the upper right side of the chest
• Use infant paddles or self-adhesive pads for children <10 kg; adult size for children >10 kg

Notify all participating personnel before discharging paddles so that no one is in contact with patient or bed
Begin with 2 J/kg; resume chest compressions immediately
If unsuccessful, increase to 4 J/kg and repeat
Higher energy levels may be considered, not to exceed 10 J/kg or the adult maximum dose

CARDIOVERSION

Consider sedation if possible

For symptomatic supraventricular tachycardia* or ventricular tachycardia with a pulse, synchronize signal with ECG

Choose paddles, position pads, and notify personnel as above

Begin with 0.5–1 J/kg

If unsuccessful, use 2 J/kg

ECG, Electrocardiogram.
*Consider adenosine first (see Table 38-4)

Table 38-4	Drug Doses for Cardiopulmonary Resuscitation	
DRUG	**INDICATION**	**DOSE**
Adenosine	Supraventricular tachycardia	0.1 mg/kg (maximum 6 mg); second dose: 0.2 mg/kg (maximum 12 mg)
Amiodarone	Pulseless VF/VT	5 mg/kg; may repeat twice up to 15 mg/kg; maximum single dose 300 mg
	Perfusing tachyarrhythmias	Dose as above but administer slowly over 20 to 60 minutes. Expert consultation strongly recommended.
Atropine	Supraventricular or junctional bradycardia	0.02 mg/kg (minimum dose 0.1 mg); up to 0.5 mg; higher doses needed in organophosphate poisoning
Bicarbonate	Hyperkalemia, some toxidromes	1 mEq/kg bolus; ensure adequate ventilation; monitor ABGs; can repeat every 10 min
Calcium chloride	Hypocalcemia, calcium channel blocker overdose, hypermagnesemia, hyperkalemia	20 mg/kg; maximum single dose 2 g; administer slowly
Epinephrine	Hypotension, chronotropy, inotropy	0.01 mg/kg IV/IO; 0.1 mg/kg ET; may repeat every 3–5 minutes; may promote arrhythmias
Fluid	Hypovolemia, sepsis	Administer crystalloid in 20 mL/kg boluses titrated to patient's physiologic needs
Glucose	Hypoglycemia	Newborns: 5–10 mL/kg 10% dextrose; infants and children: 2–4 mL/kg 25% dextrose; adolescents: 1–2 mL/kg 50% dextrose
Lidocaine	VT	1 mg/kg/bolus followed by 20–50 mcg/kg/min continuous infusion

Data from 2010 American Heart Association Guidelines for Cardiopulmonary Resuscitation and Emergency Cardiovascular Care. Part 14: Pediatric Advanced Life Support, Circulation 122 [suppl 3]:S876-S908, 2010.
ABG, Arterial blood gas; ET, endotracheal; IO, intraosseous; IV, intravenous; VF, ventricular fibrillation; VT, ventricular tachycardia.

Chapter 39

RESPIRATORY FAILURE

ETIOLOGY

Acute respiratory failure occurs when the pulmonary system is unable to maintain adequate gas exchange to meet metabolic demands. The resulting failure can be classified as hypercarbic ($Paco_2$ >50 mm Hg in previously healthy children), hypoxemic (Pao_2 <60 mm Hg in previously healthy children without an intracardiac shunt), or both. **Hypoxemic respiratory failure** is frequently caused by ventilation-perfusion mismatch (perfusion of lung that is not adequately ventilated) and shunting (deoxygenated blood bypasses ventilated alveoli). **Hypercarbic respiratory failure** results from inadequate alveolar ventilation secondary to decreased minute ventilation (tidal volume × respiratory rate) or an increase in dead space ventilation (ventilation of areas receiving no perfusion).

Respiratory failure may occur with **acute lung injury (ALI)** or **acute respiratory distress syndrome (ARDS)**. The definitions of these are in the process of revision; however, currently ALI is defined as having the following four clinical features: acute onset, bilateral pulmonary edema, no clinical evidence of elevated left atrial pressure, and a ratio of Pao_2 to Fio_2 ≤ 300 mm Hg regardless of the level of positive end-expiratory pressure (PEEP). ARDS is a subset of ALI with more severe hypoxemia (Pao_2/Fio_2 of ≤ 200 mm Hg). These syndromes can be triggered by a variety of insults, including sepsis, pneumonia, shock, burns, or traumatic injury, all resulting in inflammation and increased vascular permeability leading to pulmonary edema. Numerous mediators of inflammation (tumor necrosis factor, interferon-γ, nuclear factor κB, and adhesion molecules) may be involved in the development of ARDS. Surfactant action also may be affected.

EPIDEMIOLOGY

Respiratory failure is frequently caused by bronchiolitis (often caused by respiratory syncytial virus), asthma, pneumonia, upper airway obstruction, and sepsis/ARDS. Respiratory failure requiring mechanical ventilation develops in 7% to 21% of patients hospitalized for respiratory syncytial virus.

Asthma is increasing in prevalence and is the most common reason for unplanned hospital admissions in children 3 to 12 years of age in the United States. Environmental factors (exposure to cigarette smoke) and prior disease characteristics (severity of asthma, exercise intolerance, delayed start of therapy, and previous intensive care unit admissions) affect hospitalization and near-fatal episodes. The mortality rate of asthma for children younger than 19 years of age has increased by nearly 80% since 1980. Deaths are more common in African-American children.

Chronic respiratory failure (with acute exacerbations) is often due to chronic lung disease (bronchopulmonary dysplasia, cystic fibrosis), neurologic or neuromuscular abnormalities, and congenital anomalies.

CLINICAL MANIFESTATIONS

Early signs of hypoxic respiratory failure include **tachypnea and tachycardia** in attempt to improve minute ventilation and cardiac output and to maintain delivery of oxygenated blood to the tissues. Further progression of disease may result in dyspnea, nasal flaring, grunting, use of accessory muscles of respiration, and diaphoresis. Late signs of inadequate oxygen delivery include **cyanosis** and **altered mental status** (initially confusion and agitation). Signs and symptoms of hypercarbic respiratory failure include attempts to increase minute ventilation (tachypnea and increased depth of breathing) and altered mental status (somnolence).

LABORATORY AND IMAGING STUDIES

A chest radiograph may show evidence of the etiology of respiratory failure. The detection of atelectasis, hyperinflation, infiltrates, or pneumothoraces assists with ongoing management. Diffuse infiltrates or pulmonary edema may suggest ARDS. The chest radiograph may be normal when upper airway obstruction or impaired respiratory controls are the etiology. In patients presenting with stridor or other evidence of upper airway obstruction, a lateral neck film or computed tomography (CT) may delineate anatomic defects. Direct visualization through flexible bronchoscopy allows identification of dynamic abnormalities of the anatomic airway. Helical CT helps diagnose a pulmonary embolus.

Pulse oximetry allows noninvasive, continuous assessment of oxygenation but is unable to provide information about ventilation abnormalities. Determination of CO_2 levels requires a blood gas measurement (arterial, venous, or capillary). An **arterial blood gas** allows measurement of CO_2 levels and analysis of the severity of oxygenation defect through calculation of an alveolar-arterial oxygen difference. A normal Pco_2 in a patient who is hyperventilating should heighten concern about the risk of further deterioration.

DIFFERENTIAL DIAGNOSIS

Hypoxic respiratory failure resulting from impairment of alveolar-capillary function is seen in ARDS; cardiogenic pulmonary edema; interstitial lung disease; aspiration pneumonia; bronchiolitis; bacterial, fungal, or viral pneumonia; and sepsis. It also can be due to intracardiac or intrapulmonary shunting seen with atelectasis and embolism.

Hypercarbic respiratory failure can occur when the respiratory center fails as a result of drug use (opioids, barbiturates, anesthetic agents), neurologic or neuromuscular junction abnormalities (cervical spine trauma, demyelinating diseases, anterior horn cell disease, botulism), chest wall injuries, or diseases that cause increased resistance to airflow (croup, vocal cord paralysis, post-extubation edema). Maintenance of ventilation requires adequate function of the chest wall and diaphragm. Disorders of the neuromuscular pathways, such as muscular dystrophy, myasthenia gravis, and botulism, result in inadequate chest wall movement, development of atelectasis, and respiratory failure. Scoliosis rarely results in significant chest deformity that leads to restrictive pulmonary function. Similar impairments of air exchange may result from distention of the abdomen (postoperatively or due to ascites, obstruction, or a mass) and thoracic trauma (flail chest).

Mixed forms of respiratory failure are common and occur when disease processes result in more than one pathophysiologic change. Increased secretions seen in asthma often lead to atelectasis and hypoxia, whereas restrictions of expiratory airflow may lead to hypercarbia. Progression to respiratory failure results from peripheral airway obstruction, extensive atelectasis, and resultant hypoxemia and retention of CO_2.

TREATMENT

Initial treatment of patients in respiratory distress includes addressing the ABCs (see Chapter 38). **Bag/mask ventilation** must be initiated for patients with apnea. In other patients, oxygen therapy is administered using appropriate methods (e.g., simple mask). Administration of oxygen by nasal cannula allows the patient to entrain room air and oxygen, making it an insufficient delivery method for most children in respiratory failure. Delivery methods, including intubation and mechanical ventilation, should be escalated if there is inability to increase oxygen saturation appropriately.

Patients presenting with hypercarbic respiratory failure are often hypoxic as well. When oxygenation is established, measures should be taken to address the underlying cause of hypercarbia (reversal of drug action, control of fever, or seizures). Patients who are hypercarbic without signs of respiratory fatigue or somnolence may not require intubation based on the Pco_2 alone; however, patients with marked increase in the work of breathing or inadequate respiratory effort may require assistance with ventilation.

After identification of the etiology of respiratory failure, specific interventions and treatments are tailored to the needs of the patient. External support of oxygenation and ventilation may be provided by **noninvasive ventilation** methods (heated humidified high-flow nasal cannula, continuous positive airway pressure, biphasic positive airway pressure, or negative pressure ventilation) or through invasive methods (traditional **mechanical ventilation,** high-frequency oscillatory ventilation, or extracorporeal membrane oxygenation). Elimination of CO_2 is achieved through manipulation of minute ventilation (tidal volume and respiratory rate). Oxygenation is improved by altering variables that affect oxygen delivery (fraction of inspired oxygen) or mean airway pressure (PEEP, peak inspiratory pressure, inspiratory time, gas flow).

COMPLICATIONS

The major complication of hypoxic respiratory failure is the development of organ dysfunction. **Multiple organ dysfunction** includes the development of two or more of the following: respiratory failure, cardiac failure, renal insufficiency/failure, gastrointestinal or hepatic insufficiency, disseminated intravascular coagulation, and hypoxic-ischemic brain injury. Mortality rates increase with increasing numbers of involved organs (see Table 38-3).

Complications associated with mechanical ventilation include pressure-related and volume-related lung injury. Both overdistention and insufficient lung distention (loss of functional residual capacity) are associated with lung injury. Pneumomediastinum and pneumothorax are potential complications of the disease process and overdistention. Inflammatory mediators may play a role in the development of chronic fibrotic lung diseases in ventilated patients.

PROGNOSIS

Prognosis varies with the etiology of respiratory failure. Fewer than 1% of previously healthy children with bronchiolitis die. Asthma mortality rates, although still low, have increased. Despite advances in support and understanding of the pathophysiology of ARDS, the mortality rate remains approximately 30%.

PREVENTION

Prevention strategies are explicit to the etiology of respiratory failure. Some infectious causes can be prevented through active immunization against organisms causing primary respiratory disease (pertussis, pneumococcus, *Haemophilus influenzae* type b) and sepsis (pneumococcus, *H. influenzae* type b). Passive immunization with respiratory syncytial virus immunoglobulins prevents severe illness in highly susceptible patients (prematurity, bronchopulmonary dysplasia). Primary prevention of traumatic injuries may decrease the incidence of ARDS. Compliance with appropriate therapies for asthma may decrease the number of episodes of respiratory failure (see Chapter 78).

Chapter **40**

SHOCK

ETIOLOGY AND EPIDEMIOLOGY

Shock is the inability to provide sufficient perfusion of oxygenated blood and substrate to tissues to meet metabolic demands. **Oxygen delivery** is directly related to the arterial oxygen content (oxygen saturation and hemoglobin concentration) and to cardiac output (stroke volume and heart rate). Changes in metabolic needs are met primarily by adjustments in cardiac output. Stroke volume is related to myocardial end-diastolic fiber length (preload), myocardial contractility (inotropy), and resistance of blood ejection from the ventricle (afterload) (see Chapter 145). In a young infant whose myocardium possesses relatively less contractile tissue, increased demand for cardiac output is met primarily by a neurally mediated increase in heart rate. In older children and adolescents, cardiac output is most efficiently augmented by increasing stroke volume through neurohormonally mediated changes in vascular tone, resulting in increased venous return to the heart (increased preload), decreased arterial resistance (decreased afterload), and increased myocardial contractility.

HYPOVOLEMIC SHOCK

Acute hypovolemia is the most common cause of shock in children. It results from loss of fluid from the intravascular space secondary to inadequate intake or excessive losses (vomiting and diarrhea, blood loss, capillary leak syndromes, or pathologic renal fluid losses) (Table 40-1). Reduced blood volume decreases preload, stroke volume, and cardiac output. Hypovolemic shock results in increased sympathoadrenal activity, producing an increased heart rate and enhanced myocardial

Table 40-1	Classification of Shock and Common Underlying Causes	
TYPE	**PRIMARY CIRCULATORY DERANGEMENT**	**COMMON CAUSES**
Hypovolemic	Decreased circulating blood volume	Hemorrhage
		Diarrhea
		Diabetes insipidus, diabetes mellitus
		Burns
		Adrenogenital syndrome
		Capillary leak
Distributive	Vasodilation → venous pooling → decreased preload	Sepsis
	Maldistribution of regional blood flow	Anaphylaxis
		CNS/spinal injury
		Drug intoxication
Cardiogenic	Decreased myocardial contractility	Congenital heart disease
		Arrhythmia
		Hypoxic/ischemic injuries
		Cardiomyopathy
		Metabolic derangements
		Myocarditis
		Drug intoxication
		Kawasaki disease
Obstructive	Mechanical obstruction to ventricular filling or outflow	Cardiac tamponade
		Massive pulmonary embolus
		Tension pneumothorax
		Cardiac tumor
Dissociative	Oxygen not appropriately bound or released from hemoglobin	Carbon monoxide poisoning Methemoglobinemia

CNS, Central nervous system.

contractility. Neurohormonally mediated constriction of the arterioles and capacitance vessels maintains blood pressure, augments venous return to the heart to improve preload, and redistributes blood flow from nonvital to vital organs. If hypovolemic shock remains untreated, the increased heart rate may impair coronary blood flow and ventricular filling, while elevated systemic vascular resistance increases myocardial oxygen consumption, resulting in worsening myocardial function. Ultimately, intense systemic vasoconstriction and hypovolemia produce tissue ischemia, impairing cell metabolism and releasing potent vasoactive mediators from injured cells. Cytokines and other vasoactive peptides can change myocardial contractility and vascular tone and promote release of other inflammatory mediators that increase capillary permeability and impair organ function further.

DISTRIBUTIVE SHOCK

Abnormalities in the distribution of blood flow may result in profound inadequacies in tissue perfusion, even in the presence of a normal or high cardiac output. This maldistribution of flow usually results from abnormalities in vascular tone. Septic shock is the most common type of distributive shock in children. Other causes include anaphylaxis, neurologic injury, and drug-related causes (see Table 40-1).

Distributive shock may present with the **systemic inflammatory response syndrome** (SIRS), defined as two or more of the following: temperature greater than 38° C or less than 36° C; heart rate greater than 90 beats/min or more than two standard deviations above normal for age; tachypnea; or white blood count greater than 12,000 cells/mm^3, less than 4000 cells/mm^3, or greater than 10% immature forms.

CARDIOGENIC SHOCK

Cardiogenic shock is caused by an abnormality in myocardial function and is expressed as depressed myocardial contractility and cardiac output with poor tissue perfusion. Compensatory mechanisms may contribute to the progression of shock by depressing cardiac function further. Neurohormonal vasoconstrictor responses increase afterload and add to the work of the failing ventricle. Tachycardia may impair coronary blood flow, which decreases myocardial oxygen delivery. Increased central blood volume caused by sodium and water retention and by incomplete emptying of the ventricles during systole results in elevated left ventricular volume and pressure, which impair subendocardial blood flow. As compensatory mechanisms are overcome, the failing left ventricle produces increased ventricular end-diastolic volume and pressure, which leads to increased left atrial pressure, resulting in pulmonary edema. This sequence also contributes to right ventricular failure because of increased pulmonary artery pressure and increased right ventricular afterload.

Primary cardiogenic shock may occur in children who have congenital heart disease. Cardiogenic shock also may occur in previously healthy children secondary to viral myocarditis, dysrhythmias, or toxic or metabolic abnormalities or after hypoxic-ischemic injury (see Chapters 142, 145, and 147, as well as Table 40-1).

OBSTRUCTIVE SHOCK

Obstructive shock results from mechanical obstruction of ventricular outflow. Causes include congenital lesions such as coarctation of the aorta, interrupted aortic arch, and severe aortic valvular stenosis, along with acquired diseases (e.g., hypertrophic cardiomyopathy) (see Table 40-1). For neonates presenting in shock, obstructive lesions must be considered.

DISSOCIATIVE SHOCK

Dissociative shock refers to conditions in which tissue perfusion is normal, but cells are unable to use oxygen because the hemoglobin has an abnormal affinity for oxygen, preventing its release to the tissues (see Table 40-1).

CLINICAL MANIFESTATIONS

All forms of shock produce evidence that tissue perfusion and oxygenation are insufficient (increased heart rate, abnormal blood pressure, alterations of peripheral pulses). The etiology of shock may alter the initial presentation of these signs and symptoms.

Hypovolemic Shock

Hypovolemic shock is distinguished from other causes of shock by history and the absence of signs of heart failure or sepsis. In addition to the signs of sympathoadrenal activity (tachycardia, vasoconstriction), clinical manifestations include signs of dehydration (dry mucous membranes, decreased urine output) or blood loss (pallor). Recovery depends on the degree of hypovolemia, the patient's preexisting status, and rapid diagnosis and treatment. The prognosis is good, with a low mortality in uncomplicated cases.

Distributive Shock

Patients with distributive shock usually have tachycardia and alterations of peripheral perfusion. In early stages, when cytokine release results in vasodilation, pulses may be bounding, and vital organ function may be maintained (an alert patient, with rapid capillary refill and some urine output in *warm shock*). As the disease progresses untreated, extremities become cool and mottled with a delayed capillary refill time. At this stage, the patient has hypotension and vasoconstriction. If the etiology of distributive shock is sepsis, the patient often has fever, lethargy, petechiae, or purpura, and he or she may have an identifiable source of infection.

Cardiogenic Shock

Cardiogenic shock results when the myocardium is unable to supply the cardiac output required to support tissue perfusion and organ function. Because of this self-perpetuating cycle, heart failure progressing to death may be rapid. Patients with cardiogenic shock have tachycardia and tachypnea. The liver is usually enlarged, a gallop is often present, and jugular venous distention may be noted. Because renal blood flow is poor, sodium and water are retained, resulting in oliguria and peripheral edema.

Obstructive Shock

Restriction of cardiac output results in an increase in heart rate and an alteration of stroke volume. The pulse pressure is narrow (making pulses harder to feel), and capillary refill is delayed. The liver is often enlarged, and jugular venous distention may be evident.

Dissociative Shock

The principal abnormality in dissociative shock is the inability to deliver oxygen to tissues. Symptoms include tachycardia, tachypnea, alterations in mental status, and ultimately cardiovascular collapse.

LABORATORY AND IMAGING STUDIES

Shock requires immediate resuscitation before obtaining laboratory or diagnostic studies. Following initial stabilization (including glucose administration if hypoglycemia is present), the type of shock dictates the necessary laboratory studies. All patients with shock may benefit from determination of a baseline arterial blood gas and blood lactate level to assess the impairment of tissue oxygenation. Measurement of **mixed venous oxygen saturation** aids in the assessment of the adequacy of oxygen delivery. In contrast to other forms of shock, patients with sepsis often have high mixed venous saturation values because of impairment of mitochondrial function and inability of tissues to extract oxygen. A complete blood count can potentially assess intravascular blood volume after equilibration following a hemorrhage. Electrolyte measurements in patients with hypovolemic shock may identify abnormalities from losses. Patients presenting in distributive shock require appropriate bacterial and viral cultures to identify a cause of infection. If cardiogenic or obstructive shock is suspected, an echocardiogram assists with the diagnosis and, in the case of tamponade, assists with placement of a pericardial drain to relieve the fluid. Patients with dissociative shock require detection of the causative agent (carbon monoxide, methemoglobin). The management of shock also requires monitoring of arterial blood gases for oxygenation, ventilation (CO_2), and acidosis, and frequently assessing the levels of serum electrolytes, calcium, magnesium, phosphorus, and blood urea nitrogen (BUN).

DIFFERENTIAL DIAGNOSIS

SEE TABLE 40-1.

TREATMENT
General Principles

The key to therapy is the recognition of shock in its early, partially compensated state, when many of the hemodynamic and metabolic alterations may be reversible. Initial therapy for shock follows the ABCs of resuscitation. Later therapy can then be directed at the underlying cause. Therapy should minimize cardiopulmonary work, while ensuring cardiac output, blood pressure, and gas exchange. Intubation, combined with mechanical ventilation with oxygen supplementation, improves oxygenation and decreases or eliminates the work of breathing but may impede venous return if distending airway pressures (positive end-expiratory pressure [PEEP] or peak inspiratory pressure) are excessive. Blood pressure support is crucial because the vasodilation in sepsis may reduce perfusion despite supranormal cardiac output.

Monitoring a child in shock requires maintaining access to the arterial and central venous circulation to record pressure measurements, perform blood sampling, and measure systemic blood pressure continuously. These measurements facilitate the estimation of preload and afterload. Regional monitoring with near infrared spectroscopy may allow early, noninvasive detection of alterations in perfusion.

Organ-Directed Therapeutics
Fluid Resuscitation

Alterations in preload have a dramatic effect on cardiac output. In hypovolemic and distributive shock, decreased preload significantly impairs cardiac output. In these cases, early and aggressive fluid resuscitation is important and greatly affects outcome. In cardiogenic shock, an elevated preload contributes to pulmonary edema.

Selection of fluids for resuscitation and ongoing use is dictated by clinical circumstances. Crystalloid volume expanders generally are recommended as initial choices because they are effective and inexpensive. Most acutely ill children with signs of shock may safely receive, and usually benefit greatly from, a 20-mL/kg bolus of an isotonic crystalloid over 5 to 15 minutes. This dose may be repeated until a response is noted. Colloids contain larger molecules that may stay in the intravascular space longer than crystalloid solutions and exert oncotic pressure, drawing fluid out of the tissues into the vascular compartment. However, long-term risks of colloids may exceed benefits. Care must be exercised in treating cardiogenic shock with volume expansion because the ventricular filling pressures may rise without improvement of the cardiac performance. Carefully monitoring cardiac output or central venous pressure guides safe volume replacement.

Cardiovascular Support

In an effort to improve cardiac output after volume resuscitation or when further volume replacement may be dangerous, a variety of inotropic and vasodilator drugs may be useful (Table 40-2). Therapy is directed first at increasing myocardial contractility, then at decreasing left ventricular afterload. The hemodynamic status of the patient dictates the choice of the agent.

Therapy may be initiated with dopamine at 3 to 15 mcg/kg/min; however, epinephrine or norepinephrine may be preferable in patients with decompensated shock. In addition to improving contractility, certain catecholamines cause an increase in systemic vascular resistance. The addition of a vasodilator drug may improve cardiac performance by decreasing the resistance against which the heart must pump (afterload). Afterload reduction may be achieved with dobutamine, milrinone, amrinone, nitroprusside, nitroglycerin, and angiotensin-converting enzyme inhibitors. The use of these drugs may be particularly important in late shock, when vasoconstriction is prominent.

Respiratory Support

The lung is a target organ for inflammatory mediators in shock and SIRS. Respiratory failure may develop rapidly and become progressive. Intervention requires endotracheal intubation and mechanical ventilation accompanied by the use of supplemental oxygen and PEEP. Care must be taken with the process of intubation, because a child with compensated shock may suddenly decompensate on administration of sedative medications that reduce systemic vascular resistance. Severe cardiopulmonary failure may be managed with inhaled nitric oxide and, if necessary, extracorporeal membrane oxygenation.

Renal Salvage

Poor cardiac output accompanied by decreased renal blood flow may cause prerenal azotemia and oliguria/anuria. Severe hypotension may produce **acute tubular necrosis** and **acute renal failure.** Prerenal azotemia is corrected when blood volume deficits are replaced or myocardial contractility is improved, but acute tubular necrosis does not improve immediately when shock is corrected. Prerenal azotemia is associated with a serum BUN-to-creatinine ratio of greater than 10:1 and a urine sodium level less than 20 mEq/L; acute tubular necrosis has a BUN-to-creatinine ratio of 10:1 or less and a urine sodium level between 40 and 60 mEq/L (see Chapter 165). Aggressive fluid replacement is often necessary to improve oliguria associated with prerenal azotemia. Because the management of shock requires administering large volumes of fluid, maintaining urine output greatly facilitates patient management.

Prevention of acute tubular necrosis and the subsequent complications associated with acute renal failure (hyperkalemia, acidosis, hypocalcemia, fluid overload) is important. The use of pharmacologic agents to augment urine output is indicated when the intravascular volume has been replaced. The use of loop diuretics, such as furosemide, or combinations of a loop diuretic and a thiazide agent may enhance urine output. Infusion of low-dose dopamine, which produces renal artery vasodilation, also may improve urine output. Nevertheless, if hyperkalemia, refractory acidosis, hypervolemia, or altered mental status associated with uremia occurs, dialysis or hemofiltration should be initiated.

COMPLICATIONS

Shock results in impairment of tissue perfusion and oxygenation and activation of inflammation and cytokine pathways. The major complication of shock is multiple organ system failure, defined as the dysfunction of more than one organ, including respiratory failure, renal failure, liver dysfunction, coagulation abnormalities, or cerebral dysfunction. Patients with shock and multiple organ failure have a higher mortality rate and, for survivors, a longer hospital stay.

PROGNOSIS

Early recognition and **goal-directed intervention** in patients with shock improve survival. However, delays in treatment of hypotension increase the incidence of multiple organ failure and mortality. Goal-directed therapy focused on maintaining mixed venous oxygen saturation may improve survival.

Table 40-2	Medications Used to Improve Cardiac Output				
	POSITIVE INOTROPE	**POSITIVE CHRONOTROPE**	**DIRECT PRESSOR**	**VASOCONSTRICTOR**	**VASODILATOR**
Dopamine	++	+	±	++ (high dose)	+ (low dose)*
Dobutamine	++	±	–	–	+
Epinephrine	+++	+++	+++	++ (high dose)	+ (low dose)†
Norepinephrine	+++	+++	+++	+++	–
Milrinone	+	-	-	-	+

*Primarily splanchnic and renal in low doses (3–5 mcg/kg/min).
†Low dose (<0.3 mcg/kg/min).

PREVENTION

Prevention strategies for shock are focused, for the most part, on shock associated with sepsis and hypovolemia. Some forms of septic shock can be prevented through use of immunizations (*Haemophilus influenzae* type b, meningococcal, pneumococcal vaccines). Decreasing the risk of sepsis in a critically ill patient requires adherence to strict hand washing, isolation practices, and minimizing the duration of indwelling catheters. Measures to decrease pediatric trauma do much to minimize hemorrhage-induced shock.

lower incidence of traumatic brain injury and death. Enforcement of seatbelt laws increases seatbelt use and may decrease injuries.

Automatic strategies require no action on the part of the population and often change the environment (speed bumps) or involve engineering (child-resistant pill bottles, air bags). Automatic strategies have more consistently resulted in a significant reduction in injuries. The most successful approaches to preventing injury have combined strategies (education, environmental changes, and engineering changes focused on the host, agent, and environment in all three time phases).

Chapter 41

INJURY PREVENTION

EPIDEMIOLOGY AND ETIOLOGY

Unintentional injury is the leading cause of death in children 1 to 18 years of age. In 2010, approximately 52% of these deaths were caused by motor vehicle crashes. Most remaining unintentional injury-related deaths were the result of drowning (15%), poisoning (9%), burns (5%), and suffocation (4%). Geography, climate, population density (access to care), and population traits vary by region and affect the frequency, etiology, and severity of injuries.

Injury occurs through interaction of the **host** (child) with the **agent** (e.g., car and driver) through a vector and an **environment** (e.g., roadways, weather) that is conducive to exposure. The age of the child may determine the exposure to various agents and environments. For example, most injuries in infants and toddlers occur in the home as the result of exposure to agents found there (water heaters, bathtubs, soft bedding). Gender affects exposure to injury, with boys having a fatal injury rate greater than that of girls.

EDUCATION FOR PREVENTING INJURIES

The recognition that much of the morbidity and mortality are determined at the scene of an injury has stimulated the development of prevention measures. The **Haddon matrix** combines the epidemiologic components (host, agent, physical and social environments) with time factors (before, during, and after the event) to identify effective interventions focused on different aspects of the injury event. Primary strategies (preventing the event), secondary strategies (minimizing the severity of injury), and tertiary strategies (minimizing long-term impact) can be targeted for each epidemiologic component. Such strategies typically fall into one of three areas: education, enforcement, and environment (including engineering).

Education is often the first strategy considered but requires behavioral change and actions on the part of people. Most educational strategies are not well evaluated.

Despite the reliance on an action by the individuals involved, some active strategies benefit from enforcement. Children wearing bicycle helmets experience a significantly

Chapter 42

MAJOR TRAUMA

ASSESSMENT AND RESUSCITATION

The general goal of **prehospital trauma care** is rapid assessment, support of the ABCs, immobilization, and transportation. Outcomes of patients with major or life-threatening trauma are significantly improved in a pediatric trauma center or in an adult center with pediatric trauma certification compared with level I or II adult trauma centers.

Once the injured child arrives at the emergency department, the trauma team must initiate an organized and synchronized response. The initial assessment of a seriously injured child should involve a systematic approach, including a primary survey, resuscitation, secondary survey, postresuscitation monitoring, and definitive care. The **primary survey** focuses on the **ABCDEs** of emergency care, as modified for trauma from the ABCs of cardiopulmonary resuscitation (see Chapter 38). The assessment of the airway and breathing components should include meticulous control of the cervical spine (especially if the patient has an altered mental status), evaluation for anatomic injuries that could impair air entry or gas exchange, and consideration of the likelihood of a full stomach (risk of aspiration pneumonia). Circulation can be assessed via observation (heart rate, skin color, mental status) and palpation (pulse quality, capillary refill, skin temperature) and restored (via two large peripheral intravenous lines, when possible) while control of bleeding is accomplished through the use of direct pressure. Assessment for **disabilities** (D), including neurologic status, includes examination of pupil size and reactivity, a brief mental status assessment (*AVPU—a*lert; responds to *v*oice; responds to *p*ain; *u*nresponsive), and examination of extremity movement to assess for spinal cord injury. The **Glasgow Coma Scale** can direct decisions regarding the initiation of cerebral resuscitation in patients with suspected closed head injuries (Table 42-1). **E,** which stands for *exposure,* requires a full assessment of the patient by completely disrobing the child for a detailed examination of the entire body. The examiner should ensure a neutral thermal environment to prevent hypothermia.

Table 42-1	Glasgow Coma Scales	
ACTIVITY	**BEST RESPONSE**	**SCORE**
Eye opening	Spontaneous	4
	To verbal stimuli	3
	To pain	2
	None	1
Verbal	Oriented • Infant: coos, babbles	5
	Confused • Infant: irritable, cries	4
	Inappropriate words • Infant: cries to pain	3
	Nonspecific sounds • Infant: moans to pain	2
	None	1
Motor	Follows commands • Infant: spontaneous movement	6
	Localizes pain • Infant: withdraws to touch	5
	Withdraws to pain	4
	Flexion to pain • Infant: abnormal flexion	3
	Extension to pain • Infant: abnormal extension	2
	None	1

Table 42-2	Initial Laboratory Evaluation of the Major Trauma Patient
HEMATOLOGY	
Complete blood count	
Platelet count	
Type and cross-match	
URINALYSIS	
Gross	
Microscopic	
CLINICAL CHEMISTRY	
Amylase	
AST/ALT	
RADIOLOGY	
Cervical spine films	
Anteroposterior chest radiograph	
Radiographs of all apparent fractures	
Computed tomography scans where indicated for head, chest, and abdominal trauma	

AST/ALT, Aspartate aminotransferase/alanine aminotransferase.

On completion of the primary survey, a more detailed head-to-toe examination (the **secondary survey**) should ensue along with efforts to obtain a more complete history. The purpose of this careful re-examination is to identify life-threatening and limb-threatening injuries as well as less serious injuries. Coincident with the secondary survey and depending, in part, on the assessed physiologic status of the patient, certain procedures and resuscitative measures are initiated. The prioritization of definitive care needs is determined by the injury findings collected from the primary and secondary surveys, the child's physiologic response to resuscitation, and data from continuous monitoring. A **tertiary survey,** including repeat primary and secondary surveys along with review of laboratory tests and radiologic studies, should be performed within 24 hours.

ETIOLOGY AND EPIDEMIOLOGY
SEE CHAPTER 41.

LABORATORY AND IMAGING STUDIES
Screening laboratory studies during initial resuscitation often include the tests listed in Table 42-2. Radiographic studies are determined by the pattern of injuries. A head computed tomography (CT) scan should be obtained in patients with evidence of head trauma or a history of loss of consciousness. Patients with obvious injury to the thorax or abdomen or who have pulmonary or abdominal symptoms may benefit from a CT scan. The focused abdominal sonography for trauma is gaining popularity because of concerns about radiation exposure. Diagnostic peritoneal lavage has limited utility. A spiral enhanced CT scan should be performed if there is concern about aortic injuries.

CLINICAL MANIFESTATIONS AND TREATMENT
Head injuries and injuries to the limbs are the most common. Multiple organ involvement is also common, and penetrating trauma is becoming more frequent. After the initial evaluation and stabilization, the team focuses on the involved organ systems.

Head Trauma
SEE CHAPTER 184.

Spinal Cord Trauma
Although spinal cord injury is not common in pediatric trauma patients, it is potentially devastating when it occurs. Cervical spine immobilization should be maintained until a spinal cord injury is ruled out. Cervical spine radiographs are not sufficient to rule out a spinal cord injury because the immature vertebral column in children may allow stretching of the cord or nerve roots with no radiologic abnormality (spinal cord injury without radiologic abnormality [SCIWORA]). SCIWORA may occur in a significant percentage of children with a spinal cord injury; when it is suspected, magnetic resonance imaging should be performed.

Thoracic Trauma
Thoracic injury is the second leading cause of trauma death. Pulmonary contusion, pneumothorax, and rib fractures occur most commonly, and patients may present without external signs of trauma. Patients with pulmonary parenchymal injury should receive supportive treatment to ensure adequate

oxygenation and ventilation. Most pediatric blunt thoracic injuries can be managed without surgery. Injury to the heart and great vessels is rare but requires urgent diagnosis and treatment. Great vessel injury should be suspected if a widened mediastinum is seen on chest radiograph.

Abdominal Trauma

Injury to the abdomen occurs in approximately 8% of pediatric trauma patients and is the third leading cause of trauma death. The relative size and closer proximity of intra-abdominal organs in children increase the risk of significant injury after blunt trauma. Penetrating trauma may result in a child who is asymptomatic or who presents in hypovolemic shock.

Imaging studies such as abdominal CT and serial physical examinations are the primary methods of obtaining information on which to base decisions regarding operative intervention. Abdominal wall bruising is an important physical examination finding and is associated with significant intra-abdominal injury in more than 10% of patients. Operative intervention may be required in patients whose vital signs are persistently unstable in the face of aggressive fluid resuscitation, even in the absence of extravascular volume loss or an enlarging abdomen. The presence of peritoneal irritation or abdominal wall discoloration, together with signs of intravascular volume loss, indicates the need for laparotomy.

Most blunt solid organ injury is handled nonoperatively. Clinical observation is important, because most failures with nonoperative management occur in the first 12 hours.

Injury to the Spleen

The most frequently injured abdominal organ in children is the spleen. Suspicion of a splenic injury should be heightened if there are left upper quadrant abrasions or tenderness. A positive *Kehr sign* (pressure on the left upper quadrant eliciting left shoulder pain) is due to diaphragmatic irritation by the ruptured spleen and strongly suggests splenic injury. CT scans are used to identify and grade splenic injury.

Nonoperative management is the treatment of choice for most serious splenic injuries, unless there is continued large blood loss or hemodynamic instability. If a splenectomy is performed, patients should receive penicillin prophylaxis and should receive pneumococcal and *Haemophilus influenzae* vaccines to decrease the increased risk of overwhelming sepsis.

Liver Trauma

Major trauma to the liver is a serious cause of morbidity. Severe hemorrhage is more common in patients with liver injury than with other abdominal injuries because of its dual blood supply. Without significant vascular injury, hepatic injury presents and behaves clinically like a splenic injury. Nonoperative management is recommended but requires close clinical observation for signs of ongoing blood loss or hemodynamic instability. As with splenic injury, there is a grading system based on the pattern of injury.

Renal Injury

The kidney is less frequently injured than the liver or spleen, and when injured is often associated with other injuries. A young child's kidney is more vulnerable to trauma than an adult's because of a more compliant rib cage and relatively immature abdominal muscle development. The diagnosis of renal injury is based on history and physical examination coupled with urinalysis showing blood and increased protein levels. An ultrasound or CT may also be useful. Low-grade renal injury is usually managed conservatively, with bed rest, catheter drainage, and monitoring for resolution of injury by ultrasound or CT. Surgery may be required for falling hemoglobin levels, refractory shock, or urinary obstruction caused by clots.

Pancreatic Injury

Injuries of the pancreas are less common in children than in adults but are seen in bicycle handlebar injuries, motor vehicle crashes, and nonaccidental trauma. The diagnosis is difficult unless there is obvious injury to overlying structures, such as the stomach or duodenum. Diffuse abdominal tenderness, pain, and vomiting may be accompanied by elevations of amylase and lipase but may not occur until several days after the injury. Hemodynamic instability secondary to retroperitoneal hemorrhage may be the presenting sign. Nasogastric suction and parenteral nutrition are indicated in the management of these patients. Nonoperative management is appropriate for contusions, but surgical intervention may be required in patients with distal transection. Drainage of pseudocysts, in patients who develop them, may be required if they are unresponsive to bowel rest and parenteral nutrition.

Intestinal Injury

Injury to the intestine occurs less frequently than injury to solid intra-abdominal organs and varies with the amount of intestinal contents. A full bowel is likely to shear more easily than an empty bowel. Shearing occurs at points of fixation (the ligament of Treitz, the ileocecal valve, and the ascending and descending peritoneal reflections). Pneumoperitoneum should prompt surgical exploration. Serial physical examinations are useful when the clinical picture is uncertain.

Duodenal hematoma can occur in the absence of perforation. Duodenal hematomas result from blunt injury to the abdomen, and affected patients often present with persistent pain and bilious emesis. Most hematomas respond to nonoperative management with gastric decompression and parenteral nutrition.

COMPLICATIONS

Patients requiring hospitalization for multiple trauma are at risk for a variety of complications based on the type and severity of injury. Sepsis and multiple organ failure may occur in children with multiple trauma. Delays in enteral nutrition because of an ileus may further increase the risk of sepsis secondary to translocation of bacteria across the intestinal mucosa.

Renal failure secondary to myoglobinuria may be seen in children who sustain crushing or electrical injuries and burns. Deep venous thrombosis is less common in the pediatric population, but prophylaxis for children who will be immobilized because of injury is often provided.

PROGNOSIS

Unintentional injury is the leading cause of death for children ages 1 to 18; however, many of these deaths occur in the field, immediately after the injury. Once admitted to the hospital, mortality rates are much lower. Morbidities are numerous and include hypoxic-ischemic brain injury, loss of limbs, and psychological dysfunction.

PREVENTION
SEE CHAPTER 41.

Chapter 43

DROWNING

ETIOLOGY

Drowning, as defined by the World Congress on Drowning in 2002, is the process of experiencing respiratory impairment from submersion/immersion in liquid. Drowning can further be categorized as fatal or nonfatal, but other terms such as near-drowning, secondary drowning, or dry drowning should be abandoned.

Initially, submersion or immersion results in aspiration of small amounts of fluid into the larynx, triggering breath holding or laryngospasm. In many cases, the laryngospasm resolves, and larger volumes of water or gastric contents are aspirated into the lungs, destroying surfactant and causing alveolitis and dysfunction of the alveolar-capillary gas exchange. The resulting hypoxemia leads to hypoxic brain injury that is exacerbated by ischemic injury after circulatory collapse.

EPIDEMIOLOGY

Drowning deaths overall have decreased over the past decade; however, drowning is still a significant cause of morbidity and mortality. In 2010, drowning was the leading cause of injury death for children 1 to 4 years of age and the second leading cause of injury death for children 1 to 18 years of age. Boys are four times more likely than girls to drown. The most common location of drowning varies by age, with drowning in natural bodies of water becoming more frequent in older age groups.

CLINICAL MANIFESTATIONS

Hypoxemia is the result of laryngospasm and aspiration during drowning. Victims may also develop respiratory distress secondary to **pulmonary endothelial injury, increased capillary permeability,** and **destruction of surfactant.** Clinical manifestations include tachypnea, tachycardia, increased work of breathing, and decreased breath sounds with or without crackles. The hypoxic-ischemic injury that may occur can lead to depressed myocardial function resulting in tachycardia, impaired perfusion, and potentially cardiovascular collapse. After resuscitation, acute respiratory distress syndrome is common. Altered mental status may be present and requires frequent monitoring of neurologic status. Following submersion in cold water, hypothermia may result in relative bradycardia and hypotension and place the child at risk for cardiac dysrhythmias.

LABORATORY AND IMAGING STUDIES

After resuscitation, arterial blood gas measurement assists in assessing pulmonary gas exchange. A chemistry profile may reveal elevated liver enzymes if hypoxemia and ischemia were of long duration and provide baseline renal functions. Electrolytes are often obtained, although alterations of serum electrolytes are minimal, even in freshwater drowning.

TREATMENT

Resuscitation of a drowning victim includes the basic ABCs (see Chapter 38). Victims of unwitnessed drowning require stabilization of the cervical spine because of the possibility of a fall or diving injury. Optimizing oxygenation and maintaining cerebral perfusion are two of the major foci of treatment. Rewarming the hypothermic patient requires careful attention to detail, including acid-base and cardiac status. Further treatment is based on the patient response to initial resuscitation. Some children begin breathing spontaneously and awaken before arrival at an emergency department. If the episode was significant, these children still require careful observation for pulmonary complications over the subsequent 6 to 12 hours. Children who have evidence of lung injury, cardiovascular compromise, or neurologic compromise should be monitored in an intensive care unit. Pulmonary dysfunction often results in hypoxemia. Oxygen supplementation should be implemented to maintain normal oxygen saturations. Mechanical ventilation may be needed in patients with significant pulmonary or neurologic dysfunction. Cardiovascular compromise is often the result of impaired contractility because of hypoxic-ischemic injury. The use of intracranial pressure monitoring devices and medical management with hypothermia and sedation is controversial and has not been shown to improve outcomes. Prophylactic antibiotics have not been shown to be beneficial and may increase the selection of resistant organisms.

PROGNOSIS

The outcome of drowning is determined by the success of immediate resuscitation efforts and the severity of the **hypoxic-ischemic injury** to the brain. Patients who have regained consciousness on arrival to the hospital will likely survive with intact neurologic function. Unfavorable prognostic markers include the need for CPR for more than 25 minutes, continued CPR at the hospital, Glasgow Coma Scale of 5 or less, fixed and dilated pupils, seizures, and coma for more than 72 hours.

PREVENTION

Despite the decreased incidence of drowning since the 1990s, few prevention strategies have been shown to be effective. Exceptions include implementation of mandatory four-sided fencing around pools (decreasing the number of children <5 years of age who drown) and immediate provision of CPR to children who drown. The use of safety flotation devices in older children during water sport activities may be beneficial. Enhanced supervision is required to reduce the incidence of infants drowning in bathtubs.

Chapter **44**

BURNS

ETIOLOGY

The pathophysiology of burn injury is caused by disruption of the three key functions of the skin: regulation of heat loss, preservation of body fluids, and barrier to infection. Burn injury releases inflammatory and vasoactive mediators resulting in increased capillary permeability, decreased plasma volume, and decreased cardiac output. The body then becomes hypermetabolic with increased resting energy expenditure and protein catabolism. This hypermetabolic state may continue for up to a year after injury.

Burns usually are classified on the basis of four criteria:
1. Depth of injury
2. Percent of body surface area involved
3. Location of the burn
4. Association with other injuries

EPIDEMIOLOGY

More than 100,000 children sustain a burn injury each year. Burns are the third leading cause of injury-related death for children ages 1 to 9 and are a major cause of morbidity. Boys are more likely to sustain a burn injury, as are children age 6 and under. Scald burns are more common in younger children as compared to older children. Overall, thermal burns secondary to scald or flame are much more common than electrical or chemical burns. Most fire-related childhood deaths and injuries occur in homes.

CLINICAL MANIFESTATIONS

The depth of injury should be assessed by the clinical appearance. Categories of first-degree, second-degree, and third-degree are commonly used; however, classification by depth (superficial, superficial partial-thickness, deep partial-thickness, and full-thickness) conveys more information about the structures injured and the likely need for surgical treatment and may be more clinically useful.

Superficial (first-degree) burns are red, painful, and dry. Commonly seen with sun exposure or mild scald injuries, these burns involve injury to the epidermis only. They heal in 2 to 5 days without scarring and are not included in burn surface area calculations. **Superficial partial-thickness** (second-degree) burns involve the entire epidermis and superficial dermis. These burns have fluid-containing blisters.

PERCENTAGE OF SURFACE AREA OF HEAD AND LEGS AT VARIOUS AGES

	AGE IN YEARS				
AREA IN DIAGRAM	0	1	5	10	15
A = ½ of head	9½	8½	6½	5½	4½
B = ½ of one thigh	2¾	3¼	4	4¼	4½
C = ½ of one lower leg	2½	2½	2¾	3	3¼

Figure 44-1 This chart of body areas, together with the table inserted in the figure showing the percentage of surface area of head and legs at various ages, can be used to estimate the surface area burned in a child. *From Solomon JR: Pediatric burns*, Crit Care Clin 1:159–174, 1985.

After debridement the underlying dermis will appear erythematous and wet, will be painful, and will blanch under pressure. Healing is dependent on the uninjured dermis and usually occurs within about 2 weeks without the need for skin grafting and without scarring. **Deep partial-thickness** (also second-degree) burns involve the entire epidermis and deeper portions of the dermis. These burns may also have blistering, but the dermal base is less blanching, mottled pink or white, and less painful than superficial partial-thickness burns. They behave more like full-thickness burns and will often require excision and grafting. **Full-thickness** (third-degree and fourth-degree) burns involve all skin layers. They appear dry, white, dark red, brown, or black in color. They do not blanch and are usually insensate. Full-thickness burns require surgical management. Fourth-degree burns involve underlying fascia, muscle, or bone and may require reconstruction in addition to grafting. **Inhalation injuries** should be suspected if there are facial burns, singed nasal hairs, or carbonaceous sputum. Hoarseness on vocalization also is consistent with a supraglottic injury. Inhalation injuries may result in bronchospasm, airway inflammation, and impaired pulmonary function.

There are multiple methods and charts available for calculating the percentage of skin surface involved in a burn. One method that may be used for children of various ages is presented in Figure 44-1. The extent of skin involvement of older adolescent and adult patients may be estimated as follows: each upper extremity, 9%; each lower extremity, 18%; anterior trunk, 18%; posterior trunk, 18%; head, 9%; and perineum, 1%.

The location of the burn is important in assessing the risk of disability. The risk is greatest when the face, eyes, ears, feet, perineum, or hands are involved. Inhalation injuries not only cause respiratory compromise but also may result in difficulty in eating and drinking.

LABORATORY AND IMAGING STUDIES

Initial laboratory testing, including complete blood count, type and crossmatch for blood, coagulation studies, basic chemistry profile, arterial blood gas, and chest radiograph, can be helpful for patients with major burns. A carboxyhemoglobin assessment should be performed for any suspected inhalation exposure (a house or closed-space fire or a burn victim who requires cardiopulmonary resuscitation). Cyanide levels should be considered in children who sustain smoke inhalation and have altered mental status. Unusual patterns of burns may increase suspicion of child abuse and result in appropriate evaluation to assess for nonaccidental trauma to the skeleton or central nervous system.

TREATMENT

For severe burns, care is best managed by a multidisciplinary team in a qualified burn center. The American Burn Association criteria for patients who should be transferred to a burn center are: partial and full-thickness burns greater than 10% total body surface area (TBSA) in patients less than 10 years old or more than 50 years old, or greater than 20% TBSA in other age groups; partial and full-thickness burns involving the face, hands, feet, genitalia, perineum, or major joints; electrical burns; chemical burns; inhalation injury; burn injury in patients with preexisting medical conditions that could complicate management, prolong recovery, or increase mortality rate; any burn with concomitant trauma in which the burn injury poses the greatest risk; burn injury in children admitted to hospitals without qualified personnel or equipment for pediatric care; burn injury in patients requiring special social, emotional, or rehabilitative support, including child abuse cases.

Initial treatment should follow the ABCs of resuscitation. **Airway management** should include assessment for the presence of airway or inhalation injury, with early intubation if such an injury is suspected. Smoke inhalation may be associated with carbon monoxide toxicity; 100% humidified oxygen should be given if hypoxia or inhalation is suspected.

The systemic capillary leak that occurs after a serious burn makes initial fluid and electrolyte support of a burned child crucial. The first priority is to support the circulating blood volume, which requires the administration of intravenous fluids to provide maintenance fluid and electrolyte requirements and to replace ongoing burn-related losses. Formulas exist to help guide **fluid management**; however, no formula accurately predicts the fluid needs of every burn patient. Children with a significant burn should receive a rapid bolus of 20 mL/kg of lactated Ringer solution. Thereafter, the resuscitation formula for fluid therapy is determined by the percent of body surface burned. Total fluids are 2 to 4 mL/kg/percent burn/24 hours, with half the estimated burn requirement administered during the first 8 hours. (If resuscitation is delayed, half of the fluid replacement should be completed by the end of the eighth hour post-injury.) Fluids should be titrated to achieve adequate perfusion, one marker of which is urine output greater than 1 mL/kg/hour. Controversy exists over whether and when to administer colloid during fluid resuscitation. Colloid therapy may be needed for patients with extensive burns.

Because burn injury produces a **hypermetabolic** response, children with significant burns require immediate nutritional support. Enteral feeds should be started early unless there is a specific contraindication. Children with critical burn injury may require parenteral nutrition if unable to tolerate full enteral feeds. Consider supplementation of vitamins and trace elements. Factors that may modify the hypermetabolic state such as beta blockers, androgenic steroids, and others are being investigated.

Wound care starts with cleaning and debriding the wound. Effective pain control is important to allow for complete debridement. Topical agents and dressings are then applied to control bacterial colonization, decrease evaporative losses, and aid in pain control. Commonly used topical agents include silver sulfadiazine (Silvadene) or, if the burn is shallow, polymyxin B/bacitracin/neomycin (Neosporin) ointment. Silver nitrate and mafenide acetate (Sulfamylon) are alternative antimicrobial agents. Sulfamylon has the benefit of penetrating eschar, but it is painful and can cause metabolic acidosis. Silver nitrate is used less commonly because of poor tissue penetration and potential for electrolyte abnormalities. These agents

Table 44-1	Complications of Burns
PROBLEM	**TREATMENT**
Sepsis	Monitor for infection, avoid prophylactic antibiotics
Hypovolemia	Fluid replacement
Hypothermia	Adjust ambient temperature: dry blankets in field
Laryngeal edema	Endotracheal intubation, tracheostomy
Carbon monoxide poisoning	100% oxygen, hyperbaric oxygen
Cyanide poisoning	100% O_2 plus amyl nitrate, sodium nitrate, and sodium thiosulfate
Cardiac dysfunction	Inotropic agents, diuretics
Gastric ulcers	H_2-receptor antagonist, antacids
Compartment syndrome	Escharotomy incision
Contractures	Physical therapy
Hypermetabolic state	Enteral and parenteral nutritional support
Renal failure	Supportive care, dialysis
Transient antidiuresis	Expectant management
Anemia	Transfusions as indicated
Psychological trauma	Psychological rehabilitation
Pulmonary infiltrates	PEEP, ventilation, oxygen
Pulmonary edema	Avoid overhydration, give diuretics
Pneumonia	Antibiotics
Bronchospasm	β-Agonist aerosols

PEEP, Positive end-expiratory pressure.

inhibit but do not prevent bacterial growth. Various grafts, such as cadaver allografts, porcine xenografts, or skin substitutes, have been used initially to cover wounds. For full-thickness burns, skin autografting and skin substitutes are required for eventual closure.

COMPLICATIONS
SEE TABLE 44-1.

PROGNOSIS
Most children who sustain burns recover without significant disability; however, burns remain the third leading cause of injury-related deaths in children ages 1 to 9. Estimation of morbidity is difficult to ascertain from databases. Physical scarring and emotional impact of disfiguring burns are long-term consequences of burn injuries.

PREVENTION
About 92% of burns occur in the home. Prevention is possible by using smoke and fire alarms, having identifiable escape routes and a fire extinguisher, and reducing hot water temperature to 49°C (120°F). Immersion full-thickness burns develop after 1 second at 70°C (158°F), after 5 seconds at 60°C (140°F), after 30 seconds at 54.5°C (130°F), and after 10 minutes at 49°C (120°F).

Chapter **45**

POISONING

ETIOLOGY AND EPIDEMIOLOGY
The most common agents ingested by young children include cosmetics, personal care products, analgesics, and cleaning solutions. Fatal childhood poisonings are commonly caused by analgesics, antihistamines, sedative/hypnotics, and fumes/gases/vapors.

More than 2 million human exposures are called in to poison control centers in the United States each year. More than half of all exposures are in children (63% in 2010) with a male predominance in children under 13, but a female predominance in adolescence. Most ingestions in young children are unintentional, with intentional ingestions becoming more common in children 13 and older. Most ingestions occur at home (91%) and are single substance (90%).

CLINICAL MANIFESTATIONS
Any child who presents with unexplained symptoms including altered mental status, seizure, cardiovascular compromise, or metabolic abnormality should be considered to have ingested a poison until proven otherwise. A history and physical examination by someone who understands the signs and symptoms of various ingestions often provide sufficient clues to distinguish between toxic ingestion and organic disease (Table 45-1). Determination of all substances that the child was exposed to, type of medication, amount of medication, and time of exposure is crucial in directing interventions. Available data often are incomplete or inaccurate, requiring a careful physical examination and laboratory approach. A complete physical examination, including vital signs, is necessary. Certain complexes of symptoms and signs are relatively specific to a given class of drugs (toxidrome) (Table 45-2).

COMPLICATIONS
A poisoned child can exhibit any one of six basic clinical patterns: coma, toxicity, metabolic acidosis, heart rhythm aberrations, gastrointestinal symptoms, and seizures.

Coma
Coma is perhaps the most striking symptom of a poison ingestion, but it also may be seen as a result of several other causes including trauma, a cerebrovascular accident, asphyxia, or meningitis. A careful history and clinical examination are needed to distinguish among these alternatives.

Direct Toxicity
Hydrocarbon ingestion occasionally may result in systemic toxicity, but more often it leads to pulmonary toxicity. Hydrocarbons with low viscosity, low surface tension, and high volatility pose the greatest risk of producing aspiration pneumonia; however, when swallowed, they pose no risk unless emesis is induced. Emesis or lavage should *not* be initiated in a child who has ingested volatile hydrocarbons.

Caustic ingestions may cause dysphagia, epigastric pain, oral mucosal burns, and low-grade fever. Patients with esophageal lesions may have no oral burns or may have significant signs and symptoms. Treatment depends on the agent ingested and the presence or absence of esophageal injury. Alkali agents may be solid, granular, or liquid. Liquid agents are tasteless and produce full-thickness liquefaction necrosis of the esophagus or oropharynx. When the esophageal lesions heal, strictures form. Ingestion of these agents also creates a long-term risk of esophageal carcinoma. Treatment includes antibiotics if there are signs of infection and dilation of late-forming (2 to 3 weeks later) strictures.

Ingested button batteries also may produce a caustic mucosal injury. Batteries that remain in the esophagus may cause esophageal burns and erosion and should be removed with an endoscope. Acid agents can injure the lungs (with hydrochloric acid fumes), oral mucosa, esophagus, and stomach. Because acids taste sour, children usually stop drinking the solution, limiting the injury. Acids produce a coagulation necrosis, which limits the chemical from penetrating into deeper layers of the mucosa and damages tissue less severely than alkali. The signs, symptoms, and therapeutic measures are similar to those for alkali ingestion.

Metabolic Acidosis
A poisoned child may also have a high anion gap metabolic acidosis (mnemonic *MUDPILES*) (Table 45-3), which

Table 45-1	Historical and Physical Findings in Poisoning
ODOR	
Bitter almonds	Cyanide
Acetone	Isopropyl alcohol, methanol, paraldehyde, salicylate
Alcohol	Ethanol
Wintergreen	Methyl salicylate
Garlic	Arsenic, thallium, organophosphates, selenium
Violets	Turpentine
OCULAR SIGNS	
Miosis	Narcotics (except propoxyphene, meperidine, and pentazocine), organophosphates, muscarinic mushrooms, clonidine, phenothiazines, chloral hydrate, barbiturates (late)
Mydriasis	Atropine, cocaine, amphetamines, antihistamines, cyclic antidepressants, PCP, LSD
Nystagmus	Phenytoin, barbiturates, ethanol, carbamazepine, PCP, ketamine, dextromethorphan
Lacrimation	Organophosphates, irritant gas or vapors
Retinal hyperemia	Methanol
Poor vision	Methanol, botulism, carbon monoxide
CUTANEOUS SIGNS	
Needle tracks	Heroin, PCP, amphetamine
Dry, hot skin	Anticholinergic agents, botulism
Diaphoresis	Organophosphates, muscarinic mushrooms, aspirin, cocaine
Alopecia	Thallium, arsenic, lead, mercury
Erythema	Boric acid, mercury, cyanide, anticholinergics
ORAL SIGNS	
Salivation	Organophosphates, salicylate, corrosives, strychnine, ketamine
Dry mouth	Amphetamine, anticholinergics, antihistamine
Burns	Corrosives, oxalate-containing plants
Gum lines	Lead, mercury, arsenic
Dysphagia	Corrosives, botulism
INTESTINAL SIGNS	
Diarrhea	Antimicrobials, arsenic, iron, boric acid, cholinergics
Constipation	Lead, narcotics, botulism
Hematemesis	Corrosives, iron, salicylates, NSAIDs
CARDIAC SIGNS	
Tachycardia	Atropine, aspirin, amphetamine, cocaine, cyclic antidepressants, theophylline
Bradycardia	Digitalis, narcotics, clonidine, organophosphates, β-blockers, calcium channel blockers
Hypertension	Amphetamine, LSD, cocaine, PCP
Hypotension	Phenothiazines, barbiturates, cyclic antidepressants, iron, β-blockers, calcium channel blockers, clonidine, narcotics
RESPIRATORY SIGNS	
Depressed respiration	Alcohol, narcotics, barbiturates
Increased respiration	Amphetamines, aspirin, ethylene glycol, carbon monoxide, cyanide
Pulmonary edema	Hydrocarbons, organophosphates
CENTRAL NERVOUS SYSTEM SIGNS	
Ataxia	Alcohol, barbiturates, anticholinergics, narcotics
Coma	Sedatives, narcotics, barbiturates, salicylate, cyanide, carbon monoxide, cyclic antidepressants, alcohol
Hyperpyrexia	Anticholinergics, salicylates, amphetamine, cocaine
Muscle fasciculation	Organophosphates, theophylline
Muscle rigidity	Cyclic antidepressants, PCP, phenothiazines, haloperidol
Peripheral neuropathy	Lead, arsenic, mercury, organophosphates
Altered behavior	LSD, PCP, amphetamines, cocaine, alcohol, anticholinergics

LSD, Lysergic acid diethylamide; *MSG,* monosodium glutamate; *NSAID,* nonsteroidal anti-inflammatory drug; *PCP,* phencyclidine.

Table 45-2 | Toxic Syndromes

AGENT	MANIFESTATIONS
Acetaminophen	Nausea, vomiting, pallor, delayed jaundice–hepatic failure (72–96 hr)
Amphetamine, cocaine, and sympathomimetics	Tachycardia, hypertension, hyperthermia, psychosis and paranoia, seizures, mydriasis, diaphoresis, piloerection, aggressive behavior
Anticholinergics	Mania, delirium, fever, red dry skin, dry mouth, tachycardia, mydriasis, urinary retention
Carbon monoxide	Headache, dizziness, coma, other systems affected
Cyanide	Coma, convulsions, hyperpnea, bitter almond odor
Ethylene glycol (antifreeze)	Metabolic acidosis, hyperosmolarity, hypocalcemia, oxalate crystalluria
Iron	Vomiting (bloody), diarrhea, hypotension, hepatic failure, leukocytosis, hyperglycemia, radiopaque pills on KUB, late intestinal stricture, *Yersinia* sepsis
Narcotics	Coma, respiratory depression, hypotension, pinpoint pupils, bradycardia
Cholinergics (organophosphates, nicotine)	Miosis, salivation, urination, diaphoresis, lacrimation, bronchospasm (bronchorrhea), muscle weakness and fasciculations, emesis, defecation, coma, confusion, pulmonary edema, bradycardia
Salicylates	Tachypnea, fever, lethargy, coma, vomiting, diaphoresis, alkalosis (early), acidosis (late)
Cyclic antidepressants	Coma, convulsions, mydriasis, hyperreflexia, arrhythmia (prolonged Q-T interval), cardiac arrest, shock

KUB, Kidney-ureter-bladder radiograph.

Table 45-3 | Screening Laboratory Clues in Toxicologic Diagnosis

ANION GAP METABOLIC ACIDOSIS (MNEMONIC = MUDPILES)

Methanol,* metformin

Uremia*

Diabetic ketoacidosis*

Paraldehyde,* phenformin

Isoniazid, iron

Lactic acidosis (cyanide, carbon monoxide)

Ethanol,* ethylene glycol*

Salicylates, starvation, seizures

HYPOGLYCEMIA

Ethanol

Isoniazid

Insulin

Propranolol

Oral hypoglycemic agents

HYPERGLYCEMIA

Salicylates

Isoniazid

Iron

Phenothiazines

Sympathomimetics

HYPOCALCEMIA

Oxalate

Ethylene glycol

Fluoride

RADIOPAQUE SUBSTANCE ON KUB (MNEMONIC = CHIPPED)

Chloral hydrate, calcium carbonate

Heavy metals (lead, zinc, barium, arsenic, lithium, bismuth as in Pepto-Bismol)

Iron

Phenothiazines

Play-Doh, potassium chloride

Enteric-coated pills

Dental amalgam

KUB, Kidney-ureter-bladder radiograph.
*Indicates hyperosmolar condition.

is assessed easily by measuring arterial blood gases, serum electrolyte levels, and urine pH. An osmolar gap, if present, strongly suggests the presence of an unmeasured component, such as methanol or ethylene glycol. These ingestions require thorough assessment and prompt intervention.

Dysrhythmias

Dysrhythmias may be prominent signs of a variety of toxic ingestions, although ventricular arrhythmias are rare. Prolonged Q-T intervals may suggest phenothiazine or antihistamine ingestion, and widened QRS complexes are seen with ingestions of cyclic antidepressants and quinidine. Because many drug and chemical overdoses may lead to sinus tachycardia, this is not a useful or discriminating sign; however, sinus bradycardia suggests digoxin, cyanide, a cholinergic agent, or β-blocker ingestion (Table 45-4).

Gastrointestinal Symptoms

Gastrointestinal symptoms of poisoning include emesis, nausea, abdominal cramps, and diarrhea. These symptoms may be the result of direct toxic effects on the intestinal mucosa or of systemic toxicity after absorption.

Seizures

Seizures are the sixth major mode of presentation for children with toxic ingestions, but poisoning is an uncommon cause of afebrile seizures. When seizures do occur with intoxication, they may be life-threatening and require aggressive therapeutic intervention.

LABORATORY AND IMAGING STUDIES

Laboratory studies helpful in initial management include specific toxin-drug assays; measurement of arterial blood gases and electrolytes, osmoles, and glucose; and calculation of the

Table 45-4	Drugs Associated with Major Modes of Presentation

COMMON TOXIC CAUSES OF CARDIAC ARRHYTHMIA	Hypoglycemic agents
Amphetamine	Lead
Antiarrhythmics	Lithium
Anticholinergics	Methemoglobinemia*
Antihistamines	Methyldopa
Arsenic	Narcotics
Carbon monoxide	Phencyclidine
Chloral hydrate	Phenothiazines
Cocaine	Salicylates
Cyanide	COMMON AGENTS CAUSING SEIZURES (MNEMONIC = CAPS)
Cyclic antidepressants	**C**amphor
Digitalis	Carbamazepine
Freon	Carbon monoxide
Phenothiazines	Cocaine
Physostigmine	Cyanide
Propranolol	**A**minophylline
Quinine, quinidine	Amphetamine
Theophylline	Anticholinergics
CAUSES OF COMA	Antidepressants (cyclic)
Alcohol	**P**b (lead) (also lithium)
Anticholinergics	Pesticide (organophosphate)
Antihistamines	Phencyclidine
Barbiturates	Phenol
Carbon monoxide	Phenothiazines
Clonidine	Propoxyphene
Cyanide	**S**alicylates
Cyclic antidepressants	Strychnine

*Causes of methemoglobinemia: amyl nitrite, aniline dyes, benzocaine, bismuth subnitrate, dapsone, primaquine, quinones, spinach, sulfonamides.

anion or osmolar gap. A full 12-lead electrocardiogram should be part of the initial evaluation in all patients suspected of ingesting toxic substances. Urine screens for drugs of abuse or to confirm suspected ingestion of medications in the home may be revealing.

Quantitative toxicology assays are important for some agents (Table 45-5), not only for identifying the specific drug, but also for providing guidance for therapy, anticipating complications, and estimating the prognosis.

TREATMENT

The four foci of treatment for poisonings are supportive care, decontamination, enhanced elimination, and specific antidotes.

Supportive Care

Supportive care is the mainstay of treatment in most cases. Prompt attention must be given to protecting and maintaining the airway, establishing effective breathing, and supporting the circulation. This management sequence takes precedence over other diagnostic or therapeutic procedures. If the level of consciousness is depressed, and a toxic substance is suspected, glucose (1 g/kg intravenously), 100% oxygen, and naloxone should be administered.

Gastrointestinal Decontamination

The intent of gastrointestinal decontamination is to prevent the absorption of a potentially toxic ingested substance and, in theory, to prevent the poisoning. There has been great controversy about which methods are the safest and most efficacious. Recommendations from the American Academy of Clinical Toxicology (AACT) and the European Association of Poison Centres and Clinical Toxicologists (EAPCCT) follow. **Syrup of ipecac** should not be administered routinely to poisoned patients because of potential complications and lack of evidence that it improves outcome. Likewise, **gastric lavage** should not be used routinely, if ever, in the management of poisoned patients because of lack of efficacy and potential complications. **Single-dose activated charcoal** decreases drug absorption when used within 1 hour of ingestion; however, it has not been shown to improve outcome. Thus, it should be used selectively in the management of a poisoned patient. Charcoal is ineffective against caustic or corrosive agents, hydrocarbons, heavy metals (arsenic, lead, mercury, iron, lithium), glycols, and water-insoluble compounds.

The administration of a cathartic (sorbitol or magnesium citrate) alone has no role in the management of the poisoned patient. The AACT has stated that based on available data, the use of a cathartic in combination with activated charcoal is not recommended.

Whole-bowel irrigation using polyethylene glycol (GoLYTELY) as a nonabsorbable cathartic may be effective for toxic ingestion of sustained-release or enteric-coated drugs.

Table 45-5	Drugs Amenable to Therapeutic Monitoring for Drug Toxicity

ANTIBIOTICS

Aminoglycosides—gentamicin, tobramycin, and amikacin

Chloramphenicol

Vancomycin

IMMUNOSUPPRESSION

Methotrexate

Cyclosporine

ANTIPYRETICS

Acetaminophen

Salicylate

OTHER

Digoxin

Lithium

Theophylline

Anticonvulsant drugs

Serotonin uptake inhibitor agent

The AACT does not recommend the routine use of whole-bowel irrigation. However, there is theoretical benefit in its use for potentially toxic ingestions of iron, lead, zinc, or packets of illicit drugs.

Enhanced Elimination
Multiple-dose activated charcoal should be considered only if a patient has ingested a life-threatening amount of carbamazepine, dapsone, phenobarbital, quinine, or theophylline. **Alkalinization of urine** may be helpful for salicylate or methotrexate ingestion. **Dialysis** may be used for substances that have a low volume of distribution, low molecular weight, low protein binding, and high degree of water solubility, such as methanol, ethylene glycol, salicylates, theophylline, bromide, and lithium.

Specific Antidotes
SEE TABLE 45-6.

When in doubt about therapy, contacting one of the U.S. Poison Control Centers (1-800-222-1222) can help to determine what additional treatment is necessary.

PROGNOSIS
Most poisonings result in minimal or no toxicity. Major toxicity is seen in fewer than 1% of ingestions, with fatality in fewer than 0.1%. Only 12% of children 12 and under with poisoning require treatment in a health care facility, compared with 48% of adolescents.

PREVENTION
Properly educating parents regarding safe storage of medications and household toxins is necessary for preventing ingestions. If a child has ingested poison, a poison control center should be called.

Table 45-6	Specific Antidotes			
POISON	**ANTIDOTE**	**DOSAGE**		**COMMENTS**
Acetaminophen	N-Acetylcysteine	140 mg/kg PO initial dose, then 70 mg/kg PO q4hr × 17 doses 150 mg/kg IV over 1 hr, followed by 50 mg/kg IV over 4 hr, followed by 100 mg/kg IV over 16 hr		Most effective within 16 h of ingestion
Benzodiazepine	Flumazenil	0.2 mg IV, may repeat to 1 mg max		Possible seizures, arrhythmias, DO NOT USE FOR UNKNOWN INGESTIONS
β-Blocking agents	Glucagon	0.15 mg/kg IV, followed by infusion of 0.05–0.15 mg/kg/hr		
Carbon monoxide	Oxygen	100%; hyperbaric O_2		Half-life of carboxyhemoglobin is 5 hr in room air but 1.5 hr in 100% O_2
Cyclic antidepressants	Sodium bicarbonate	1–2 mEq/kg IV, followed by continuous infusion; titrated to produce pH of 7.5–7.55		Follow potassium levels and replace as needed
Iron	Deferoxamine	Infusion of 5–15 mg/kg/hr IV (max 6 g/24 hr)		Hypotension (worse with rapid infusion rates)

Continued

Table 45-6	Specific Antidotes—cont'd		
POISON	**ANTIDOTE**	**DOSAGE**	**COMMENTS**
Lead	Edetate calcium disodium (EDTA)	35–50 mg/kg/day IV × 5 days; continuous infusion or divided q 12 hours	
	BAL (British anti-Lewisite [dimercaprol])	3–5 mg/kg/dose IM q4h × 4–11 days	May cause sterile abscesses. Prepared in peanut oil, do not use in patients with peanut allergy.
	Succimer (2,3-dimercaptosuccinic acid ([DMSA])	10 mg/kg/dose PO tid × 5 days, then 10 mg/kg/dose PO bid × 14 days	Few toxic effects, requires lead-free home plus compliant family
Nitrites/ methemoglobinemia*	Methylene blue	1–2 mg/kg IV, repeat q 30–60 min if needed; treat for levels >30%	Exchange transfusion may be needed for severe methemoglobinemia; methylene blue overdose also causes methemoglobinemia
Opiates	Naloxone	0.1 mg/kg IV, ET, SC, IM for children, up to 2 mg, repeat as needed	Naloxone causes no respiratory depression
Organophosphates	Atropine	0.05–0.1 mg/kg IV/ET, repeat every 5–10 minutes as needed	Physiologic: blocks acetylcholine
	Pralidoxime (2 PAM; Protopam)	25–50 mg/kg IV over 5–10 min (max 200 mg/min); may repeat after 1–2 hr, then q10–12 h as needed	Specific: disrupts phosphate-cholinesterase bond

From Kliegman RM, Stanton BF, St. Geme JW, et al., editors: Nelson Textbook of Pediatrics, ed 19, Philadelphia, 2011, Saunders, pp 256–257.
ET, Endotracheal; IM, intramuscular; IV, intravenous; PO, oral; SC, subcutaneous.
*See Table 45-4 for causes of methemoglobinemia.

Chapter 46

SEDATION AND ANALGESIA

An acutely ill pediatric patient may have pain, discomfort, and anxiety resulting from injury, surgery, and invasive procedures (intubation, bone marrow aspiration, venous access placement) or during life-sustaining mechanical ventilation. Clear goals should be identified to allow provision of optimal analgesia or sedation without compromising the physiologic status of the patient. Anxiolysis, cooperation, amnesia, immobility, and lack of awareness all are goals of sedation and can be accomplished with various drugs (Table 46-1). Many of these goals can be achieved with behavioral techniques (preprocedural teaching), but sedation is often a necessary adjunct for painful procedures. Pain may be expressed by verbal or visible discomfort, crying, agitation, tachycardia, hypertension, and tachypnea. A variety of scales have been developed in an attempt to quantify pain and allow more directed therapy. Few of these scales are well validated, especially in populations of acutely ill children with physiologic derangements secondary to the underlying pathology. Pain caused by procedural interventions should always be treated with analgesics in addition to sedation (Table 46-2).

ASSESSMENT
Procedural Sedation
A medical evaluation must be performed for any patient receiving procedural sedation to identify underlying medical conditions that may affect the choice of sedative agents. Specific attention must be paid to assessment of the airway (for ability to maintain a patent airway) and respiratory system (asthma, recent respiratory illness, loose teeth), cardiovascular status (especially adequacy of volume status), factors affecting drug metabolism (renal or liver disease), and risk of aspiration (adequate nothing-by-mouth status, gastroesophageal reflux). During the administration of procedural sedation, assessment of status must include monitoring of oxygen saturation, heart rate, and respiratory rate, as well as some assessment of effectiveness of ventilation. This assessment must be performed by someone who is not involved in the procedure; this person is also responsible for recording vital signs and drugs administered on a time-based graph. Monitoring must be continued until the child has returned to baseline. Patients who are receiving long-term sedation (e.g., to maintain endotracheal tube placement) may need only local anesthesia for painful procedures but may benefit from additional sedation or analgesia as well.

Nonprocedural Sedation
Many ventilated pediatric patients require sedation and some analgesia while intubated. The most common choice is a combination of a longer acting benzodiazepine and an opioid. Avoidance of oversedation is important. Use of appropriate pain and sedation scores allows for titration of medications to achieve goals of the sedation plan. Long-term use of benzodiazepines and opioids leads to tolerance, a problematic occurrence that must be considered as medications are added and weaned. True addiction is a rare occurrence, especially when medications are provided at the minimum level needed to achieve adequate sedation and pain control.

Table 46-1 | Agents that Produce Sedation

SEDATIVES	EFFECT	CONCERNS
Midazolam	Anxiolysis, sedation, muscle relaxation, amnesia	Tolerance is possible; apnea, hypotension, depressed myocardial function; short action
Lorazepam	Anxiolysis, sedation, muscle relaxation, amnesia	Same as midazolam; long action
Dexmedetomidine	Sedation without respiratory depression	May cause bradycardia
Ketamine	Anesthesia, analgesia, amnesia	Dissociative reactions, tachycardia, hypertension, increased bronchial secretions, emergent delirium, hallucinations; increases intracranial pressure
Chloral hydrate	Sedative	Emesis, hypotension, arrhythmias, hepatic dysfunction
Propofol	Rapid-onset sedative for induction and maintenance of anesthesia	Metabolic acidosis in children; may depress cardiac function

Table 46-2 | Agents that Produce Analgesia

ANALGESIC	EFFECT	COMPLICATIONS
Acetaminophen and NSAIDs	Moderate analgesia, antipyresis	Ceiling effect, requires PO administration; NSAIDs—gastrointestinal bleed, ulceration
Opioids		No ceiling effect; respiratory depression, sedation, pruritus, nausea/vomiting, decreased gastric motility, urinary retention, tolerance with abuse potential
Morphine	Analgesia	May cause myocardial depression
Codeine	Analgesia	Nausea/vomiting
Fentanyl, alfentanil, sufentanil	Analgesia, sedation	No adverse effects on cardiovascular system; stiff chest syndrome
Methadone	Analgesia	

NSAIDs, Nonsteroidal anti-inflammatory drugs; *PO*, oral.

PAIN AND ANALGESIA

The subjective aspect of pain requires that self-reporting be used for assessment. Visual analog scales, developed for adult patients (allowing patients to rate pain on a scale of 1 to 10), have been used for older children. Pain scales for younger children often incorporate behavioral and physiologic parameters, despite the imprecision of physiologic responses.

Local anesthetics, such as lidocaine, can be used for minor procedures. However, lidocaine requires subcutaneous or intradermal injection. The use of EMLA, a cream containing lidocaine and prilocaine, is less effective than intradermal lidocaine but is preferred by many patients.

Patient-controlled analgesia is an effective method for providing balanced analgesia care in older children and adolescents. Children using patient-controlled analgesia have better pain relief and experience less sedation than patients receiving intermittent, nurse-controlled, bolus analgesics. Analgesics can be administered through the patient-controlled analgesia pump with continuous basal infusions, bolus administration, or both. Morphine is the most frequent opioid used for patient-controlled analgesia.

Monitoring of oxygen saturations and respiratory rate are crucial with continuous opioid infusions because of the shift in CO_2 response curve and potential to decrease ventilatory response to hypoxia.

Epidural analgesia decreases the need for inhalation anesthetics during surgery and can provide significant analgesia without sedation in the postoperative period. Decreased costs and length of stay also may be benefits of epidural analgesic approaches. Medications used in epidurals include bupivacaine and morphine. Adverse effects include nausea and vomiting, motor blockade, and technical problems requiring catheter removal. Infection and permanent neurologic deficits are rare.

Suggested Reading
Kleinman ME, Chameides L, Schexnayder SM, et al: Part 14: pediatric advanced life support: 2010 American Heart Association guidelines for cardiopulmonary resuscitation and emergency cardiovascular care, *Circulation* 122(Suppl 3):S876–S908, 2010.
Kliegman RM, Stanton BF, St. Geme JW, et al, editors: *Nelson Textbook of Pediatrics*, ed 19, Philadelphia, 2011, Elsevier.

Human Genetics and Dysmorphology

Paul A. Levy and Robert W. Marion

SECTION
9

Chapter 47

PATTERNS OF INHERITANCE

TYPES OF GENETIC DISORDERS

Among infants born in the United States, 2% to 4% have **congenital malformations**, abnormalities of form or function identifiable at birth. At 1 year of age, the number approaches 7%, because some anomalies may not be identifiable until after the neonatal period. The prevalence of congenital malformations is much greater in inpatient pediatric populations; 30% to 50% of hospitalized children have congenital anomalies or genetic disorders.

The clinical geneticist attempts to identify the etiology, mode of inheritance, and risk that a disorder might occur in the affected child's siblings. In evaluating children with congenital malformations, the patient's condition may be classified into one of five different categories:

1. Single-gene mutations, accounting for 6% of children with congenital anomalies
2. Chromosomal disorders, accounting for approximately 7.5%
3. Multifactorially inherited conditions, accounting for 20%
4. Disorders that show an unusual pattern of inheritance, accounting for 2% to 3%
5. Conditions caused by exposure to teratogens, accounting for 6%

INTRODUCTION TO GENETICS AND GENOMICS

DNA is composed of four nucleotide building blocks: adenine, guanine, cytosine, and thymine. Each nucleotide is linked to other nucleotides, forming a chain. The DNA molecule consists of two chains of nucleotides held together by hydrogen bonds. The purine nucleotides, adenine and guanine, cross-link by hydrogen bonds to the pyrimidines, thymine and cytosine. Because of this cross-linking, the nucleotide sequence of one strand sets the other strand's sequence. Separating the two strands permits complementary nucleotides to bind to each DNA strand; this copies the DNA and replicates the sequence.

DNA exists as multiple fragments that, together with a protein skeleton (chromatin), form chromosomes. Human cells have 23 pairs of chromosomes, with one copy of each chromosome inherited from each parent. Twenty-two pairs of chromosomes are **autosomes**; the remaining pair is called the **sex chromosomes**. Females have two X chromosomes; males have one X and one Y.

Spread along the chromosomes, like beads on a string, DNA sequences form **genes,** the basic units of heredity. A typical gene contains a promoter sequence, an untranslated region, and an open reading frame, all arrayed from the 5′ to the 3′ end of the DNA. In the open reading frame, every three nucleotides represent a single **codon**, coding for a particular amino acid. In this way, the sequence of bases dictates the sequence of amino acids in the corresponding protein. Some codons, rather than coding for a specific amino acid, act as a "start" signal, whereas others serve as "stop" signals. Between the start and stop codons, genes consist of two major portions: **exons**, regions containing the code that ultimately corresponds to a sequence of amino acids, and **introns** (intervening sequence), which do not become part of the amino acid sequence.

Genes are **transcribed** into messenger RNA (mRNA), then **translated** into proteins. During transcription, RNA is processed to remove introns. The mRNA serves as a template to construct the protein.

Human genetic material contains 3.1 billion bases. Less than 2% of the DNA codes for proteins, comprising the genome's approximately 21,000 genes. Through a mechanism called **alternative splicing**, these 21,000 genes may create more than 100,000 proteins. The remainder of the DNA, the portion not involved in protein formation, had been termed *junk DNA*, but a project called ENCODE (Encyclopedia of DNA Elements) found that much of this presumed *junk DNA* is functional and likely serves some regulatory function.

Disease may be caused by changes or **mutations** in the DNA sequence, with the **point mutation**, a change in a single DNA base, being the most common type. A point mutation that changes a codon and the resulting amino acid that goes into the protein is referred to as a **missense mutation**. A **nonsense mutation** is a point mutation that changes the codon to a "stop" codon so that transcription stops prematurely. A **frameshift mutation** often stems from the loss or addition of one or more DNA bases; this causes a shift in how the DNA is transcribed and generally leads to premature stop codons.

Pedigree Drawing

To identify specific patterns of inheritance, geneticists construct and analyze pedigrees, which are pictorial representations of a family history. Males are represented by squares and females by circles. Matings are connected with a solid line between each partner's symbols. Unmarried couples are often connected by a dashed line. Children from a couple are represented below their parents and are the next generation.

Grandparents, uncles, and aunts are added in similar fashion. Children of aunts and uncles also may be included. Ages or birthdays may be written next to or underneath each symbol. The proband (the patient who is the initial contact) is indicated with an arrow. Affected individuals are indicated by shading, or some other technique, which should be explained in a key. Carriers for a disorder (e.g., sickle cell disease) usually are indicated by a dot in the center of their symbol (Fig. 47-1).

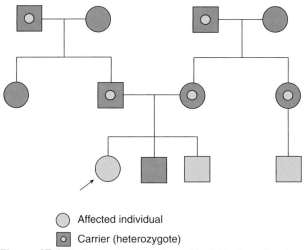

○ Affected individual
⊡ Carrier (heterozygote)

Figure 47-1 Pedigree showing affected individuals and carriers.

To be useful, pedigrees should include representatives of at least three generations of family members.

Autosomal Dominant Disorders (AD)

If a single copy of a gene bearing a mutation is sufficient to cause disease and that gene is not on one of the sex chromosomes, that condition is inherited in an AD fashion (Table 47-1). In AD disorders, an affected parent has a 50% chance of passing the mutated gene to each child (Fig. 47-2; Table 47-2). Possessing one *working* gene and one *nonworking* gene is termed **heterozygous.** If both copies are the same, they are referred to as **homozygous**.

Some people who are obligate carriers of a mutation known to cause an AD disorder may not show clinical signs of the disorder, whereas other such individuals manifest symptoms. This phenomenon is referred to as **penetrance.** If all individuals who carry a mutation for an AD disorder show signs of that disorder, the gene is said to have complete penetrance. Many AD disorders show decreased penetrance.

Often, AD disorders show variability in symptoms expressed in different individuals carrying the same mutated gene. Some individuals have only mild clinical symptoms, whereas others have more severe disease. This phenomenon is referred to as **variable expressivity.**

AD disorders sometimes appear in a child of unaffected parents because of a **spontaneous mutation.** Known in some cases to be associated with advanced paternal age (>35 years of age), spontaneous mutations may account for most individuals with some disorders. Approximately 80% of patients with achondroplasia have a spontaneous mutation in the fibroblast growth factor receptor type 3 *(FGFR3)* gene. The following are examples of autosomal dominant disorders.

Table 47-1	Autosomal Dominant Diseases	
DISEASE	**FREQUENCY**	**COMMENTS**
Achondroplasia Thanatophoric dysplasia Crouzon syndrome with acanthosis nigricans Nonsyndromic craniosynostosis	~1:12,000	Mutations are in the gene for *fibroblast growth factor receptor-3* on chromosome 4p16.3. 40% of cases are new mutations (different mutations in the same gene cause achondroplasia, thanatophoric dysplasia, Crouzon syndrome with acanthosis, and nonsyndromic craniosynostosis)
Neurofibromatosis 1	1:3500	About 50% of cases result from new mutations in the gene for neurofibromin, a tumor suppressor gene located at 17q11.2. Expression is quite variable
Neurofibromatosis 2 (NF2, bilateral acoustic neuromas, Merlin)	Genotype at birth, 1:33,000 Phenotype prevalence, 1:200,000	The NF2 gene is a tumor suppressor gene located at 22q12.2. The protein is called "Merlin"
Huntington disease (HD)	Variable in populations, 1:5000–1:20,000	The disease is caused by a (CAG) repeat expansion in the "Huntington" protein gene on chromosome 4p16.3
Myotonic dystrophy (DM, Steinert disease)	1:500 in Quebec 1:25,000 Europeans	The disease is caused by a (CTG) repeat expansion in the DM kinase gene at chromosome 19q13.2. The condition shows genetic anticipation with successive generations
Marfan syndrome (FBN-1)	1:10,000	The syndrome is caused by mutations in the fibrillin 1 (FBN 1) gene on chromosome 15q21.1; there is variable expression
Hereditary angioneurotic edema (HANE) (C-1 esterase inhibitor that regulates the C-1 component of complement)	1:10,000	The gene is located on chromosome 11q11-q13.2. The phenotype of episodic and variable subcutaneous and submucosal swelling and pain is caused by diminished or altered esterase inhibitor protein, which can result from any one of many mutations in the gene

Achondroplasia

Caused by a defect in cartilage-derived bone, achondroplasia (ACH) is the most common skeletal dysplasia in humans. The bony abnormalities lead to short stature, macrocephaly, a flat midface with a prominent forehead, and rhizomelic shortening of the limbs. The disorder occurs in approximately 1 in 12,000 births.

ACH is caused by mutations in the *FGFR3* gene. Early in development, *FGFR3* is expressed during endochondral bone formation. More than 95% of cases of ACH are caused by one of two mutations in the same base pair (site 1138). This site, extremely active for mutations, is known as a mutational **hot spot.**

As they grow, children with ACH often develop associated medical and psychological problems. Hydrocephalus and central apnea may occur because of narrowing of the foramen magnum and compression of the brainstem and may present a life-threatening complication in infancy. Bowing of the legs may occur later in childhood because of unequal growth of the tibia and fibula. Dental malocclusion, obstructive apnea, and hearing loss due to middle ear dysfunction are common in later childhood. During later childhood and adolescence, the psychological effects of the short stature may manifest. In adulthood, further complications include compression of nerve roots and sciatica. People with ACH have normal life spans and normal intelligence.

The diagnosis of ACH is made on the basis of clinical findings; characteristic x-ray abnormalities confirm the diagnosis. Molecular testing is available but is usually reserved for cases that are difficult to diagnose or those in which prenatal diagnosis is requested. Prenatal diagnosis is possible by molecular testing, using fetal cells obtained through amniocentesis or chorionic villus sampling.

Neurofibromatosis Type 1

One of the most common AD disorders, NF1 is estimated to be present in 1 in 3500 individuals. NF1 is caused by a mutation in the gene *NF1*, which codes for the protein neurofibromin.

Although the penetrance of NF1 is 100%, the expression is extremely variable. Many affected individuals have features so mild that they are never diagnosed.

SEE CHAPTER 186.

Marfan Syndrome (MFS)

A condition that occurs in approximately 1 in 10,000 individuals, MFS shows pleiotropy, the condition in which abnormalities in multiple organ systems are caused by a mutation in a single gene. Caused by a mutation in the *FBN1* gene, clinical symptoms in MFS mostly involve three systems: **cardiac, ophthalmologic,** and **skeletal.** Skeletal findings include a tall, thin body habitus (dolichostenomelia), spider-like fingers and toes (arachnodactyly), abnormalities of the sternum (pectus excavatum or carinatum), scoliosis, pes planus, and joint laxity. Eye findings include high myopia, which can lead to vitreoretinal degeneration; an abnormal suspensory ligament of the lens, which can lead to ectopia lentis (dislocation of the lens); and cataracts. Cardiac findings include progressive dilatation of the aortic root. Aortic insufficiency followed by aortic dissection is a common complication. Other clinical features of MFS include dural ectasia, abnormal pulmonary septation, and striae. Diagnostic criteria for MFS are summarized in Table 47-3.

New mutations in *FBN1* account for 25% of cases of MFS. The gene is large and complex; more than 600 mutations have been identified in affected individuals. Many of the symptoms of MFS are caused not by the defect in the fibrillin protein itself but rather by an excess in transforming growth factor-beta (TGF-β), a protein usually bound by fibrillin. Losartan, an angiotensin II receptor antagonist that also lowers levels of TGF-β, may prevent aneurysms in patients with MFS.

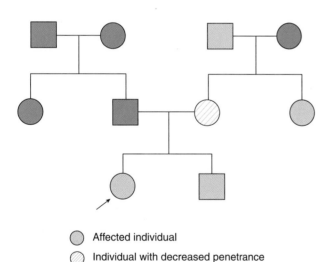

○ Affected individual

⦸ Individual with decreased penetrance

Figure 47-2 Pedigree showing decreased penetrance for an autosomal dominant disorder. Proband *(arrow)* is affected. Maternal grandfather also is affected. The individual's mother is presumed to be the carrier of the gene, even though she may show only slight symptoms of disease.

Autosomal Recessive Disorders (AR)

Disorders that are inherited in an AR manner manifest only when *both* copies of a gene pair located on a non-sex chromosome have a mutation (Tables 47-4, 47-5). Affected children usually are born to unaffected parents, each of whom carries one copy of the mutation. If both members of a couple are carriers (or heterozygotes) for this mutation, each of their offspring has a 25% chance of being affected (Fig. 47-3).

Table 47-2	Rules of Autosomal Dominant Inheritance
Trait appears in every generation
Each child of an affected parent has a one in two chance of being affected
Males and females are equally affected
Male-to-male transmission occurs
Traits generally involve mutations in genes that code for regulatory or structural proteins (collagen)

Sickle Cell Disease

SEE CHAPTER 150.

Table 47-3	Revised Ghent Nosology for the Diagnosis of Marfan Syndrome

WITHOUT FAMILY HISTORY

AORTIC ROOT DILATATION* (Z ≥2SD) or AORTIC DISSECTION	ECTOPIA LENTIS	SYSTEMIC ≥7 POINTS	*FBN1* MUTATION	DIAGNOSIS
+	+	- or +		MFS†
+			+	MFS
+	-	+	(unknown or neg)	MFS†
-	+		+	MFS
-	+			Ectopia Lentis syndrome
-	-	≥5		MASS
MVP	-	<5		MVPS

WITH FAMILY HISTORY

	+			MFS
		+		MFS†
+ (Z ≥2, if >20 years) (Z ≥3, if <20 years)				MFS†

SCORING SYSTEM FOR SYSTEMIC FEATURES‡

Thumb AND Wrist Sign	3
Thumb OR Wrist Sign	1
Pectus Carinatum	2
Pectus Excavatum or Chest Asymmetry	1
Hindfoot Deformity	2
Pes Planus	1
Pneumothorax (History)	2
Dural Ectasia	2
Protrusio acetabluli	2
Decreased US/LS ratio AND increased Arm/Height BUT NO SCOLIOSIS	1
Scoliosis or Thoracolumbar kyphosis	1
Reduced Elbow Extension	1
Facial features (3 of 5)§	1
Skin Striae	1
Myopia >3 diopters	1
Mitral Valve Prolapse	1

Data from Loeys BL, et al. The revised Ghent nosology for the Marfan syndrome. J Med Genet 47.476-405, 2010.
FBN1, Fibrillin-1; *MASS*, myopia, mitral valve prolapse, borderline aortic root dilatation (Z <2), striae, skeletal findings; *MVPS*, mitral valve prolapse syndrome.
*Aortic root dilatation (measured at the Sinuses of Valsalva);
†Loeys-Dietz syndrome (LDS), Shprintzen-Goldberg syndrome (SGS), and the vascular form of Ehlers Danlos (vEDS) should be excluded. If clinical features are suggestive, then DNA testing for *TGFBR1*, *TGFBR2* (LDS), *COL3A1* (vEDS) or collagen biochemistry should be done to help rule out these disorders.
‡Maximum Total: 20 points; more than 7 points indicates systemic involvement.
§Facial Features: Dolicocephaly, enophthalmos, downslanting palpebral fissures, malar hypoplasia, retrognathia.

Tay-Sachs Disease
SEE CHAPTERS 55 AND 185.

X-Linked Disorders
More than 1000 genes have been identified on the X chromosome, whereas only about 200 are believed to be present on the Y chromosome. Females, whose cells have two copies of an X chromosome, possess two copies of each gene on the X chromosome, whereas males, who have one X chromosome and a Y chromosome, have only one copy of these genes. Early in female embryonic development, one X chromosome is randomly inactivated in each cell. There are many X-linked disorders (colorblindness, Duchenne muscular dystrophy, hemophilia A) in which heterozygous (carrier) females show some manifestations of the disorder due to skewed X chromosome inactivation.

Table 47-4	Autosomal Recessive Diseases	
DISEASE	**FREQUENCY**	**COMMENTS**
Adrenal hyperplasia, congenital (CAH, 21-hydroxylase deficiency, CA21H, CYP21, cytochrome P450, subfamily XXI)	1:5000	Phenotype variation corresponds roughly to allelic variation. A deficiency causes virilization in females. The gene is located at 6p21.3 within the HLA complex and within 0.005 centimorgans (cM) of HLA B
Phenylketonuria (PKU, phenylalanine hydroxylase deficiency, PAH)	1:12,000-1:17,000	There are hundreds of disease-causing mutations in the PAH gene located on chromosome 12q22-q24.1. The first population-based newborn screening was a test for PKU because the disease is treatable by diet. Women with elevated phenylalanine have infants with damage to the central nervous system because high phenylalanine is neurotoxic and teratogenic
Cystic fibrosis (CF)	1:2500 whites	The gene *CF transmembrane conductance regulator* (CFTR) is on chromosome 7q31.2
Friedreich ataxia (FA, frataxin)	1:25,000	Frataxin is a mitochondrial protein involved with iron metabolism and respiration. The gene is on chromosome 9q13-q21, and the common mutation is a GAA expanded triplet repeat located in the first *intron* of the gene. FA does not show anticipation
Gaucher disease, all types (glucocerebrosidase deficiency, acid β-glucosidase deficiency) (a lysosomal storage disease)	1:2500 Ashkenazi Jews	The gene is located on chromosome 1q21. There are many mutations; some mutations lead to neuropathic disease, but most are milder in expression. The phenotypes correspond to the genotypes, but the latter are difficult to analyze
Sickle cell disease (hemoglobin beta locus, beta 6 glu → val mutation)	1:625 African Americans	This is the first condition with a defined molecular defect (1959). A single base change results in an amino acid substitution of valine for glutamic acid at position 6 of the beta chain of hemoglobin, with resulting hemolytic anemia. The gene is on chromosome 11p15.5. Penicillin prophylaxis reduces death from pneumococcal infections in affected persons, especially in infants

Table 47-5	Rules of Autosomal Recessive Inheritance
Trait appears in siblings, not in their parents or their offspring	
On average, 25% of siblings of the proband are affected (at the time of conception, each sibling has a 25% chance of being affected)	
A *normal* sibling of an affected individual has a two thirds chance of being a carrier (heterozygote)	
Males and females are likely to be affected equally	
Rare traits are likely to be associated with parental consanguinity	
Traits generally involve mutations in genes that code for enzymes (e.g., phenylalanine hydroxylase–deficient in PKU) and are associated with serious illness and shortened life span	

PKU, Phenylketonuria.

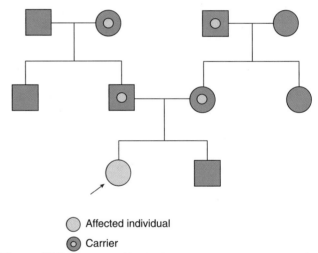

○ Affected individual
◉ Carrier

Figure 47-3 Pedigree of family showing autosomal recessive inheritance.

X-Linked Recessive Inheritance

Most disorders involving the X chromosome are recessive. With only one copy of the X chromosome, males are more likely to manifest these diseases than females. Each son born to a female carrier of an X-linked recessive trait has a 50% chance of inheriting the trait, but none of this woman's daughters would be affected (each daughter has a 50% chance of being a carrier). An affected father transmits the mutation to all of his daughters, who are carriers, but not to his sons; having received their father's Y chromosome, they would not be affected (thus there is no male-to-male transmission) (Tables 47-6, 47-7 and Fig. 47-4).

Duchenne Muscular Dystrophy
SEE CHAPTER 182.

Hemophilia A
SEE CHAPTER 151.

X-Linked Dominant Inheritance

Only a few X-linked dominant disorders have been described. Both males and females are affected by this group of disorders, but females have less severe symptoms due to X-chromosome inactivation. This is the case for **X-linked vitamin D–resistant rickets** (hypophosphatemic rickets), a disorder in which the kidney's ability to reabsorb phosphate is impaired. Phosphate levels and resulting rickets are not as severe in females as in males.

However, many X-linked dominant disorders are lethal in males. Affected mothers can have affected or normal daughters but only normal sons. Affected sons die in utero. This is the case in **incontinentia pigmenti**, which has a characteristic swirling skin pattern of hyperpigmentation that develops after a perinatal skin rash with blistering. Affected females also have variable involvement of the central nervous system, hair, nails,

Table 47-6	X-Linked Recessive Diseases	
DISEASE	**FREQUENCY**	**COMMENTS**
Fragile X syndrome (FRAXA; numerous other names)	1:4000 males	The gene is located at Xq27.3 The condition is attributable to a CGG triplet expansion that is associated with localized methylation (inactivation) of distal genes. Females may have some expression. Instability of the site may lead to tissue mosaicism; lymphocyte genotype and phenotype may not correlate
Duchenne muscular dystrophy (DMD, pseudohypertrophic progressive MD, dystrophin, Becker variants)	1:4000 males	The gene is located at Xp21 The gene is relatively large, with 79 exons, and mutations and deletions may occur anywhere. The gene product is called *dystrophin*. Dystrophin is absent in DMD but abnormal in Becker MD
Hemophilia A (factor VIII deficiency, classic hemophilia)	1:5000–1:10,000; males	The gene is located at Xq28 Factor VIII is essential for normal blood clotting. Phenotype depends on genotype and the presence of any residual factor VIII activity
Rett syndrome (RTT, RTS autism, dementia, ataxia, and loss of purposeful hand use); gene MECP2 (methyl-CpG- binding protein 2)	1:10,000–1:15,000; girls	The gene is located at locus Xq28 These diseases are a subset of autism. There is a loss of regulation (repression) for other genes, including those in *trans* positions. The disease is lethal in males. Cases represent new mutations or parental gonadal mosaicism
Color blindness (partial deutan series, green color blindness [75%]; partial protan series, red color blindness [25%])	1:12; males	The gene is located at Xq28 (proximal) for deutan color blindness and at Xq28 (distal) for protan color blindness
Adrenoleukodystrophy (ALD, XL-ALD, Addison disease, and cerebral sclerosis)	Uncommon	The gene is located at Xq28 The disease involves a defect in peroxisome function relating to *very long-chain fatty acid CoA synthetase* with accumulation of C-26 fatty acids. Phenotype is variable, from rapid childhood progression to later onset and slow progression
Glucose-6-phosphate dehydrogenase deficiency (G6PD)	1:10 African Americans 1:5 Kurdish Jews A heteromorphism in these and other populations	The gene is located at Xq28 There are numerous variants in which oxidants cause hemolysis. Variants can confer partial resistance to severe malaria

Table 47-7	Rules of X-Linked Recessive Inheritance

Incidence of the trait is higher in males than in females

Trait is passed from carrier females, who may show mild expression of the gene, to half of their sons, who are more severely affected

Each son of a carrier female has a one in two chance of being affected

Trait is transmitted from affected males to all of their daughters; it is never transmitted father to son

Because the trait can be passed through multiple carrier females, it may *skip* generations

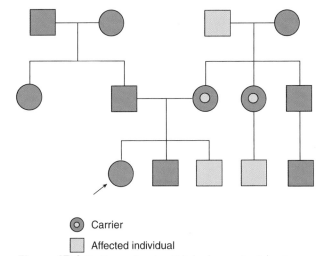

⊙ Carrier

▨ Affected individual

Figure 47-4 Pedigree showing X-linked recessive inheritance.

teeth, and eyes. In **Rett syndrome**, caused by mutations in the *MECP2* gene, females are normal at birth, but later in the first year of life develop microcephaly and developmental regression and plateau. About 50% of patients develop seizures. Girls often are diagnosed with autism and, by 2 years of age, adopt a *hand-washing* posture that causes them to lose all purposeful hand movements.

OTHER TYPES OF GENETIC DISORDERS
Multifactorial Disorders

Often termed **polygenic inheritance**, multifactorially inherited disorders result from the interplay of genetic and environmental

factors. In addition to 20% of congenital malformations, including cleft lip and palate and spina bifida, most common disorders of childhood and adult life, such as asthma, atherosclerosis, diabetes, and cancer, result from an interaction between genes and the environment. These disorders do not follow simple mendelian modes of inheritance; rather, affected individuals tend to cluster in families. The disorders occur more often in first- and second-degree relatives than would be expected by chance, and they are more likely to be concordant (although not 100%) in monozygotic twins than in dizygotic twins.

Hypertrophic Pyloric Stenosis

Decision-Making Algorithms
Available @ StudentConsult.com

Vomiting
Gastrointestinal Bleeding
Alkalemia

Occurring in about 1 in 300 children, hypertrophic pyloric stenosis (HPS) is five times more likely to occur in males than in females. When a child with HPS is born, the recurrence risk in future progeny is 5% to 10% for males and 1.5% to 2% for females. In adulthood, the risk of an affected male having an affected child is markedly increased over the general population: 4% of sons and 1% of daughters of such men would be likely to be affected. Even more striking is the risk to children born to affected females: 17% to 20% of sons and 7% of daughters are affected.

The thickness of the pyloric muscle may be distributed across a bell-shaped curve; the position on the bell-shaped curve is determined by many factors, including the expression of multiple, unknown genes. HPS may result when an individual's genetic and environmental influences cause him or her to fall to an extreme position on this curve, past a certain point, which is called a **threshold**. In HPS, this threshold is farther to the left for males than it is for females.

Neural Tube Defects

Before 1998, myelomeningocele affected 1 in 1000 liveborn infants in the United States. Anencephaly occurred with a similar frequency, although most infants were either stillborn or died in the neonatal period. Since 1998, because of the supplementation of food staples with folic acid, both of these conditions have become far less frequent. Multiple genetic and nongenetic factors dictate the speed with which the neural tube closes, as follows:

1. The frequency of neural tube defects (NTDs) varies greatly in different ethnic groups. NTDs are more common in the British Isles, where, in 1990, they occurred in 1 in 250 live births, and far less common in Asia, where the frequency was 1 in 4000. These ethnic differences suggest a **genetic** component.
2. Couples from the British Isles who move to the United States have a risk intermediate between the risks in the United Kingdom and the United States, suggesting an **environmental** component.
3. The occurrence of NTDs exhibits seasonality. In the United States, affected infants are more likely to be born during late fall and early winter, again suggesting an **environmental** component.
4. Periconceptual supplementation with folic acid has significantly lowered the risk of having an infant with an NTD. This nutritional influence suggests an **environmental** component.
5. Parents who have one child with an NTD are 20 to 40 times more likely to have a second affected child; this provides further evidence of a **genetic** component.

Disorders with Unusual Patterns of Inheritance
Mitochondrial Inheritance

Human cells contain non-nuclear DNA; a single chromosome is present in each mitochondrion, and mutations within this DNA are associated with a group of diseases.

Mitochondrial DNA (mtDNA), which is circular and 16.5 kb in length, replicates independently of nuclear DNA. Involved in energy production used to run the cell, mtDNA codes for a few respiratory chain proteins (most mitochondrial proteins are coded on nuclear DNA) and for a set of transfer RNAs unique to mitochondrial protein synthesis. Virtually all mitochondria are supplied by the oocyte, which means that mtDNA is maternally derived. A woman with a mutation in mtDNA passes this mutation to all of her children. More than one population of mitochondria may be present in the oocyte, a phenomenon called **heteroplasmy**. The mtDNA mutation may be present in a few or many mitochondria. When the fertilized egg divides, mitochondria are distributed randomly. The presence of symptoms in the offspring, and their severity, depends on the ratio of mutant to wild-type mtDNA present in a particular tissue. If an abundance of mutant mitochondria exists in tissue that has high energy requirements (brain, muscle, and liver), clinical symptoms occur. If fewer mutant mitochondria are present, few clinical symptoms may be seen.

MELAS (**m**itochondrial **e**ncephalomyopathy with **l**actic **a**cidosis and **s**trokelike episodes) is an example of a mitochondrial disorder. Normal in early childhood, individuals affected with MELAS develop episodic vomiting, seizures, and recurrent cerebral insults that resemble strokes between 5 and 10 years of age. In 80% of cases, analysis of the mtDNA reveals a specific mutation (A3242G) in *MTTL1*, a gene that codes for a mitochondrial transfer RNA.

In families in which MELAS occurs, a range of symptoms is seen in first-degree relatives, including **progressive external ophthalmoplegia**, hearing loss, cardiomyopathy, and diabetes mellitus. Although all offspring of a woman who carries a mutation would be affected, because of heteroplasmy, the severity of disease varies, depending on the percentage of mitochondria bearing the mutation that are present.

Uniparental Disomy

Evaluation of a child with uniparental disomy (UPD) reveals a normal karyotype. However, chromosomal markers for one particular chromosome are identical to the markers found on the chromosomes of the patient's mother or father (but not both). In UPD, the individual inherits two copies of one parent's chromosome and no copy from the other parent.

UPD probably occurs through a few mechanisms, but the most common results from a spontaneous *rescue* mechanism. At the time of conception, through nondisjunction, the fertilized egg is trisomic for a particular chromosome, with two copies of one parent's chromosome and one copy of the other parent's chromosome; conceptuses with trisomy often miscarry early in development. Fetuses with UPD survive because they spontaneously lose one of three copies of the affected chromosome. If the single chromosome from one parent is lost, the patient has UPD.

An alternate explanation involves monosomy for a chromosome rather than trisomy. Had the conceptus, at the time of conception, inherited only a single copy of a chromosome, spontaneous duplication of the single chromosome would lead to UPD.

Prader-Willi and Angelman Syndromes

Decision-Making Algorithms
Available @ StudentConsult.com

Hypotonia and Weakness
Short Stature
Pubertal Delay
Obesity
Polyuria

Prader-Willi syndrome (PWS), which occurs in approximately 1 in 10,000 infants, is characterized by hypotonia of prenatal onset; postnatal growth delay; a characteristic appearance, including almond-shaped eyes and small hands and feet; developmental disability; hypogonadotropic hypogonadism; and obesity after infancy. Early in life, affected infants are so hypotonic that they cannot consume enough calories to maintain their weight. Nasogastric feeding is invariably necessary, and failure to thrive is common. During the first year of life, muscle tone improves and children develop a voracious appetite. Some 60% to 70% of individuals with PWS have a small deletion of chromosome 15 (15q11). In individuals without a deletion, 20% have UPD of chromosome 15.

Angelman syndrome (AS) is a condition with moderate to severe mental retardation, absence of speech, ataxic movements of the arms and legs, a characteristic craniofacial appearance, and a seizure disorder that is characterized by inappropriate laughter. AS is also characterized by a deletion in the 15q11 region in 70% of affected individuals; UPD for chromosome 15 can be demonstrated in approximately 10% of AS patients.

If the deletion occurs in paternal chromosome 15, the affected individual has PWS, whereas AS results from a deletion occurring only in the maternal chromosome 15. When UPD is responsible, maternal UPD results in PWS, whereas paternal UPD results in AS. To summarize, if a copy of paternal chromosome 15q11.2 is lacking, PWS occurs; if maternal chromosome 15q11.2 is lacking, AS results.

This phenomenon is explained by **genomic imprinting**. Imprinting is an **epigenetic** phenomenon, a nonheritable change in the DNA that causes an alteration in gene expression based on parental origin of the gene. PWS is caused by deficiency of the protein product of the gene *SNRPN* (small nuclear ribonucleoprotein). Although present on both maternally and paternally derived chromosome 15, *SNRPN* is expressed only in the paternally derived chromosome. Expression is blocked in the maternal chromosome because the bases of the open reading frame are methylated; this physical change in the DNA prevents gene expression. PWS results whenever a paternal chromosome 15 is missing, either through deletion or through UPD.

AS results from a lack of expression of ubiquitin-protein ligase E3A *(UBE3A)*, a second gene in the chromosome 15q11.2 region. *UBE3A* is normally expressed only in the maternally derived chromosome 15. Although present in paternal chromosome 15, *UBE3A* is methylated, and gene expression is blocked. Therefore, if either the critical region of maternal chromosome 15 is deleted, or paternal UPD occurs, the individual will manifest symptoms of AS.

Expansion of a Trinucleotide Repeat

Decision-Making Algorithm
Available @ StudentConsult.com

Ataxia

More than 50% of human DNA appears as repeat sequences, two or three bases repeated over and over again. Disorders caused by expansion of trinucleotide repeats include **Fragile X syndrome**, **Huntington disease**, **myotonic dystrophy**, **Friedreich ataxia**, and the **spinocerebellar ataxias**. Although an increase in the number of the three repeated bases is at the heart of each disorder, the molecular mechanism differs.

Fragile X syndrome (FRAX), which occurs with a frequency of approximately 1 in 2000 children, is the most common cause of inherited intellectual disability. Features include characteristic craniofacial findings (large head; prominent forehead, jaw, and ears); macro-orchidism with testicular volume twice normal in adulthood; a mild connective tissue disorder, including joint laxity, patulous eustachian tubes, and mitral valve prolapse; and a characteristic neurobehavioral profile, including intellectual disability (ranging from mild to profound) and autism spectrum disorders.

Positional cloning in the Xq27 region identified a triplet repeat region composed of one cytosine and two guanine residues (CGG). These repeats occur in the CpG island, a part of the promoter region of a gene that has been called *FMR1*. Unaffected individuals who have no family history of FRAX have 0 to 45 CGG repeats (most have 25 to 35). In individuals with FRAX, the number of repeats is greater than 200; such people are said to have a *full mutation*. Between these two categories, a third group has 56 to 200 repeats; always phenotypically normal, these individuals are **premutation carriers**.

FRAX results from a failure to express FMRP, the protein product of the *FMR1* gene. "Fragile X Mental Retardation Protein" (FMRP) shuttles mRNA between the nucleus and cytoplasm in the central nervous system and other areas (e.g., the developing testis) during early embryonic development. Although FMRP is produced in unaffected individuals and premutation carriers, in those with the full mutation, FMRP transcription of the protein is blocked because the large number of CGG repeats in the CPG island become methylated (an epigenetic phenomenon). Thus, FRAX occurs as a consequence of a **loss-of-function mutation**—the failure of expression of FMRP because of methylation of the promoter sequence.

In female premutation carriers, an expansion in the number of repeats from the premutation to the full mutation range may occur during gametogenesis. The cause of this expansion is not understood. Although these females do not have symptoms and signs of FRAX, premutation carriers may manifest premature ovarian failure and/or a neurologic condition known as fragile X tremor/ataxia syndrome later in life.

TERATOGENIC AGENTS

Approximately 6.5% of all birth defects are attributed to teratogens—chemical, physical, or biologic agents that have the potential to damage embryonic tissue and result in congenital malformations. Agents known to be teratogenic include drugs (prescription and nonprescription); intrauterine infections (rubella); maternal diseases, such as diabetes mellitus; and environmental substances, such as alcohol and heavy metals. Knowledge of teratogenic agents and their effect on the developing fetus is important, because limiting exposure to these agents is an effective way to prevent birth defects (see Chapters 58, 59, and 60).

Maternal Infections

Rubella was the first maternal infection known to cause a pattern of malformations in fetuses affected in utero. Cytomegalovirus, *Toxoplasma gondii*, herpes simplex, and varicella are additional potentially teratogenic in utero infections (see Chapter 66).

Maternal Disease

Maternal diabetes mellitus and maternal phenylketonuria can result in congenital anomalies in the fetus. Strict control of these disorders before and during pregnancy protects the developing child (see Chapter 59).

Medications and Chemicals

Fetal alcohol spectrum disorder, which occurs in 10 to 20 per 1000 children, may be the most common teratogenic syndrome. Features include prenatal and postnatal growth deficiency, developmental disabilities, microcephaly, skeletal and cardiac anomalies, and a characteristic facial appearance. To cause the full-blown fetal alcohol syndrome, pregnant women must drink alcohol throughout the pregnancy. Lesser consumption during all or part of the gestation will lead to milder symptoms.

Warfarin, retinoic acid, and phenytoin are additional teratogenic agents (see Chapter 59).

Radiation

High-dose radiation exposure during pregnancy in Hiroshima and Nagasaki, Japan, was shown to increase the rate of spontaneous abortion and result in children born with microcephaly, mental retardation, and skeletal malformations. Estimates of exposure to cause these effects were approximately 25 rad. *The dose from routine radiologic diagnostic examinations is in the millirad range.*

Chapter 48

GENETIC ASSESSMENT

Individuals referred to a geneticist because of suspicion of a genetic disorder are called **probands**; individuals who come for genetic counseling are **consultands**. Referral for genetic evaluation may be made for a wide variety of reasons and at different stages of life (fetus, neonate, childhood, pregnancy).

PRECONCEPTION AND PRENATAL COUNSELING
Familial Factors

Families with relatives affected with genetic disorders may have questions about how a disorder is inherited. The inheritance pattern and the risk of having an affected child can be discussed with a geneticist.

In some cultures, it is common for relatives to mate. This relatedness or **consanguinity** does not increase the likelihood of offspring having any particular single genetic disorder, but it may increase the chance that a child will be born with a rare autosomal recessive (AR) condition, as the mutated gene segregates through that family. Generally, the closer the relation between the partners, the greater the chance that the couple shares one or more mutated genes in common, increasing the risk that offspring will have an AR disorder. The risk of first cousins producing a child with an AR disorder is 1 in 64. In evaluating these couples, it is important to determine which ethnic group they belong to and to test for conditions commonly found in that group.

Screening

It is common for couples to be screened for disorders that may occur more commonly in their particular ethnic group. People of Ashkenazi Jewish background may choose to be screened for heterozygosity for a panel of AR disorders, including Tay-Sachs disease, Niemann-Pick disease, Bloom syndrome, Canavan disease, Gaucher syndrome, cystic fibrosis, Fanconi anemia, and familial dysautonomia. People of African-American ancestry may choose to be screened for sickle cell anemia. People whose ancestors originated in the Mediterranean basin may be screened for thalassemia.

Historically, prenatal screening involved maternal serum screening for α-fetoprotein (AFP), a protein secreted during fetal life by the liver, gastrointestinal tract, and yolk sac. Some of the AFP crosses the placenta and enters the maternal circulation. Although maternal serum screening was initially used to detect high levels of AFP associated with neural tube defects (NTDs) and the disruption of fetal integument such as omphalocele or gastroschisis, low levels of AFP were found to be associated with fetal aneuploidy. Approximately 50% of fetuses with autosomal trisomies (Down syndrome, trisomy 18, trisomy 13) will be detected by low maternal serum AFP levels. Three other proteins—unconjugated estriol (uE3), inhibin A, and human chorionic gonadotropin (HCG)—were added to the maternal serum screening to create the **quad screen**. The addition of these compounds increased the detection rate to about 80%.

The quad screen is done in the second trimester. During the first trimester, measurement of a fluid collection of the posterior neck of the developing fetus is termed nuchal translucency. An increase in the nuchal translucency is a marker for chromosomal anomalies as well as genetic and structural abnormalities in the fetus. This association provided a noninvasive first trimester marker. Once standardization of nuchal translucency measurements was done, the detection rate for aneuploidy approached 70%. Testing for abnormalities with two first trimester analytes, free β-HCG and PAPP-A (pregnancy associated plasma protein) has enhanced first trimester screening to a detection rate of almost 90%.

Although the risk of nondisjunction resulting in aneuploidy rises as a woman gets older (and more so for women older than 35 years of age), all pregnant women should be individually counseled as to their risk for aneuploidy and other fetal abnormalities. A combination of first and second trimester screening together with the women's age produces an individualized risk factor. It is important to emphasize that both of these first and second trimester screening tests are just screens to identify increased risk. If this risk is high, or if there is concern about fetal anomalies from family history, ultrasound, or serum screening, then a more definitive test, either chorionic villus sampling (CVS) or amniocentesis, is offered as further testing. Fetal cells are usually tested for chromosomal abnormalities by cytogenetic techniques, but the use of chromosomal microarray is becoming more common. Biochemical testing for a known family history of an inherited metabolic disorder can also be done on the fetal cells, as well as molecular screening for familial mutations for known disorders

Historically, serum screening has required the use of invasive testing follow-up to confirm findings. Because invasive testing carries a small but real risk of pregnancy loss, many women were not willing to submit to an amniocentesis or CVS. What has been needed is a noninvasive definitive test, one in which fetal risk is negligible. Recently, the search for such a noninvasive test has been successful.

Prenatal diagnosis using cell-free fetal DNA in maternal blood offers the ability to detect trisomies in fetuses using nothing more than a sample of the mother's blood. Although still in the research stage, this technique is being piloted in high-risk pregnancies.

It is common for pregnant women to have a *screening* sonogram at 18 weeks' gestation. An anatomy scan is done to look for congenital anomalies. Brain, heart, kidneys, lungs, and spine are examined.

Maternal Factors

The presence of either acute or chronic maternal illness during pregnancy may lead to complications in the developing fetus. Chronic conditions may expose the fetus to maternal medications that are potentially teratogenic. Acute illnesses such as varicella, Lyme disease, and cytomegalovirus expose the fetus to infectious agents that may cause birth defects. Other factors, such as maternal smoking, alcohol use, and maternal exposure to radiation or chemicals, also may necessitate genetic counseling.

Postnatal—Newborn and Infant

Two percent to four percent of newborns have a genetic abnormality or birth defect. This broad definition of a birth defect includes not only a visible malformation but also functional defects that might not be apparent at birth.

Birth defects have a significant impact on childhood morbidity and mortality. Almost 11% of childhood deaths can be traced to a genetic cause. If contributing genetic factors related to childhood deaths are considered, this increases to almost 25%. Consultation with a geneticist for a newborn or infant may be prompted by many different findings, including the presence of a malformation, abnormal results on a routine newborn screening test, abnormalities in growth (e.g., failure to gain weight, increase in length, or abnormal head growth), developmental delay, blindness or deafness, and the knowledge of a family history of a genetic disorder or chromosomal abnormality or (as a result of prenatal testing) the presence of a genetic disorder or chromosomal abnormality in the infant.

Adolescent and Adult

Adolescents and adults may be seen by a geneticist for evaluation of a genetic disorder that has late onset. Some neurodegenerative disorders, such as Huntington disease and adult-onset spinal muscular atrophy, present later in life. Some forms of hereditary blindness (retinal degenerative diseases) and deafness (Usher syndrome, neurofibromatosis type 2) may not show significant symptoms until adolescence or early adulthood. Genetic consultation also may be prompted for a known family history of a **hereditary cancer syndrome** (breast, thyroid, colon, and ovarian cancers). Individuals may wish to have testing done to determine if they carry a mutation for these syndromes and would be at risk for developing certain types of cancers. A known family history or personal history of a genetic disorder or chromosomal abnormality might prompt testing in anticipation of pregnancy planning.

GENERAL APPROACH TO PATIENTS
Family History

A pedigree usually is drawn to help visualize various inheritance patterns. Answers to questions about the family help determine if there is an autosomal dominant, AR, X-linked, or sporadic disorder. When a child is affected with the new onset of an AD disorder, it is necessary to closely examine the parents to check for the presence of manifestations. If the parents are unaffected, the child's condition is most likely the result of a new mutation; the risk of recurrence is extremely low (although not 0, because of the possibility of gonadal mosaicism in one of the parents). When one parent is affected (even mildly so due to varying penetrance), the recurrence risk rises to 50%. With X-linked disorders, the focus is on the maternal family history to determine if there is a significant enough risk to warrant testing.

Questions about the couple's age are important to ascertain the risk related to maternal age for chromosome abnormalities and paternal age for new mutations leading to AD and X-linked disorders. A history of more than two spontaneous abortions increases the risk that one of the parents has a balanced translocation and the spontaneous abortions are due to chromosomal abnormalities in the fetus.

Pregnancy

During a genetic consultation, it is important to gather information about the pregnancy (see Chapters 58, 59, and 60). A maternal history of a chronic medical condition, such as a seizure disorder or diabetes, has known consequences in the fetus. Medication used in pregnancy can be teratogenic; the pregnant woman's exposure to toxic chemicals (work related) or use of alcohol, cigarettes, or drugs of abuse can have serious effects on the developing fetus. Maternal infection during pregnancy with varicella, *Toxoplasma,* cytomegalovirus, and parvovirus B19, among others, has been found to cause malformations in the fetus.

Follow-up is needed if an amniocentesis or CVS reveals abnormal results. A fetal ultrasound may detect a malformation that needs follow-up when the infant is born. Often hydronephrosis is detected prenatally. These infants need a repeat ultrasound soon after birth.

Delivery and Birth

An infant born prematurely is likely to have more complications than a term infant. An infant can be small, appropriate, or large for his or her gestational age; each of these has implications for the child (see Chapters 58, 59, and 60). In general, the finding that an infant is small for gestational age is suggestive of exposure to a teratogen or the presence of a chromosomal abnormality.

Medical History

Children with inborn errors of metabolism who have intermittent symptoms often have a history of multiple hospitalizations for dehydration or vomiting. Children with neuromuscular disorders may have a normal period followed by increasing weakness or ataxia. Children with lysosomal storage diseases, such as the mucopolysaccharidoses, often have recurrent ear infections and can develop sleep apnea.

Development

Many genetic disorders are associated with developmental disabilities. However, the onset of the disability may not always be present from the newborn period; many inborn errors of metabolism, including storage disorders, cause developmental manifestations after a period of normal development (see Chapters 7 and 8). Some adult-onset disorders have no symptoms until the teens or later. Assessing school problems is important. The type of learning problem, age at onset, and whether there is improvement with intervention or continued decline all are important for proper assessment.

Physical Examination

A careful and thorough physical examination is necessary for all patients with signs, symptoms, or suspicion of genetic disease. Sometimes subtle clues may lead to an unsuspected diagnosis. Features suggestive of a syndrome are discussed in more detail in Chapter 50.

Laboratory Evaluation

Chromosome Analysis

An individual's chromosomal material, known as the karyotype, can be analyzed using cells capable of dividing. In pediatrics, lymphocytes obtained from peripheral blood are the usual source for such cells, but cells obtained from bone marrow aspiration, skin biopsy (fibroblasts), or, prenatally, from amniotic fluid or chorionic villi also can be used. Cells are placed in culture medium and stimulated to grow, their division is arrested in either metaphase or prophase, slides are made, the chromosomes are stained with Giemsa or other dyes, and the chromosomes are analyzed.

In metaphase, chromosomes are short, squat, and easy to count. Metaphase analysis should be ordered in children whose features suggest a known aneuploidy syndrome, such as a trisomy or monosomy. Chromosomes analyzed in prophase are long, thin, and drawn out; analysis gives far more details than are seen in metaphase preparations. Prophase analysis is ordered in individuals with multiple congenital anomalies without an obvious disorder.

Fluorescent In Situ Hybridization

Fluorescent in situ hybridization (FISH) allows the identification of the presence or absence of a specific region of DNA. A complementary DNA probe specific for the region in question is generated, and a fluorescent marker is attached. The probe is incubated with cells from the subject and viewed under a microscope. The bound probe fluoresces, allowing the number of copies of the DNA segment in question to be counted. This technique is useful in Prader-Willi syndrome and Angelman syndrome, in which a deletion in a segment of 15q11.2 occurs, and in velocardiofacial (DiGeorge) syndrome, which is associated with a deletion of 22q11.2.

Microarray Comparative Genomic Hybridization

Microarray comparative genomic hybridization (array CGH) has supplanted prophase analysis in cases in which a subtle chromosomal deletion or duplication (copy number variant) is suspected. In array CGH, DNA from the individual being studied and a normal control is labeled with fluorescent markers and hybridized to thousands of FISH-like probes for sequences spread around the genome. The probes are derived from known genes and noncoding regions. By analyzing the ratio of intensity of the fluorescent marker at each site, it is possible to determine whether the individual in question has any difference in copy number compared with the control DNA.

Direct DNA Analysis

Direct DNA analysis allows identification of mutations in a growing number of genetic disorders. Using polymerase chain reaction, the specific gene in question can be amplified and analyzed. The website www.genetests.org lists disorders in which direct DNA analysis is available and identifies laboratories performing such testing.

Chapter 49

CHROMOSOMAL DISORDERS

Errors that occur in meiosis during the production of gametes can lead to abnormalities of chromosome structure or number. Syndromes caused by chromosomal abnormalities include trisomy 21 (Down syndrome or DS), trisomy 13, trisomy 18, Turner syndrome (TS), and Klinefelter syndrome (KS), as well as rarer chromosomal duplications, deletions, or inversions.

Chromosomal abnormalities occur in approximately 8% of fertilized ova but in only 0.6% of liveborn infants. Fifty percent of spontaneous abortuses have chromosomal abnormalities, the most common being 45,X (TS); an estimated 99% of 45,X fetuses are spontaneously aborted. The fetal loss rate for DS, the most viable of the autosomal aneuploidies, approaches 80%. Most other chromosomal abnormalities also adversely affect fetal viability. In newborns and older children, features that suggest the presence of a chromosome anomaly include low birth weight (small for gestational age), failure to thrive, developmental delay, and the presence of three or more congenital malformations.

ABNORMALITIES IN NUMBER (ANEUPLOIDY)

During meiosis or mitosis, failure of a chromosomal pair to separate properly results in nondisjunction. **Aneuploidy** is a change in the number of chromosomes that results from nondisjunction. A cell may have one (**monosomy**) or three (**trisomy**) copies of a particular chromosome.

Trisomies
Down Syndrome

Decision-Making Algorithms
Available @ StudentConsult.com

Stiff or Painful Neck
Hypotonia and Weakness
Pancytopenia

DS is the most common abnormality of chromosomal number. It occurs in 1 of every 1000 births. Most cases (92.5%) are due to nondisjunction; in 68%, the nondysjunctional event occurs in maternal meiosis phase I. As a result of nondisjunction, there are three copies of chromosome 21 (trisomy 21); using standard cytogenetic nomenclature, trisomy 21 is designated 47,XX,+21 or 47,XY,+21. In 4.5% of cases, the extra chromosome is part of a **robertsonian translocation**, which occurs when the long arms (q) of two acrocentric chromosomes (numbers 13, 14, 15, 21, or 22) fuse at the centromeres, and the short arms (p), containing copies of ribosomal RNA, are lost. The most common robertsonian translocation leading to DS involves chromosomes 14 and 21; standard nomenclature is 46,XX,t(14q21q) or 46,XY,t(14q21q). The parents of DS infants with translocations should have a karyotype to exclude a balanced translocation.

In approximately 1% to 2% of children with DS, **mosaicism** occurs. These individuals have two populations of cells: one with trisomy 21 and one with a normal chromosome complement. Mosaicism results from a either a nondisjunctional event that occurs after fertilization and after a few cell divisions, or from **trisomic rescue**. The loss of this aneuploidy returns the cell to 46,XX or 46,XY. In either case, the individual is referred to as a mosaic for these two populations of cells and is designated 47,XX, +21/46XX or 47,XY,+21/46,XY. Although it is widely believed that individuals with mosaic DS are more mildly affected, there are wide variations in the clinical findings.

Children with DS are most likely diagnosed in the newborn period. These infants tend to have normal birth weight and length, but are hypotonic. The characteristic facial appearance, with brachycephaly, flattened occiput, hypoplastic midface, flattened nasal bridge, upslanting palpebral fissures, epicanthal folds, and large protruding tongue, is apparent at birth. Infants also have short broad hands, often with a single transverse palmar crease, and a wide gap between the first and second toes. The severe hypotonia may cause feeding problems and decreased activity.

Approximately 50% of children with DS have **congenital heart disease**, including atrioventricular canal, ventriculoseptal or atrioseptal defects, and valvular disease. Approximately 10% of newborns with DS have **gastrointestinal tract anomalies**. The three most common defects are duodenal atresia, annular pancreas, and imperforate anus.

Four percent to 18% of infants with DS are found to have congenital hypothyroidism, which is identified as part of the newborn screening program. Acquired hypothyroidism is a more common problem. Thyroid function testing must be monitored periodically during the child's life.

Polycythemia at birth (hematocrit levels >70%) is common and may require treatment. Some infants with DS show a leukemoid reaction, with markedly elevated white blood cell counts. Although this resembles congenital leukemia, it is a self-limited condition, resolving on its own over the first month of life. Nonetheless, children with DS also have an increased risk of **leukemia**, with a 10- to 20-fold increase in risk compared with individuals without DS. In children with DS younger than 2 year of age, the type is generally acute megakaryoblastic leukemia; in individuals older than 3 years of age, the types of leukemia are similar to those of other children, with acute lymphoblastic leukemia being the predominant type.

Children with DS are more susceptible to infection, more likely to develop cataracts, and approximately 10% have atlantoaxial instability, an increased distance between the first and second cervical vertebrae that may predispose to spinal cord injury. Many individuals older than 35 years of age develop Alzheimer-like features.

The recurrence risk for parents who have had a child with DS depends on the child's cytogenetic findings. If the child has trisomy 21, the empiric recurrence risk is 1% (added to the age-specific risk for women up to 40 years of age; after 40, the age-specific risk alone is used for subsequent pregnancies). If the child has a robertsonian translocation, chromosomal analysis of both parents must be performed. In approximately 65% of cases, the translocation is found to have arisen de novo (i.e., spontaneously, with both parents having normal karyotypes), and in 35% of cases, one parent has a balanced translocation. The recurrence risk depends on which parent is the carrier: if the mother is the carrier, the risk is 10% to 15%; if the father is the carrier, the recurrence risk is 2% to 5%.

Trisomy 18

Trisomy 18 (47,XX,+18 or 47,XY,+18) is the second most common autosomal trisomy, occurring in approximately 1 in 7500 live births. More than 95% of conceptuses with trisomy 18 are spontaneously aborted in the first trimester. Trisomy 18 is usually lethal; fewer than 10% of affected infants survive until their first birthday. Most infants with trisomy 18 are small for gestational age. Clinical features include hypertonia, prominent occiput, micrognathia, low-set and malformed ears, short

Table 49-1	Possible Clinical Findings in Trisomy 13 and Trisomy 18	
	TRISOMY 13	**TRISOMY 18**
Head and face	Scalp defects (e.g., cutis aplasia) Microphthalmia, corneal abnormalities Cleft lip and palate in 60%–80% of cases Microcephaly Sloping forehead Holoprosencephaly (arrhinencephaly) Capillary hemangiomas Deafness	Small and premature appearance Tight palpebral fissures Narrow nose and hypoplastic nasal alae Narrow bifrontal diameter Prominent occiput Micrognathia Cleft lip or palate
Chest	Congenital heart disease (e.g., VSD, PDA, and ASD) in 80% of cases Thin posterior ribs (missing ribs)	Congenital heart disease (e.g., VSD, PDA, and ASD) Short sternum, small nipples
Extremities	Overlapping of fingers and toes (clinodactyly) Polydactyly Hypoplastic nails, hyperconvex nails	Limited hip abduction Clinodactyly and overlapping fingers; index over third, fifth over fourth Rocker-bottom feet Hypoplastic nails
General	Severe developmental delays and prenatal and postnatal growth retardation Renal abnormalities Nuclear projections in neutrophils Only 5% live >6 mo	Severe developmental delays and prenatal and postnatal growth retardation Premature birth, polyhydramnios Inguinal or abdominal hernias Only 5% live >1yr

ASD, Atrial septal defect; *PDA*, patent ductus arteriosus; *VSD*, ventricular septal defect.

sternum, rocker-bottom feet, hypoplastic nails, and characteristic clenching of fists—the second and fifth digits overlap the third and fourth digits (Table 49-1).

Trisomy 13

The third of the common trisomies, trisomy 13 (47,XX,+13 or 47,XY,+13) occurs in 1 in 12,000 live births. It is usually fatal in the first year of life; only 8.6% of infants survive beyond their first birthday.

Infants with trisomy 13 have numerous malformations (see Table 49-1). These infants are small for gestational age and microcephalic. Midline facial defects such as cyclopia (single orbit), cebocephaly (single nostril), and cleft lip and palate are common, as are midline central nervous system anomalies, such as alobar holoprosencephaly. The forehead is generally sloping, ears are often small and malformed, and microphthalmia or anophthalmia may occur. Postaxial polydactyly of the hands is common, as is clubfeet or rocker-bottom feet. Hypospadias and cryptorchidism are common in boys, whereas girls generally have hypoplasia of the labia minora. Most infants with trisomy 13 also have congenital heart disease. Many infants with this condition have a punched-out scalp lesion over the occiput called **aplasia cutis congenita;** when seen in conjunction with polydactyly and some or all of the facial findings, this finding is essentially pathognomonic for the diagnosis of trisomy 13.

Klinefelter Syndrome

Decision-Making Algorithms
Available @ StudentConsult.com

Short Stature
Pubertal Delay
Gynecomastia

Occurring in 1 in 500 male births, KS is the most common genetic cause of hypogonadism and infertility in men. It is caused by the presence of an extra X chromosome (47,XXY) (see Chapter 174). The extra X chromosome arises from a nondisjunction in either the sperm or the egg. About 15% of boys with features of KS are found to be mosaic, with 46,XY/47,XXY mosaicism being the most common. Before puberty, boys with KS are phenotypically indistinguishable from the rest of the population.

The diagnosis is often made when the boy is 15 or 16 years of age. At that point, the finding of the progressive development of pubic and axillary hair in the presence of testes that remain infantile in volume should alert the clinician to the disorder. Adolescents and young adults with KS tend to be tall, with long limbs. During adolescence or adulthood, gynecomastia occurs.

Because of failure of growth and maturation of the testes, males with KS have testosterone deficiency and failure to produce viable sperm. Low production of testicular testosterone results in failure to develop later secondary sexual characteristics, such as facial hair, deepening of the voice, and libido. In adulthood, osteopenia and osteoporosis develop. Because of these findings, testosterone supplementation is indicated.

Most men with KS are infertile because they produce few viable sperm. Through the use of isolation of viable sperm through testicular biopsy, coupled with in vitro fertilization and intracytoplasmic sperm injection, it is possible for men with KS to father children; all children born to these men using this technology have had a normal chromosome complement.

Monosomies
Turner Syndrome

Decision-Making Algorithms
Available @ StudentConsult.com

Amenorrhea
Short Stature
Pubertal Delay
Obesity

TS is the only condition in which a monosomic conceptus survives to term; however, 99% of embryos with 45,X are spontaneously aborted. The most common aneuploidy found in conceptuses (accounting for 1.4%,), 45,X is seen in 13% of first-trimester pregnancy losses. Occurring in 1 in 3200 live-born females, TS is notable for its spectrum of relatively mild physical and developmental findings. Affected women tend to have normal intelligence and life expectancy.

Females with TS typically have a characteristic facial appearance with low-set, mildly malformed ears, triangular face, flattened nasal bridge, and epicanthal folds. There is webbing of the neck, with or without cystic hygroma, a shield-like chest with widened internipple distance, and puffiness of the hands and feet. Internal malformations may include congenital heart defect (in 45%, coarctation of the aorta is the most common anomaly, followed by bicuspid aortic valve; later in life, post-stenotic aortic dilation with aneurysm may develop). Renal anomalies, including horseshoe kidney, are seen in more than 50% of patients. Short stature is a cardinal feature of this condition, and acquired hypothyroidism is estimated to occur five times more frequently in women with TS than in the general population.

The presence of streak gonads (gonadal dysgenesis) instead of well-developed ovaries leads to estrogen deficiency, which prevents these women from developing secondary sexual characteristics and results in amenorrhea. Although 10% of women with TS may have normal pubertal development and are even fertile, most affected women require estrogen replacement to complete secondary sexual development.

Infertility in these women is not corrected by estrogen replacement. Assisted reproductive technology using donor ova has allowed women with TS to bear children. During pregnancy, these women must be followed carefully, because poststenotic dilatation of the aorta, leading to dissecting aneurysm, may occur.

Many girls with TS escape detection during the newborn period because phenotypic features are subtle. About 33% of children with TS are diagnosed in the newborn period because of the presence of heart disease and physical features; another 33% are diagnosed in childhood, often during a workup for short stature (and receive growth hormone therapy); the final 33% are diagnosed during adolescence when they fail to develop secondary sexual characteristics.

The karyotypic spectrum in girls with TS is wide. Only 50% have a 45,X karyotype; 15% have an isochromosome Xq [46,X,i(Xq)], in which one X chromosome is represented by two copies of the long arm (leading to a trisomy of Xq and a monosomy of Xp); and approximately 25% are mosaic (45,X/46,XX or 45,X/46,XY). Deletions involving the short (p) arm of the X chromosome (Xp22) produce short stature and congenital malformations, whereas deletions of the long arm (Xq) cause gonadal dysgenesis.

Although monosomy X is caused by nondisjunction, TS is not associated with advanced maternal age. Rather, it is believed that the 45,X karyotype results from a loss of either an X or a Y chromosome after conception; that is, it is a postconceptual mitotic (rather than meiotic) nondisjunctional event.

SYNDROMES INVOLVING CHROMOSOMAL DELETIONS

Cri du Chat Syndrome
A deletion in the short arm of chromosome 5 is responsible for cri du chat syndrome, with its characteristic catlike cry during early infancy, the result of tracheal hypoplasia. Other clinical features include low birth weight and postnatal failure to thrive, hypotonia, developmental disability, microcephaly, and craniofacial dysmorphism, including ocular hypertelorism, epicanthal folds, downward obliquity of the palpebral fissures, and low-set malformed ears. Clefts of the lip and palate, congenital heart disease, and other malformations may be seen.

The clinical severity of cri du chat syndrome depends on the size of the chromosomal deletion. Larger deletions are associated with more severe expression. Most cases arise de novo; the deletion is usually in the chromosome 5 inherited from the father.

Williams Syndrome

Decision-Making Algorithm
Available @ StudentConsult.com

Hypercalcemia

Williams syndrome is due to a small deletion of chromosome 7q11.2. Congenital heart disease is seen in 80% of affected children, with supravalvar aortic-valve and pulmonic-valve stenosis and peripheral pulmonic stenosis being the most common anomalies. Although these children often have normal birth weight, they have growth delay, manifesting short stature. They have a distinctive facial appearance ("elfin facies"), with median flare of the eyebrows, fullness of the perioral and periorbital region, blue irides with a stellate pattern of pigment, and depressed nasal bridge with anteversion of the nares. Moderate intellectual disability (average IQ in the 50 to 60 range) is common, but developmental testing reveals strength in personal social skills and deficiencies in cognitive areas. Hypercalcemia is present in neonates.

Individuals with Williams syndrome often have a striking personality. Loquacious and gregarious, they are frequently described as having a *cocktail party* personality. However, approximately 10% of children with Williams syndrome have features of autism spectrum disorder. Patients occasionally have unusual musical ability (about 20% have absolute or perfect pitch). Most children with Williams syndrome have a de novo deletion. In rare cases, the deletion is inherited from a parent in an autosomal dominant pattern.

Aniridia Wilms Tumor Association
WAGR syndrome (**W**ilms tumor, **a**niridia, **g**enitourinary anomalies, and mental **r**etardation) is caused by a deletion of 11p13 and is generally a de novo deletion. Genitourinary abnormalities include cryptorchidism and hypospadias. Patients often have short stature, and half may have microcephaly. Wilms tumor develops in 50% of patients with aniridia, genitourinary abnormalities, and mental retardation (see Chapter 159).

Prader-Willi Syndrome
SEE CHAPTER 47.

Angelman Syndrome
SEE CHAPTER 47.

Chromosome 22q11.2 Deletion Syndromes

Decision-Making Algorithm
Available @ StudentConsult.com

Hypocalcemia

Deletions of chromosome 22q11.2 are responsible for a group of findings that have been called by several names, including **velocardiofacial syndrome**, **conotruncal anomaly face syndrome**, **Shprintzen syndrome**, and **DiGeorge syndrome**.

These conditions represent a continuum of findings, virtually all of which are due to the chromosomal deletion.

Although chromosome 22q11.2 deletions can be inherited in an autosomal dominant fashion, most cases arise de novo. Common features include clefting of the palate with velopharyngeal insufficiency; conotruncal cardiac defects (including truncus arteriosus, ventriculoseptal defect, tetralogy of Fallot, and right-sided aortic arch); and a characteristic facial appearance, including a prominent nose and a broad nasal root. Speech and language difficulties are common, as is mild intellectual impairment. More than 200 additional abnormalities have been identified in individuals with these conditions. About 70% have immunodeficiencies, largely related to T-cell dysfunction. A wide spectrum of psychiatric disturbances, including schizophrenia and bipolar disorder, has been seen in more than 33% of affected adults.

Damage to the third and fourth pharyngeal pouches, embryonic structures that form parts of the cranial portion of the developing embryo, leads to abnormalities in the developing face (clefting of the palate, micrognathia), the thymus gland, the parathyroid glands, and the conotruncal region of the heart. This spectrum of findings, called the **DiGeorge malformation sequence**, is an important chromosome 22 deletion syndrome.

The deletion that occurs in chromosome 22q11 is usually too small to be seen by standard chromosome analysis; either fluorescent in situ hybridization or chromosomal microarray is needed to identify the deletion. A gene called *TBX1* is within the deleted sequence. It is believed that deletion of one copy of *TBX1* is responsible for many of the features of the various 22q11 deletion syndromes.

SYNDROMES INVOLVING CHROMOSOME DUPLICATION

Duplications and deletions occur secondary to misalignment and unequal crossing over during meiosis. Small extra chromosomes are found in a small percentage of the population (0.06%). These "marker" chromosomes sometimes are associated with mental retardation and other abnormalities, and other times they have no apparent phenotypic effects.

Inverted Duplication Chromosome 15

Chromosome 15 is the most common of all marker chromosomes, and its inverted duplication accounts for almost 40% of this group of chromosomal abnormalities. Features seen in children with 47,XX,+inv dup (15q) or 47,XY,inv dup(15q) depend on the size of the extra chromosomal material present: the larger the region, the worse the prognosis. Children with this disorder tend to have a variable degree of developmental disability and autism spectrum disorders; seizures are common, as are behavior problems. The phenotype shows minimal dysmorphic features, with a sloping forehead, short and downward-slanting palpebral fissures, a prominent nose with a broad nasal bridge, a long and well-defined philtrum, a midline crease in the lower lip, and micrognathia.

Cat Eye Syndrome

Named for the iris coloboma that gives patients' eyes a catlike appearance, cat eye syndrome is due to a small, supernumerary chromosome with an inversion duplication of 22q11. The two copies of 22q11 on this extra chromosome plus the two normal copies of chromosome 22 result in four copies of this region. Although the colobomas name the syndrome, they occur in fewer than 50% of individuals with the marker chromosome. Other clinical features include mild mental retardation, behavioral disturbances, mild ocular hypertelorism, downward-slanting palpebral fissures, micrognathia, auricular pits and/or tags, anal atresia with rectovestibular fistula, and renal agenesis.

Chapter **50**

THE APPROACH TO THE DYSMORPHIC CHILD

Dysmorphology is the recognition of the pattern of congenital malformations (often multiple congenital malformations) and dysmorphic features that characterize a particular syndrome. **Syndromes** are collections of abnormalities, including **malformations**, **deformations**, dysmorphic features, and abnormal behaviors that have a unifying, identifiable etiology. This etiology may be the presence of a mutation in a single gene, as is the case in **Rett syndrome**, a disorder that is caused by a mutation in the *MECP2* gene on Xq28; by the deletion or duplication of chromosomal material, as is the case in **Prader-Willi syndrome**, which is caused by the deletion of the paternal copy of the imprinted *SNRPN* gene on chromosome 15q11.2; or by exposure to a teratogenic substance during embryonic development, as in fetal alcohol spectrum disorder.

DEFINITIONS

Congenital **malformations** are defined as clinically significant abnormalities in either form or function. They result from localized **intrinsic** defects in morphogenesis, which were caused by an event that occurred in embryonic or early fetal life. This event may have been a disturbance of development from some unknown cause, but often mutations in developmental genes led to the abnormality. **Extrinsic** factors may cause **disruptions** of development by disturbing the development of apparently normal tissues. These disruptions may include amniotic bands, disruption of blood supply to developing tissues, or exposure to teratogens. A **malformation sequence** is the end result of a malformation that has secondary effects on later developmental events. An example is the **Pierre Robin sequence**. The primary malformation, failure of the growth of the mandible during the first weeks of gestation, results in micrognathia, which forces the normal-sized tongue into an unusual position. The abnormally placed tongue blocks the fusion of the palatal shelves, which normally come together in the midline to produce the hard and soft palate; this leads to the presence of a U-shaped cleft palate. After delivery, the normal-sized tongue in the smaller than normal oral cavity leads to airway obstruction, a potentially life-threatening complication. Pierre Robin sequence comprises a triad of anomalies (micrognathia, U-shaped cleft palate, and obstructive apnea) which results from a single malformation, the failure of the jaw to grow at a critical time during gestation. Many children with Pierre Robin syndrome have Stickler syndrome, an autosomal dominant disorder caused by mutations in collagen genes. Stickler syndrome also manifests with ocular and musculoskeletal abnormalities.

Deformations arise as a result of environmental forces acting on normal structures. They occur later in pregnancy or after delivery. For instance, plagiocephaly (rhomboid shaped head) may result from intrauterine positioning or from torticollis experienced in the newborn period. Deformations often resolve with minimal intervention, but malformations often require surgical and medical management.

Minor malformations, variants of normal that occur in less than 3% of the population, include findings such as single transverse palmar creases, low-set ears, or hypertelorism; when isolated, they have no clinical significance. A **multiple malformation syndrome** is the recognizable pattern of anomalies that results from a single identifiable underlying cause. It may involve a series of malformations, malformation sequences, and deformations. These syndromes often prompt a consultation with a clinical geneticist. **Dysmorphology** is the specialty focusing on recognition of patterns of malformations that occur in syndromes (Table 50-1).

An **association** differs from a syndrome in that in the former, no single underlying etiology explains the recognizable pattern of anomalies that occur together more often than would be expected by chance alone. The **VACTERL** association (**v**ertebral anomalies, **a**nal atresia, **c**ardiac defects, **t**racheo**e**sophageal fistula, **r**enal anomalies, and **l**imb anomalies) is an example of a group of malformations that occur more commonly together than might be expected by chance. No single unifying etiology explains this condition, so it is considered an association.

In approximately 50% of children noted to have one or more congenital malformations, only a single malformation is identifiable; in the other 50%, multiple malformations are present. About 6% of infants with congenital malformations have chromosomal defects, 7.5% have a single gene disorder, 20% have conditions that are due to multifactorial effects (an interplay between genetic and environmental factors), and approximately 7% are due to exposure to a teratogen. In more than 50% of cases, no cause can be identified.

HISTORY AND PHYSICAL EXAMINATION
Pregnancy History

The history of the pregnancy and birth can reveal multiple risk factors that are associated with dysmorphology. Small for gestational age infants may have a chromosome anomaly or may have been exposed to a teratogen. Large for gestational age infants may be infants of diabetic mothers or have an overgrowth syndrome, such as Beckwith-Wiedemann syndrome. When evaluating an older child with intellectual disabilities, complications of extreme prematurity may account for the child's problems. Postmaturity also is associated with some chromosome anomalies (e.g., trisomy 18) and anencephaly. Infants born from breech presentation are more likely to have congenital malformations.

As a woman gets older there is increased risk of nondisjunction leading to trisomies. Advanced paternal age may be

Table 50-1	Glossary of Selected Terms Used in Dysmorphology

TERMS PERTAINING TO THE FACE AND HEAD

Brachycephaly: Condition in which head shape is shortened from front to back along the sagittal plane; the skull is rounder than normal

Canthus: The lateral or medial angle of the eye formed by the junction of the upper and lower lids

Columella: The fleshy tissue of the nose that separates the nostrils

Glabella: Bony midline prominence of the brows

Nasal alae: The lateral flaring of the nostrils

Nasolabial fold: Groove that extends from the margin of the nasal alae to the lateral aspects of the lips

Ocular hypertelorism: Increased distance between the pupils of the two eyes

Palpebral fissure: The shape of the eyes based on the outline of the eyelids

Philtrum: The vertical groove in the midline of the face between the nose and the upper lip

Plagiocephaly: Condition in which head shape is asymmetric in the sagittal or coronal planes; can result from asymmetry in suture closure or from asymmetry of brain growth

Scaphocephaly: Condition in which the head is elongated from front to back in the sagittal plane; most normal skulls are scaphocephalic

Synophrys: Eyebrows that meet in the midline

Telecanthus: A wide space between the medial canthi

TERMS PERTAINING TO THE EXTREMITIES

Brachydactyly: Condition of having short digits

Camptodactyly: Condition in which a digit is bent or fixed in the direction of flexion (a "trigger finger"–type appearance)

Clinodactyly: Condition in which a digit is crooked and curves toward or away from adjacent digits

Hypoplastic nail: An unusually small nail on a digit

Melia: Suffix meaning "limb" (e.g., amelia—missing limb; brachymelia—short limb)

Polydactyly: The condition of having six or more digits on an extremity

Syndactyly: The condition of having two or more digits at least partially fused (can involve any degree of fusion, from webbing of skin to full bony fusion of adjacent digits)

associated with the risk of a new mutation leading to an autosomal dominant trait. Maternal medical problems and exposures (medications, drugs, cigarette smoking, and alcohol use) are associated with malformations (see Chapters 47 and 48).

An increased amount of amniotic fluid may be associated with intestinal obstruction or a central nervous system anomaly that leads to poor swallowing. A decreased amount of fluid may be the result of a chronic amniotic fluid leak or point to a urinary tract abnormality that results in a failure to produce urine.

Family History

A pedigree comprising at least three generations should be constructed, searching for similar or dissimilar abnormalities in first- and second-degree relatives. A history of pregnancy or neonatal losses should be documented. For a more detailed discussion of pedigrees, see Chapter 47.

Physical Examination

When examining children with dysmorphic features, the following approach should be used.

Growth

The height (length), weight, and head circumference should be measured carefully and plotted on appropriate growth curves. Small size or growth restriction may be secondary to a chromosomal abnormality, skeletal dysplasia, or exposure to toxic or teratogenic agents. Larger than expected size suggests an **overgrowth syndrome** (Sotos or Beckwith-Wiedemann syndrome) or, in the newborn period, might suggest a diabetic mother.

The clinician should note if the child is proportionate. Limbs that are too short for the head and trunk imply the presence of a short-limbed bone dysplasia, such as achondroplasia. A trunk and head that are too short for the extremities suggest a disorder affecting the vertebrae, such as spondyloepiphyseal dysplasia.

Craniofacial

Decision-Making Algorithm
Available @ StudentConsult.com

Abnormal Head Size, Shape, and Fontanels

Careful examination of the head and face is crucial for the diagnosis of many congenital malformation syndromes. Head shape should be carefully assessed; if the head is not normal in size and shape (normocephalic), it may be long and thin (**dolichocephalic**), short and wide (**brachycephalic**), or asymmetric or lopsided (**plagiocephalic**).

Any asymmetry of facial features should be noted. Asymmetry may be due to a deformation related to intrauterine position or a malformation of one side of the face. The face should be divided into four regions, which are evaluated separately. The **forehead** may show overt prominence (achondroplasia) or deficiency (often described as a sloping appearance, which occurs in children with primary microcephaly). The **midface,** extending from the eyebrows to the upper lip and from the outer canthi of the eyes to the commissures of the mouth, is especially important. Careful assessment of the distance between the eyes (inner canthal distance) and the pupils (interpupillary distance) may confirm the impression of hypotelorism (eyes that are too close together), which suggests a defect in midline brain formation, or **hypertelorism** (eyes that are too far apart). The length of the palpebral fissure should be noted and may help define whether the opening for the eye is short, as is found with fetal alcohol syndrome, or excessively long, as in Kabuki makeup syndrome (short stature, mental retardation, long palpebral fissures with eversion of lateral portion of lower lid).

Other features of the eyes should be noted. The obliquity (slant) of the palpebral fissures may be upward (as seen with Down syndrome) or downward (as in Treacher Collins syndrome). The presence of epicanthal folds (Down syndrome and fetal alcohol syndrome) is also important. Features of the nose—especially the nasal bridge, which can be flattened in Down syndrome, fetal alcohol syndrome, and many other syndromes, or prominent as in velocardiofacial syndrome—should be noted.

The **malar** region of the face is examined next. It extends from the ear to the midface. The ears should be checked for size (measured and checked against appropriate growth charts), shape, position (low-set ears are below a line drawn from the outer canthus to the occiput), and orientation (posterior rotation is where the ear appears turned toward the rear of the head). Ears may be low set because they are small (or microtic) or because of a malformation of the mandibular region.

The **mandibular region** is the area from the lower portion of the ears bounded out to the chin by the mandible. In most newborns, the chin is often slightly retruded (that is, slightly behind the vertical line extending from the forehead to the philtrum). If this retrusion is pronounced, the child may have the Pierre Robin malformation sequence. In addition, the mouth should be examined. The number and appearance of the teeth should be noted, the tongue should be observed for abnormalities, and the palate and uvula checked for defects.

Neck

Examination of the neck may reveal webbing, a common feature in Turner syndrome and Noonan syndrome, or shortening, as is seen occasionally in some skeletal dysplasias and in conditions in which anomalies of the cervical spine occur, such as Klippel-Feil syndrome. The position of the posterior hairline also should be evaluated. The size of the thyroid gland should be assessed.

Trunk

The chest may be examined for shape (shield-like chest in Noonan syndrome and Turner syndrome) and for symmetry. The presence of a pectus deformity should be noted and is common in Marfan syndrome. The presence of scoliosis should be assessed; it is common in Marfan syndrome and many other syndromes.

Extremities

Many congenital malformation syndromes are associated with anomalies of the extremities. All joints should be examined for range of motion. The presence of single or multiple joint contractures suggests either intrinsic neuromuscular dysfunction, as in some forms of muscular dystrophy, or external deforming forces that limited motion of the joint in utero. Multiple contractures also are found with **arthrogryposis multiplex congenita** and are due to a variety of causes. **Radioulnar synostosis**, an inability to pronate or supinate the elbow, occurs in fetal alcohol spectrum disorder and in some X chromosome aneuploidy syndromes.

Examination of the hands is important. **Polydactyly** (the presence of extra digits) usually occurs as an isolated autosomal dominant trait but also can be seen in trisomy 13. **Oligodactyly** (a deficiency in the number of digits) is seen in Fanconi syndrome (anemia, leukopenia, thrombocytopenia, and associated heart, renal, and limb anomalies—usually radial aplasia and thumb malformation or aplasia), in which it is generally part of a more severe limb reduction defect, or secondary to intrauterine amputation, which may occur with amniotic band disruption sequence. **Syndactyly** (a joining of two or more digits) is common to many syndromes, including Smith-Lemli-Opitz syndrome (see Chapters 199 and 201).

Dermatoglyphics include palmar crease patterns. A transverse palmar crease, indicative of hypotonia during early fetal life, is seen in approximately 50% of children with Down syndrome (and 10% of individuals in the general population). A characteristic palmar crease pattern is also seen in fetal alcohol spectrum disorder.

Genitalia

Decision-Making Algorithm
Available @ StudentConsult.com

Ambiguous Genitalia

Genitalia should be examined closely for abnormalities in structure. In boys, if the penis appears short, it should be measured and compared with known age-related data. Ambiguous genitalia often are associated with endocrinologic disorders, such as congenital adrenal hyperplasia (girls have masculinized external genitalia, but male genitalia may be unaffected), or chromosomal disorders such as 45,X/46,XY mosaicism or possibly secondary to a multiple congenital anomaly syndrome (see Chapters 174 and 177). Although hypospadias, which occurs in 1 in 300 newborn boys, is a common congenital malformation that often occurs as an isolated defect, if it is associated with other anomalies, especially cryptorchidism, there is a strong possibility of a syndrome.

LABORATORY EVALUATION

Chromosome analysis should be ordered for children with multiple congenital anomalies, the involvement of one major organ system and the presence of multiple dysmorphic features, or the presence of mental retardation. In recent years, microarray comparative genomic hybridization has supplanted routine or high-resolution chromosome analysis in most situations. For a complete discussion of chromosome analysis, see Chapter 48.

Direct DNA analysis can be performed to identify specific mutations. It is necessary to use Web-based resources to keep up-to-date. An extremely helpful website is www.genetests.org, which provides information about the availability of testing for specific conditions and identifies laboratories performing the testing.

Radiologic imaging plays an important role in the evaluation of children with dysmorphic features. Individuals found to have multiple external malformations should have a careful evaluation to search for the presence of internal malformations. Testing might include **ultrasound evaluations** of the head and abdomen to look for anomalies in the brain, kidney, bladder, liver, and spleen. **Skeletal radiographs** should be performed if there is concern about a possible skeletal dysplasia. The presence of a heart murmur should trigger a cardiology consultation; an **electrocardiogram** and **echocardiogram** may be indicated. **Magnetic resonance imaging** may be indicated in children with neurologic abnormalities or a spinal

defect. The presence of craniosynostosis may indicate a **computed tomography scan** of the head.

For those patients for whom testing does not yield a diagnosis, whole-exome sequencing or whole-genome sequencing is becoming a powerful tool.

DIAGNOSIS

Although the presence of characteristic findings may make the diagnosis of a malformation syndrome straightforward, in most cases no specific diagnosis is immediately evident. Some constellations of findings are rare, and finding a "match" may prove difficult. In many cases, all laboratory tests are normal, and confirmation relies on subjective findings. Clinical geneticists have attempted to resolve this difficulty by developing scoring systems, cross-referenced tables of anomalies that help in the development of a differential diagnosis, and computerized diagnostic programs. An accurate diagnosis is important for the following reasons:

1. It offers an explanation to the family why their child was born with congenital anomalies. This may help allay guilt for parents, who often believe they are responsible for their child's problem.
2. With well-described natural histories of many disorders, a diagnosis allows anticipation of medical problems associated with a particular syndrome and appropriate screening. It also provides reassurance that other medical problems are no more likely to occur than they might with other children who do not have the diagnosis.
3. It permits genetic counseling to be done to identify the risk to future children and permits prenatal testing to be done for the disorders for which it is available.

Diagnosis enables the clinician to provide the family with educational materials about the diagnosis and facilitate contact with support groups for particular disorders. The Internet has become an important source for such information. Care should be exercised, as information on the Internet is not subject to editorial control and may be inaccurate. A good site is the National Organization for Rare Disorders (www.rarediseases.org), a clearinghouse for information about rare diseases and their support groups. Genetic testing information is available at the Genetests website (www.genetests.org). This site provides information on available clinical and research testing for many diseases.

Suggested Reading

Brent RL: Environmental causes of human congenital malformations, *Pediatrics* 113:957–968, 2004.

Crissman BG, Worley G, Roizen N, et al: Current perspectives on Down syndrome: selected medical and social issues, *Am J Med Genet C Semin Med Genet* 142C:127–130, 2006.

Encode Project Consortium: An integrated encyclopedia of DNA elements in the human genome, *Nature* 489:57–74, 2012.

Hobbs CA, Cleves MA, Simmons CJ: Genetic epidemiology and congenital malformations: from the chromosome to the crib, *Arch Pediatr Adolesc Med* 156:315–320, 2002.

Holmes LB, Westgate MN: Inclusion and exclusion criteria for malformations in newborns exposed to potential teratogens, *Birth Defects Research (Part A)* 91:807–812, 2011.

Kliegman RM, Stanton B, St. Geme J, et al: *Nelson Textbook of Pediatrics*, 19th ed, Philadelphia, 2011, Saunders.

Online Mendelian Inheritance in Man (website): http://www.ncbi.nlm.nih.gov/sites/entrez?db=omim.

Metabolic Disorders

David Dimmock

Chapter **51**

METABOLIC ASSESSMENT

Optimal outcomes for children with inborn errors of metabolism (IEMs) depend upon recognition of the signs and symptoms of metabolic disease, and prompt evaluation and referral to a center familiar with their management. Delay in diagnosis may result in end organ damage including progressive neurologic injury or death.

With the exception of phenylketonuria (PKU), and medium chain acyl-CoA dehydrogenase (MCAD) deficiency, most metabolic disorders are individually rare, having an incidence of less than 1 per 100,000 births in the United States. When considered collectively, the incidence may approach 1 in 800 to 2500 births (Table 51-1) with the prevalence of a confirmed metabolic disorder detected by newborn screening in 1 in 4000 live births (about 12,500 diagnoses each year) in the United States. This is comparable with the 1 in 1000 infants who have early-onset bacterial sepsis and the 1 in 3000 infants who have invasive group B streptococcal infections.

IEMs are frequent causes of sepsis-like presentations, mental retardation, seizures, sudden infant death, and neurologic impairment; 20% of admissions to a regional children's hospital are for genetic disorders.

Metabolic disorders can be classified using a variety of schemes based on the clinical presentation, including the age of onset, the tissues or organ systems involved, the defective metabolic pathways, or the subcellular localization of the underlying defect. These classification schemes have differing utility when considering approach to diagnosis, management, and screening strategies. The clinical presentation and long-term prognosis have the most bearing on management of children with genetic metabolic disorders.

Genetic metabolic disorders result from the deficiency of an enzyme, its cofactors, or biochemical transporters that lead to the deficiency of a required metabolite, the buildup of a toxic compound, or a combination of both processes (Fig. 51-1, Table 51-2). Understanding which of these mechanisms is involved and if the effects are systemic or restricted to the local tissue enables a rational approach to diagnosis, therapy, and management.

SIGNS AND SYMPTOMS

Decision-Making Algorithms
Available @ StudentConsult.com

Seizures and Other Paroxysmal Disorders
Altered Mental Status
Irritable Infant

The signs and symptoms of an inborn error are diverse and can involve any organ system. The presentation varies among age groups. Inborn errors of metabolism often present a few hours to weeks after birth, often mimicking late-onset sepsis. Infants who survive the neonatal period without developing recognized symptoms often experience intermittent illness separated by periods of being well. While pursuing the evaluation of the specific clinical presentations (e.g., the approach to the sick newborn, irritable child, or child with liver dysfunction), the hypoglycemic and intoxicating (encephalopathy) metabolic disorders should be considered in all neonates presenting with lethargy, poor tone, poor feeding, hypothermia, irritability, or seizures. In most cases these should be evaluated for by assessment of plasma ammonia, blood glucose, and anion gap (Fig. 51-2). Significant ketosis in the neonate is unusual and suggests

Table 51-1	Estimates of Incidence of Various Classes of Disorders Diagnosed or Followed at Specialized Clinics per 100,000 Population*	
	BRITISH COLUMBIA 1969–1996	**WEST MIDLANDS 1999–2003**
Amino acid disorders (excluding phenylketonuria)	7.5	19
Lysosomal storage diseases	7.5	19
Phenylketonuria	7.5	8
Organic acidemias	4	12.5
Peroxisomal disorders	3.5	7.5
Mitochondrial diseases	3	20
Glycogen storage diseases	2	7
Urea cycle diseases	2	4.5

*Populations in British Columbia, Canada (a predominantly white population), between 1969 and 1996, and in the West Midlands of the United Kingdom (which has a diverse ethnic breakdown) between 1999 and 2003.

an organic acid disorder. Similarly specific metabolic disorders predispose to cardiomyopathy, myopathy, hepatopathy, developmental delay, sepsis and developmental regression; appropriate evaluation should be tailored to the clinical presentation.

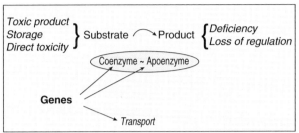

Figure 51-1 Depiction of the basic paradigm in inherited disorders of metabolism. Deficiency of an enzyme complex results in accumulation of metabolites proximal to the blocked metabolism and deficiency of the product of the reaction. Sites of genetic control are indicated.

Introduction of new foods or metabolic stress associated with fasting or fever may unmask an inborn error of metabolism during infancy or in older children. The introduction of fructose or sucrose in the diet may lead to decompensation in hereditary fructose intolerance. In older children, increased protein intake may unmask disorders of ammonia detoxification.

TYPES OF CLINICAL PRESENTATION OF INBORN ERRORS
Toxic Presentation

Decision-Making Algorithms
Available @ StudentConsult.com

Vomiting
Altered Mental Status
Acidemia

DISORDER	DEFICIENCY OF A REQUIRED COMPOUND	ACCUMULATION OF TOXIC COMPOUND	RESULT
HYPOGLYCEMIC DISORDERS			
Medium-chain fatty acid oxidation defects	Fat for energy		Use of glucose with consequent hypoglycemia
Long-chain fatty acid oxidation defects	Fat for energy	Long-chain fats	Use of glucose with consequent hypoglycemia; mitochondrial dysfunction in liver, heart, etc., leading to organ dysfunction
Glycogen storage disease	Glucose to prevent fasting hypoglycemia	Glycogen resulting in storage in liver, muscle, heart	Risk of hypoglycemic brain injury and storage tissue dysfunction
Ketone utilization disorders	Fat for energy	Ketones	Risk of hypoglycemic brain injury; profound metabolic acidosis and reversible neurologic dysfunction
Galactosemia		Galactose	Elevated galactose leads to severe hepatic dysfunction, neurologic injury, and impaired immune response
INTOXICATING DISORDERS (ENCEPHALOPATHY)			
Urea cycle defects		Ammonia	Central nervous system dysfunction, probably mediated through glutamine
Propionic acidemia, methymalonic acidemia, other organic acidemias		Organic acids	Systemic or local impairment of mitochondrial function; impaired neurotransmission; impairment of urea cycle
Phenylketonuria	Tyrosine	Phenylalanine	Impairment of tryptophan metabolism leading to serotonin deficiency; defective neurotransmission and white matter damage
Maple syrup urine disease		Leucine	Leucine toxicity leading to cerebral edema
CELLULAR COMPARTMENT DISORDERS			
Mitochondrial disease	Deficiency of ATP (energy) in affected tissues		Failure of affected tissues to carry out normal functions, e.g., muscle weakness, failure of relaxation of blood vessel muscles
Peroxisomal disorders	Deficiency of VLCFA and steroid hormones necessary for signaling		Aberrant embryonic patterning and hormone deficiency, defects in maintenance of myelin and white matter
Lysosomal storage disorders		Tissue-specific accumulation of compound not metabolized by lysosome	Cell type–specific damage and dysfunction as a result of lysosomal failure and reaction to waste product buildup
OTHER			
Disorders of creatine biosynthesis	Deficiency of cerebral creatine	Accumulation of guanidinoacetate in AGAT deficiency leads to seizures	Global brain energy defect leads to severe cognitive delays
Cholesterol biosynthesis disorders	Deficiency of steroid hormones		Endocrinopathies; disordered cellular signaling

Table 51-2 | Primary Underlying Pathophysiologic Mechanisms for Select Metabolic Disorders

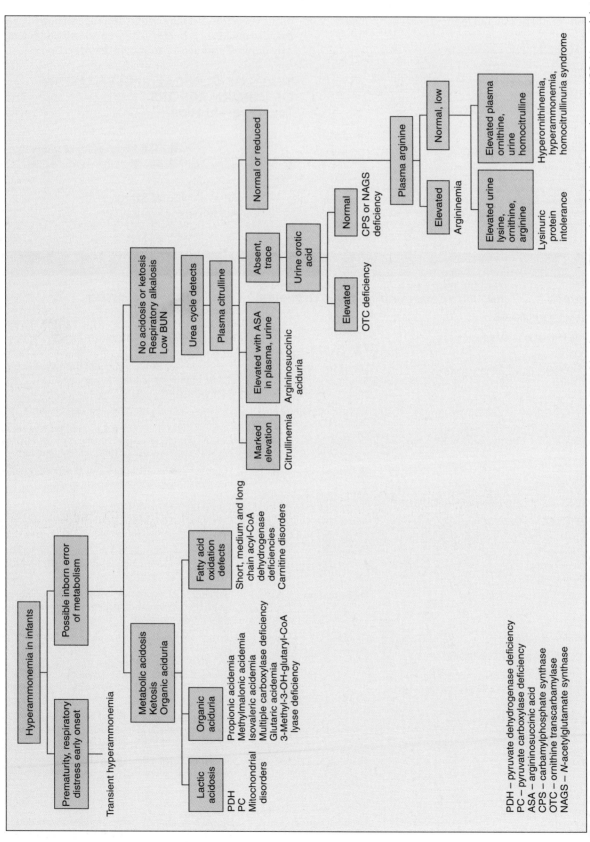

Figure 51-2 Algorithm for the approach to hyperammonemia infants. *ASA,* Argininosuccinic acid; *BUN,* blood urea nitrogen; *CPS,* carbamylphosphate synthase; *NAGS, N*-acetylglutamate synthase; *OTC,* ornithine transcarbamylase; *PC,* pyruvate carboxylase deficiency; *PDH,* pyruvate dehydrogenase deficiency.

The toxic presentation often presents as an **encephalopathy.** Fever, infection, fasting, or other catabolic stresses may precipitate the symptom complex. A **metabolic acidosis,** vomiting, lethargy, and other neurologic findings may be present. Diagnostic testing is most effective when metabolites are present in highest concentration in blood and urine at presentation. Abnormal metabolism of amino acids, organic acids, ammonia, or carbohydrates may be at fault. **Hyperammonemia** is an important diagnostic possibility if an infant or child presents with features of toxic encephalopathy (see Fig. 51-2). Symptoms and signs depend on the underlying cause of the hyperammonemia, the age at which it develops, and its degree. The severity of hyperammonemia may provide a clue to the etiology (Tables 51-3 and 51-4).

Severe Neonatal Hyperammonemia

Decision-Making Algorithms
Available @ StudentConsult.com

Apnea
Vomiting
Hypotonia and Weakness
Alkalemia

Infants with genetic defects in urea synthesis, transient neonatal hyperammonemia, and impaired synthesis of urea and glutamine secondary to genetic disorders of organic acid metabolism can have levels of blood ammonia (>1000 µmol/L) more than 10 times normal in the neonatal period. Poor feeding, hypotonia, apnea, hypothermia, and vomiting rapidly give way to **coma** and occasionally to intractable seizures.

Respiratory alkalosis is common. Death occurs in hours to days if the condition remains untreated.

Moderate Neonatal Hyperammonemia

Decision-Making Algorithms
Available @ StudentConsult.com

Vomiting
Altered Mental Status

Moderate neonatal hyperammonemia (range, 200 to 400 µmol/L) is associated with depression of the central nervous system, poor feeding, and vomiting. Seizures are not characteristic. Respiratory alkalosis may occur. This type of hyperammonemia may be caused by partial or more distal blocks in urea synthesis and commonly is caused by disorders of organic acid metabolism (producing a metabolic acidosis) that secondarily interfere with the elimination of nitrogen.

Clinical Hyperammonemia in Later Infancy and Childhood

Infants who are affected by defects in the urea cycle may continue to do well while receiving the low-protein intake of breast milk, developing clinical hyperammonemia when dietary protein is increased or when catabolic stress occurs. Vomiting and lethargy may progress to coma. Seizures are not typical. During a crisis, the plasma ammonia level is usually 200 to 500 µmol/L. However, as the ammonia level decreases with decreased protein intake, the condition may go unrecognized for years, especially in the absence of central nervous system symptoms. If a crisis occurs during an epidemic of influenza, the child mistakenly may be thought to have **Reye syndrome.**

Table 51-3	Inborn Errors of Metabolism Presenting with Neurologic Signs in Infants <3 Months of Age
GENERALIZED SEIZURES	**ENCEPHALOPATHIC COMA WITH OR WITHOUT SEIZURES**
All disorders that cause hypoglycemia: Most hepatic glycogen storage diseases Galactosemia, hereditary fructose intolerance Fructose-1,6-bisphosphatase deficiency Disorders of fatty acid beta oxidation Glucose transporter deficiency Disorders of the propionate pathway HMG-CoA lyase deficiency Menkes disease Pyruvate carboxylase deficiency (PCD) Maple syrup urine disease **SEIZURES AND/OR POSTURING** Nonketotic hyperglycinemia Maple syrup urine disease	Mitochondrial disease: *POLG* deficiency Iron-sulfur cluster disease Maple syrup urine disease Nonketotic-hyperglycinemia Diseases producing extreme hyperammonemia: Disorders of the urea cycle Disorders of the propionate pathway Disorders of beta oxidation Congenital lactic acidosis (PCD)

HMG-CoA, 3-hydroxy-3-methylglutaryl-CoA.

Table 51-4	Etiologies of Hyperammonemia in Infants
ETIOLOGY OF HYPERAMMONEMIA	**COMMENTS**
Disorders of the urea cycle	Lethal hyperammonemia is common
Disorders of the propionate pathway	Severe hyperammonemia may precede acidosis
Disorders of fatty acid catabolism and of ketogenesis	Reye-like syndrome possible
Transient neonatal hyperammonemia	Idiopathic, self-limited
Portal-systemic shunting	Thrombosis of portal vein, cirrhosis, hepatitis
Mitochondrial DNA depletion	Typically associated with elevated lactate level
Drug intoxication: salicylate, valproic acid, acetaminophen	Obtain drug levels
Hyperinsulinism/hyperammonemia syndrome	Clinical hypoglycemia, subclinical hyperammonemia
Non-metabolic liver disease including infections such as herpes, cytomegalovirus	Ensure evaluation of hepatic function and appropriate infectious disease workup

Older children may have neuropsychiatric or behavioral abnormalities (see Fig. 51-2).

Specific Organ Presentation

Decision-Making Algorithms
Available @ StudentConsult.com

Ocular
Hepatomegaly
Seizures and Other Paroxysmal Disorders
Ataxia

Any organ or system can be injured by toxic accumulation of any of the metabolites involved in inborn errors. Symptoms relate to organ-specific or system-specific toxicity and injury. Examples include nervous system (seizures, coma, ataxia), liver (hepatocellular damage), eye (cataracts, dislocated lenses), renal (tubular dysfunction, cysts), and heart (cardiomyopathy, pericardial effusion) (Table 51-5).

Energy Deficiency

Disorders whose pathophysiology results in energy deficiency (e.g., disorders of fatty acid oxidation, mitochondrial function/oxidative phosphorylation, or carbohydrate metabolism) may manifest myopathy; central nervous system dysfunction, including mental retardation and seizures; cardiomyopathy; vomiting; hypoglycemia; or renal tubular acidosis.

Ketosis and Ketotic Hypoglycemia

Decision-Making Algorithm
Available @ StudentConsult.com

Acidemia

Acidosis is often found in children without metabolic diseases and may be due to fasting associated with anorexia, vomiting, diarrhea, and dehydration in the course of a viral illness. In this normal result of fasting, the blood glucose is relatively low; a mild acidosis and ketonuria may be present. Administration of carbohydrate restores balance. Severe ketosis may also be the result of disorders of ketone utilization such as ketothiolase deficiency or SCOT (succinyl-CoA:3 ketoacid CoA transferase)

deficiency. In these conditions, which frequently present in the context of fasting, infection with fever, or decreased intake secondary to vomiting and diarrhea, hypoglycemia may be profound; the ketosis resolves slowly. As ketone bodies accumulate, cyclic vomiting may ensue. **Ketotic hypoglycemia** is a common condition in which tolerance for fasting is impaired. Symptomatic hypoglycemia with seizures or coma occurs when the child encounters a catabolic stress. The stress may be significant (viral infection with vomiting) or minor (a prolongation by several hours of the normal overnight fast). Ketotic hypoglycemia first appears in the second year of life and occurs in otherwise healthy children. It is treated by frequent snacks and the provision of glucose during periods of stress. The pathophysiology is poorly understood (see Chapter 172). Although ketonuria is a normal response to prolonged (not overnight) fasting in older infants and children, it indicates metabolic disease in neonates. **A high anion gap metabolic acidosis with or without ketosis** suggests a metabolic disorder (Table 51-6). Although ketone production may be reduced in some fatty acid oxidation disorders, the presence of ketonuria does not exclude this group of disorders.

Disorders Associated with Dysmorphic Findings

Congenital malformations or dysmorphic features are not intuitively thought of as symptoms and signs of inborn errors. Conditions that cause congenital malformations include carbohydrate-deficient glycoprotein syndrome, disorders of cholesterol biosynthesis (Smith-Lemli-Opitz syndrome), disorders of copper transport (Menkes syndrome, occipital horn syndrome), maternal phenylketonuria syndrome, glutaric aciduria II (also called multiple acyl-coenzyme A [CoA] dehydrogenase deficiency), and several storage diseases.

Storage Disorders

Decision-Making Algorithm
Available @ StudentConsult.com

Hepatomegaly

Storage disorders are caused by accumulation of incompletely metabolized macromolecules. This storage often occurs in subcellular organelles, such as lysosomes. The glycogen storage diseases and mucopolysaccharide disorders are examples of storage disorders.

Table 51-5	Inborn Errors of Metabolism Presenting with Hepatomegaly or Hepatic Dysfunction in Infants	
HEPATOMEGALY	**HEPATIC FAILURE**	**JAUNDICE**
GSD I	Citrin deficiency Galactosemia	Citrin deficiency Galactosemia
GSD III	Hereditary fructose intolerance	Hereditary fructose intolerance
Mucopolysaccharidosis I and II	Tyrosinemia type 1 (fumarylacetoacetate hydrolase deficiency)	Infantile tyrosinemia (fumarylacetoacetate hydrolase deficiency)
Gaucher and Niemann-Pick diseases	GSD IV (slowly evolving)	Crigler-Najjar disease Rotor, Dubin-Johnson syndromes

GSD, Glycogen storage disease.

Table 51-6	Etiologies of Metabolic Acidosis Caused by Inborn Errors of Metabolism in Infants

DISORDER	COMMENT
Methylmalonic acidemia (MMA)	Hyperammonemia, ketosis, neutropenia, thrombocytopenia
Propionic acidemia	Similar to MMA
Isovaleric acidemia	Similar to MMA; odor of *sweaty feet*
Pyruvate dehydrogenase deficiency	Lactic acidosis, hyperammonemia
Pyruvate carboxylase deficiency	Lactic acidosis, hypoglycemia, and ketosis
Respiratory chain (mitochondrial) disorders	Lactic acidosis, ketosis occasionally seen
Medium-chain acyl-CoA dehydrogenase deficiency (MCAD)	Moderate acidosis, hypoglycemia, decreased ketosis, possible hyperammonemia
Other fatty acid oxidation defects	Similar to MCAD, with potential hepatic and cardiac disease
Galactosemia	Renal tubular acidosis, *Escherichia coli* neonatal sepsis, hypoglycemia
3-Hydroxy-3-methyl-glutaryl-CoA lyase deficiency	Severe lactic acidosis, hyperammonemia, hypoglycemia
Multiple acyl-CoA dehydrogenase deficiency (glutaric aciduria 2)	Metabolic acidosis, hypoglycemia, lethal renal malformations

Table 51-7	Initial Diagnostic Evaluation for a Suspected Inborn Error of Metabolism*

BLOOD AND PLASMA	URINE
Arterial blood gas	Glucose
Electrolytes—anion gap	pH
Glucose	Ketones
Ammonia	Reducing substances
Liver enzymes	Organic acids
Complete blood count, differential,† and platelet count	Acylglycines
Lactate, pyruvate	Orotic acid
Organic acids	
Amino acids	
Acylcarnitines	
Carnitine	

*Organ-specific evaluation is indicated for specific symptoms (e.g., cranial magnetic resonance imaging for coma or seizures; echocardiography for cardiomyopathy; cerebrospinal fluid amino acids by column chromatography if nonketotic hyperglycemia is suspected).
†Thrombocytopenia and neutropenia are seen in organic acidurias; vacuolated lymphocytes and metachromatic granules are seen in lysosomal disorders.

feature of fatty acid oxidation disorders. In some disorders, such as urea cycle disorders, ketone utilization disorders, milder forms of fatty acid oxidation defects, and intermittent maple syrup urine disease, the laboratory abnormalities may be present only during an acute presentation. Therefore, normal testing in the well state does not rule out a metabolic disorder.

CLINICAL ASSESSMENT AND LABORATORY TESTING

The assessment begins with a careful history (family and individual) and clinical evaluation. Clinical laboratory testing can define the metabolic derangement (Table 51-7). The results generate a differential diagnosis and a list of more specific laboratory testing to confirm the diagnosis.

The combination of symptoms and abnormal clinical laboratory findings demands urgent metabolic evaluation. A metabolic emergency often presents with vomiting, acidosis, hypoglycemia, ketosis (or *lack of appropriate ketosis*), intercurrent infection, anorexia/failure to feed, lethargy proceeding to coma, and hyperventilation or hypoventilation. Clinical evaluation should focus on the cardiac, renal, neurologic, and developmental assessment as well as looking for changes in mental status, seizures, abnormal tone, visual symptoms, poor developmental progress, global developmental delay, loss of developmental milestones (regression), cardiomyopathy, cardiac failure, cystic renal malformation, and renal tubular dysfunction.

Clinical laboratory testing should begin with tests that are available in most hospital clinical laboratories. Care in the collection and handling of laboratory specimens is crucial to obtaining accurate results. Plasma measurements of lactate and ammonia are particularly subject to spurious results if not handled correctly. Significant ketosis in the neonate is unusual and suggests an organic acid disorder. Ketosis out of proportion to fasting status in an older child occurs in disorders of ketone usage. Lack of severe ketosis in an older child under conditions of metabolic stress is a

GENETIC ASPECTS OF INBORN ERRORS
Mechanisms of Inheritance

Although all of the classic mechanisms of inheritance are represented, most inborn errors of metabolism are autosomal recessive. Isolation or founder effect may make a specific recessive condition common in some populations (e.g., maple syrup urine disease in the Old Order Mennonite population in Pennsylvania). X-linked conditions exhibit increased presentation in males. In general, carriers of recessive or X-linked (females) diseases are asymptomatic. However, in ornithine transcarbamylase deficiency, females can be symptomatic if they have a low proportion of normal cells in the liver. Most mitochondrial disorders in children are a result of mutations in autosomal genes, although there are X-linked forms. Mutations in the mitochondrial DNA also lead to mitochondrial disease. In this situation the type and severity of the presentation depend on the specific defects and the tissue specific ratio of normal to abnormal copies of the mitochondrial DNA (*the degree of heteroplasmy*).

Identification of Molecular Pathology

If the molecular basis of an inborn error of metabolism is known (i.e., the gene or genes have been mapped and mutations defined), specific genetic testing may be clinically available. In some disorders, there is a good correlation between specific mutations and clinical outcome. Genetic testing in other at-risk family members can provide important genetic information for them, enabling decision making throughout the rest of the family.

Table 51-8	Disorders Identified by Newborn Screening Programs in the United States	
DISORDER	**METHODS**	**CONFIRMATORY TESTING**
AMINO ACID		
Phenylketonuria (PKU)	Guthrie*, MS/MS	Plasma phenylalanine, mutation testing
Tyrosinemia	Guthrie, MS/MS	Plasma amino acid profile, urine succinylacetone
Maple syrup urine disease (MSUD)	Guthrie, MS/MS	Plasma amino acid profile, look for alloisoleucine
ORGANIC ACID		
Propionic acidemia	MS/MS	Urine organic acid profile
Methylmalonic acidemias	MS/MS	Urine organic acid profile, plasma amino acid profile, plasma homocysteine
Isovaleric acidemia	MS/MS	Urine organic acid profile
Biotinidase deficiency	Enzyme measurement	Quantitative biotinidase measurement, DNA mutations
FATTY ACID		
Medium-chain acyl-CoA dehydrogenase deficiency (MCAD)	MS/MS	Urine organic acid profile, urine acylglycine profile, plasma acylcarnitine profile
Long-chain 3-hydroxyacyl-CoA dehydrogenase deficiency (LCHAD)	MS/MS	Urine organic acid profile, urine acylglycine profile, plasma acylcarnitine profile
Very long-chain acyl-CoA dehydrogenase deficiency (VLCAD)	MS/MS	Urine organic acid profile, urine acylglycine profile, plasma acylcarnitine profile
CARBOHYDRATE		
Galactosemia	GALT enzyme measurement	GALT enzyme measurement, DNA mutations, galactose-1-P measurement
UREA CYCLE		
	MS/MS	Plasma amino acid profile, DNA mutations

IDENTIFICATION OF INBORN ERRORS BY NEONATAL SCREENING
Disorders Identified by Neonatal Screening
In the United States the majority of infants diagnosed with a treatable metabolic disorder will be identified as a result of an abnormal newborn screen. Most states use tandem mass spectrometry to screen for a core panel of 29 disorders (Table 51-8). In most states, biotinidase deficiency and galactosemia are typically screened for by evaluating enzyme function.

Strategy of Neonatal Screening
The purpose of neonatal screening is the early detection and rapid treatment of disorders before the onset of symptoms, thus preventing morbidity and mortality. In most states, infants are tested at 24 to 48 hours (see Chapter 58). A positive test demands prompt evaluation. Specific follow-up testing and treatment of an affected child depends on the disorder. Consistent with most screening tests, a significant proportion of infants who have a positive neonatal screening test do not have a metabolic disorder.

Confirmatory Testing Principles
Neonatal screening is designed to maximize detection of affected infants but is not diagnostic. "Cutoff values" for each test are established carefully to identify infants with an elevated concentration of the substance or decreased activity of an enzyme with an acceptable number of false-positive results. A positive screening test must be followed by prompt clinical assessment as recommended by the screening program and metabolic specialist. In many cases children will also be provided therapy until the completion of definitive testing.

A positive screening test result causes anxiety for new parents; management of such anxiety is essential to minimize the harm of the program. In addition, definitive testing must be carried out promptly and accurately. If an inborn error of metabolism is excluded, parents need a thorough explanation of the results and reassurance that the infant is well. Such explanations will frequently require the expertise of a metabolic specialist or genetic counselor in the newborn period but may require reassessment by the primary care physician in the long term.

Specialized Laboratory and Clinical Testing
Specialized testing for inherited disorders of metabolism is effective in confirming a diagnosis suspected on the basis of an abnormal newborn screening result or on the basis of clinical suspicion. The tests that are helpful and examples of diagnoses made using these measurements depend on the deficient pathway in the disorder under consideration (Table 51-9).

Amino acid analysis is performed in plasma, urine, and cerebrospinal fluid. The plasma amino acid profile is most useful in identifying disorders of amino acid catabolism. Amino acids in the deficient pathway of the organic acid disorders may be abnormal, but often they are normal or may not be diagnostic.

Table 51-9	Specialized Metabolic Testing	
TEST	**ANALYTES MEASURED**	**TEST HELPFUL IN IDENTIFYING DISORDERS**
Plasma amino acid profile	Amino acids, including alloisoleucine	PKU, urea cycle defects, tyrosinemias, MSUD, homocystinuria
Plasma total homocysteine	Protein-bound and free homocysteine	Homocystinuria, some forms of methylmalonic acidemia
Urine amino acid profile	Amino acids	Disorders of amino acid renal transport
Plasma acylcarnitine profile	Acylcarnitine derivatives of organic and fatty acid catabolism	Organic acid disorders, fatty acid oxidation disorders
Urine acylglycine profile	Acylglycine derivatives of organic and fatty acid catabolism	Organic acid disorders, fatty acid oxidation disorders
Plasma carnitines	Free, total, and acylated carnitine	Primary and secondary carnitine deficiency; abnormal in many organic acid and fatty acid disorders
Urine organic acid profile	Organic acids	Organic acid, mitochondrial and fatty acid disorders
Urine or blood succinylacetone	Succinylacetone	Tyrosinemia I
Urine oligosaccharide chromatography	Glycosaminoglycans, mucopolysaccharides	Lysosomal storage disorders

MSUD, Maple syrup urine disease; *PKU,* phenylketonuria.

The urine amino acid profile is helpful in diagnosing primary disorders of renal tubular function, such as Lowe syndrome and cystinuria, as well as secondary disorders of renal tubular function, such as cystinosis and Fanconi syndrome of any cause. The urine amino acid profile is not the test of choice for diagnosing disorders of amino acid or organic acid metabolism.

Markers of disordered fatty acid oxidation are measured in urine and plasma. Excessive intermediates of fatty acid oxidation and organic acid catabolism are conjugated with glycine and carnitine. The **urine acylglycine profile** and the **plasma acylcarnitine profile** reflect this accumulation. In organic acid disorders and fatty acid oxidation disorders, measurement of plasma carnitine may reveal a secondary deficiency of carnitine and abnormal distribution of free and acylated carnitine. The plasma free fatty acid profile is helpful in diagnosis of disorders of fatty acid oxidation. Excess 3-OH-butyrate suggests a disorder of ketone metabolism; absence of ketones or decreased amounts of 3-OH-butyrate suggests a fatty acid oxidation disorder. Profiling of fatty acid intermediates in cultured skin fibroblasts may be informative.

Disorders of organic acid metabolism, such as propionic acidemia and methylmalonic acidemia, have typical urine organic acid profiles. Although analysis of blood and urine usually suggest the specific diagnosis, more targeted testing is typically needed by measuring enzymatic activity in the pathway or establishing DNA changes in the gene.

Disorders of creatine biosynthesis are reflected by a reduction in creatine in cerebrospinal fluid (CSF) and, in one form, an increase in guanidinoacetic acid in blood and urine. Disorders of purine and pyrimidine metabolism are suggested by the presence of an abnormal urinary profile of purines, such as xanthine, hypoxanthine, inosine, guanosine, adenosine, adenine, or succinyladenosine. Similarly, disorders of pyrimidine metabolism are identified by an abnormal profile of pyrimidines, including uracil, uridine, thymine, thymidine, orotic acid, orotidine, dihydrouracil, dihydrothymine, pseudouridine, N-carbamoyl-β-alanine, or N-carbamoyl-β-aminoisobutyrate, in the urine.

Storage disorders show abnormalities in urine mucopolysaccharides (glycosaminoglycans, glycoproteins), sialic acid, heparan sulfate, dermatan sulfate, or chondroitin sulfate. Specific enzymology depends on the disorder; tissue can be either white blood cells or cultured skin fibroblasts, depending on assay. In several disorders, CSF is the most helpful specimen, including glycine encephalopathy (CSF amino acid profile when compared to concurrent plasma amino acids), disorders of neurotransmitter synthesis (biogenic amine profile), glucose transporter (GLUT1) deficiency (plasma-to–cerebrospinal fluid glucose ratio), and serine synthesis defect (amino acid profile).

In many disorders, an abnormal metabolic profile is consistently present during illness and when the child is well. In some cases, it is only diagnostic during an episode of illness.

OVERVIEW OF TREATMENT

There are several basic principles for treatment of inborn errors of metabolism. Syndromes with toxicity often present with encephalopathy; removal of toxic compounds is the first goal of therapy. Strategies include hemodialysis, hemovenovenous filtration, and administration of alternate pathway agents (see Chapter 53). A second strategy is to enhance deficient enzyme activity through administration of enzyme cofactors (e.g., pyridoxine in homocystinuria, tetrahydrobiopterin in PKU). If deficiency of a pathway product plays an important role, providing missing products is helpful (e.g., tyrosine in the treatment of phenylketonuria). A major principle is to decrease flux through the deficient pathway by restricting precursors in the diet. Examples include the restriction of protein in disorders of ammonia detoxification and of amino acid precursors in the organic acid disorders.

CARBOHYDRATE DISORDERS

GLYCOGEN STORAGE DISEASES

Many glycogen storage diseases are characterized by **hypoglycemia** and **hepatomegaly** (Table 52-1). Glycogen, the storage form of glucose, is found most abundantly in the liver (where it modulates blood glucose levels) and in muscles (where it facilitates anaerobic work). Glycogen is synthesized from uridine diphosphoglucose through the concerted action of glycogen synthetase and brancher enzyme (Fig. 52-1). The accumulation of glycogen is stimulated by insulin. Glycogenolysis occurs through a cascade initiated by epinephrine or glucagon. It results in rapid phosphorolysis of glycogen to yield glucose 1-phosphate, accompanied by, to a lesser degree, hydrolysis of glucose residues from the branch points in glycogen molecules. In the liver and kidneys, glucose 1-phosphate is converted to glucose 6-phosphate through the actions of phosphoglucomutase; glucose-6-phosphatase hydrolyses glucose 6-phosphate to produce glucose. The latter enzyme is not present in muscles. Glycogen storage diseases fall into the following four categories:

1. Diseases that predominantly affect the liver and have a direct influence on blood glucose (types I, VI, and VIII)
2. Diseases that predominantly involve muscles and affect the ability to do anaerobic work (types V and VII)
3. Diseases that can affect the liver and muscles and directly influence blood glucose and muscle metabolism (type III)
4. Diseases that affect various tissues but have no direct effect on blood glucose or on the ability to do anaerobic work (types II and IV)

The **diagnosis** of type I or type III glycogen storage disease is suggested by an elevated uric acid, lactate, and triglycerides in blood. For all forms, a diagnosis can normally be confirmed by DNA mutation testing in white blood cells. When this is feasible, invasive procedures, such as muscle and liver biopsy, can be avoided. When mutation testing is not available or is inconclusive, enzyme measurements in tissue from the affected organ confirm the diagnosis. If the diagnosis cannot be established, metabolic challenge and exercise testing may be needed. **Treatment** of hepatic glycogen storage disease is aimed at maintaining satisfactory

Table 52-1	Glycogen Storage Diseases*				
DISEASE	**AFFECTED ENZYME**	**ORGANS AFFECTED**	**CLINICAL SYNDROME**	**NEONATAL MANIFESTATIONS**	**PROGNOSIS**
Type 1a: von Gierke	Glucose-6-phosphatase	Liver, kidney, GI tract, platelets	Hypoglycemia, lactic acidosis, ketosis, hepatomegaly, hypotonia, slow growth, diarrhea, bleeding disorder, gout, hypertriglyceridemia, xanthomas	Hypoglycemia, lactic acidemia, liver may not be enlarged	Early death from hypoglycemia, lactic acidosis; do well with early diagnosis and strict adherence to dietary therapy; hepatomas may occur in late childhood
Type 1b	Glucose-6-phosphate translocase	Liver, kidney, GI tract, platelets, white blood cells	As Type 1a, but in addition have clinically significant neutropenia	As type 1a but also may present with infections	In addition to risks for type 1a, children have significant GI dysfunction. Historically death due to infections has occurred in the second decade.
Type II: Pompe	Lysosomal α-glucosidase	All; notably striated muscle, nerve cells	Symmetrical profound muscle weakness, cardiomegaly, heart failure, shortened P-R interval	May have muscle weakness, cardiomegaly, or both	Very poor in neonatal form; death in the first year of life is usual; variants exist; therapy with recombinant human α-glucosidase is promising
Type III: Forbes	Debranching enzyme	Liver, muscles	Early in course hypoglycemia, ketonuria, hepatomegaly that resolves with age; may show muscle fatigue	Usually none	Very good for hepatic disorder; if myopathy present, it tends to be like that of type I and V
Type IV: Andersen	Branching enzyme	Liver, other tissues	Hepatic cirrhosis beginning at several months of age; early liver failure	Usually none	Very poor; death from hepatic failure in first decade is typical
Type V: McArdle	Muscle phosphorylase	Muscle	Muscle fatigue beginning in adolescence	None	Good, with sedentary lifestyle
Type VI: Hers	Liver phosphorylase	Liver	Mild hypoglycemia with hepatomegaly, ketonuria	Usually none	Probably good
Type VII: Tarui	Muscle phosphofructokinase	Muscle	Clinical findings similar to type V	None	Similar to that of type V
Type VIII	Phosphorylase kinase	Liver	Clinical findings similar to type III, without myopathy	None	Good

GI, Gastrointestinal.
*Except for one form of hepatic phosphorylase kinase, which is X-linked, these disorders are autosomal recessive.

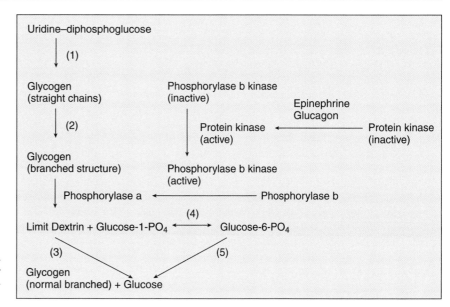

Figure 52-1 Glycogen synthesis and degradation. (1) Glycogen synthetase, (2) brancher enzyme, (3) debrancher enzyme, (4) phosphoglucomutase, (5) glucose-6-phosphatase.

blood glucose levels or supplying alternative energy sources to muscle. In glucose-6-phosphatase deficiency (type I), the treatment usually requires nocturnal intragastric feedings of glucose during the first 1 or 2 years of life. Thereafter, snacks or nocturnal intragastric feedings of uncooked cornstarch may be satisfactory; hepatic tumors (sometimes malignant) are a threat in adolescence and adult life. No specific treatment exists for the diseases of muscle that impair skeletal muscle ischemic exercise. Enzyme replacement early in life is effective in Pompe disease (type II), which involves cardiac and skeletal muscle.

GALACTOSEMIA

 Decision-Making Algorithms
Available @ StudentConsult.com

Visual Impairment and Leukocoria
Jaundice
Hepatomegaly
Alkalemia

Galactosemia is an autosomal recessive disease caused by deficiency of galactose-1-phosphate uridyltransferase (Fig. 52-2). Clinical manifestations are most striking in a neonate who, when fed milk, generally exhibits evidence of **liver failure** (hyperbilirubinemia, disorders of coagulation, hypoglycemia), disordered **renal tubular function** (acidosis, glycosuria, aminoaciduria), and **cataracts**. The neonatal screening test must have a rapid turnaround time because affected infants may die in the first week of life. Affected infants are at increased risk for severe neonatal *Escherichia coli* sepsis. Major effects on liver and kidney function and the development of cataracts are limited to the first few years of life; older children may have learning disorders despite dietary compliance. Girls usually develop premature ovarian failure despite treatment.

Laboratory manifestations of galactosemia depend on dietary galactose intake. When galactose is ingested (as lactose), levels of plasma galactose and erythrocyte galactose

Figure 52-2 Pathway of galactose metabolism. (1) Lactase (intestinal), (2) galactokinase, (3) galactose-1-phosphate uridyltransferase, (4) uridine diphosphoglucose 4-epimerase.

1-phosphate are elevated. Hypoglycemia is frequent, and albuminuria is present. Galactose frequently is present in the urine and can be detected by a positive reaction for reducing substances without a reaction with glucose oxidase on urine strip tests. The absence of urinary reducing substances cannot be relied on to exclude the diagnosis. The diagnosis is made by showing extreme reduction in erythrocyte galactose-1-phosphate uridyltransferase activity. DNA testing for the mutations in galactose-1-phosphate uridyltransferase confirms the diagnosis and may be useful in predicting prognosis. Renal tubular dysfunction may be evidenced by a normal–anion-gap hyperchloremic metabolic acidosis. **Treatment** by the elimination of dietary galactose results in rapid correction of abnormalities, but infants who are extremely ill before treatment may die before therapy is effective.

Galactokinase deficiency, an autosomal recessive disorder, also leads to the accumulation of galactose in body fluids (see Fig. 52-2), which results in the formation of galactitol (dulcitol) through the action of aldose reductase. Galactitol, acting as an osmotic agent, can be responsible for cataract formation and, rarely, for increased intracranial pressure. These are the only clinical manifestations. Individuals homozygous for galactokinase deficiency usually develop cataracts after the neonatal period, whereas heterozygous individuals may be at risk for cataracts as adults.

Hereditary fructose intolerance, in many ways, is analogous to galactosemia. When fructose is ingested, deficiency of fructose-1-phosphate aldolase leads to the intracellular accumulation of fructose 1-phosphate with resultant emesis, hypoglycemia, and severe liver and kidney disease. Elimination of fructose and sucrose from the diet prevents clinical disease. **Fructosuria** is caused by fructokinase deficiency, but its deficiency is not associated with clinical consequences.

Chapter 53

AMINO ACID DISORDERS

DISORDERS OF AMINO ACID METABOLISM

Disorders of amino acid metabolism are the result of the inability to catabolize specific amino acids derived from protein. Usually a single amino acid pathway is involved. This amino acid accumulates in excess and is toxic to various organs, such as the brain, eyes, skin, or liver. Treatment is directed at the specific pathway and usually involves dietary restriction of the offending amino acid and supplementation with special medical foods (formulas) that provide the other amino acids and other nutrients. Confirmatory testing includes quantitative specific plasma amino acid profiles along with specific mutation testing and sometimes enzymology.

PHENYLKETONURIA

Phenylketonuria (PKU), an autosomal recessive disease, primarily affects the brain and occurs in 1 in 10,000 persons. Classic PKU is the result from a defect in the hydroxylation of phenylalanine to form tyrosine (Fig. 53-1); the activity of phenylalanine hydroxylase in the liver is absent or greatly reduced. Affected infants are normal at birth, but if untreated, severe mental retardation (IQ 30) develops in the first year of life. A positive newborn screening test must be followed up by performing quantitative plasma amino acid analysis. A plasma phenylalanine value of greater than 360 μM (6 mg/dL) is consistent with the diagnosis of one of the hyperphenylalaninemias and demands prompt evaluation and treatment. Untreated, classic PKU is characterized by blood phenylalanine concentrations higher than 600 μM. Milder forms of hyperphenylalaninemia are indicated by values of plasma phenylalanine lower than this but higher than 360 μM. A significant percentage of premature infants and a few full-term infants have transient elevations in phenylalanine. Short-term follow-up usually identifies these infants promptly. A small percentage of infants diagnosed with PKU (≤2% in the United States) have a defect in the synthesis or metabolism of tetrahydrobiopterin, the cofactor for phenylalanine hydroxylase and for other enzymes involved in the intermediary metabolism of aromatic amino acids. Such disorders in biopterin metabolism are diagnosed by measuring dihydrobiopterin reductase in erythrocytes and by analyzing biopterin metabolites in urine. This testing should be carried out in all hyperphenylalaninemic infants.

Treatment is designed to maintain plasma phenylalanine values in the therapeutic range of 120 to 360 mM using a diet specifically restricted in phenylalanine but otherwise nutritionally complete. Since the early 1980s, treatment for life is recommended to reduce the risks of long-term neuropsychiatric problems and reduce the risk of maternal PKU syndrome.

Outcome of treatment in classic PKU is excellent. Most infants with classic PKU who are treated within the first

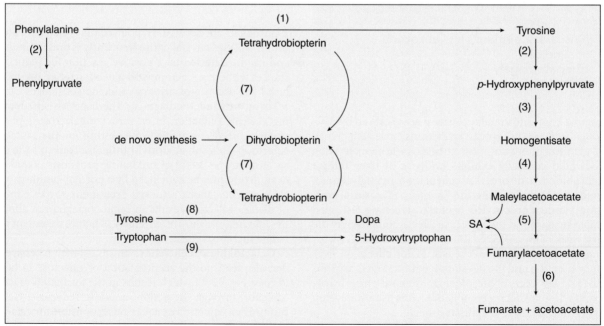

Figure 53-1 Metabolism of aromatic amino acids. (1) Phenylalanine hydroxylase, (2) transaminase, (3) *p*-hydroxyphenylpyruvate oxidase, (4) homogentisate oxidase, (5) maleylacetoacetate isomerase, (6) fumarylacetoacetate hydrolase, (7) dihydrobiopterin reductase, (8) tyrosine hydroxylase, (9) tryptophan hydroxylase. *SA*, Succinylacetone.

10 days of life achieve normal intelligence. However, learning problems and problems with executive function are more frequent than in unaffected peers. The safe concentration of phenylalanine in older children and adults with PKU has not been clearly established. Reversible cognitive dysfunction is associated with acute elevations of plasma phenylalanine in adults and children with PKU. If the elevated level has been sustained, the dysfunction may not be reversible. Treatment with modified preparation of tetrahydrobiopterin has shown good responses in some individuals with PKU.

Females with PKU and their families must be educated on the risks and prevention of "maternal PKU syndrome." **Maternal hyperphenylalaninemia** requires rigorous management before conception and throughout pregnancy to prevent fetal brain damage, congenital heart disease, and microcephaly.

TYROSINEMIAS

Tyrosinemia is identified in neonatal screening programs using tandem mass spectrometry methods to detect elevated tyrosine and/or succinylacetone. Elevated tyrosine levels also occur as a nonspecific consequence of severe liver disease or transient tyrosinemia of the newborn, which responds to ascorbic acid treatment. The inherited disorders of tyrosine metabolism are the target of neonatal screening. **Tyrosinemia Type I,** which is due to fumarylacetoacetate hydrolase deficiency (see Fig. 53-1), is a rare disease in which accumulated metabolites produce severe liver disease associated with bleeding disorder, hypoglycemia, hypoalbuminemia, elevated transaminases, and defects in renal tubular function. Hepatocellular carcinoma may eventually occur. Quantitative measurement of plasma tyrosine and blood or urine succinylacetone is performed after a positive neonatal screen. The **diagnosis** of tyrosinemia I is confirmed by an increased concentration of succinylacetone; DNA testing is available for some mutations. **Treatment** with nitisinone (NTBC) (an inhibitor of the oxidation of parahydroxyphenylpyruvic acid) effectively eliminates the production of the toxic succinylacetone. A low-phenylalanine, low-tyrosine diet may also play a role. These treatments have obviated the immediate need for liver transplantation in children identified by neonatal screening. Whether they completely eliminate the occurrence of hepatocellular carcinoma is unknown.

Tyrosinemias II and **III** are more benign forms of hereditary tyrosinemia. Blocked metabolism of tyrosine at earlier steps in the pathway is responsible, and succinylacetone is not produced. The clinical features include **hyperkeratosis** of palms and soles and **keratitis,** which can cause severe visual disturbance. Poor dietary compliance with type II tyrosinemia is associated with mild cognitive impairment. Treatment with a phenylalanine- and tyrosine-restricted diet is effective.

HOMOCYSTINURIA

Homocystinuria, an autosomal recessive disease (1:200,000 live births) involving connective tissue, the brain, and the vascular system, is caused by a deficiency of cystathionine β-synthase. In the normal metabolism of the sulfur amino acids, methionine gives rise to cystine; homocysteine is a pivotal intermediate (Fig. 53-2). When cystathionine β-synthase is deficient, homocysteine accumulates in the blood and appears in the

urine. Another result is enhanced reconversion of homocysteine to methionine, resulting in an increase in the concentration of methionine in the blood. The neonatal screening test most commonly used measures methionine. An excess of homocysteine produces a slowly evolving **clinical syndrome** that includes dislocated ocular lenses; long, slender extremities; malar flushing; and livedo reticularis. Arachnodactyly, scoliosis, pectus excavatum or carinatum, and genu valgum are skeletal features. Mental retardation, psychiatric illness, or both may be present. Major arterial or venous thromboses are a constant threat.

Confirmation of the **diagnosis** requires demonstration of elevated total homocysteine in the blood. A plasma amino acid profile reveals hypermethioninemia. Measurement of cystathionine β-synthase is not clinically available, but numerous mutations in the gene are known and can be tested.

There are two clinical forms of homocystinuria. In one form, activity of the deficient enzyme can be enhanced by the administration of large doses of pyridoxine (100 to 1000 mg/day). Folate supplementation is added to overcome folate deficiency if folate is trapped in the process of remethylation of homocysteine to methionine. This pyridoxine-responsive form comprises about 50% of cases and is the more likely form to be missed by neonatal screening because the methionine concentrations are not always above the screening cutoff. The second form is not responsive to pyridoxine therapy. The accumulation of homocysteine is controlled with a methionine-restricted diet and cystine and folate supplementation. The use of supplemental betaine (trimethylglycine), a donor of methyl groups for remethylation of homocysteine to methionine, also has a role in the management of pyridoxine-unresponsive patients. Diet and betaine are sometimes required to control plasma homocysteine, even in pyridoxine-responsive patients. The prognosis is good for infants whose plasma homocysteine concentration is controlled.

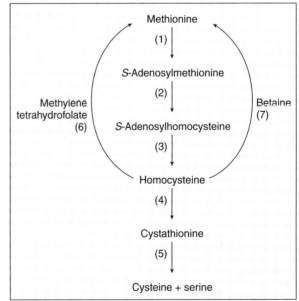

Figure 53-2 Metabolism of methionine and homocysteine. (1) Methionine adenosyltransferase, (2) S-methyltransferase, (3) S-adenosylhomocysteine hydrolase, (4) cystathionine β-synthase, (5) cystathionase, (6) homocysteine methyltransferase, (7) betaine-homocysteine methyltransferase.

MAPLE SYRUP URINE DISEASE

Maple syrup urine disease (MSUD) is an autosomal recessive disease, also called **branched chain ketoaciduria**. A deficiency of the decarboxylase initiates the degradation of the keto-acid analogs of the three branched chain amino acids—leucine, isoleucine, and valine (Fig. 53-3). Classic MSUD is rare (1:250,000) in the general population but much more common in some population isolates (Pennsylvania Mennonites 1:150). The American College of Medical Genetics neonatal screening panel includes MSUD.

Although MSUD does have intermittent-onset and late-onset forms, **clinical manifestations** of the classic form typically begin within 1 to 4 weeks of birth. Poor feeding, vomiting, and tachypnea commonly are noted, but the hallmark of the disease is profound depression of the central nervous system, associated with alternating hypotonia and hypertonia (**extensor spasms**), opisthotonos, and seizures. The urine has the odor of maple syrup.

Laboratory manifestations of MSUD include hypoglycemia and a variable presence of metabolic acidosis, with elevation of the undetermined anions; the acidosis is caused, in part, by plasma branched chain organic acids and, in part, by the usual *ketone bodies,* β-hydroxybutyrate and acetoacetate. Branched-chain ketoacids in urine (but not β-hydroxybutyrate or acetoacetate) react immediately with 2,4-dinitrophenylhydrazine to form a copious, white precipitate.

The **definitive diagnosis** of MSUD generally is made by showing large increases in plasma leucine, isoleucine, and valine concentrations and identification of alloisoleucine in the plasma in excess. The urinary organic acid profile is usually abnormal and shows the ketoacid derivatives of the branched chain amino acids.

Provision of adequate calories and protein, **with restriction of leucine**, is crucial for acute and chronic management. Hemodialysis, hemofiltration, or peritoneal dialysis can be lifesaving during acidotic crises in addition to close monitoring and therapy for cerebral edema. Ordinary catabolic stresses, such as moderate infections or labor and delivery in a pregnant mother with MSUD, can precipitate clinical crises. Liver transplantation effectively treats MSUD.

DISORDERS OF AMMONIA DISPOSAL

Inherited enzymatic deficiencies have been described for each of the steps of urea synthesis (Fig. 53-4). Neonatal screening does not currently detect all of the disorders in the urea cycle.

Figure 53-3 Metabolism of the branched chain amino acids. (1) Aminotransferases, (2) α-ketoacid dehydrogenase complex.

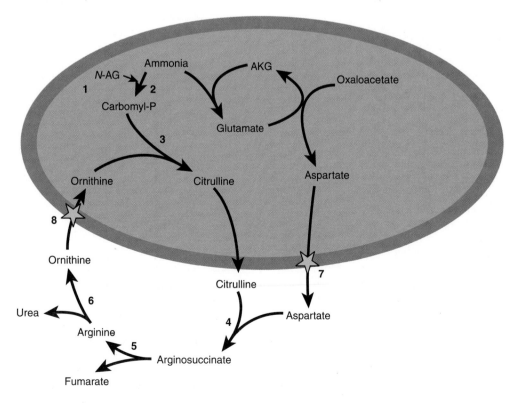

Figure 53-4 The urea cycle. Site of enzymatic defects: (1) *N*-acetylglutamate synthase (*N*-AG), (2) carbamoyl phosphate synthetase, (3) ornithine carbamoyltransferase, (4) argininosuccinate acid synthetase, (5) argininosuccinate acid lyase, (6) arginase. Transporters (*star*). (7) citrin, (8) ornithine translocator (*star*). *AKG,* Alpha ketoglutarate.

Clinically the two most frequent disorders in the United States are ornithine carbamoyltransferase (OTC) deficiency and argininosuccinate lyase (ASL) deficiency.

Ornithine carbamoyltransferase (OTC) deficiency is X-linked. Gene mutations include both deletions and point mutations. If the enzyme is nonfunctional, there is no OTC activity in affected males, who are likely to die in the neonatal period. Affected females are heterozygous and, because of lyonization, may have a significant degree of enzyme deficiency and may be clinically affected at any time in life. **Clinical manifestations** range from lethal disease in the male (coma, encephalopathy) to clinical normalcy in a high percentage of females. Late-onset forms in males also occur. Manifestations in clinically affected females include recurrent emesis, lethargy, seizures, developmental delay, mental retardation, or episodic confusion. Affected females may spontaneously limit their protein intake.

Confirmatory testing for OTC includes a plasma amino acid profile, which may show reduced citrulline and arginine concentrations with increased glutamate and alanine. A urine organic acid profile shows increased excretion of orotic acid after protein loading or with concurrent administration of allopurinol. Mutation testing, deletion testing, and sequencing of the entire coding region of the related genes are available as clinical tests.

Argininosuccinate lyase (ASL) deficiency is autosomal recessive, and most children in the United States are detected as a result of an elevated citrulline on newborn screening. The diagnosis is confirmed by the detection of elevated argininosuccinic acid in the urine.

Treatment of Hyperammonemia

During episodes of symptomatic hyperammonemia, protein intake is reduced, and intravenous glucose is given in sufficient quantity to suppress catabolism of endogenous protein. Ammonia can be eliminated by use of the **alternate pathway** agents, **sodium benzoate** and **sodium phenylacetate**, which are excreted in the urine as conjugates of glycine and glutamine. Arginine, which is usually deficient, is supplied. When ammonia levels are very high (>1000 μM) or refractory to therapy, direct removal of ammonia using hemodialysis or hemofiltration, but not peritoneal dialysis, is required. The neurologic status must be followed closely and cerebral edema treated promptly. Despite successful management of hyperammonemic crises, the long-term outcome for males with severe neonatal OTC deficiency and all children with severe ASL deficiency is guarded. Early liver transplantation has increased survival, especially in males with severe OTC deficiency.

Restriction of dietary protein intake to daily needs is the mainstay of ongoing treatment for urea cycle defects. Crystalline essential amino acids can be supplied in amounts just sufficient to support protein synthesis. Arginine is an essential amino acid when arginine synthesis via the urea cycle is grossly impaired; thus arginine must be supplied except in the case of arginase deficiency. Citrulline needs to be supplied for some urea cycle disorders. For OTC deficiency and carbamoyl phosphate synthase deficiency, treatment with phenylbutyrate (which is metabolized to phenylacetate) prevents accumulation of ammonia.

DISORDERS OF AMINO ACID TRANSPORT THAT AFFECT SPECIFIC TRANSPORT MECHANISMS IN THE KIDNEY AND INTESTINE

Cystinuria is a disorder of renal tubular transport of cystine, lysine, arginine, and ornithine. Although intestinal transport is affected in some genetic forms, the symptoms are largely due to the renal transport abnormality. The concentration of cystine exceeds its solubility product and results in significant renal stones. Evaluation and diagnosis are based on the pattern of amino acid excretion in the urine. Mutation testing can be done. **Treatment** is based on increasing the solubility of cystine by complexing it with compounds such as penicillamine.

Intestinal transport of tryptophan is impaired in **Hartnup syndrome**; pellagra-like symptoms result from this deficiency. Diagnosis is based on the amino acid pattern in urine. Treatment with tryptophan is successful.

ORGANIC ACID DISORDERS

DISORDERS OF ORGANIC ACID METABOLISM

Organic acid disorders result from a block in the pathways of amino acid catabolism. Occurring after the amino moiety has been removed, they result in the accumulation of specific organic acids in the blood and urine. Treatment is directed at the specific abnormality, with restriction in precursor substrates and administration of enzyme cofactors, when available. Outcome is generally poor for children with neonatal-onset propionic or methylmalonic acidemia but is influenced by frequency and severity of crises and is optimal when diagnosis is made before the onset of the first episode. Liver transplantation has been used in some patients with early indicators of success. Confirmatory testing begins with a urine organic acid profile and plasma amino acid profile. More specific testing often requires enzyme measurements in appropriate tissues. When abnormal results suggest a specific disorder, DNA testing may identify the mutations involved.

PROPIONIC ACIDEMIA AND METHYLMALONIC ACIDEMIA

Propionic acidemia and methylmalonic acidemia result from defects in a series of reactions called the propionate pathway (Fig. 54-1). Defects in these steps produce **ketosis** and **hyperglycinemia**. Propionic acidemia and methylmalonic acidemia are identified by neonatal screening with tandem mass spectrometry methods. The **clinical manifestations** of both of these disorders in the neonatal period consist of tachypnea, vomiting, lethargy, coma, intermittent ketoacidosis, hyperglycinemia, neutropenia, thrombocytopenia, hyperammonemia,

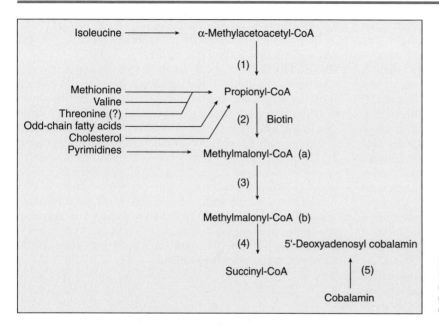

Figure 54-1 The propionate pathway. (1) β-Ketothiolase, (2) propionyl-CoA carboxylase, (3) methylmalonyl-CoA isomerase, (4) methylmalonyl-CoA mutase, (5) cobalamin metabolic pathway. *CoA,* Coenzyme A.

and hypoglycemia. If these disorders are not identified by neonatal screening, intermittent episodes of metabolic acidosis occur. Crises occur during periods of catabolic stress, such as fever, vomiting, and diarrhea; they also may occur without an apparent precipitating event. During periods of neutropenia, the risk of serious bacterial infection is increased. Failure to thrive and impaired development are common.

Propionic acidemia results from deficiency in propionyl CoA-carboxylase, an enzyme that has two pairs of identical subunits. All forms of propionic acidemia are inherited in an autosomal recessive manner and are due to mutations in one of the subunits. **Methylmalonic acidemia** results from deficiency in methylmalonyl mutase; this may be caused by mutations in the gene for the mutase protein itself or in one of the steps of the synthesis of the cobalamin cofactors for the enzyme. A complex set of defects in cobalamin metabolism results in other forms of methylmalonic acidemia, some of which are associated with hyperhomocystinemia. **Treatment** with massive doses of hydroxocobalamin (the active form of vitamin B_{12}) is helpful in some cases of methylmalonic acidemia.

For propionic acidemia and the vitamin B_{12}–unresponsive forms of methylmalonic acidemia, management includes the restriction of dietary protein and addition of a medical food deficient in the specific amino acid precursors of propionyl-CoA (isoleucine, valine, methionine, and threonine). Carnitine supplementation is often needed because it is lost in the urine as acylcarnitines. Intestinal bacteria produce a significant quantity of propionate; thus, antibacterial treatment to reduce the population of bacteria in the gut has some beneficial effect in propionic acidemia and vitamin B_{12}–unresponsive methylmalonic acidemia.

ISOVALERIC ACIDEMIA

Isovaleric acidemia results from a block in the catabolism of leucine. Its clinical manifestations are similar to those of defects in the propionate pathway. The strong odor of isovaleric acid results in **sweaty feet odor** in untreated infants. Therapy involves restricting the intake of leucine, and providing glycine

Figure 54-2 Metabolism in isovaleric acidemia. (1) Leucine catabolic pathway (transamination and decarboxylation), (2) isovaleryl-CoA dehydrogenase, (3) glycine acyltransferase. *CoA,* Coenzyme A.

as an alternate pathway therapy that conjugates isovaleric acid (Fig. 54-2) and is then excreted in the urine.

GLUTARIC ACIDEMIA I

Glutaric acidemia I results from a deficiency at the end of the lysine catabolic pathway. It is an autosomal recessive disease produced by deficiency of glutaryl-CoA dehydrogenase activity (Fig. 54-3). **Clinical manifestations** include **macrocephaly**, which may be present at birth, with fever and metabolic distress. Before the advent of newborn screening, more than 70% of children had *metabolic stroke-like episodes* associated with infarction of the basal ganglia and **dystonia**, which characteristically develops after an episode of intercurrent illness, although it may reflect birth stress or prenatal insults. **Treatment** includes a protein-restricted diet accompanied by a medical food deficient in lysine and aggressive management of intercurrent illness. Despite this treatment as many as one third of children still develop neurologic symptoms.

BIOTINIDASE DEFICIENCY AND HOLOCARBOXYLASE DEFICIENCY

Biotin is a ubiquitous vitamin that is covalently linked to many carboxylases and cannot be recycled from its attachment to

Figure 54-3 Scheme of flavoprotein metabolism with reference to glutaric aciduria types I and II. (1) Glutaryl-CoA dehydrogenase (deficient in glutaric aciduria type1), (2) fatty acyl-CoA dehydrogenases, (3) other flavoprotein dehydrogenases, (4) ETF (deficiency results in glutaric aciduria type II), (5) ETF-ubiquinone oxidoreductase (deficiency results in glutaric aciduria type II). *CoA*, Coenzyme A; *ETF*, electron transfer flavoprotein.

the carboxylases. Thus, inherited biotinidase deficiency greatly increases the dietary requirement for biotin. Affected individuals become biotin deficient while consuming normal diets. Clinical disease can appear in the neonatal period or be delayed until later infancy, depending on the degree of deficiency.

Clinical manifestations of biotin deficiency vary greatly (seizures, hypotonia, sensory neural deafness, alopecia, skin rash, metabolic acidosis, immune deficits) and depend on which enzymes in which tissues have the most biotin depletion. Carboxylation is a crucial reaction in the metabolism of organic acids; most patients with biotinidase deficiency excrete abnormal amounts of several organic acids, among which β-methyl-crotonylglycine is prominent. In addition to biotinidase deficiency, an inherited deficiency of holocarboxylase synthetase gives rise to severe disease and to similar patterns of organic aciduria. Both conditions respond well to **treatment** with large doses of biotin (10 to 40 mg/day). Confirmatory testing is accomplished with quantitative measurement of biotinidase activity.

Chapter **55**

FAT METABOLIC DISORDERS

DISORDERS OF FATTY ACID OXIDATION

Fatty acids are derived from hydrolysis of triglycerides and catabolism of fat. The catabolism of fatty acids (Fig. 55-1) proceeds through the serial, oxidative removal of two carbons at a time as acetyl groups (each as acetyl-CoA). The reactions are catalyzed by a group of enzymes that exhibit specificities related to the chain length and other properties of the fatty acids: very long chain acyl-CoA dehydrogenase (VLCAD), long-chain hydroxyacyl-CoA dehydrogenase (LCHAD) or trifunctional protein, medium-chain acyl-CoA dehydrogenase (MCAD), and short-chain acyl-CoA dehydrogenase (SCAD).

MCAD deficiency is the most common inborn error of β-oxidation. Hypoketotic hypoglycemia is a common

manifestation, as is Reye syndrome–like illness with hypoglycemia and elevated liver enzymes. Fatty infiltration of the liver also occurs. True hepatic failure is rare. Episodes may be recurrent in the patient or the family. **Sudden infant death syndrome** is reported in infants with MCAD deficiency, perhaps related to hypoglycemia. **Treatment** requires avoidance of fasting and provision of calories with fever or other metabolic stress. Medium-chain triglycerides must be avoided.

VLCAD deficiency and LCHAD (trifunctional protein) deficiency result in significant myopathy and cardiomyopathy. LCHAD deficiency is accompanied by a retinopathy in later childhood. In all of the disorders of β-oxidation, carnitine depletion can occur through excessive urinary excretion of carnitine esters of the incompletely oxidized fatty acids. Measurement of plasma carnitine is helpful in monitoring for this deficiency, which results in weakness and muscle pain, along with myoglobinuria in some people.

Hydroxymethylglutaryl-CoA lyase deficiency, although not a disorder of β-oxidation, interferes profoundly with hepatic adaptation to fasting by impairing ketogenesis (see Fig. 55-1). The clinical manifestations are those of MCAD deficiency, except that carnitine depletion is less prominent.

The diagnosis of disorders involving a deficiency of β-oxidation is suggested by the clinical picture and by **hypoketotic hypoglycemia**. The diagnosis is confirmed by analysis of urinary organic acid and acylglycine profiles, along with plasma acylcarnitine and free fatty acid profiles. Enzyme measurements and DNA testing complete the confirmatory testing. The profile of acylcarnitines in cultured skin fibroblasts may be helpful if other testing is not conclusive. In MCAD deficiency, a single mutation 985 A→G accounts for a significant percentage of cases. **Treatment** includes avoidance of fasting, as well as fluid and calorie supplementation during periods of metabolic stress, such as fever. In MCAD deficiency, medium-chain triglycerides must be avoided. In the long-chain fatty acid metabolic disorders, provision of medium-chain fatty acids improves muscle energy metabolism.

GLUTARIC ACIDURIA TYPE II

Glutaric aciduria type II (multiple acyl-CoA dehydrogenase deficiency) is a clinical disease produced by a defect in the transfer of electrons from flavine adenine nucleotides to the electron transport chain (electron transfer flavoprotein [ETF], or ETF dehydrogenase); this defect results in a deficiency of multiple fatty acyl CoA dehydrogenases (see Fig. 55-1).

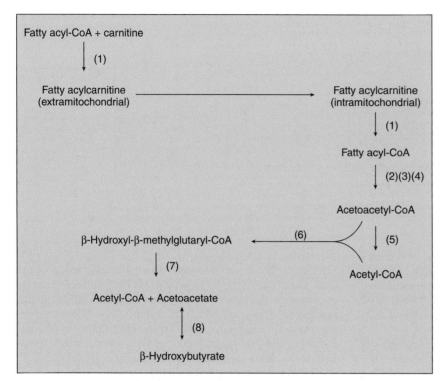

Fatty acyl-CoA + carnitine

(1)

Fatty acylcarnitine (extramitochondrial) ⟶ Fatty acylcarnitine (intramitochondrial)

(1)

Fatty acyl-CoA

(2)(3)(4)

Acetoacetyl-CoA

β-Hydroxyl-β-methylglutaryl-CoA ⟵ (6) (5)

(7) Acetyl-CoA

Acetyl-CoA + Acetoacetate

(8)

β-Hydroxybutyrate

FIGURE 55-1 Scheme of fatty acid and catabolism and ketone body formation. (1) Carnitine acyl-CoA dehydrogenases, (2) long-chain fatty acyl-CoA dehydrogenase (trifunctional protein), (3) medium-chain fatty acyl-CoA dehydrogenase, (4) short-chain fatty acyl-CoA dehydrogenase, (5) β-ketothiolase, (6) β-hydroxy-β-methylglutaryl-CoA synthase, (7) β-hydroxy-β-methylglutaryl-CoA lyase, (8) β-hydroxybutyrate dehydrogenase. *CoA,* Coenzyme A.

It should not be confused with glutaric acidemia type I (see Chapter 54). When the enzyme essentially is nonfunctional, congenital anomalies are common, including renal cysts, facial abnormalities, rocker-bottom feet, and hypospadias. Severely affected infants have nonketotic hypoglycemia, metabolic acidosis, and the odor of sweaty feet soon after birth; these infants may die within the neonatal period. Less severely affected infants may have a more episodic, Reye syndrome–like illness. Skeletal and cardiac myopathy can be prominent in this complex, multisystemic disease. Onset in later childhood may be marked by recurrent hypoglycemia and myopathy. **Treatment** has not been effective in infants with complete deficiency. Milder forms respond to avoidance of fasting and caloric support during metabolic stress. Some patients respond to administration of riboflavin. Glutaric aciduria type II exhibits autosomal recessive inheritance. Confirmatory testing is similar to that for the other fatty acid oxidation disorders.

CARNITINE DEFICIENCY

Carnitine is a crucial cofactor in the transport of long-chain fatty acids across the mitochondrial inner membrane (see Fig. 55-1). It is synthesized from lysine by humans and is present in dietary red meat and dairy products. Carnitine deficiency is either primary (caused by failure of intake, synthesis, or transport of carnitine) or secondary (caused by the excretion of excessive amounts of carnitine as carnityl esters in patients with other inborn errors of metabolism; treatment with drugs that complex carnitine, such as valproic acid; or as a result of renal replacement therapy). Primary systemic carnitine deficiency is rare and results from inadequate renal reabsorption of carnitine secondary to a mutation in the sodium-dependent carnitine transporter. It responds well to carnitine supplementation. There are numerous examples of secondary carnitine deficiency among the organic acidurias, most prominently in disorders of the propionate pathway and in disorders of the β-oxidation of long-chain and medium-chain fatty acids. Clinical manifestations of carnitine deficiency include hypoketotic hypoglycemia, lethargy, lassitude, muscle weakness, sudden death, and cardiomyopathy.

Chapter **56**

LYSOSOMAL AND PEROXISOMAL DISORDERS

PEROXISOMAL DISORDERS

Peroxisomes are subcellular organelles involved in metabolism and biosynthesis of bile acids, membrane phospholipids, and some β-oxidation of long-chain fatty acids. Disorders include conditions caused by abnormal peroxisomal enzyme function and abnormal peroxisomal biogenesis. **Clinical symptoms** are diverse and frequently include **developmental delay** and **dysmorphic features** that can involve the skeleton and the head. Zellweger syndrome, neonatal adrenoleukodystrophy, and infantile Refsum disease are examples of disorders of peroxisome biogenesis. **Zellweger syndrome,** an autosomal recessive disease (1:100,000 births), is also called *cerebrohepatorenal syndrome*. Peroxisomes are virtually absent, as are normal peroxisomal functions, which include the oxidation of very long chain fatty acids. Affected infants have high

Table 56-1 | Lysosomal Storage Diseases

DISEASE (EPONYM)	ENZYME DEFICIENCY	CLINICAL ONSET	DYSOSTOSIS MULTIPLEX	CORNEA	RETINA	LIVER, SPLEEN	CNS FINDINGS	STORED MATERIAL IN URINE	WBC/BONE MARROW	COMMENT	MULTIPLE FORMS
MUCOPOLYSACCHARIDOSES (MPS)											
MPS I (Hurler)	α-L-Iduronidase	~1 yr	Yes	Cloudy	—	Both enlarged	Profound loss of function	Acid mucopolysaccharide	Alder-Reilly bodies (WBC)	Kyphosis	Yes—Scheie and compounds
MPS II (Hunter)	Iduronate-2-sulfatase	1-2 yr	Yes	Clear	Retinal degeneration, papilledema	Both enlarged	Slow loss of function	Acid mucopolysaccharide	Alder-Reilly bodies (WBC)	X-linked	Yes
MPS III (Sanfilippo)	One of several degrading heparan SO₄s	2-6 yr	Mild	Clear	—	Liver ± enlarged	Rapid loss of function	Acid mucopolysaccharide	Alder-Reilly bodies (WBC)	—	Several types biochemically
MPS IV (Morquio)	Galactose-6-sulfatase or β-galactosidase	2 yr	No, dwarfism deformities	Faint clouding	—	—	Normal	Acid mucopolysaccharide	Alder-Reilly bodies (WBC)	—	Yes
MPS VI (Maroteaux-Lamy)	N-Acetylgalactosamine-4-sulfatase	2 yr	Yes	Cloudy	—	Normal in size	Normal	Acid mucopolysaccharide	Alder-Reilly bodies (WBC)	—	Yes
MPS VII (Sly)	β-Glucuronidase	Variable neonatal	Yes	± Cloudy	—	Both enlarged	± Affected	Acid mucopolysaccharide	Alder-Reilly bodies (WBC)	Nonimmune hydrops	Yes
LIPIDOSES											
Glucosylceramide lipidosis (Gaucher 1)	Glucocerebrosidase	Any age	No	Clear	Normal	Both enlarged	Normal	No	Gaucher cells in marrow	Bone pain fractures	Variability is the rule
Glucosylceramide lipidosis 2 (Gaucher 2)	Glucocerebrosidase	Fetal life to 2nd year	No	Clear	Normal	Both enlarged	Profound loss of function	No	Gaucher cells in marrow	—	Yes
Sphingomyelin lipidosis A (Niemann-Pick A)	Sphingomyelinase	1st mo	No	Clear	Cherry-red spots (50%)	Both enlarged	Profound loss of function	No	Foam cells in marrow	—	No
Sphingomyelin lipidosis B (Niemann-Pick B)	Sphingomyelinase	1st mo or later	No	Clear	Normal	Both enlarged	Normal	No	Foam cells in marrow	—	Yes
Niemann-Pick C	Lysosomal cholesterol; trafficking (NPC1 gene)	Fetal life to adolescence	No	Clear	Normal	Enlarged	Vertical ophthalmoplegia, dystonia, cataplexy, seizures	No	Foam cells and sea-blue histiocytes in marrow	Pathogenesis not as for NP-A and NP-B	Lethal neonatal to adolescent onset
GM₂ gangliosidosis (Tay-Sachs)	Hexosaminidase A	3-6 mo	No	Clear	Cherry-red spots	Normal	Profound loss of function	No	Normal	Sandhoff disease related	Yes
Generalized gangliosidosis (infantile) (GM₁)	β-Galactosidase	Neonatal to 1st mo	Yes	Clear	Cherry-red spots (50%)	Both enlarged	Profound loss of function	No	Inclusion in WBC	—	Yes
Metachromatic leukodystrophy	Arylsulfatase A	1-2 yr	No	Clear	Normal	Normal	Profound loss of function	No	Normal	—	Yes
Fabry disease	α-Galactosidase A (cerebrosidase)	Childhood, adolescence	No	Cloudy by slit lamp	—	Liver may be enlarged	Normal	No	Normal	X-linked	No
Galactosylceramide lipidosis (Krabbe)	Galactocerebroside β-galactosidase	Early months	No	Clear	Optic atrophy	Normal	Profound loss of function	No	Normal	Storage not lysosomal	Yes
Wolman disease	Acid lipase	Neonatal	No	Clear	Normal	Both enlarged	Profound loss of function	No	Inclusion in WBC	—	Yes

Table 56-1 Lysosomal Storage Diseases—cont'd

DISEASE (EPONYM)	ENZYME DEFICIENCY	CLINICAL ONSET	DYSOSTOSIS MULTIPLEX	CORNEA	RETINA	LIVER, SPLEEN	CNS FINDINGS	STORED MATERIAL IN URINE	WBC/BONE MARROW	COMMENT	MULTIPLE FORMS
Farber lipogranulomatosis	Acid ceramidase	1st 4 mo	No	Usually clear	Cherry-red spots (12%)	May be enlarged	Normal or impaired	Usually not	—	Arthritis, nodules	Yes
MUCOLIPIDOSES (ML) AND CLINICALLY RELATED DISEASE											
Sialidosis II (formerly ML I)	Neuraminidase	Neonatal	Yes	Cloudy	Cherry-red spot	Both enlarged	Yes	Oligosaccharides	Vacuolated lymphocytes	—	Yes (also see galactosialidosis)
Sialidosis I (formerly ML I)	Neuraminidase	Usually second decade	No	Fine opacities	Cherry-red spot	Normal	Myoclonus, seizures	Oligosaccharides	Usually none	Cherry-red spot/myoclonus syndrome	Severity varies
Galactosialidosis	Absence of PP/CathA causes loss of neuraminidase and β-galactosidase	Usually second decade	Frequent	Clouding	Cherry-red spot	Occasionally enlarged	Myoclonus, seizures Mental retardation	Oligosaccharides	Foamy lymphocytes	Onset from 1 to 40 yr	Congenital and infantile forms such as sialidosis 2
ML II (I-cell disease)	Mannosyl phosphotransferase	Neonatal	Yes	Clouding	—	Liver often enlarged	Profound loss of function	Oligosaccharides	No	Gingival hyperplasia	No
ML III (pseudo-Hurler polydystrophy)	Mannosyl phosphotransferase	2–4 yr	Yes	Late clouding	Normal	Normal in size?	Modest loss of function	Oligosaccharides	No	—	No
Multiple sulfatase deficiency	Many sulfatases	1–2 yr	Yes	Usually clear	Usually normal	Both enlarged	Profound loss of function	Acid mucopolysaccharide	Alder-Reilly bodies (WBC)	Ichthyosis	Yes
Aspartylglycosaminuria	Aspartylglucosaminidase	6 mo	Mild	Clear	Normal	Early, not late	Profound loss of function	Aspartylglucosamine	Inclusions in lymphocytes	Develop cataracts	No
Mannosidosis	α-Mannosidase	1st mo	Yes	Cloudy	—	Liver enlarged	Profound loss of function	Generally no	Inclusions in lymphocytes	Cataracts	Yes
Fucosidosis	α-L-Fucosidase	1st mo	Yes	Clear	May be pigmented	Both enlarged commonly	Profound loss of function	Oligosaccharides	Inclusions in lymphocytes	—	Yes
STORAGE DISEASES CAUSED BY DEFECTS IN LYSOSOMAL PROTEOLYSIS											
Neuronal ceroid lipofuscinosis (NCL), Batten disease	Impaired lysosomal proteolysis—various specific etiologies	6 mo–10 yr, adult form	No	Normal	May have brown pigment	Normal, distinct	Optic atrophy, seizures, dementia			Clinical picture consistent, time course variable	Etiologies for age-related forms
STORAGE DISEASES CAUSED BY DEFECTIVE SYNTHESIS OF THE LYSOSOMAL MEMBRANE											
Cardiomyopathy, myopathy, mental retardation, Danon disease	Lamp-2, a structural protein of lysosomes, is deficient	Usually 5–6 yr	No	Normal	Normal	Hepatomegaly	Delayed development, seizures	No	Normal	X-linked pediatric disease in males only	Variability in time course of signs
STORAGE DISEASES CAUSED BY DYSFUNCTION OF LYSOSOMAL TRANSPORT PROTEINS											
Nephropathic cystinosis	Defect in cystine transport from lysosome to cytoplasm	6 mo–1 yr	No	Cystine crystals	Pigmentary retinopathy	Hepatomegaly common	Normal CNS function	Generalized aminoaciduria	Elevated cystine in WBCs	Treatment with cysteamine is effective	Yes
Salla disease	Defect in sialic acid transport from lysosome to cytoplasm	6–9 mo	No	Normal	Normal	Normal	Delayed development, ataxia, nystagmus, exotropia	Sialic aciduria	Vacuolated lymphocytes may be found	Growth retarded in some	Lethal infantile form

CNS, Central nervous system; WBC, white blood cell.

foreheads, flat orbital ridges, widely open fontanelles, hepatomegaly, and hypotonia. Other anomalies are common. Failure to thrive, seizures, and nystagmus develop early, and death occurs within the first year. Refsum disease, neonatal adrenoleukodystrophy, and malonic aciduria are examples of peroxisomal single-enzyme disorders. Diagnostic testing includes measurement of very long chain fatty acids in plasma and pipecolic acid in urine. Specific molecular testing, particularly for the disorders involving one in the series of *PEX* genes, is available for some disorders. Most of these conditions are untreatable; however, bone marrow transplant can be helpful in X-linked adrenoleukodystrophy before the onset of severe symptoms.

LYSOSOMAL STORAGE DISORDERS

Lysosomes are subcellular organelles that contain degradative enzymes for complex **glycosaminoglycans**, also called **mucopolysaccharides**. Glycosaminoglycans are macromolecules that play a number of roles within cells. Genetic disorders result from abnormal formation of the lysosome itself or from deficiency in specific hydrolytic enzymes, in the mechanisms that protect intralysosomal enzymes from hydrolytic destruction, or in the transport of materials into the lysosome and of metabolites out of the lysosome. These materials are stored in cells and ultimately result in their destruction, especially in the nervous system. The clinical disorders are diverse, reflecting tissue specificity of lysosomal function and the intrinsic turnover rates of the compounds whose cycling is affected (Table 56-1). Some disorders affect many tissues but spare the brain. Some are apparent only during adult life. Storage in solid organs results in organomegaly. In many of these disorders, developmental delay, corneal clouding, and limitation of joint mobility are common features. Storage in tissues of the upper and lower airways may result in respiratory compromise. Nonimmune hydrops fetalis occurs in several lysosomal disorders.

DIAGNOSTIC TESTING

Diagnostic testing includes measurement of glycosaminoglycans in urine and specific assays for lysosomal enzyme activity in white blood cells. If the urine test is positive, it helps direct specific enzyme measurement. If it is negative, it does not exclude a lysosomal storage disorder, and other testing modalities are needed if clinical signs are convincing. In disorders in which specific mutations are known, molecular testing refines the diagnosis. Specific diagnosis, carrier testing, and evaluation of at-risk family members require one of these approaches. Making a specific diagnosis is assuming increasing importance because specific treatment for some lysosomal disorders is very effective.

TREATMENT STRATEGIES

Specific treatment directed at the metabolic abnormality is available for some lysosomal disorders. In specific disorders (Gaucher disease) oral medication may be successful in reducing the accumulation of the metabolite that cannot be catabolized. For some disorders, bone marrow (stem cell) transplantation can restore lysosomal function. For others, replacement of the missing hydrolytic enzyme by systemic administration of the enzyme allows degradation of stored material. The disorders caused by deficient α-L-iduronidase (Hurler syndrome, Scheie syndrome, and their variants) respond to treatment with intravenous human recombinant α-L-iduronidase (laronidase). Other disorders for which enzyme therapy is available include MPS VI (Maroteaux-Lamy syndrome), Gaucher disease, Fabry disease, and MPS II (Hunter syndrome). Stem cell transplantation has been helpful or is under investigation in the following disorders: MPS type IH (Hurler syndrome), MPS type VI (Maroteaux-Lamy syndrome), MPS type VII (Sly syndrome), Krabbe disease, metachromatic leukodystrophy, alpha-fucosidosis, alpha-mannosidosis, Gaucher disease, and Niemann-Pick disease type B. However, treatment for many of these conditions is supportive, with careful attention to respiratory status and physical therapy. As a result of the rapidly changing therapeutic options, geneticists with a special interest in these disorders should be consulted when a diagnosis is suspected. Treatment decisions should be made by the family in the light of the potential therapeutic benefits and burdens of therapy and typically should be resolved before the onset of central nervous system manifestations, which are typically not improved by these approaches.

Chapter **57**

MITOCHONDRIAL DISORDERS

MITOCHONDRIAL FUNCTION

Mitochondria are very complex organelles located in virtually all cells of the body. They perform a variety of functions such as intracellular signaling of oxygen tension and key roles in programmed cell death. From a biochemical perspective, mitochondria are the key site of energy production in the cell. Indeed they are the site of beta oxidation (see Chapter 55), the Krebs cycle, and parts of the urea cycle (see Figure 53-4). This complexity requires more than 1000 proteins localized specifically to the mitochondrion. Only 13 of these are encoded by the mitochondrial DNA (mtDNA); the remainder are nuclear encoded (on the chromosomes) and require import into the mitochondrion. In addition, the mitochondrial DNA needs its own set of proteins to allow for its maintenance, transcription, and translation.

Mitochondrial disorders are typically defined as defects in the ability to generate energy from oxidative phosphorylation to produce ATP by transferring electrons formed by glycolysis and the Krebs cycle to a cascade that generates NADH and $FADH_2$ (Fig. 57-1) and are also known as phosphorylation disorders or respiratory chain disorders. The more dependent on energy production an organ is, the more profound the symptoms of deficiency of mitochondrial function in that organ. Certain proteins are only expressed in specific tissues, and defects in these will lead to differing patterns of disease. Taken together, mitochondrial disorders may affect as many as 1 in 2500 people.

Figure 57-1 The mammalian mitochondrial genome and its protein-coding gene repertoire involved in the oxidative phosphorylation pathway. **(A)** Schematic representation of genes within mammalian mitochondrial genome (~7000 bp). Genes on the outer circle are transcribed from the light strand. Location of the tRNAs *(red boxes)* conforms to the canonical placental mammalian arrangement. **(B)** Simplified view of the mitochondrial oxidative phosphorylation machinery. Complexes I (NADH dehydrogenase) and II (succinate dehydrogenase) receive electrons from either NADH or FADH2. Electrons are then carried between complexes by the carrier molecules coenzyme Q/ubiquinone (UQ) and cytochrome c (CYC). The potential energy of these electron transfer events is used to pump protons against the gradient, from the mitochondrial matrix into the intermembrane space [complexes I and III (cytochrome bc₁) and IV (cytochrome c oxidase)]. ATP synthesis by complex V (ATP synthase) is driven by the proton gradient and occurs in the mitochondrial matrix. *HSP,* Putative heavy-strand promoter; *IM,* intermembrane space; *MM,* mitochondrial matrix; *OHR,* origin of heavy-strand replication; *OLR,* origin of light-strand replication. *(From da Fonseca RR, Johnson WE, O'Brien SJ, et al: The adaptive evolution of the mammalian mitochondrial genome,* BMC Genomics 9:119, 2008.)

SIGNS AND SYMPTOMS OF GENETIC DISORDERS OF MITOCHONDRIAL FUNCTION

The signs and symptoms of mitochondrial disorders are varied. Symptoms depend on how an organ is affected by energy deficiency. Muscle function that is compromised will result in muscle fatigue and weakness. Myopathy is common and may show **ragged red fibers** on a muscle biopsy. **Rhabdomyolysis** can occur. Brain dysfunction may be expressed as seizures, loss of intellectual function, headache, or signs consistent with stroke. Spastic paraplegia may occur. Ataxia and basal ganglia symptoms are features of some disorders. Vision and eye muscle movement may be compromised, with **progressive external ophthalmoplegia** being almost diagnostic of an oxidative phosphorylation defect. **Cardiomyopathy** is frequent, and cardiac rhythm disturbances occur. Liver dysfunction may be expressed as both synthetic deficiencies and liver failure. Diabetes may signal pancreatic involvement. Renal tubular abnormalities and renal failure both occur. Gastrointestinal symptoms include both diarrhea and constipation that are difficult to treat. **Alper disease** (cerebral degeneration and liver disease) and **Leigh disease** (subacute necrotizing encephalomyelopathy) show similar brain lesions but in distinctly different areas of the brain. Because the signs and symptoms may involve multiple organs and may seem nonspecific, physicians may not suspect a mitochondrial disorder until significant progression has occurred.

BIOCHEMICAL ABNORMALITIES IN MITOCHONDRIAL FUNCTION

Defects in the mitochondrial respiratory chain may produce **lactic acidosis**. Given the complexity of the respiratory chain, it is not surprising that the described defects are varied as to cause, intensity, and tissues affected. The metabolism of glucose to carbon dioxide and water, with pyruvate as an intermediate (Fig. 57-2), occurs as part of the energy cycle in many tissues. Interference with mitochondrial oxidative metabolism may result in the accumulation of pyruvate. Because lactate dehydrogenase is ubiquitous, and because the equilibrium catalyzed by this enzyme greatly favors lactate over pyruvate, the accumulation of pyruvate results in lactic acidosis. The most common cause of such lactic acidosis is oxygen deficiency caused by hypoxia or poor perfusion. Lactic acidosis also occurs when specific reactions of pyruvate are impaired. In the liver, pyruvate undergoes carboxylation to form oxaloacetate using the enzyme pyruvate carboxylase; deficiency in this enzyme causes severe lactic acidosis. In many tissues, lactate is catabolized to form acetyl coenzyme A (CoA) by the pyruvate dehydrogenase complex; deficiency in pyruvate dehydrogenase also can cause lactic acidosis. Because these reactions also play a role in gluconeogenesis, hypoglycemia can be a feature of these disorders. These disorders comprise forms of **primary lactic acidosis**. They frequently present as intractable, lethal acidosis in the first days or weeks of life and are difficult to treat. Some of the enzymes in this pathway can be measured

Figure 57-2 Metabolism of pyruvate and lactate. (1) Alanine aminotransferase, (2) lactate dehydrogenase, (3) pyruvate dehydrogenase, (4) pyruvate carboxylase, (5) Krebs cycle, (6) phosphoenolpyruvate carboxykinase, (7) reverse glycolysis. *CoA*, Coenzyme A.

and specific diagnosis can be made. This may require white blood cells or tissue biopsy.

GENETICS OF MITOCHONDRIAL DISORDERS

Mitochondrial function is carried out by proteins that are coded for by both nuclear and mitochondrial genes. These enzymes are extremely complicated, and several are quite large. The mitochondrial genome encodes 13 subunits of the enzymes involved in mitochondrial oxidative phosphorylation. More than 85 autosomal genes code for the rest of the subunits of these enzymes. In children, only about 15% of cases of mitochondrial disease are caused by mutations in mitochondrial DNA (mtDNA); the rest are due to mutations in nuclear genes. The most frequent cases in several large series have been mutations that lead to a reduction in the ability of the mtDNA to maintain itself. Large population studies show carrier rates of about 2% of the population for mutations in polymerase (DNA directed), gamma (*POLG*), and deoxyguanosine kinase (*DGUOK*). Most disorders show autosomal recessive inheritance. A few are X linked or passed on by maternal mtDNA

mutations, such as mitochondrial encephalopathy with lactic acidosis (**MELAS**) and mitochondrial encephalopathy with ragged red fibers (**MERRF**), or deletions such as maternally inherited diabetes and deafness (MIDD).

TREATMENT OF MITOCHONDRIAL DISORDERS

Repairing the basic energy deficit and getting the appropriate drugs and cofactors to the appropriate location within the mitochondrion are difficult. Nevertheless, a number of strategies are used, including judicious physical therapy and exercise with adequate rest, adequate nutrition, and cofactors for the deficient pathway. Specific treatment is limited for most mitochondrial defects. Vitamin cofactors for the respiratory chain, such as riboflavin and pharmaceutical forms of coenzyme Q, are often used. When a single organ bears most of the damage, organ transplant may be effective. Identification of family members at risk may allow earlier diagnosis and treatment.

The author would like to acknowledge Dr. Margretta R. Seashore for her superb work in the last edition. Hers was an excellent analysis of the topic and has informed much of the present discussion.

Suggested Reading

de Baulny HO, Benoist JF, Rigal O, et al: Methylmalonic and propionic acidaemias: management and outcome, *J Inherit Metab Dis* 28(3):415–423, 2005.

Heese BA: Current strategies in the management of lysosomal storage diseases, *Semin Pediatr Neurol* 15(3):119–126, 2008.

Kayser MA: Inherited metabolic diseases in neurodevelopmental and neurobehavioral disorders, *Semin Pediatr Neurol* 15(3):127–131, 2008.

Kliegman RM, Stanton BF, St. Geme JW, et al: *Nelson Textbook of Pediatrics,* ed 19, Philadelphia, 2011, Elsevier Science.

Koeberl DD, Kishnani PS, Chen YT: Glycogen storage disease types I and II: treatment updates, *J Inherit Metab Dis* 30(2):159–164, 2007.

Kompare M, Rizzo WB: Mitochondrial fatty-acid oxidation disorders, *Semin Pediatr Neurol* 15(3):140–149, 2008.

Tuchman M, Lee B, Lichter-Konecki U, et al: Cross-sectional multicenter study of patients with urea cycle disorders in the United States, *Mol Genet Metab* 94(4):397–402, 2008.

Fetal and Neonatal Medicine

Clarence W. Gowen, Jr.

Chapter 58

ASSESSMENT OF THE MOTHER, FETUS, AND NEWBORN

ASSESSMENT OF THE MOTHER

Pregnancies associated with perinatal morbidity or mortality are considered high risk. Identification of high-risk pregnancies is essential to the care of the infant because they may result in intrauterine fetal death, intrauterine growth restriction (IUGR), congenital anomalies, excessive fetal growth, birth asphyxia and trauma, prematurity (birth at <38 weeks) or postmaturity (birth at ≥42 weeks), neonatal disease, or long-term risks of cerebral palsy, mental retardation, and chronic sequelae of neonatal intensive care. Ten percent to 20% of women may be high risk at some time during their pregnancy. Although some obstetric complications are first seen during labor and delivery and cannot be predicted, more than 50% of perinatal mortality and morbidity results from problems identified before delivery as high risk. After a high-risk pregnancy is identified, measures can be instituted to prevent complications, provide intensive fetal surveillance, and initiate appropriate treatments of the mother and fetus.

A history of previous premature birth, intrauterine fetal death, multiple gestation, IUGR, congenital malformation, explained or unexplained neonatal death (e.g., group B streptococcal sepsis), birth trauma, preeclampsia, gestational diabetes, grand multipara status (five or more pregnancies), or cesarean section is associated with additional risk in subsequent pregnancies.

Pregnancy complications that increase the risk of a poor outcome can be secondary to maternal or fetal causes or both. Complications include placenta previa; abruptio placentae; preeclampsia; diabetes; oligohydramnios or polyhydramnios; multiple gestation; blood group sensitization; abnormal levels of unconjugated estriols, chorionic gonadotropin, or alpha-fetoprotein; abnormal fetal ultrasound; hydrops fetalis; maternal trauma or surgery; abnormal fetal presentation (breech); exposure to prescribed or illicit drugs; prolonged labor; cephalopelvic disproportion; prolapsed cord; fetal distress; prolonged or premature rupture of membranes; short cervical length (<25 mm) and the presence of fetal fibronectin in cervical secretions at less than 35 weeks' gestation (a predictor of preterm labor); cervical infections and vaginosis; and congenital infections, including rubella, cytomegalovirus, herpes simplex, human immunodeficiency virus (HIV), toxoplasmosis, syphilis, and gonorrhea.

Maternal medical complications associated with increased risk of maternal and fetal morbidity and mortality include diabetes, chronic hypertension, congenital heart disease (especially with right-to-left shunting and Eisenmenger complex), glomerulonephritis, collagen vascular disease (especially systemic lupus erythematosus with or without antiphospholipid antibodies), lung disease (cystic fibrosis), severe anemia (sickle cell anemia), hyperthyroidism, myasthenia gravis, idiopathic thrombocytopenic purpura, inborn errors of metabolism (maternal phenylketonuria), and malignancy.

Obstetric complications often are associated with increased fetal or neonatal risk. Vaginal bleeding in the first trimester or early second trimester may be caused by a threatened or actual spontaneous abortion and is associated with increased risk of congenital malformations or chromosomal disorders. Painless vaginal bleeding that is not associated with labor and occurs in the late second or (more likely) third trimester often is the result of **placenta previa.** Bleeding develops when the placental mass overlies the internal cervical os; this may produce maternal hemorrhagic shock, necessitating transfusions. Bleeding also may result in premature delivery. Painful vaginal bleeding is often the result of retroplacental hemorrhage or **placental abruption.** Associated findings may be advanced maternal age and parity, maternal chronic hypertension, maternal cocaine use, preterm rupture of membranes, polyhydramnios, twin gestation, and preeclampsia. Fetal asphyxia ensues as the retroplacental hematoma causes placental separation that interferes with fetal oxygenation. Both types of bleeding are associated with fetal blood loss. Neonatal anemia may be more common with placenta previa.

Abnormalities in the volume of amniotic fluid, resulting in oligohydramnios or polyhydramnios, are associated with increased fetal and neonatal risk. **Oligohydramnios** (amniotic ultrasound fluid index ≤2 cm) is associated with IUGR and major congenital anomalies, particularly of the fetal kidneys, and with chromosomal syndromes. Bilateral renal agenesis results in diminished production of amniotic fluid and a specific deformation syndrome (**Potter syndrome**), which includes clubfeet, characteristic compressed facies, low-set ears, scaphoid abdomen, and diminished chest wall size accompanied by pulmonary hypoplasia and, often, pneumothorax. Uterine compression in the absence of amniotic fluid retards lung growth, and patients with this condition die of respiratory failure rather than renal insufficiency. Twin-to-twin transfusion syndrome (donor) and complications from amniotic fluid leakage also are associated with oligohydramnios. Oligohydramnios increases the risk of fetal distress during labor (meconium-stained fluid and variable decelerations); the risk may be reduced by saline amnioinfusion during labor.

Polyhydramnios may be acute and associated with premature labor, maternal discomfort, and respiratory compromise. More often, polyhydramnios is chronic and is associated with diabetes, immune or nonimmune hydrops fetalis, multiple gestation, trisomy 18 or 21, and major congenital anomalies. Anencephaly, hydrocephaly, and meningomyelocele are associated with reduced fetal swallowing of amniotic fluid. Esophageal and duodenal atresia as well as cleft palate interfere with swallowing and gastrointestinal fluid dynamics. Additional causes of polyhydramnios include Werdnig-Hoffmann and Beckwith-Wiedemann syndromes, conjoined twins, chylothorax, cystic adenomatoid lung malformation, diaphragmatic hernia, gastroschisis, sacral teratoma, placental chorioangioma, and myotonic dystrophy. **Hydrops fetalis** may be a result of Rh or other blood group incompatibilities and anemia caused by intrauterine hemolysis of fetal erythrocytes by maternal IgG-sensitized antibodies crossing the placenta. Hydrops is characterized by fetal edema, ascites, hypoalbuminemia, and congestive heart failure. Causes of **nonimmune hydrops** include fetal arrhythmias (supraventricular tachycardia, congenital heart block), fetal anemia (bone marrow suppression, nonimmune hemolysis, or twin-to-twin transfusion), severe congenital malformation, intrauterine infections, congenital neuroblastoma, inborn errors of metabolism (storage diseases), fetal hepatitis, nephrotic syndrome, and pulmonary lymphangiectasia. Twin-to-twin transfusion syndrome (recipient) also may be associated with polyhydramnios. Polyhydramnios is often the result of unknown causes. If severe, polyhydramnios may be managed with bed rest, indomethacin, or serial amniocenteses.

Premature rupture of the membranes, which occurs in the absence of labor, and **prolonged rupture of the membranes** (>24 hours) are associated with an increased risk of maternal or fetal infection (chorioamnionitis) and preterm birth. In the immediate newborn period, group B streptococcus and *Escherichia coli* are the two most common pathogens associated with sepsis. *Listeria monocytogenes* is a less common cause. *Mycoplasma hominis, Ureaplasma urealyticum, Chlamydia trachomatis,* and anaerobic bacteria of the vaginal flora also have been implicated in infection of the amniotic fluid. Infection with community-acquired methicillin-resistant *Staphylococcus aureus* must be considered for infants with skin infections or with known exposures. The risk of serious fetal infection increases as the duration between rupture and labor (latent period) increases, especially if the period is greater than 24 hours. Intrapartum antibiotic therapy decreases the risk of neonatal sepsis.

Multiple gestations are associated with increased risk resulting from polyhydramnios, premature birth, IUGR, abnormal presentation (breech), congenital anomalies (intestinal atresia, porencephaly, and single umbilical artery), intrauterine fetal demise, birth asphyxia, and twin-to-twin transfusion syndrome. **Twin-to-twin transfusion syndrome** is associated with a high mortality and is seen only in monozygotic twins who share a common placenta and have an arteriovenous connection between their circulations. The fetus on the arterial side of the shunt serves as the blood donor, resulting in fetal anemia, growth retardation, and oligohydramnios for this fetus. The recipient, or venous-side twin, is larger or discordant in size, is plethoric and polycythemic, and may show polyhydramnios. Weight differences of 20% and hemoglobin differences of 5 g/dL suggest the diagnosis. Ultrasonography in the second trimester reveals discordant amniotic fluid volume with oliguria/oligohydramnios and hypervolemia/polyuria/polyhydramnios with a distended bladder, with or without hydrops and heart failure. Treatment includes amniocentesis and attempts to ablate the arteriovenous connection (using a laser). The birth order of twins also affects morbidity by increasing the risk of the second-born twin for breech position, birth asphyxia, birth trauma, and respiratory distress syndrome.

Overall, twinning is observed in 1 of 80 pregnancies; 80% of all twin gestations are dizygotic twins. The diagnosis of the type of twins can be determined by placentation, sex, fetal membrane structure, and, if necessary, tissue and blood group typing or DNA analysis.

Toxemia of pregnancy, or **preeclampsia/eclampsia**, is a disorder of unknown but probably vascular etiology that may lead to maternal hypertension, uteroplacental insufficiency, IUGR, intrauterine asphyxia, maternal seizures, and maternal death. Toxemia is more common in nulliparous women and in women with twin gestation, chronic hypertension, obesity, renal disease, positive family history of toxemia, or diabetes mellitus. A subcategory of preeclampsia, the *HELLP* syndrome (**h**emolysis, **e**levated **l**iver enzyme levels, **l**ow **p**latelets), is more severe and is often associated with a fetal inborn error of fatty acid oxidation (long-chain hydroxyacyl–coenzyme A dehydrogenase of the trifunctional protein complex).

FETUS AND NEWBORN

The late fetal–early neonatal period has the highest mortality rate of any age interval. **Perinatal mortality** refers to fetal deaths occurring from the 20th week of gestation until the 28th day after birth and is expressed as number of deaths per 1000 live births. Intrauterine fetal death accounts for 40% to 50% of the perinatal mortality rate. Such infants, defined as **stillborn**, are born without a heart rate and are apneic, limp, pale, and cyanotic. Many stillborn infants exhibit evidence of maceration; pale, peeling skin; corneal opacification; and soft cranial contents.

Mortality rates around the time of birth are expressed as number of deaths per 1000 live births. The **neonatal mortality rate** includes all infants dying during the period from after birth to the first 28 days of life. Modern neonatal intensive care allows many newborns with life-threatening diseases to survive the neonatal period, only to die of their original diseases or of complications of therapy after 28 days of life. This delayed mortality and mortality caused by acquired illnesses occur during the **postneonatal period**, which begins after 28 days of life and extends to the end of the first year of life.

The **infant mortality rate** encompasses the neonatal and the postneonatal periods. In the United States, it declined to 6.15:1000 in 2010. The rate for African American infants was approximately 11.6:1000. The most common causes of

Table 58-1	Major Causes of Perinatal and Neonatal Mortality

FETUS

Abruptio placentae

Chromosomal anomalies

Congenital malformations (heart, CNS, renal)

Hydrops fetalis

Intrauterine asphyxia*

Intrauterine infection*

Maternal underlying disease (chronic hypertension, autoimmune disease, diabetes mellitus)

Multiple gestation*

Placental insufficiency*

Umbilical cord accident

PRETERM INFANT

Respiratory distress syndrome/bronchopulmonary dysplasia (chronic lung disease)*

Severe immaturity*

Congenital anomalies

Infection

Intraventricular hemorrhage*

Necrotizing enterocolitis

FULL-TERM INFANT

Birth asphyxia*

Birth trauma

Congenital anomalies*

Infection*

Macrosomia

Meconium aspiration pneumonia

Persistent pulmonary hypertension

CNS, Central nervous system.
*Common.

perinatal and neonatal death are listed in Table 58-1. Overall, congenital anomalies and diseases of the premature infant are the most significant causes of neonatal mortality.

Low birth weight (LBW) infants, defined as infants having birth weights of less than 2500 g, represent a disproportionately large component of the neonatal and infant mortality rates. Although LBW infants make up only about 6% to 7% of all births, they account for more than 70% of neonatal deaths. IUGR is the most common cause of LBW in developing countries, whereas prematurity is the cause in developed countries.

Very low birth weight (VLBW) infants, weighing less than 1500 g at birth, represent about 1% of all births but account for 50% of neonatal deaths. Compared with infants weighing 2500 g or more, LBW infants are 40 times more likely to die in the neonatal period; VLBW infants have a 200-fold higher risk of neonatal death. The LBW rate has not improved in recent years and is one of the major reasons that the U.S. infant mortality rate is high compared with other large, modern, industrialized countries.

Maternal factors associated with a LBW caused by premature birth or IUGR include a previous LBW birth, low

socioeconomic status, low level of maternal education, no antenatal care, maternal age younger than 16 years or older than 35 years, short interval between pregnancies, cigarette smoking, alcohol and illicit drug use, physical (excessive standing or walking) or psychological (poor social support) stresses, unmarried status, low pre-pregnancy weight (<45 kg), poor weight gain during pregnancy (<10 lb), and African American race. LBW and VLBW rates for African American women are twice the rates for white women. The neonatal and infant mortality rates are nearly twofold higher among African American infants. These racial differences are only partly explained by poverty.

ASSESSMENT OF THE FETUS

Fetal size can be determined accurately by ultrasound techniques. **Fetal growth** can be assessed by determining the fundal height of the uterus through bimanual examination of the gravid abdomen. Ultrasound measurements of the fetal biparietal diameter, femur length, and abdominal circumference are used to estimate fetal growth. A combination of these measurements predicts fetal weight. Deviations from the normal fetal growth curve are associated with high-risk conditions.

IUGR is present when fetal growth stops and, over time, declines to less than the 5th percentile of growth for gestational age or when growth proceeds slowly, but absolute size remains less than the 5th percentile. Growth restriction may result from fetal conditions that reduce the innate growth potential, such as fetal rubella infection, primordial dwarfing syndromes, chromosomal abnormalities, and congenital malformation syndromes. Reduced fetal production of insulin and insulin-like growth factor I is associated with fetal growth restriction. Placental causes of IUGR include villitis (congenital infections), placental tumors, chronic abruptio placentae, twin-to-twin transfusion syndrome, and placental insufficiency. Maternal causes include severe peripheral vascular diseases that reduce uterine blood flow (chronic hypertension, diabetic vasculopathy, and preeclampsia/eclampsia), reduced nutritional intake, alcohol or drug abuse, cigarette smoking, and uterine constraint (noted predominantly in mothers of small stature with a low prepregnancy weight) and reduced weight gain during pregnancy. The outcome of IUGR depends on the cause of the reduced fetal growth and the associated complications after birth (Table 58-2). Fetuses subjected to chronic intrauterine hypoxia as a result of uteroplacental insufficiency are at an increased risk for the comorbidities of birth asphyxia, polycythemia, and hypoglycemia. Fetuses with reduced tissue mass due to chromosomal, metabolic, or multiple congenital anomaly syndromes have poor outcomes based on the prognosis for the particular syndrome. Fetuses born to small mothers and fetuses with poor nutritional intake usually show catch-up growth after birth.

Fetal size does not always correlate with functional or structural maturity. Determining **fetal maturity** is crucial when making a decision to deliver a fetus because of fetal or maternal disease. Fetal gestational age may be determined accurately on the basis of a correct estimate of the last menstrual period. Clinically relevant landmark dates can be used to determine gestational age; the first audible heart tones by fetoscope are detected at 18 to 20 weeks (12 to 14 weeks by Doppler methods), and quickening of fetal movements usually is perceived at 18 to 20 weeks. However, it is not always

Table 58-2	Problems of Intrauterine Growth Restriction and Small for Gestational Age
PROBLEM*	**PATHOGENESIS**
Intrauterine fetal demise	Placental insufficiency, hypoxia, acidosis, infection, lethal anomaly
Temperature instability	Cold stress, ↓ fat stores, hypoxia, hypoglycemia
Perinatal asphyxia	↓ Uteroplacental perfusion during labor with or without chronic fetal hypoxia-acidosis, meconium aspiration syndrome
Hypoglycemia	↓ Tissue glycogen stores; ↓ gluconeogenesis, hyperinsulinism, ↑ glucose needs of hypoxia, hypothermia, relatively large brain
Polycythemia-hyperviscosity	Fetal hypoxia with ↑ erythropoietin production
Reduced oxygen consumption/hypothermia	Hypoxia, hypoglycemia, starvation effect, poor subcutaneous fat stores
Dysmorphology	Syndrome anomalads, chromosomal-genetic disorders, oligohydramnios-induced deformations
Pulmonary hemorrhage	Hypothermia, polycythemia, hypoxia

Modified from Carlo WA: The high-risk infant. In Kliegman RM, Stanton BF, St. Geme JW, et al, editors: Nelson Textbook of Pediatrics, ed 19, Philadelphia, 2011, Elsevier Science.
*Other problems are common to the gestational age–related risks of prematurity if born before 37 weeks.

possible to determine fetal maturity by such dating, especially in a high-risk situation, such as preterm labor or a diabetic pregnancy.

Surfactant, a combination of surface-active phospholipids and proteins, is produced by the maturing fetal lung and eventually is secreted into the amniotic fluid. The amount of surfactant in amniotic fluid is a direct reflection of surface-active material in the fetal lung and can be used to predict the presence or absence of **pulmonary maturity**. Because phosphatidylcholine, or lecithin, is a principal component of surfactant, the determination of lecithin in amniotic fluid is used to predict a mature fetus. Lecithin concentration increases with increasing gestational age, beginning at 32 to 34 weeks.

Methods used to assess **fetal well-being** before the onset of labor are focused on identifying a fetus at risk for asphyxia or a fetus already compromised by uteroplacental insufficiency. The **oxytocin challenge test** simulates uterine contractions through an infusion of oxytocin sufficient to produce three contractions in a 10-minute period. The development of periodic fetal bradycardia out of phase with uterine contractions (late deceleration) is a positive test result and predicts an at-risk fetus.

The **nonstress test** examines the heart rate response to fetal body movements. Heart rate increases of more than 15 beats/min lasting 15 seconds, are reassuring. If two such episodes occur in 30 minutes, the test result is considered reactive (versus nonreactive), and the fetus is not at risk. Additional signs of fetal well-being are fetal breathing movements, gross body movements, fetal tone, and the presence of amniotic fluid pockets more than 2 cm in size, detected by ultrasound. The **biophysical profile** combines the nonstress test with these four parameters and offers the most accurate fetal assessment.

Doppler examination of the fetal aorta or umbilical arteries permits identification of decreased or reversed diastolic blood flow associated with increased peripheral vascular resistance, fetal hypoxia with acidosis, and placental insufficiency. **Cordocentesis** (percutaneous umbilical blood sampling) can provide fetal blood for P_{O_2}, pH, lactate, and hemoglobin measurements to identify a hypoxic, acidotic, or anemic fetus who is at risk for intrauterine fetal demise or birth asphyxia. Cordocentesis also can be used to determine fetal blood type, platelet count, microbial testing, antibody titer, and rapid karyotype.

In a high-risk pregnancy, the fetal heart rate should be monitored continuously during labor, as should uterine contractions. Fetal heart rate abnormalities may indicate baseline tachycardia (>160 beats/min as a result of anemia, β-sympathomimetic drugs, maternal fever, hyperthyroidism, arrhythmia, or fetal distress), baseline **bradycardia** (<120 beats/min as a result of fetal distress, complete heart block, or local anesthetics), or reduced beat-to-beat variability (flattened tracing resulting from fetal sleep, tachycardia, atropine, sedatives, prematurity, or fetal distress). Periodic changes of the heart rate relative to uterine pressure help determine the presence of hypoxia and acidosis caused by uteroplacental insufficiency or maternal hypotension (late or type II decelerations) or by umbilical cord compression (variable decelerations). In the presence of severe decelerations (late or repeated prolonged variable), a fetal scalp blood gas level should be obtained to assess **fetal acidosis**. A scalp pH of less than 7.20 indicates fetal hypoxic compromise. A pH between 7.20 and 7.25 is in a borderline zone and warrants repeat testing.

Fetal anomalies may be detected by ultrasonography. Emphasis should be placed on visualization of the genitourinary tract; the head (for anencephaly or hydrocephaly), neck (for thickened nuchal translucency), and back (for spina bifida); skeleton; gastrointestinal tract; and heart. Four-chamber and great artery views are required for detection of heart anomalies. **Chromosomal anomaly syndromes** are often associated with an abnormal "triple test" (low estriols, low maternal serum alpha-fetoprotein levels, and elevated placental chorionic gonadotropin levels). If a fetal abnormality is detected, fetal therapy or delivery with therapy in the neonatal intensive care unit may be lifesaving.

ASSESSMENT OF THE NEWBORN

The approach to the birth of an infant requires a detailed history (Table 58-3). Knowing the mother's risk factors enables the delivery room team to anticipate problems that may occur after birth. The history of a woman's labor and delivery can reveal events that might lead to complications affecting either the mother or the neonate, even when the pregnancy was previously considered low risk. Anticipating the need to resuscitate a newborn as a result of fetal distress increases the likelihood of successful resuscitation.

The **transition from fetal to neonatal physiology** occurs at birth. Oxygen transport across the placenta results in a gradient between the maternal and fetal Pa_{O_2}. Although fetal oxygenated blood has a low Pa_{O_2} level compared with that of adults and infants, the fetus is not anaerobic. Fetal oxygen uptake and consumption are similar to neonatal rates, even though the thermal environments and activity levels of fetuses and neonates differ. The oxygen content of fetal blood

Table 58-3	Components of the Perinatal History

DEMOGRAPHIC SOCIAL INFORMATION	Fetal surveillance (OCT, NST, biophysical profile)
Age	Ultrasonography (anomalies, hydrops)
Race	Amniotic fluid analysis (L/S ratio)
Sexually transmitted infections, hepatitis, AIDS	Oligohydramnios-polyhydramnios
Illicit drugs, cigarettes, ethanol, cocaine	Vaginal bleeding
Immune status (syphilis, rubella, hepatitis B, HIV, blood group)	Preterm labor
Occupational exposure	Premature (prolonged) rupture of membranes (duration)
PAST MEDICAL DISEASES	Preeclampsia
Chronic hypertension	Urinary tract infection
Heart disease	Colonization status (herpes simplex, group B streptococcus)
Diabetes mellitus	Medications/drugs
Thyroid disorders	Acute medical illness/exposure to infectious agents
Hematologic/malignancy	Fetal therapy
Collagen-vascular disease (SLE)	**LABOR AND DELIVERY**
Genetic history—inborn errors of metabolism, bleeding, jaundice	Duration of labor
Drug therapy	Presentation—vertex, breech
PRIOR PREGNANCY	Vaginal versus cesarean section
Abortion/stillbirths	Spontaneous labor versus augmented or induced with oxytocin (Pitocin)
Intrauterine fetal demise	Forceps delivery
Congenital malformation	Presence of meconium-stained fluid
Incompetent cervix	Maternal fever/amnionitis
Birth weight	Fetal heart rate patterns (distress)
Prematurity	Scalp pH
Twins	Maternal analgesia, anesthesia
Blood group sensitization/neonatal jaundice	Nuchal cord
Hydrops	Apgar score/methods of resuscitation
Infertility	Gestational age assessment
PRESENT PREGNANCY	Growth status (AGA, LGA, SGA)
Current gestational age	
Method of assessing gestational age	

AGA, Average for gestational age; *AIDS,* acquired immunodeficiency syndrome; *LGA,* large for gestational age; *L/S,* lecithin-to-sphingomyelin ratio; *NST,* nonstress test; *OCT,* oxytocin challenge test; *SGA,* small for gestational age; *SLE,* systemic lupus erythematosus.

is almost equal to the oxygen content in older infants and children because fetal blood has a much higher concentration of hemoglobin.

Fetal hemoglobin (two alpha and two gamma chains) has a higher affinity for oxygen than adult hemoglobin, facilitating oxygen transfer across the placenta. The fetal hemoglobin-oxygen dissociation curve is shifted to the left of the adult curve (Fig. 58-1); at the same Pao_2 level, fetal hemoglobin is more saturated than adult hemoglobin. Because fetal hemoglobin functions on the steep, lower end of the oxygen saturation curve (Pao_2, 20 to 30 mm Hg), however, oxygen unloading to the tissue is not deficient. In contrast, at the higher oxygen concentrations present in the placenta, oxygen loading is enhanced. In the last trimester, fetal hemoglobin production begins to decrease as adult hemoglobin production begins to increase, becoming the only hemoglobin available to the infant by 3 to 6 months of life. At this time, the fetal hemoglobin dissociation curve has shifted to the adult position.

A portion of well-oxygenated umbilical venous blood returning to the heart from the placenta perfuses the liver. The remainder bypasses the liver through a shunt (the **ductus venosus**) and enters the inferior vena cava. This oxygenated blood in the vena cava constitutes 65% to 70% of venous return to the right atrium. The crista dividens in the right atrium directs one third of this blood across the patent foramen ovale to the left atrium, where it subsequently is pumped to the coronary, cerebral, and upper extremity circulations by the left ventricle. Venous return from the upper body combines with the remaining two thirds of the vena caval blood in the right atrium and is directed to the right ventricle. This mixture of venous low-oxygenated blood from the upper and lower body enters the pulmonary artery. Only 8% to 10% of it is pumped to the pulmonary circuit; the remaining 80% to 92% of the right ventricular output bypasses the lungs through a **patent ductus arteriosus** and enters the descending aorta. The amount of blood flowing to the pulmonary system is low because vasoconstriction produced by medial muscle

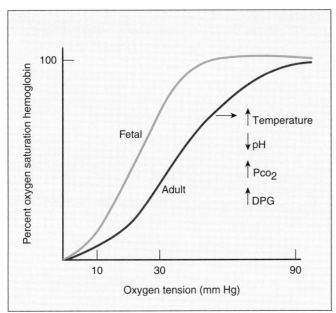

Figure 58-1 Hemoglobin-oxygen dissociation curves. The position of the adult curve depends on the binding of adult hemoglobin to 2,3-diphosphoglycerate (DPG), temperature, P_{CO_2}, and hydrogen ion concentration (pH).

hypertrophy of the pulmonary arterioles and fluid in the fetal lung increases resistance to blood flow. Pulmonary artery tone also responds to hypoxia, hypercapnia, and acidosis with vasoconstriction, a response that may increase pulmonary vascular resistance further. The ductus arteriosus remains patent in the fetus because of low Pa_{O_2} levels and dilating prostaglandins. In utero, the right ventricle is the dominant ventricle, pumping 65% of the combined ventricular output, which is a high volume (450 mL/kg/min) compared with that pumped by an older infant's right ventricle (200 mL/kg/min).

The **transition of the circulation**, occurring between the fetal and neonatal periods, involves the removal of the low-resistance circulation of the placenta, the onset of breathing, reduction of pulmonary arterial resistance, and closure of in utero shunts. Clamping the umbilical cord eliminates the low-pressure system of the placenta and increases systemic blood pressure. Decreased venous return from the placenta decreases right atrial pressure. As breathing begins, air replaces lung fluid, maintaining the functional residual capacity. Fluid leaves the lung, in part, through the trachea; it is either swallowed or squeezed out during vaginal delivery. The pulmonary lymphatic and venous systems reabsorb the remaining fluid.

Most normal infants require little pressure to spontaneously open the lungs after birth (5 to 10 cm H_2O). With the onset of breathing, pulmonary vascular resistance decreases, partly a result of the mechanics of breathing and partly a result of the elevated arterial oxygen tensions. The increased blood flow to the lungs increases the volume of pulmonary venous blood returning to the left atrium; left atrial pressure now exceeds right atrial pressure, and the foramen ovale closes. As the flow through the pulmonary circulation increases and arterial oxygen tensions rise, the ductus arteriosus begins to constrict. In a term infant, this constriction functionally closes the ductus arteriosus within 1 day after birth. A permanent closure requires thrombosis and fibrosis, a process that may take several weeks. In a premature infant, the ductus arteriosus is less

sensitive to the effects of oxygen; if circulating levels of vasodilating prostaglandins are elevated, the ductus arteriosus may remain patent. This patency is a common problem in a premature infant with respiratory distress syndrome.

Ventilation, oxygenation, and normal pH and P_{CO_2} levels immediately reduce pulmonary artery vasoconstriction by causing smooth muscle relaxation. Remodeling of the medial muscle hypertrophy begins at birth and continues for the next 3 months, resulting in a further reduction of pulmonary vascular resistance and a further increase of pulmonary blood flow. Persistence or aggravation of pulmonary vasoconstriction caused by acidosis, hypoxia, hypercapnia, hypothermia, polycythemia, asphyxia, shunting of blood from the lungs, or pulmonary parenchymal hypoplasia results in **persistent pulmonary hypertension of the newborn (PPHN)**. Failure to replace pulmonary alveolar fluid completely with air can lead to respiratory distress (**transient tachypnea of the newborn**).

Routine Delivery Room Care and Resuscitation

Silver nitrate (1%) instilled into both eyes without being washed out is an indicated effective therapy for the prevention of neonatal gonococcal ophthalmia, which can result in severe panophthalmitis and subsequent blindness. Silver nitrate may produce a chemical conjunctivitis with a mucopurulent discharge and is not effective against *C. trachomatis*. Many hospitals use erythromycin drops to prevent neonatal gonococcal and chlamydial eye disease.

Bacterial colonization of a newborn may begin in utero if the fetal membranes have been ruptured. Most infants undergo colonization after birth and acquire the bacteria present in the mother's genitourinary system, such as group B streptococci, staphylococci, *E. coli*, and clostridia. Antiseptic skin or cord care is routine in most nurseries to prevent the spread of pathologic bacteria from one infant to another and to prevent disease in the individual infant. Staphylococcal bullous impetigo, omphalitis, diarrhea, and systemic disease may result from colonization with virulent *S. aureus*. Triple antibiotic ointment (polymyxin B, neomycin, and bacitracin) or bacitracin may be applied to the umbilical cord to reduce its colonization with gram-positive bacteria. Epidemics of *S. aureus* nursery infections are managed with strict infectious disease control measures (cohorting, hand washing, and monitoring for colonization).

Vitamin K prophylaxis (intramuscular) should be given to all infants to prevent hemorrhagic disease of the newborn. Before discharge, infants should receive the hepatitis B vaccine and be screened for various diseases (Tables 58-4 and 58-5).

Fetal or neonatal hypoxia, hypercapnia, poor cardiac output, and a metabolic acidosis can result from numerous conditions affecting the fetus, the placenta, or the mother. Whether in utero or after birth, asphyxia-caused **hypoxic-ischemic brain injury** is the result of reduced gaseous exchange through the placenta or through the lungs. Asphyxia associated with severe bradycardia or cardiac insufficiency reduces or eliminates tissue blood flow, resulting in ischemia. The fetal and neonatal circulatory systems respond to reduced oxygen availability by shunting the blood preferentially to the brain, heart, and adrenal glands and away from the intestine, kidneys, lungs, and skin.

Table 58-4	Core Disorders Recommended for Screening by American College of Medical Genetics

DISORDER	ACRONYM	PRIMARY MARKER
METABOLIC DISORDERS DETECTED USING TANDEM MASS SPECTROMETRY		
Organic Acid Disorders		
Beta-ketothiolase deficiency (mitochondrial acetoacetyl CoA thiolase deficiency)	BKT	C5:1/C5OH
Cobalamin defects A, B	CBL (A,B)	C3
Isovaleric acidemia*	IVA	C5
Glutaric aciduria I	GA-I	C5DC
3-Hydroxy 3-methylglutaryl-CoA lyase deficiency*	HMG	C5OH/C5-3M-DC
Multiple carboxylase deficiency*	MCD	C3/C5OH
3-Methylcrotonyl-CoA carboxylase deficiency	3MCC	C5OH
Methylmalonic aciduria (mutase)*	MMA	C3
Propionic acidemia*	PA	C3
Fatty Acid Oxidation Defects		
Carnitine uptake defect (carnitine transporter defect)	CUD	C0
Long-chain hydroxyacyl-CoA dehydrogenase deficiency*	LCHAD/D	C16OH/C18:1OH
Medium-chain acyl-CoA dehydrogenase deficiency	MCAD/D	C8
Trifunctional protein deficiency*	TFP	C16OH/C18:1OH
Very long chain acyl-CoA dehydrogenase deficiency	VLCAD/D	C14:1/C14
Amino Acid Disorders		
Argininosuccinic aciduria (argininosuccinate lyase deficiency)*	ASA	ASA
Citrullinemia I (argininosuccinate synthase deficiency)*	CIT-I	Citrulline
Phenylketonuria	PKU	Phenylalanine
Maple syrup urine disease*	MSUD	Leucine
Homocystinuria	HCY	Methionine
Tyrosinemia type I	TYR-I	Tyrosine
OTHER METABOLIC DISORDERS		
Biotinidase deficiency	BIOT	Biotinidase activity
Galactosemia*	GALT	Total galactose, GALT activity
ENDOCRINE DISORDERS		
Congenital adrenal hyperplasia*	CAH	17-Hydroxyprogesterone
Congenital hypothyroidism	CH	T_4, TSH
HEMOGLOBIN DISORDERS		
Sickle cell anemia	HbSS	Hb variants
Sickle cell disorder	HbS/C	Hb variants
Hemoglobin S/β-thalassemia	HbS/betaTh	Hb variants
OTHER DISORDERS		
Cystic fibrosis	CF	Immunoreactive trypsinogen
Hearing	HEAR	

From Sahai I, Levy H: Newborn screening. In Gleason C, Devasker D editors: Avery's diseases of the newborn, ed 9, Philadelphia, 2012, Saunders.
*Can manifest acutely in the first week of life.

Metabolic acidosis during asphyxia is caused by the combined effects of poor cardiac output secondary to hypoxic depression of myocardial function, systemic hypoxia, and tissue anaerobic metabolism. With severe or prolonged intrauterine or neonatal asphyxia, multiple vital organs are affected (Table 58-6).

Many conditions that contribute to **fetal or neonatal asphyxia** are the same medical or obstetric problems associated with high-risk pregnancy (Table 58-7). Maternal diseases that interfere with uteroplacental perfusion (chronic hypertension, preeclampsia, and diabetes mellitus) place the fetus at risk for intrauterine asphyxia. Maternal epidural anesthesia and the development of the vena caval compression syndrome may produce maternal hypotension, which decreases uterine perfusion. Maternal medications given to relieve pain during labor may cross the placenta and depress the infant's respiratory center, resulting in apnea at the time of birth.

Table 58-5	Abnormal Newborn Screening Results: Possible Implications and Initial Action to Be Taken

NEWBORN SCREENING FINDING	DIFFERENTIAL DIAGNOSIS	INITIAL ACTION
↑ Phenylalanine	PKU, non-PKU hyperphenylalaninemia, pterin defect, galactosemia, transient hyperphenylalaninemia	Repeat blood specimen
↓ T_4, ↑ TSH	Congenital hypothyroidism, iodine exposure	Repeat blood specimen or thyroid function testing, begin thyroxine treatment
↓ T_4, normal TSH	Maternal hyperthyroidism, thyroxine-binding globulin deficiency, secondary hypothyroidism, congenital hypothyroidism with delayed TSH elevation	Repeat blood specimen
↑ Galactose (1-P) transferase	Galactosemia, liver disease, reducing substance, repeat deficiency variant (Duarte), transient	Clinical evaluation, urine for blood specimen. If reducing substance positive, begin lactose-free formula
↓ Galactose-1-phosphate uridyltransferase	Galactosemia, transferase deficiency variant (Duarte), transient	Clinical evaluation, urine for reducing substance, repeat blood specimen. If reducing substance positive, begin lactose-free formula
↑ Methionine	Homocystinuria, isolated liver dysfunction, tyrosinemia type I, transient hypermethioninemia	Repeat blood and urine specimen
↑ Leucine	Maple syrup urine disease, transient elevation	Clinical evaluation including urine for ketones, acid-base status, amino acid studies, immediate neonatal ICU care if urine ketones positive
↑ Tyrosine	Tyrosinemia type I or type II, transient tyrosinemia, liver disease	Repeat blood specimen
↑ 17α- Hydroxyprogesterone	Congenital adrenal hyperplasia, prematurity, transient (residual fetal adrenal cortex), stress in neonatal period, early specimen collection	Clinical evaluation including genital examination, serum electrolytes, repeat blood specimen
S-hemoglobin	Sickle cell disease, sickle cell trait	Hemoglobin electrophoresis
↑ Trypsinogen	Cystic fibrosis, transient, intestinal anomalies, perinatal stress, trisomies 13 and 18, renal failure	Repeat blood specimen, possible sweat test and DNA testing
↑ Creatinine phosphokinase	Duchenne muscular dystrophy, other type of muscular dystrophy, birth trauma, invasive procedure	Repeat blood test
↓ Biotinidase	Biotinidase deficiency	Serum biotinidase assay, biotin therapy
↓ G6PD	G6PD deficiency	Complete blood count, bilirubin determination
↓ α_1-Antitrypsin	α_1-Antitrypsin deficiency	Confirmatory test
Toxoplasma antibody (IgM)	Congenital toxoplasmosis	Infectious disease consultation
HIV antibody (IgG)	Maternally transmitted HIV, possible AIDS	Infectious disease consultation
↑ Organic acids	Fatty acid oxidation defects (medium-chain acyl-CoA dehydrogenase deficiency)	Perform specific assay (tandem mass spectroscopy); frequent feeds

From Kim SZ, Levy HL: Newborn screening. In Taeusch HW, Ballard RA, editors: Avery's Diseases of the Newborn, ed 7, Philadelphia, 1998, Saunders.
AIDS, Acquired immunodeficiency syndrome; G6PD, glucose-6-phosphate dehydrogenase; HIV, human immunodeficiency virus; ICU, intensive care unit; PKU, phenylketonuria; T_4, thyroxine; TSH, thyroid-stimulating hormone.

Table 58-6	Effects of Asphyxia

SYSTEM	EFFECT
Central nervous system	Hypoxic-ischemic encephalopathy, IVH, PVL, cerebral edema, seizures, hypotonia, hypertonia
Cardiovascular	Myocardial ischemia, poor contractility, tricuspid insufficiency, hypotension
Pulmonary	Persistent pulmonary hypertension, respiratory distress syndrome
Renal	Acute tubular or cortical necrosis
Adrenal	Adrenal hemorrhage
Gastrointestinal	Perforation, ulceration, necrosis
Metabolic	Inappropriate ADH, hyponatremia, hypoglycemia, hypocalcemia, myoglobinuria
Integument	Subcutaneous fat necrosis
Hematology	Disseminated intravascular coagulation

ADH, Antidiuretic hormone; IVH, intraventricular hemorrhage; PVL, periventricular leukomalacia.

Table 58-7	Etiology of Birth Asphyxia
TYPE	**EXAMPLE**
INTRAUTERINE	
Hypoxia-ischemia	Uteroplacental insufficiency, abruptio placentae, prolapsed cord, maternal hypotension, unknown
Anemia-shock	Vasa previa, placenta previa, fetomaternal hemorrhage, erythroblastosis
INTRAPARTUM	
Birth trauma	Cephalopelvic disproportion, shoulder dystocia, breech presentation, spinal cord transection
Hypoxia-ischemia	Umbilical cord compression, tetanic contraction, abruptio placentae
POSTPARTUM	
Central nervous system	Maternal medication, trauma, previous episodes of fetal hypoxia-acidosis
Congenital neuromuscular disease	Congenital myasthenia gravis, myopathy, myotonic dystrophy
Infection	Consolidated pneumonia, shock
Airway disorder	Choanal atresia, severe obstructing goiter or tumor, laryngeal webs
Pulmonary disorder	Severe immaturity, pneumothorax, pleural effusion, diaphragmatic hernia, pulmonary hypoplasia
Renal disorder	Pulmonary hypoplasia, pneumothorax

Table 58-8	Apgar Score		
	POINTS		
SIGNS	**0**	**1**	**2**
Heart rate	0	<100/min	>100/min
Respiration	None	Weak cry	Vigorous cry
Muscle tone	None	Some extremity flexion	Arms, legs well flexed
Reflex irritability	None	Some motion	Cry, withdrawal
Color of body	Blue	Pink body, blue extremities	Pink all over

Fetal conditions associated with asphyxia usually do not become manifested until delivery, when the infant must initiate and sustain ventilation. In addition, the upper and lower airways must be patent and unobstructed. Alveoli must be free from foreign material, such as meconium, amniotic fluid debris, and infectious exudates, which increases airway resistance, reduces lung compliance, and leads to respiratory distress and hypoxia. Some extremely immature infants weighing less than 1000 g at birth may be unable to expand their lungs, even in the absence of other pathology. Their compliant chest walls and surfactant deficiency may result in poor air exchange, retractions, hypoxia, and apnea.

The newborn (particularly a preterm infant) responds paradoxically to hypoxia with apnea rather than tachypnea as occurs in adults. Episodes of intrauterine asphyxia also may depress the neonatal central nervous system. If recovery of the fetal heart rate occurs as a result of improved uteroplacental perfusion, fetal hypoxia and acidosis may resolve. Nonetheless, if the effect on the respiratory center is more severe, a newborn may not initiate an adequate ventilatory response at birth and may undergo another episode of asphyxia.

The **Apgar examination**, a rapid scoring system based on physiologic responses to the birth process, is a good method for assessing the need to resuscitate a newborn (Table 58-8). At intervals of 1 minute and 5 minutes after birth, each of the five physiologic parameters is observed or elicited by a qualified examiner. Full-term infants with a normal cardiopulmonary adaptation should score 8 to 9 at 1 and 5 minutes. Apgar scores of 4 to 7 warrant close attention to determine whether the infant's status will improve and to ascertain whether any pathologic condition is contributing to the low Apgar score.

By definition, an Apgar score of 0 to 3 represents either a cardiopulmonary arrest or a condition caused by severe bradycardia, hypoventilation, or central nervous system depression. Most low Apgar scores are caused by difficulty in establishing adequate ventilation and not by primary cardiac pathology. In addition to an Apgar score of 0 to 3, most infants with asphyxia severe enough to cause neurologic injury also manifest fetal acidosis (pH <7); seizures, coma, or hypotonia; and multiorgan dysfunction. Low Apgar scores may be caused by fetal hypoxia or other factors listed in Table 58-7. Most infants with low Apgar scores respond to assisted ventilation by face mask or by endotracheal intubation and usually do not need emergency medication.

Resuscitation of a newborn with a low Apgar score follows the same systematic sequence as that for resuscitation of older patients, but in the newborn period this simplified *ABCD* approach requires some qualification (Fig. 58-2). In the ABCD approach, **A** stands for securing a patent airway by clearing amniotic fluid or meconium by suctioning; **A** is also a reminder of *anticipation* and the need for knowing the events of pregnancy, labor, and delivery. Evidence of a diaphragmatic hernia and a low Apgar score indicate that immediate endotracheal intubation is required. If a mask and bag are used, gas enters the lung and the stomach, and the latter may act as an expanding mass in the chest that compromises respiration. If fetal hydrops has occurred with pleural effusions, bilateral thoracentesis to evacuate the pleural effusions may be needed to establish adequate ventilation.

B represents **breathing**. If the neonate is apneic or hypoventilating and remains cyanotic, artificial ventilation should be initiated. Ventilation should be performed with a well-fitted mask attached to an anesthesia bag and a manometer to prevent extremely high pressures from being given to the newborn; 100% oxygen should be administered through the mask.

Newborn Resuscitation

Figure 58-2 New Guidelines and Algorithm for Neonatal Resuscitation. *CPAP*, Continuous positive airway pressure; *PPV*, positive-pressure ventilation. *(From Kattwinkel J, Perlman JM, Aziz K, et al: Special Report—Neonatal Resuscitation: 2010 American Heart Association Guidelines for Cardiopulmonary Resuscitation and Emergency Cardiovascular Care, Pediatrics 126(5):e1400–e1413, 2010. Erratum in Neoreviews 128(1):176, 2011. doi: 10.1542/peds.2011-1260.)*

If the infant does not revive, an endotracheal tube should be placed, attached to the anesthesia bag and manometer, and 100% oxygen should be administered. The pressure generated should begin at 20 to 25 cm H_2O, with a rate of 40 to 60 breaths/minute. An adequate response to ventilation includes good chest rise, return of breath sounds, well-oxygenated color, heart rate returning to the normal range (120 to 160 beats/minute), normal end-tidal carbon dioxide, and, later, increased muscle activity and wakefulness. The usual recovery after a cardiac arrest first involves a return to a normal heart rate, followed by disappearance of cyanosis and noticeably improved perfusion. An infant may remain limp and be apneic for a prolonged time after return of cardiac output and correction of acidosis.

Breathing initially should be briefly delayed if meconium-stained amniotic fluid is present to avoid dissemination of meconium into the lungs, producing severe aspiration pneumonia. If meconium is noted in the amniotic fluid, the oropharynx should be suctioned when the head is delivered. After the birth of a **depressed infant**, the oral cavity should be

Table 58-9	Life-Threatening Congenital Anomalies
NAME	**MANIFESTATIONS**
Choanal atresia (stenosis)	Respiratory distress in delivery room, apnea, unable to pass nasogastric tube through nares
Pierre Robin syndrome	Micrognathia, cleft palate, airway obstruction
Diaphragmatic hernia	Scaphoid abdomen, bowel sounds present in left chest, heart shifted to right, respiratory distress, polyhydramnios
Tracheoesophageal fistula	Polyhydramnios, aspiration pneumonia, excessive salivation, unable to place nasogastric tube in stomach
Intestinal obstruction: volvulus, duodenal atresia, ileal atresia	Polyhydramnios, bile-stained emesis, abdominal distention
Gastroschisis/omphalocele	Polyhydramnios; intestinal obstruction
Renal agenesis/Potter syndrome	Oligohydramnios, anuria, pulmonary hypoplasia, pneumothorax
Hydronephrosis	Bilateral abdominal masses
Neural tube defects: anencephaly, meningomyelocele	Polyhydramnios, elevated α-fetoprotein; decreased fetal activity
Down syndrome (trisomy 21)	Hypotonia, congenital heart disease, duodenal atresia
Ductal-dependent congenital heart disease	Cyanosis, murmur, shock

suctioned again; the vocal cords should be visualized and the infant intubated.

C represents **circulation** and external cardiac massage. If artificial ventilation does not improve bradycardia, if asystole is present, or if peripheral pulses cannot be palpated, external cardiac massage should be performed at a rate of 120 compressions/minute with compressions and breaths given at a ratio of 3:1. External cardiac massage usually is not needed because most infants in the delivery room respond to ventilation.

D represents the **administration of drugs**. If bradycardia is unresponsive to ventilation or if asystole is present, epinephrine should be administered. Intravenous (IV) epinephrine (1:10,000), 0.1 to 0.3 mL/kg, should be given through an umbilical venous line or injected into the endotracheal tube. However, when epinephrine is administered through the endotracheal tube, the result is often unpredictable. Before medications are administered in the presence of electrical cardiac activity with poor pulses, it is important to determine whether there is a **pneumothorax**. Transillumination of the thorax, involving the use of a bright light through each side of the thorax and over the sternum, may suggest pneumothorax if one side transmits more light than the other. Breath sounds may be decreased over a pneumothorax and there may be a shift of the heart tones away from the side of a tension pneumothorax.

If central nervous system depression in the infant may be due to a narcotic medication given to the mother, 0.1 mg/kg of naloxone (Narcan) can be given to the infant intravenously or endotracheally. Before this drug is administered, the ABCs should be followed carefully. Naloxone should not be given to a newborn of a mother who is suspected of being addicted to narcotics or is on methadone maintenance because the newborn may experience severe withdrawal seizures.

In babies of more than 35 weeks' gestation suffering hypoxic ischemic injury at birth, induced therapeutic **hypothermia** (33.0°C to 34.0°C) for 72 hours has been shown in clinical studies to be efficacious in reducing the severity of brain injury. Brain hypothermia, whether induced by whole-body or selective head cooling, provides neuroprotection against encephalopathy presumably due to hypoxic ischemia.

Physical Examination and Gestational Age Assessment

The first physical examination of a newborn may be a general physical examination of a well infant or an examination to confirm fetal diagnoses or to determine the cause of various manifestations of neonatal diseases. Problems in the transition from fetal to neonatal life may be detectable immediately in the delivery room or during the first day of life. Physical examination also may reveal effects of the labor and delivery resulting from asphyxia, drugs, or birth trauma. The first newborn examination is an important way to detect congenital malformations or deformations (Table 58-9). Significant congenital malformations may be present in 1% to 3% of all births.

Appearance

Signs such as cyanosis, nasal flaring, intercostal retractions, and grunting suggest pulmonary disease. Meconium staining of the umbilical cord, nails, and skin suggest fetal distress and the possibility of aspiration pneumonia. The level of spontaneous activity, passive muscle tone, quality of the cry, and apnea are useful screening signs to evaluate the state of the nervous system.

Vital Signs

The examination should proceed with an assessment of vital signs, particularly heart rate (normal rate, 120 to 160 beats/min); respiratory rate (normal rate, 30 to 60 breaths/min); temperature (usually done per rectum and later as an axillary measurement); and blood pressure (often reserved for sick infants). Length, weight, and head circumference should be measured and plotted on growth curves to determine whether growth is normal, accelerated, or retarded for the specific gestational age.

Physical maturity	−1	0	1	2	3	4	5
Skin	Sticky, friable, transparent	Gelatinous, red, translucent	Smooth, pink, visible veins	Superficial peeling or rash, few veins	Cracking, pale areas, rare veins	Parchment, deep cracking, no vessels	Leathery, cracked, wrinkled
Lanugo	None	Sparse	Abundant	Thinning	Bald areas	Mostly bald	
Plantar surface	Heel–toe 40-50 mm: −1 Less than 40 mm: −2	<50 mm, no crease	Faint red marks	Anterior transverse crease only	Creases on anterior 2/3	Creases over entire sole	
Breast	Imperceptible	Barely perceptible	Flat areola– no bud	Stripped areola, 1-2 mm bud	Raised areola, 3-4 mm bud	Full areola, 5-10 mm bud	
Eye/ear	Lids fused, loosely (−1), tightly (−2)	Lids open, pinna flat, stays folded	Slightly curved pinna; soft, slow recoil	Well-curved pinna, soft but ready recoil	Formed and firm; instant recoil	Thick cartilage, ear stiff	
Genitals male	Scrotum flat, smooth	Scrotum empty, faint rugae	Testes in upper canal, rare rugae	Testes descending, few rugae	Testes down, good rugae	Testes pendulous, deep rugae	
Genitals female	Clitoris prominent, labia flat	Prominent clitoris, small labia minora	Prominent clitoris, enlarging minora	Majora and minora equally prominent	Majora large, minora small	Majora cover clitoris and minora	

Figure 58-3 Physical criteria for assessment of maturity and gestational age. Expanded New Ballard Score (NBS) includes extremely premature infants and has been refined to improve accuracy in more mature infants. *(From Ballard JL, Khoury JC, Wedig K, et al: New Ballard Score, expanded to include extremely premature infants, J Pediatr 119:417-423, 1991.)*

Gestational Age

Gestational age is determined by an assessment of various physical signs (Fig. 58-3) and neuromuscular characteristics (Fig. 58-4) that vary according to fetal age and maturity. **Physical criteria** mature with advancing fetal age, including increasing firmness of the pinna of the ear; increasing size of the breast tissue; decreasing fine, immature lanugo hair over the back; and decreasing opacity of the skin. **Neurologic criteria** mature with gestational age, including increasing flexion of the legs, hips, and arms; increasing tone of the flexor muscles of the neck; and decreasing laxity of the joints. These signs are determined during the first day of life and are assigned scores. The cumulative score is correlated with a gestational age, which is usually accurate to within 2 weeks (Fig. 58-5).

Gestational age assessment permits the detection of abnormal fetal growth patterns, aiding in predicting the neonatal complications of largeness or smallness for gestational age (Fig. 58-6). Infants born at a weight greater than the 90th percentile for age are considered **large for gestational age.** Among the risks associated with being large for gestational age are all the risks of the infant of a diabetic mother and risks associated with postmaturity. Infants born at a weight less than 10th percentile for age (some growth curves use <2 standard deviations or the 5th percentile) are **small for gestational age** and have IUGR. Problems associated with small for gestational age

infants include congenital malformations, in addition to the problems listed in Table 58-2.

Skin

The skin should be evaluated for pallor, plethora, jaundice, cyanosis, meconium staining, petechiae, ecchymoses, congenital nevi, and neonatal rashes. Vasomotor instability with cutis marmorata, telangiectasia, phlebectasia (intermittent mottling with venous prominence), and acrocyanosis (feet and hands) is normal in a premature infant. Acrocyanosis also may be noted in a healthy term infant in the first days after birth.

The skin is covered with lanugo hair, which disappears by term gestation. **Hair tufts** over the lumbosacral spine suggest a spinal cord defect. **Vernix caseosa**, a soft, white, creamy layer covering the skin in preterm infants, disappears by term. Postterm infants often have peeling, parchment-like skin. **Mongolian spots** are transient, dark blue to black pigmented macules seen over the lower back and buttocks in 90% of African American, Indian, and Asian infants. **Nevus simplex** (*salmon patch*), or pink macular hemangioma, is common, usually transient, and noted on the back of the neck, eyelids, and forehead. **Nevus flammeus**, or **port-wine stain**, is seen on the face and should cause the examiner to consider Sturge-Weber syndrome (trigeminal angiomatosis, convulsions, and ipsilateral intracranial *tram-line* calcifications).

Neuromuscular maturity

	−1	0	1	2	3	4	5
Posture							
Square window (wrist)	< 90°	90°	60°	45°	30°	0°	
Arm recoil		180°	140–180°	110–140°	90–110°	< 90°	
Popliteal angle	180°	160°	140°	120°	100°	90°	< 90°
Scarf sign							
Heel to ear							

Figure 58-4 Neuromuscular criteria for assessment of maturity and gestational age. Expanded New Ballard Score (NBS) includes extremely premature infants and has been refined to improve accuracy in more mature infants. *(From Ballard JL, Khoury JC, Wedig K, et al: New Ballard Score, expanded to include extremely premature infants, J Pediatr 119:417-423, 1991.)*

Maturity rating

Score	Weeks
−10	20
−5	22
0	24
5	26
10	28
15	30
20	32
25	34
30	36
35	38
40	40
45	42
50	44

Figure 58-5 Maturity rating as calculated by adding the physical and neurologic scores, calculating the gestational age. *(From Ballard JL, Khoury JC, Wedig K, et al: New Ballard Score, expanded to include extremely premature infants, J Pediatr 119:417-423, 1991.).*

Congenital melanocytic nevi are pigmented lesions of varying size noted in 1% of neonates. **Giant pigmented nevi** are uncommon but have malignant potential. **Capillary hemangiomas** are raised, red lesions, whereas **cavernous hemangiomas** are deeper, blue masses. Both lesions increase in size after birth, then resolve when the child is 1 to 4 years of age. When enlarged, these hemangiomas may produce high-output heart failure or platelet trapping and hemorrhage. **Erythema toxicum** is an erythematous, papular-vesicular rash common in neonates that develops after birth and involves eosinophils in the vesicular fluid. **Pustular melanosis**, more common in African American infants, may be seen at birth and consists of a small, dry vesicle on a pigmented brown macular base. Erythema toxicum and pustular melanosis are benign lesions but may mimic more serious conditions, such as the vesicular rash of disseminated herpes simplex or the bullous eruption of *S. aureus* impetigo. Tzanck smear, Gram stain, Wright stain, direct fluorescent antibody stain, polymerase chain reaction for herpes DNA, and appropriate cultures may be needed to distinguish these rashes. Other common characteristic rashes are **milia** (yellow-white epidermal cysts of the pilosebaceous follicles that are noted on the nose) and **miliaria** (prickly heat), which is caused by obstructed sweat glands. **Edema** may be present in preterm infants, but also suggests hydrops fetalis, sepsis, hypoalbuminemia, or lymphatic disorders.

Skull

The skull may be elongated and molded after a prolonged labor; this resolves 2 to 3 days after birth. The sutures should be palpated to determine the width and the presence of premature fusion or cranial synostosis. The anterior and posterior

Figure 58-6 Birth weight–specific and estimated gestational age–specific mortality rates. The dashed lines of the figure represent the 10th and 90th percentile weights. The grid lines are plotted by each gestational age and in 250-g weight increments. Each number in the box is the percent mortality rate for the grid defined by gestational age and birth weight range. *(From Thomas P, Peabody J, Turnier V, et al: A new look at intrauterine growth and impact of race, attitude, and gender, Pediatrics 106:E21, 2000.)*

fontanelles should be soft and nonbulging, with the anterior larger than the posterior. A large fontanelle is associated with hydrocephalus, hypothyroidism, rickets, and other disorders. Soft areas away from the fontanelle are **craniotabes**; these lesions feel like a Ping-Pong ball when they are palpated. They may be a result of in utero compression. The skull should be examined carefully for signs of trauma or lacerations from internal fetal electrode sites or fetal scalp pH sampling; abscesses may develop in these areas.

Face, Eyes, and Mouth
The face should be inspected for dysmorphic features, such as epicanthal folds, hypertelorism, preauricular tags or sinuses, low-set ears, long philtrum, and cleft lip or palate. Facial asymmetry may be a result of seventh nerve palsy; head tilt may be caused by torticollis.

The eyes should open spontaneously, especially in an upright position. Before 28 weeks' gestational age, the eyelids may be fused. Coloboma, megalocornea, and microphthalmia suggest other malformations or intrauterine infections. A cloudy cornea greater than 1 cm in diameter also may be seen in congenital glaucoma, uveal tract dysgenesis, and storage diseases. Conjunctival and retinal hemorrhages are common and usually of no significance. The pupillary response to light is present at 28 weeks of gestation. The **red reflex** of the retina is shown easily. A white reflex, or **leukokoria**, is abnormal and may be the result of cataracts, ocular tumor, severe chorioretinitis, persistent hyperplastic primary vitreous, or retinopathy of prematurity.

The mouth should be inspected for the presence of natal teeth, clefts of the soft and hard palate and uvula, and micrognathia. A bifid uvula suggests a submucosal cleft. White, shiny, multiple transient epidermal inclusion cysts (Epstein pearls)

on the hard palate are normal. Hard, marble-sized masses in the buccal mucosa are usually transient idiopathic fat necrosis. The **tympanic membranes** are dull, gray, opaque, and immobile in the first 1 to 4 weeks. These findings should not be confused with otitis media.

Neck and Chest
The neck appears short and symmetrical. Abnormalities include midline clefts or masses caused by thyroglossal duct cysts or by goiter and lateral neck masses (or sinuses), which are the result of branchial clefts. Cystic hygromas and hemangiomas may be present. Shortening of the sternocleidomastoid muscle with a fibrous tumor over the muscle produces head tilt and asymmetrical facies (neonatal torticollis). Arnold-Chiari malformation and cervical spine lesions also produce torticollis. Edema and webbing of the neck suggest Turner syndrome. Both clavicles should be palpated for fractures.

Examination of the **chest** includes inspection of the chest wall to identify asymmetry resulting from absence of the pectoralis muscle and inspection of the breast tissue to determine gestational age and detect a breast abscess. Boys and girls may have breast engorgement and produce milk; milk expression should not be attempted. **Supernumerary nipples** may be bilateral and may be associated with renal anomalies.

Lungs
Examination of the lungs includes observations of the rate, depth, and nature of intercostal or sternal retractions. Breath sounds should be equal on both sides of the chest, and rales should not be heard after the first 1 to 2 hours of life. Diminished or absent breath sounds on one side suggest

pneumothorax, collapsed lung, pleural effusion, or diaphragmatic hernia. Shift of the cardiac impulse away from a tension pneumothorax and diaphragmatic hernia and toward the collapsed lung is a helpful physical finding for differentiating these disorders. Subcutaneous emphysema of the neck or chest also suggests a pneumothorax or pneumomediastinum, whereas bowel sounds auscultated in the chest in the presence of a scaphoid abdomen suggest a diaphragmatic hernia.

Heart

The position of the heart in infants is more midline than in older children. The first heart sound is normal, whereas the second heart sound may not be split in the first day of life. Decreased splitting of the second heart sound is noted in PPHN, transposition of the great vessels, and pulmonary atresia. Heart murmurs in newborns are common in the delivery room and during the first day of life. Most of these murmurs are transient and are due to closure of the ductus arteriosus, peripheral pulmonary artery stenosis, or a small ventral septal defect. Pulses should be palpated in the upper and lower extremities (over the brachial and femoral arteries). Blood pressure in the upper and lower extremities should be measured in all patients with a murmur or heart failure. An upper-to-lower extremity gradient of more than 10 to 20 mm Hg suggests coarctation of the aorta.

Abdomen

The liver may be palpable 2 cm below the right costal margin. The spleen tip is less likely to be palpable. A left-sided liver suggests situs inversus and asplenia syndrome. Both kidneys should be palpable in the first day of life with gentle, deep palpation. The first urination occurs during the first day of life in more than 95% of normal term infants.

Abdominal masses usually represent hydronephrosis or dysplastic-multicystic kidney disease. Less often, masses indicate ovarian cysts, intestinal duplication, neuroblastoma, or mesoblastic nephroma. Masses should be evaluated immediately with ultrasound. Abdominal distention may be caused by intestinal obstructions, such as ileal atresia, meconium ileus, midgut volvulus, imperforate anus, or Hirschsprung disease. Meconium stool is passed normally within 48 hours of birth in 99% of term infants. The anus should be patent. An imperforate anus is not always visible; the first temperature taken with a rectal thermometer should be taken carefully. The abdominal wall musculature may be absent, as in prune-belly syndrome, or weak, resulting in diastasis recti. **Umbilical hernias** are common in African American infants. The umbilical cord should be inspected to determine the presence of two arteries and one vein and the absence of an urachus or a herniation of abdominal contents, as occurs with an **omphalocele**. The latter is associated with extraintestinal problems, such as genetic trisomies and hypoglycemia (Beckwith-Wiedemann syndrome). Bleeding from the cord suggests a coagulation disorder, and a chronic discharge may be a granuloma of the umbilical stump or, less frequently, a draining omphalomesenteric cyst or urachus. Erythema around the umbilicus is **omphalitis** and may cause portal vein thrombophlebitis and subsequent extrahepatic portal hypertension. The herniation of bowel through the abdominal wall 2 to 3 cm lateral to the umbilicus is a **gastroschisis**.

Genitalia

Decision-Making Algorithm
Available @ StudentConsult.com

Ambiguous Genitalia

At term, the testes should be descended into a well-formed pigmented and rugated scrotum. The testes occasionally are in the inguinal canal; this is more common among preterm infants, as is cryptorchidism. Scrotal swelling may represent a hernia, transient hydrocele, in utero torsion of the testes, or, rarely, dissected meconium from meconium ileus and peritonitis. Hydroceles are clear and readily seen by transillumination, whereas testicular torsion in the newborn may present as a painless, dark swelling. The urethral opening should be at the end of the penis. Epispadias or hypospadias alone should not raise concern about pseudohermaphroditism. However, if no testes are present in the scrotum and hypospadias is present, problems of sexual development should be suspected. Circumcision should be deferred with hypospadias because the foreskin is often needed for the repair. The normal prepuce is often too tight to retract in the neonatal period.

The female genitalia normally may reveal a milky white or blood-streaked vaginal discharge as a result of maternal hormone withdrawal. Mucosal tags of the labia majora are common. Distention of an imperforate hymen may produce hydrometrocolpos and a lower midline abdominal mass as a result of an enlarged uterus. Clitoral enlargement with fusion of the labial-scrotal folds (labia majora) suggests adrenogenital syndrome or exposure to masculinizing maternal hormones.

Extremities

Examination of the extremities should involve assessment of length, symmetry, and presence of hemihypertrophy, atrophy, polydactyly, syndactyly, simian creases, absent fingers, overlapping fingers, rocker-bottom feet, clubfoot, congenital bands, fractures, and amputations.

Spine

The spine should be examined for evidence of sacral hair tufts, a dermal sinus tract above the gluteal folds, congenital scoliosis (a result of hemivertebra), and soft tissue masses such as lipomas or meningomyeloceles.

Hips

The hips should be examined for congenital dysplasia (dislocation). Gluteal fold asymmetry or leg length discrepancy is suggestive of dysplasia, but the examiner should perform the Barlow test and the Ortolani maneuver to evaluate the stability of the hip joint. These tests determine whether the femoral head can be displaced from the acetabulum (**Barlow test**) and then replaced (**Ortolani maneuver**).

NEUROLOGIC ASSESSMENT

The neurologic examination should include assessment of active and passive tone, level of alertness, primary neonatal

Table 58-10	Differential Diagnosis of Neonatal Cyanosis
SYSTEM/DISEASE	**MECHANISM**
PULMONARY	
Respiratory distress syndrome	Surfactant deficiency
Sepsis, pneumonia	Inflammation, pulmonary hypertension, ARDS
Meconium aspiration pneumonia	Mechanical obstruction, inflammation, pulmonary hypertension
Persistent pulmonary hypertension of the newborn	Pulmonary hypertension
Diaphragmatic hernia	Pulmonary hypoplasia, pulmonary hypertension
Transient tachypnea	Retained lung fluid
CARDIOVASCULAR	
Cyanotic heart disease with decreased pulmonary blood flow	Right-to-left shunt as in pulmonary atresia, tetralogy of Fallot
Cyanotic heart disease with increased pulmonary blood flow	Mixing lesion as in single ventricle or truncus arteriosus
Cyanotic heart disease with congestive heart failure	Pulmonary edema and poor cardiac output as in hypoplastic left heart and coarctation of aorta
Heart failure alone	Pulmonary edema and poor cardiac contractility as in sepsis, myocarditis, supraventricular tachycardia, or complete heart block; high-output failure as in PDA or vein of Galen or other arteriovenous malformations
CENTRAL NERVOUS SYSTEM (CNS)	
Maternal sedative drugs	Hypoventilation, apnea
Asphyxia	CNS depression
Intracranial hemorrhage	CNS depression, seizure
Neuromuscular disease	Hypotonia, hypoventilation, pulmonary hypoplasia
HEMATOLOGIC	
Acute blood loss	Shock
Chronic blood loss	Heart failure
Polycythemia	Pulmonary hypertension
Methemoglobinemia	Low-affinity hemoglobin or red blood cell enzyme defect
METABOLIC	
Hypoglycemia	CNS depression, congestive heart failure
Adrenogenital syndrome	Shock (salt-losing)

ARDS, Acute respiratory distress syndrome; *CNS,* central nervous system; *PDA,* patent ductus arteriosus.

(primitive) reflexes, deep tendon reflexes, spontaneous motor activity, and cranial nerves (involving retinal examination, extraocular muscle movement, masseter power as in sucking, facial motility, hearing, and tongue function). The Moro reflex, present at birth and gone in 3 to 6 months, is one of the primary newborn reflexes. It is elicited by sudden, slight dropping of the supported head from a slightly raised supine position, which should elicit opening of the hands and extension and abduction of the arms, followed by upper extremity flexion and a cry. The palmar grasp is present by 28 weeks' gestation and gone by 4 months of age. Deep tendon reflexes may be brisk in a normal newborn; 5 to 10 beats of ankle clonus are normal. The Babinski sign is extensor (upgoing). The sensory examination can be evaluated by withdrawal of an extremity, grimace, and cry in response to painful stimuli. The rooting reflex (turning of the head toward light tactile stimulation of the perioral area) is present by 32 weeks' gestation.

Special Conditions Requiring Resuscitation in the Delivery Room
Cyanosis

Decision-Making Algorithm
Available @ StudentConsult.com

Cyanosis

Acrocyanosis (blue color of the hands and feet with pink color of the rest of the body) is common in the delivery room and is usually normal. **Central cyanosis** of the trunk, mucosal membranes, and tongue can occur at any time after birth and is always a manifestation of a serious underlying condition. Cyanosis is noted with 4 to 5 g/dL of deoxygenated hemoglobin. Central cyanosis can be caused by problems in many different organ systems, although cardiopulmonary diseases are the most common (Table 58-10). Respiratory distress syndrome, sepsis, and cyanotic heart disease are the three most common causes of cyanosis in infants admitted to a neonatal intensive care unit. A systematic evaluation of these and other causes of cyanosis is required for every cyanotic infant after prompt administration of oxygen, with or without assisted ventilation.

Life-Threatening Congenital Malformations

Various congenital anomalies can interfere with vital organ function after birth (see Table 58-9). Some malformations, such as choanal atresia and other lesions obstructing the airway, may complicate ventilation. Intrathoracic lesions, such as cysts or diaphragmatic hernia, interfere with respiration. Other malformations that obstruct the gastrointestinal system at the level of the esophagus, duodenum, ileum, or colon may lead to aspiration pneumonia, intestinal perforation, or gangrene. Gastroschisis and omphalocele are associated with exposed bowel on the abdominal wall. Omphalocele is often associated with other malformations, whereas intestinal necrosis is more common in gastroschisis.

Shock

Shock in the delivery room is manifested by pallor, poor capillary refill time, lack of palpable pulses, hypotonia, cyanosis, and eventually cardiopulmonary arrest. Blood loss before or during labor and delivery is a common cause of shock in the delivery room. Blood loss may be caused by fetal-maternal hemorrhage, placenta previa, vasa previa, twin-to-twin transfusion syndrome, or displacement of blood from the fetus to the placenta as during asphyxia (*asphyxia pallida*). Hemorrhage into a viscus, such as the liver or spleen, may be noted in macrosomic infants, and hemorrhage into the cerebral ventricles may produce shock and apnea in preterm infants. Anemia, hypoalbuminemia, hypovolemia, and shock at birth are common manifestations of Rh immune hydrops.

Severe intrauterine bacterial sepsis may present with shock in the delivery room or immediately after the infant is transferred to the nursery. Typically these infants are mottled, hypotonic, and cyanotic and have diminished peripheral pulses. They have a normal hemoglobin concentration but may manifest neutropenia, thrombocytopenia, and disseminated intravascular coagulation. Peripheral symmetrical gangrene (purpuric rash) often is a sign of hypotensive shock in infants with severe congenital bacterial infections. Congenital left ventricular cardiac obstruction (critical aortic stenosis or hypoplastic left heart syndrome) also produces shock, although not usually in the delivery room.

Treatment of newborn infants with shock should involve the management approaches used for the sick infant. Problems may be anticipated through knowledge of the infant's immune status, evidence of hydrops, or suspicion of intrauterine infection or anomalies. Stabilization of the airway and institution of respiratory support are essential. Hypovolemic shock should be managed with repeated boluses of 10 to 15 mL/kg of normal saline or lactated Ringer solution. If severe immune hemolysis is predicted, blood typed against the mother's blood should be available in the delivery room and should be given to the newborn if signs of anemia and shock are present. Thereafter, all blood should be crossmatched with the infant's and mother's blood before transfusion. Drugs such as dopamine, epinephrine, or cortisol may improve cardiac output and tissue perfusion.

Birth Injury

Birth injury refers to avoidable and unavoidable injury to the fetus during the birth process. **Caput succedaneum** is a diffuse, edematous, often dark swelling of the soft tissue of the scalp that extends across the midline and suture lines. In infants delivered from a face presentation, soft tissue edema of the eyelids and face is an equivalent phenomenon. Caput succedaneum may be seen after prolonged labor in full-term and preterm infants. Molding of the head often is associated with caput succedaneum and is the result of pressure that is induced from overriding the parietal and frontal bones against their respective sutures.

A **cephalhematoma** is a subperiosteal hemorrhage that does not cross the suture lines surrounding the respective bones. A linear skull fracture rarely may be seen underlying a cephalhematoma. With time, the cephalhematoma may organize, calcify, and form a central depression.

Infants with cephalhematoma and caput succedaneum require no specific treatment. Occasionally a premature infant may develop a massive scalp hemorrhage. This **subgaleal bleeding** and the bleeding noted from a cephalhematoma may cause indirect hyperbilirubinemia requiring phototherapy. **Retinal and subconjunctival hemorrhages** are common but usually are small and insignificant. No treatment is necessary.

Spinal cord or **spine injuries** may occur in the fetus as a result of the hyperextended *star gazing* posture. Injuries also may occur in infants after excessive rotational (at C3–4) or longitudinal (at C7–T1) force is transmitted to the neck during vertex or breech delivery. Fractures of vertebrae are rare; trauma may cause direct damage to the spinal cord, leading to transection and permanent sequelae, hemorrhage, edema, and neurologic signs. Rarely, a snapping sound indicating cord transection rather than vertebral displacement is heard at the time of delivery. Neurologic dysfunction usually involves complete flaccid paralysis, absence of deep tendon reflexes, and absence of responses to painful stimuli below the lesion. Painful stimuli may elicit reflex flexion of the legs. Infants with spinal cord injury often are flaccid, apneic, and asphyxiated, all of which may mask the underlying spinal cord transection.

Injury to the nerves of the **brachial plexus** may result from excessive traction on the neck, producing paresis or complete paralysis. The mildest injury (neurapraxia) is edema; axonotmesis is more severe and consists of disrupted nerve fibers with an intact myelin sheath; neurotmesis, or complete nerve disruption or root avulsion, is most severe. **Erb-Duchenne paralysis** involves the fifth and sixth cervical nerves and is the most common and usually mildest injury. The infant cannot abduct the arm at the shoulder, externally rotate the arm, or supinate the forearm. The usual picture is one of painless adduction, internal rotation of the arm, and pronation of the forearm. The **Moro reflex** is absent on the involved side, and the hand grasp is intact. **Phrenic nerve palsy** (C3, C4, and C5) may lead to diaphragmatic paralysis and respiratory distress. Elevation of the diaphragm caused by nerve injury must be differentiated from elevation caused by eventration resulting from congenital weakness or absence of diaphragm muscle. **Klumpke paralysis** is caused by injury to the seventh and eighth cervical nerves and the first thoracic nerve, resulting in a paralyzed hand and, if the sympathetic nerves are injured, an ipsilateral **Horner syndrome** (ptosis, miosis). Complete arm and hand paralysis is noted with the most severe form of damage to C5, C6, C7, C8, and T1. **Treatment** of brachial plexus injury is supportive and includes positioning to avoid contractures. Active and passive range of motion exercises also may be beneficial. If the deficit persists, nerve grafting may be beneficial.

Facial nerve injury may be the result of compression of the seventh nerve between the facial bone and the mother's pelvic bones or the physician's forceps. This peripheral nerve injury is characterized by an asymmetric crying face whose normal side, including the forehead, moves in a regular manner. The affected side is flaccid, the eye does not close, the nasolabial fold is absent, and the side of the mouth droops at rest. If there is a central injury to the facial nerve, only the lower two thirds of the face (not the forehead) are involved. Complete agenesis of the facial nucleus results in a central facial paralysis; when this is bilateral, as in **Möbius syndrome**, the face appears expressionless.

Skull fractures are rare, are usually linear, and require no treatment other than observation for very rare, delayed (1 to 3 months) complications (e.g., leptomeningeal cyst). Depressed skull fractures are unusual, but may be seen with complicated forceps delivery and may need surgical elevation. Fractures of the **clavicle** usually are unilateral and are noted in macrosomic infants after shoulder dystocia. Often a snap is heard after a difficult delivery, and the infant exhibits an asymmetrical Moro response and decreased movement of the affected side. The prognosis is excellent; many infants require no treatment or a simple figure of eight bandage to immobilize the bone.

Extremity fractures are less common than fractures of the clavicle and involve the humerus more often than the femur. **Treatment** involves immobilization and a triangular splint bandage for the humerus and traction suspension of the legs for femoral fractures. The prognosis is excellent.

Fractures of the **facial bones** are rare, but dislocation of the cartilaginous part of the nasal septum out of the vomeral groove and columella is common. Clinical manifestations include feeding difficulty, respiratory distress, asymmetrical nares, and a flattened, laterally displaced nose. Treatment reduces the dislocation by elevating the cartilage back into the vomeral groove.

Visceral trauma to the liver, spleen, or adrenal gland occurs in macrosomic infants and in extremely premature infants, with or without breech or vaginal delivery. Rupture of the liver with subcapsular hematoma formation may lead to anemia, hypovolemia, shock, hemoperitoneum, and disseminated intravascular coagulation. Infants with anemia and shock who are suspected to have an intraventricular hemorrhage but with a normal head ultrasound examination should be evaluated for hepatic or splenic rupture. Adrenal hemorrhage may be asymptomatic, detected only by finding calcified adrenal glands in normal infants. Infants with severe adrenal hemorrhage may exhibit a flank mass, jaundice, and hematuria, with or without shock.

Temperature Regulation

After birth, a newborn remains covered by amniotic fluid and situated in a cold environment (20° C to 25° C). An infant's skin temperature may decrease 0.3° C/min, and the core temperature may decrease 0.1º C/min in the delivery room. In the absence of an external heat source, the infant must increase metabolism substantially to maintain body temperature.

Heat loss occurs through four basic mechanisms. In the cold delivery room, the wet infant loses heat predominantly by **evaporation** (cutaneous and respiratory loss when wet or in low humidity), **radiation** (loss to nearby cold, solid surfaces), and **convection** (loss to air current). When the infant is dry, radiation, convection, and **conduction** (loss to object in direct contact with infant) are important causes of heat loss. After birth, all high-risk infants should be dried immediately to eliminate evaporative heat losses. A radiant or convective heat source should be provided for these high-risk infants. Normal term infants should be dried and wrapped in a blanket.

The ideal environmental temperature is the **neutral thermal environment,** the ambient temperature that results in the lowest rate of heat being produced by the infant and maintains normal body temperature. The neutral thermal environmental temperature decreases with increasing gestational and postnatal age. Ambient temperatures less than the neutral thermal environment result in increasing rates of oxygen consumption for heat production, which is designed to maintain normal body temperature. If the ambient temperature decreases further or if oxygen consumption cannot increase sufficiently (due to hypoxia, hypoglycemia, or drugs), the core body temperature decreases.

Heat production by a newborn is created predominantly by nonshivering thermogenesis in specialized areas of tissue containing brown adipose tissue. Brown fat is highly vascular, contains many mitochondria per cell, and is situated around large blood vessels, resulting in rapid heat transfer to the circulation. The vessels of the neck, thorax, and interscapular region are common locations of brown fat. These tissues also are innervated by the sympathetic nervous system, which serves as a primary stimulus for heat production by brown adipose cells. Shivering does not occur in newborns.

Severe **cold injury** in an infant is manifested by acidosis, hypoxia, hypoglycemia, apnea, bradycardia, pulmonary hemorrhage, and a pink skin color. The color is caused by trapping of oxygenated hemoglobin in the cutaneous capillaries. Many of these infants appear dead, but most respond to treatment and recover. Milder degrees of cold injury in the delivery room may contribute to metabolic acidosis and hypoxia after birth. Conversely, hypoxia delays heat generation in cold-stressed infants.

Treatment of severe hypothermia should involve resuscitation and rapid warming of core (e.g., lung and stomach) and external surfaces. Fluid resuscitation also is needed to treat hypovolemia seen in many of these infants. Reduced core temperature (32° C to 35° C) in the immediate newborn period often requires only external warming with a radiant warmer, incubator, or both.

Elevated Temperature

Exposure to ambient temperatures above the neutral thermal environment results in *heat stress* and an elevated core temperature. Sweating is uncommon in newborns and may be noted only on the forehead. In response to moderate heat stress, infants may increase their respiratory rate to dissipate heat. Excessive environmental temperatures may result in heatstroke or in hemorrhagic shock encephalopathy syndrome.

MISCELLANEOUS DISORDERS
Hypocalcemia

Decision-Making Algorithm
Available @ StudentConsult.com

Hypocalcemia

Hypocalcemia is common in sick and premature newborns. Calcium levels are higher in cord blood than in maternal blood because of active placental transfer of calcium to the fetus. Fetal calcium accretion in the third trimester approaches 150 mg/kg/24 hr; fetal bone mineral content doubles between 30 and 40 weeks of gestation. All infants show a slight decline of serum calcium levels after birth, reaching a trough level at 24 to 48 hours, the point at which hypocalcemia usually occurs. Total serum calcium levels of less than 7 mg/dL and ionized calcium levels of less than 3 to 3.5 mg/dL are considered hypocalcemia.

The etiology of hypocalcemia varies with the time of onset and the associated illnesses of the child. **Early neonatal hypocalcemia** occurs in the first 3 days of life and is often asymptomatic. Transient hypoparathyroidism and a reduced parathyroid response to the usual postnatal decline of serum calcium levels may be responsible for hypocalcemia in premature infants and infants of diabetic mothers. Congenital absences of the parathyroid gland with DiGeorge syndrome is a cause of hypocalcemia. **Hypomagnesemia** (<1.5 mg/dL) may be seen simultaneously with hypocalcemia, especially in infants of diabetic mothers. Treatment with calcium alone does not relieve symptoms or increase serum calcium levels until hypomagnesemia is also treated. Sodium bicarbonate therapy, phosphate release from cell necrosis, transient hypoparathyroidism, and hypercalcitoninemia may be responsible for early neonatal hypocalcemia associated with asphyxia. Early-onset hypocalcemia associated with asphyxia often occurs with seizures as a result of hypoxic-ischemic encephalopathy

Late neonatal hypocalcemia, or **neonatal tetany**, often is the result of ingestion of high phosphate–containing milk or the inability to excrete the usual phosphorus in commercial infant formula. Hyperphosphatemia (>8 mg/dL) usually occurs in infants with hypocalcemia after the first week of life. Vitamin D deficiency states and malabsorption also have been associated with late-onset hypocalcemia.

The clinical manifestations of hypocalcemia and hypomagnesemia include apnea, muscle twitching, seizures, laryngospasm, **Chvostek sign** (facial muscle spasm when the side of the face over the seventh nerve is tapped), and **Trousseau sign** (carpopedal spasm induced by partial inflation of a blood pressure cuff). The latter two signs are rare in the immediate newborn period.

Neonatal hypocalcemia may be prevented in high-risk neonates by administration of IV or oral calcium supplementation at a rate of 25 to 75 mg/kg/24 hr. Early asymptomatic hypocalcemia of preterm infants and infants of diabetic mothers often resolves spontaneously. Symptomatic hypocalcemia should be treated with 2 to 4 mL/kg of 10% calcium gluconate given intravenously and slowly over 10 to 15 minutes, followed by a continuous infusion of 75 mg/kg/24 hr of elemental calcium. If hypomagnesemia is associated with hypocalcemia, 50% magnesium sulfate, 0.1 mL/kg, should be given by intramuscular injection and repeated every 8 to 12 hours.

The **treatment** of late hypocalcemia includes immediate management, as in early hypocalcemia, plus the initiation of feedings with low-phosphate formula. Subcutaneous infiltration of IV calcium salts can cause tissue necrosis; oral supplements are hypertonic and may irritate the intestinal mucosa.

Neonatal Drug Addiction and Withdrawal

Infants may become passively and physiologically addicted to medications or to drugs of abuse (heroin, methadone, barbiturates, tranquilizers, amphetamines) taken chronically by the mother during pregnancy; these infants subsequently may have signs and symptoms of drug withdrawal. Many of these pregnancies are at high risk for other complications related to IV drug abuse, such as hepatitis, acquired immunodeficiency syndrome (AIDS), and syphilis. In addition, the LBW rate and the long-term risk for sudden infant death syndrome are higher in the infants of these high-risk women.

Opiates

Neonatal withdrawal signs and symptoms usually begin at 1 to 5 days of life with maternal heroin use and at 1 to 4 weeks with maternal methadone addiction. Clinical manifestations of withdrawal include sneezing, yawning, ravenous appetite, emesis, diarrhea, fever, diaphoresis, tachypnea, high-pitched cry, tremors, jitteriness, poor sleep, poor feeding, and seizures. The illness tends to be more severe during methadone withdrawal. The initial treatment includes swaddling in blankets in a quiet, dark room. When hyperactivity is constant, and irritability interferes with sleeping and feeding, or when diarrhea or seizures are present, pharmacologic treatment is indicated. Seizures usually are treated with phenobarbital. The other symptoms may be managed with replacement doses of a narcotic (usually tincture of opium) to calm the infant; weaning from narcotics may be prolonged over 1 to 2 months.

Cocaine

Cocaine use during pregnancy is associated with preterm labor, abruptio placentae, neonatal irritability, and decreased attentiveness. Infants may be small for gestational age and have small head circumferences. Usually no treatment is needed.

Chapter 59

MATERNAL DISEASES AFFECTING THE NEWBORN

Maternal diseases during pregnancy can affect the fetus directly or indirectly (Table 59-1). Autoantibody-mediated diseases can have direct consequences on the fetus and neonate because the antibodies are usually of the IgG type and can cross the placenta to the fetal circulation.

| Table 59-1 | Maternal Disease Affecting the Fetus or Neonate |

MATERNAL DISORDER	FETAL EFFECTS	MECHANISM
Cyanotic heart disease	Intrauterine growth restriction	Low fetal oxygen delivery
Diabetes mellitus		
Mild	Large for gestational age, hypoglycemia	Fetal hyperglycemia—produces hyperinsulinemia promoting growth
Severe	Growth retardation	Vascular disease, placental insufficiency
Drug addiction	Intrauterine growth restriction, neonatal withdrawal	Direct drug effect, plus poor diet
Endemic goiter	Hypothyroidism	Iodine deficiency
Graves disease	Transient thyrotoxicosis	Placental immunoglobulin passage of thyrotropin receptor antibody
Hyperparathyroidism	Hypocalcemia	Maternal calcium crosses to fetus and suppresses fetal parathyroid gland
Hypertension	Intrauterine growth restriction, intrauterine fetal demise	Placental insufficiency, fetal hypoxia
Idiopathic thrombocytopenic purpura	Thrombocytopenia	Nonspecific platelet antibodies cross placenta
Infection	Neonatal sepsis (see Chapter 66)	Transplacental or ascending infection
Isoimmune neutropenia or thrombocytopenia	Neutropenia or thrombocytopenia	Specific antifetal neutrophil or platelet antibody crosses placenta after sensitization of mother
Malignant melanoma	Placental or fetal tumor	Metastasis
Myasthenia gravis	Transient neonatal myasthenia	Immunoglobulin to acetylcholine receptor crosses the placenta
Myotonic dystrophy	Neonatal myotonic dystrophy	Autosomal dominant with genetic anticipation
Phenylketonuria	Microcephaly, retardation, ventricular septal defect	Elevated fetal phenylalanine levels
Rh or other blood group sensitization	Fetal anemia, hypoalbuminemia, hydrops, neonatal jaundice	Antibody crosses placenta directed at fetal cells with antigen
Systemic lupus erythematosus	Congenital heart block, rash, anemia, thrombocytopenia, neutropenia, cardiomyopathy, stillbirth	Antibody directed at fetal heart, red and white blood cells, and platelets; lupus anticoagulant

From Stoll BJ, Kliegman RM: The fetus and neonatal infant. In Behrman RE, Kliegman RM, Jenson HB, editors: Nelson textbook of pediatrics, ed 16, Philadelphia, WB Saunders, 2000.

ANTIPHOSPHOLIPID SYNDROME

Antiphospholipid syndrome is associated with thrombophilia and recurrent pregnancy loss. Antiphospholipid antibodies are found in 2% to 5% of the general healthy population, but they also may be associated with systemic lupus erythematosus and other rheumatic diseases. Obstetric complications arise from the prothrombotic effects of the antiphospholipid antibodies on placental function. Vasculopathy, infarction, and thrombosis have been identified in mothers with antiphospholipid syndrome. Antiphospholipid syndrome can include fetal growth impairment, placental insufficiency, maternal preeclampsia, and premature birth.

IDIOPATHIC THROMBOCYTOPENIA

Idiopathic thrombocytopenic purpura (ITP) is seen in approximately 1 to 2 per 1000 live births and is an immune process in which antibodies are directed against platelets. Platelet-associated IgG antibodies can cross the placenta and cause thrombocytopenia in the fetus and newborn. The severely thrombocytopenic fetus is at increased risk for intracranial hemorrhage. ITP during pregnancy requires close maternal and fetal management to reduce the risks of life-threatening maternal hemorrhage and trauma to the fetus at delivery. Postnatal management involves observation of the infant's platelet count. For infants who have evidence of hemorrhage, single-donor irradiated platelets may be administered to control the bleeding. The infant may benefit from an infusion of intravenous immunoglobulin. Neonatal thrombocytopenia usually resolves within 4 to 6 weeks.

SYSTEMIC LUPUS ERYTHEMATOSUS

Immune abnormalities in systemic lupus erythematosus (SLE) can lead to the production of anti-Ro (SS-A) and anti-La (SS-B) antibodies that can cross the placenta and injure fetal tissue. The most serious complication is damage to the cardiac conducting system, which results in **congenital heart block**. The heart block observed in association with maternal SLE tends to be complete (third degree), although less advanced blocks have been observed. The mortality rate is approximately 20%; most surviving infants require pacing. Neonatal lupus may occur and is characterized by skin lesions (sharply demarcated erythematous plaques or central atrophic macules with peripheral scaling with predilection for the eyes, face, and scalp), thrombocytopenia, autoimmune hemolysis, and hepatic involvement.

Table 59-2	Problems of Diabetic Pregnancy

MATERNAL

Ketoacidosis

Hyperglycemia/hypoglycemia

Nephritis

Preeclampsia

Polyhydramnios

Retinopathy

NEONATAL

Birth asphyxia

Birth injury (macrosomia, shoulder dystocia)

Congenital anomalies (lumbosacral dysgenesis—caudal regression)

Congenital heart disease (ventricular and atrial septal defects, transposition of the great arteries, truncus arteriosus, double-outlet right ventricle, coarctation of the aorta)

Hyperbilirubinemia (unconjugated)

Hypocalcemia

Hypoglycemia

Hypomagnesemia

Neurologic disorders (neural tube defects, holoprosencephaly)

Organomegaly

Polycythemia (hyperviscosity)

Renal disorders (double ureter, renal vein thrombosis, hydronephrosis, renal agenesis)

Respiratory distress syndrome

Small left colon syndrome

Transient tachypnea of the newborn

NEONATAL HYPERTHYROIDISM

Graves disease is associated with thyroid-stimulating antibodies. The prevalence of clinical hyperthyroidism in pregnancy has been reported to be about 0.1% to 0.4%; it is the second most common endocrine disorder during pregnancy (after diabetes). Neonatal hyperthyroidism is due to the transplacental passage of thyroid-stimulating antibodies; hyperthyroidism can appear rapidly within the first 12 to 48 hours. Symptoms may include intrauterine growth restriction, prematurity, goiter (may cause tracheal obstruction), exophthalmos, stare, craniosynostosis (usually coronal), flushing, heart failure, tachycardia, arrhythmias, hypertension, hypoglycemia, thrombocytopenia, and hepatosplenomegaly. Treatment includes propylthiouracil, iodine drops, and propranolol. Autoimmune induced neonatal hyperthyroidism usually resolves in 2 to 4 months.

DIABETES MELLITUS

Diabetes mellitus that develops during pregnancy (*gestational diabetes* is noted in about 5% of women) or diabetes that is present before pregnancy adversely influences fetal and neonatal well-being. The effect of diabetes on the fetus depends, in part, on the severity of the diabetic state: age of onset of diabetes, duration of treatment with insulin, and presence of vascular disease. Poorly controlled maternal diabetes leads to maternal and fetal hyperglycemia that stimulates the fetal pancreas, resulting in hyperplasia of the islets of Langerhans. Fetal

Table 59-3	Common Teratogenic Drugs	
DRUG	**RESULTS**	
Alcohol	Fetal alcohol syndrome, microcephaly, congenital heart disease	
Aminopterin	Mesomelia, cranial dysplasia	
Coumarin	Hypoplastic nasal bridge, chondrodysplasia punctata	
Fluoxetine	Minor malformations, low birth weight, poor neonatal adaptation	
Folic acid antagonists*	Neural tube, cardiovascular, renal, and oral cleft defects	
Isotretinoin and vitamin A	Facial and ear anomalies, congenital heart disease	
Lithium	Ebstein anomaly	
Methyl mercury	Microcephaly, blindness, deafness, retardation (Minamata disease)	
Misoprostol	Arthrogryposis	
Penicillamine	Cutis laxa syndrome	
Phenytoin	Hypoplastic nails, intrauterine growth restriction, typical facies	
Radioactive iodine	Fetal hypothyroidism	
Radiation	Microcephaly	
Stilbestrol (DES)	Vaginal adenocarcinoma during adolescence	
Streptomycin	Deafness	
Testosterone-like drugs	Virilization of female	
Tetracycline	Enamel hypoplasia	
Thalidomide	Phocomelia	
Toluene (solvent abuse)	Fetal alcohol–like syndrome, preterm labor	
Trimethadione	Congenital anomalies, typical facies	
Valproate	Spina bifida	
Vitamin D	Supravalvular aortic stenosis	

*Trimethoprim, triamterene, phenytoin, primidone, phenobarbital, carbamazepine.

hyperinsulinemia results in increased fat and protein synthesis, producing a fetus that is large for gestational age. After birth, hyperinsulinemia persists, resulting in fasting neonatal hypoglycemia. Strictly controlling maternal diabetes during pregnancy and preventing hyperglycemia during labor and delivery prevent macrosomic fetal growth and neonatal hypoglycemia. Additional problems of the diabetic mother and her fetus and newborn are summarized in Table 59-2.

OTHER CONDITIONS

Other maternal illnesses, such as severe pulmonary disease (cystic fibrosis), cyanotic heart disease, and sickle cell anemia, may reduce oxygen availability to the fetus. Severe hypertensive or diabetic vasculopathy can result in uteroplacental insufficiency. The fetus and the newborn may also be adversely affected by the medications used to treat maternal illnesses. These effects may appear as teratogenesis (Table 59-3) or as an adverse metabolic, neurologic, or cardiopulmonary adaptation to extrauterine life (Table 59-4). Acquired infectious diseases of the mother also may affect the fetus or newborn adversely.

Table 59-4	Agents Acting on Pregnant Women That May Adversely Affect the Newborn Infant
AGENT	**POTENTIAL CONDITION(S)**
Acebutolol	IUGR, hypotension, bradycardia
Acetazolamide	Metabolic acidosis
Adrenal corticosteroids	Adrenocortical failure (rare)
Amiodarone	Bradycardia, hypothyroidism
Anesthetic agents (volatile)	CNS depression
Aspirin	Neonatal bleeding, prolonged gestation
Atenolol	IUGR, hypoglycemia
Blue cohosh herbal tea	Neonatal heart failure
Bromides	Rash, CNS depression, IUGR
Captopril, enalapril	Transient anuric renal failure, oligohydramnios
Caudal-paracervical anesthesia with mepivacaine (accidental introduction of anesthetic into scalp of infant)	Bradypnea, apnea, bradycardia, convulsions
Cholinergic agents (edrophonium, pyridostigmine)	Transient muscle weakness
CNS depressants (narcotics, barbiturates, benzodiazepines) during labor	CNS depression, hypotonia
Cephalothin	Positive direct Coombs test reaction
Fluoxetine	Possible transient neonatal withdrawal, hypertonicity, minor anomalies
Haloperidol	Withdrawal
Hexamethonium bromide	Paralytic ileus
Ibuprofen	Oligohydramnios, PPHN
Imipramine	Withdrawal
Indomethacin	Oliguria, oligohydramnios, intestinal perforation, PPHN
Intravenous fluids during labor (e.g., salt-free solutions)	Electrolyte disturbances, hyponatremia, hypoglycemia
Iodide (radioactive)	Goiter
Iodides	Neonatal goiter
Lead	Reduced intellectual function
Magnesium sulfate	Respiratory depression, meconium plug, hypotonia
Methimazole	Goiter, hypothyroidism
Morphine and its derivatives (addiction)	Withdrawal symptoms (poor feeding, vomiting, diarrhea, restlessness, yawning and stretching, dyspnea and cyanosis, fever and sweating, pallor, tremors, convulsions)
Naphthalene	Hemolytic anemia (in G6PD-deficient infants)
Nitrofurantoin	Hemolytic anemia (in G6PD-deficient infants)
Oxytocin	Hyperbilirubinemia, hyponatremia
Phenobarbital	Bleeding diathesis (vitamin K deficiency), possible long-term reduction in IQ, sedation
Primaquine	Hemolytic anemia (in G6PD-deficient infants)
Propranolol	Hypoglycemia, bradycardia, apnea
Propylthiouracil	Goiter, hypothyroidism
Reserpine	Drowsiness, nasal congestion, poor temperature stability
Sulfonamides	Interfere with protein binding of bilirubin; kernicterus at low levels of serum bilirubin, hemolysis with G6PD deficiency
Sulfonylurea	Refractory hypoglycemia
Sympathomimetic (tocolytic–β agonist) agents	Tachycardia
Thiazides	Neonatal thrombocytopenia (rare)

Stoll BJ, Kliegman RM: The fetus and neonatal infant. In Behrman RE, Kliegman RM, Jenson HB, editors: Nelson textbook of pediatrics, ed 16, Philadelphia, WB Saunders, 2000.
CNS, Central nervous system; G6PD, glucose-6-phosphate dehydrogenase; IUGR, intrauterine growth restriction; PPHN, persistent pulmonary hypertension of the newborn.

DISEASES OF THE FETUS

The principal determinants of fetal disease include the fetal genotype and the in utero environment. Variation in environmental factors rather than the fetal genetics plays a more significant role in determining overall fetal well-being, although a genetically abnormal fetus may not thrive as well or survive. The ability to assess a fetus genetically, biochemically, and physically is greatly enhanced through the development of amniocentesis, fetoscopy, chorionic villus sampling, fetal blood sampling, genetic testing of circulating fetal DNA in the mother's blood, and real-time ultrasonography.

INTRAUTERINE GROWTH RESTRICTION AND SMALL FOR GESTATIONAL AGE

Fetuses subjected to abnormal maternal, placental, or fetal conditions that restrain growth are a high-risk group and traditionally classified as having intrauterine growth restriction (IUGR). The terms *IUGR* and *SGA* (small for gestational age) are not synonymous. IUGR represents a deviation from expected growth patterns. The decreased fetal growth associated with IUGR is an adaptation to unfavorable intrauterine conditions that result in permanent alterations in metabolism, growth, and development. IUGR most frequently occurs with a variety of maternal conditions that are associated with preterm delivery. SGA describes an infant whose birth weight is statistically less than the 10th percentile or two standard deviations below the mean birth weight for gestational age. The cause of SGA may be pathologic, as in an infant with IUGR, or nonpathologic, as in an infant who is small but otherwise healthy (Table 60-1).

Only about 50% of IUGR infants are identified before delivery. Measurement and recording of maternal fundal height in conjunction with serial ultrasound assessment of the fetus (growth rate, amniotic fluid volume, malformations, anomalies, and Doppler velocimetry of uterine, placental, and fetal blood flow) can aid detection. When suspected and identified, IUGR and SGA fetuses must be monitored for fetal well-being, and appropriate maternal care needs to be instituted (see Chapter 58).

At birth, infants who are mildly to moderately SGA appear smaller than normal with decreased subcutaneous fat. More severely affected infants may present with a *wasted appearance* with asymmetrical findings, including larger heads for the size of the body (central nervous system sparing), widened anterior fontanelles, small abdomen, thin arms and legs, decreased subcutaneous fat, dry and redundant skin, decreased muscle mass, and thin (often meconium-stained) umbilical cord. Gestational age is often difficult to assess when based on physical appearance and perceived advanced neurologic maturity. Physical examination should detail the presence of dysmorphic features, abnormal extremities, or gross anomalies that might suggest underlying congenital malformations, chromosomal defects, or exposure to teratogens. Hepatosplenomegaly, jaundice, and skin rashes in addition to ocular disorders,

Table 60-1	Etiologies for Intrauterine Growth Restriction and Small for Gestational Age at Birth
MATERNAL FACTORS	
Age (young and advanced)	
Cigarette smoking	
Genetics (short stature, weight)	
Illnesses during pregnancy (preeclampsia, severe diabetes, chronic hypertension, connective tissue disease)	
Infections (intrauterine)	
Lack of good prenatal care	
Oligohydramnios	
Poor nutrition	
Race (African American)	
FETAL FACTORS	
Chromosomal abnormality and nonchromosomal syndromes	
Congenital infections	
Inborn errors of metabolism	
Multiple gestations	
Insulin resistance or reduced insulin or insulin-like growth factor-1 production	
MATERNAL MEDICATIONS	
Antimetabolites (methotrexate)	
Heavy metals (mercury, lead)	
Hydantoin	
Narcotics (morphine, methadone)	
Steroids (prednisone)	
Substance and illicit drug use (alcohol, cocaine)	
Warfarin	
PLACENTAL AND UTERINE ABNORMALITIES	
Abruptio placentae	
Abnormal implantation	
Abnormal placental vessels	
Chorioangioma	
Circumvallate placenta	
Fetal vessel thrombosis	
Ischemic villus necrosis	
Multiple gestations	
True knots in umbilical cord	
Villitis (congenital infection)	

such as chorioretinitis, cataracts, glaucoma, and cloudy cornea, suggest the presence of a congenital infection or inborn error of metabolism. Infants with severe IUGR or SGA, particularly in conjunction with fetal distress, may have problems at birth that include respiratory acidosis, metabolic acidosis, asphyxia, hypoxemia, hypotension, hypoglycemia, polycythemia, meconium aspiration syndrome, and persistent pulmonary hypertension of the newborn.

Management of IUGR and SGA infants is usually symptomatic and supportive. The diagnostic evaluation at birth should be directed at identifying the cause of the IUGR and SGA, if possible. The consequences of IUGR and SGA depend on the etiology, severity, and duration of growth retardation. The mortality rates of infants who are severely affected are 5 to 20 times those of infants who are appropriate for gestational age. Postnatal growth and development depend in part on the etiology, the postnatal nutritional intake, and the social environment. Infants who have IUGR and SGA secondary to congenital infection, chromosomal abnormalities, or constitutional syndromes remain small throughout life. Infants who have growth inhibited late in gestation because of uterine constraints, placental insufficiency, or poor nutrition have catch-up growth and, under optimal environmental conditions, approach their inherited growth and development potential.

HYDROPS FETALIS

Decision-Making Algorithm
Available @ StudentConsult.com

Anemia

Hydrops fetalis is caused by immune and nonimmune conditions. Hydrops fetalis is a fetal clinical condition of excessive fluid accumulation in the skin and one or more other body compartments, including the pleural space, peritoneal cavity, pericardial sac, or placenta with resultant high morbidity and mortality. Hydrops initially was described in association with Rhesus blood group isoimmunization. The use of Rho (D) immune globulin has reduced the incidence of isoimmune fetal hydrops. Concurrently the incidence of nonimmune hydrops has increased as a cause of this severe clinical condition.

Fetal hydrops results from an imbalance of interstitial fluid accumulation and decreased removal of fluid by the capillaries and lymphatic system. Fluid accumulation can be secondary to congestive heart failure, obstructed lymphatic flow, or decreased plasma oncotic pressure (hypoproteinemic states). Edema formation is the final common pathway for many disease processes that affect the fetus, including fetal cardiac, genetic, hematologic, metabolic, infection, or malformation syndromes.

The diagnostic workup of the hydropic fetus should focus on discovering the underlying cause. Maternal findings may include hypertension, anemia, multiple gestation, thickened placenta, and polyhydramnios, whereas fetal findings may include tachycardia, ascites, scalp and body wall edema, and pleural and pericardial effusion. Invasive fetal testing may be indicated. Amniocentesis provides amniotic fluid samples for karyotype, culture, alpha-fetoprotein, and metabolic and enzyme analysis. Percutaneous umbilical cord blood sampling can provide fetal blood for chromosomal analysis and hematologic and metabolic studies and provide a source for intervention (fetal transfusion for profound anemia).

Management depends on the underlying cause and the gestational age of the fetus. Resuscitative efforts at delivery are often required. It is often necessary to remove ascitic fluid from the abdomen or pleural fluid to improve ventilation. Profound anemia necessitates immediate transfusion with packed red blood cells.

The overall mortality for infants with nonimmune hydrops is approximately 50%. If the diagnosis is made before 24 weeks

of gestation with subsequent premature delivery, the survival rate is approximately 4% to 6%.

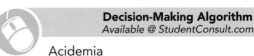

Chapter 61

RESPIRATORY DISEASES OF THE NEWBORN

Decision-Making Algorithm
Available @ StudentConsult.com

Acidemia

Respiratory distress that becomes manifested by tachypnea, intercostal retractions, reduced air exchange, cyanosis, expiratory grunting, and nasal flaring is a nonspecific response to serious illness. The differential diagnosis of respiratory distress includes pulmonary, cardiac, hematologic, infectious, anatomic, and metabolic disorders that may involve the lungs directly or indirectly. Surfactant deficiency causes **respiratory distress syndrome (RDS)**, resulting in cyanosis and tachypnea; **infection** produces pneumonia, shown by interstitial or lobar infiltrates; **meconium aspiration** results in a chemical pneumonitis with hypoxia and pulmonary hypertension; **hydrops fetalis** causes anemia and hypoalbuminemia with high-output heart failure and pulmonary edema; and congenital or acquired **pulmonary hypoplasia** causes pulmonary hypertension and pulmonary insufficiency. It also is clinically useful to differentiate the common causes of respiratory distress according to gestational age (Table 61-1).

In addition to the specific therapy for the individual disorder, supportive care and evaluation of the infant with respiratory distress can be applied to all the problems mentioned earlier (Table 61-2). Blood gas monitoring and interpretation are key components of general respiratory care.

Treatment of hypoxemia requires knowledge of normal values. In term infants, the arterial Pao_2 level is 55 to 60 mm Hg at 30 minutes of life, 75 mm Hg at 4 hours, and 90 mm Hg at 24 hours. Preterm infants have lower values. $Paco_2$ levels should be 35 to 40 mm Hg, and the pH should be 7.35 to 7.40. It is imperative that arterial blood gas analysis be performed in all infants with significant respiratory distress, whether or not cyanosis is perceived. Cyanosis becomes evident when there is 5 g of unsaturated hemoglobin; anemia may interfere with the perception of cyanosis. Jaundice also may interfere with the appearance of cyanosis. Capillary blood gas determinations are useful in determining blood pH and the $Paco_2$ level but may result in falsely low blood Pao_2 readings. Serial blood gas levels may be monitored by an indwelling arterial catheter placed in a peripheral artery or through the umbilical artery. Another method for monitoring blood gas levels is to combine capillary blood gas techniques with noninvasive methods used

Table 61-1	Etiology of Respiratory Distress

PRETERM INFANT

Respiratory distress syndrome (RDS)*

Erythroblastosis fetalis

Nonimmune hydrops

Pulmonary hemorrhage

FULL-TERM INFANT

Primary pulmonary hypertension of the neonate*

Meconium aspiration pneumonia*

Polycythemia

Amniotic fluid aspiration

PRETERM AND FULL-TERM INFANT

Bacterial sepsis (GBS)*

Transient tachypnea*

Spontaneous pneumothorax

Congenital anomalies (e.g., congenital lobar emphysema, cystic adenomatoid malformation, diaphragmatic hernia)

Congenital heart disease

Pulmonary hypoplasia

Viral infection (e.g., herpes simplex, CMV)

Inborn metabolic errors

CMV, Cytomegalovirus; *GBS*, group B streptococcus.
*Common.

Table 61-2	Initial Laboratory Evaluation of Respiratory Distress

TEST	RATIONALE
Chest radiograph	To determine reticular granular pattern of RDS; to determine presence of pneumothorax, cardiomegaly, life-threatening congenital anomalies
Arterial blood gas	To determine severity of respiratory compromise, hypoxemia, and hypercapnia and type of acidosis; severity determines treatment strategy
Complete blood count	Hemoglobin/hematocrit to determine anemia and polycythemia; white blood cell count to determine neutropenia/sepsis; platelet count and smear to determine DIC
Blood culture	To recover potential pathogen
Blood glucose	To determine presence of hypoglycemia, which may produce or occur simultaneously with respiratory distress; to determine stress hyperglycemia
Echocardiogram, ECG	In the presence of a murmur, cardiomegaly, or refractory hypoxia; to determine structural heart disease or PPHN

DIC, Disseminated intravascular coagulation; *ECG*, electrocardiogram; *PPHN*, primary pulmonary hypertension of the newborn; *RDS*, respiratory distress syndrome.

to monitor oxygen (pulse oximetry or transcutaneous oxygen diffusion).

Metabolic acidosis, defined as a reduced pH (<7.25) and bicarbonate concentration (<18 mEq/L) accompanied by a normal or low Pco_2 level, may be caused by hypoxia or by insufficient tissue perfusion. The origin of the disorder may be pulmonary, cardiac, infectious, renal, hematologic, nutritional, metabolic, or iatrogenic. The initial approach to metabolic acidosis is to determine the cause and treat the pathophysiologic problem. This approach may include, as in the sequence of therapy for hypoxia, increasing the inspired oxygen concentration; applying continuous positive airway pressure nasally; or initiating mechanical ventilation using positive end-expiratory pressure. Patients with hypotension produced by hypovolemia require fluids and may need inotropic or vasoactive drug support. If metabolic acidosis persists despite specific therapy, sodium bicarbonate (1 mEq/kg/dose) may be given by slow intravenous infusion. Near-normal or low Pco_2 levels should be documented before sodium bicarbonate infusion. The buffering effect of sodium bicarbonate results in increased Pco_2 levels, unless adequate ventilation is maintained.

Respiratory acidosis, defined as an elevated Pco_2 level and reduced pH without a reduction in the bicarbonate concentration, may be caused by pulmonary insufficiency or central hypoventilation. Most disorders producing respiratory distress can lead to hypercapnia. Treatment involves assisted ventilation but not sodium bicarbonate. If central nervous system depression of respirations is caused by placental passage of narcotic analgesics, assisted ventilation is instituted first, then the central nervous system depression is reversed by naloxone.

RESPIRATORY DISTRESS SYNDROME (HYALINE MEMBRANE DISEASE)

RDS occurs after the onset of breathing and is associated with an insufficiency of pulmonary surfactant.

Lung Development

The lining of the alveolus consists of 90% type I cells and 10% type II cells. After 20 weeks of gestation, the type II cells contain vacuolated, osmophilic, lamellar inclusion bodies, which are packages of surface-active material (Fig. 61-1). This lipoprotein surfactant is 90% lipid and is composed predominantly of saturated phosphatidylcholine (lecithin), but also contains phosphatidylglycerol, other phospholipids, and neutral lipids. The surfactant proteins, SP-A, SP-B, SP-C, and SP-D, are packaged into the lamellar body and contribute to surface-active properties and recycling of surfactant. Surfactant prevents atelectasis by reducing surface tension at low lung volumes when it is concentrated at end expiration as the alveolar radius decreases; surfactant contributes to lung recoil by increasing surface tension at larger lung volumes when it is diluted during inspiration as the alveolar radius increases. Without surfactant, surface tension forces are not reduced, and atelectasis develops during end expiration as the alveolus collapses.

The timing of surfactant production in quantities sufficient to prevent atelectasis depends on an increase in fetal cortisol levels that begins between 32 and 34 weeks of gestation. By 34 to 36 weeks, sufficient surface-active material is produced by the type II cells in the lung, is secreted into the alveolar lumen, and is excreted into the amniotic fluid. The concentration of

Air

Water

MLB

LMF

MLB

MVB

SLB

GZ

N

ER

Figure 61-1 Proposed pathway of synthesis, transport, secretion, and reuptake of surfactant in the type II alveolar cell. Phospholipids are synthesized in the smooth endoplasmic reticulum (ER). The glucose/glycerol precursor may be derived from lung glycogen or circulating glucose. Phospholipids and surfactant proteins are packaged in the Golgi apparatus (GZ), emerge as small lamellar bodies (SLB), coalesce to mature lamellar bodies (MLB), migrate to the apical membrane, and are released by exocytosis into the liquid hypophase below the air-liquid interface. The tightly coiled lamellar body unravels to form the lattice (tubular) myelin figure (LMF), the immediate precursor to the phospholipid monolayer at the alveolar surface. Reuptake by endocytosis forms multivesicular bodies (MVB) that recycle surfactant. The enzymes, receptors, transporters, and surfactant proteins are controlled by regulatory processes at the transcriptional level in the nucleus (N). Corticosteroid and thyroid hormones are regulatory ligands that may accelerate surfactant synthesis. *(From Hansen T, Corbet A: Lung development and function. In Taeusch HW, Ballard R, Avery ME, editors: Diseases of the Newborn, ed 6, Philadelphia, 1991, Saunders, p 465.)*

lecithin in amniotic fluid indicates fetal pulmonary maturity. Because the amount of lecithin is difficult to quantify, the ratio of lecithin (which increases with maturity) to sphingomyelin (which remains constant during gestation) (L/S ratio) is determined. An L/S ratio of 2:1 usually indicates pulmonary maturity. The presence of minor phospholipids, such as phosphatidylglycerol, also is indicative of fetal lung maturity and may be useful in situations in which the L/S ratio is borderline or possibly affected by maternal diabetes, which reduces lung maturity. The absence of phosphatidylglycerol suggests that surfactant might not be mature.

Clinical Manifestations

A deficiency of pulmonary surfactant (most often due to prematurity) results in atelectasis, decreased functional residual capacity, arterial hypoxemia, and respiratory distress. Surfactant synthesis may also be reduced as a result of hypovolemia, hypothermia, acidosis, hypoxemia, and rare genetic disorders of surfactant synthesis. These factors also produce pulmonary

artery vasospasm, which may contribute to RDS in larger premature infants who have developed sufficient pulmonary arteriole smooth muscle to produce vasoconstriction. Surfactant deficiency–induced atelectasis causes alveoli to be perfused but not ventilated, which results in a pulmonary shunt and hypoxemia. As atelectasis increases, the lungs become increasingly difficult to expand, and lung compliance decreases. Because the chest wall of the premature infant is very compliant, the infant attempts to overcome decreased lung compliance with increasing inspiratory pressures, resulting in retractions of the chest wall. The sequence of decreased lung compliance and chest wall retractions leads to poor air exchange, an increased physiologic dead space, alveolar hypoventilation, and hypercapnia. A cycle of hypoxia, hypercapnia, and acidosis acts on type II cells to reduce surfactant synthesis and, in some infants, on the pulmonary arterioles to produce pulmonary hypertension.

Infants at greatest risk for RDS are premature and have an immature L/S ratio. The incidence of RDS increases with decreasing gestational age. RDS develops in 30% to 60% of infants between 28 and 32 weeks of gestation. Other risk factors include delivery of a previous preterm infant with RDS, maternal diabetes, hypothermia, fetal distress, asphyxia, male sex, white race, being the second-born of twins, and delivery by cesarean section without labor.

RDS may develop immediately in the delivery room in extremely immature infants at 26 to 30 weeks of gestation. Some more mature infants (34 weeks' gestation) may not show signs of RDS until 3 to 4 hours after birth, correlating with the initial release of stored surfactant at the onset of breathing accompanied by the ongoing inability to replace the surfactant owing to inadequate stores. **Manifestations** of RDS include cyanosis, tachypnea, nasal flaring, intercostal and sternal retractions, and grunting. Grunting is caused by closure of the glottis during expiration, the effect of which is to maintain lung volume (decreasing atelectasis) and gas exchange during exhalation. Atelectasis is well documented by radiographic examination of the chest, which shows a ground-glass haze in the lung surrounding air-filled bronchi (the air bronchogram) (Fig. 61-2). Severe RDS may show an airless lung field (*whiteout*) on a radiograph, even obliterating the distinction between the atelectatic lungs and the heart.

During the first 72 hours, infants with untreated RDS have increasing distress and hypoxemia. In infants with severe RDS, the development of edema, apnea, and respiratory failure necessitates assisted ventilation. Thereafter, uncomplicated cases show a spontaneous improvement that often is heralded by diuresis and a marked resolution of edema. Complications include the development of a pneumothorax, a patent ductus arteriosus (PDA), and bronchopulmonary dysplasia (BPD). The differential diagnosis of RDS includes diseases associated with cyanosis and respiratory distress (see Table 58-10).

Prevention and Treatment

Strategies to prevent preterm birth include maternal cervical cerclage, bed rest, treatment of infections, and administration of tocolytic medications. In addition, prevention of neonatal cold stress, birth asphyxia, and hypovolemia reduces the risk of RDS. If premature delivery is unavoidable, the antenatal administration of corticosteroids (e.g., betamethasone) to the

Figure 61-2 Respiratory distress syndrome. The infant is intubated, and the lungs show a dense reticulonodular pattern with air bronchograms (**A**). To evaluate rotation on the frontal chest, the lengths of the posterior ribs are compared from left to right (*arrows*). Because the infant is supine, the side of the longer ribs indicates to which side the thorax is rotated. In this case, the left ribs are longer, and this radiograph is a left posterior oblique view. Surfactant was administered, resulting in significant improvement in the density of the lung (**B**). The right lung is slightly better aerated than the left. Uneven distribution of clearing is common. (*From Hilton S, Edwards D:* Practical Pediatric Radiology, *ed 2, Philadelphia, 1994, Saunders.*)

Table 61-3	Potential Causes of Neonatal Apnea
Central nervous system	IVH, drugs, seizures, hypoxic injury
Respiratory	Pneumonia, obstructive airway lesions, atelectasis, extreme prematurity (<1000 g), laryngeal reflex, phrenic nerve paralysis, severe RDS, pneumothorax
Infectious	Sepsis, necrotizing enterocolitis, meningitis (bacterial, fungal, viral)
Gastrointestinal	Oral feeding, bowel movement, gastroesophageal reflux, esophagitis, intestinal perforation
Metabolic	↓ Glucose, ↓ calcium, ↓ Po_2, ↓↑ sodium, ↑ ammonia, ↑ organic acids, ↑ ambient temperature, hypothermia
Cardiovascular	Hypotension, hypertension, heart failure, anemia, hypovolemia, change in vagal tone
Idiopathic	Immaturity of respiratory center, sleep state, upper airway collapse

IVH, Intraventricular hemorrhage; *RDS,* respiratory distress syndrome.

mother (and thus to the fetus) stimulates fetal lung production of surfactant; this approach requires multiple doses for at least 48 hours.

After birth, RDS may be prevented or its severity reduced by intratracheal administration of exogenous surfactant immediately after birth in the delivery room or within a few hours of birth. A mammalian-derived surfactant is currently preferred. Exogenous surfactant can be administered repeatedly during the course of RDS in patients receiving endotracheal intubation, mechanical ventilation, and oxygen therapy. Additional management includes the general supportive and ventilation care presented in Table 61-3.

The Pao_2 level should be maintained between 60 and 70 mm Hg (oxygen saturation 90%), and the pH should be maintained above 7.25. An increased concentration of warm and humidified inspired oxygen administered by a nasal cannula or an oxygen hood may be all that is needed for larger premature infants. If hypoxemia (Pao_2 <50 mm Hg) is present, and the needed inspired oxygen concentration is 70% to 100%, nasal continuous positive airway pressure should be added at

a distending pressure of 8 to 10 cm H_2O. If respiratory failure ensues (Pco_2 >60 mm Hg, pH <7.20, and Pao_2 <50 mm Hg with 100% oxygen), assisted ventilation using a ventilator is indicated. Conventional rate (25 to 60 breaths/min), high-frequency jet (150 to 600 breaths/min), and oscillatory (900 to 3000 breaths/min) ventilators all have been successful in managing respiratory failure caused by severe RDS. Suggested starting settings on a conventional ventilator are fraction of inspired oxygen, 0.60 to 1.0; peak inspiratory pressure, 20 to 25 cm H_2O; positive end-expiratory pressure, 5 cm H_2O; and respiratory rate, 30 to 50 breaths/min.

In response to persistent hypercapnia, alveolar ventilation (tidal volume − dead space × rate) must be increased. Ventilation can be increased by an increase in the ventilator's rate or an increase in the tidal volume (the gradient between peak inspiratory pressure and positive end-expiratory pressure using a pressure-controlled ventilator). In response to hypoxia, the inspired oxygen content may be increased. Alternatively, the degree of oxygenation depends on the mean airway pressure. Mean airway pressure is directly related to positive end-expiratory pressure, flow, and inspiratory time. Increased mean airway pressure may improve oxygenation by improving lung volume, enhancing ventilation-perfusion matching. Because of the difficulty in distinguishing sepsis and pneumonia from RDS, broad-spectrum parenteral antibiotics (ampicillin and gentamicin) are administered for 48 to 72 hours, pending the recovery of an organism from a previously obtained blood culture.

COMPLICATIONS OF RESPIRATORY DISTRESS SYNDROME
Patent Ductus Arteriosus

Decision-Making Algorithm
Available @ StudentConsult.com

Heart Murmurs

PDA is a common complication that occurs in many low birth weight infants who have RDS. The incidence of PDA is inversely related to the maturity of the infant. In term newborns, the ductus closes within 24 to 48 hours after birth. However, in preterm newborns, the ductus frequently fails to close, requiring medical or surgical closure. The ductus arteriosus in a preterm infant is less responsive to vasoconstrictive stimuli, which, when complicated with hypoxemia during RDS, may lead to a persistent PDA that creates a shunt between the pulmonary and systemic circulations.

During the acute phase of RDS, hypoxia, hypercapnia, and acidosis lead to pulmonary arterial vasoconstriction. The pulmonary and systemic pressures may be equal, and flow through the ductus may be small or bidirectional. When RDS improves and pulmonary vascular resistance declines, flow through the ductus arteriosus increases in a left-to-right direction. Significant systemic-to-pulmonary shunting may lead to heart failure and pulmonary edema. Excessive intravenous fluid administration may increase the incidence of symptomatic PDA. The infant's respiratory status deteriorates because of increased lung fluid, hypercapnia, and hypoxemia.

Clinical manifestations of a PDA usually become apparent on day 2 to 4 of life. Because the left-to-right shunt directs flow to a low-pressure circulation from one of high pressure, the pulse pressure widens; a previously inactive precordium shows an extremely active precordial impulse, and peripheral pulses become easily palpable and bounding. The murmur of a PDA may be continuous in systole and diastole, but usually only the systolic component is auscultated. Heart failure and pulmonary edema result in rales and hepatomegaly. A chest radiograph shows cardiomegaly and pulmonary edema; a two-dimensional echocardiogram shows ductal patency; and Doppler studies show markedly increased left-to-right flow through the ductus.

Treatment of a PDA during RDS involves initial fluid restriction and diuretic administration. If there is no improvement after 24 to 48 hours, a prostaglandin synthetase inhibitor, indomethacin or ibuprofen, is administered. Contraindications to using indomethacin include thrombocytopenia (platelets <50,000/mm³), bleeding, serum creatinine measuring more than 1.8 mg/dL, and oliguria. Because 20% to 30% of infants do not respond initially to indomethacin and because the PDA reopens in 10% to 20% of infants, a repeat course of indomethacin or surgical ligation is required in some patients.

Pulmonary Air Leaks

Assisted ventilation with high peak inspiratory pressures and positive end-expiratory pressures may cause overdistention of alveoli in localized areas of the lung. Rupture of the alveolar epithelial lining may produce pulmonary interstitial emphysema as gas dissects along the interstitial space and the peribronchial lymphatics. Extravasation of gas into the parenchyma reduces lung compliance and worsens respiratory failure. Gas dissection into the mediastinal space produces a pneumomediastinum, occasionally dissecting into the subcutaneous tissues around the neck, causing subcutaneous emphysema.

Alveolar rupture adjacent to the pleural space produces a **pneumothorax** (Fig. 61-3). If the gas is under tension, the pneumothorax shifts the mediastinum to the opposite side of the chest, producing hypotension, hypoxia, and hypercapnia.

Figure 61-3 Pneumothorax. Right-sided hyperlucent pleural air is obvious. The findings of linear interstitial air and the resultant noncompliant but collapsed lung are noted. *(From Heller RM, Kirchner SG: Advanced exercises in diagnostic radiology: the newborn, Philadelphia, WB Saunders, 1979.)*

The diagnosis of a pneumothorax may be based on unequal transillumination of the chest and may be confirmed by chest radiograph. Treatment of a symptomatic pneumothorax requires insertion of a pleural chest tube connected to negative pressure or to an underwater drain. Prophylactic or therapeutic use of exogenous surfactant has reduced the incidence of pulmonary air leaks.

Pneumothorax also is observed after vigorous resuscitation, meconium aspiration pneumonia, pulmonary hypoplasia, and diaphragmatic hernia. Spontaneous pneumothorax is seen in fewer than 1% of deliveries and may be associated with renal malformations.

Bronchopulmonary Dysplasia (Chronic Lung Disease)

BPD is a clinical diagnosis defined by oxygen dependence at 36 weeks' postconceptual age and accompanied by characteristic clinical and radiographic findings that correspond to anatomic abnormalities. Oxygen concentrations greater than 40% are toxic to the neonatal lung. Oxygen-mediated lung injury results from the generation of superoxides, hydrogen peroxide, and oxygen free radicals, which disrupt membrane lipids. Assisted ventilation with high peak pressures produces barotrauma, compounding the damaging effects of highly inspired oxygen levels. In most patients, BPD develops after ventilation for RDS that may have been complicated by PDA or pulmonary interstitial emphysema. Inflammation from prolonged assisted ventilation and repeated systemic and pulmonary infections may play a major role. Failure of RDS to improve after 2 weeks, the need for prolonged mechanical ventilation, and oxygen therapy required at 36 weeks' postconceptual age are characteristic of patients with RDS in whom BPD develops. BPD also may develop in infants weighing less than 1000 g who require mechanical ventilation for poor respiratory drive in the absence of RDS. Fifty percent of infants of 24 to 26 weeks' gestational age require oxygen at 36 weeks' corrected age.

The **radiographic appearance** of BPD is characterized initially by lung opacification and subsequently by development of cysts accompanied by areas of overdistention and atelectasis, giving the lung a spongelike appearance. The histopathology of BPD reveals interstitial edema, atelectasis, mucosal metaplasia, interstitial fibrosis, necrotizing obliterative bronchiolitis, and overdistended alveoli.

The **clinical manifestations** of BPD are oxygen dependence, hypercapnia with a compensatory metabolic alkalosis, pulmonary hypertension, poor growth, and development of right-sided heart failure. Increased airway resistance with reactive airway bronchoconstriction also is noted and is treated with bronchodilating agents. Severe chest retractions produce negative interstitial pressure that draws fluid into the interstitial space. Together with cor pulmonale, these chest retractions cause fluid retention, necessitating fluid restriction and the administration of diuretics.

Patients with severe BPD may need treatment with mechanical ventilation for many months. To reduce the risk of subglottic stenosis, a tracheotomy may be indicated. To reduce oxygen toxicity and barotrauma, ventilator settings are reduced to maintain blood gases with slightly lower Pao_2 (50 mm Hg) and higher $Paco_2$ (50 to 75 mm Hg) levels than for infants during the acute phase of RDS. Dexamethasone therapy may reduce inflammation, improve pulmonary function, and enhance weaning of patients from assisted ventilation. However, dexamethasone may increase the risk of cerebral palsy or abnormal neuromotor developmental outcome. Older survivors of BPD have hyperinflation, reactive airways, and developmental delay. They are at risk for severe respiratory syncytial virus pneumonia and as infants should receive prophylaxis against respiratory syncytial virus.

Retinopathy of Prematurity (Retrolental Fibroplasia)

Decision-Making Algorithm
Available @ StudentConsult.com

Visual Impairment and Leukocoria

Retinopathy of prematurity (ROP) is caused by the acute and chronic effects of oxygen toxicity on the developing blood vessels of the premature infant's retina. The completely vascularized retina of the term infant is not susceptible to ROP. ROP is a leading cause of blindness in very low birth weight infants (<1500 g). Excessive arterial oxygen tensions produce vasoconstriction of immature retinal vasculature in the first stage of this disease. Vaso-obliteration follows if the duration and extent of hyperoxia are prolonged beyond the time when vasoconstriction is reversible. Hypercarbia and hypoxia may contribute to ROP. The subsequent proliferative stages are characterized by extraretinal fibrovascular proliferation, forming a ridge between the vascular and avascular portions of the retina, and by the development of neovascular tufts. In mild cases, vasoproliferation is noted at the periphery of the retina. Severe cases may have neovascularization involving the entire retina, retinal detachment resulting from traction on vessels as they leave the optic disc, fibrous proliferation behind the lens producing leukokoria, and synechiae displacing the lens

forward, leading to glaucoma. Both eyes usually are involved, but severity may be asymmetrical.

The incidence of ROP may be reduced by careful monitoring of arterial blood gas levels in all patients receiving oxygen. Although there is no absolutely safe Pao_2 level, it is wise to keep the arterial oxygen level between 50 and 70 mm Hg in premature infants. Infants who weigh less than 1500 g or who are born before 28 weeks' gestational age (some authors say 32 weeks) should be screened when they are 4 weeks of age or more than 34 weeks' corrected gestational age, whichever comes first. Laser therapy or (less often) cryotherapy may be used for vitreous hemorrhage or for severe, progressive vasoproliferation. Surgery is indicated for retinal detachment. Less severe stages of ROP resolve spontaneously and without visual impairment in most patients.

TRANSIENT TACHYPNEA OF THE NEWBORN

Transient tachypnea of the newborn is a self-limited condition characterized by tachypnea, mild retractions, hypoxia, and occasional grunting, usually without signs of severe respiratory distress. Cyanosis, when present, usually requires treatment with supplemental oxygen in the range of 30% to 40%. Transient tachypnea of the newborn usually is noted in larger premature infants and in term infants born by precipitous delivery or cesarean section without prior labor. Infants of diabetic mothers and infants with poor respiratory drive as a result of placental passage of analgesic drugs are at risk. Transient tachypnea of the newborn may be caused by retained lung fluid or slow resorption of lung fluid. Chest radiographs show prominent central vascular markings, fluid in the lung fissures, overaeration, and occasionally a small pleural effusion. Air bronchograms and a reticulogranular pattern are not seen; their presence suggests another pulmonary process, such as RDS or pneumonia.

MECONIUM ASPIRATION SYNDROME

Meconium-stained amniotic fluid is seen in 15% of predominantly term and post-term deliveries. Although the passage of meconium into amniotic fluid is common in infants born in the breech presentation, meconium-stained fluid should be considered clinically as a sign of fetal distress in all infants. The presence of meconium in the amniotic fluid suggests in utero distress with asphyxia, hypoxia, and acidosis.

Aspiration of amniotic fluid contaminated with particulate meconium may occur in utero in a distressed, gasping fetus; more often, meconium is aspirated into the lung immediately after delivery. Affected infants have abnormal chest radiographs, showing a high incidence of pneumonia and pneumothoraces.

Meconium aspiration pneumonia is characterized by tachypnea, hypoxia, hypercapnia, and small airway obstruction causing a ball-valve effect, leading to air trapping, overdistention, and extra-alveolar air leaks. Complete small airway obstruction produces atelectasis. Within 24 to 48 hours, a chemical pneumonitis develops in addition to the mechanical effects of airway obstruction. Abnormal pulmonary function may be caused by the meconium, in part, through inactivation of surfactant. Primary pulmonary hypertension of the newborn (PPHN) frequently accompanies meconium aspiration, with right-to-left shunting caused by increased pulmonary vascular resistance. The chest radiograph reveals patchy infiltrates, overdistention, flattening of the diaphragm, increased anteroposterior diameter, and a high incidence of pneumomediastinum and pneumothoraces. Comorbid diseases include those associated with in utero asphyxia that initiated the passage of meconium.

Treatment of meconium aspiration includes general supportive care and assisted ventilation. Infants with a PPHN-like presentation should be treated for PPHN. If severe hypoxia does not subside with conventional or high-frequency ventilation, surfactant therapy, and inhaled nitric oxide, extracorporeal membrane oxygenation (ECMO) may be beneficial.

Prevention of meconium aspiration syndrome involves careful in utero monitoring to prevent asphyxia. When meconium-stained fluid is observed, the obstetrician should suction the infant's oropharynx before delivering the rest of the infant's body. If the infant is depressed with poor tone, minimal respiratory effort, and cyanosis, the infant's oropharynx should be suctioned, the vocal cords visualized, and the area below the vocal cords suctioned to remove any meconium from the trachea. Saline intrauterine amnioinfusion during labor may reduce the incidence of aspiration and pneumonia.

PRIMARY PULMONARY HYPERTENSION OF THE NEWBORN

PPHN occurs in post-term, term, or near-term infants. PPHN is characterized by severe hypoxemia, without evidence of parenchymal lung or structural heart disease. PPHN is often seen with asphyxia or meconium-stained fluid. The chest radiograph usually reveals normal lung fields rather than the expected infiltrates and hyperinflation that may accompany meconium aspiration. Additional problems that may lead to PPHN are congenital pneumonia, hyperviscosity-polycythemia, congenital diaphragmatic hernia, pulmonary hypoplasia, congenital cyanotic heart disease, hypoglycemia, and hypothermia. Total anomalous venous return associated with obstruction of blood flow may produce a clinical picture that involves severe hypoxia and that is initially indistinguishable from PPHN; however, a chest radiograph reveals severe pulmonary venous engorgement and a small heart. Echocardiography or cardiac catheterization confirms the diagnosis.

Significant right-to-left shunting through a patent foramen ovale, through a PDA, and through intrapulmonary channels is characteristic of PPHN. The pulmonary vasculature often shows hypertrophied arterial wall smooth muscle, suggesting that the process of or predisposition to PPHN began in utero as a result of previous periods of fetal hypoxia. After birth, hypoxia, hypercapnia, and acidosis exacerbate pulmonary artery vasoconstriction, leading to further hypoxia and acidosis. Some infants with PPHN have extrapulmonary manifestations as a result of asphyxia. Myocardial injuries include heart failure, transient mitral insufficiency, and papillary muscle or myocardial infarction. Thrombocytopenia, right atrial thrombi, and pulmonary embolism also may be noted.

The **diagnosis** is confirmed by echocardiographic examination, which shows elevated pulmonary artery pressures and sites of right-to-left shunting. Echocardiography also rules out structural congenital heart disease and transient myocardial dysfunction.

Treatment involves general supportive care; correction of hypotension, anemia, and acidosis; and management of complications associated with asphyxia. If myocardial dysfunction is present, dopamine or dobutamine is needed. The most important therapy for PPHN is assisted ventilation. Reversible mild pulmonary hypertension may respond to conventional assisted ventilation. Patients with severe PPHN do not always respond to conventional therapy. Paralysis with a muscle relaxant may be needed to assist vigorous ventilation. Surfactant replacement seems to have no effect when PPHN is the primary diagnosis. If mechanical ventilation and supportive care are unsuccessful in improving oxygenation, inhaled nitric oxide, a selective pulmonary artery vasodilating agent, should be administered. If hypoxia persists, the patient may be a candidate for ECMO. Infants who require extremely high ventilator settings, marked by an alveolar-to-arterial oxygen gradient greater than 620 mm Hg, have a high mortality rate and benefit from ECMO if they do not respond to nitric oxide. In addition, the oxygenation index (OI) is used to assess the severity of hypoxemia and to guide the timing of interventions such as inhaled nitric oxide and ECMO. The OI is calculated using the equation OI = [(mean airway pressure × fraction of inspired oxygen)/Pao$_2$] × 100. A high OI indicates severe hypoxemic respiratory failure.

APNEA OF PREMATURITY

Decision-Making Algorithm
Available @ StudentConsult.com

Apnea

Although apnea typically is associated with immaturity of the respiratory control system, it also may be the presenting sign of other diseases or pathophysiologic states that affect preterm infants (see Table 61-3). A thorough consideration of possible causes is always warranted, especially with the onset or unexpected increase in the frequency of episodes of apnea (or bradycardia).

Apnea is defined as the cessation of pulmonary airflow for a specific time interval, usually longer than 10 to 20 seconds. Bradycardia often accompanies prolonged apnea. **Central apnea** refers to a complete cessation of airflow and respiratory efforts with no chest wall movement. **Obstructive apnea** refers to the absence of noticeable airflow but with the continuation of chest wall movements. **Mixed apnea**, a combination of these two events, is the most frequent type. It may begin as a brief episode of obstruction followed by a central apnea. Alternatively, central apnea may produce upper airway closure (passive pharyngeal hypotonia), resulting in mixed apnea.

A careful evaluation to determine the cause of apnea should be performed immediately in any infant with apnea. The incidence of apnea increases as gestational age decreases. Idiopathic apnea, a disease of premature infants, appears in the absence of any other identifiable disease states during the first week of life and usually resolves by 36 to 40 weeks of postconceptual age (gestational age at birth + postnatal age). The premature infant's process of regulating respiration is especially vulnerable to apnea. Preterm infants respond paradoxically to hypoxia by developing apnea rather than by increasing respirations as in mature infants. Poor tone of the laryngeal muscles also may lead to collapse of the upper airway, causing obstruction. Isolated obstructive apnea also may occur as a result of flexion or extreme lateral positioning of the premature infant's head, which obstructs the soft trachea.

Treatment of apnea of prematurity involves administration of oxygen to hypoxic infants, transfusion of anemic infants, and physical cutaneous stimulation for infants with mild apnea. Methylxanthines (caffeine or theophylline) are the mainstay of pharmacologic treatment of apnea. Xanthine therapy increases minute ventilation, improves the carbon dioxide sensitivity, decreases hypoxic depression of breathing, enhances diaphragmatic activity, and decreases periodic breathing. Treatment usually is initiated with a loading dose followed by maintenance therapy. High-flow nasal cannula therapy and nasal continuous positive airway pressure of 4 to 6 cm H_2O also are effective and relatively safe methods of treating obstructive or mixed apneas; they may work by stimulating the infant and splinting the upper airway. Continuous positive airway pressure also probably increases functional residual capacity, improving oxygenation.

Chapter **62**

ANEMIA AND HYPERBILIRUBINEMIA

ANEMIA

Embryonic hematopoiesis begins by the 20th day of gestation and is evidenced as blood islands in the yolk sac. In midgestation, erythropoiesis occurs in the liver and spleen; the bone marrow becomes the predominant site in the last trimester. Hemoglobin concentration increases from 8 to 10 g/dL at 12 weeks to 16.5 to 18 g/dL at 40 weeks. Fetal red blood cell (RBC) production is responsive to erythropoietin; the concentration of this hormone increases with fetal hypoxia and anemia.

After birth, hemoglobin levels increase transiently at 6 to 12 hours, then decline to 11 to 12 g/dL at 3 to 6 months. A premature infant (<32 weeks' gestational age) has a lower hemoglobin concentration and a more rapid postnatal decline of hemoglobin level, which achieves a nadir 1 to 2 months after birth. Fetal and neonatal RBCs have a shorter life span (70 to 90 days) and a higher mean corpuscular volume (110 to 120 fL) than adult cells. In the fetus, hemoglobin synthesis in the last two trimesters of pregnancy produces fetal hemoglobin (hemoglobin F), composed of two alpha chains and two gamma chains. Immediately before term, the infant begins to synthesize beta-hemoglobin chains; the term infant should have some adult hemoglobin (two alpha chains and two beta chains). Fetal hemoglobin represents 60% to 90% of hemoglobin at term birth. The levels decline to adult levels of less than 5% by 4 months of age.

For a term infant, blood volume is 72 to 93 mL/kg, and for a preterm infant, blood volume is 90 to 100 mL/kg. The placenta and umbilical vessels contain approximately 20 to 30 mL/kg

of additional blood that can increase neonatal blood volume and hemoglobin levels transiently for the first 3 days of life if clamping or milking (*stripping*) of the umbilical cord is delayed at birth. Delayed clamping may increase the risk of polycythemia and jaundice, but it improves glomerular filtration. Early clamping may lead to anemia, a cardiac murmur, poor peripheral perfusion, and less tachypnea. Hydrostatic pressure affects blood transfer between the placenta and the infant at birth. An undesired fetal-to-placental transfusion occurs if the infant is situated above the level of the placenta.

The physiologic anemia noted at 2 to 3 months of age in term infants and at 1 to 2 months of age in preterm infants is a normal process that does not result in signs of illness and does not require any treatment. It is a physiologic condition believed to be related to several factors, including increased tissue oxygenation experienced at birth, shortened RBC life span, and low erythropoietin levels.

Etiology

Decision-Making Algorithms
Available @ StudentConsult.com

Gastrointestinal Bleeding
Anemia
Bleeding
Petechiae/Purpura
Pancytopenia

Symptomatic anemia in the newborn period (Fig. 62-1) may be caused by decreased RBC production, increased RBC destruction, or blood loss.

Decreased Red Blood Cell Production

Anemia caused by decreased production of RBCs appears at birth with pallor, a low reticulocyte count, and absence of erythroid precursors in the bone marrow. Potential causes of neonatal decreased RBC production include bone marrow failure syndromes (congenital RBC aplasia [Diamond-Blackfan anemia]), infection (congenital viral infections [parvovirus, rubella], acquired bacterial or viral sepsis), nutritional deficiencies (protein, iron, folate, vitamin B_{12}), and congenital leukemia.

Increased Red Blood Cell Destruction

Immunologically mediated hemolysis in utero may lead to **erythroblastosis fetalis,** or the fetus may be spared and **hemolytic disease** may appear in the newborn. Hemolysis of fetal erythrocytes is a result of blood group differences between the sensitized mother and fetus, which causes production of maternal IgG antibodies directed against an antigen on fetal cells.

ABO blood group incompatibility with neonatal hemolysis develops only if the mother has IgG antibodies from a previous exposure to A or B antigens. These IgG antibodies cross the placenta by active transport and affect the fetus or newborn. Sensitization of the mother to fetal antigens may have occurred by previous transfusions or by conditions of pregnancy that result in transfer of fetal erythrocytes into the

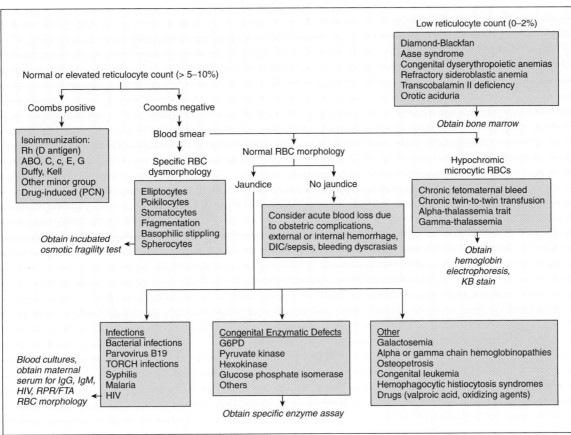

Figure 62-1 Differential diagnosis of neonatal anemia. The physician obtains information from the family, maternal and labor and delivery histories, and laboratory tests, including hemoglobin, reticulocyte count, blood type, direct Coombs test, peripheral smear, red blood cell (RBC) indices, and bilirubin concentration. *DIC,* Disseminated intravascular coagulation; *FTA,* fluorescent treponemal antibody test; *G6PD,* glucose-6-phosphate dehydrogenase; *HIV,* human immunodeficiency virus; *KB,* Kleihauer-Betke; *PCN,* penicillin; *RPR,* rapid plasma reagin tests; *TORCH,* toxoplasmosis, other, rubella, cytomegalovirus, herpes simplex. *(From Ohls RK: Anemia in the neonate. In Christensen RD, editor:* Hematologic problems of the neonate, *Philadelphia, 2000, Saunders, p 162.)*

maternal circulation, such as first-trimester abortion, ectopic pregnancy, amniocentesis, manual extraction of the placenta, version (external or internal) procedures, or normal pregnancy.

ABO incompatibility with sensitization usually does not cause fetal disease other than extremely mild anemia. It may produce **hemolytic disease of the newborn,** which is manifested as significant anemia and hyperbilirubinemia. Because many mothers who have blood group O have IgG antibodies to A and B before pregnancy, the firstborn infant of A or B blood type may be affected. In contrast to Rh disease, ABO hemolytic disease does not become more severe with subsequent pregnancies. Hemolysis with ABO incompatibility is less severe than hemolysis in Rh-sensitized pregnancy, either because the anti-A or anti-B antibody may bind to nonerythrocytic cells that contain A or B antigen or because fetal erythrocytes have fewer A or B antigenic determinants than they have Rh sites. With the declining incidence of Rh hemolytic disease, ABO incompatibility has become the most common cause of neonatal hyperbilirubinemia requiring therapy—currently accounting for approximately 20% of clinically significant jaundice in the newborn.

Erythroblastosis fetalis classically is caused by Rh blood group incompatibility. Most Rh-negative women have no anti-Rh antibodies at the time of their first pregnancy. The Rh antigen system consists of five antigens: C, D, E, c, and e;

the d type is not antigenic. In most Rh-sensitized cases, the D antigen of the fetus sensitizes the Rh-negative (d) mother, resulting in IgG antibody production during the first pregnancy. Because most mothers are not sensitized to Rh antigens at the start of pregnancy, Rh erythroblastosis fetalis is usually a disease of the second and subsequent pregnancies. The first affected pregnancy results in an antibody response in the mother, which may be detected during antenatal screening with the Coombs test and determined to be anti D antibody. The first affected newborn may show no serious fetal disease and may manifest hemolytic disease of the newborn only by the development of anemia and hyperbilirubinemia. Subsequent pregnancies result in an increasing severity of response because of an earlier onset of hemolysis in utero. Fetal anemia, heart failure, elevated venous pressure, portal vein obstruction, and hypoalbuminemia result in **fetal hydrops,** which is characterized by ascites, pleural and pericardial effusions, and anasarca (see Chapter 60). The risk of fetal death is high.

The **management** of a pregnancy complicated by Rh sensitization depends on the severity of hemolysis, its effects on the fetus, and the maturity of the fetus at the time it becomes affected. The severity of the hemolysis can be assessed by the quantity of bilirubin transferred from the fetus to the amniotic fluid, quantified by spectrophotometric analysis of the optical density (at 450 nm) of amniotic fluid.

Three zones of optical densities with decreasing slopes toward term gestation have been developed to predict the severity of the illness. The high optical density zone 3 is associated with severe hemolysis. Fetuses in the lower zones probably are not affected. If a fetus's optical density measurement for bilirubin falls into zone 3, and the fetus has pulmonary maturity as determined by the lecithin-to-sphingomyelin ratio, the infant should be delivered and treated in the neonatal intensive care unit. If the lungs are immature and the fetus is between 22 and 33 weeks of gestational age, an ultrasound-guided intrauterine transfusion with O-negative blood into the umbilical vein is indicated and may have to be repeated until pulmonary maturity is reached or fetal distress is detected. Indications for fetal intravascular transfusion in sensitized fetuses between 22 and 32 weeks of gestational age include a fetal hematocrit of less than 25% to 30%, fetal hydrops, and fetal distress too early in gestation for delivery. Intravascular intrauterine transfusion corrects fetal anemia, improves the outcome of severe hydrops, and reduces the need for postnatal exchange transfusion, but is associated with neonatal anemia as a result of continued hemolysis plus suppressed erythropoiesis.

Prevention of sensitization of the mother carrying an Rh-positive fetus is possible by treating the mother during gestation (>28 weeks' gestational age) and within 72 hours after birth with anti-Rh-positive immune globulin (RhoGAM). The dose of RhoGAM (300 µg) is based on the ability of this amount of anti-Rh-positive antibody to bind all the possible fetal Rh-positive erythrocytes entering the maternal circulation during the fetal-to-maternal transfusion at birth (approximately 30 mL). RhoGAM may bind Rh-positive fetal erythrocytes or interfere with maternal anti-Rh-positive antibody production by another, unknown mechanism. RhoGAM is effective only in preventing sensitization to the D antigen. Other blood group antigens that can cause immune hydrops and erythroblastosis include Rh C, E, Kell, and Duffy. Anti-Kell alloimmunity produces lower amniotic bilirubin levels and a lower reticulocyte count because, in addition to hemolysis, it inhibits erythropoiesis.

Nonimmune causes of hemolysis in the newborn include RBC enzyme deficiencies of the Embden-Meyerhof pathway, such as pyruvate kinase or glucose-6-phosphate dehydrogenase deficiency. RBC membrane disorders are another cause of nonimmune hemolysis. Hereditary spherocytosis is inherited as a severe autosomal recessive form or less severe autosomal dominant form and is the result of a deficiency of spectrin, a protein of the RBC membrane. Hemoglobinopathies, such as thalassemia, are another cause of nonimmunologically mediated hemolysis.

Blood Loss

Decision-Making Algorithms
Available @ StudentConsult.com

Gastrointestinal Bleeding
Bleeding

Anemia from blood loss at birth is manifested by two patterns of presentation, depending on the rapidity of blood loss. **Acute blood loss** after fetal-maternal hemorrhage, rupture of the umbilical cord, placenta previa, or internal hemorrhage

(hepatic or splenic hematoma; retroperitoneal) is characterized by pallor, diminished peripheral pulses, and shock. There are no signs of extramedullary hematopoiesis and no hepatosplenomegaly. The hemoglobin content and serum iron levels initially are normal, but the hemoglobin levels decline during the subsequent 24 hours. Newborns with **chronic blood loss** caused by chronic fetal-maternal hemorrhage or a twin-to-twin transfusion present with marked pallor, heart failure, hepatosplenomegaly with or without hydrops, a low hemoglobin level at birth, a hypochromic microcytic blood smear, and decreased serum iron stores. Fetal-maternal bleeding occurs in 50% to 75% of all pregnancies, with fetal blood losses ranging from 1 to 50 mL; most blood losses are 1 mL or less, 1 in 400 are approximately 30 mL, and 1 in 2000 are approximately 100 mL.

The diagnosis of fetal-maternal hemorrhage is confirmed by the Kleihauer-Betke acid elution test. Pink fetal RBCs are observed and counted in the mother's peripheral blood smear because fetal hemoglobin is resistant to acid elution; adult hemoglobin is eluted, leaving discolored maternal cells (patients with sickle cell anemia or hereditary persistence of fetal hemoglobin may have a false-positive result, and ABO incompatibility may produce a false-negative result).

Diagnosis and Management

Hemolysis in utero resulting from any cause may produce a spectrum of clinical manifestations at birth. Severe hydrops with anasarca, heart failure, and pulmonary edema may prevent adequate ventilation at birth, resulting in asphyxia. Infants affected with hemolysis in utero have hepatosplenomegaly and pallor and become jaundiced within the first 24 hours after birth. Less severely affected infants manifest pallor and hepatosplenomegaly at birth and become jaundiced subsequently. Patients with ABO incompatibility often are asymptomatic and show no physical signs at birth; mild anemia with jaundice develops during the first 24 to 72 hours of life.

Because hydrops, anemia, or jaundice are secondary to many diverse causes of hemolysis, a laboratory evaluation is needed in all patients with suspected hemolysis. A complete blood count, blood smear, reticulocyte count, blood type, and direct Coombs test (to determine the presence of antibody-coated RBCs) should be performed in the initial evaluation of all infants with hemolysis. Reduced hemoglobin levels, reticulocytosis, and a blood smear characterized by polychromasia and anisocytosis are expected with isoimmune hemolysis. Spherocytes commonly are observed in ABO incompatibility. The determination of the blood type and the Coombs test identify the responsible antigen and antibody in immunologically mediated hemolysis.

In the absence of a positive Coombs test and blood group differences between the mother and fetus, other causes of nonimmune hemolysis must be considered. RBC enzyme assays, hemoglobin electrophoresis, or RBC membrane tests (osmotic fragility, spectrin assay) should be performed. Internal hemorrhage also may be associated with anemia, reticulocytosis, and jaundice when the hemorrhage reabsorbs; ultrasound evaluation of the brain, liver, spleen, or adrenal gland may be indicated when nonimmune hemolysis is suspected. Shock is more typical in patients with internal hemorrhage, whereas in hemolytic diseases, heart failure may be seen with severe anemia. Evaluation of a possible fetal-maternal hemorrhage should include the Kleihauer-Betke test.

The **treatment** of *symptomatic* neonatal anemia is transfusion of cross-matched packed RBCs. If immune hemolysis is present, the cells to be transfused must be cross-matched against maternal and neonatal plasma. Acute volume loss may necessitate resuscitation with nonblood products, such as saline if blood is not available; packed RBCs can be given subsequently. To correct anemia and any remaining blood volume deficit, 10 to 15 mL/kg of packed RBCs should be sufficient. Cytomegalovirus-seronegative blood should be given to cytomegalovirus-seronegative infants, and all blood products should be irradiated to reduce the risk of graft-versus-host disease; blood should be screened for HIV, hepatitis B and C, and syphilis. Recombinant erythropoietin may improve the hematocrit in infants with a hyporegenerative anemia after in utero transfusion.

HYPERBILIRUBINEMIA

Hemolytic disease of the newborn is a common cause of neonatal jaundice. Nonetheless, because of the immaturity of the pathways of bilirubin metabolism, many newborn infants without evidence of hemolysis become jaundiced.

Bilirubin is produced by the catabolism of hemoglobin in the reticuloendothelial system. The tetrapyrrole ring of heme is cleaved by heme oxygenase to form equivalent quantities of biliverdin and carbon monoxide. Because no other biologic source of carbon monoxide exists, the excretion of this gas is stoichiometrically identical to the production of bilirubin. Biliverdin is converted to bilirubin by biliverdin reductase. One gram of hemoglobin produces 35 mg of bilirubin. Sources of bilirubin other than circulating hemoglobin represent 20% of bilirubin production; these sources include inefficient (shunt) hemoglobin production and lysis of precursor cells in bone marrow. Compared with adults, newborns have a twofold to threefold greater rate of bilirubin production (6 to 10 mg/kg/24 hr versus 3 mg/kg/24 hr). This increased production is caused, in part, by an increased RBC mass (higher hematocrit) and a shortened erythrocyte life span of 70 to 90 days compared with the 120-day erythrocyte life span in adults.

Bilirubin produced after hemoglobin catabolism is lipid soluble and unconjugated and reacts as an indirect reagent in the van den Bergh test. Indirect-reacting, unconjugated bilirubin is toxic to the central nervous system and is insoluble in water, limiting its excretion. Unconjugated bilirubin binds to albumin on specific bilirubin binding sites; 1 g of albumin binds 8.5 mg of bilirubin in a newborn. If the binding sites become saturated or if a competitive compound binds at the site, displacing bound bilirubin, free bilirubin becomes available to enter the central nervous system. Organic acids such as free fatty acids and drugs such as sulfisoxazole can displace bilirubin from its binding site on albumin.

Bilirubin dissociates from albumin at the hepatocyte and becomes bound to a cytoplasmic liver protein Y (ligandin). Hepatic conjugation results in the production of bilirubin diglucuronide, which is water soluble and capable of biliary and renal excretion. The enzyme glucuronosyltransferase represents the rate-limiting step of bilirubin conjugation. The concentrations of ligandin and glucuronosyltransferase are lower in newborns, particularly in premature infants, than in older children.

Conjugated bilirubin gives a direct reaction in the van den Bergh test. Most conjugated bilirubin is excreted through the bile into the small intestine and eliminated in the stool. Some bilirubin may undergo hydrolysis back to the unconjugated fraction by intestinal glucuronidase, however, and may be reabsorbed (enterohepatic recirculation). In addition, bacteria in the neonatal intestine convert bilirubin to urobilinogen and stercobilinogen, which are excreted in urine and stool and usually limit bilirubin reabsorption. Delayed passage of meconium, which contains bilirubin, also may contribute to the enterohepatic recirculation of bilirubin.

Bilirubin is produced in utero by the normal fetus and by the fetus affected by erythroblastosis fetalis. Indirect, unconjugated, lipid-soluble fetal bilirubin is transferred across the placenta and becomes conjugated by maternal hepatic enzymes. The placenta is impermeable to conjugated water-soluble bilirubin. Fetal bilirubin levels become only mildly elevated in the presence of severe hemolysis, but may increase when hemolysis produces fetal hepatic inspissated bile stasis and conjugated hyperbilirubinemia. Maternal indirect (but not direct) hyperbilirubinemia also may increase fetal bilirubin levels.

Etiology of Indirect Unconjugated Hyperbilirubinemia

Decision-Making Algorithm
Available @ StudentConsult.com

Jaundice

Physiologic jaundice is a common cause of hyperbilirubinemia among newborns. It is a diagnosis of exclusion, made after careful evaluation has ruled out more serious causes of jaundice, such as hemolysis, infection, and metabolic diseases. Physiologic jaundice is the result of many factors that are normal physiologic characteristics of newborns: increased bilirubin production resulting from an increased RBC mass, shortened RBC life span, and hepatic immaturity of ligandin and glucuronosyltransferase. Physiologic jaundice may be exaggerated among infants of Greek and Asian ancestry.

The clinical pattern of physiologic jaundice in term infants includes a peak indirect-reacting bilirubin level of no more than 12 mg/dL on day 3 of life. In premature infants, the peak is higher (15 mg/dL) and occurs later (fifth day). The peak level of indirect bilirubin during physiologic jaundice may be higher in breast milk–fed infants than in formula-fed infants (15 to 17 mg/dL versus 12 mg/dL). This higher level may be partly a result of the decreased fluid intake of infants fed breast milk. Jaundice is unphysiologic or pathologic if it is clinically evident on the first day of life, if the bilirubin level increases more than 0.5 mg/dL/hr, if the peak bilirubin is greater than 13 mg/dL in term infants, if the direct bilirubin fraction is greater than 1.5 mg/dL, or if hepatosplenomegaly and anemia are present.

Crigler-Najjar syndrome is a serious, rare, autosomal recessive, permanent deficiency of glucuronosyltransferase that results in severe indirect hyperbilirubinemia. Type II responds to enzyme induction by phenobarbital, producing an increase in enzyme activity and a reduction of bilirubin levels. Type I does not respond to phenobarbital and manifests as persistent indirect hyperbilirubinemia, often leading to kernicterus. **Gilbert disease** is caused by a mutation of the promoter region of glucuronosyltransferase and results in a mild indirect hyperbilirubinemia. In the presence of another icterogenic factor (hemolysis), more severe jaundice may develop.

Table 62-1	Etiology of Unconjugated Hyperbilirubinemia	
	HEMOLYSIS PRESENT	**HEMOLYSIS ABSENT**
Common	*Blood group incompatibility:* ABO, Rh, Kell, Duffy infection	Physiologic jaundice, breast milk jaundice, internal hemorrhage, polycythemia, infant of diabetic mother
Rare	*Red blood cell enzyme defects:* glucose-6-phosphate dehydrogenase, pyruvate kinase *Red blood cell membrane disorders:* spherocytosis, ovalocytosis *Hemoglobinopathy:* thalassemia	Mutations of glucuronyl transferase enzyme (Crigler-Najjar syndrome, Gilbert disease), pyloric stenosis, hypothyroidism, immune thrombocytopenia

Table 62-2	Etiology of Conjugated Hyperbilirubinemia
COMMON	
Hyperalimentation cholestasis	
CMV infection Other perinatal congenital infections (TORCH)	
Inspissated bile from prolonged hemolysis	
Neonatal hepatitis	
Sepsis	
UNCOMMON	
Hepatic infarction	
Inborn errors of metabolism (galactosemia, tyrosinemia)	
Cystic fibrosis	
Biliary atresia	
Choledochal cyst	
α_1-Antitrypsin deficiency	
Neonatal iron storage disease	
Alagille syndrome (arteriohepatic dysplasia)	
Byler disease	

CMV, Cytomegalovirus; *TORCH,* toxoplasmosis, other, rubella, cytomegalovirus, herpes simplex.

Breast milk jaundice may be associated with unconjugated hyperbilirubinemia without evidence of hemolysis during the first to second week of life. Bilirubin levels rarely increase to more than 20 mg/dL. Interruption of breastfeeding for 1 to 2 days results in a rapid decline of bilirubin levels, which do not increase significantly after breastfeeding resumes. Breast milk may contain an inhibitor of bilirubin conjugation or may increase enterohepatic recirculation of bilirubin because of breast milk glucuronidase.

Jaundice on the first day of life is always pathologic, and immediate attention is needed to establish the cause. Early onset often is a result of hemolysis, internal hemorrhage (cephalhematoma, hepatic or splenic hematoma), or infection (Table 62-1). Infection also is often associated with direct-reacting bilirubin resulting from perinatal congenital infections or from bacterial sepsis.

Physical evidence of jaundice is observed in infants when bilirubin levels reach 5 to 10 mg/dL (versus 2 to 3 mg/dL in adults). When jaundice is observed, the laboratory evaluation for hyperbilirubinemia should include a total bilirubin measurement to determine the magnitude of hyperbilirubinemia. Bilirubin levels greater than 5 mg/dL on the first day of life or greater than 13 mg/dL thereafter in term infants should be evaluated further with measurement of indirect and direct bilirubin levels, blood typing, Coombs test, complete blood count, blood smear, and reticulocyte count. These tests must be performed before treatment of hyperbilirubinemia with phototherapy or exchange transfusion. In the absence of hemolysis or evidence for either the common or the rare causes of nonhemolytic indirect hyperbilirubinemia, the diagnosis is either physiologic or breast milk jaundice. Jaundice present after 2 weeks of age is pathologic and suggests a direct-reacting hyperbilirubinemia.

Etiology of Direct Conjugated Hyperbilirubinemia

Decision-Making Algorithm
Available @ StudentConsult.com

Jaundice

Direct-reacting hyperbilirubinemia (defined as a direct bilirubin level >2 mg/dL or >20% of the total bilirubin) is never physiologic and should always be evaluated thoroughly according to the diagnostic categories (Table 62-2). Direct-reacting bilirubin (composed mostly of conjugated bilirubin) is not neurotoxic to the infant but signifies a serious underlying disorder involving cholestasis or hepatocellular injury. The diagnostic evaluation of patients with direct-reacting hyperbilirubinemia involves the determination of the levels of liver enzymes (aspartate aminotransferase, alkaline phosphatase, alanine aminotransferase, and γ-glutamyl transpeptidase), bacterial and viral cultures, metabolic screening tests, hepatic ultrasound, sweat chloride test, and occasionally liver biopsy. In addition, the presence of dark urine and gray-white (acholic) stools with jaundice after the second week of life strongly suggests biliary atresia. The treatment of disorders manifested by direct bilirubinemia is specific for the diseases that are listed in Table 62-2. These diseases do not respond to phototherapy or exchange transfusion.

Kernicterus (Bilirubin Encephalopathy)

Lipid-soluble, unconjugated, indirect bilirubin fraction is toxic to the developing central nervous system, especially when indirect bilirubin concentrations are high and exceed the binding capacity of albumin. Kernicterus results when indirect bilirubin is deposited in brain cells and disrupts neuronal metabolism and function, especially in the basal ganglia. Indirect bilirubin may cross the blood-brain barrier because of its lipid solubility. Other theories propose that a disruption of the blood-brain barrier permits entry of a bilirubin-albumin or free bilirubin–fatty acid complex.

Kernicterus usually is noted when the bilirubin level is excessively high for gestational age. It usually does not develop in term infants when bilirubin levels are less than 20 to

25 mg/dL, but the incidence increases as serum bilirubin levels exceed 25 mg/dL. Kernicterus may be noted at bilirubin levels less than 20 mg/dL in the presence of sepsis, meningitis, hemolysis, asphyxia, hypoxia, hypothermia, hypoglycemia, bilirubin-displacing drugs (sulfa drugs), and prematurity. Other risks for kernicterus in term infants are hemolysis, jaundice noted within 24 hours of birth, and delayed diagnosis of hyperbilirubinemia. Kernicterus has developed in extremely immature infants weighing less than 1000 g when bilirubin levels are less than 10 mg/dL because of a more permeable blood-brain barrier associated with prematurity.

The earliest clinical manifestations of kernicterus are lethargy, hypotonia, irritability, poor Moro response, and poor feeding. A high-pitched cry and emesis also may be present. Early signs are noted after day 4 of life. Later signs include bulging fontanelle, opisthotonic posturing, pulmonary hemorrhage, fever, hypertonicity, paralysis of upward gaze, and seizures. Infants with severe cases of kernicterus die in the neonatal period. Spasticity resolves in surviving infants, who may manifest later nerve deafness, choreoathetoid cerebral palsy, mental retardation, enamel dysplasia, and discoloration of teeth as permanent sequelae. Kernicterus may be prevented by avoiding excessively high indirect bilirubin levels and by avoiding conditions or drugs that may displace bilirubin from albumin. Early signs of kernicterus occasionally may be reversed by immediately instituting an exchange transfusion (see later).

Therapy of Indirect Hyperbilirubinemia

Phototherapy is an effective and safe method for reducing indirect bilirubin levels, particularly when initiated before serum bilirubin increases to levels associated with kernicterus. In term infants, phototherapy is begun when indirect bilirubin levels are between 16 and 18 mg/dL. Phototherapy is initiated in premature infants when bilirubin is at lower levels, to prevent bilirubin from reaching the high concentrations necessitating exchange transfusion. Blue lights and white lights are effective in reducing bilirubin levels.

Under the effects of phototherapy light with maximal irradiance in the 425- to 475-nm wavelength band, bilirubin is transformed into isomers that are water soluble and easily excreted. Unconjugated bilirubin (IX) is in the 4Z, 15Z configuration. Phototherapy causes a photochemical reaction producing the reversible, more water-soluble isomer 4Z, 15E bilirubin IX. This isomer can be excreted easily, bypassing the liver's conjugation system. Another photochemical reaction results in the rapid production of lumirubin, a more water-soluble isomer than the aforementioned isomer, which does not spontaneously revert to unconjugated native bilirubin and can be excreted in urine.

Complications of phototherapy include an increased insensible water loss, diarrhea, and dehydration. Additional problems are macular-papular red skin rash, lethargy, masking of cyanosis, nasal obstruction by eye pads, and potential for retinal damage. Skin bronzing may be noted in infants with direct-reacting hyperbilirubinemia. Infants with mild hemolytic disease of the newborn occasionally may be managed successfully with phototherapy for hyperbilirubinemia, but care must be taken to follow these infants for the late occurrence of anemia from continued hemolysis.

Exchange transfusion usually is reserved for infants with dangerously high indirect bilirubin levels who are at risk for kernicterus. As a rule of thumb, a level of 20 mg/dL for indirect-reacting bilirubin is the *exchange number* for infants *with hemolysis* who weigh more than 2000 g. Asymptomatic infants with physiologic or breast milk jaundice may not require exchange transfusion, unless the indirect bilirubin level exceeds 25 mg/dL. The exchangeable level of indirect bilirubin for other infants may be estimated by calculating 10% of the birth weight in grams: the level in an infant weighing 1500 g would be 15 mg/dL. Infants weighing less than 1000 g usually do not require an exchange transfusion until the bilirubin level exceeds 10 mg/dL.

The exchange transfusion usually is performed through an umbilical venous catheter placed in the inferior vena cava or, if free flow is obtained, at the confluence of the umbilical vein and the portal system. The level of serum bilirubin immediately after the exchange transfusion declines to levels that are about half of those before the exchange; levels rebound 6 to 8 hours later as a result of continued hemolysis and redistribution of bilirubin from tissue stores.

Complications of exchange transfusion include problems related to the blood (transfusion reaction, metabolic instability, or infection), the catheter (vessel perforation or hemorrhage), or the procedure (hypotension or necrotizing enterocolitis [NEC]). Unusual complications include thrombocytopenia and graft-versus-host disease. Continuation of phototherapy may reduce the necessity for subsequent exchange transfusions.

Polycythemia (Hyperviscosity Syndrome)

Polycythemia is an excessively high hematocrit (≥65%), which may lead to hyperviscosity that produces symptoms related to vascular stasis, hypoperfusion, and ischemia. As the hematocrit increases from 40% to 60%, there is a small increase in blood viscosity. When the central hematocrit increases to greater than 65%, the blood viscosity begins to increase markedly, and symptoms may appear. Neonatal erythrocytes are less filterable or deformable than adult erythrocytes, which further contributes to hyperviscosity. A central venous hematocrit of 65% or greater is noted in 3% to 5% of infants. Infants at special risk for polycythemia are term and post-term small for gestational age infants, infants of diabetic mothers, infants with delayed cord clamping, and infants with neonatal hyperthyroidism, adrenogenital syndrome, trisomy 13, trisomy 18, trisomy 21, twin-to-twin transfusion syndrome (recipient), or Beckwith-Wiedemann syndrome. In some infants, polycythemia may reflect a compensation for prolonged periods of fetal hypoxia caused by placental insufficiency; these infants have increased erythropoietin levels at birth.

Polycythemic patients appear plethoric or ruddy and may develop acrocyanosis. Symptoms are a result of the increased RBC mass and of vascular compromise. Seizures, lethargy, and irritability reflect abnormalities of microcirculation of the brain, whereas hyperbilirubinemia may reflect the poor hepatic circulation or the increased amount of hemoglobin that is being broken down into bilirubin. Additional problems include respiratory distress and primary pulmonary hypertension of the newborn (PPHN) that result in part from elevated pulmonary vascular resistance. The chest radiograph often reveals cardiomegaly, increased vascular markings, pleural effusions, and interstitial edema. Other problems are NEC, hypoglycemia, thrombocytopenia, priapism, testicular infarction, hemiplegic stroke, and feeding intolerance. Many of these complications also are related to the primary condition associated with polycythemia (small for gestational age infants are at risk for hypoglycemia and PPHN after periods of hypoxia in utero).

Long-term sequelae of neonatal polycythemia relate to neurodevelopmental abnormalities that may be prevented by treatment of symptomatic infants with partial exchange transfusion after birth. A partial exchange transfusion removes whole blood and replaces it with normal saline. The equation used to calculate the volume exchanged is based on the central venous hematocrit because peripheral hematocrits may be falsely elevated:

$$\text{Volume to exchange (mL)} =$$
$$[\text{blood volume} \times (\text{observed hematocrit}$$
$$- \text{desired hematocrit})]/\text{observed hematocrit}$$

The desired hematocrit is 50%, and the blood volume 85 mL/kg.

COAGULATION DISORDERS

Disorders of coagulation are common in the neonatal period. Hemorrhage during this time may be a result of trauma, inherited permanent deficiency of coagulation factors, transient deficiencies of vitamin K–dependent factors, disorders of platelets, and disseminated intravascular coagulation (DIC) seen in sick newborns with shock or hypoxia. Thrombosis also is a potential problem in the newborn because of developmentally lower circulating levels of antithrombin III, protein C (a vitamin K–dependent protein that inhibits factors VIII and V), and the fibrinolytic system.

Coagulation factors do not pass through the placenta to the fetus, and newborn infants have relatively low levels of the vitamin K–dependent factors II, VII, IX, and X. Contact factors XI and XII, prekallikrein, and kininogen also are lower in newborns than in adults. Fibrinogen (factor I); plasma levels of factors V, VIII, and XIII; and platelet counts are within the adult normal range.

Because of the transient, relative deficiencies of the contact and vitamin K–dependent factors, the *partial thromboplastin time* (PTT), which is dependent on factors XII, IX, VIII, X, V, II, and I, is prolonged in the newborn period. Preterm infants have the most marked prolongation of the PTT (50 to 80 seconds) compared with term infants (35 to 50 seconds) and older, more mature infants (25 to 35 seconds). The administration of heparin and the presence of DIC, hemophilia, and severe vitamin K deficiency prolong the PTT.

The *prothrombin time* (PT), which is dependent on factors X, VII, V, II, and I, is a more sensitive test for vitamin K deficiency. The PT is only slightly prolonged in term infants (13 to 20 seconds) compared with preterm infants (13 to 21 seconds) and more mature patients (12 to 14 seconds). Abnormal prolongations of the PT occur with vitamin K deficiency, hepatic injury, and DIC. Levels of *fibrinogen* and *fibrin degradation products* are similar in infants and adults. The *bleeding time,* which reflects platelet function and number, is normal during the newborn period in the absence of maternal salicylate therapy.

Vitamin K is a necessary cofactor for the carboxylation of glutamate on precursor proteins, converting them into the more active coagulation factors II, VII, IX, and X; γ-carboxyglutamic acid binds calcium, which is required for the immediate activation of factors during hemorrhage. There is no congenital deficiency of hepatic synthesis of these precursor proteins, but in the absence of vitamin K their conversion to the active factor is not possible. Levels of *protein induced by vitamin K absence* increase in vitamin K deficiency and are helpful diagnostic markers; vitamin K administration rapidly corrects the coagulation defects, reducing protein induced by vitamin K absence to undetectable levels.

Although most newborns are born with reduced levels of vitamin K–dependent factors, hemorrhagic complications develop only rarely. Infants at risk for **hemorrhagic disease of the newborn** have the most profound deficiency of vitamin K–dependent factors, and these factors decline further after birth. Because breast milk is a poor source of vitamin K, breastfed infants are at increased risk for hemorrhage that usually occurs between days 3 and 7 of life. Bleeding usually ensues from the umbilical cord, circumcision site, intestines, scalp, mucosa, and skin, but internal hemorrhage places the infant at risk for fatal complications, such as intracranial bleeding.

Hemorrhage on the first day of life resulting from a deficiency of the vitamin K–dependent factors often is associated with administration to the mother of drugs that affect vitamin K metabolism in the infant. This early pattern of hemorrhage has been seen with maternal warfarin or antibiotic (e.g., isoniazid or rifampin) therapy and in infants of mothers receiving phenobarbital and phenytoin. Bleeding also may occur 1 to 3 months after birth, particularly among breastfed infants. Vitamin K deficiency in breastfed infants also should raise suspicion about the possibility of vitamin K malabsorption resulting from cystic fibrosis, biliary atresia, hepatitis, or antibiotic suppression of the colonic bacteria that produce vitamin K.

Bleeding associated with vitamin K deficiency may be **prevented** by administration of vitamin K to all infants at birth. Before routine administration of vitamin K, 1% to 2% of all newborns had hemorrhagic disease of the newborn. One intramuscular dose (1 mg) of vitamin K prevents vitamin K–deficiency bleeding. **Treatment** of bleeding resulting from vitamin K deficiency involves intravenous administration of 1 mg of vitamin K. If severe, life-threatening hemorrhage is present, fresh frozen plasma also should be given. Unusually high doses of vitamin K may be needed for hepatic disease and for maternal warfarin or anticonvulsant therapy.

Clinical Manifestations and Differential Diagnoses of Bleeding Disorders

Decision-Making Algorithms
Available @ StudentConsult.com

Bleeding
Petechiae/Purpura

Bleeding disorders in a newborn may be associated with cutaneous bleeding, such as cephalhematoma, subgaleal hemorrhage, ecchymosis, and petechiae. Facial petechiae are common in infants born by vertex presentation, with or without a nuchal cord, and usually are insignificant. Mucosal bleeding may appear as hematemesis, melena, or epistaxis.

Internal hemorrhage results in organ-specific dysfunction, such as seizures associated with intracranial hemorrhage. Bleeding from venipuncture or heel-stick sites, circumcision sites, or the umbilical cord also is common.

The differential diagnosis depends partly on the clinical circumstances associated with the hemorrhage. In a **sick newborn**, the differential diagnosis should include DIC, hepatic failure, and thrombocytopenia. Thrombocytopenia in an ill neonate may be secondary to consumption by trapping of platelets in a hemangioma (**Kasabach-Merritt syndrome**) or may be associated with perinatal, congenital, or bacterial infections; NEC; thrombotic endocarditis; PPHN; organic acidemia; maternal preeclampsia; or asphyxia. Thrombocytopenia also may be due to peripheral washout of platelets after an exchange transfusion. Treatment of a sick infant with thrombocytopenia should be directed at the underlying disorder, supplemented by infusions of platelets, blood, or both.

The etiology of DIC in a newborn includes hypoxia, hypotension, asphyxia, bacterial or viral sepsis, NEC, death of a twin while in utero, cavernous hemangioma, nonimmune hydrops, neonatal cold injury, neonatal neoplasm, and hepatic disease. The treatment of DIC should be focused primarily on therapy for the initiating or underlying disorder. Supportive management of consumptive coagulopathy involves platelet transfusions and factor replacement with fresh frozen plasma. Heparin and factor C concentrate should be reserved for infants with DIC who also have thrombosis.

Disorders of hemostasis in a well child are not associated with systemic disease in a newborn but reflect coagulation factor or platelet deficiency. Hemophilia initially is associated with cutaneous or mucosal bleeding and no systemic illness. If bleeding continues, hypovolemic shock may develop. Bleeding into the brain, liver, or spleen may result in organ-specific signs and shock.

In a well child, thrombocytopenia may be part of a syndrome such as Fanconi anemia syndrome (involving hypoplasia and aplasia of the thumb), radial aplasia-thrombocytopenia syndrome (thumbs present), or Wiskott-Aldrich syndrome. Various maternal drugs also may reduce the neonatal platelet count without producing other adverse effects. These drugs include sulfonamides, quinidine, quinine, and thiazide diuretics.

The most common causes of thrombocytopenia in well newborns are transient isoimmune thrombocytopenia and transient neonatal thrombocytopenia. **Isoimmune thrombocytopenia** is caused by antiplatelet antibodies produced by the HPLA1-negative mother after her sensitization to specific paternal platelet antigen (HPA-1a and HPA-5b represent 85% and 10% of cases, respectively) expressed on the fetal platelet. The incidence is 1 in 1000 to 1 in 2000 births. This response to maternal-sensitized antibodies that produce isoimmune thrombocytopenia is analogous to the response that produces erythroblastosis fetalis. The maternal antiplatelet antibody does not produce maternal thrombocytopenia, but after crossing the placenta this IgG antibody binds to fetal platelets that are trapped by the reticuloendothelial tissue, resulting in thrombocytopenia. Infants with thrombocytopenia produced in this manner are at risk for development of petechiae, purpura, and intracranial hemorrhage (an incidence of 10% to 15%) before or after birth. Vaginal delivery may increase the risk of neonatal bleeding; cesarean section may be indicated.

Specific **treatment** for severe thrombocytopenia (<20,000 platelets/mm^3) or significant bleeding is transfusion of ABO-compatible and RhD-compatible, HPA-1a-negative and HPA-5b-negative maternal platelets. Because the antibody in isoimmune thrombocytopenia is directed against the fetal rather than the maternal platelet, thrombocytapheresis of the mother yields sufficient platelets to treat the affected infant. After one platelet transfusion, the infant's platelet count dramatically increases and usually remains in a safe range. Without treatment, thrombocytopenia resolves during the first month of life as the maternal antibody level declines. *Treatment* of the mother with intravenous immunoglobulin or the thrombocytopenic fetus with intravascular platelet transfusion (cordocentesis) is also effective. Cesarean section reduces the risk of intracranial hemorrhage.

Neonatal thrombocytopenia in infants born to women with idiopathic thrombocytopenic purpura (ITP) also is a result of placental transfer of maternal IgG antibodies. In ITP, these autoantibodies are directed against all platelet antigens; mother and newborn may have low platelet counts. The risks of hemorrhage in an infant born to a mother with ITP may be lessened by cesarean section and by treatment of the mother with corticosteroids.

Treatment of an affected infant born to a mother with ITP may involve prednisone and intravenous immunoglobulin. In an emergency, random donor platelets may be used and may produce a transient increase in the infant's platelet count. Thrombocytopenia resolves spontaneously during the first month of life as maternal-derived antibody levels decline. Elevated levels of platelet-associated antibodies also have been noted in thrombocytopenic infants with sepsis and thrombocytopenia of unknown cause who were born to mothers without demonstrable platelet antibodies.

The laboratory evaluation of an infant (well or sick) with bleeding must include a platelet count, blood smear, and evaluation of PTT and PT. Isolated thrombocytopenia in a well infant suggests immune thrombocytopenia. Laboratory evidence of DIC includes a markedly prolonged PTT and PT (minutes rather than seconds), thrombocytopenia, and a blood smear suggesting a microangiopathic hemolytic anemia (burr or fragmented blood cells). Further evaluation reveals low levels of fibrinogen (<100 mg/dL) and elevated levels of fibrin degradation products. Vitamin K deficiency prolongs the PT more than the PTT, whereas hemophilia resulting from factors VIII and IX deficiency prolongs only the PTT. Specific factor levels confirm the diagnosis of hemophilia.

Chapter 63

NECROTIZING ENTEROCOLITIS

Necrotizing enterocolitis (NEC) is a syndrome of intestinal injury and is the most common intestinal emergency occurring in preterm infants admitted to the neonatal intensive care unit. NEC occurs in 1 to 3 per 1000 live births and 1% to 8%

of admissions to the neonatal intensive care unit. Prematurity is the most consistent and significant factor associated with neonatal NEC. The disease occurs in 4% to 13% of infants who weigh less than 1500 g at birth. NEC is infrequent in term infants (<10% of affected infants).

Most cases of NEC occur in premature infants born before 34 weeks' gestation who have been fed enterally. Prematurity is associated with immaturity of the gastrointestinal tract, including decreased integrity of the intestinal mucosal barrier, depressed mucosal enzymes, suppressed gastrointestinal hormones, suppressed intestinal host defense system, decreased coordination of intestinal motility, and differences in blood flow autoregulation, which is thought to play a significant role in the pathogenesis of NEC. More than 90% of infants diagnosed with NEC have been fed enterally, but NEC has been reported in infants who have never been fed. Feeding with human milk has shown a beneficial role in reducing the incidence of NEC. In addition, probiotics may offer potential benefits for the preterm infant by increasing mucosal barrier function, improving nutrition, upregulating the immune system, and reducing mucosal colonization by potential pathogens. It also is theorized that compromised intestinal blood flow contributes to NEC.

Early clinical signs of NEC include abdominal distention, feeding intolerance/increased gastric residuals, emesis, rectal bleeding, and occasional diarrhea. As the disease progresses, patients may develop marked abdominal distention, bilious emesis, ascites, abdominal wall erythema, lethargy, temperature instability, increased episodes of apnea/bradycardia, disseminated intravascular coagulation, and shock. With abdominal perforation, the abdomen may develop a bluish discoloration.

The white blood cell count can be elevated, but often it is depressed. Thrombocytopenia is common. In addition, infants may develop coagulation abnormalities along with metabolic derangements, including metabolic acidosis, electrolyte imbalance, and hypoglycemia and hyperglycemia. No unique infectious agent has been associated with NEC; bacteriologic and fungal cultures may prove helpful but not conclusive.

Radiographic imaging is essential to the diagnosis of NEC. The earliest radiographic finding is intestinal ileus, often associated with thickening of the bowel loops and air-fluid levels. The pathognomonic radiographic finding is **pneumatosis intestinalis** caused by hydrogen gas production from pathogenic bacteria present between the subserosal and muscularis layers of the bowel wall. Radiographic findings also may include a fixed or persistent dilated loop of bowel, intrahepatic venous gas, and *pneumoperitoneum* seen with bowel perforation.

The **differential diagnosis** of NEC includes sepsis with intestinal ileus or a volvulus. Both conditions can present with systemic signs of sepsis and abdominal distention. The absence of pneumatosis on abdominal radiographs does not rule out the diagnosis of NEC; other causes of abdominal distention and perforation (gastric or ileal perforation) should be considered and investigated. Patients diagnosed with Hirschsprung enterocolitis or severe gastroenteritis may present with pneumatosis intestinalis.

The **management** of NEC includes the discontinuation of enteral feedings, gastrointestinal decompression with nasogastric suction, fluid and electrolyte replacement, total parenteral nutrition, and systemic broad-spectrum antibiotics. When the diagnosis of NEC is made, consultation with a pediatric surgeon should be obtained. Even with aggressive and appropriate medical management, 25% to 50% of infants with NEC require surgical intervention. The decision to perform surgery is obvious when the presence of a pneumoperitoneum is observed on abdominal radiograph. Other, not so obvious indications for surgical intervention include rapid clinical deterioration despite medical therapy, rapid onset and progression of pneumatosis, abdominal mass, and intestinal obstruction. The surgical procedure of choice is laparotomy with removal of the frankly necrotic and nonviable bowel. Many extremely small infants are managed initially with primary peritoneal drainage followed by surgical intervention as needed later, when the infant is stable and a laparotomy can be performed safely. The long-term outcome includes intestinal strictures requiring further surgical intervention, short bowel syndrome with poor absorption of enteral fluids and nutrients, associated cholestasis with resultant cirrhosis and liver failure from prolonged parenteral nutrition, and neurodevelopmental delay from prolonged hospitalization.

Chapter **64**

HYPOXIC-ISCHEMIC ENCEPHALOPATHY, INTRACRANIAL HEMORRHAGE, AND SEIZURES

The human newborn spends more time asleep (predominantly in rapid eye movement or active sleep) than in a wakeful state and is totally dependent on adults. Primitive reflexes, such as the Moro, grasp, stepping, rooting, sucking, and crossed extensor reflexes, are readily elicited and are normal for this age. In addition, the newborn has a wealth of cortical functions that are less easily shown (e.g., the ability to extinguish repetitive or painful stimuli). The newborn also has the capacity for attentive eye fixation and differential responses to the mother's voice. During the perinatal period, many pathophysiologic mechanisms can adversely and permanently affect the developing brain, including prenatal events, such as hypoxia, ischemia, infections, inflammation, malformations, maternal drugs, and coagulation disorders, as well as postnatal events, such as birth trauma, hypoxia-ischemia, inborn errors of metabolism, hypoglycemia, hypothyroidism, hyperthyroidism, polycythemia, hemorrhage, and meningitis.

NEONATAL SEIZURES

Decision-Making Algorithms
Available @ StudentConsult.com

Seizures and Other Paroxysmal Disorders
Hypocalcemia

Table 64-1	Clinical Characteristics of Neonatal Seizures
DESIGNATION	**CHARACTERIZATION**
Focal clonic	Repetitive, rhythmic contractions of muscle groups of the limbs, face, or trunk May be unilateral or multifocal May appear synchronously or asynchronously in various body regions Cannot be suppressed by restraint
Focal tonic	Sustained posturing of single limbs Sustained asymmetric posturing of the trunk Sustained eye deviation Cannot be provoked by stimulation or suppressed by restraint
Myoclonic	Arrhythmic contractions of muscle groups of the limbs, face, or trunk Typically not repetitive or may recur at a slow rate May be generalized, focal, or fragmentary May be provoked by stimulation
Generalized tonic	Sustained symmetric posturing of limbs, trunk, and neck May be flexor, extensor, or mixed extensor/flexor May be provoked by stimulation May be suppressed by restraint or repositioning
Ocular signs	Random and roving eye movements or nystagmus Distinct from tonic eye deviation
Orobuccolingual movements	Sucking, chewing, tongue protrusions May be provoked by stimulation
Progression movements	Rowing or swimming movements of the arms Pedaling or bicycling movements of the legs May be provoked by stimulation May be suppressed by restraint or repositioning

From Mizrahi EM: Neonatal seizures. In Shinnar S, Branski D, editors: Pediatric and adolescent medicine, vol 6, Childhood seizures, Basel, 1995, S. Karger.

Seizures during the neonatal period may be the result of multiple causes, with characteristic **historical and clinical manifestations**. Seizures caused by **hypoxic-ischemic encephalopathy** (postasphyxial seizures), a common cause of seizures in the full-term infant, usually occur 12 to 24 hours after a history of birth asphyxia and often are refractory to conventional doses of anticonvulsant medications. Postasphyxial seizures also may be caused by metabolic disorders associated with neonatal asphyxia, such as hypoglycemia and hypocalcemia. **Intraventricular hemorrhage (IVH)** is a common cause of seizures in premature infants and often occurs between 1 and 3 days of age. Seizures with IVH are associated with a bulging fontanelle, hemorrhagic spinal fluid, anemia, lethargy, and coma. Seizures caused by hypoglycemia often occur when blood glucose levels decline to the lowest postnatal value (at 1 to 2 hours of age or after 24 to 48 hours of poor nutritional intake). Seizures caused by **hypocalcemia** and **hypomagnesemia** develop in high-risk infants and respond well to therapy with calcium, magnesium, or both.

Seizures noted in the delivery room often are caused by direct *injection of local anesthetic agents* into the fetal scalp (associated with transient bradycardia and fixed dilated pupils), severe *anoxia*, or *congenital brain malformation*. Seizures after the first 5 days of life may be the result of *infection* or *drug withdrawal*. Seizures associated with lethargy, acidosis, and a family history of infant deaths may be the result of an *inborn error of metabolism*. An infant whose parent has a history of a neonatal seizure also is at risk for *benign familial seizures*. In an infant who appears well, a sudden onset on day 1 to 3 of life of seizures that are of short duration and that do not recur may be the result of a *subarachnoid hemorrhage*. Focal seizures often are the result of local cerebral infarction.

Seizures may be difficult to differentiate from benign jitteriness or from tremulousness in infants of diabetic mothers, in infants with narcotic withdrawal syndrome, and in any infants after an episode of asphyxia. In contrast to seizures, jitteriness and tremors are sensory dependent, elicited by stimuli, and interrupted by holding the extremity. Seizure activity becomes manifested as coarse, fast and slow clonic activity, whereas jitteriness is characterized by fine, rapid movement. Seizures may be associated with abnormal eye movements, such as tonic deviation to one side. The electroencephalogram often shows seizure activity when the clinical diagnosis is uncertain. Identifying seizures in the newborn period is often difficult because the infant, especially the low birth weight infant, usually does not show the tonic-clonic major motor activity typical of the older child (Table 64-1). Subtle seizures are a common manifestation in newborns. The subtle signs of seizure activity include apnea, eye deviation, tongue thrusting, eye blinking, fluctuation of vital signs, and staring. Continuous bedside electroencephalographic monitoring can help identify subtle seizures.

The **diagnostic evaluation** of infants with seizures should involve an immediate determination of capillary blood glucose levels with a Chemstrip. In addition, blood concentrations of sodium, calcium, glucose, and bilirubin should be determined. When infection is suspected, cerebrospinal fluid and blood specimens should be obtained for culture. After the seizure has stopped, a careful examination should be done to identify signs of increased intracranial pressure, congenital malformations, and systemic illness. If signs of elevated intracranial pressure are absent, a lumbar puncture should be performed. If the diagnosis is not apparent at this point, further evaluation should involve magnetic resonance imaging, computed tomography, or cerebral ultrasound and tests to determine the presence of an inborn error of metabolism. Determinations of inborn errors of metabolism are especially important in infants with unexplained lethargy, coma, acidosis, ketonuria, or respiratory alkalosis.

The **treatment** of neonatal seizures may be specific, such as treatment of meningitis or the correction of **hypoglycemia**, **hypocalcemia**, **hypomagnesemia**, **hyponatremia**, or **vitamin B$_6$ deficiency** or **dependency**. In the absence of an identifiable cause, therapy should involve an anticonvulsant agent, such as 20 to 40 mg/kg of phenobarbital, 10 to 20 mg/kg of phenytoin, or 0.1 to 0.3 mg/kg of diazepam. Treatment of status epilepticus requires repeated doses of phenobarbital and may require diazepam or midazolam, titrated to clinical signs. The long-term outcome for neonatal seizures usually is related to the underlying cause and to the primary pathology, such as hypoxic-ischemic encephalopathy, meningitis, drug withdrawal, stroke, or hemorrhage.

INTRACRANIAL HEMORRHAGE

Intracranial hemorrhage may be confined to one anatomic area of the brain, such as the subdural, subarachnoid, periventricular, intraventricular, intraparenchymal, or cerebellar region. **Subdural hemorrhages** are seen in association with birth trauma, cephalopelvic disproportion, forceps delivery, large for gestational age infants, skull fractures, and postnatal head trauma. The subdural hematoma does not always cause symptoms immediately after birth; with time, however, the RBCs undergo hemolysis and water is drawn into the hemorrhage because of the high oncotic pressure of protein, resulting in an expanding symptomatic lesion. Anemia, vomiting, seizures, and macrocephaly may occur in an infant who is 1 to 2 months of age and has a subdural hematoma. **Child abuse** in this situation should be suspected and appropriate diagnostic evaluation undertaken to identify other possible signs of skeletal, ocular, or soft tissue injury. Occasionally, a massive subdural hemorrhage in the neonatal period is caused by rupture of the vein of Galen or by an inherited coagulation disorder, such as hemophilia. Infants with these conditions exhibit shock, seizures, and coma. The **treatment** of all symptomatic subdural hematomas is surgical evacuation.

Subarachnoid hemorrhages may be spontaneous, associated with hypoxia, or caused by bleeding from a cerebral arteriovenous malformation. Seizures are a common presenting manifestation, and the *prognosis* depends on the underlying injury. Treatment is directed at the seizure and the rare occurrence of posthemorrhagic hydrocephalus.

Periventricular hemorrhage and **IVH** are common in very low birth weight infants; the risk decreases with increasing gestational age. Fifty percent of infants weighing less than 1500 g have evidence of intracranial bleeding. The pathogenesis for these hemorrhages is unknown (they usually are not caused by coagulation disorders), but the initial site of bleeding may be the weak blood vessels in the periventricular germinal matrix. The vessels in this area have poor structural support. These vessels may rupture and hemorrhage because of passive changes in cerebral blood flow occurring with the variations of blood pressure that sick premature infants often exhibit (failure of autoregulation). In some sick infants, these blood pressure variations are the only identifiable etiologic factors. In others, the disorders that may cause the elevation or depression of blood pressure or that interfere with venous return from the head (venous stasis) increase the risk of IVH; these disorders include asphyxia, pneumothorax, mechanical ventilation, hypercapnia, hypoxemia, prolonged labor, breech delivery, patent ductus arteriosus, heart failure, and therapy with hypertonic solutions such as sodium bicarbonate.

Most periventricular hemorrhages and IVHs occur in the first 3 days of life. It is unusual for IVH to occur after day 5 of life. The clinical manifestations of IVH include seizures, apnea, bradycardia, lethargy, coma, hypotension, metabolic acidosis, anemia not corrected by blood transfusion, bulging fontanelle, and cutaneous mottling. Many infants with small hemorrhages (grade 1 or 2) are asymptomatic; infants with larger hemorrhages (grade 4) often have a catastrophic event that rapidly progresses to shock and coma.

The diagnosis of IVH is confirmed and the severity graded by ultrasound through the anterior fontanelle or computed tomography examination. Grade 1 IVH is confined to the germinal matrix; grade 2 is an extension of grade 1, with blood noted in the ventricle without ventricular enlargement; grade 3 is an extension of grade 2 with ventricular dilation; and grade 4 has blood in dilated ventricles and in the cerebral cortex, either contiguous with or distant from the ventricle. Grade 4 hemorrhage has a poor prognosis, as does the development of periventricular, small, echolucent cystic lesions, with or without porencephalic cysts and posthemorrhagic hydrocephalus. Periventricular cysts often are noted after the resolution of echodense areas in the periventricular white matter. The cysts may correspond to the development of **periventricular leukomalacia**, which may be a precursor to cerebral palsy. Extensive intraparenchymal echodensities represent hemorrhagic necrosis. They are associated with a high mortality rate and have a poor neurodevelopmental prognosis for survivors.

Treatment of an acute hemorrhage involves standard supportive care, including ventilation for apnea and blood transfusion for hemorrhagic shock. Posthemorrhagic hydrocephalus may be managed with serial daily lumbar punctures, an external ventriculostomy tube, or a permanent ventricular-peritoneal shunt. Implementation of the shunt often is delayed because of the high protein content of the hemorrhagic ventricular fluid.

HYPOXIC-ISCHEMIC ENCEPHALOPATHY

Conditions known to reduce uteroplacental blood flow or to interfere with spontaneous respiration lead to perinatal hypoxia, lactic acidosis, and, if severe enough to reduce cardiac output or cause cardiac arrest, ischemia. The combination of the reduced availability of oxygen for the brain resulting from hypoxia and the diminished or absent blood flow to the brain resulting from ischemia leads to reduced glucose for metabolism and to an accumulation of lactate that produces local tissue acidosis. After reperfusion, hypoxic-ischemic injury also may be complicated by cell necrosis and vascular endothelial edema, reducing blood flow distal to the

Table 64-2	Hypoxic-Ischemic Encephalopathy in Term Infants		
SIGNS	**STAGE 1**	**STAGE 2**	**STAGE 3**
Level of consciousness	Hyperalert	Lethargic	Stuporous
Muscle tone	Normal	Hypotonic	Flaccid
Tendon reflexes/clonus	Hyperactive	Hyperactive	Absent
Moro reflex	Strong	Weak	Absent
Pupils	Mydriasis	Miosis	Unequal, poor light reflex
Seizures	None	Common	Decerebration
Electroencephalography	Normal	Low voltage changing to seizure activity	Burst suppression to isoelectric
Duration	>24 h if progresses, otherwise may remain normal	24 h to 14 days	Days to weeks

Modified from Sarnat HB, Sarnat MS: Neonatal encephalopathy following fetal distress, Arch Neurol 33:696, 1976.

involved vessel. Typically, hypoxic-ischemic encephalopathy in the term infant is characterized by cerebral edema, cortical necrosis, and involvement of the basal ganglia, whereas in the preterm infant it is characterized by periventricular leukomalacia. Both lesions may result in cortical atrophy, mental retardation, and spastic quadriplegia or diplegia.

The clinical manifestations and characteristic course of hypoxic-ischemic encephalopathy vary according to the severity of the injury (Table 64-2). Infants with severe stage 3 hypoxic-ischemic encephalopathy are usually hypotonic, although occasionally they initially appear hypertonic and hyperalert at birth. As cerebral edema develops, brain functions are affected in a descending order; cortical depression produces coma, and brainstem depression results in apnea. As cerebral edema progresses, refractory seizures begin 12 to 24 hours after birth. Concurrently the infant has no signs of spontaneous respirations, is hypotonic, and has diminished or absent deep tendon reflexes.

Survivors of stage 3 hypoxic-ischemic encephalopathy have a high incidence of seizures and serious neurodevelopmental handicaps. The prognosis of severe asphyxia also depends on other organ system injury (see Table 58-6). Another indicator of poor prognosis is time of onset of spontaneous respiration as estimated by Apgar score. Infants with Apgar scores of 0 to 3 at 10 minutes have a 20% mortality and a 5% incidence of cerebral palsy; if the score remains this low by 20 minutes, the mortality increases to 60%, and the incidence of cerebral palsy increases to 57%.

Chapter 65

SEPSIS AND MENINGITIS

Systemic and local infections (lung, cutaneous, ocular, umbilical, kidney, bone-joint, and meningeal) are common in the newborn period. Infection may be acquired in utero through the transplacental or transcervical routes and during or after birth. Ascending infection through the cervix, with or without rupture of the amniotic fluid membranes, may result in amnionitis, funisitis (infection of the umbilical cord), congenital pneumonia, and sepsis. The bacteria responsible for ascending infection of the fetus are common bacterial organisms of the maternal genitourinary tract, such as group B streptococci, *Escherichia coli*, *Haemophilus influenzae*, and *Klebsiella*. Herpes simplex virus (HSV)-1 or, more often, HSV-2 also causes ascending infection that at times may be indistinguishable from bacterial sepsis. Syphilis and *Listeria monocytogenes* are acquired by transplacental infection.

Maternal humoral immunity may protect the fetus against some neonatal pathogens, such as group B streptococci and HSV. Nonetheless, various deficiencies of the neonatal antimicrobial defense mechanism probably are more important than maternal immune status as a contributing factor for neonatal infection, especially in the low birth weight infant. The incidence of sepsis is approximately 1:1500 in full-term infants and 1:250 in preterm infants. The sixfold-higher rate of sepsis in preterm infants relates to the more immature immunologic systems of preterm infants and to their prolonged periods of hospitalization, which increase risk of nosocomially acquired infectious diseases.

Preterm infants before 32 weeks of gestational age have not received the full complement of maternal antibodies (IgG), which cross the placenta by active transport predominantly in the latter half of the third trimester. In addition, although low birth weight infants may generate IgM antibodies, their own IgG response to infection is reduced. These infants also have deficiencies of the alternate and, to a smaller degree, the classic complement activation pathways, which results in diminished complement-mediated opsonization. Newborn infants also show a deficit in phagocytic migration to the site of infection (to the lung) and in the bone marrow reserve pool of leukocytes. In addition, in the presence of suboptimal activation of complement, neonatal neutrophils ingest and kill bacteria less effectively than adult neutrophils do. Neutrophils from sick infants seem to have an even greater deficit in bacterial killing capacity compared with phagocytic cells from normal neonates.

Defense mechanisms against viral pathogens also may be deficient in a newborn. Neonatal antibody-dependent, cell-mediated immunity by the natural killer lymphocytes is deficient in the absence of maternal antibodies and in the presence of reduced interferon production; reduced antibody levels occur in premature infants and in infants born during a primary viral infection of the mother, such as with enteroviruses, HSV-2, or cytomegalovirus. In addition, antibody-independent cytotoxicity may be reduced in lymphocytes of newborns.

Bacterial sepsis and meningitis often are linked closely in neonates. Despite this association, the incidence of meningitis relative to neonatal sepsis has been on a steady decline. The incidence of meningitis is approximately 1 in 20 cases of sepsis. The causative organisms isolated most frequently are the same as for neonatal sepsis: group B streptococci, *E. coli*, and *L. monocytogenes*. Gram-negative organisms, such as *Klebsiella*, *Salmonella*, and *Serratia marcescens*, are more common in less developed countries, and coagulase-negative staphylococcus needs to be considered in very low birth weight infants. Male infants seem to be more susceptible to neonatal infection than female infants. Severely premature infants are at even greater risk secondary to less effective defense mechanisms and deficient transfer of antibodies from the mother to the fetus (which occurs mostly after 32 weeks' gestation). Neonates in the neonatal intensive care unit live in a hostile environment, with exposure to endotracheal tubes, central arterial and venous catheters, and blood draws, all predisposing to bacteremia and meningitis. Genetic factors have been implicated in the ability of bacteria to cross the blood-brain barrier. This penetration has been noted for group B streptococci, *E. coli*, *Listeria*, *Citrobacter*, and *Streptococcus pneumoniae*.

Neonatal sepsis presents during three periods. **Early-onset sepsis** often begins in utero and usually is a result of infection caused by the bacteria in the mother's genitourinary tract. Organisms related to this sepsis include group B streptococci, *E. coli*, *Klebsiella*, *L. monocytogenes*, and nontypeable *H. influenzae*. Most infected infants are premature and show nonspecific cardiorespiratory signs, such as grunting, tachypnea, and cyanosis at birth. Risk factors for early-onset sepsis include vaginal colonization with group B streptococci, prolonged rupture of the membranes (>24 hours), amnionitis, maternal fever or leukocytosis, fetal tachycardia, and preterm birth. African American race and male sex are unexplained additional risk factors for neonatal sepsis.

Early-onset sepsis (birth to 7 days) is an overwhelming multiorgan system disease frequently manifested as respiratory failure, shock, meningitis (in 30% of cases), disseminated intravascular coagulation, acute tubular necrosis, and symmetrical peripheral gangrene. Early manifestations—grunting, poor feeding, pallor, apnea, lethargy, hypothermia, or an abnormal cry—may be nonspecific. Profound neutropenia, hypoxia, and hypotension may be refractory to treatment with broad-spectrum antibiotics, mechanical ventilation, and vasopressors such as dopamine and dobutamine. In the initial stages of early-onset septicemia in a preterm infant, it is often difficult to differentiate sepsis from respiratory distress syndrome. Because of this difficulty, premature infants with respiratory distress syndrome receive broad-spectrum antibiotics.

The clinical manifestations of sepsis are difficult to separate from the manifestations of meningitis in the neonate. Infants with early-onset sepsis should be evaluated by blood and cerebrospinal fluid (CSF) cultures, CSF Gram stain, cell count, and protein and glucose levels. Normal newborns generally have an elevated CSF protein content (100 to 150 mg/dL) and may have 25 to 30/mm^3 white blood cells (mean, 9/mm^3), which are 75% lymphocytes in the absence of infection. Some infants with neonatal meningitis caused by group B streptococci do not have an elevated CSF leukocyte count but are seen to have microorganisms in the CSF on Gram stain. In addition to culture, other methods of identifying the pathogenic bacteria are the determination of bacterial antigen in samples of blood, urine, or CSF. In cases of neonatal meningitis, the ratio of CSF glucose to blood glucose usually is less than 50%. The polymerase chain reaction test primarily is used to identify viral infections. Serial complete blood counts should be performed to identify neutropenia, an increased number of immature neutrophils (bands), and thrombocytopenia. C-reactive protein levels are often elevated in neonatal patients with bacterial sepsis.

A chest radiograph also should be obtained to determine the presence of pneumonia. In addition to the traditional neonatal pathogens, pneumonia in very low birth weight infants may be the result of acquisition of maternal genital mycoplasmal agent (e.g., *Ureaplasma urealyticum* or *Mycoplasma hominis*). Arterial blood gases should be monitored to detect hypoxemia and metabolic acidosis that may be caused by hypoxia, shock, or both. Blood pressure, urine output, and peripheral perfusion should be monitored to determine the need to treat septic shock with fluids and vasopressor agents.

The mainstay of treatment for sepsis and meningitis is antibiotic therapy. Antibiotics are used to suppress bacterial growth, allowing the infant's defense mechanisms time to respond. In addition, support measures, such as assisted ventilation and cardiovascular support, are equally important to the management of the infant. A combination of ampicillin and an aminoglycoside (usually gentamicin) for 10 to 14 days is effective treatment against most organisms responsible for early-onset sepsis. The combination of ampicillin and cefotaxime also is proposed as an alternative method of treatment. If meningitis is present, the treatment should be extended to 21 days or 14 days after a negative result from a CSF culture. Persistently positive results from CSF cultures are common with neonatal meningitis caused by gram-negative organisms, even with appropriate antibiotic treatment, and may be present for 2 to 3 days after antibiotic therapy. If gram-negative meningitis is present, some authorities continue to treat with an effective penicillin derivative combined with an aminoglycoside, whereas most change to a third-generation cephalosporin. High-dose penicillin (250,000 to 450,000 U/kg/24 hr) is appropriate for group B streptococcal meningitis. Inhaled nitric oxide, extracorporeal membrane oxygenation (in term infants), or both may improve the outcome of sepsis-related pulmonary hypertension. Intratracheal surfactant may reverse respiratory failure. Intrapartum penicillin empirical prophylaxis for group B streptococcal colonized mothers or mothers with risk factors (fever, preterm labor, previous infant with group B streptococci, and amnionitis) has reduced the rate of early-onset infection.

Late-onset sepsis (8 to 28 days) usually occurs in a healthy full-term infant who was discharged in good health from the normal newborn nursery. Clinical manifestations may include lethargy, poor feeding, hypotonia, apathy, seizures, bulging fontanelle, fever, and direct-reacting hyperbilirubinemia. In addition to bacteremia, hematogenous seeding may result in focal infections, such as meningitis (in 75% of cases), osteomyelitis (group B streptococci, *Staphylococcus aureus*), arthritis (gonococcus, *S. aureus*, *Candida albicans*, gram-negative bacteria), and urinary tract infection (gram-negative bacteria).

The evaluation of infants with late-onset sepsis is similar to that for infants with early-onset sepsis, with special attention given to a careful physical examination of the bones (infants with osteomyelitis may exhibit pseudoparalysis) and to the laboratory examination and culture of urine obtained by sterile suprapubic aspiration or urethral catheterization. Late-onset sepsis may be caused by the same pathogens as early-onset sepsis, but infants exhibiting sepsis late in the neonatal period also may have infections caused by the pathogens usually found in older infants (*H. influenzae*, *S. pneumoniae*, and *Neisseria meningitidis*). In addition, viral agents (HSV, cytomegalovirus, or enteroviruses) may manifest with a late-onset, sepsis-like picture.

Because of the increased rate of resistance of *H. influenzae* and pneumococcus to ampicillin, some centers begin treatment with ampicillin and a third-generation cephalosporin (and vancomycin if meningitis is present) when sepsis occurs in the last week of the first month of life. The treatment of late-onset neonatal sepsis and meningitis is the same as that for early-onset sepsis.

Chapter 66

CONGENITAL INFECTIONS

An infection acquired transplacentally during gestation is a congenital infection. Numerous pathogens that produce mild or subclinical disease in older infants and children can cause severe disease in neonates who acquire such infections prenatally or perinatally. Sepsis, meningitis, pneumonia, and other infections caused by numerous perinatally acquired pathogens are the cause of significant neonatal morbidity and mortality. Congenital infections include a well-known group of fungal, bacterial, and viral pathogens: toxoplasmosis, rubella, cytomegalovirus (CMV), herpes simplex virus (HSV), varicella-zoster virus, congenital syphilis, parvovirus, human immunodeficiency virus (HIV), hepatitis B, *Neisseria gonorrhoeae*, *Chlamydia*, and *Mycobacterium tuberculosis*.

Many of the clinical manifestations of congenital infections are similar, including intrauterine growth restriction, nonimmune hydrops, anemia, thrombocytopenia, jaundice, hepatosplenomegaly, chorioretinitis, and congenital malformations. Some unique manifestations and epidemiologic characteristics of these infections are listed in Table 66-1. Evaluation of patients thought to have a congenital infection should include attempts to isolate the organism by culture (for rubella, CMV, HSV, gonorrhea, and *M. tuberculosis*), to identify the antigen of the pathogen (for hepatitis B and *Chlamydia trachomatis*), to identify the pathogen's genome with polymerase chain reaction (PCR), and to identify specific fetal production of antibodies (IgM or increasing titer of IgG for *Toxoplasma*, syphilis, parvovirus, HIV, or *Borrelia*).

Treatment is not always available, specific, or effective. Nonetheless, some encouraging results have been reported for preventing the disease and for specifically treating the infant when the correct diagnosis is made (see Table 66-1).

TOXOPLASMOSIS

Decision-Making Algorithms
Available @ StudentConsult.com

Abnormal Head Size, Shape, and Fontanels
Visual Impairment and Leukocoria
Petechiae/Purpura

Vertical transmission of *Toxoplasma gondii* occurs by transplacental transfer of the organism from the mother to the fetus after an acute maternal infection. Fetal infection rarely can occur after reactivation of disease in an immunocompromised pregnant mother. Transmission from an acutely infected mother to her fetus occurs in about 30% to 40% of cases, but the rate varies directly with gestational age. Transmission rates and the timing of fetal infection correlate directly with placental blood flow; the risk of infection increases throughout gestation to 90% or greater near term, and the time interval between maternal and fetal infection decreases.

The severity of fetal disease varies inversely with the gestational age at which maternal infection occurs. Most infants have subclinical infection with no overt disease at birth; however, specific ophthalmologic and central nervous system (CNS) evaluations may reveal abnormalities. The classic findings of hydrocephalus, chorioretinitis, and intracerebral calcifications suggest the diagnosis of congenital toxoplasmosis. Affected infants tend to be small for gestational age, develop early-onset jaundice, have hepatosplenomegaly, and present with a generalized maculopapular rash. Seizures are common, and skull films may reveal diffuse cortical calcifications in contrast to the periventricular pattern observed with CMV. These infants are at increased risk for long-term neurologic and neurodevelopmental complications.

Serologic tests are the primary means of diagnosis. IgG-specific antibodies achieve a peak concentration 1 to 2 months after infection and remain positive indefinitely. For infants with seroconversion or a fourfold increase in IgG titers, specific IgM antibody determinations should be performed to confirm disease. Especially for congenital infections, measurement of IgA and IgE antibodies can be useful to confirm the disease. Thorough ophthalmologic, auditory, and neurologic evaluations (head computed tomography and cerebrospinal fluid [CSF] examination) are indicated.

For symptomatic and asymptomatic congenital infections, initial therapy should include pyrimethamine (supplemented with folic acid) combined with sulfadiazine. Duration of therapy is often prolonged, even up to 1 year. Optimal dosages of medications and duration of therapy should be determined in consultation with appropriate specialists.

RUBELLA

Decision-Making Algorithms
Available @ StudentConsult.com

Abnormal Head Size, Shape, and
    Fontanelles
Visual Impairment and Leukocoria
Heart Murmurs
Hearing Loss

Table 66-1	Perinatal Congenital Infections (TORCH)	
AGENT	**MATERNAL EPIDEMIOLOGY**	**NEONATAL FEATURES**
Toxoplasma gondii	Heterophil-negative mononucleosis Exposure to cats or raw meat or immunosuppression High-risk exposure at 10–24 wk gestation	Hydrocephalus, abnormal spinal fluid, intracranial calcifications, chorioretinitis, jaundice, hepatosplenomegaly, fever Many infants asymptomatic at birth *Treatment:* pyrimethamine plus sulfadiazine
Rubella virus	Unimmunized seronegative mother; fever ± rash Detectable defects with infection: by 8 wk, 85% 9–12 wk, 50% 13–20 wk, 16% Virus may be present in infant's throat for 1 yr *Prevention:* vaccine	Intrauterine growth restriction, microcephaly, microphthalmia, cataracts, glaucoma, "salt and pepper" chorioretinitis, hepatosplenomegaly, jaundice, PDA, deafness, blueberry muffin rash, anemia, thrombocytopenia, leukopenia, metaphyseal lucencies, B-cell and T-cell deficiency Infant may be asymptomatic at birth
CMV	Sexually transmitted disease: primary genital infection may be asymptomatic Heterophil-negative mononucleosis; infant may have viruria for 1–6 yr	Sepsis, intrauterine growth restriction, chorioretinitis, microcephaly, periventricular calcifications, blueberry muffin rash, anemia, thrombocytopenia, neutropenia, hepatosplenomegaly, jaundice, deafness, pneumonia Many asymptomatic at birth *Prevention:* CMV-negative blood products *Possible treatment:* ganciclovir
Herpes simplex type 2 or 1 virus	Sexually transmitted disease: primary genital infection may be asymptomatic; intrauterine infection rare, acquisition at time of birth more common	*Intrauterine infection:* chorioretinitis, skin lesions, microcephaly *Postnatal:* encephalitis, localized or disseminated disease, skin vesicles, keratoconjunctivitis *Treatment:* acyclovir
Varicella-zoster virus	Intrauterine infection with chickenpox Infant develops severe neonatal varicella with maternal illness 5 days before or 2 days after delivery	Microphthalmia, cataracts, chorioretinitis, cutaneous and bony aplasia/hypoplasia/atrophy, cutaneous scars Zoster as in older child *Prevention of neonatal condition* with VZIG *Treatment of ill neonate:* acyclovir
Treponema pallidum (syphilis)	Sexually transmitted disease Maternal primary asymptomatic: painless "hidden" chancre Penicillin, not erythromycin, prevents fetal infection	Presentation *at birth* as nonimmune hydrops, prematurity, anemia, neutropenia, thrombocytopenia, pneumonia, hepatosplenomegaly *Late neonatal* as snuffles (rhinitis), rash, hepatosplenomegaly, condylomata lata, metaphysitis, cerebrospinal fluid pleocytosis, keratitis, periosteal new bone, lymphocytosis, hepatitis *Late onset:* teeth, eye, bone, skin, central nervous system, ear *Treatment:* penicillin
Parvovirus	Etiology of fifth disease; fever, rash, arthralgia in adults	Nonimmune hydrops, fetal anemia *Treatment:* in utero transfusion
HIV	AIDS; most mothers are asymptomatic and HIV positive; high-risk history; prostitute, drug abuse, married to bisexual, or hemophiliac	AIDS symptoms develop between 3 and 6 mo of age in 10%–25%; failure to thrive, recurrent infection, hepatosplenomegaly, neurologic abnormalities *Management:* trimethoprim/sulfamethoxazole, AZT, other antiretroviral agents *Prevention:* prenatal, intrapartum, postpartum AZT; avoid breastfeeding
Hepatitis B virus	Vertical transmission common; may result in cirrhosis, hepatocellular carcinoma	Acute neonatal hepatitis; many become asymptomatic carriers *Prevention:* HBIG, vaccine
Neisseria gonorrhoeae	Sexually transmitted disease, infant acquires at birth *Treatment:* cefotaxime, ceftriaxone	Gonococcal ophthalmia, sepsis, meningitis *Prevention:* silver nitrate, erythromycin eye drops *Treatment:* ceftriaxone
Chlamydia trachomatis	Sexually transmitted disease, infant acquires at birth *Treatment:* oral erythromycin	Conjunctivitis, pneumonia *Prevention:* erythromycin eye drops *Treatment:* oral erythromycin
Mycobacterium tuberculosis	Positive PPD skin test, recent converter, positive chest radiograph, positive family member *Treatment:* INH and rifampin ± ethambutol	Congenital rare septic pneumonia; acquired primary pulmonary TB; asymptomatic, follow PPD *Prevention:* INH, BCG, separation Treatment: INH, rifampin, pyrazinamide
Trypanosoma cruzi (Chagas disease)	Central South American native, immigrant, travel Chronic disease in mother	Failure to thrive, heart failure, achalasia *Treatment:* nifurtimox

AZT, Zidovudine (azidothymidine); *BCG,* bacille Calmette-Guerin; *CMV,* cytomegalovirus; *HBIG,* hepatitis B immune globulin; *INH,* isoniazid; *PDA,* patent ductus arteriosus; *PPD,* purified protein derivative; *TB,* tuberculosis; *VZIG,* varicella-zoster immune globulin.

With the widespread use of vaccination, congenital rubella is rare in developed countries. Acquired in utero during early gestation, rubella can cause severe neonatal consequences. The occurrence of congenital defects approaches 85% if infection is acquired during the first 4 weeks of gestation; close to 40% spontaneously abort or are stillborn. If infection occurs during weeks 13 to 16, 35% of infants can have abnormalities. Infection after 4 months' gestation does not seem to cause disease.

The most common characteristic abnormalities associated with congenital rubella include ophthalmologic (cataracts, retinopathy, and glaucoma), cardiac (patent ductus arteriosus and peripheral pulmonary artery stenosis), auditory (sensorineural hearing loss), and neurologic (behavioral disorders, meningoencephalitis, and mental retardation) conditions. In addition, infants can present with growth retardation, hepatosplenomegaly, early-onset jaundice, thrombocytopenia, radiolucent bone disease, and purpuric skin lesions ("blueberry muffin" appearance from dermal erythropoiesis).

Detection of rubella-specific IgM antibody usually indicates recent infection. Measurement of rubella-specific IgG over several months can be confirmatory. Rubella virus can be isolated from blood, urine, CSF, and throat swab specimens. Infants with congenital rubella are chronically and persistently infected and tend to shed live virus in urine, stools, and respiratory secretions for 1 year. Infants should be isolated while in the hospital and kept away from susceptible pregnant women when sent home.

CYTOMEGALOVIRUS

Decision-Making Algorithms
Available @ StudentConsult.com

Visual Impairment and Leukocoria
Hepatomegaly
Hearing Loss
Petechiae/Purpura

CMV is the most common congenital infection and the leading cause of sensorineural hearing loss, mental retardation, retinal disease, and cerebral palsy. Congenital CMV occurs in about 0.5% to 1.5% of births. When primary infection occurs in mothers during a pregnancy, the virus is transmitted to the fetus in approximately 35% of cases. Rates of CMV infection are three to seven times greater in infants born to adolescent mothers compared to others. The risk of transmission of CMV to the fetus is independent of gestational age at the time of maternal infection. The earlier in gestation that the primary maternal infection occurs, the more symptomatic the infant will be at birth. The most common sources of CMV for primary infections occurring in mothers during pregnancy are sexual contacts and contact with young children. It is well known that CMV can be transmitted to the fetus even when maternal infection occurred long before conception. This transmission can occur as the result of virus reactivation, chronic infection, or reinfection with a new strain.

More than 90% of infants who have congenital CMV infection exhibit no clinical evidence of disease at birth. Approximately 10% of infected infants are small for gestational age and have symptoms at birth. Findings include microcephaly, thrombocytopenia, hepatosplenomegaly, hepatitis,

intracranial calcifications, chorioretinitis, and hearing abnormalities. Some infants can present with a blueberry muffin appearance as the result of dermal erythropoiesis. Skull films may reveal periventricular calcifications. An additional 10% of infected infants may not present until later in infancy or early childhood, when they are found to have sensorineural hearing loss and developmental delays. Mortality is 10% to 15% in symptomatic newborns. Perinatal CMV infection acquired during birth or from mother's milk is not associated with newborn illness or CNS sequelae.

Congenital CMV infection is diagnosed by detection of virus in the urine or saliva. Detection is often accomplished by traditional virus culture methods but can take several weeks to obtain a result. Rapid culture methods using centrifugation to enhance infectivity and monoclonal antibody to detect early antigens in infected tissue culture can give results in 24 hours. PCR also can be used to detect small amounts of CMV DNA in the urine. Detection of CMV within the first 3 weeks after birth is considered proof of congenital CMV infection.

Trial studies in severely symptomatic newborns of the antiviral agent ganciclovir have shown a lack of progression of hearing loss.

HERPES SIMPLEX VIRUS

HSV-2 accounts for 90% of primary genital herpes. About 70% to 85% of neonatal herpes simplex infections are caused by HSV-2. Most commonly, neonatal infections are acquired from the mother shortly before (ascending infection) or during passage through the birth canal at delivery. The incidence of neonatal HSV is estimated to range from 1 in 3000 to 1 in 20,000 live births. Infants with HSV infections are more likely to be born prematurely (40% of affected infants are <36 weeks' gestation). The risk of infection at delivery in an infant born vaginally to a mother with primary genital herpes is about 33% to 50%. The risk to an infant born to a mother with a reactivated infection is less than 5%. More than 75% of infants who acquire HSV infection are born to mothers who have no previous history or clinical findings consistent with HSV infection.

Most infants are normal at birth, and symptoms of infection develop at 5 to 10 days of life. Symptoms of neonatal HSV infection include disseminated disease involving multiple organ systems, most notably the liver and lungs; localized infection to the CNS; or localized infection to the skin, eyes, and mouth. Symptoms may overlap, and in many cases of disseminated disease, skin lesions are a late finding. Disseminated infection should be considered in any infant with symptoms of sepsis, liver dysfunction, and negative bacteriologic cultures. HSV infection also should be suspected in any neonate who presents with fever, irritability, abnormal CSF findings, and seizures. Initial symptoms can occur anytime between birth and 4 weeks of age, although disseminated disease usually occurs during the first week of life. HSV infections are often severe, and a delay in treatment can result in significant morbidity and mortality.

For the diagnosis of neonatal HSV infection, specimens for culture should be obtained from any skin vesicle, nasopharynx, eyes, urine, blood, CSF, stool, or rectum. Positive cultures obtained from these sites more than 48 hours after birth indicate intrapartum exposure. PCR is a sensitive method for detecting HSV DNA in blood, urine, and CSF.

Parenteral acyclovir is the treatment of choice for neonatal HSV infections. Acyclovir should be administered to all infants suspected to have infection or diagnosed with HSV. The most benign outcome with regard to morbidity and mortality is observed in infants with disease limited to the skin, eyes, and mouth.

CONGENITAL SYPHILIS

Decision-Making Algorithms
Available @ StudentConsult.com

Rhinorrhea
Abnormal Head Size, Shape, and Fontanels
Red Eye
Hoarseness
Hepatomegaly
Hearing Loss
Lymphadenopathy

Congenital syphilis most commonly results from transplacental infection of the fetus, although the fetus can acquire infection by contact with a chancre at birth. In addition, hematogenous infection can occur throughout pregnancy. The longer the time elapsed between the mother's infection and pregnancy, the less likely she is to transmit the disease to the fetus.

Intrauterine infection can result in stillbirth, hydrops fetalis, or prematurity. Clinical symptoms vary but include hepatosplenomegaly, snuffles, lymphadenopathy, mucocutaneous lesions, osteochondritis, rash, hemolytic anemia, and thrombocytopenia. Untreated infants, regardless of whether they manifest symptoms at birth, may develop late symptoms, which usually appear after 2 years of age and involve the CNS, bones, joints, teeth, eyes, and skin. Some manifestations of disease may not become apparent until many years after birth, such as interstitial keratitis, eighth cranial nerve deafness, Hutchinson teeth, bowing of the shins, frontal bossing, mulberry molars, saddle nose, rhagades, and Clutton joints. The combination of interstitial keratitis, eighth cranial nerve deafness, and Hutchinson teeth is commonly referred to as the *Hutchinson triad* (see Table 66-1).

Many infants are asymptomatic at the time of diagnosis. If untreated, most infants develop symptoms within the first 5 weeks of life. The most striking lesions affect the mucocutaneous tissues and bones. Early signs of infection may be poor feeding and snuffles (syphilitic rhinitis). Snuffles are more severe and persistent than the common cold and are often bloody. A maculopapular desquamative rash develops over the palms and soles and around the mouth and anus. The rash may progress to become vesicular with bullae. Severely ill infants may be born with hydrops and have profound anemia. Severe consolidated pneumonia may be present at birth, and there may be laboratory findings consistent with a glomerulonephritis. CSF evaluation may reveal a pleocytosis and elevated protein. More than 90% of symptomatic infants exhibit radiographic abnormalities of the long bones consistent with osteochondritis and perichondritis.

No newborn should be discharged from the hospital without knowledge or determination of the mother's serologic status for syphilis. All infants born to seropositive mothers require a careful examination and a quantitative nontreponemal syphilis test. Dark-field examination of direct fluorescent antibody staining of organisms obtained by scraping a skin or mucous membrane lesion is the quickest and most direct method of diagnosis. More commonly, serologic testing is used. The nontreponemal reaginic antibody assays—the Venereal Disease Research Laboratory (VDRL) and the rapid plasma reagin—are helpful as indicators of disease. The test performed on the infant should be the same as that performed on the mother to enable comparison of results. An infant should be evaluated further if the maternal titer has increased fourfold, if the infant's titer is fourfold greater than the mother's titer, if the infant is symptomatic, or if the mother has inadequately treated syphilis. A mother infected later in pregnancy may deliver an infant who is incubating active disease. The mother and infant may have negative serologic testing at birth. When clinical or serologic tests suggest congenital syphilis, CSF should be examined microscopically, and a CSF VDRL test should be performed. An increased CSF white blood cell count and protein concentration suggests neurosyphilis; a positive CSF VDRL is diagnostic.

Parenteral penicillin is the preferred drug of choice for treatment of syphilis. Penicillin G for 10 to 14 days is the only documented effective therapy for infants who have congenital syphilis and neurosyphilis. Infants should have repeat nontreponemal antibody titers repeated at 3, 6, and 12 months to document falling titers. Infants with neurosyphilis must be followed carefully with serologic testing and CSF determinations every 6 months for at least 3 years or until CSF findings are normal.

HUMAN IMMUNODEFICIENCY VIRUS
(SEE CHAPTER 125)

HEPATITIS B
(SEE CHAPTER 113)

NEISSERIA GONORRHOEAE

Decision-Making Algorithm
Available @ StudentConsult.com

Hepatomegaly

N. gonorrhoeae infection in a newborn usually involves the eyes (ophthalmia neonatorum). Other sites of infection include scalp abscesses (often associated with fetal monitoring with scalp electrodes), vaginitis, and disseminated disease with bacteremia, arthritis, or meningitis. Transmission to the infant usually occurs during passage through the birth canal when mucous membranes come in contact with infected secretions.

Infection usually is present within the first 5 days of life and is characterized initially by a clear, watery discharge, which rapidly becomes purulent. There is marked conjunctival hyperemia and chemosis. Infection tends to be bilateral; however, one eye may be clinically worse than the other. Untreated infections can spread to the cornea (keratitis) and anterior chamber of the eye. This extension can result in corneal perforation and blindness.

Recommended treatment for isolated infection, such as ophthalmia neonatorum, is one intramuscular dose of ceftriaxone. Infants with gonococcal ophthalmia should receive eye irrigations with saline solution at frequent intervals before discharge. Topical antibiotic therapy alone is inadequate and is unnecessary when recommended systemic antimicrobial therapy is given. Infants with gonococcal ophthalmia should be hospitalized and evaluated for disseminated disease (sepsis, arthritis, meningitis). Disseminated disease should be treated with antimicrobial therapy (ceftriaxone or cefotaxime) for 7 days. Cefotaxime can be used in infants with hyperbilirubinemia. If documented, infants with meningitis should be treated for 10 to 14 days.

Tests for concomitant infection with *C. trachomatis,* congenital syphilis, and HIV should be performed. Results of the maternal test for hepatitis B surface antigen should be confirmed. Topical prophylaxis with silver nitrate, erythromycin, or tetracycline is recommended for all newborns for the prevention of gonococcal ophthalmia.

CHLAMYDIA

Decision-Making Algorithm
Available @ StudentConsult.com

Hepatomegaly

C. trachomatis is the most common reportable sexually transmitted infection, with a high rate of infection among sexually active adolescents and young adults. Prevalence of the organism in pregnant women ranges from 6% to 12% and can be 40% in adolescents. *Chlamydia* can be transmitted from the genital tract of an infected mother to her newborn. Acquisition occurs in about 50% of infants born vaginally to infected mothers. Transmission also has been reported in some infants delivered by cesarean section with intact membranes. In infected infants, the risk of conjunctivitis is 25% to 50%, and the risk of pneumonia is 5% to 20%. The nasopharynx is the most commonly infected anatomic site.

Neonatal chlamydial conjunctivitis is characterized by ocular congestion, edema, and discharge developing 5 to 14 days to several weeks after birth and lasting for 1 to 2 weeks. Clinical manifestations vary from mild conjunctivitis to intense inflammation and swelling. Both eyes are almost always involved; however, one eye may appear to be more swollen and infected than the other. The cornea is rarely involved, and preauricular adenopathy is rare.

Pneumonia in a young infant can occur between 2 and 19 weeks of age and is characterized by an afebrile illness with a repetitive staccato cough, tachypnea, and rales. Wheezing is uncommon. Hyperinflation with diffuse infiltrates can be seen on chest radiograph. Nasal stuffiness and otitis media can occur.

Diagnosis can be made by scraping the conjunctiva and culturing the material. Giemsa staining of the conjunctival scrapings revealing the presence of blue-stained intracytoplasmic inclusions within the epithelial cells is diagnostic. PCR is also available. Infants with conjunctivitis and pneumonia are treated with oral erythromycin for 14 days. Topical treatment of conjunctivitis is ineffective and unnecessary. The recommended topical prophylaxis with silver nitrate, erythromycin, or tetracycline for all newborns for the prevention of gonococcal ophthalmia does not prevent neonatal chlamydial conjunctivitis.

MYCOBACTERIUM TUBERCULOSIS
(SEE CHAPTER 124)

Suggested Reading

Engle WE: Infants born late preterm: definition, physiologic and metabolic immaturity, and outcomes, *NeoReviews* 10:e280, 2009.

Frankovich J, Sandborg C, Barnes P, et al: Neonatal lupus and related autoimmune disorders of infants, *NeoReviews* 9:e207–217, 2008.

HAPO Study Cooperative Research Group: Hyperglycemia and adverse pregnancy outcomes, *N Engl J Med* 358(19):1991–2002, 2008.

Jesse N, Neu J: Necrotizing enterocolitis: relationship to innate immunity, clinical features and strategies for prevention, *NeoReviews* 7:e143, 2006.

Kates EH, Kates JS: Anemia and polycythemia in the newborn, *Pediatr Rev* 28:33–34, 2007.

Kattwinkel J, Perlman J: The neonatal resuscitation program: the evidence evaluation process and anticipating edition 6, *NeoReviews* 11:e673, 2010.

Shankaran S: Neonatal encephalopathy: treatment with hypothermia, *NeoReviews* 11:e85, 2010.

Silva RA, Moshfeghi DM: Interventions in retinopathy of prematurity, *NeoReviews* 13:e476, 2012.

Steinhorn RH, Farrow KN: Pulmonary hypertension in the neonate, *NeoReviews* 8:e14–e21, 2007.

Wong RJ, Stevenson DK, Ahlfors CE, et al: Neonatal jaundice: bilirubin physiology and clinical chemistry, *NeoReviews* 8:e58–e67, 2007.

Adolescent Medicine

Kim Blake and Lisa M. Allen

Chapter 67

OVERVIEW AND ASSESSMENT OF ADOLESCENTS

The leading causes of mortality (Table 67-1) and morbidity (Table 67-2) in adolescents in the United States are behaviorally mediated. Motor vehicle injuries and other injuries account for more than 75% of all deaths. Unhealthy dietary behaviors and inadequate physical activity result in adolescent obesity with associated health complications (e.g., diabetes, hypertension).

It is the physician's responsibility to use every opportunity to inquire about risk-taking behaviors (Fig. 67-1), regardless of the presenting issue. Physical symptoms in adolescents are often related to psychosocial problems.

INTERVIEWING ADOLESCENTS

The adolescent interview shifts from information gathering from the parent to the adolescent. Interviewing an adolescent alone and discussing confidentiality are the cornerstones of obtaining information regarding risk-taking behaviors, anticipatory guidance, and protective factors (see Chapters 7 and 9).

The interview should take into account the developmental age of the adolescent (Table 67-3). Conversations about sports, friends, movies, and activities outside of school can be useful for all ages and help build rapport (Fig. 67-2).

Confidentiality is a key element when interviewing an adolescent (Table 67-4). The vital, open discussion about risk-taking behavior is more likely to happen when the adolescent is alone (Table 67-5). Some issues cannot be kept confidential, such as suicidal intent and disclosure of sexual or physical abuse. If there is an ambiguous situation, it is wise to obtain legal, ethical, or social work consultation. When caring for a young adolescent, the health care provider should encourage open discussions with a parent, guardian, or other adult.

The law confers certain rights on adolescents, depending on their health condition and personal characteristics, allowing them to receive health services without parental permission (Table 67-6). Usually adolescents can seek health care without parental consent for reproductive, mental, and emergency health services. Emancipated adolescents and *mature minors* may be treated without parental consent; such status should be documented in the record. The key characteristics of mature minors are their competence and capacity to understand, not their chronologic age. There must be a reasonable judgment that the health intervention is in the best interests of the minor.

Table 67-1	Leading Causes of Death in Adolescents	
RANK	**CAUSE**	**RATE (PER 100,000)**
1	Unintentional injuries	30.3
2	Assault (homicide)	10.4
3	Suicide	6.9
4	Malignant neoplasms (cancer)	3.2
5	Diseases of the heart	1.6

From Centers for Disease Control and Prevention, National Center for Health Statistics: National Vital Statistics 2007.

Table 67-2	Prevalence of Common Chronic Illnesses of Children and Adolescents
ILLNESS	**PREVALENCE**
PULMONARY	
Asthma	8%–12%
Cystic fibrosis	1:2500 white, 1:17,000 black
NEUROMUSCULAR	
Cerebral palsy	2–3:1000
Mental retardation	1%–2%
Seizure disorder	3.5:1000
Any seizure	3%–5%
Auditory-visual defects	2%–3%
Traumatic paralysis	2:1000
Scoliosis	3% males, 5% females
Migraine	6%–27% (↑ with increasing age)
ENDOCRINE/NUTRITION	
Diabetes mellitus	1.8:1000
Obesity	25%–30%
Anorexia nervosa	0.5%–1%
Bulimia	1% (young adolescence), 5%–10% (19–20 yr)
Dysmenorrhea	20%
Acne	65%

Structured Communication Adolescent Guide (SCAG)

Instructions for scoring this form

After your check-up, please score your doctor (or medical student) using this form.

Examples:

0 = Did Not	1 = Did	2 = Did Well
Dr. didn't ask at all.	Dr. asked as if reading a list.	Dr. established a relationship.
	Dr. asked as if embarrassed.	Dr. comfortable with questions.
	I felt judged.	Dr. did not judge.
	I felt a bit uncomfortable.	I felt comfortable.

General Rating: Give a general impression of each section.
A = Excellent, B = Good, C = Average, D = Poor, F = Fail

	Did Not 0	Did 1	Did Well 2	Give examples of things that stood out in your interview, one positive and one negative.
A. GETTING STARTED				*Example: I liked that you talked to me and not just my mom.*
1. Greeted me.	0	1	2	
2. Introduced self.	0	1	2	
3. Discussed confidentiality.	0	1	2	
GENERAL RATING A B C D F				

	Did Not 0	Did 1	Did Well 2	Give examples of things that stood out in your interview, one positive and one negative.
B. GATHERING INFORMATION				*Example: I felt bad when you asked about smoking with my mom in the room.*
4. Good body language.	0	1	2	
5. Encouraged me to speak by asking questions other than ones with a yes/no answer.	0	1	2	
6. Encouraged parent to speak *(leave out if no parent present)*.	0	1	2	
7. Listened and did not judge me.	0	1	2	
8. Established relationship with me by appropriate choice of words.	0	1	2	
GENERAL RATING A B C D F				

Figure 67-1 The Structured Communication Adolescent Guide (SCAG). The SCAG is an interviewing tool developed for learners to use with real or standardized adolescent patients. It incorporates the four major interview components: confidentiality, separation of the adolescent from the adult, psychosocial data gathering (using the HEADDSS mnemonic), and a nonjudgmental approach. The SCAG is at a grade 5 reading level and has demonstrated reliability and validity. A printable version is available through MedEdPORTAL.

Continued

	Did Not 0	Did 1	Did Well 2	Give examples of things that stood out in your interview, one positive and one negative.
C. TEEN ALONE				*Example: I was glad you talked about confidentially. I need lots of reassurance that you won't tell my mom.*
9. Separated me and parent. *(Leave out if no parent present.)*	0	1	2	
10. Discussed confidentiality.	0	1	2	
11. Gave me a chance to talk about things other than what I came in to discuss.	0	1	2	
12. Reflected on my feelings or concerns (example: You seem...)	0	1	2	
LIFESTYLES: Physician asks or talks about the following:				
13. **Home:** Family	0	1	2	
14. **Education:** School	0	1	2	
15. Friends	0	1	2	
16. **Activities**	0	1	2	
17. **Alcohol:** Beer and hard liquor	0	1	2	
18. **Drugs:** Cigarettes	0	1	2	
19. Marijuana	0	1	2	
20. Street drugs	0	1	2	
21. **Diet:** Weight/diet/eating habits	0	1	2	
22. **Sex:** Boyfriend/girlfriend	0	1	2	
23. Sexual activity	0	1	2	
24. Safe sex/ contraception	0	1	2	
25. **Self:** Body image, self-esteem	0	1	2	*Example: You weren't embarrassed to talk about sex. OR You seemed embarrassed to talk about sex.*
26. Moods/depression/ suicide	0	1	2	
GENERAL RATING A B C D F				

	Did Not 0	Did 1	Did Well 2	Comments: Please give examples of things that stood out in your interview.
D. WRAP UP				*Example: I wasn't sure what the next step would be.*
27. Summary, recapped issues	0	1	2	
28. Kept the confidentiality	0	1	2	
29. Asked if there were any questions	0	1	2	
30. Talked about what to do next (plan and follow-up)	0	1	2	
GENERAL RATING A B C D F				

Figure 67-1, cont'd

Table 67-3	Adolescent Psychological Development		
STAGE	**AGE**	**THINKING**	**CHARACTERISTICS**
Early teens	10–14	Concrete ↓	Appearance–"Am I normal?"
			Invincible
			Peer group
			No tomorrow
Middle teens	15–17		Risk-taking increased
			Limit testing
			"Who am I?"
			Experiment with ideas
Late teens	18–21	Formal operational	Future
			Planning
			Partner
			Separation

Table 67-5	Interviewing the Adolescent Alone: Discussion of HEADDSS Topics*
HOME/friends	Family, relationships, and activities. "What do you do for fun?"
EDUCATION	"What do you like best at school?" "How's school going?"
ALCOHOL	"Are any of your friends drinking?" "Are you drinking?"
DRUGS	Cigarettes, marijuana, street drugs. "Have you ever smoked?" "Many adolescents experiment with different drugs and substances. . . . Have you tried anything?"
DIET*	Weight, diet/eating habits. "Many adolescents worry about their weight and try dieting. Have you ever done this?"
SEX	Sexual activity, contraception. "Are you going out with anybody?" "Have you dated in the past?"
SUICIDE/ DEPRESSION	Mood swings, depression, suicide attempts or thoughts, self-image. "Feeling down or depressed is common for everyone. Have you ever felt so bad that you wanted to harm yourself?"

*The acronym HEADDSS can represent other terms, that is, A = Activities, D = Depression. Also see Figure 67-1.

SETTING ~ TOPICS ~ EXPLORE ~ PLAN

Figure 67-2 STEP guide for adolescent interviewing.

Table 67-6	Legal Rights of Minors

Age of majority (≥18 years of age in most states)

Exceptions in which health care services can be provided to a minor*:

Emergency care (e.g., life-threatening condition or condition in which a delay in treatment would increase significantly the likelihood of morbidity)

Diagnosis and treatment of sexuality-related health care

Diagnosis and treatment of drug-related health care

Emancipated minors (physically and financially independent of family; Armed Forces; married; childbirth)

Mature minors (able to comprehend the risks and benefits of evaluation and treatment)

All exceptions should be documented clearly in the patient's health record.

*Determined by individual state laws.

During the physical examination, a choice between the parent and a chaperone being present needs to be offered.

PHYSICAL GROWTH AND DEVELOPMENT OF ADOLESCENTS
Girls

Breast budding under the areola (**thelarche**) and fine straight pubic hair over the mons pubis (**adrenarche** or **pubarche**) are early pubertal changes occurring around 11 years of age (range, 8 to 13 years) (see Chapter 174). These changes mark the sexual maturity rating, or Tanner stage, II of pubertal development (Figs. 67-3 and 67-4). Completion of the Tanner stages should take 4 to 5 years. The peak growth spurt usually

Table 67-4	Guidelines for Confidentiality

Prepare the preadolescent and parent for confidentiality and being interviewed alone.

Discuss confidentiality at the start of the interview.

Conversations with parents/guardians/adolescent are confidential (with exceptions*).

Reaffirm confidentiality when alone with your adolescent patient.

*Exceptions to confidentiality include major or impending harm to any person (i.e., abuse, suicide, homicide).

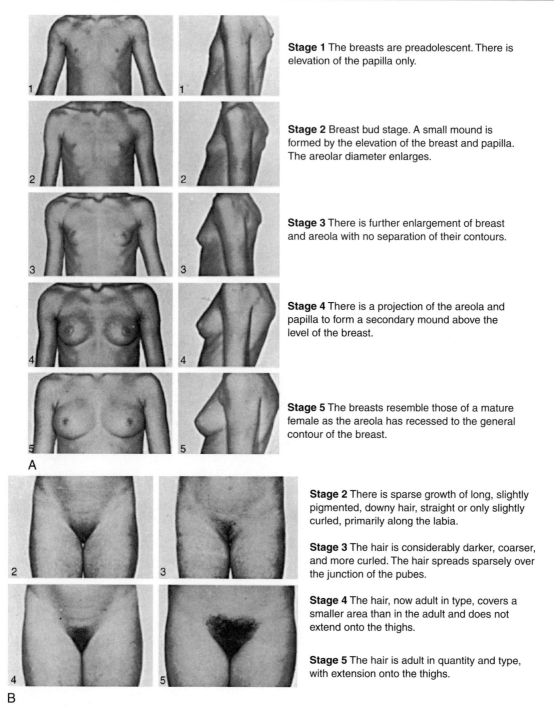

Stage 1 The breasts are preadolescent. There is elevation of the papilla only.

Stage 2 Breast bud stage. A small mound is formed by the elevation of the breast and papilla. The areolar diameter enlarges.

Stage 3 There is further enlargement of breast and areola with no separation of their contours.

Stage 4 There is a projection of the areola and papilla to form a secondary mound above the level of the breast.

Stage 5 The breasts resemble those of a mature female as the areola has recessed to the general contour of the breast.

Stage 2 There is sparse growth of long, slightly pigmented, downy hair, straight or only slightly curled, primarily along the labia.

Stage 3 The hair is considerably darker, coarser, and more curled. The hair spreads sparsely over the junction of the pubes.

Stage 4 The hair, now adult in type, covers a smaller area than in the adult and does not extend onto the thighs.

Stage 5 The hair is adult in quantity and type, with extension onto the thighs.

Figure 67-3 Typical progression of female pubertal development, stages 1 to 5. **A**, Pubertal development in the size of female breasts. **B**, Pubertal development of female pubic hair. Note that in stage 1 (not shown) there is no pubic hair. *(Courtesy of J.M. Tanner, MD, Institute of Child Health, Department of Growth and Development, University of London, London, England.)*

occurs approximately 1 year after thelarche at sexual maturity rating stage III to IV breast development and before the onset of menstruation **(menarche).** Menarche is a relatively late pubertal event. Females grow only 2 to 5 cm in height before menarche (see Chapter 174).

The mean ages of thelarche and adrenarche are approximately 9 and 10 years for African American and white girls, respectively. The mean ages of menarche are 12.2 and 12.9 years for African American and white girls, respectively. The interval from the initiation of thelarche to the onset of menses (menarche) is 2.3 ± 1 years. Pubertal changes before 6 years of age in African American and 7 years of age in white girls are considered precocious.

Boys
Testicular enlargement (≥2.5 cm) corresponds to sexual maturity rating, or Tanner, stages I to II (Figs. 67-5 and 67-6). Testicular enlargement is followed by pubic hair development at the base of the penis **(adrenarche)** and then axillary hair within the year. The growth spurt is a relatively late event; it can occur from 10½ years of age to 16 years of age. Deepening of the

Figure 67-4 Sequence of pubertal events in the average American female. More recent studies suggest that onset of breast development may be 9 years of age for African American girls and 10 years of age for white girls. *(From Brookman RR, Rauh JL, Morrison JA, et al: The Princeton maturation study, 1976, unpublished data for adolescents in Cincinnati, Ohio. Reprinted from* Assessment of Pubertal Development, *Columbus, Ohio, 1986, Ross Laboratories.)*

Figure 67-6 Sequence of pubertal events in the average American male. Testicular volume less than 4 mL using an orchidometer (Prader Beads) represents prepubertal stage. *(From Brookman RR, Rauh JL, Morrison JA, et al: The Princeton maturation study, 1976, unpublished data for adolescents in Cincinnati, Ohio. Reprinted from* Assessment of Pubertal Development, *Columbus, Ohio, 1986, Ross Laboratories.)*

Stage 1 The penis, testes, and scrotum are of childhood size.

Stage 2 There is enlargement of the scrotum and testes, but the penis usually does not enlarge. The scrotal skin reddens.

Stage 3 There is further growth of the testes and scrotum and enlargement of the penis, mainly in length.

Stage 4 There is still further growth of the testes and scrotum and increased size of the penis, especially in breadth.

Stage 5 The genitalia are adult in size and shape.

A

Stage 2 There is sparse growth of long, slightly pigmented, downy hair, straight or only slightly curled, primarily at the base of the penis.

Stage 3 The hair is considerably darker, coarser, and more curled. The hair spreads sparsely over the junction of the pubes.

Stage 4 The hair, now adult in type, covers a smaller area than in the adult and does not extend onto the thighs.

Stage 5 The hair is adult in quantity and type, with extension onto the thighs.

B

Figure 67-5 Typical progression of male pubertal development. **A,** Pubertal development in the size of male genitalia. **B,** Pubertal development of male pubic hair. Note that in stage 1 there is no pubic hair. *(Courtesy of J.M. Tanner, MD, Institute of Child Health, Department of Growth and Development, University of London, London, England.)*

voice, facial hair, and acne indicate the early stages of puberty. See Chapter 174 for discussion of disorders of puberty.

Changes Associated with Physical Maturation

Tanner stages mark biologic maturation that can be related to specific laboratory value changes and certain physical conditions. The higher hematocrit values in adolescent boys than in adolescent girls are the result of greater androgenic stimulation of the bone marrow and not loss through menstruation. Alkaline phosphatase levels in boys and girls increase during puberty because of rapid bone turnover, especially during the growth spurt. Worsening of mild scoliosis is common in adolescents during their growth spurt.

PSYCHOLOGICAL GROWTH AND DEVELOPMENT OF ADOLESCENTS
SEE TABLE 67-3 AND CHAPTERS 7 AND 9.

Chapter **68**

WELL-ADOLESCENT CARE

When interviewing an adolescent, use a nonjudgmental approach and find some common ground to get the adolescent talking about himself or herself. The HEADDSS (home, education, alcohol, drugs, diet, sex, suicide/depression) mnemonic addresses important risk-taking elements of the history (see Table 67-5). Adolescents who experiment in one area of risk-taking often have contemplated or tried multiple other risk-taking behaviors. When all of the risk-taking information has been gathered, the physician should choose one or two health care issues to discuss, making it clear that the information is confidential and that he or she is there to help the adolescent in a partnership way. Although the focus in adolescent care is on psychosocial issues, a general examination also needs to be performed (Table 68-1). Pediatric issues, such as immunization (see Chapter 94) and health screening, should be included (see Table 9-5).

EARLY ADOLESCENCE (AGES 10 TO 14 YEARS)

Rapid changes in physical appearance and behavior are the major characteristics of early adolescence, leading to a great deal of self-consciousness and need for privacy. The history focuses on the early adolescent's physical and psychosocial health.

MIDDLE ADOLESCENCE (AGES 15 TO 17 YEARS)

Autonomy and a global sense of identity are the major characteristics of middle adolescence. The history focuses on

Table 68-1	Examination of the Adolescent

PHYSICAL EXAMINATION—CHECKLIST

Explain to your patient what you are going to do.

Explain how you are going to do it.

Ask whether your adolescent wants his or her parent in the room.*

Be sensitive to the adolescent's needs.

Always use a sheet or blanket to provide privacy.

Let the adolescent remain dressed and work around the clothing.

Ask some questions as you go through the physical to keep the adolescent at ease. Give reassurance that elements of the physical are normal for this age.

ASSESSMENT

Examination can be used to offer reassurance about normalcy.†

Assess the following:

   Height/weight/body mass index and plot on percentile charts

   Skin for acne

   Mouth for periodontal disease

   Tanner staging

   Breasts and testicles

   Thyroid (palpation)

   Skeletal: scoliosis, Osgood-Schlatter disease, slipped capital femoral epiphysis

   Mental status for depression; use screening tools

   Signs of substance abuse, risk-taking behaviors, and trauma

*If not, you will need a chaperone.
†For example, 70% of boys can have breast enlargement (gynecomastia), and girls often have one breast larger than the other.

the middle adolescent's interactions with family, school, and peers. High-risk behaviors as a result of experimentation are common.

LATE ADOLESCENCE (AGES 18 TO 21 YEARS)

Individuality and planning for the future are the major characteristics of late adolescence. Greater emphasis is placed on the late adolescent's responsibility for his or her health.

PELVIC EXAMINATION

A full pelvic examination is rarely required in a virginal adolescent girl. A bimanual rectal-abdominal examination (all midline internal genitalia are immediately anterior to the rectal wall) is as efficient as a vaginal-abdominal examination. In some girls, anesthesia may be required for a full pelvic examination.

Before a pelvic examination, the patient should be informed about the importance of the assessment and what maneuvers will take place; she should be encouraged to ask questions before, during, or after the examination. A chaperone should be offered when a family caregiver is not present. Assuring the patient that she has complete control over the examination and allowing participating by using a mirror or guiding the examiner is important. The examiner should maintain

Table 68-2	Etiology of Breast Masses in Adolescents

Classic or juvenile fibroadenoma (70%)

Fibrocystic disease

Breast cyst

Abscess/mastitis

Intraductal papilloma

Fat necrosis/lipoma

Cystosarcoma phyllodes (low-grade malignancy)

Adenomatous hyperplasia

Hemangioma, lymphangioma, lymphoma (rare)

Carcinoma (<1%)

Table 68-3	Etiology of Gynecomastia

Idiopathic

Hypogonadism (primary or secondary)

Liver disease

Renal disease

Hyperthyroidism

Neoplasms

  Adrenal

  Ectopic human chorionic gonadotropin secreting

  Testicular

Drugs

  Antiandrogens

  Antibiotics (isoniazid, ketoconazole, metronidazole)

  Antacids (H$_2$ blockers)

  Cancer chemotherapy (especially alkylating agents)

  Cardiovascular drugs

Drugs of abuse

  Alcohol

  Amphetamines

  Heroin

  Marijuana

Hormones (for female sex)

Psychoactive agents (e.g., diazepam, phenothiazines, tricyclics)

eye contact during the examination. Before all maneuvers, the patient must be informed of what to expect and the sensations.

A padded examination table with the patient in a frog-leg position maximizes comfort of a pelvic examination. Stirrups can be used but are less comfortable. The examination room, lubricants, and instruments should be warm. The examination should be unhurried but efficient.

Inspection of the genitalia includes evaluation of the pubic hair, labia majora and minora, clitoris, urethra, and hymenal ring. When a **speculum examination** is required, it must be performed before bimanual palpation of internal genitalia because lubricants interfere with the evaluation of microscopic and microbiologic samples. The speculum allows visualization of the vaginal walls and cervical os for collection of appropriate specimens, such as cultures or Papanicolaou (Pap) smears. A Pap smear is not needed until the adolescent is sexually active, unless there is a history of sexual abuse or vulvar infection with human papillomavirus. In the rare circumstance that a vaginal examination is necessary in a virginal girl, a Huffman (0.5 in. × 4.5 in.) or Pederson (0.9 in. × 4.5 in.) speculum should be used. A nonvirginal introitus frequently admits a small to medium-sized adult speculum.

NORMAL VARIANTS OF PUBERTY
Breast Asymmetry and Masses
It is not unusual for one breast to begin growth before (or to grow more rapidly than) the other, with resulting asymmetry. Reassurance that after full maturation the asymmetry will be less obvious and that all women have some degree of asymmetry is needed by some. The breast bud is a pea-sized mass below the nipple that is often tender. Occasionally young women present with a breast mass; usually these are **benign fibroadenomas** or cysts (Table 68-2). Breast cancer is extremely rare in this age group. An ultrasound evaluation is better for the evaluation of young, dense breasts and avoids the radiation exposure of mammography.

Physiologic Leukorrhea
Peripubertal girls (sexual maturity rating stage III) often complain of vaginal discharge. If the discharge is clear without

symptoms of pruritus or odor, it is most likely physiologic leukorrhea, due to ovarian estrogen stimulation of the uterus and vagina. A physical examination should reveal evidence of an estrogenized vulva and hymen without erythema or excoriation. The physician should always be alert for signs of abuse. If there are symptoms, cultures should be obtained. In these circumstances, vaginal cultures can be obtained without a speculum because **sexually transmitted infections** are vaginal until menarche, when cervical infections are the rule. Inspection of physiologic leukorrhea shows few white blood cells, estrogen maturation of vaginal epithelial cells, and no pathogens on a culture.

Irregular Menses
Menarche typically occurs approximately 2 years after thelarche, at the average age of 12.6 years. The initial menses are anovulatory and tend to be irregular in duration. This irregularity may persist for 2 to 5 years, so reassurance may be required. During this phase, estrogen feedback on the hypothalamus decreases gonadotropin secretion, which reduces estrogen production and induces an estrogen withdrawal bleed that can be prolonged and heavy. Anovulatory bleeding is usually painless. As the hypothalamic-pituitary-gonadal axis matures, the cycle becomes ovulatory, and menses are secondary to progesterone withdrawal. When ovulation is established, the average cycle length is 21 to 45 days. Some adolescents ovulate with their first cycle, as indicated by pregnancy before menarche.

Gynecomastia

Breast enlargement in boys is usually a benign, self-limited condition. Gynecomastia is noted in 50% to 60% of boys during early adolescence. It is often idiopathic, but it may be noted in various conditions (Table 68-3). Typical findings include the appearance of a 1- to 3-cm, round, freely mobile, often tender, and firm mass immediately beneath the areola during sexual maturity rating stage III. Large, hard, or fixed enlargements and masses associated with any nipple discharge warrant further investigation. Reassurance is usually the only treatment required. If the condition worsens and is associated with psychological morbidity, it may be treated with bromocriptine. Surgical treatment with reduction mammoplasty can be helpful with massive hypertrophy.

Chapter 69

ADOLESCENT GYNECOLOGY

MENSTRUAL DISORDERS

Irregular menses is the most common complaint of early adolescent girls. As regular, ovulatory cycles become established, pain with menstruation (**dysmenorrhea**) is a frequent complaint.

Amenorrhea

Primary amenorrhea is the complete absence of menstruation by 16 years of age in the presence of breast development or by 14 years of age in the absence of breast development. However 98% of adolescents have onset of menarche by age 15; therefore, investigations should begin at that age in young women without menses. **Secondary amenorrhea** refers to the cessation of menses for more than 3 consecutive months, any time after menarche.

Primary amenorrhea may be a result of functional or anatomic abnormalities of the hypothalamus, pituitary gland, ovaries, uterus, or vagina. Physiologic immaturity, stress, excessive exercise, and abnormal dietary patterns (anorexia/bulimia) are the most common causes of amenorrhea. Pregnancy should be considered in all cases of secondary amenorrhea, even if the patient denies sexual activity.

The **history** and **physical examination** should guide the investigation. An outflow tract obstruction should be ruled out in adolescents with primary amenorrhea, abdominal pain, and secondary sexual characteristics. An abdominal mass resulting from accumulated blood may be present. Low outflow tract obstructions, such as an imperforate hymen, are visible on examination. An endocrine evaluation is indicated for girls with primary amenorrhea without secondary sexual characteristics and an unremarkable history and physical examination. Elevated follicle-stimulating hormone (FSH) and luteinizing hormone (LH) indicate primary ovarian insufficiency, which may reflect ovarian dysgenesis or ovarian agenesis and warrants a karyotype. **Turner syndrome** is a common cause, but other chromosomal anomalies, fragile X premutation carriers, and autoimmune etiologies should be ruled out. Low levels of FSH and LH suggest hypothalamic dysfunction, which may be due to physiologic immaturity (often familial), isolated gonadotropin deficiency, or hypogonadotropic hypogonadism (chronic illness, low body weight, stressful life events). Additional hormone evaluation includes thyroid-stimulating hormone and prolactin. Hypothyroidism is a common cause of menstrual dysfunction. A prolactinoma, although rare, must be ruled out.

Girls with secondary amenorrhea have secondary sexual characteristics. The most common causes are pregnancy, anorexia/stress (low LH, FSH, and estradiol), and **polycystic ovary syndrome (PCOS)**. In PCOS there may be symptoms of androgen excess, such as acne and hirsutism, and weight gain and, with insulin resistance, acanthosis. If hirsutism or virilization is present, free and total testosterone, androstenedione, and dihydroepiandrosterone sulfate should be measured to rule out ovarian or adrenal tumors. A normal 17-hydroxyprogesterone level rules out late-onset **congenital adrenal hyperplasia**. PCOS is diagnosed with two of the following: infrequent menstrual bleeding or secondary amenorrhea, clinical or biochemical hyperandrogenism, and polycystic morphology of ovaries on ultrasound. Estradiol may be normal or low; and androgens, including dihydroepiandrosterone sulfate, may be elevated, although not to the extent that a tumor produces. Patients may have impaired glucose tolerance or hypercholesterolemia.

In a patient with amenorrhea (primary or secondary), normal secondary sex characteristics, negative pregnancy test, normal prolactin and thyroid-stimulating hormone, and no evidence of outflow tract obstruction, the total effect of estrogen on the uterus (rather than a single point estradiol level) can be determined by a **progesterone withdrawal test.** To achieve this, 5 to 10 mg of medroxyprogesterone (depending on body weight) is given daily for 5 days. If the uterus is normal and primed by estrogen (an intact hypothalamic-pituitary-gonadal axis) with no outflow tract obstruction, there should be bleeding within 1 week after the last progesterone tablet. If there is bleeding, the amenorrhea is secondary to anovulation. If there is no progesterone withdrawal bleeding, the uterus has been insufficiently exposed to estrogen, and there is systemic estrogen deficiency.

Therapy for the amenorrhea should be directed at the cause. Anovulation can be managed with either cyclic progesterone withdrawal or combined hormonal contraceptives (CHCs). In hypothalamic amenorrhea and ovarian failure, there is an associated hypoestrogenism; therapy is directed at replacing estrogen and progesterone, usually with a CHC. PCOS usually can be treated effectively with weight loss, exercise, progesterone withdrawal, or CHC. If there is evidence of androgen excess, CHCs reduce androgen production from the ovaries and increases sex hormone–binding globulin to reduce the amount of available androgen. Spironolactone helps treat hirsutism, and when there is evidence of insulin insensitivity, metformin can restore ovulatory cycles. Contraception should be prescribed, if applicable.

Abnormal Uterine Bleeding

Decision-Making Algorithm
Available @ StudentConsult.com

Abnormal Vaginal Bleeding

Normal, ovulatory menses can occur 21 to 45 days apart, measuring from the first day of menstruation to the first day of the next menstruation. The average duration of flow is 3 to 7 days, with more than 7 days considered prolonged. More than 8 well-soaked pads or 12 tampons per day may be considered excessive, although classically blood loss is difficult to estimate. Table 69-1 defines menstrual disorders according to the new International Federation of Gynecology and Obstetrics nomenclature and classification of **abnormal uterine bleeding (AUB)**. If the menstrual problem is unclear and nonacute, observation and charting on a menstrual calendar are warranted. Excessively heavy, prolonged, or infrequent bleeding in the first year after menarche is often physiologic but should be investigated, especially if there is associated iron deficiency anemia.

Approximately 20% of adolescents with heavy or prolonged menses, especially those presenting in early menarche, have a coagulation disorder and 10% have other pathology. If an underlying pathology is discovered, treatment should be directed at the primary disorder and the secondary menstrual dysfunction.

The differential diagnosis of AUB is found in Table 69-2. **Anovulation** is the most common etiology of AUB in adolescents. Without progesterone from the corpus luteum, unopposed estrogen causes endometrial hyperplasia and irregular endometrial shedding, which can be prolonged and heavy, sometimes life threatening. Progesterone induces a secretory endometrium. When progesterone is withdrawn, the endometrium sheds in a synchronous fashion with myometrial and vascular contractions (causing dysmenorrhea but limiting blood loss). For the first 1 to 2 years post-menarche, the majority of adolescent cycles are anovulatory. After 1 year of regular cycles, irregular bleeding usually indicates an organic abnormality.

A thorough history with a menstrual calendar indicating the amount of flow and associated symptoms is followed by physical examination, including a pelvic examination in a nonvirginal adolescent or an ultrasound in a virginal adolescent. Physical examination should also assess for signs of anemia, bruising or petechia, signs of hyperandrogenism or thyroid disease. A complete blood count, pregnancy test, thyroid function tests, and coagulation screen should be performed. In sexually active adolescents, **sexually transmitted infections (STIs)** should be ruled out.

Unpredictable, heavy, and prolonged menses may impair school attendance and social functioning; iron deficiency anemia is associated with lower academic scores. **Treatment** is indicated for heavy menses. Chronic and acute bleeding can be managed with CHCs; multiple daily doses may be required until blood loss is controlled. Occasionally uncontrollable bleeding requires hospitalization for intravenous fluids and high-dose estrogen. Uterine curettage is rarely indicated in adolescents. Iron therapy is also important. Use of CHCs to regulate menstruation and allow the hypothalamic-pituitary-gonadal axis to mature is appropriate; only 6 to 12 months of therapy may be required. CHCs are paramount in the management of heavy menstrual bleeding in individuals with **bleeding disorders** (von Willebrand disease), although adjuvant therapy with tranexamic acid may be needed for management of any scheduled withdrawal bleeds. Parents are often concerned that CHC use will cause their daughter to become sexually active, but literature and experience do not support this.

Table 69-1	Definition of Menstrual Disorders	
CLINICAL DIMENSION	**DESCRIPTIVE TERM**	**DEFINITION**
Frequency	Frequent menstrual bleeding	<21 days/cycle
	Infrequent menstrual bleeding	>35 days/cycle
Regularity	Amenorrhea	Absent for 6 months or more
	Irregular menstrual bleeding	>20 day variation in cycle length
Duration	Prolonged menstrual bleeding	>8 days of flow
	Shortened menstrual bleeding	<2 days of flow
Flow	Heavy menstrual bleeding	>80 cc loss
	Light menstrual bleeding	<5 cc loss
Intermenstrual bleeding		Bleeding between normally timed periods

Table 69-2	Differential Diagnosis of Abnormal Vaginal Bleeding*
Pregnancy, including ectopic pregnancy
Infection—usually sexually transmitted
Endocrine disorder—thyroid disorder, PCOS, pituitary disorder
Blood dyscrasia
Systemic disease
Trauma
Medications
Contraception
Vaginal, cervical, or uterine disorders
Ovarian tumor/cyst
Foreign body

PCOS, Polycystic ovary syndrome.
*When all excluded, the diagnosis of dysfunctional uterine bleeding can be made.

Dysmenorrhea

Decision-Making Algorithm
Available @ StudentConsult.com

Dysmenorrhea

The most common gynecologic complaint of young women is painful menstruation, or dysmenorrhea, during the first 1 to 3 days of bleeding. **Primary dysmenorrhea** is defined as pelvic pain during menstruation in the absence of pelvic pathology and is a feature of ovulation, typically developing 1 to 3 years after menarche, with an increasing incidence to the age of 24, as ovulatory cycles are established. The release of prostaglandins and leukotrienes from the degenerating endometrium after progesterone levels decline causes increased uterine tone and increased frequency and dysrhythmia of uterine contractions. This creates excessive uterine pressures and ischemia that heightens the sensitivity of pain fibers to bradykinin and other physical stimuli.

Secondary dysmenorrhea is menstrual pain associated with pelvic pathology and is caused most frequently by **endometriosis** or **pelvic inflammatory disease**. Adolescents with endometriosis usually have mild to moderate disease, but girls with obstructed outflow tracts tend to have severe endometriosis soon after menarche. The types of dysmenorrhea usually can be distinguished by history and physical examination. Ultrasound is preferred as the initial screen for obstructing genital tract lesions. Magnetic resonance imaging may be useful in complex reproductive tract anomalies. Laparoscopy is required to diagnose endometriosis and pelvic inflammatory disease with certainty, although it usually is reserved for patients who fail medical therapy.

Treatment of primary dysmenorrhea should be considered with symptoms causing significant distress. First-line therapy is nonsteroidal anti-inflammatory drugs (NSAIDs) (Table 69-3). To maximize pain relief, NSAIDs should be taken before or as soon as menstruation begins, and the dosing schedule should be followed closely. Typically NSAIDs are needed for 2 to 3 days. If NSAIDs fail to provide adequate relief, CHCs or long-acting reversible contraceptives (LARCs) may be added.

Table 69-3	Treatment of Dysmenorrhea
NSAIDs	
Over-the-counter	
Ibuprofen or naproxen sodium taken every 4 h	
Prescription	
Ibuprofen 400 mg PO qid	
Naproxen 500 mg PO stat then 250 PO to 500 mg PO bid	
Mefenamic acid 500 mg PO stat then 250 mg qid or 500 mg PO tid	
Diclofenac 100 mg PO stat then 50 mg tid	
Combined hormonal contraceptives—cyclic or continuous	
Progestogen-only pill	
Depo-Provera—150 mg IM every 12–14 wk	
LNG Intrauterine System	

LNG, Levonorgestrel; *NSAIDs*, nonsteroidal anti-inflammatory drugs.

These contraceptives may be first-line therapy, depending on need for pregnancy prevention.

If dysmenorrhea persists despite an adequate trial of CHCs (>4 months), an alternative diagnosis, such as endometriosis, should be considered. When CHCs fail, a laparoscopy may be performed before advancing therapy to confirm the diagnosis and excise endometriotic lesions. Extended CHC therapy (84 days of active CHC followed by a 5- to 7-day hormone-free interval) may control symptoms. Alternatives are depot medroxyprogesterone acetate (150 mg) every 2 months until symptoms are controlled, then every 3 months of levonorgestrel-releasing intrauterine system. Endometriosis may be treated with gonadotropin-releasing hormone agonists (nafarelin or leuprolide) and hormonal therapy, in older adolescents (>16 years of age) when symptom relief is required.

PREGNANCY

The median age of first intercourse in the United States is 17 years for girls and 16 years for boys; this is similar to other developed countries. Although the age of coital initiation is similar among different socioeconomic groups, the prevalence of adolescent childbearing is greatest in the lower socioeconomic strata. Risk factors for adolescent pregnancy include lower socioeconomic status, lower education, low self-esteem, lack of access to contraception, alcohol and drug use, and adverse early life experiences in the adolescent home. Approximately 900,000 U.S. females 12 to 19 years of age become pregnant each year. In women younger than 20 years of age, there are 97 pregnancies, 54 births, and 29 abortions per 1000. Increased use of contraceptives has reduced adolescent pregnancy by up to 35% since the peak year of 1990. Adolescents who continue their pregnancy have an increased incidence of preterm and very preterm births, low birth weight infants, infant neonatal admission, postneonatal mortality, child abuse, subsequent maternal unemployment, and poor maternal educational achievement. These risks are influenced by behavior and socioeconomic status, as well as inherent biologic risks within adolescents. Good prenatal care, nutrition, and social support improve pregnancy outcomes.

Diagnosis

Pregnancy should be considered and ruled out in any adolescent presenting with secondary amenorrhea. Frequently pregnant adolescents delay seeking a diagnosis until several periods have been missed and initially may deny having intercourse. Early adolescents often present with other symptoms, such as vomiting, vague pains, or deteriorating behavior and may report normal periods. Because of the varied presentations of adolescent pregnancy, a thorough menstrual history should be obtained in all menstruating adolescents. Urine pregnancy tests are sensitive approximately 7 to 10 days after conception. Rape or incest should be ruled out in all cases of adolescent pregnancy.

When pregnancy is confirmed, immediate gestational dating is important to assist in planning. Options are to continue or terminate the pregnancy (if not beyond 20 to 24 weeks' gestation). With the former, the adolescent may choose to parent the child or have the child adopted. Pregnant adolescents should be encouraged to involve their families to assist with decision making; parents may be more understanding than the adolescent expects.

Continuation of the Pregnancy

Adolescents who continue the pregnancy need early, consistent, and comprehensive prenatal care by a team of health care providers. Their socioeconomic situation should be evaluated in an effort to optimize the infant's health and development. Although fewer than 5% of adolescents have their infants adopted, this option should be discussed. Pregnancy is the most common cause for females to drop out of school, so special attention should be given to keeping the adolescent in school during and after pregnancy.

Termination

If a pregnant adolescent chooses to terminate her pregnancy, she should be referred immediately to a nonjudgmental abortion service. The options for pregnancy termination depend on the gestational age. Surgical procedures include manual vacuum aspiration (<8 weeks' gestational age), suction curettage (<12 to 14 weeks' gestational age, depending on the provider), and dilation and evacuation (14 to 20 weeks' gestational age). Early pregnancy (<8 weeks' gestational age) can be terminated medically with oral mifepristone (RU-486) in combination with misoprostol, methotrexate with misoprostol, or misoprostol alone. Adolescents rarely present early enough to explore this option. In the second trimester (>12 weeks' gestational age), labor induction and delivery can be effected by vaginal misoprostol or the intra-amniotic instillation of prostaglandins or hypertonic saline. Psychosocial support and subsequent contraceptive counseling and implementation should be available for adolescents who choose abortion.

CONTRACEPTION

Adolescents often begin intercourse without adequate birth control. Because unintended pregnancy can be associated with significant psychosocial morbidity for the mother, father, and child, prevention should be a primary goal. All methods of contraception significantly reduce the risk of pregnancy when used in a consistent and correct fashion. The best form of contraception is the one an individual will use. Contraceptives can be divided into user-based methods and LARCs. It is important to remind young women that steroidal contraception or LARCs do not provide any protection from STIs, and condoms should be used to reduce the risk of infection.

Abstinence

Abstaining from sexual intercourse is the most commonly used and most effective form of adolescent birth control. A degree of self-control, self-assuredness, and self-esteem is necessary. Adolescents who choose to be sexually active should be offered birth control, because there is a 70% chance of pregnancy in 1 year of regular, unprotected intercourse.

Steroidal Contraception

Combined Oral Contraceptives

Combined oral contraceptives (COCs) contain a synthetic estrogen and progesterone that suppress gonadotropin secretion and ovarian follicle development and ovulation. COCs also produce an atrophic endometrium (inhospitable for blastocyst implantation) and thicken cervical mucus to inhibit sperm penetration. COCs are 99% effective if taken regularly and have numerous noncontraceptive benefits (decreased acne, less dysmenorrhea, and lighter menstrual flow). After a history and physical examination, COCs can be started on the first day of the next menstrual period or as a Quick Start. The Quick Start method refers to starting on any day of the cycle, usually on the day of the visit to the health care provider, as long as pregnancy has been ruled out. Contraindications and relative contraindications to COCs are listed in Tables 69-4 and 69-5. Blood pressure measurement to rule out preexisting hypertension should be obtained before prescribing a COC. Initially the adolescent should be seen monthly to reinforce good contraceptive use and safer sex. Unless adolescents show the ability to take a pill daily, contraception with COCs should be avoided. When COCs are prescribed, 28-day packets are recommended because they encourage a daily routine. One novel contraceptive regimen has packaged 84 active tablets to be taken sequentially followed by a 7-day hormone-free interval and the next package. Any COC can be used in such a fashion to induce long intervals between withdrawal bleeding.

Initial **side effects,** such as nausea (pills should be taken at night to reduce this), breast tenderness, and breakthrough bleeding (especially if pills are missed), are common and usually transient. COCs do not generally cause weight gain. Usually 3 to 4 months on one COC are needed to determine acceptability. If there is breakthrough bleeding, the physician

Table 69-4	Absolute Contraindications to Combined Hormonal Contraceptives
Smoking and age >35 yr	
Hypertension (systolic ≥160 mm Hg or diastolic ≥100 mm Hg)	
Current or history of venous thromboembolism	
Ischemic heart disease	
History of cerebrovascular accident	
Complicated valvular heart disease (pulmonary hypertension, atrial fibrillation, history of subacute bacterial endocarditis)	
Migraine with focal neurologic symptoms	
Breast cancer (current)	
Diabetes with retinopathy/nephropathy/neuropathy	
Severe cirrhosis	
Liver tumor (adenoma or hepatoma)	

Table 69-5	Relative Contraindications to Combined Hormonal Contraceptives
<1 month postpartum and breastfeeding or <21 days postpartum not breastfeeding	
Adequately controlled hypertension	
Hypertension (systolic 140–159 mm Hg, diastolic 90–99 mm Hg)	
Migraine and age >35 yr	
Currently symptomatic gallbladder disease	
Mild cirrhosis	
History of combined oral contraceptive-related cholestasis	
History of malabsorptive bariatric surgery procedure	

Table 69-6	Management of Missed Combined Oral Contraceptives
1 Active pill delayed for <24 hours in any week	Take 1 active pill as soon as possible. Continue taking 1 pill OD until end of pack.
1 or more active pills missed (Week 1)	Take 1 active pill as soon as possible. Continue taking 1 pill OD until end of pack. Back up contraception for 7 days. Consider emergency contraception.
<3 pills missed (Week 2 or 3)	Take 1 active pill as soon as possible. Continue taking 1 pill OD until end of pack. Discard any placebo pills. Start new cycle of COC without an HFI.
3 or more missed pills (Week 2 or 3)	Take 1 active pill as soon as possible. Continue taking 1 pill OD until end of pack. Discard any placebo pills and start new cycle without an HFI. Back up contraception for 7 days. Consider emergency contraception.

COC, Combined oral contraceptive; HFI, hormone-free interval; OD, once daily.

should determine how often pills are forgotten before changing pills. Adolescents should be taught the appropriate response to missed doses (Table 69-6). Health care providers usually suggest the use of additional contraception in the first month.

Progestogen-Only Pill or Minipill

Although not as widely used as COCs, the progestogen-only (or progestin-only) pill, *norethindrone (Micronor),* is a safe and effective form of contraception when used consistently. It is supplied in packages of 28 tablets, each containing norethindrone with no hormone-free interval. It prevents pregnancy through reduced volume, increased viscosity, and altered molecular structure of cervical mucus, resulting in little or no sperm penetration. In addition, endometrial changes reduce the potential for implantation, and ovulation is partially or completely suppressed. Approximately 40% of women using progestogen-only contraceptives continue to ovulate. Progestogen-only contraception is indicated for women who have a contraindication to estrogen-based contraceptives (see Table 69-4) or have estrogen-related side effects.

Contraceptive Vaginal Ring

The contraceptive vaginal ring (*NuvaRing*) is a flexible, Silastic ring. The ring releases a constant rate of 15 mg of ethinyl estradiol and 0.120 mg of etonogestrel per day. Each ring is used continuously for 3 weeks and then removed. A new ring is inserted 7 days later. The contraindications and side effects are the same as with COCs.

Contraceptive Patch

The contraceptive patch (*norelgestromin [Evra]*) is a 25-cm^2 pink patch that is applied, usually on the buttocks, for 1 week followed by removal and application of a new patch for a total of 3 weeks of patch use, then a patch-free week for a withdrawal bleed. The 4-week cycle is repeated. The daily dose is equivalent to a 35-mg ethinyl estradiol COC. In women weighing 90 kg or more, the contraceptive patch is less efficacious.

Contraindications and side effects are the same as those in COCs.

Long-Acting Reversible Contraceptives
Hormonal Injections and Implants

Intramuscular injection of 150 mg of medroxyprogesterone acetate (*Depo-Provera*) every 12 to 14 weeks is an effective form of birth control. Progestogen-only contraception is associated with menstrual irregularities (70% amenorrhea and 30% frequent menstrual bleeding). Medroxyprogesterone acetate (*Depo-SubQ Provera 104*) is designed for subcutaneous use every 12 to 14 weeks and may be self-administered with minimal training. An implant containing the progestin etonogestrel (*Implanon*) is now available on the U.S. market. This single rod implant is inserted subcutaneously and is effective for 3 years. These forms of contraception are user- and coital-independent and reduce failure secondary to missed doses.

Intrauterine Devices

Intrauterine devices (IUDs) are inserted into the uterus where they release either copper (*ParaGard*) that is spermicidal or levonorgestrel (*Mirena*) that prevents implantation by inducing an atrophic endometrium. The copper IUD, which lasts up to 10 years, may increase the amount and duration of bleeding as well as dysmenorrhea. The levonorgestrel-releasing intrauterine system is highly effective for up to 5 years while decreasing bleeding and dysmenorrhea, even causing amenorrhea. Although a small increased risk of pelvic inflammatory disease exists for 21 days after insertion of an IUD, the risk following that transient period lowers and continues at a low rate for the remainder of time that the young woman uses an IUD. Adolescents should be screened for STIs at the time of IUD insertion, with treatment provided as soon as possible for positive results or if there is a concern of compliance at the time of IUD insertion. Insertion in nulliparous women can be aided by the use of a paracervical block. IUDs require no active involvement by the user, thus eliminating error and can be considered as one of the first line options for adolescent contraception. Condoms should be encouraged to reduce the risk of STI.

Emergency Postcoital Contraception

Emergency postcoital contraception should be discussed at every visit. A prescription should be given in advance of need when no over-the-counter access is available. Emergency contraception reduces the risk of pregnancy after unprotected intercourse if used within 5 days, although efficacy is greatest when used as early as possible. Other indications and contraindications to emergency postcoital contraception are listed in Table 69-7. There are two forms of emergency contraception: (a) **Plan B** (0.75 mg of levonorgestrel), one pill taken twice, 12 hours apart, or two tablets given once and (b) using a CHC pill the equivalent of 50 mg of ethinyl estradiol and 250 μg of norgestrel, each repeated in 12 hours. Plan B is also associated with significantly less nausea and vomiting than the CHC regimen. Mifepristone is also an effective postcoital contraceptive; however it is not approved for this use in the United States. A copper IUD can be inserted 7 days from the act of unprotected intercourse and has an efficacy of greater than 99%. This method is not generally recommended for adolescents.

Table 69-7	Emergency Contraception

INDICATIONS

No method of contraception being used

Condom breaks

Diaphragm dislodged/removed <6 h

Missed birth control pills

>1 wk late for Depo-Provera

Ejaculation on external genitalia

Sexual assault

CONTRAINDICATIONS

Known pregnancy

If strong contraindications to estrogens, use progestin.

Barrier Methods
Condoms and Foam
When condoms and spermicide (foam, gel, film, sponge) are used together in a correct fashion (film must be placed 10 minutes before intercourse), they are almost as effective as COCs in the prevention of pregnancy, especially in individuals who have infrequent intercourse. This method is available over-the-counter (latex and polyurethane condoms) without the need for a physician visit or prescription and reduces the risk of STIs, including human immunodeficiency virus (HIV). The female condom (*Reality*) is an additional barrier method made of polyurethane that affords females more control, but adolescents usually do not consider it aesthetically pleasing.

Sponge, Caps, and Diaphragm
The vaginal sponge (*Protectaid*) is a spermicide-impregnated synthetic sponge that is effective for 24 hours of intercourse. The *FemCap* is a silicone cap fitted by a health care provider and then placed on the cervix by the user before intercourse. This method is technically difficult, especially for an adolescent. The *diaphragm* is fitted by a health care provider but is technically simpler to use than the cap because the edges go into the vaginal fornices. To be effective, the diaphragm should be used with spermicide applied to the cervical side and along the rim. The diaphragm needs additional spermicide with each act of intercourse. The *Lea's Shield* is a silicone device, similar to a diaphragm, that covers the cervix and adheres to the vaginal vault by a mild vacuum generated by its design. All of these methods need to be left in place for 6 hours after the last act of intercourse for optimal efficacy.

Coitus Interruptus
Withdrawal is a common method of birth control used by sexually active adolescents, but it is ineffective because sperm are released into the vagina before ejaculation, and withdrawal may occur after ejaculation has begun.

Rhythm Method (Periodic Coital Abstinence)
The rhythm method is the practice of periodic abstinence just before, during, and just after ovulation. This method requires the user to have an accurate knowledge of her cycle, awareness of clues indicating ovulation, and discipline. Adolescents tend to have unpredictable cycles and consequently less predictable ovulation, so it is difficult to determine with any accuracy a time of the month that can be considered completely safe.

Oral and Anal Sex
Some adolescents engage in oral or anal sex because they believe that it eliminates the need for contraception. Many do not consider this activity to mean "having sex." Condoms generally are not used during oral or anal sex, but the risk of acquiring an STI is still present. Adolescents should be asked specifically about nonvaginal forms of sexual activity, and adolescents who engage in oral and anal sex require STI and HIV counseling and screening.

RAPE
Rape is a legal term for nonconsensual intercourse. Almost half of rape victims are adolescents, and the perpetrator is known in 50% of cases. Although gathering historical and physical evidence for a criminal investigation is important, the physician's primary responsibility is to perform these functions in a supportive, nonjudgmental manner. The history should include details of the sexual assault, time from the assault until presentation, whether the victim cleaned herself, date of last menstrual period, and previous sexual activity, if any.

For optimal results, forensic material should be collected within 72 hours of the assault. Clothes, especially undergarments, need to be placed in a paper bag for drying (plastic holds humidity, which allows organisms to grow, destroying forensic evidence). The patient should be inspected for bruising, bites, and oral, genital, and anal trauma. Photographs are the best record to document injuries. Specimens should be obtained from the fingernails, mouth, vagina, pubic hair, and anus. The sexual assault kit provides materials to obtain DNA from semen, saliva, blood, fingernail scrapings, and pubic hair. A wet mount of vaginal fluids shows the presence or absence of sperm under the microscope. Cultures for STIs should be taken but are often negative (unless previously infected), because 72 hours are needed for the bacterial load to be sufficient for a culture. Blood should be drawn for baseline HIV and syphilis (Venereal Disease Research Laboratories test). All materials must be maintained in a "chain of evidence" that cannot be called into question in court.

Therapy after a rape includes prophylaxis for emergency contraception and STI and, if indicated, hepatitis immune globulin and hepatitis vaccine. A single oral dose of cefixime, 400 mg, and azithromycin, 1 g, treats *Chlamydia*, gonorrhea, and syphilis. An alternative regimen is a single intramuscular dose of ceftriaxone, 125 mg, with a single oral dose of azithromycin, 1 g. For prophylaxis against bacterial vaginosis and *Trichomonas*, a single oral dose of metronidazole, 2 g, is recommended. Repeat cultures, wet mounts, and a pregnancy test should be performed 3 weeks after the assault, followed by serology for syphilis, hepatitis, and HIV at 12 weeks. Long-term sequelae are common; patients should be offered immediate and ongoing psychological support, such as that offered by local rape crisis services.

Chapter 70

EATING DISORDERS

Eating disorders are common chronic diseases in adolescents, especially in females. The *Diagnostic and Statistical Manual of Mental Disorders, fifth edition (DSM-V)*, classifies these as psychiatric illnesses. The diagnosis in young adolescents (pre-growth spurt, premenstrual) may not follow the typical diagnostic criteria (Table 70-1).

ANOREXIA NERVOSA

The *prevalence* of anorexia nervosa is 1.5% in teenage girls. The female-to-male ratio is approximately 20:1, and the condition shows a familial pattern. The cause of anorexia nervosa is unknown, but it involves a complex interaction between social, environmental, psychological, and biologic events (Fig. 70-1), with risk factors having been identified (Fig. 70-2).

Clinical Manifestations and Diagnosis

Screening for eating disorders is important and is best done as a part of the larger psychosocial screen for risk-taking factors (see Fig. 67-1). Although it is recommended that the adolescent be interviewed alone, he or she may minimize the problem; thus interviewing the parent(s) alone is also important. The first event usually described by an affected patient is a behavioral change in eating or exercise (i.e., food obsession, food-related ruminations, mood changes). The patient has an unrealistic body image and feels too fat, despite appearing excessively thin. Parents' response to this situation can be anger, self-blame, focusing attention on the child, ignoring the disorder, or approving of the behavior.

The physician should be nonjudgmental, collect information, and assess the differential diagnosis. The **differential diagnosis** of weight loss includes gastroesophageal reflux, peptic ulcer, malignancy, chronic diarrhea, malabsorption, inflammatory bowel disease, increased energy demands, hypothalamic lesions, hyperthyroidism, diabetes mellitus, and Addison disease. Psychiatric disorders also need to be considered (e.g., drug abuse, depression, obsessive-compulsive disorders).

The **clinical features** of anorexia include wearing oversized layered clothing to hide appearance, fine hair on the face and trunk (lanugo-like hair), rough and scaly skin, bradycardia, hypothermia, decreased body mass index, erosion of enamel of teeth (acid from emesis), and acrocyanosis of hands and feet. Signs of hyperthyroidism should not be present (see Chapter 175). The diagnostic criteria for anorexia nervosa are listed in Table 70-2.

Treatment and Prognosis

Treatment requires a multidisciplinary approach, including a feeding program as well as individual and family therapy. Feeding is accomplished through voluntary intake of regular foods, nutritional formula orally or by nasogastric tube. When vital signs are stable, discussion and negotiation of a detailed treatment contract with the patient and the parents

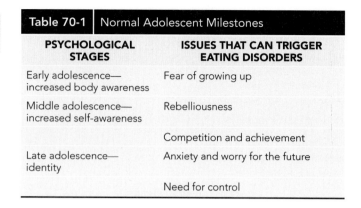

Table 70-1	Normal Adolescent Milestones	
PSYCHOLOGICAL STAGES	**ISSUES THAT CAN TRIGGER EATING DISORDERS**
Early adolescence—increased body awareness	Fear of growing up
Middle adolescence—increased self-awareness	Rebelliousness
	Competition and achievement
Late adolescence—identity	Anxiety and worry for the future
	Need for control

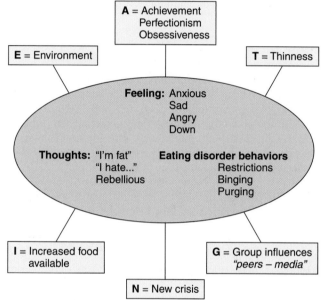

Figure 70-1 The eating disorder cycle.

are essential. The first step is to restore body weight. Hospitalization may be necessary (Table 70-3). When 80% of normal weight is achieved, the patient is given freedom to gain weight at a personal pace. The *prognosis* includes a 3% to 5% mortality (suicide, malnutrition) rate, the development of bulimic symptoms (30% of individuals), and persistent anorexia nervosa syndrome (20% of individuals).

BULIMIA NERVOSA

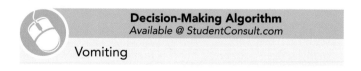

Decision-Making Algorithm
Available @ StudentConsult.com

Vomiting

Table 70-4 presents the diagnostic criteria for bulimia nervosa. The prevalence of bulimia nervosa is 5% in female college students. The female-to-male ratio is 10:1. Binge-eating episodes consist of large quantities of often forbidden foods or leftovers or both, consumed rapidly, followed by vomiting. Metabolic abnormalities result from the excessive vomiting or laxative

Clinical features
- Wearing oversized clothing
- Fine hair on the face and trunk (lanugo-like hair)
- Bradycardia, hypothermia
- Decreased body mass index
- Erosion of enamel of teeth (acid from emesis)
- Acrocyanosis of hands and feet.

Risk Factors
Familial
Personality types
Previous overweight
Affective disorders (family history)
Impulsive/negative (bulimia nervosa)
Psychiatric disease

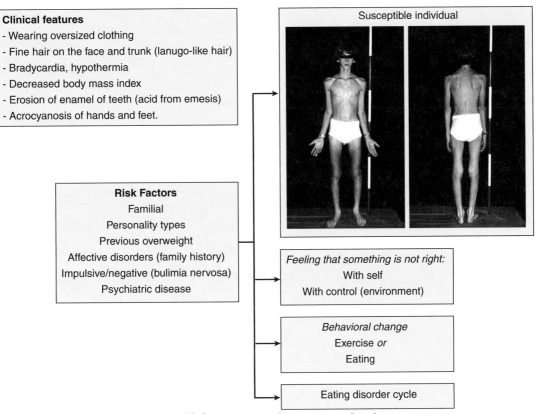

Susceptible individual

Feeling that something is not right:
With self
With control (environment)

Behavioral change
Exercise *or*
Eating

Eating disorder cycle

Figure 70-2 The slippery slope to eating disorders.

Table 70-2	Diagnostic Criteria for Anorexia Nervosa

Refusal to maintain body weight at or above a minimally normal weight for age and height (e.g., weight loss leading to body weight <85% of ideal)*

Intense fear of gaining weight or becoming fat, even though underweight

Denial of the seriousness of the low body weight—a disturbance in the way in which one's body weight or shape is experienced

Amenorrhea in postmenarche females*

*The diagnostic criteria may be difficult to meet in a young adolescent. Allow for a wide spectrum of clinical features.

Table 70-3	When to Hospitalize an Anorexic Patient

Weight loss >25% ideal body weight*

Risk of suicide

Bradycardia, hypothermia

Dehydration, hypokalemia, dysrhythmias

Outpatient treatment fails

*Less weight loss accepted in young adolescent.

Table 70-4	Diagnostic Criteria for Bulimia Nervosa

Recurrent episodes of binge eating, at least twice a week for 3 months, characterized by the following:

Eating in a discrete period an amount of food that is definitely larger than most people would eat during a similar period

A sense of lack of control over eating during the episode (e.g., a feeling that one cannot stop eating or control what or how much one is eating)

Compensatory behavior to prevent weight gain (i.e., self-induced vomiting, misuse of laxatives or diuretics, excessive exercise)

Self-evaluation unduly influenced by body shape and weight

Disturbance does not occur exclusively during episodes of anorexia nervosa.

and diuretic intake. Binge-eating episodes and the loss of control over eating often occur in young women who are slightly overweight with a history of dieting.

Nutritional, educational, and self-monitoring techniques are used to increase awareness of the maladaptive behavior, following which efforts are made to change the eating behavior. Patients with bulimia nervosa may respond to antidepressant therapy because they often have personality disturbances, impulse control difficulties, and family histories of affective disorders. Patients feel embarrassed, guilty, and ashamed of their actions. Attempted suicide and completed suicide (5%) are an important concern.

SUBSTANCE ABUSE

The age at which street drugs are first used is decreasing (<12 years), and females are overtaking males in terms of substance use. Ninety percent of adult smokers begin their habit during their adolescent years. Marijuana and stimulant drug use is increasing. Inhalant use (glue solvents, aerosol products) is prevalent in younger adolescents and in Native Americans. The use of *club drugs* by adolescents from upper income groups at rave parties (3,4-methylenedioxymethamphetamine [Ecstasy]) and so-called date-rape drugs (gamma-hydroxybutyrate or flunitrazepam [Rohypnol]) has risen sharply. Anabolic steroid use has increased in adolescent boys seeking enhanced athletic performance.

A history of drug use should be taken in a nonjudgmental and supportive manner and include the types of substances, frequency, timing, circumstances, and outcomes of substance use. Table 71-1 is a helpful screening tool. There are few physical findings even with chronic adolescent substance use. An adolescent may present in an overdose or intoxicated state, or in a psychosis triggered by a hallucinogen, such as phencyclidine ("angel dust"). Club drugs have direct (coma and seizures) and indirect (sexual assault and dehydration) adverse effects. Anabolic steroids also have direct (gynecomastia and testicular atrophy) and indirect (mood swings and violence) adverse effects.

Table 71-1	CRAFFT: A Screening Tool for Adolescent Substance Abuse	
C	Car	Driving under the influence of drugs
R	Relax	Using drugs to relax, fit in, feel better
A	Alone	Drugs/alcohol consumption while alone
F	Forgetting	Forgetting things as a result of drugs/alcohol
F	Family/Friends	Family and friends tell teen to stop/cut down
T	Trouble	Getting into trouble because of drugs/alcohol

ACUTE OVERDOSE

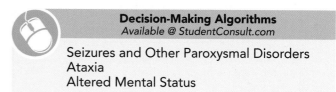

Decision-Making Algorithms
Available @ StudentConsult.com

Seizures and Other Paroxysmal Disorders
Ataxia
Altered Mental Status

Many drugs (most commonly alcohol, amphetamines, opiates, and cocaine) can result in a toxicologic emergency, often with first time use (Table 71-2). Initial management should be directed at appropriate supportive medical treatment, with follow-up counseling after the toxic effects have diminished.

Table 71-2	Substances Abused by Adolescents: Names and Acute Effects		
SUBSTANCE (STREET/ ALTERNATIVE NAME)	**EFFECTS AND FACTS**	**ROUTE OF ADMINISTRATION (TIME OF ACTION)**	**DETECTION**
Alcohol (Meths)	Disinhibition, ataxia, slurred speech, respiratory and CNS depression	Ingested (depends on amount and tolerance)	Urine and blood
Nicotine	Relaxation, CNS dependence, ↑ blood pressure, ↑ heart rate, ↓ temperature	Inhaled (minutes) Snuffed, dipped, chewed	
Marijuana (Cannabis, hashish, joints)	Euphoria, relaxation, ↑ appetite, ↓ reaction time	Inhaled (minutes) Tablets (30 min +)	Urine up to 1 mo
Stimulants	Alertness, euphoria	Inhaled and snorted	Urine up to 48 h
Cocaine (crack)	Insomnia, ↓ appetite	(Quick high) Tablets (longer effect)	
Amphetamines (ice)			
Hallucinogens	Hallucination, anxiety	Oral	
Mescaline	Psychosis, dilated pupils	Injected, sniffed, ingested	Immunoassay
Psilocybin (magic mushrooms)	Dysphoria		
LSD	"Artistic high" "Lucy in the sky with diamonds"	2–12 h "trip"	
Phencyclidine (PCP, angel dust)	Microdots in many colors Can induce suicide attempts		Immunoassay for PCP

EDMA

Table 71-2	Substances Abused by Adolescents: Names and Acute Effects—cont'd			
SUBSTANCE (STREET/ ALTERNATIVE NAME)	**EFFECTS AND FACTS**	**ROUTE OF ADMINISTRATION (TIME OF ACTION)**	**DETECTION**
Ecstasy (club drugs: combinations, i.e., of hallucinogens and amphetamines)			Ecstasy not detected by urine screen
Opiates	Euphoria, ataxia, miosis, slurred speech	Oral, IV, smoked, snorted, and sniffed	
Heroin			
Opium and heroin (freebase)	A common adolescent mix		
OxyContin (cotton, hillbilly)—new			
Tranquilizers			
Flunitrazepam (Rohypnol, "roofies," "date rape" drugs)		Small white pills; dissolve easily, odorless, colorless, tasteless (often mixed in alcohol)	Urine 1–24 h
Sedatives (barbiturates, "downers")			
Inhalants (solvents, gasoline)	Like alcohol	Inhaled	
Anabolic steroids	To enhance athletic performance	Tablets	Urine

Common side effects (treatment) of substance abuse drugs are paranoia (haloperidol), seizures (diazepam), hyperthermia (slow cooling), hypertension (β-blockers), and opiate overdose (naloxone).
From Office of the Surgeon General: Reducing tobacco use: a report of the Surgeon General, August 9, 2000 (website). http://www.surgeongeneral.gov/library/reports/tobacco_use/index.html. *Accessed October 31, 2013.*
CNS, central nervous system; *EDMA,* 3,4-ethylenedioxy-N-methylamphetamine; *LSD,* lysergic acid diethylamide; *PCP,* phencyclidine.

ACUTE AND CHRONIC EFFECTS

Heavy alcohol use can cause acute gastritis and acute pancreatitis. Intravenous drug use can result in hepatitis B, bacterial endocarditis, osteomyelitis, septic pulmonary embolism, infection, or acquired immunodeficiency syndrome (commonly known as *AIDS*). Chronic marijuana or tobacco use is associated with bronchoconstriction and bronchitis. Compulsive drug or alcohol use results in an adolescent being unable to help himself or herself out of the psychosocial sequelae that attend such habituation (e.g., stealing, prostitution, drug dealing, unemployment, school failure, social isolation).

TREATMENT

Specific management of substance use by adolescents depends on many individual patient factors. Because of the highly addictive (physical and psychological) nature of most substances, residential drug treatment facilities are suggested, especially for younger adolescents.

Suggested Reading

Black A, Fleming N, Rome E: Pregnancy in adolescents, *Adolesc Med State Art Rev Apr* 23(1):123–138, 2012.

Blake K, Mann K, Kutcher M: The structured communication adolescent guide (SCAG), *MedEdPORTAL*, 2008. https://www.mededportal.org/publication/798. Accessed October 31, 2013.

The Emergency Contraception Website, Office of Population Research: Princeton, NJ. http://ec.princeton.edu/. Updated June 2012.

Hartman L, Monasterio E, Hwang L: Adolescent contraception: review and guidance for pediatric clinicians, *Curr Probl Pediatr Adolesc Health Care* 24:221–263, 2012.

Keel PK, Brown TA: Update on course and outcome in eating disorders, *Int J Eat Disord* 43(3):195–204, 2010.

Williams C, Creighton S: Menstrual disorders in adolescents: review of current practice, *Horm Res Paediatr* 78(30):135–143, 2012.

Immunology

James W. Verbsky

Chapter 72

ASSESSMENT

The major components of host defense include anatomic barriers and the innate and adaptive immune systems. Integrity of the **anatomic** and **mucociliary barrier** (i.e., skin and mucous membranes) is essential for protection against infection, and defects in this barrier function can lead to infections (Table 72-1). The **innate immune system** acts as the first line of defense against pathogens, responding rapidly but nonspecifically before the development of the more versatile **adaptive immune system**. The **innate immune system** includes soluble factors, including acute-phase proteins, cytokines, chemokines, and complement, as well as cellular components, including neutrophils, monocytes/macrophages, and natural killer (NK) cells. The **adaptive immune system** is made up of T and B lymphocytes and their effector molecules (Table 72-2).

Recognition of pathogens by the innate immune system is facilitated by receptors on macrophages, NK cells, and neutrophils that recognize conserved pathogen motifs called **pathogen-associated molecular patterns (PAMPs),** including lipopolysaccharide of gram-negative bacteria, lipoteichoic acid of gram-positive bacteria, mannans of yeast, and specific nucleotide sequences of bacterial and viral DNA. Recognition of PAMPs by the innate immune system leads to the production of cytokines and chemokines that initiate inflammation and recruit inflammatory cells, induce an acute phase response (e.g., C-reactive protein, mannose binding lectin, complement), and activate the adaptive immune system. Complement proteins kill pathogens by facilitating uptake by phagocytic cells or by lysis of pathogens. Polymorphonuclear neutrophils ingest pyogenic bacteria and some fungi. Macrophages are effective in killing facultative intracellular organisms such as *Mycobacterium, Toxoplasma,* and *Legionella.* In addition NK lymphocytes mediate cytotoxic activity against virus-infected cells and cancer cells.

The key features of the **adaptive immune system** are antigen specificity and the development of immunologic memory, produced by expansion and maturation of antigen-specific T cells and B cells. Antibodies (immunoglobulin) produced by **B cells** neutralize toxins released by pathogens, opsonize pathogens to facilitate uptake by phagocytic cells, activate complement causing cytolysis of the pathogen, and direct NK cells to kill infected cells through antibody-mediated cytotoxicity. **T cells** kill virus-infected cells and cancer cells, activate macrophage to kill intracellular pathogens, and deliver the necessary signals for B-cell antibody synthesis and memory B-cell formation. Immunodeficiency can result from defects in one or more components of innate or adaptive immunity, leading

Table 72-1	Anatomic and Mucociliary Defects that Result in Recurrent or Opportunistic Infections
ANATOMIC DEFECTS IN UPPER AIRWAYS	
Aspiration syndromes (gastroesophageal reflux, ineffective cough, foreign body)	
Cleft palate, eustachian tube dysfunction	
Adenoidal hypertrophy	
Nasal polyps	
Obstruction of paranasal sinus drainage (osteomeatal complex disease), encephaloceles	
Posttraumatic or congenital sinus tracts (CSF rhinorrhea)	
ANATOMIC DEFECTS IN THE TRACHEOBRONCHIAL TREE	
Tracheoesophageal fistula, bronchobiliary fistula	
Pulmonary sequestration, bronchogenic cysts	
Vascular ring	
Tumor, foreign body, or enlarged lymph nodes	
PHYSIOLOGIC DEFECTS IN UPPER AND LOWER AIRWAYS	
Primary ciliary dyskinesia syndromes, Young syndrome Cystic fibrosis Bronchopulmonary dysplasia Bronchiectasis	
Allergic disease (allergic rhinitis, asthma)	
Chronic cigarette smoke exposure	
OTHER DEFECTS	
Burns	
Chronic atopic dermatitis	
Ureteral obstruction, vesicoureteral reflux	
IV drug use	
Central venous line, artificial heart value, CSF shunt, peritoneal dialysis catheter, urinary catheter	
Dermal sinus tract	

CSF, Cerebrospinal fluid.

to recurrent, opportunistic, or life-threatening infections. Primary immunodeficiency diseases are relatively rare individually, but together they cause significant chronic disease, morbidity, and mortality (Table 72-3).

HISTORY

The frequency, severity, and location of the infection and the pathogens involved can help differentiate infections in a normal host from infections in an immunodeficient patient (see Table 72-3). Although otitis media and sinopulmonary infections are common in children, recurrent infections, invasive or deep seeded infections, infections that require multiple rounds of oral antibiotics or need intravenous antibiotics, or infections with opportunistic infections suggest a primary immunodeficiency. Recurrent sinopulmonary infections with encapsulated bacteria suggest a defect in antibody-mediated immunity because these pathogens evade phagocytosis. Failure to thrive, diarrhea, malabsorption, and infections with opportunistic infections (i.e., fungi, *Candida* sp, *Pneumocystis jiroveci [carinii]*) suggest

T-cell immunodeficiency. Recurrent viral infections can result from T-cell or NK-cell deficiency. Deep-seated abscesses and infections with *Staphylococcus aureus, Serratia marcescens,* and *Aspergillus* suggest a disorder of neutrophil function, such as chronic granulomatous disease (CGD). Delayed separation of the umbilical cord, especially in the presence of omphalitis and later onset periodontal disease, in addition to poorly formed abscesses, indicates leukocyte adhesion deficiency.

Age of onset of symptoms can be helpful in defining an immune deficiency, although significant variability does occur. Neutrophil defects (e.g., congenital neutropenia, leukocyte adhesion deficiency) typically present in the first several months of life. Antibody defects (e.g., agammaglobulinemia) and T-cell defects (e.g., severe combined immunodeficiency [SCID]) typically present after 3 months of life after maternal antibody levels have waned. Presentation with symptoms of an antibody deficiency in adolescence or young adulthood suggests common variable immunodeficiency (CVID) rather than agammaglobulinemia, although milder phenotypes of primary immunodeficiency disease may not present until later

Table 72-2	Cytokines and Chemotactic Cytokines and Their Functions	
FACTOR	**SOURCE**	**FUNCTION**
IL-1	Macrophages	Co-stimulatory effect on T cells, enhances antigen presentation, acute phase response, fever
IL-2	T cells	Primary T-cell growth factor; B-cell and NK-cell growth factors; required for T regulatory cell function and survival
IL-3	T cells	Mast cell growth factor; multicolony-stimulating factor
IL-4	T cells	T-cell growth factor; enhances IgE synthesis; enhances B-cell differentiation; mast cell growth
IL-5	T cells	Enhances eosinophil differentiation; enhances immunoglobulin synthesis; enhances IgA synthesis
IL-6	T cells, macrophages, fibroblasts, endothelium	Enhances immunoglobulin synthesis, antiviral activity, induces acute phase response, fever, hematopoietic effects
IL-7	Stromal cells	Enhances growth of pre-T cells
IL-8	T cells, macrophages, epithelium	Neutrophil-activating protein; T lymphocyte and neutrophil chemotactic factor
IL-9	T cells	Acts in synergy with IL-4 to induce IgE production, mast cell growth
IL-10	T cells, including regulatory T cells, macrophages	Cytokine synthesis inhibitory factor; suppresses macrophage function; enhances B-cell growth; inhibits IL-12 production; suppresses inflammation at mucosal surfaces
IL-12	Macrophages, neutrophils	NK cell stimulatory factor; cytotoxic lymphocyte maturation factor; enhances IFN-γ synthesis; inhibits IL-4 synthesis
IL-13	T cells	Enhances IgE synthesis; enhances B-cell growth; inhibits macrophage activation; causes airway hyperreactivity
IL-17	T cells	Induces IL-1β and IL-6 synthesis, important in fungal infections
IL-18	Macrophages	Enhances IFN-γ synthesis
IFN-γ	T cells	Macrophage activation; inhibits IgE synthesis; antiviral activity
TGF-β	T cells, including regulatory T cells, many other cells	Inhibits T-cell and B-cell proliferation and activation, induces T regulatory cells
RANTES	T cells, endothelium	Chemokine for monocytes, T cells, eosinophils
MIP-1α	Mononuclear cells, endothelium	Chemokine for T cells; enhances differentiation of CD4+ T cells
Eotaxin 1, 2, and 3	Epithelium, endothelium, eosinophils, fibroblasts, macrophages	Chemokine for eosinophils, basophils, and Th2 cells
IP-10	Monocytes, macrophages, endothelium	Chemokine for activated T cells, monocytes, and NK cells

IFN, Interferon; *NK,* natural killer; *RANTES,* regulated on activation, normal T expressed and secreted; *Th2,* T helper 2.

Table 72-3	Clinical Characteristics of Primary Immunodeficiencies

B-CELL DEFECTS

Recurrent pyogenic infections with extracellular encapsulated organisms, such as *Streptococcus pneumoniae*, *Haemophilus influenzae* type b, and group A streptococcus

Otitis, sinusitis, recurrent pneumonia, bronchiectasis, and conjunctivitis

Few problems with fungal or viral infections (except enterovirus and poliomyelitis)

Diarrhea common, especially secondary to infection with *Giardia lamblia*

Minimal growth retardation

Compatible with survival to adulthood or for several years after onset unless complications occur

COMPLEMENT DEFECTS

Recurrent bacterial infections with extracellular encapsulated organisms, such as *S. pneumoniae* and *H. influenzae*

Susceptibility to recurrent infections with *Neisseria meningitides*

Increased incidence of autoimmune disease

Severe or recurrent skin and respiratory tract infection

T-CELL DEFECTS

Recurrent infections with less virulent or opportunistic organisms, such as fungi, *Candida* sp mycobacteria, viruses, and protozoa as well as bacteria

Growth retardation, malabsorption, diarrhea, and failure to thrive common

Anergy

Susceptible to graft-versus-host disease from nonirradiated blood or from maternal engraftment

Fatal reactions may occur from live virus or bacille Calmette-Guérin vaccination.

High incidence of malignancy

Poor survival beyond infancy or early childhood

NEUTROPHIL DEFECTS

Recurrent dermatologic infections with bacteria such as *Staphylococcus*, *Pseudomonas*, and *Escherichia coli*, and fungi such as *Aspergillus*

Subcutaneous, lymph node, lung, and liver abscesses Pulmonary infections common, including abscess and pneumatocele formation, contributing to chronic disease

Bone and joint infection common

Delayed separation of umbilical cord

Absence of pus at site(s) of infection
Poor wound healing

Table 72-4	Causes of Secondary Immunodeficiency

VIRAL INFECTIONS

HIV (destroys CD4 T cells)
Measles
Rubella
Influenza

METABOLIC DISORDERS

Diabetes mellitus

Malnutrition

Uremia

Sickle cell disease

Zinc and vitamin deficiency

Multiple carboxylase deficiency

Burns

PROTEIN-LOSING STATES

Nephrotic syndrome

Protein-losing enteropathy

OTHER CAUSES

Prematurity

Immunosuppressive agents (e.g., corticosteroids, radiation, and antimetabolites)

Malignancy (leukemia, Hodgkin disease, nonlymphoid cancer)

Acquired asplenia

Acquired neutropenia (autoimmune, viral, or drug-induced)

Stem cell transplantation/graft-versus-host disease

Systemic lupus erythematosus and other autoimmune diseases

Sarcoidosis

PHYSICAL EXAMINATION

Recurrent infection in immunologically deficient children is associated with pathology at sites of infection resulting in substantial morbidity, such as scarring tympanic membranes leading to hearing loss or chronic lung disease due to recurrent pneumonia. Height and weight percentiles, nutritional status, and presence of subcutaneous fat should be assessed. Oral thrush, purulent nasal or otic discharge, and chronic rales may be evidence of repeated or persistent infections. Absence of lymphoid tissue (e.g., tonsils) suggests agammaglobulinemia or SCID, whereas increased size of lymphoid tissue suggests CVID, CGD, or human immunodeficiency virus (HIV) infection. Cerebellar ataxia and telangiectasia indicate ataxia-telangiectasia. Severe eczema and inflammatory bowel disease are seen in some disorders of immune regulation with polyendocrinopathy and enteropathy that is X-linked (IPEX), whereas eczema and petechiae or bruises suggest Wiskott-Aldrich syndrome.

DIFFERENTIAL DIAGNOSIS

There are many secondary causes of immunodeficiency that should be considered, particularly if the immunologic testing is nonrevealing (Table 72-4). In patients with primary immunodeficiencies, infections develop at multiple sites (e.g., ears, sinuses, lungs, skin), whereas in individuals with anatomic

---

in life. The presence of associated problems, such as congenital heart disease and hypocalcemia (DiGeorge syndrome), abnormal gait and telangiectasia (Ataxia-telangiectasia), atopic dermatitis (hyper-IgE syndrome, Omenn syndrome), and easy bruising or a bleeding disorder (Wiskott-Aldrich syndrome) can be informative in guiding an immune workup. Finally a **family history** of a primary immune deficiency or death of a young child due to infections should prompt an immune evaluation, particularly in the setting of recurrent infections.

problems (e.g., sequestered pulmonary lobe, ureteral reflux), infections are confined to a single anatomic site. Asplenia is associated with recurrent and severe infections, even in the presence of protective antibody titers. Infection with HIV should be considered in any patient presenting with a history suggesting a T-cell immunodeficiency.

DIAGNOSTIC EVALUATION

The diagnosis of patients with primary immunodeficiency diseases depends on early recognition of signs and symptoms, followed by laboratory tests to evaluate immune function. Recognizing the patient who may have an immunodeficiency disease prompts an evaluation and referral to an immunologist (see Table 72-3).

Laboratory Tests

A diagnosis of primary immunodeficiency disease cannot be established without the use of laboratory tests based on the clinical history (Table 72-5). A **complete blood count with differential** should always be obtained to identify patients with neutropenia or lymphopenia (SCID) as well as the presence of eosinophils (allergic disease) and anemia (chronic disease). **Serum immunoglobulin levels** are essential to the workup of suspected primary immunodeficiency. Antibody levels vary with age, with normal adult values of IgG at full-term birth from transplacental transfer of maternal IgG, a physiologic nadir occurring between 3 and 6 months of age, and a gradual increase to adult values over several years. IgA and IgM are low at birth, and levels increase gradually over several years, with IgA taking the longest to reach normal adult values. Low albumin levels with low immunoglobulin levels suggest low synthetic rates for all proteins or increased loss of proteins, as in protein-losing enteropathy. High immunoglobulin levels suggest intact B-cell immunity and can be found in diseases with recurrent infections, such as CGD, immotile cilia syndrome, cystic fibrosis, HIV infection, and autoimmune diseases. Elevated IgE levels can be found in a number of immune deficiencies such as hyper-IgE syndrome, as well as in atopic dermatitis.

Specific antibody titers after childhood vaccination (tetanus, diphtheria, *Haemophilus influenzae* type b, or *Streptococcus pneumoniae* vaccines) reflect the capacity of the immune system to synthesize specific antibodies and to develop memory B cells. If titers are low, immunization with a specific vaccine and titers obtained 4 to 6 weeks later confirm response to the immunization. Poor response to bacterial polysaccharide antigens is normal before 24 months of age but is also associated with IgG subclass deficiency or specific antibody deficiency. The development of protein-conjugate polysaccharide vaccines has prevented infections with these organisms in early childhood. Antibody responses to the *S. pneumoniae* serotypes found in the 23-valent polysaccharide vaccine, but not in the conjugate vaccine, can be used to test antibody responses to polysaccharide antigens.

Delayed-type hypersensitivity skin tests to protein antigens such as tetanus, diphtheria, *Candida,* or mumps demonstrate the presence of antigen-specific T cells and functional antigen-presenting cells. If delayed-type hypersensitivity skin test results are negative, patients should receive a booster vaccination and be retested 4 weeks later.

Table 72-5	Tests for Suspected Immune Deficiency

GENERAL

Complete blood count, including hemoglobin, differential white blood cell count and morphology, and platelet count

Radiographs to document infection in chest, sinus, mastoids, and long bones, if indicated by clinical history

Cultures, if appropriate

ANTIBODY-MEDIATED IMMUNITY

Quantitative immunoglobulin levels: IgG, IgA, IgM, IgE, Isohemagglutinin titers (anti-A, anti-B, measures IgM function)

Specific antibody levels:

Protein antigens: diphtheria, tetanus

Protein-conjugated antigens: *Haemophilus influenzae, Streptococcus pneumoniae* (conjugate vaccine)

Polysaccharide antigens: *S. pneumoniae* (unconjugated vaccine)

B-cell numbers and subsets by flow cytometry

CELL-MEDIATED IMMUNITY

Lymphocyte count and morphology

Delayed hypersensitivity skin tests (*Candida,* tetanus toxoid, mumps): measure T-cell and macrophage function

T-cell and NK cell numbers and subsets by flow cytometry T-lymphocyte functional analyses (mitogen responses, cytokines)

NK cell cytotoxicity assays

PHAGOCYTOSIS

Neutrophil cell count and morphology

Nitroblue tetrazolium dye test/dihydrorhodamine 123 using flow cytometry

Staphylococcal killing, chemotaxis assay

Myeloperoxidase stain

COMPLEMENT

Total hemolytic complement CH_{50}: measures classical and common pathway activity

AH_{50}: measures alternative and common pathway activity Levels of individual complement components

Cl-inhibitor level and function

NK, Natural killer.

Lymphocyte phenotyping by flow cytometry enumerates the percentage and absolute numbers of T-cell, B-cell, and NK-cell subsets. Flow cytometry can also test for the presence of surface proteins that are necessary for normal immunity, such as major histocompatibility complex molecules or adhesion molecules, as well as intracellular analysis of signaling proteins and cytokines. **T-cell proliferation** assays to mitogens (phytohemagglutinin, concanavalin A, or pokeweed mitogen) or antigens (tetanus toxoid or *Candida*) are in vitro assays that confirm the capacity of T cells to proliferate in response to a nonspecific stimulus (mitogens) or the presence of antigen-specific memory T cells (antigens). Such presence requires prior vaccination (tetanus) or exposure (*Candida*) to the antigen. **Tests for cytokine synthesis or expression of activation markers** by T cells may be performed in specialized research laboratories and can help identify defects in T-cell function when, despite present T cells, the clinical history suggests a T-cell disorder.

Complement assays include the CH_{50} test, which measures the presence of proteins in the classical pathway of complement (C1, C2, C3, C4), and the AH_{50} test, which tests the proteins of the alternative pathway of complement (C3, factor B, properdin). If both the CH_{50} and AH_{50} levels are abnormal, a defect in the common pathway is likely (C5–C9). Specialized laboratories can measure the presence or function of specific complement proteins. Tests for C1-inhibitor antigen and function are used to diagnose hereditary or acquired angioneurotic edema.

Tests for neutrophil function include the nitroblue tetrazolium (NBT) or dihydrorhodamine 123 (DHR) test for CGD, in which oxygen radicals generated by activated neutrophils oxidize NBT to an insoluble blue dye and DHR to a fluorescent molecule. Patients with CGD have no blue-staining neutrophils with NBT and little fluorescence when DHR is used. In vitro tests for evaluation of neutrophil phagocytosis, chemotaxis, bacterial killing, and for the presence of myeloperoxidase activity are available in some laboratories. Tests for the expression of adhesion molecules such as CD18 (leukocyte function–associated antigen type 1, LFA-1) can be performed by flow cytometry.

Genetic testing to confirm the diagnosis of a primary immunodeficiency disease can be performed in specialized laboratories and may be helpful for deciding on a course of treatment, determining the natural history and prognosis of the disease, genetic counseling, and prenatal diagnosis. In patients in whom DiGeorge syndrome is suspected, fluorescent in situ hybridization studies for deletions of chromosome 22 can be helpful. In patients in whom ataxia-telangiectasia is suspected, chromosomal studies for breakage in chromosomes 7 and 14 are useful.

Diagnostic Imaging

The absence of a thymus on chest x-ray suggests DiGeorge syndrome or other defects in T-cell development. Abnormalities in the cerebellum are found in patients with ataxia-telangiectasia. Otherwise the use of diagnostic imaging in the evaluation of immunodeficiency diseases is essentially limited to the diagnosis of infectious diseases.

Chapter **73**

LYMPHOCYTE DISORDERS

Disorders that affect lymphocyte development or function result in significant immunodeficiency because lymphocytes provide antigen specificity and memory responses. Hematopoietic stem cells give rise to lymphoid precursors that develop into T lymphocytes in the thymus or B lymphocytes in the bone marrow (Fig. 73-1). Isolated B-cell disorders result in **antibody deficiency diseases,** whereas T-cell disorders usually cause **combined immunodeficiency** because they are necessary for cell-mediated immunity to clear intracellular pathogens and for antibody synthesis by B cells. NK cells are an important component of the **innate immune response,** develop from lymphoid precursors, and can kill virus-infected cells and tumor cells. Antibodies can enhance NK cell function by antibody-mediated cellular cytotoxicity.

ETIOLOGY AND CLINICAL MANIFESTATIONS
Antibody Deficiency Diseases

Decision-Making Algorithm
Available @ StudentConsult.com

Recurrent Infections

Disorders of B cells result in an increased susceptibility to infections by encapsulated bacteria.

Agammaglobulinemia results from the absence or defective function of B cells with subsequent severe decrease in immunoglobulin levels and a total absence of specific antibody. **X-linked agammaglobulinemia** affects males and is characterized by a profound deficiency of B cells, severe hypogammaglobulinemia, and absence of lymphoid tissue (Table 73-1; see Fig. 73-1). The defect is caused by mutations in a gene encoding the tyrosine kinase *Btk* on chromosome Xq22 that is involved in a signaling of the pre-B-cell receptor and the B-cell antigen receptor. **Autosomal recessive agammaglobulinemia** results from a variety of defects in the pre-B-cell and B-cell antigen receptor complexes and includes mutations in the μ heavy chain gene, λ5, Igα, Igβ, and BLNK. X-linked agammaglobulinemia is more common than the autosomal recessive forms.

Patients with agammaglobulinemia usually present during the first 6 to 12 months of life as maternally derived antibodies wane, although patients can present years later. These patients develop infections with *Streptococcus pneumoniae, Haemophilus influenzae* type b, *Staphylococcus aureus,* and *Pseudomonas,* organisms for which antibody is an important opsonin. They also have increased susceptibility to giardiasis and enteroviral infections, leading to chronic enteroviral meningoencephalitis and vaccine-associated poliomyelitis (if immunized with oral live, attenuated poliovirus vaccine).

Common variable immunodeficiency (CVID) is a heterogeneous disorder characterized by hypogammaglobulinemia developing after an initial period of normal immune function, most commonly in the second and third decades of life (see Table 73-1). Serum IgG levels are less than 500 mg/dL (usually <300 mg/dL) with IgA levels less than 10 mg/dL and/or low IgM levels. Antibody titers to protein antigens, such as tetanus and diphtheria, and to polysaccharide antigens, such as pneumococcus, are low or absent. T-cell numbers and function are highly variable, and B-cell numbers can be normal or low. Patients exhibit normal-sized or enlarged tonsils and lymph nodes and may have splenomegaly. They are susceptible to frequent respiratory tract infections due to *Streptococcus pneumoniae, Haemophilus influenzae* type b, and *Mycoplasma.* Gastrointestinal infections with *Giardia, Campylobacter, Salmonella, Helicobacter,* and enteroviruses are common. Autoimmune hemolytic anemia and thrombocytopenia occur frequently, and granulomatous disease affecting the gastrointestinal tract, liver, and lungs leads to significant morbidity. Cancer, especially lymphoma, is a major cause of mortality.

Figure 73-1 Sites of cellular abnormalities in congenital immunodeficiencies. In primary immunodeficiency diseases, the maturation or activation of B or T lymphocytes may be blocked at different stages. *τ*, Inhibition; *B*, B lymphocyte; *T*, T lymphocyte. (*Adapted from Abbas AK, Lichtman AH, Pober JS: Cellular and Molecular Immunology, ed 3, Philadelphia, 1997, Saunders.*)

The gene defects leading to the majority of cases of CVID are unknown. Some patients have a defect in the gene encoding for inducible co-stimulator (ICOS) on activated T cells, transmembrane activator and calcium-modulating cyclophilin ligand interactor (TACI), CD19, CD21, CD81, or BAFF-R. It is important to exclude X-linked agammaglobulinemia, X-linked lymphoproliferative disease, or hyper-IgM syndrome as well as other causes of hypogammaglobulinemia, such as hypogammaglobulinemia associated with thymoma, secondary to protein losing enteropathy, or secondary to medications, before making the diagnosis of CVID.

Selective **IgA deficiency** is defined as serum IgA levels less than 10 mg/dL with normal levels of other immunoglobulins. The diagnosis cannot be confirmed until the patient is at least 4 years of age when IgA levels should reach adult levels. Selective IgA deficiency occurs in approximately 1 in 500 individuals. Most patients with selective IgA deficiency are asymptomatic. In others it is associated with recurrent sinopulmonary infections, IgG_2 subclass deficiency, specific antibody deficiency, food allergy, autoimmune disease, or celiac disease. IgA deficiency occurs in families, suggesting autosomal inheritance.

IgG subclass deficiency occurs when the level of antibodies in one or more of the four IgG subclasses is selectively decreased while total IgG levels are normal. Normal individuals can express low levels of one or more subclasses, so a history of recurrent infections is important. An inability to synthesize specific antibody titers to protein or polysaccharide antigens is the best marker of IgG subclass deficiency associated with recurrent infections and requiring therapy.

Transient hypogammaglobulinemia of infancy is a temporary condition characterized by delayed immunoglobulin production. The pathogenesis of this disorder is unknown but is thought to result from a prolongation of the physiologic hypogammaglobulinemia of infancy. The immunoglobulin nadir at 6 months of age is accentuated, with immunoglobulin levels less than 200 mg/dL. Immunoglobulin levels remain diminished throughout the first year of life and usually increase to normal, age-appropriate levels, generally by 2 to 4 years of age. The incidence of sinopulmonary infection is increased in some patients. The diagnosis is supported by normal levels of both B and T cells and by normal antibody responses to protein antigens such as diphtheria and tetanus toxoids. The transient nature of this disorder cannot be confirmed, however, until immunoglobulin levels return to normal ranges.

Specific antibody deficiency syndrome is characterized by recurrent infections with normal immunoglobulin levels and

| Table 73-1 | Antibody Deficiency Diseases |

DISORDER	GENETICS	ONSET	MANIFESTATIONS	PATHOGENESIS	ASSOCIATED FEATURES
Agammaglobulinemia	X-linked, AR	Infancy (6–9 mo)	Recurrent infections, sinusitis, pneumonia, meningitis (encapsulated bacteria, enteroviruses)	Arrest in B-cell differentiation (pre-B level); mutations in: Btk gene (X-linked); μ chain, BLNK, Igα, Igβ, Vpre-B, and λ5 (AR)	Lymphoid hypoplasia
Common variable immunodeficiency	AR; AD; sporadic	Second to third decade	Sinusitis, bronchitis, pneumonia, chronic diarrhea	Arrest in plasma cell differentiation, mutations in ICOS, TACI, CD19	Autoimmune disease, RA, SLE, Graves disease, ITP, malignancy, granulomatous disease
Transient hypogammaglobulin-emia of infancy		Infancy (3–7 mo)	Recurrent viral and pyogenic infections	Unknown; delayed plasma cell maturation	Frequently in families with other immunodeficiencies
IgA deficiency	Variable	Variable	Sinopulmonary infections; can be normal	Failure of IgA expression	IgG subclass deficiency common, autoimmune diseases
IgG subclass deficiency	Variable	Variable	Sinopulmonary infections; can be normal	Defect in IgG isotype production	IgA deficiency, ataxia telangiectasia, polysaccharide antibody deficiency
IgM deficiency	Variable	First year	Variable (normal to recurrent sinopulmonary infections and meningitis)	Defective helper T cell–B cell interaction	Whipple disease, regional enteritis, lymphoid hyperplasia
Specific antibody deficiency, IgA deficiency	Variable	After 2 years of age	Sinopulmonary infections	Unknown	IgG subclass deficiency
Hyper-IgM syndrome	AR	Variable	Sinopulmonary infections	Defect in AID, UNG	Autoimmunity

AD, Autosomal dominant; *AID,* activation-induced cytidine deaminase; *AR,* autosomal recessive; *ITP,* idiopathic thrombocytopenic purpura; *RA,* rheumatoid arthritis; *SLE,* systemic lupus erythematosus; *UNG,* uracil-DNA glycosylase.

normal lymphocyte numbers and subsets, but the disorder has an inability to synthesize specific antibody to polysaccharide antigens, such as to the 23-valent pneumococcal vaccine. The pathogenesis of this disorder is unknown. Lack of specific antibody titers explains the recurrent infections and justifies therapy.

Combined Immunodeficiency Diseases

Decision-Making Algorithms
Available @ StudentConsult.com

Petechiae/Purpura
Recurrent Infections

Disorders that affect T-cell development or function usually result in combined immunodeficiency because T cells provide necessary signals for B-cell differentiation. **X-linked hyper-IgM syndrome**, the most common form of hyper-IgM syndrome, is a combined immunodeficiency with deficient T-cell function due to defects in CD40 ligand. Defects in CD40 cause **autosomal recessive hyper-IgM syndrome** and present similarly to X-linked hyper-IgM syndrome (Fig. 73-2 and Table 73-2). Hyper-IgM syndrome is characterized by a failure of immunoglobulin isotype switching from IgM and IgD to IgG, IgA, or IgE, and a lack of memory responses. Affected patients have normal or elevated serum levels of IgM with low or absent levels of IgG, IgA, and IgE. Immunoglobulin isotype switching allows a B cell to maintain antigen specificity while altering immunoglobulin function, and is directed by cytokines and

interaction between CD40 ligand on CD4 T cells and CD40 on B cells (see Fig. 73-2). Signal transduction via CD40 activates several signaling molecules and transcription factors, including nuclear factor κB (NF-κB) and two enzymes, activation-induced cytidine deaminase (AID) and uracil-DNA glycosylase (UNG), which are required for class switching. Deficiency of AID or UNG presents with a failure of immunoglobulin isotype switching without any abnormality in T-cell function. These forms of hyper-IgM are antibody deficiency diseases and not combined immunodeficiencies (see Table 73-1).

All patients with hyper-IgM syndrome have increased susceptibility to sinopulmonary infections, whereas patients with defects in CD40 ligand or CD40 are susceptible to opportunistic infections, such as *P. jiroveci (carinii) and Cryptosporidium parvum.* Signaling via CD40 on B cells and other antigen-presenting cells leads to upregulation of co-stimulatory molecules important for promoting T-cell differentiation and for activating cell-mediated immune responses. The hyper-IgM phenotype is also found in an X-linked disorder associated with ectodermal dysplasia, resulting from defects in the gene encoding the NF-κB essential modulator (NEMO). Patients with defects in NEMO are susceptible to a wider spectrum of infectious organisms, especially meningitis and infection with atypical mycobacteria, because NF-κB signaling is important for the function of both innate and adaptive immune systems.

Severe combined immunodeficiency (SCID) is characterized by a profound lack of T-cell numbers or function, and B-cell dysfunction resulting from the absence of B cells from the gene defect itself, or secondary to lack of T-cell function (see Table 73-2). T cells develop from bone marrow–derived

Figure 73-2 Schematic representation of the interaction between a CD4 T cell and a B cell. T-cell activation follows T-cell receptor (TCR) recognition of peptide antigen presented via MHC class II molecules resulting in CD40 ligand (CD40L) expression and cytokine synthesis. CD40L stimulates the B cell via CD40, resulting in expression of co-stimulatory molecules (B7) that are important in T-cell priming and cytokine synthesis that drives T-cell differentiation. CD40 and cytokine signaling in B cells activate activation-induced cytidine deaminase (AID) and uracil-DNA glycosylase (UNG) to promote immunoglobulin isotype switching and somatic hypermutation. Defects in CD40L cause X-linked hyper-IgM (X-HIM), and defects in CD40, AID, or UNG cause autosomal recessive hyper-IgM (AR-HIM). Defects in either CD40L or CD40 affect T-cell co-stimulation and priming, leading to T-cell defects, whereas defects in AID and UNG maintain normal T-cell co-stimulation and function.

Table 73-2	Combined Immunodeficiency Diseases				
DISORDER	**GENETICS**	**ONSET**	**MANIFESTATIONS**	**PATHOGENESIS**	**ASSOCIATED FEATURES**
Hyper-IgM syndrome (see Table 73-1)	X-linked, AR	First year	Sinopulmonary infections, opportunistic infections, *Pneumocystis jiroveci*	Defect in CD40 ligand (X-linked) or CD40 (AR)	Neutropenia, liver disease, cancer
DiGeorge anomaly	22q11.2 (or 10p) deletion	Newborn, early infancy	Hypocalcemic tetany, pyogenic infections, partial or complete T-cell deficiency	Hypoplasia of third and fourth pharyngeal pouch	Congenital heart disease (aortic arch anomalies), hypoparathyroidism, micrognathia, hypertelorism
Severe combined immunodeficiency (T⁻B⁺ SCID)	X-linked; AR	1–3 mo	Candidiasis, all types of infections, failure to thrive, chronic diarrhea	Mutation in IL-2Rγ chain, Jak3 kinase, ZAP-70, IL-7Ra, CD3 subunits	GVHD from maternal-fetal transfusions, severe GVHD from nonirradiated blood transfusion
Severe combined immunodeficiency (T⁻B⁻ SCID)	AR	1–3 mo	Same as T⁻ B⁺ SCID	Mutation in RAG1/2, Artemis, ADA/PNP deficiency	Same as T⁻ B⁺ SCID ADA deficiency: chondroosseous dysplasia PNP deficiency: neurologic disorders
Omenn syndrome	AR	1–3 mo	Same as T⁻ B⁻ SCID, exfoliative erythroderma, lymphadenopathy, hepatosplenomegaly	Hypomorphic mutations in SCID-causing genes (RAG1/2, Artemis)	Restricted T-cell receptor heterogeneity, eosinophilia, elevated IgE
Reticular dysgenesis (T⁻ B⁻SCID)	AR	1–3 mo	Same as T⁻ B⁻ SCID	Defective maturation of common stem cells due to *AK2* mutations	Agammaglobulinemia, alymphocytosis, agranulocytosis
Bare lymphocyte syndrome (MHC class I deficiency)	AR	First decade	Sinopulmonary infections	Mutation in TAP1 or TAP2 (transporter associated with antigen processing)	Decreased CD8 T cells, chronic lung inflammation
Bare lymphocyte syndrome (MHC class II deficiency)	AR	Early infancy	Respiratory tract infections, chronic diarrhea, viral infections in central nervous system	Mutations in CIITA, RFX5, RFXAP, and RFX-B (DNA binding factors)	Decreased CD4 T cells, autoimmune disease

AD, Autosomal dominant; *ADA,* adenosine deaminase; *AR,* autosomal recessive; *dATP,* deoxyadenosine triphosphate; *dGTP,* deoxyguanosine triphosphate; *GVHD,* graft-versus-host disease; *IL,* interleukin; *IL-2Rγ,* interleukin-2 receptor gamma chain; *MHC,* major histocompatibility complex; *PNP,* purine nucleoside phosphorylase; *SCID,* severe combined immunodeficiency; *T⁻ B⁻,* T⁻ cells absent and B cells present; *T⁻ B⁻,* T cells absent and B cells absent.

precursors in the thymus (see Fig. 73-2), where they undergo several stages of development characterized by DNA recombination of the variable region of T-cell antigen receptor genes to generate a diverse T-cell receptor repertoire. A process of positive selection occurs in the thymus to select thymocytes with antigen receptors that can interact with major histocompatibility complex (MHC) molecules to ensure their survival (see Fig. 73-2). Thymocytes differentiate into CD4 or CD8 T cells if they interact with MHC class II or class I molecules, respectively. Some of the positively selected thymocytes, however, have antigen receptors that recognize self-antigens presented by MHC molecules in the thymus. These cells are deleted in the thymus by a process of negative selection. Positive selection and negative selection in the thymus ensure that the mature T cells that leave the thymus can function with the individual's MHC molecules and recognize a multitude of foreign antigens without mounting autoimmune responses. SCID can result from any specific genetic mutation that interferes with T-cell development in the thymus or T-cell function in the periphery.

Clinical manifestations of SCID include failure to thrive, severe bacterial infections, chronic candidiasis and other fungal infections, chronic viral infections, infection with *P. jiroveci* (*carinii*) and other opportunistic organisms, and intractable diarrhea. Patients often have skin disease similar to eczema, possibly related to graft-versus-host disease (GVHD) from engraftment of maternal lymphocytes, which usually is not fatal. Patients with SCID are extremely susceptible to fatal GVHD from lymphocytes in blood transfusions and can be infected by cytomegalovirus-positive blood products. Patients with T-cell disorders always should receive irradiated blood products.

X-linked SCID, the most common form, is caused by mutations in the gene on chromosome Xq13.1 coding for the common gamma chain of the interleukin-2 (IL-2), IL-4, IL-7, IL-9, IL-15, and IL-21 receptors. Affected patients have no T cells or NK cells in the peripheral blood but have normal numbers of B cells. Immunoglobulin levels are low or undetectable because there are no CD4 T cells to stimulate B cells. The defect in T-cell development results from a failure of signaling via the IL-7 receptor, and IL-15 is required for NK-cell development. There are many causes of **autosomal recessive SCID.** Defects in Janus kinase 3 (Jak3), which binds to the common gamma chain, results in a similar phenotype as X-linked SCID. Defects in the IL-7 receptor, ZAP-70, and subunits of the CD3 molecule result in a deficiency of T cells with normal B- and NK-cell numbers. In addition there is a variety of defects that affect DNA recombination in T and B cells, including two genes called *recombinase activating gene (RAG) 1* and *2* as well as other genes important in DNA excision and repair such as *Artemis*. Defects in any of the genes that abolish DNA recombination or DNA repair result in autosomal recessive SCID with no T cells or B cells present. Mutations in *RAG1, RAG2, or Artemis* that preserve limited function result in **Omenn syndrome,** a variant form of SCID that is characterized by exfoliative erythroderma, lymphadenopathy, hepatosplenomegaly, marked eosinophilia, elevated serum IgE, and impaired T-cell function. Patients with Omenn syndrome have T cells in the periphery, but these T cells have a limited repertoire.

Deficiencies in **adenosine deaminase (ADA)** and **purine nucleoside phosphorylase,** two enzymes involved in the purine salvage pathway, also result in SCID. Accumulation of nucleoside substrates or their metabolic products in the plasma and urine is toxic to lymphocytes, including T, B, and NK cells. Most patients exhibit severe infection early in life, although the diagnosis in patients with partial enzyme function may not be established until after 5 years of age or, occasionally, in adulthood. Patients with late-onset diagnosis are generally lymphopenic; they may have B cells and normal total immunoglobulin levels but little functional antibody (**Nezelof syndrome**). All patients with ADA or purine nucleoside phosphorylase deficiency SCID have lymphopenia and loss of immune function over time.

Bare lymphocyte syndrome results from defects in transcription factors that regulate expression of class II molecules or genes that affect transport of antigen peptides, which leads to the absence of either MHC class I or MHC class II molecules. Lymphoid tissue and B cells may be present in normal amounts, but CD4 T cells are decreased or absent in class II deficiency, whereas CD8 cells are decreased or absent in class I deficiency. Some patients may have normal numbers of CD4 or CD8 T cells, but none of the T cells are functional because peptide antigens cannot be presented to T cells.

DiGeorge syndrome, also known as **velocardiofacial syndrome** or **CATCH 22 syndrome (c**ardiac anomalies, **a**bnormal facies, **t**hymic hypoplasia, **c**left palate, and **h**ypocalcemia), is the result of dysmorphogenesis of the third and fourth pharyngeal pouches, resulting in hypoplasia of the thymus required for T-cell maturation. Most, but not all, patients with DiGeorge syndrome have a defect on chromosome 22q11.2. DiGeorge syndrome is classically characterized by hypocalcemic tetany, conotruncal and aortic arch anomalies, and increased infections. The diagnosis is established by fluorescent in situ hybridization or a polymerase chain reaction with a DNA probe to detect deletions in chromosome 22q11.2. Most patients have partial immune defects with low T-cell numbers and function that generally improve with age. Severe T-cell deficiency is rare, but it results in SCID due to a complete lack of T cells. Most important, DiGeorge syndrome and bare lymphocyte syndrome do not respond well to bone marrow transplantation as do other forms of SCID because the defects are in the thymus, although transfer of mature T cells during transplant may confer some immune function.

Wiskott-Aldrich syndrome is an X-linked disorder characterized by thrombocytopenia, eczema, defects in cell-mediated and humoral immunity, and a predisposition to lymphoproliferative disease (Table 73-3). It is caused by mutations of the gene on chromosome Xp11.22 coding for the Wiskott-Aldrich syndrome protein (WASP), expressed in lymphocytes, platelets, and monocytes. Deficiency of this protein results in elevated levels of IgE and IgA, decreased IgM, poor responses to polysaccharide antigens, waning T-cell function, and profound thrombocytopenia. Opportunistic infections and autoimmune cytopenias become problematic in older children. **Isolated X-linked thrombocytopenia** also results from mutations of the identical gene. One third of patients with Wiskott-Aldrich syndrome die as a result of hemorrhage, and two thirds die as a result of recurrent infection caused by bacteria, cytomegalovirus, *P. jiroveci* (*carinii*)*,* or herpes simplex virus. Stem cell transplantation has corrected the immunologic and hematologic problems in some patients.

Ataxia-telangiectasia is a syndrome caused by the *ATM* (ataxia-telangiectasia, mutated) gene on chromosome 11q22.3 (see Table 73-3). Patients have cutaneous and conjunctival

Table 73-3	Other Immunodeficiency Diseases				
DISORDER	**GENETICS**	**ONSET**	**MANIFESTATIONS**	**PATHOGENESIS**	**ASSOCIATED FEATURES**
Wiskott-Aldrich syndrome	X-linked, (Xp11.22)	Early infancy	Thrombocytopenia, atopic dermatitis, recurrent infections	53-kD protein (WASP) defect	Polysaccharide antibody deficiency, small platelets, decreased cell-mediated immunity, lymphoproliferation
Ataxia-telangiectasia	AR (11q22.3)	2–5 yr	Recurrent otitis media, pneumonia, meningitis with encapsulated organisms	*ATM* gene mutation Disorder of cell cycle checkpoint and of DNA double-strand break repair	Neurologic and endocrine dysfunction, malignancy, telangiectasis; sensitivity to radiation
Nijmegen breakage syndrome	AR (8q21)	Infancy	Sinopulmonary infections, bronchiectasis, urinary tract infections	Defect in chromosomal repair mechanisms; hypomorphic mutation in *NBS1* (Nibrin)	Sensitivity to ionizing radiation; microcephaly with mild neurologic impairment; malignancy
Cartilage-hair hypoplasia (short-limbed dwarf)	AR (9p13–21)	Birth	Variable susceptibility to infections	Mutation in *RMRP*	Metaphyseal dysplasia, short extremities
Chronic mucocutaneous candidiasis (APECED)	AR	3–5 yr	Candidal infections of mucous membranes, skin, and nails	Mutations in *AIRE* gene	Autoimmune endocrinopathies
X-linked-lymphoproliferative syndromes	X-linked	Variable	Variable decrease in T, B, and NK cell function, hypogammaglobulinemia	Mutation in *SH2D1A* (SAP: SLAM-associated protein) or *XIAP*	Life-threatening Epstein-Barr virus infection, lymphoma or Hodgkin disease, aplastic anemia, lymphohistiocytic disorder
Hyper-IgE syndrome	AD, AR	Variable	Skin and pulmonary abscesses, fungal infections, eczema, elevated IgE	Mutation in STAT3 (AD), TYK2 (AR), and DOCK8 (AR)	Coarse facial features, failure to shed primary teeth, frequent fractures (STAT3), viral and other infections (TYK2 and DOCK8)

AD, Autosomal dominant; *AR,* autosomal recessive; *NK,* natural killer.

telangiectasias and progressive cerebellar ataxia with degeneration of Purkinje cells. IgA deficiency, IgG$_2$ subclass deficiency of variable severity, low IgE levels, and variably depressed T-cell function may be seen. The normal function of the *ATM* gene is not clear but appears to be involved in detecting DNA damage, blocking cell growth division until the damage is repaired, or both. Ataxia-telangiectasia cells are exquisitely sensitive to irradiation. Leukemias, lymphomas, and diabetes also may be present. Sexual maturation is delayed. There is no uniformly effective therapy, but antimicrobial therapy and intravenous immunoglobulin (IVIG) replacement therapy may be helpful.

Decision-Making Algorithms
Available @ StudentConsult.com

Involuntary Movements
Ataxia
Recurrent Infections

Chronic mucocutaneous candidiasis (autoimmune-polyendocrinopathy-candidiasis-ectodermal dystrophy [APECED]) is characterized by chronic or recurrent candidal infections of the mucous membranes, skin, and nails (see Table 73-3). There is normal antibody production but significantly decreased or absent lymphocyte proliferation and delayed skin reactivity to

Candida. Patients usually do not respond to topical antifungal therapy and must be treated with oral antifungal agents. In most patients, an autoimmune endocrine disorder, such as hypoparathyroidism and Addison disease, develops by early adulthood. Other autoimmune disorders have been reported. The insidious onset requires the need for frequent evaluation for autoimmune endocrine disorders. This disease results from a defect in the gene for the transcription factor autoimmune regulator *(AIRE),* which is necessary for expression of peripheral tissue antigens in the thymus, resulting in a negative selection in the thymus and in tolerance to these tissues in normal individuals.

Patients with **X-linked lymphoproliferative disease** (see Table 73-3) have a defect in immune responsiveness to Epstein-Barr virus (EBV). Boys with this disease are normal until infected with EBV, which is acutely fatal in 80% of patients. The disease is caused by a mutation in the gene called *SH2D1A* at chromosome Xq25, which codes for an adapter protein involved in signal transduction of lymphocytes. With EBV infection, the mutation results in an extensive expansion of CD8 T cells, hepatic necrosis, and death. Boys who survive initial EBV infection have significant hypogammaglobulinemia and are at high risk for developing aplastic anemia and lymphoma. A similar disorder is seen in boys with mutations in *XIAP,* which results in X-linked lymphoproliferative disorder type 2.

Table 73-4 | General Management of Patients with Immunodeficiency

Avoid transfusions with blood products unless they are irradiated and cytomegalovirus-negative.

Avoid live virus vaccines, especially in patients with severe T-cell deficiencies or agammaglobulinemia, and in household members.

Use prophylaxis to *Pneumocystis jiroveci* (*carinii*) in T-cell immunodeficiency, and in X-linked hyper-IgM, consider antifungal prophylaxis in T-cell immunodeficiency.

Follow pulmonary function in patients with recurrent pneumonia.

Use chest physiotherapy and postural drainage in patients with recurrent pneumonia.

Consider using prophylactic antibiotics because minor infections can quickly disseminate.

Examine diarrheal stools for *Giardia lamblia* and *Clostridium difficile*.

Avoid unnecessary exposure to individuals with infection. Boil water for T-cell defects and hyper-IgM syndrome (*Cryptosporidium* risk).

Use immunoglobulin for severe antibody deficiency states (400–600 mg/kg q3–4 wk IV).

Hyper-IgE syndrome is characterized by markedly elevated serum IgE levels, a rash that resembles atopic dermatitis, eosinophilia, and staphylococcal abscesses of the skin, lungs, joints, and viscera (see Table 73-3). Infections with *H. influenzae* type b, *Candida*, and *Aspergillus* also may occur. These patients have coarse facial features, develop osteopenia, and may have giant pneumatoceles in the lungs after staphylococcal pneumonias. Although serum IgG, IgA, and IgM levels are normal, humoral immune responses to specific antigens are reduced, as is cell-mediated immunity. Long-term treatment with antistaphylococcal medications is indicated, and immunoglobulin replacement therapy may be helpful. Most patients have an autosomal dominant form of inheritance, whereas some patients appear to have an autosomal recessive inheritance. Defects in the *TYK2* and *DOCK8* genes have been found in a patient with an autosomal recessive hyper-IgE syndrome, and defects in the *STAT3* (signal transducer and activator of transcription 3) gene were identified in autosomal dominant hyper-IgE syndrome.

TREATMENT

The approach to therapy of lymphocyte disorders depends on the diagnosis, clinical findings, and laboratory findings (Table 73-4). When immunodeficiency is suspected and while the evaluation is in process, all blood products need to be irradiated and negative for cytomegalovirus. Lymphocytes present in blood products can cause fatal **GVHD** in patients with SCID. Cytomegalovirus infection can be fatal in an immunodeficiency patient undergoing stem cell transplantation. Live virus vaccines should be withheld from patients and household members until a diagnosis is established.

Infections should be treated with appropriate antibiotics; prophylactic antibiotics can be used to prevent recurrent infections, provide a better quality of life, and decrease possible consequences. **Antibiotic prophylaxis** can be provided with once-daily administration of trimethoprim-sulfamethoxazole or amoxicillin at one half of the total daily therapeutic dose. Patients with severe T-cell deficiencies should receive prophylaxis against *Pneumocystis* and fungi until treated with stem cell transplantation. Patients with milder forms of antibody deficiency diseases may benefit from **vaccination** with protein-conjugate vaccines to *H. influenzae* type b and *S. pneumoniae*, assaying post vaccination titers at least 1 month later. These vaccines are administered routinely to young children; older children and adults with antibody deficiency syndrome should also receive them to generate protective antibody levels.

Immunoglobulin replacement therapy, intravenously or subcutaneously, is a lifesaving therapy for patients with severe antibody deficiency diseases and SCIDs. It provides passive immunity against common microorganisms and reduces the frequency and severity of infection in most patients. Immunoglobulin replacement therapy is usually administered at a total monthly dose of 400 to 600 mg/kg of body weight administered intravenously every 3 to 4 weeks, or subcutaneously by infusion pump every 1 to 2 weeks. IVIG therapy should be monitored by regularly measuring trough immunoglobulin levels and, more important, the patient's clinical course. Patients who continue to have recurrent infections, especially in the last week before the administration of IVIG, may require higher doses or more frequent administration. A combination of prophylactic antibiotics and immunoglobulin replacement therapy may be indicated in patients who continue to have recurrent infections. **Complications of IVIG** therapy include transfusion reactions with chills, fever, and myalgias. They usually can be prevented in subsequent infusions by pretreatment with an antihistamine, an antipyretic, and by a slower rate of infusion. Headache from aseptic meningitis can develop after IVIG therapy, usually in the first 24 hours. It most often responds to treatment with ibuprofen. Allergic reactions to IVIG can occur in patients with absent IgA. Allergic reactions are rare and should not occur in patients who have detectable serum IgA levels or patients who cannot synthesize any antibodies. Subcutaneous administration of immunoglobulin has fewer adverse effects but may be complicated by local reactions at the site(s) of infusion. The risk of transmission of infectious agents, despite preparation from large numbers of selected donors, is extremely low.

Therapy for severe T-cell disorders is stem cell transplantation, preferably from a human leukocyte antigen–matched sibling (see Chapter 76). Immunoglobulin replacement provides passive antibody-mediated immunity. Some patients continue to have poor B-cell function after stem cell transplantation and require lifelong immunoglobulin replacement therapy. **GVHD,** in which the transplanted cells initiate an immune response against the host tissues, is the main complication of stem cell transplantation. Patients with the ADA deficiency form of SCID who lack matched sibling donors can receive repeated intramuscular replacement doses of ADA, stabilized by coupling to polyethylene glycol. Gene therapy has been performed in several patients with common gamma chain deficiency and ADA deficiency by transfer of a normal gene into bone marrow stem cells, which are infused into the patient. Gene therapy for common gamma chain deficiency was successful in most of the treated patients; however, it was complicated by the development of leukemia in some patients.

PREVENTION AND NEWBORN SCREENING

Population-based screening programs for SCID is underway because early identification of SCID prior to infectious complications improves outcomes. Polymerase chain reaction amplification of T-cell receptor excision circles (TRECs) formed during T-cell receptor recombination can be performed on newborn screening blood spots to detect severe T-cell lymphopenia. Newborn screening for TRECs has been shown to detect SCID at birth, and this test has been recommended for universal screening.

Chapter **74**

NEUTROPHIL DISORDERS

Neutrophils play important roles in immunity and wound healing; their primary function is ingesting and killing pathogens. Neutrophil disorders can result from deficient cell numbers or defective function (Table 74-1). Patients with neutrophil disorders are susceptible to a variety of bacterial infections and certain fungi. Suggestive signs include mucous membrane infections (gingivitis), abscesses in the skin and viscera, lymphadenitis, poor wound healing, delayed umbilical cord separation, or absence of pus. Neutrophils develop in the bone marrow from hematopoietic stem cells by the action of several colony-stimulating factors, including stem cell factor, granulocyte-monocyte colony-stimulating factor, granulocyte colony-stimulating factor (G-CSF), and interleukin-3. On leaving the bone marrow, mature neutrophils are found in the circulation or reside in the marginating pool. Adhesion molecules are necessary for neutrophils to roll and adhere to vascular endothelium and extravasate from the blood into sites of infection, where they phagocytose and kill pathogens, especially those coated by complement or antibodies. Chemotactic factors, including the complement fragment C5a, interleukin-8, and bacterial formulated peptides, mobilize neutrophils to enter tissues and sites of infections. Neutrophils kill ingested pathogens using granular enzymes or by activation of oxygen radicals.

ETIOLOGY AND CLINICAL MANIFESTATIONS
Disorders of Neutrophil Numbers

Decision-Making Algorithms
Available @ StudentConsult.com

Diarrhea
Neutropenia
Failure to Thrive

The normal neutrophil count varies with age. **Neutropenia** is defined as an absolute neutrophil count (ANC) less than 1500/mm³ for white children 1 year of age or older. African American children normally have lower total white blood cell and neutrophil counts. The effect of neutropenia depends on its severity. The susceptibility to infection is minimally increased until the ANC is less than 1000/mm³. Most patients do well with an ANC greater than 500/mm³. At these levels, localized infections are more common than generalized bacteremia. Serious bacterial infections are more common with an ANC less than 200/mm³. The major types of infections associated with neutropenia are cellulitis, pharyngitis, gingivitis, lymphadenitis, abscesses (cutaneous or perianal), enteritis (typhlitis), and pneumonia. The sites of the infection usually are colonized heavily with normal bacterial flora that becomes invasive in the presence of neutropenia. Neutropenia may be congenital or acquired (Table 74-2) and may be associated with specific diseases, especially infections (Table 74-3), or result from drug reactions (Table 74-4).

There are several forms of congenital neutropenia. **Severe congenital neutropenia (Kostmann syndrome)** is an autosomal recessive disorder in which myeloid cells fail to mature beyond the early stages of the promyelocyte due to mutations in the *HAX-1* gene. The peripheral blood may show an impressive monocytosis. Although endogenous G-CSF levels are increased, exogenous G-CSF produces a rise in the neutrophil count, improving the care of these children. Acute myeloid leukemia has developed in a few patients who have survived into adolescence. Stem cell transplantation may be curative. Defects in *G6PC3* and *GFI1* have also been shown to cause severe congenital neutropenia. **Cyclic neutropenia** is a stem cell disorder in which all marrow elements cycle. It may be transmitted as an autosomal dominant, recessive, or sporadic disorder. Because of the short half-life of neutrophils in the blood (6 to 7 hours) compared to platelets (10 days) and red blood cells (120 days), neutropenia is the only clinically significant abnormality. The usual cycle is 21 days, with neutropenia lasting 4 to 6 days, accompanied by monocytosis and often by eosinophilia. Severe, debilitating bone pain is common when the neutrophil count is low. G-CSF results in increasing neutrophil numbers and a shorter duration of neutropenia. Defects in *ELA2,* the gene encoding for neutrophil elastase, has been found in patients with cyclic neutropenia. Further analysis has demonstrated *ELA2* mutations in some cases of severe congenital neutropenia.

Severe congenital neutropenia that may be either persistent or cyclic also is a component of **Shwachman-Diamond syndrome,** an autosomal recessive syndrome of pancreatic insufficiency accompanying bone marrow dysfunction. This is a panmyeloid disorder in which neutropenia is the most prominent manifestation. Metaphyseal dysostosis and dwarfism may occur. Patients usually respond to G-CSF. Other congenital neutropenia caused by deficient neutrophil production vary in severity and are poorly characterized. A gain of function mutation in the Wiskott-Aldrich syndrome protein has also been associated with an X-linked form of severe congenital neutropenia. **Benign congenital neutropenia** is a functional diagnosis for patients with significant neutropenia in whom major infectious complications do not develop. Many patients whose ANC ranges from 100 to 500/mm³ have an increased frequency of infections, particularly respiratory infections, but the major problem is the slow resolution of infections that develop. These disorders may be sporadic or familial and, in some instances, are transmitted as an autosomal dominant disorder. Severe congenital neutropenia may be associated with severe combined immunodeficiency in **reticular dysgenesis,** a

Table 74-1	Phagocytic Disorders	
NAME	**DEFECT**	**COMMENT**
Chronic granulomatous disease	Bactericidal	X-linked recessive (66%), autosomal recessive (33%); eczema, osteomyelitis, granulomas, abscesses caused by *Staphylococcus aureus*, *Burkholderia cepacia*, *Aspergillus fumigatus*
Chédiak-Higashi syndrome (1q42l-44)	Bactericidal plus chemotaxis; poor natural killer function	Autosomal recessive; oculocutaneous albinism, neuropathy, giant neutrophilic cytoplasmic inclusions; malignancy, neutropenia
Hyperimmunoglobulin E (Job syndrome)	Chemotaxis, opsonization	Autosomal dominant (STAT3 mutation), autosomal recessive (TYK2, DOCK8 mutation), eczema, staphylococcal abscesses, granulocyte and monocyte chemotaxis affected
Myeloperoxidase deficiency	Bactericidal, fungicidal	Reduced chemiluminescence; autosomal recessive (1:4000); persistent candidiasis in diabetic patients
Glucose-6-phosphate dehydrogenase deficiency	Bactericidal	Phenotypically similar to chronic granulomatous disease
Burns, malnutrition	Bactericidal plus chemotaxis	Reversible defects
Lazy leukocyte syndrome	Chemotaxis	Normal bone marrow cells but poor migration; granulocytopenia
Leukocyte adhesion deficiency	Adherence, chemotaxis, phagocytosis; reduced lymphocyte cytotoxicity	Delayed separation or infection of umbilical cord; lethal bacterial infections without pus; autosomal recessive; neutrophilia; deficiency of LFA-1, Mac-1, CR3
Shwachman-Diamond syndrome	Chemotaxis, neutropenia	Pancreatic insufficiency, metaphyseal chondrodysplasia; autosomal recessive

CR3, Complement receptor 3; *LFA-1*, leukocyte function-associated antigen type 1; *Mac-1*, macrophage 1 antigen.

disorder of hematopoietic stem cells affecting all bone marrow lineages due to mutations in the *AK2* gene.

Isoimmune neutropenia occurs in neonates as the result of transplacental transfer of maternal antibodies to fetal neutrophil antigens. The mother is sensitized to specific neutrophil antigens on fetal leukocytes that are inherited from the father and are not present on maternal cells. Isoimmune neonatal neutropenia, similar to isoimmune anemia and thrombocytopenia, is a transient process (see Chapters 62 and 151). Cutaneous infections are common, and sepsis is rare. Early treatment of infection while the infant is neutropenic is the major goal of therapy. Intravenous immune globulin may decrease the duration of neutropenia.

Autoimmune neutropenia usually develops in children 5 to 24 months of age and often persists for prolonged periods. Neutrophil autoantibodies may be IgG, IgM, IgA, or a combination of these. Usually the condition resolves in 6 months to 4 years. Although intravenous immune globulin and corticosteroids have been used, most patients respond to G-CSF. Autoimmune neutropenia rarely may be an early manifestation of systemic lupus erythematosus, rheumatoid arthritis, or autoimmune lymphoproliferative disease.

Disorders of Neutrophil Migration

Neutrophils normally adhere to endothelium and migrate to areas of inflammation by the interaction of membrane proteins, called *integrins* and *selectins*, with endothelial cell adhesion molecules. A hallmark of defects in neutrophil migration is the absence of pus at sites of infection. In **leukocyte adhesion deficiency type I (LAD-I),** infants lacking the β_2 integrin CD18 exhibit the condition early in infancy with failure of separation of the umbilical cord (often 2 months after birth) with attendant omphalitis and sepsis (see Table 74-1). The neutrophil count usually is greater than 20,000/mm³ because of failure of the neutrophils to adhere normally to vascular

endothelium and to migrate out of blood to the tissues (Fig. 74-1). Cutaneous, respiratory, and mucosal infections occur. Children with this condition often have severe gingivitis. Sepsis usually leads to death in early childhood. This disorder is transmitted as an autosomal recessive trait. Stem cell transplantation can be lifesaving.

LAD-II results from impairment of neutrophil rolling along the vascular wall, which is the first step in neutrophil migration into tissues and sites of infection. Rolling is mediated by sialylated and fucosylated tetrasaccharides related to the sialylated Lewis X (S-LeX) blood group found on the surface of neutrophils, monocytes, and activated lymphocytes binding to selectin molecules on vascular endothelium (see Fig. 74-1). LAD-II results from a general defect in fucose metabolism leading to the absence of S-LeX blood group on the surface of neutrophils and other leukocytes. LAD-III is a rare disorder caused by defects in the KINDLIN-3 protein resulting in defective neutrophil adhesion as well as platelet defects. Defective migration of neutrophils has also been described in **Hyper-IgE syndrome** and with mutations in the *RAC2* gene (see Chapter 73 and Table 74-1).

Disorders of Neutrophil Function

Decision-Making Algorithms
Available @ StudentConsult.com

Jaundice
Neutropenia
Recurrent Infections

Defects in neutrophil function are relatively rare inherited disorders and tend to be associated with a marked susceptibility to bacterial and fungal infection. **Chronic granulomatous disease (CGD)** is a disorder of white blood cells that results

Table 74-2	Mechanisms of Neutropenia

ABNORMAL BONE MARROW

Marrow Injury

Drugs: idiosyncratic, cytotoxic (myelosuppressive)

Radiation

Chemicals: DDT, benzene

Immune-mediated: T and B cell and immunoglobulin

Infections (viruses, rickettsia)

Infiltrative processes: tumor, storage disease

Myelodysplasia

Aplastic anemia

Maturation Defects

Folic acid deficiency

Vitamin B_{12}

Copper

Congenital Disorders

Kostmann syndrome (HAX-1, G6PC3, ELA-2, G-CSF, GFI-1)

Cyclic neutropenia (ELA-2)

Cartilage hair hypoplasia

Shwachman-Diamond syndrome

Diamond-Blackfan syndrome

Griscelli syndrome

Chédiak-Higashi syndrome

WHIM syndrome (warts, hypogammaglobulinemia, infections, myelokathexis)
Glycogen storage disease type Ib
Methylmalonicacidemia

PERIPHERAL CIRCULATION

Pseudoneutropenia: Shift to Bone Marrow

Hereditary

Severe infection

Intravascular

Destruction: neonatal isoimmune, autoimmune, hypersplenism
Autoimmune diseases (systemic lupus erythematosus, rheumatoid arthritis, Sjögren syndrome)

Leukoagglutination. lung, after cardiac bypass surgery

ELA-2, Elastase 2; G6PC3, glucose-6-phosphatase catalytic subunit 3; G-CSF, granulocyte colony-stimulating factor; GFI-1, growth factor independent 1; HAX-1, HS1-associated protein X-1.

Table 74-3	Infection-Associated Neutropenia

BACTERIAL

Typhoid-paratyphoid

Brucellosis

Neonatal sepsis

Meningococcemia

Overwhelming sepsis

Congenital syphilis

Tuberculosis

VIRAL

Measles

Hepatitis B

HIV

Rubella

Cytomegalovirus

Influenza

Epstein-Barr virus

RICKETTSIAL

Rocky Mountain spotted fever

Typhus

Ehrlichiosis

Rickettsialpox

HIV, human immunodeficiency virus.

Table 74-4	Drug-Associated Neutropenia

CYTOTOXIC

Myelosuppressive, chemotherapeutic agents

Immunosuppressive agents

IDIOSYNCRATIC

Indomethacin

Para-aminophenol derivatives

Pyrazolone derivatives (aminopyrine, dipyrone, oxyphenbutazone)

Chloramphenicol

Sulfonamides

Antithyroid drugs (propylthiouracil, methimazole, carbimazole)

Phenothiazines (chlorpromazine, phenothiazines)

Penicillins and semisynthetic penicillins

Adapted from Dale DC: Neutropenia. In Lichtman MA, Kipps TJ, Seligsohn U, et al, editors: Williams Hematology, ed 8, New York, 2010, McGraw-Hill.

from defective intracellular killing of bacteria and intracellular pathogens by neutrophils and macrophages because of an inability to activate the "respiratory burst," the catalytic conversion of molecular oxygen to superoxide (O_2^-). Reduced nicotinamide adenine dinucleotide phosphate oxidase, the enzyme that catalyzes the respiratory burst, consists of four subunits; gp91^{phox}, p22^{phox}, p47^{phox}, and p67^{phox}. Defects in any of these enzymes lead to an inability to kill catalase-positive pathogens such as *S. aureus* and enteric gram-negative bacteria (*Burkholderia*) and fungi (*Aspergillus fumigatus, Candida albicans*). The gp91^{phox} gene is located on chromosome Xp21.1 and is responsible for the most common form of the disease. The other gene defects are inherited in an autosomal recessive manner. The chromosome locations for

these genes are 16q24 for p22^{phox}, 7q11.23 for p47^{phox}, and 1q25 for p67^{phox}. Glucose-6-phosphate dehydrogenase also is involved in the production of superoxide, and severe forms of glucose-6-phosphate dehydrogenase deficiency also result in CGD. Patients characteristically have lymphadenopathy, hypergammaglobulinemia, hepatosplenomegaly, dermatitis, failure to thrive, anemia, chronic diarrhea, and abscesses. Infections occur in the lungs, the middle ear, gastrointestinal tract, skin, urinary tract, lymph nodes, liver, and bones.

Figure 74-1 Schematic representation of neutrophil migration from the vascular space across the vascular endothelium into tissues. Neutrophils bind to selectin (E- or P-selectin) molecules on the surface of vascular endothelium via sialylated and fucosylated tetrasaccharides related to the S-LeX blood group found on the surface of neutrophils. The bound neutrophils roll along the endothelium and become tightly bound by the interaction of the adhesion molecule leukocyte function-associated antigen type 1 (LFA-1) on the neutrophil and intercellular adhesion molecule type 1 on vascular endothelium, allowing neutrophils to move through the endothelium and into the tissue spaces. *(Adapted from Janeway CA, Travers P, Walport M, et al: Immunobiology: the Immune System in Health and Disease, ed 4, New York, 1999, Elsevier.)*

Granulomas are prominent and may obstruct the pylorus or ureters.

Chédiak-Higashi syndrome, an abnormality of secondary granules, is an autosomal recessive disorder caused by a mutation in a cytoplasmic protein (CHS1) thought to be involved in organellar protein trafficking, resulting in a fusion of the primary and secondary granules in neutrophils. Giant granules are present in many cells, including lymphocytes, platelets, and melanocytes. Patients usually have partial oculocutaneous albinism. The defect in Chédiak-Higashi syndrome results in defective neutrophil and natural killer cell function, leading to recurrent and sometimes fatal infections with streptococci and staphylococci. Most patients progress to an accelerated phase associated with Epstein-Barr virus infection and characterized by a **lymphoproliferative syndrome** with generalized lymphohistiocytic infiltrates, fever, jaundice, hepatomegaly, lymphadenopathy, and pancytopenia. The condition resembles hemophagocytic lymphohistiocytosis.

LABORATORY DIAGNOSIS

The evaluation of a neutropenic child depends on clinical signs of infection, family and medication history, age of the patient, cyclic or persistent nature of the condition, signs of bone marrow infiltration (malignancy or storage disease), and evidence of involvement of other cell lines. Neutropenia is confirmed by a complete blood count and differential. A bone marrow aspirate and biopsy may be necessary to determine whether the neutropenia is due to a failure of production in the bone marrow, infiltration of the bone marrow, or loss of neutrophils in the periphery. Antineutrophil antibodies help diagnose autoimmune neutropenia.

Neutrophil chemotactic defects can be excluded by the presence of neutrophils at the site of infection. The **Rebuck skin window** is a 4-hour in vivo test for neutrophil chemotaxis that is not performed routinely by most laboratories. In vitro studies

of neutrophil migration are available in specialized laboratories. Flow cytometry for the presence of adhesion molecules, such as CD18 or CD15, can help diagnose leukocyte adhesion defects. Point mutations that affect the function of the adhesion molecule but do not alter antibody binding are missed using flow cytometry. CGD can be diagnosed by the flow cytometry-based test using dihydrorhodamine 123 or the **nitroblue tetrazolium** test (see Chapter 72). Light microscopy of neutrophils for the presence of giant granules can help diagnose Chédiak-Higashi syndrome.

TREATMENT

Therapy for neutropenia depends on the underlying cause. Patients with severe bacterial infections require broad-spectrum antibiotics; the resolution of neutropenia is the most important prognostic factor. Most patients with severe congenital neutropenia or autoimmune neutropenia respond to therapy with G-CSF. Granulocyte transfusion should be reserved for life-threatening infection. Chronic mild neutropenia not associated with immunosuppression can be managed expectantly with prompt antimicrobial treatment of soft tissue infections, which usually are caused by *S. aureus* or group A streptococcus.

Frequent courses of antibiotics, including trimethoprim-sulfamethoxazole prophylaxis, and surgical débridement of infections are required in **CGD.** Because *A. fumigatus* can cause serious infection in patients with CGD, moldy hay, decomposing compost, and other nests of fungi must be avoided, and prophylactic antifungals can be helpful. The frequency of infection in CGD is lessened by treatment with **recombinant interferon-γ** administered subcutaneously three times a week. Stem cell transplantation (see Chapter 76) may be lifesaving in CGD, LAD-1, and Chédiak-Higashi syndrome.

PROGNOSIS AND PREVENTION

The prognosis depends on the particular defect. Milder and transient defects in neutrophil numbers have a better prognosis. Prolonged absence of neutrophils or their function has a poor prognosis, especially with the risk of bacterial and fungal sepsis. Treatment with prophylactic antibiotics and interferon-γ has improved the prognosis of patients with CGD. Stem cell transplantation is the only currently available mode of therapy that can reverse the poor prognosis of severe neutrophil defects. As in other genetic defects, prenatal diagnosis and genetic counseling are possible for all known gene mutations.

Chapter **75**

COMPLEMENT SYSTEM

The **complement system** consists of plasma and membrane proteins that function in the innate immune response as well as facilitate adaptive immunity. **Complement proteins** can kill pathogens with or without antibodies, opsonize pathogens

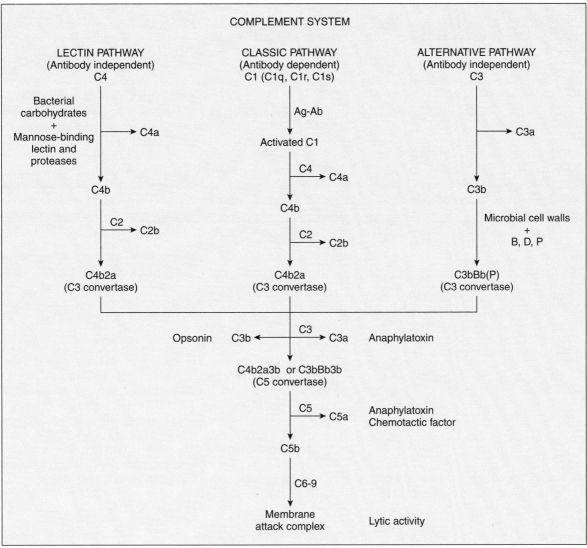

Figure 75-1 Complement component cascade involving the classic, alternative, and lectin pathways. The initiating events for the pathways differ, but they result in the production of C3 cleaving enzyme activity, which is the pivotal step as the three pathways converge to the terminal activation sequences. *Ag-Ab*, Antigen-antibody complex; *B*, factor B; *D*, factor D (factor B clearing enzyme); *P*, properdin.

to facilitate their uptake by phagocytes, or mediate inflammation. The complement system can be activated through three pathways—classic, alternative, or lectin—that involve a cascade-like, sequential activation of complement factors resulting in an amplified response (Fig. 75-1). Disorders of the complement system predispose to recurrent infection, autoimmunity, and angioedema (Table 75-1).

ETIOLOGY

The three pathways for complement activation are initiated by different mechanisms. The **classic pathway** is activated by antigen-antibody complexes or by C-reactive protein. The **alternative pathway** may be activated by C3b generated through classic complement activation or by spontaneous hydrolysis of C3 on microbial surfaces. The **lectin pathway** is initiated by the interaction of mannose-binding lectin with microbial carbohydrate. Activation of the classic pathway by an antigen-antibody complex is initiated by the binding of C1q to the Fc portion of an antibody molecule in the immune complex. C1r auto-activates and cleaves C1s, which cleaves

C4 and then C2, forming the C3 convertase, C4b2a. C4b2a is activated by the lectin pathway when mannose-binding protein binds to sugar residues on the surface of pathogens, and mannose-binding protein–associated proteases (MASP) cleave C4 and C2. The alternative pathway is always active at a low level and is amplified when active C3 binds to a surface that lacks regulatory proteins. C3b generated from C3 binds to factor B, which is cleaved by factor D to form the alternative pathway C3 convertase, C3bBb. Properdin binds to and stabilizes the C3 convertase (see Fig. 75-1). The C3 convertase can cleave C3 resulting in further C3b deposition and activation of the alternative pathway that acts as an amplification loop by generating more C3b, or it can form the C5 convertase which initiates the formation of a **membrane attack complex (MAC).** The MAC is a complex of C5b, C6, C7, C8, and several C9 molecules that is common to all three pathways (see Fig. 75-1). The MAC generates pores in the cell membrane, leading to lysis of the cells. C3a and C5a, produced by cleavage of C3 and C5 respectively, can release histamine from mast cells and basophils, leading to increased vascular permeability and smooth muscle contraction. In addition, C5a has chemotactic

Table 75-1	Deficiency of Complement and Associated Disease
DEFICIENT PROTEIN	**ASSOCIATED DISEASE**
C1q, C1r	SLE, glomerulonephritis; encapsulated bacterial infections
C2	SLE, glomerulonephritis; encapsulated bacterial infections
C3	Recurrent bacterial infections, rare glomerulonephritis, or SLE
C4	SLE, glomerulonephritis; encapsulated bacterial infections
C5	Recurrent meningococcal infections
C6	Recurrent meningococcal infections
C7	Recurrent meningococcal infections
C8	Recurrent meningococcal infections
C9	Occasional meningococcal infection
Properdin	Recurrent infections, severe meningococcal infection
MBL	Increased susceptibility to infections
Factor H	Glomerulonephritis, atypical HUS
Factor I	Recurrent infections, glomerulonephritis
MCP	Glomerulonephritis, atypical HUS
C1 inhibitor	Hereditary angioedema

HUS, hemolytic uremic syndrome; *MBL,* mannose binding lectin; *MCP,* membrane cofactor protein; *SLE,* systemic lupus erythematosus.

activity, attracting phagocytes to the site of complement activation, and it can cause degranulation of phagocytic cells. C3b acts as an opsonin when attached to the surface of a pathogen by binding to phagocytes via complement receptor 1 (CR1). Its degradation product, iC3b, can bind to CR3 on the surface of phagocytes leading to the ingestion of the C3b-coated or iC3b-coated pathogen. iC3b and its breakdown product C3dg can bind complement receptor 2 (CR2) on B cells leading to activation and differentiation.

The complement system is under tight regulation because it has potent inflammatory activity and the potential to cause significant damage to host cells. The complement cascade is inherently regulated by the short half-life C4b and C3b and by instability of the C3 convertases, C4b2a, and C3bBb. C1-inhibitor regulates the cascade by blocking active sites on C1r, C1s, and the MASP. Factor I destabilizes C3 convertase complexes and degrades the active fragments. Other inhibitors include membrane proteins, such as decay accelerating factor, CR1, membrane cofactor protein (MCP), and plasma proteins such as C4b-binding protein and factor H. Formation of the MAC can be blocked by cell surface CD59, protein S, and other plasma proteins. Deficiency of any of these regulatory proteins can result in an inflammatory response, tissue damage, or excessive complement consumption.

Disorders of complement proteins can result from inherited deficiency or can be secondary to increased consumption. The consequences of decreased complement depend on the affected factor (see Table 75-1). **Deficiencies of early components** of the classic pathway (C1, C2, or C4) are not usually associated with severe infections, although patients with

C2 deficiency may present with milder recurrent infections. Patients with C1, C2, or C4 deficiency are susceptible to autoimmune diseases, especially systemic lupus erythematosus. The exact mechanism of this susceptibility is not known but is thought to arise from the role of these early components in clearing immune complexes.

Deficiency of properdin, C3, or the terminal components predisposes patients to severe recurrent infections. Deficiency of C3, the major opsonin, due to a genetic defect or secondary to excessive consumption, predisposes patients to infections, especially with encapsulated organisms. Deficiency of one of the terminal components that compose the MAC predisposes patients to infection with *Neisseria meningitidis.* Complement deficiency may be found in 40% of patients presenting with recurrent neisserial infections. Deficiency of mannose-binding lectin also is associated with an increased frequency of bacterial infections, including sepsis.

Congenital deficiency of C1-inhibitor results in **hereditary angioedema,** characterized by recurrent episodes of nonpruritic angioedema lasting 48 to 72 hours, which occur spontaneously or after minor trauma, stress, or anxiety. Abdominal edema can cause acute abdominal pain; edema of the upper airway can be life threatening and may necessitate emergency tracheostomy. The disorder is inherited as an autosomal dominant disease and results from a heterozygous deficiency of C1-inhibitor leading to serum levels less than 30% of normal values. Some mutations (type II hereditary angioedema) result in normal levels of C1-inhibitor with defective function. An acquired form of angioedema results from autoantibodies to C1-inhibitor in lymphoid malignancies or autoimmune disorders but is uncommon in childhood. C1-inhibitor is a regulator of Hageman factor (clotting factor XIIa), clotting factor XIa, plasma kallikrein, and plasmin in addition to C1r and C1s. Lack of inhibition of the contact system, Hageman factor and plasma kallikrein, is responsible for the development of angioedema. Deficiencies in the complement regulatory proteins factor H, factor I, and MCP result in **atypical hemolytic uremic syndrome, membranoproliferative glomerulonephritis type II,** and have been linked to **age-related macular degeneration.**

LABORATORY STUDIES

The **CH₅₀ test** is a widely available test of classic complement pathway function, based on an antibody-dependent hemolytic assay, which measures the serum dilution that results in lysis of 50% of sheep red blood cells. The CH₅₀ test depends on the function of all nine complement proteins, C1 through C9. The **AH₅₀ test,** which measures complement activation using red blood cells from different species (e.g., rabbit) that can activate the alternative pathway without antibody, is less widely available than the CH₅₀ test and requires the alternative pathway components and C5 to C9. Abnormal results of both tests indicate a deficiency in a terminal component common to both pathways, whereas an abnormal result of one or the other test indicates a deficiency of an early component of the respective pathway. If the CH₅₀ or AH₅₀ levels are abnormal, individual components can be analyzed in specialized laboratories.

Determination of C1-inhibitor levels and function is needed to diagnose hereditary angioedema. Some functional tests miss rare mutations that allow C1-inhibitor to bind C1s, but not one or more of the other enzymes with which it interacts. Low C1-inhibitor levels or function results in chronically decreased

C4 levels and decreased C2 levels during acute attacks. Low C1q levels are found in acquired C1-inhibitor deficiency, which distinguishes it from hereditary angioedema. Tests for autoantibodies to C1-inhibitor and C1q can be performed by enzyme-linked immunosorbent assay.

TREATMENT

Specific treatment of complement deficiencies with component replacement is not available. Long, frequent courses of antibiotics constitute the primary therapy. Immunization of patients and close contacts with pneumococcal and meningococcal vaccines may be useful, but infections may still occur in immunized complement-deficient patients. Replacement of complement proteins by plasma transfusion has been used in some patients with C2 deficiency, factor H deficiency, or factor I deficiency. MCP deficiency is treated with renal transplantation because it is a membrane protein.

Patients with C1-inhibitor deficiency and frequent episodes of angioedema respond to prophylactic use of an oral attenuated androgen (**stanozolol** or **danazol**), which increases serum concentrations of C1-inhibitor. Adverse effects, including masculinization in females, growth arrest, and hepatitis, limit their use. Prophylactic administration of fresh frozen plasma before surgery can prevent angioedema, but administration during an acute episode may exacerbate the episode. Angioedema of the airway can present as an acute emergency, necessitating a tracheostomy because administration of epinephrine, antihistamines, or corticosteroids is ineffective in reversing this type of angioedema. Purified C1-inhibitor is available and can be used prophylactically (before surgery) and during acute episodes of angioedema. Angiotensin-converting enzyme inhibitors, such as captopril, should be avoided in patients with C1-inhibitor deficiency because these drugs can precipitate episodes of angioedema by inhibiting degradation of kinins that mediate edema formation. Novel therapeutic agents, including a kallikrein inhibitor and a bradykinin receptor 2 antagonist, are being investigated as potential therapy for hereditary angioedema.

Chapter **76**

HEMATOPOIETIC STEM CELL TRANSPLANTATION

Hematopoietic stem cell transplantation (HSCT) can cure some patients with primary immunodeficiency disease (Table 76-1). Use of HSCT is limited to immunodeficiency diseases with T-cell defects, some metabolic storage diseases (see Chapters 55 and 56), malignancies (see Chapter 154), aplastic anemia (see Chapter 150), hemoglobinopathies (Chapter 150), and a few other disorders.

Table 76-1	Immunodeficiency Diseases Curable by Stem Cell Transplantation

Severe combined immunodeficiency (SCID)

    X-linked SCID (γ_c deficiency)

    Jak 3 kinase deficiency

    ZAP 70 deficiency and other T-cell activation defects

    RAG1/RAG2 deficiency and other T^- B^- SCID

    Omenn syndrome

    Adenosine deaminase deficiency

    Purine nucleoside phosphorylase deficiency

    Reticular dysgenesis

    Bare lymphocyte syndrome

Wiskott-Aldrich syndrome

X-linked hyper-IgM

X-linked lymphoproliferative syndromes

Cartilage hair hypoplasia

Autoimmune lymphoproliferative syndrome (Fas defect)

Severe congenital neutropenia

Shwachman-Diamond syndrome

Immune dysregulation, polyendocrinopathy, enteropathy, X-linked (IPEX)

Cyclic neutropenia

Chédiak-Higashi syndrome

Leukocyte adhesion deficiency type I

Familial hemophagocytic lymphohistiocytosis

The principle of HSCT is to replace a patient's defective bone marrow stem cells with normal stem cells. Hematopoietic stem cells reside in the bone marrow but can also be obtained from peripheral blood or cord blood. Peripheral blood does not contain a significant proportion of stem cells unless the donor's bone marrow is actively stimulated to generate stem cells. Cord blood is a good source of stem cells and is used for sibling and unrelated HSCT.

Major histocompatibility complex (MHC) compatibility is crucial in the choice of a stem cell donor to avoid rejection of the donor cells by the host immune system and to prevent graft-versus-host disease (GVHD) caused by contaminating mature T cells. The donor stem cells give rise to T cells that develop in the host thymus and need to interact with donor and host antigen-presenting cells. In cases with MHC mismatched donors, mature T cells need to be removed from the donor to reduce the risk of **GVHD;** this complication outweighs the disadvantage of a prolonged time of 90 to 120 days before T-cell development. Patients are at risk for developing **B-cell lymphoproliferative disease,** usually associated with Epstein-Barr virus, when T-cell–depletion techniques are used, likely due to the delay in T-cell engraftment.

The most important factor affecting outcomes in HSCT is the similarity of the donor MHC. The best outcomes are obtained using MHC-identical siblings (25% chance of a matched sibling) as donors, followed by matched unrelated donors. Unlike transplantation for other disorders, MHC haploidentical bone marrow from a parent (preferred) or a sibling can be used to treat severe combined immunodeficiency (SCID), likely the result of these patients lacking functioning T cells. Stem cells from a partially mismatched donor, such as a parent, can give rise to a functioning immune system because the patient shares at least half of the MHC molecules with the donor stem cells.

MHC molecules are highly polymorphic, and typing is currently performed on DNA rather than by serology. Bone marrow and cord blood registries are available worldwide. Searching and identifying a donor can be a lengthy process, especially for some underrepresented ethnic backgrounds. Finding a suitable cord blood donor is faster because the cord blood already has been obtained and stored, whereas bone marrow donors have to be identified, located, and tested. A matched sibling, if available, is the preferred source of hematopoietic stem cells.

Patients with SCID are ideal candidates for HSCT, which is the only option for treatment of SCID at this time. Patients are unlikely to survive beyond 1 to 2 years of age without transplantation, and they have no T-cell function to reject donor cells. Thus they may not need to undergo conditioning with chemotherapy or irradiation before transplantation. The development of transplantation using T-cell–depleted, haploidentical bone marrow from a parent for SCID has provided almost every patient with SCID a potential donor. The mother is the preferred source for haploidentical bone marrow, if she is able to donate, because some transfer of maternal T cells can occur during pregnancy, and these maternal T cells can reject cells obtained from the father. The survival rate after HSCT for SCID is approximately 90% with MHC-identical and 60% with haploidentical bone marrow transplantation. Early transplant before the acquisition of infection improves outcomes. Because newborn screening for SCID is now possible, stem cell transplantation can occur as early as possible when the infants are healthy, providing the best opportunity for a cure.

The decision to treat other primary immunodeficiency diseases with HSCT is more difficult because it is difficult to predict the prognosis of a particular patient because of the variability in clinical course of most primary immunodeficiency diseases. This must be weighed with the risks of transplantation. In addition, HSCT for other primary immunodeficiencies is less successful than for SCID because patients typically have some T-cell function and require conditioning with the risks that it entails. The availability of a matched related sibling favors the decision to perform HSCT. Disorders of B cells have not been treated with HSCT because, in many cases, donor B cells do not engraft, and patients usually do well with intravenous immunoglobulin. Regardless a variety of primary immunodeficiencies have been treated with HSCT (see Table 76-1)

COMPLICATIONS

Rejection of the grafted cells is the first potential complication of HSCT and depends on the immunocompetence of the patient, the degree of MHC incompatibility, and the number of cells administered. Preconditioning with myeloablative drugs, such as busulfan and cyclophosphamide, can prevent graft rejection but may be complicated by pulmonary toxicity and by venoocclusive disease of the liver, which results from damage to the hepatic vascular endothelium and can be fatal. Myeloablation results in anemia, leukopenia, and thrombocytopenia, making patients susceptible to infection and bleeding disorders. Neutropenic precautions should be maintained and patients supported with red blood cell and platelet transfusions until the red blood cell, platelet, and neutrophil lineages engraft. Reduced intensity preconditioning has been used recently to prevent graft rejection and decrease the adverse effects of myeloablation. **B-cell lymphoproliferative** disorder can develop after T-cell depleted bone marrow transplantation. **GVHD** can arise from an MHC-mismatched transplantation or from mismatch in minor histocompatibility antigens that are not tested for before transplantation. T-cell depletion of haploidentical bone marrow reduces the risk of GVHD. Patients with SCID transplanted with T-cell–depleted haploidentical bone marrow do not usually develop severe GVHD. **Acute GVHD** begins 6 or more days after transplantation and can result from transfusion of nonirradiated blood products in patients with no T-cell function. Acute GVHD presents with fever, skin rash, and severe diarrhea. Patients develop a high, unrelenting fever; a morbilliform maculopapular erythematous rash that is painful and pruritic; hepatosplenomegaly and abnormal liver function tests; and nausea, vomiting, abdominal pain, and watery diarrhea. Acute GVHD is staged from grades 1 to 4, depending on the degree of skin, fever, gastrointestinal, and liver involvement. **Chronic GVHD** results from acute GVHD lasting longer than 100 days and can develop without acute GVHD or after acute GVHD has resolved. Chronic GVHD is characterized by skin lesions (hyperkeratosis, reticular hyperpigmentation, fibrosis, and atrophy with ulceration), limitation of joint movement, interstitial pneumonitis, and immune dysregulation with autoantibody and immune complex formation.

Suggested Reading

Klein C: Genetic defects in severe congenital neutropenia: emerging insights into life and death of human neutrophil granulocytes, *Annu Rev Immunol* 29:399–413, 2011.

Ricklin D, Hajishengallis G, Yang K, et al: Complement: a key system for immune surveillance and homeostasis, *Nat Immunol* 11:785–797, 2010.

Szabolcs P, Cavazzana-Calvo M, Fischer A, et al: Bone marrow transplantation for primary immunodeficiency diseases, *Pediatr Clin N Am* 57:207–237, 2010.

Waleed A, Bousfiha A, Casanova JL, et al: Primary immunodeficiency diseases: an update on the classification from the International Union of Immunological Societies Expert Committee for Primary Immunodeficiency, *Front Immunol* 2:1–26, 2011.

Allergy

Asriani M. Chiu

14

 Chapter 77

ASSESSMENT

Atopy is a result of a complex interaction between multiple genes and environmental factors. It implies specific IgE-mediated diseases, including allergic rhinitis, asthma, and atopic dermatitis. An **allergen** is an antigen that triggers an IgE response in genetically predisposed individuals.

Hypersensitivity disorders of the immune system are classified into four groups, based on the mechanism that leads to tissue inflammation (Table 77-1). **Type I reactions** are triggered by the binding of antigen to high-affinity IgE receptors on the surface of tissue mast cells, circulating basophils, or both, causing the release of preformed chemical mediators, such as histamine and tryptase, and newly generated mediators, such as leukotrienes, prostaglandins, and platelet-activating factor. These mediators contribute to the development of allergic symptoms, with anaphylaxis as the most profound symptom. Several hours after the initial response, a **late-phase reaction** may develop with an influx of other inflammatory cells such as basophils, eosinophils, monocytes, lymphocytes, and neutrophils, and their inflammatory mediators. Recruitment of these cells leads to more persistent and chronic symptoms.

Type II (antibody cytotoxicity) reactions involve IgM, IgG, or IgA antibodies binding to the cell surface and activating the entire complement pathway resulting in lysis of the cell or release of anaphylatoxins, such as C3a, C4a, and C5a (see Chapter 75). These anaphylatoxins trigger mast cell degranulation, resulting in inflammatory mediator release. The target can be cell surface membrane antigens, such as red blood cells (hemolytic anemia); platelet cell surface molecules (thrombocytopenia); basement membrane molecules in the kidney (Goodpasture syndrome); the alpha chain of the acetylcholine receptor at the neuromuscular junction (myasthenia gravis); and thyroid-stimulating hormone receptor on thyroid cells (Graves disease).

Type III (immune complex) reactions involve the formation of antigen-antibody or immune complexes that enter into the circulation and are deposited in tissues such as blood vessels and filtering organs (i.e., liver, spleen, and kidney). These complexes initiate tissue injury by activating the complement cascade and recruiting neutrophils that release their toxic mediators. Local reactions caused by the injection of antigen

Table 77-1	Gell and Coombs Classification of Hypersensitivity Disorders				
TYPE	**INTERVAL BETWEEN EXPOSURE AND REACTION**	**EFFECTOR CELL**	**TARGET OR ANTIGEN**	**EXAMPLES OF MEDIATORS**	**EXAMPLES**
I—Anaphylactic immediate late phase	<30 min 2–12 h	IgE	Pollens, food, venom, drugs	Histamine, tryptase, leukotrienes, prostaglandins, platelet-activating factor	Anaphylaxis, urticaria, allergic rhinitis, allergic asthma
II—Cytotoxic antibody	Variable (minutes to hours)	IgG, IgM, IgA	Red blood cells, platelets	Complement	Rh hemolytic anemia, thrombocytopenia, hemolysis (quinidine), Goodpasture syndrome
III—Immune complex reactions	1–3 weeks after drug exposure	Antigen-antibody/ aggregates	Blood vessels, liver, spleen, kidney, lung	Complement, anaphylatoxin	Serum sickness (cefaclor), hypersensitivity pneumonitis
IV—Delayed type	2–7 days after drug exposure	Lymphocytes	*Mycobacterium tuberculosis*, chemicals	Cytokines (IFN-γ, TNF-α, GM-CSF)	TB skin test reactions, contact dermatitis (neomycin), graft-versus-host disease

CSF, Cerebrospinal fluid; *GM-CSF,* granulocyte-macrophage colony-stimulating factor; *IFN-γ,* interferon-γ; *TB,* tuberculosis; *TNF-α,* tumor necrosis factor-α.

271

into tissue are called **Arthus reactions.** The administration of large amounts of antigen leads to **serum sickness,** a classic example of a type III reaction. Other type III–mediated reactions include hypersensitivity pneumonitis and some vasculitic syndromes.

Type IV (cellular immune–mediated or delayed-hypersensitivity) reactions involve recognition of antigen by sensitized T cells. Antigen-presenting cells form peptides that are expressed on the cell surface in association with major histocompatibility complex class II molecules. Memory T cells recognize the antigen peptide/major histocompatibility complex class II complexes. Cytokines, such as interferon-γ, tumor necrosis factor-α, and granulocyte-macrophage colony-stimulating factor, are secreted from this interaction, which activates and attracts tissue macrophages. **Contact allergies** (nickel, poison ivy, topical medications) and immunity to tuberculosis are type IV reactions.

HISTORY

Decision-Making Algorithm
Available @ StudentConsult.com

Recurrent Infections

A family history of allergic disease is often present in affected patients. Multiple genes predispose to atopy. If one parent has allergies, the risk that a child will develop an allergic disease is 25%. If both parents have allergies, the risk increases to 50% to 70%. Similar atopic diseases tend to occur in families.

PHYSICAL EXAMINATION

Decision-Making Algorithm
Available @ StudentConsult.com

Recurrent Infections

Children with allergic rhinitis exhibit frequent nasal itching and rubbing of the nose with the palm of the hand, the **allergic salute,** which can lead to a transverse nasal crease found across the lower bridge of the nose. **Allergic shiners,** blue-gray to purple discoloration below the lower eyelids that is attributed to venous congestion, along with swollen eyelids or conjunctival injection are often present in children. Dermatologic findings of atopy include hyperlinearity of the palms and soles, white dermatographism, pityriasis alba, prominent creases under the lower eyelids **(Dennie–Morgan folds** or **Dennie lines),** and **keratosis pilaris** (asymptomatic horny follicular papules on the extensor surfaces of the arms).

COMMON MANIFESTATIONS

Cutaneous manifestations are most common and range from generalized **xerosis** (dry skin) to urticaria to the pruritic, erythematous papules, and vesicles of atopic dermatitis. There may be involvement of the upper respiratory tract with allergic rhinitis and the lower respiratory tract with asthma. Allergic disease may involve only the skin or the nose, eyes, lungs, and gastrointestinal tract alone or in combination. It is

Table 77-2	Disorders Associated with Elevated Serum Immunoglobulin E
Allergic disease	
Atopic dermatitis (eczema)	
Tissue-invasive helminthic infections	
Hyperimmunoglobulin-E syndromes	
Allergic bronchopulmonary aspergillosis	
Wiskott-Aldrich syndrome	
Bone marrow transplantation	
Hodgkin disease	
Bullous pemphigoid	
Idiopathic nephrotic syndrome	

distinguished by environmental exposure to an inciting trigger and usually a history of previous similar disease or development of symptoms after a suspected trigger. Many patients have more than one allergic symptom.

INITIAL DIAGNOSTIC EVALUATION
Screening Tests
Atopy is characterized by elevated levels of IgE (Table 77-2)

Decision-Making Algorithms
Available @ StudentConsult.com

Eosinophilia
Recurrent Infections

and **eosinophilia** (3% to 10% of white blood cells or an absolute eosinophil count of >250 eosinophils/mm³) with a predominance of Th2 cytokines, including interleukin (IL)-4, IL-5, and IL-13. Extreme eosinophilia suggests a nonallergic disorder such as infections with tissue-invasive parasites, drug reactions, or malignancies (Table 77-3). A classic example of a type IV reaction is the tuberculin skin test. A small amount of purified protein derivative from *Mycobacterium tuberculosis* is injected intradermally (see Chapter 124). In a previously sensitized individual, a type IV inflammatory reaction (induration) develops over the next 24 to 72 hours.

There are two methods for identifying allergen-specific IgE: in vivo skin testing and in vitro serum testing (Table 77-4). **In vivo skin testing** introduces allergen into the skin via a prick/puncture or intradermal injection. The allergen diffuses through the skin to interact with IgE that is bound to mast cells. Cross-linking of IgE causes mast cell degranulation, which results in a histamine release; this prompts the development of a **central wheal and erythematous flare.** The wheal and flare are measured 15 to 20 minutes after the allergen has been placed. Properly performed skin tests are the best available method for detecting the presence of allergen-specific IgE.

In vitro serum testing, such as immunoassays like the **radioallergosorbent test** (also known as **RAST**) and enzyme-linked immunosorbent assay (also known as **ELISA**), measures levels of antigen-specific IgE. Many allergists and laboratories regard the ImmunoCAP System as the method of choice. This method uses a solid phase and shows higher sensitivity,

| Table 77-3 | Disorders Associated with Eosinophilia |

ALLERGIC DISEASE
Allergic rhinitis

Atopic dermatitis

Asthma

GASTROINTESTINAL
Eosinophilic gastroenteritis

Allergic colitis

Inflammatory bowel disease

INFECTIOUS
Tissue-invasive helminthic infections

NEOPLASTIC
Eosinophilic leukemia

Hodgkin disease

RESPIRATORY
Eosinophilic pneumonia

Allergic bronchopulmonary aspergillosis

SYSTEMIC
Idiopathic hypereosinophilic syndrome

Adrenal insufficiency

Mastocytosis

IATROGENIC
Drug-induced

| Table 77-4 | Comparison of In Vivo Skin Tests and In Vitro Serum IgE Antibody Immunoassay in Allergic Diagnosis |

IN VIVO SKIN TEST	IN VITRO SERUM IMMUNOASSAY
Less expensive	No patient risk
Greater sensitivity	Patient/physician convenience
Wide allergen selection	Not suppressed by antihistamines
Results available immediately	Preferable to skin testing for dermatographism Widespread dermatitis Uncooperative children

From Skoner DP: Allergic rhinitis: definition, epidemiology, pathophysiology, detection, and diagnosis, J Allergy Clin Immunol 108:S2–S8, 2001.

specificity, and reproducibility. The assay uses a quantitative fluorescent immunoassay (FEIA); FEIA is more sensitive than other assays. These tests are indicated for patients who have dermatographism or extensive dermatitis; who cannot discontinue medications, such as antihistamines, that interfere with skin test results; who are very allergic by history, where anaphylaxis is a possible risk; or who are noncompliant for skin testing. The presence of specific IgE antibodies alone is not sufficient for the diagnosis of allergic diseases. Diagnosis must be based on the physician's assessment of the entire clinical picture, including the history and physical examination, the presence of specific IgE antibodies, and the correlation of symptoms to IgE-mediated inflammation.

DIAGNOSTIC IMAGING
Diagnostic imaging has a limited role in the evaluation of allergic disease. Chest radiography is helpful with the differential diagnosis of asthma. Sinus radiography and computed tomography may be useful, but when these images are abnormal, they do not distinguish allergic disease from nonallergic disease.

Chapter **78**

ASTHMA

ETIOLOGY
Inflammatory cells (mast cells, eosinophils, T lymphocytes, neutrophils), chemical mediators (histamine, leukotrienes, platelet-activating factor, bradykinin), and chemotactic factors (cytokines, eotaxin) mediate the underlying inflammation found in asthmatic airways. Inflammation contributes to **airway hyperresponsiveness** (airways constricting in response to allergens, irritants, viral infections, and exercise). It also results in edema, increased mucus production in the lungs, influx of inflammatory cells into the airway, and epithelial cell denudation. Chronic inflammation can lead to **airway remodeling,** which results from a proliferation of extracellular matrix proteins and vascular hyperplasia and may lead to irreversible structural changes and a progressive loss of pulmonary function.

EPIDEMIOLOGY
Asthma is the most common chronic disease of childhood in industrialized countries, affecting nearly 7 million children younger than 18 years of age in the United States. The number of people with asthma continues to grow. One in 11 children (7 million) had asthma, and 1 in 12 (18.7 million) adults (totaling over 25 million or 8% of U.S. population) had asthma in 2010 compared to 1 in 14 people (about 20 million, or 7%) in 2001. One in 5 children went to the emergency department for an asthma-related visit in 2009. Women are more likely than men to have asthma, and boys are more likely than girls to have asthma.

CLINICAL MANIFESTATIONS

Decision-Making Algorithms
Available @ StudentConsult.com

Rhinorrhea
Cough
Wheezing
Chest Pain

Children with asthma have symptoms of coughing, wheezing, shortness of breath or rapid breathing, and chest tightness. The history should elicit the frequency, severity, and factors that worsen the child's symptoms as well as a family history of

Table 78-1	Differential Diagnosis of Cough and Wheeze in Infants and Children	
UPPER RESPIRATORY TRACT	**MIDDLE RESPIRATORY TRACT**	**LOWER RESPIRATORY TRACT**
Allergic rhinitis	Bronchial stenosis	Asthma
Adenoid/tonsillar hypertrophy	Enlarged lymph nodes	Bronchiectasis
Foreign body	Epiglottitis	Bronchopulmonary dysplasia
Infectious rhinitis	Foreign body	*Chlamydia trachomatis*
Sinusitis	Laryngeal webs	Chronic aspiration
	Laryngomalacia	Cystic fibrosis
	Laryngotracheobronchitis	Foreign body
	Mediastinal lymphadenopathy	Gastroesophageal reflux
	Pertussis	Hyperventilation syndrome
	Toxic inhalation	Obliterative bronchiolitis
	Tracheoesophageal fistula	Pulmonary hemosiderosis
	Tracheal stenosis	Toxic inhalation, including smoke
	Tracheomalacia	Tumor
	Tumor	Viral bronchiolitis
	Vascular rings	
	Vocal cord dysfunction	

From Lemanske RF Jr, Green CG: Asthma in infancy and childhood. In Middleton E Jr, Reed CE, Ellis EF, et al, editors: Allergy: Principles and Practice, ed 5, St Louis, 1998, Mosby–Year Book, p 878.

asthma and allergy. Exacerbating factors include viral infections, exposure to allergens and irritants (e.g., smoke, strong odors, fumes), exercise, emotions, and change in weather/humidity. Nighttime symptoms are common. Rhinosinusitis, gastroesophageal reflux, and nonsteroidal anti-inflammatory drugs (especially aspirin) can aggravate asthma. Treatment of these conditions may lessen the frequency and severity of the asthma.

During acute episodes, tachypnea, tachycardia, cough, wheezing, and a prolonged expiratory phase may be present. Physical findings may be subtle. Classic wheezing may not be prominent if there is poor air movement from airway obstruction. As the attack progresses, cyanosis, diminished air movement, retractions, agitation, inability to speak, tripod sitting position, diaphoresis, and pulsus paradoxus (decrease in blood pressure of >15 mm Hg with inspiration) may be observed. Physical examination may show evidence of other atopic diseases such as eczema or allergic rhinitis.

LABORATORY AND IMAGING STUDIES

Objective measurements of pulmonary function (**spirometry**) help establish the diagnosis and direct the treatment of asthma. Spirometry is used to monitor response to treatment, assess degree of reversibility with therapeutic intervention, and measure the severity of an asthma exacerbation. Children older than 5 years of age can perform spirometry maneuvers. Variability in predicted peak flow reference values make spirometry preferred to peak flow measures in the diagnosis of asthma. For younger children who cannot perform spirometry maneuvers or peak flow, a therapeutic trial of controller medications helps in the diagnosis of asthma.

Allergy skin testing should be included in the evaluation of all children with persistent asthma but not during an exacerbation of wheezing. Positive skin tests results, identifying

immediate hypersensitivity to **aeroallergens** (e.g., as tree and grass pollens, and dust), correlate strongly with bronchial allergen provocative challenges. In vitro serum tests, such as radioallergosorbent test (also known as *RAST*), fluorescent enzyme immunoassay (also known as FEIA), or enzyme-linked immunosorbent assay, are generally less sensitive in defining clinically pertinent allergens, are more expensive, and require several days for results compared to several minutes for skin testing (see Table 77-4).

A **chest radiograph** should be performed with the first episode of asthma or with recurrent episodes of undiagnosed cough or wheeze to exclude anatomic abnormalities. Repeat chest radiographs are not needed with new episodes unless there is fever (suggesting pneumonia) or localized findings on physical examination.

Two novel forms of monitoring asthma and airway inflammation directly include **exhaled nitric oxide analysis** and quantitative analysis of expectorated sputum for eosinophilia.

DIFFERENTIAL DIAGNOSIS

Many childhood conditions can cause wheezing and coughing of asthma (Table 78-1) but not all cough and wheeze is asthma. Misdiagnosis delays correcting the underlying cause and exposes children to inappropriate asthma therapy (Table 78-2).

Allergic bronchopulmonary aspergillosis is a hypersensitivity type of reaction to antigens of the mold *Aspergillus fumigatus*. It occurs primarily in patients with steroid-dependent asthma and in patients with cystic fibrosis.

TREATMENT

Optimal medical treatment of asthma includes several key components: environmental control, pharmacologic therapy, and patient education, including attainment of

Table 78-2	Mnemonic of Causes of Cough in the First Months of Life

C—Cystic fibrosis

R—Respiratory tract infections

A—Aspiration (swallowing dysfunction, gastroesophageal reflux, tracheoesophageal fistula, foreign body)

D—Dyskinetic cilia

L—Lung and airway malformations (laryngeal webs, laryngotracheomalacia, tracheal stenosis, vascular rings and slings)

E—Edema (heart failure, congenital heart disease)

From Schidlow DV: Cough. In Schidlow DV, Smith DS, editors: A Practical Guide to Pediatric Disease, Philadelphia, 1994, Hanley & Belfus.

self-management skills. Because many children with asthma have coexisting allergies, steps to minimize allergen exposure should be taken (Table 78-3). For all children with asthma, exposures to tobacco and wood smoke and to persons with viral infections should be minimized. Influenza immunizations are indicated. Asthma medications can be divided into long-term control medications and quick-relief medications.

Long-Term Control Medications
Inhaled Corticosteroids
Inhaled corticosteroids are the most effective anti-inflammatory medications for the treatment of chronic, persistent asthma and are the preferred therapy when initiating long-term control therapy. Early intervention with inhaled corticosteroids reduces morbidity but does not alter the natural history of asthma. Regular use reduces airway hyperreactivity, the need for rescue bronchodilator therapy, risk of hospitalization, and risk of death from asthma. Inhaled corticosteroids are available as an inhalation aerosol, dry powder inhaler, and nebulizer solution.

The potential risks of inhaled corticosteroids are favorably balanced with their benefits. A reduction in growth velocity may occur with poorly controlled asthma or inhaled corticosteroids use. Low-to-medium dose inhaled corticosteroids may decrease growth velocity, although these effects are small (approximately 1 cm in the first year of treatment), generally not progressive, and may be reversible. Regularly scheduled height measurements should be monitored. Inhaled corticosteroids do not have clinically significant adverse effects on hypothalamic-pituitary-adrenal axis function, glucose metabolism, or subcapsular cataracts or glaucoma when used at low-to-medium doses in children. Rinsing the mouth after inhalation and using spacers help lessen the local adverse effects of dysphonia and candidiasis and decrease systemic absorption from the gastrointestinal tract. Inhaled corticosteroids should be titrated to the lowest dose needed to maintain control of a child's asthma. For children with severe asthma, higher dose inhaled corticosteroids may be needed to minimize the oral corticosteroid dose, but other "add-on" therapy should be considered (see the following sections).

Leukotriene Modifiers
Leukotrienes, synthesized via the arachidonic acid metabolism cascade, are potent mediators of inflammation and smooth

Table 78-3	Controlling Factors Contributing to Asthma Severity	
MAJOR INDOOR TRIGGERS FOR ASTHMA	**SUGGESTIONS FOR REDUCING EXPOSURE**	
Viral upper respiratory tract (RSV, influenza virus)	Limit exposure to viral infections (day care with fewer children)	
	Annual influenza immunization for children with persistent asthma	
Tobacco smoke, wood smoke	No smoking around the child or in child's home	
	Help parents and caregivers quit smoking	
	Eliminate use of wood stoves and fireplaces	
Dust mites	Essential actions	
	Encase pillow, mattress, and box spring in allergen-impermeable encasement	
	Wash bedding in hot water weekly	
	Desirable actions	
	Avoid sleeping or lying on upholstered furniture	
	Minimize number of stuffed toys in child's bedroom	
	Reduce indoor humidity to <50%	
	If possible, remove carpets from bedroom and play areas; if not possible, vacuum frequently	
Animal dander	Remove the pet from the home or keep outdoors (if removal is not acceptable)	
	Keep pet out of bedroom	
	Use a filter on air ducts in child's room	
	Wash pet weekly (the evidence to support this has not been firmly established)	
Cockroach allergens	Do not leave food or garbage exposed	
	Use boric acid traps	
	Reduce indoor humidity to <50%	
	Fix leaky faucets, pipes	
Indoor mold	Avoid vaporizers	
	Reduce indoor humidity to <50%	
	Fix leaky faucets, pipes	

From American Academy of Allergy Asthma & Immunology: Pediatric Asthma: Promoting Best Practice, Milwaukee, Wisconsin, 1999, American Academy of Allergy Asthma & Immunology, p 50.
RSV, Respiratory syncytial virus.

muscle bronchoconstriction. Leukotriene modifiers are oral, daily-use medications that inhibit these biologic effects in the airway. Two classes of leukotriene modifiers include cysteinyl leukotriene receptor antagonists (zafirlukast and montelukast) and leukotriene synthesis inhibitors (zileuton). The leukotriene receptor antagonists have much wider appeal than zileuton. Zafirlukast is approved for children older than 5 years of age and is given twice daily. Montelukast is dosed once daily, at night, as 4-mg granules or chewable tablets (for children 6 months to 5 years), 5-mg chewable tablets (6 to 14 years), and 10-mg tablets (15 years of age or older). Pediatric studies show the usefulness of leukotriene modifiers in mild asthma and the attenuation of exercise-induced bronchoconstriction. These agents may be helpful as steroid-sparing agents in patients with asthma that is more difficult to control.

Long-Acting β₂-Agonists

Long-acting β₂-agonists, formoterol and salmeterol, have twice-daily dosing and relax airway smooth muscle for 12 hours but do not have any significant anti-inflammatory effects. Adding a long-acting bronchodilator to inhaled corticosteroid therapy is more beneficial than doubling the dose of inhaled corticosteroids. Multiple formulations are available. Formoterol is approved for use in children older than 5 years of age for maintenance asthma therapy and for prevention of exercise-induced asthma. It has a rapid onset of action similar to albuterol (15 minutes). Salmeterol is approved for children 4 years of age or older and has an onset of 30 minutes. Because combination agents administer two medications simultaneously, compliance is generally improved.

Theophylline

Theophylline was more widely used previously, but, because current management is aimed at inflammatory control, its popularity has declined. It is mildly to moderately effective as a bronchodilator and is considered an alternative, add-on treatment to low- and medium-dose inhaled corticosteroids.

Omalizumab

Omalizumab (Xolair) is a humanized anti-IgE monoclonal antibody that prevents binding of IgE to high-affinity receptors on basophils and mast cells. It is approved for moderate to severe allergic asthma in children 12 years of age and older. Xolair is delivered by subcutaneous injection every 2 to 4 weeks, depending on body weight and pretreatment serum IgE level.

Quick-Relief Medications
Short-Acting β₂-Agonists

Short-acting β₂-agonists, such as albuterol, levalbuterol, and pirbuterol, are effective bronchodilators that exert their effect by relaxing bronchial smooth muscle within 5 to 10 minutes of administration. They last for 4 to 6 hours. Generally a short-acting β₂-agonist is prescribed for acute symptoms and as prophylaxis before allergen exposure and exercise. The inhaled route is preferred because adverse effects—tremor, prolonged tachycardia, and irritability—are less. **Overuse** of β₂-agonists implies inadequate control; a change in medications may be warranted. The definition of *overuse* depends on the severity of the child's asthma; use of more than one metered dose inhaler canister per month or more than eight puffs per day suggests poor control.

Anticholinergic Agent

Ipratropium bromide is an anticholinergic bronchodilator that relieves bronchoconstriction, decreases mucus hypersecretion, and counteracts cough-receptor irritability by binding acetylcholine at the muscarinic receptors found in bronchial smooth muscle. It seems to have an additive effect with β₂-agonists when used for acute asthma exacerbations. Long-term use of anticholinergic medications in asthma is not supported by the literature.

Oral Corticosteroids

Short bursts of oral corticosteroids (3 to 10 days) are administered to children with acute exacerbations. The initial starting dose is 1 to 2 mg/kg/day of prednisone followed by 1 mg/kg/day over the next 2 to 5 days. Oral corticosteroids are available in liquid or tablet formulations. Prolonged use of oral corticosteroids can result in systemic adverse effects such as hypothalamic-pituitary-adrenal suppression, cushingoid features, weight gain, hypertension, diabetes, cataracts, glaucoma, osteoporosis, and growth suppression. Children with severe asthma may require oral corticosteroids over extended periods. The dose should be tapered as soon as possible to the minimum effective dose, preferably administered on alternate days.

Approach to Therapy

Therapy is based on the concept that chronic inflammation is a fundamental feature of asthma and that the processes underlying asthma can vary in intensity over time, requiring treatment to be adjusted accordingly. Classification of asthma severity is emphasized for initiation of therapy in patients not currently receiving controller medications. Assessing control is emphasized for monitoring and adjusting therapy. A stepwise approach is used for management of infants and young children 0 to 4 years, children 5 to 11 years (Fig. 78-1), youths 12 years or older, and adults (Fig. 78-2). Medication type, amount, and scheduling are determined by the level of asthma severity or asthma control. Therapy is then increased (**stepped up**) as necessary and decreased (**stepped down**) when possible. A short-acting bronchodilator should be available for all children with asthma. A child with intermittent asthma has asthma symptoms less than two times per week. To determine whether a child is having more persistent asthma, using the **Rules of Two** is helpful: daytime symptoms occurring two or more times per week or nighttime awakening two or more times per month implies a need for daily anti-inflammatory medication.

Inhaled corticosteroids are the preferred initial long-term control therapy for children of all ages (Fig. 78-3). Daily long-term control therapy is recommended for infants and young children 0 to 4 years of age who had four or more episodes of wheezing in the previous year that lasted more than 1 day, affected sleep, and who have a positive asthma predictive index. For children over 5 years of age with moderate persistent asthma, combining long-acting bronchodilators with low-to-medium doses of inhaled corticosteroids improves lung function and reduces rescue medication use. For children with severe persistent asthma, a high-dose inhaled corticosteroid and a long-acting bronchodilator are the preferred therapy. The guidelines also recommend that treatment be reevaluated within 2 to 6 weeks of initiating therapy. Once asthma is under control, control should be assessed on an ongoing basis every 1 to 6 months. The asthma should be well controlled for at least 3 months before stepping down therapy. Note that asthma management guidelines are based on review of the published evidence, not solely on age recommendations and dosages approved by the U.S. Food and Drug Administration.

Figure 78-1 Stepwise long-term approach for managing asthma in children, 0 to 4 years of age and 5 to 11 years of age. *(From National Heart Lung Blood Institute, National Asthma Education and Prevention Program: Expert panel report 3: guidelines for the diagnosis and management of asthma. Summary report 2007, NIH Publication No. 08-5846, Bethesda, MD, 2007, U.S. Department of Health and Human Services, p 42, http://www.nhlbi.nih.gov/guidelines/asthma/asthsumm.pdf.)*

| Intermittent asthma | **Persistent asthma: Daily medication**
Consult with asthma specialist if Step 4 care or higher is required.
Consider consultation at Step 3. |

Step 1

Preferred:
SABA PRN

Step 2

Preferred:
Low-dose ICS

Alternative:
Cromolyn, LTRA, Nedocromil, or Theophylline

Step 3

Preferred:
Low-dose ICS + LABA
OR
Medium-dose ICS

Alternative:
Low-dose ICS + either LTRA, Theophylline, or Zileuton

Step 4

Preferred:
Medium-dose ICS + LABA

Alternative:
Medium-dose ICS + either LTRA, Theophylline, or Zileuton

Step 5

Preferred:
High-dose ICS + LABA

AND

Consider Omalizumab for patients who have allergies

Step 6

Preferred:
High-dose ICS + LABA + oral corticosteroid

AND

Consider Omalizumab for patients who have allergies

Step up if needed

(first, check adherence, environmental control, and comorbid conditions)

Assess control

Step down if possible

(and asthma is well controlled at least 3 months)

Key: Alphabetical order is used when more than one treatment option is listed within either preferred or alternative therapy. *ICS,* Inhaled corticosteroid; *LABA,* long-acting inhaled beta₂-agonist; *LTRA,* leukotriene receptor antagonist; *SABA,* inhaled short-acting beta₂-agonist

Notes:

- The stepwise approach is meant to assist, not replace, the clinical decision making required to meet individual patient needs.
- If alternative treatment is used and response is inadequate, discontinue it and use the preferred treatment before stepping up.
- Zileuton is a less desirable alternative due to limited studies as adjunctive therapy and the need to monitor liver function. Theophylline requires monitoring of serum concentration levels.
- In Step 6, before oral corticosteroids are introduced, a trial of high-dose ICS + LABA + either LTRA, Theophylline, or Zileuton may be considered, although this approach has not been studied in clinical trials.
- Step 1, 2, and 3 preferred therapies are based on Evidence A; Step 3 alternative therapy is based on Evidence A for LTRA, Evidence B for Theophylline, and Evidence D for Zileuton. Step 4 preferred therapy is based on Evidence B, and alternative therapy is based on Evidence B for LTRA and Theophylline and Evidence D Zileuton. Step 5 preferred therapy is based on Evidence B. Step 6 preferred therapy is based on (EPR–2 1997) and Evidence B for Omalizumab.
- Immunotherapy for Steps 2–4 is based on Evidence B for house-dust mites, animal danders, and pollens; evidence is weak or lacking for molds and cockroaches. Evidence is strongest for immunotherapy with single allergens. The role of allergy in asthma is greater in children than in adults.
- Clinicians who administer immunotherapy or Omalizumab should be prepared and equipped to identify and treat anaphylaxis that may occur.

Each step: Patient education, environmental control, and management of comorbidities.

Steps 2–4: Consider subcutaneous allergen immunotherapy for patients who have allergic asthma (see Notes).

Quick-relief medication for all patients

- SABA as needed for symptoms. Intensity of treatment depends on severity of symptoms: up to 3 treatments at 20-minute intervals as needed. Short course of oral systemic corticosteroids may be needed.
- Use of SABA >2 days a week for symptom relief (not prevention of EIB) generally indicates inadequate control and the need to step up treatment.

Figure 78-2 Stepwise approach for managing asthma in youths 12 years of age or older and adults. *(From National Heart Lung Blood Institute, National Asthma Education and Prevention Program: Expert panel report 3: guidelines for the diagnosis and management of asthma. Summary report 2007, NIH Publication No. 08-5846, Bethesda, MD, 2007, U.S. Department of Health and Human Services, p 45, http://www.nhlbi.nih.gov/guidelines/asthma/asthsumm.pdf.)*

COMPLICATIONS

Most asthma exacerbations can be successfully managed at home. **Status asthmaticus** is an acute exacerbation of asthma that does not respond adequately to therapeutic measures and may require hospitalization. Exacerbations may progress over several days or occur suddenly and can range in severity from mild to life threatening. Significant respiratory distress, dyspnea, wheezing, cough, and a decrease in **peak expiratory flow rate (PEFR)** characterize deterioration in asthma control. During severe episodes of wheezing, pulse oximetry is helpful in monitoring oxygenation. In status asthmaticus, arterial blood gases may be necessary for measurement of ventilation. As airway obstruction worsens and chest compliance decreases, carbon dioxide retention can occur. In the face of tachypnea, a *normal* pCO_2 (40 mm Hg) indicates impending respiratory arrest.

First-line management of asthma exacerbations includes supplemental oxygen, repetitive, or continuous administration of short-acting bronchodilators. Early administration of oral or intravenous corticosteroids (Fig. 78-4) is important in treating the underlying inflammation. Administration of anticholinergic agents (ipratropium) with bronchodilators decreases rates of hospitalization and duration of time in the emergency department. Intravenous magnesium sulfate is given in the emergency department if there is clinical deterioration, despite treatment with β_2-agonists, ipratropium, and systemic glucocorticoids. The typical dose is 25 to 75 mg/kg (maximum 2.0 g) intravenously administered over 20 minutes. Epinephrine (intramuscular) or terbutaline (subcutaneous) is rarely used except when severe asthma is associated with anaphylaxis or unresponsive to continuous administration of short-acting bronchodilators.

PROGNOSIS

For some children, symptoms of wheezing with respiratory infections subside in the preschool years, whereas others have more persistent asthma symptoms. Prognostic indicators for children younger than 3 years of age who are at risk for asthma include eczema, parental asthma, or two of the

Drug	Low Daily Dose			Medium Daily Dose			High Daily Dose		
	Child 0–4 Years of Age	Child 5–11 Years of Age	≥12 Years of Age and Adults	Child 0–4 Years of Age	Child 5–11 Years of Age	≥12 Years of Age and Adults	Child 0–4 Years of Age	Child 5–11 Years of Age	≥12 Years of Age and Adults
Beclomethasone HFA 40 or 80 µg/puff	NA	80–160 µg	80–240 µg	NA	>160–320 µg	>240–480 µg	NA	>320 µg	>480 µg
Budesonide DPI 90, 180, or 200 µg/inhalation	NA	180–400 µg	180–600 µg	NA	>400–800 µg	>600–1,200 µg	NA	>800 µg	>1,200 µg
Budesonide Inhaled Inhalation suspension for nebulization	0.25–0.5 mg	0.5 mg	NA	>0.5–1.0 mg	1.0 mg	NA	>1.0 mg	2.0 mg	NA
Flunisolide 250 µg/puff	NA	500–750 µg	500–1,000 µg	NA	1,000–1,250 µg	>1,000–2,000 µg	NA	>1,250 µg	>2,000 µg
Flunisolide HFA 80 µg/puff	NA	160 µg	320 µg	NA	320 µg	>320–640 µg	NA	≥640 µg	>640 µg
Fluticasone HFA/MDI: 44, 110, or 220 µg/puff	176 µg	88–176 µg	88–264 µg	>176–352 µg	>176–352 µg	>264–440 µg	>352 µg	>352 µg	>440 µg
DPI: 50, 100, or 250 µg/inhalation	NA	100–200 µg	100–300 µg	NA	>200–400 µg	>300–500 µg	NA	>400 µg	>500 µg
Mometasone DPI 200 µg/inhalation	NA	NA	200 µg	NA	NA	400 µg	NA	NA	>400 µg
Triamcinolone acetonide 75 µg/puff	NA	300–600 µg	300–750 µg	NA	>600–900 µg	>750–1,500 µg	NA	>900 µg	>1,500 µg

Key: *DPI*, Dry power inhaler; *HFA*, hydrofluoroalkane; *MDI*, metered-dose inhaler; *NA*, not available (either not approved, no data available, or safety and efficacy not established for this age group)

Therapeutic Issues:

- The most important determinant of appropriate dosing is the clinician's judgment of the patient's response to therapy. The clinician must monitor the patient's response on several clinical parameters and adjust the dose accordingly. Once control of asthma is achieved, the dose should be carefully titrated to the minimum dose required to maintain control.

- Preparations are not interchangeable on a µg or per puff basis. This figure presents estimated comparable daily doses. See EPR–3 Full Report 2007 for full discussion.

- Some doses may be outside package labeling, especially in the high-dose range. Budesonide nebulizer suspension is the only inhaler corticosteroid (ICS) with FDA-approved labeling for children <4 years of age.

- For children <4 years of age: The safety and efficacy of ICSs in children <1 year has not been established. Children <4 years of age generally require delivery of ICS (budesonide and fluticasone HFA) through a face mask that should fit snugly over nose and mouth and avoid nebulizing in the eyes. Wash face after each treatment to prevent local corticosteroid side effects. For budesonide, the dose may be administered 1–3 times daily. Budesonide suspension is compatible with Albuterol, Ipratropium, and Levalbuterol nebulizer solutions in the same nebulizer. Use only jet nebulizers, as ultrasonic nebulizers are ineffective for suspensions. For Fluticasone HFA, the dose should be divided 2 times daily; the low dose for children <4 years of age is higher than for children 5–11 years of age due to lower dose delivered with face mask and data on efficacy in young children.

Potential Adverse Effects of Inhaled Corticosteroids:

- Cough, dysphonia, oral thrush (candidiasis).

- Spacer or valved holding chamber with non-breath-actuated MDIs and mouthwashing and spitting after inhalation decrease local side effects.

- A number of the ICSs, including Fluticasone, Budesonide, and Mometasone, are metabolized in the gastrointestinal tract and liver by CYP 3A4 isoenzymes. Potent inhibitors of CYP 3A4, such as Ritonavir and Ketoconazole, have the potential for increasing systemic concentrations of these ICSs by increasing oral availability and decreasing systemic clearance. Some cases of clinically significant Cushing syndrome and secondary adrenal insufficiency have been reported

- In high doses, systemic effects may occur, although studies are not conclusive, and clinical significance of these effects has not been established (e.g., adrenal suppression, osteoporosis, skin thinning, and easy bruising). In low-to-medium doses, suppression of growth velocity has been observed in children, but this effect may be transient, and the clinical significance has not been established.

Figure 78-3 Estimated comparative daily dosages for inhaled corticosteroids. (*From National Heart Lung Blood Institute, National Asthma Education and Prevention Program: Expert panel report 3: guidelines for the diagnosis and management of asthma. Summary report 2007, NIH Publication No. 08-5846, Bethesda, MD, 2007, U.S. Department of Health and Human Services, p 49, http://www.nhlbi.nih.gov/guidelines/asthma/asthsumm.pdf.*)

following: allergic rhinitis, wheezing with a cold, or eosinophilia of greater than 4%. Atopy is the strongest predictor for wheezing continuing into persistent asthma (Table 78-4).

PREVENTION

Education plays an important role in helping patients and their families adhere to the prescribed therapy and needs to begin at the time of diagnosis. Successful education involves teaching basic asthma facts, explaining the role of medications, teaching environmental control measures, and improving patient skills in the use of spacer devices for metered dose inhalers and peak flow monitoring. Families should have an asthma management plan (Fig. 78-5) for daily care and for exacerbations.

Peak flow monitoring is a self-assessment tool that is helpful for children over 5 years of age. It is advisable for children who are *poor perceivers* of airway obstruction, have moderate

Figure 78-4 Management of asthma exacerbations: emergency department and hospital-based care. *(From National Heart Lung Blood Institute, National Asthma Education and Prevention Program: Expert panel report 3: guidelines for the diagnosis and management of asthma. Summary report 2007, NIH Publication No. 08-5846, Bethesda, MD, 2007, U.S. Department of Health and Human Services, p 55, http://www.nhlbi.nih.gov/guidelines/asthma/asthsumm.pdf.)*

Asthma Action Plan

For: _____

Doctor's Phone Number _____

Doctor: _____ Date: _____

Hospital/Emergency Department Phone Number _____

GREEN ZONE

Doing Well
- No cough, wheeze, chest tightness, or shortness of breath during the day or night
- Can do usual activities

And, if a peak flow meter is used,

Peak flow: more than _____
(80 percent or more of my best peak flow)

My best peak flow is: _____

Take these long-term-control medicines each day (include an anti-inflammatory).

Medicine	How much to take	When to take it

Identify and avoid and control the things that make your asthma worse, like (list here): _____

Before exercise, if prescribed, take: □ 2 or □ 4 puffs   5 to 60 minutes before exercise

YELLOW ZONE

Asthma Is Getting Worse
- Cough, wheeze, chest tightness, or shortness of breath, or
- Waking at night due to asthma, or
- Can do some, but not all, usual activities

-Or-

Peak flow: _____ to _____
(50 to 79 percent of my best peak flow)

First → **Add: quick-relief medicine—and keep taking your GREEN ZONE medicine.**

□ 2 or □ 4 puffs, every 20 minutes for up to 1 hour
□ Nebulizer, once

_____ (short-acting beta₂-agonist)

If applicable, remove yourself from the thing that made your asthma worse.

If your symptoms (and peak flow, if used) return to GREEN ZONE after 1 hour of above treatment:
□ Continue monitoring to be sure you stay in the green zone.

-Or-

Second → If your symptoms (and peak flow, if used) do not return to GREEN ZONE after 1 hour of above treatment:

□ Take: _____ □ 2 or □ 4 puffs or □ Nebulizer
(short-acting beta₂-agonist)

□ Add: _____ _____ mg per day. For _____ (3–10) days
(oral corticosteroid)

□ Call the doctor □ before/ □ within _____ hours after taking the oral corticosteroid.
_____ (phone)

RED ZONE

Medical Alert!
- Very short of breath, or
- Quick-relief medicines have not helped, or
- Cannot do usual activities, or
- Symptoms are same or get worse after 24 hours in Yellow Zone.

-Or-

Peak flow: less than _____
(50 percent of my best peak flow)

Take this medicine:

□ _____ □ 4 or □ 6 puffs or □ Nebulizer
(short-acting beta₂-agonist)

□ _____ _____ mg
(oral corticosteroid)

Then call your doctor NOW. Go to the hospital or call an ambulance if
- You are still in the red zone after 15 minutes AND
- You have not reached your doctor.

DANGER SIGNS
- Trouble walking and talking due to shortness of breath
- Lips or fingernails are blue

→ ■ Take □ 4 or □ 6 puffs of your quick-relief medicine **AND**
■ Go to the hospital or call for an ambulance _____ **NOW!**
(phone)

Figure 78-5 Asthma self-management guideline. *(From National Heart Lung Blood Institute, National Asthma Education and Prevention Program: Expert panel report 3: guidelines for the diagnosis and management of asthma. Summary report 2007, NIH Publication No. 05-5251, Bethesda, MD, 2007, U.S. Department of Health and Human Services, p 119, http://www.nhlbi.nih.gov/guidelines/asthma/asthgdln.pdf.)*

Table 78-4	Risk Factors for Persistent Asthma

Allergy

    Atopic dermatitis

    Allergic rhinitis

    Elevated total serum IgE levels (first year of life)

    Peripheral blood eosinophilia >4% (2–3 yr of age)

    Food and inhalant allergen sensitization

Gender

    Boys

        Transient wheezing

        Persistent allergy-associated asthma

    Girls

        Asthma associated with obesity and early-onset puberty

        Triad asthma (adulthood)

Parental asthma

Lower respiratory tract infection

    Respiratory syncytial virus, parainfluenza

    Severe bronchiolitis (e.g., requiring hospitalization)

    Pneumonia

Environmental tobacco smoke exposure (including prenatal)

From Liu A, Martinez FD, Taussig LM: Natural history of allergic diseases and asthma. In Leung DYM, Sampson HA, Geha RS, et al, editors: Pediatric Allergy: Principles and Practice. St Louis, 2003, Mosby, p 15.

to severe asthma, or have a history of severe exacerbations. Peak flow monitoring also can be useful in children who are still learning to recognize asthma symptoms.

To use a peak flow meter, a child should be standing with the indicator placed at the bottom of the scale. The child must inhale deeply, place the device in the mouth, seal the lips around the mouthpiece, and blow out forcefully and rapidly. The indicator moves up the numeric scale. The PEFR is the highest number achieved. The test is repeated three times to obtain the best possible effort. Peak flow meters are available as low range (<300 L/sec) and high range (<700 L/sec). It is important to provide the appropriate range meter so that accurate measurements can be obtained and children do not become discouraged because their exhalations barely move the indicator.

A child's personal best is the highest PEFR achieved over a 2-week period when stable. Based on the child's personal best, a **written action plan** can be established, which is divided into three zones, similar to a stoplight. The green zone indicates a PEFR 80% to 100% of the child's personal best value. In this zone, the child is likely asymptomatic and should continue with medications as usual. The yellow zone indicates a PEFR 50% to 80% of the child's personal best value, which generally coincides with more asthma symptoms. Rescue medications, such as albuterol, are added. A call to the physician may be warranted if the peak flows do not return to the green zone within 24 to 48 hours or if asthma symptoms are increasing. The red zone indicates a PEFR below 50% and is a medical emergency. Rescue medication should be taken immediately. If the PEFR remains in the red zone or the child has significant airway compromise, a call to the physician or emergency care is needed.

Children with asthma should be seen not only when they are ill but also when they are healthy. Regular office visits allow the health care team to review **adherence** to medication and control measures and to determine whether doses of medications need adjustment.

Chapter 79

ALLERGIC RHINITIS

ETIOLOGY

Rhinitis describes diseases that involve inflammation of the nasal epithelium and is characterized by sneezing, itching, rhinorrhea, and congestion. There are many different causes of rhinitis in children, but approximately half of all cases of rhinitis are caused by allergies.

Allergic rhinitis, commonly known as **hay fever,** is caused by an IgE-mediated allergic response. During the early allergic phase, mast cells degranulate and release preformed chemical mediators, such as histamine and tryptase, and newly generated mediators, such as leukotrienes, prostaglandins, and platelet-activating factor. After a quiescent phase in which other cells are recruited, a late phase occurs approximately 4 to 8 hours later. Eosinophils, basophils, CD4 T cells, monocytes, and neutrophils release their chemical mediators, which leads to the development of chronic nasal inflammation.

Allergic rhinitis can be seasonal, perennial, or episodic depending on the particular allergen and the exposure. Some children experience perennial symptoms with seasonal exacerbations. **Seasonal allergic rhinitis** is caused by airborne pollens, which have seasonal patterns. Typically trees pollinate in the spring, grasses in late spring to summer, and weeds in the summer and fall. The pollen, microscopic in size, can travel airborne hundreds of miles and be inhaled easily into the respiratory tract. **Perennial allergic rhinitis** is primarily caused by indoor allergens, such as house dust mites, animal dander, mold, and cockroaches. **Episodic rhinitis** occurs with intermittent exposure to allergens, such as visiting a friend's home where a pet dwells.

EPIDEMIOLOGY

Chronic rhinitis is one of the most common disorders encountered in infants and children. Overall allergic rhinitis is observed in 10% to 25% of the population, with children and adolescents more commonly affected than adults. The prevalence of physician-diagnosed allergic rhinitis may be 40%.

CLINICAL MANIFESTATIONS

Decision-Making Algorithms
Available @ StudentConsult.com

Rhinorrhea
Red Eye
Cough
Hoarseness

Table 79-1	Classification of the Etiology of Rhinitis in Children

	NONALLERGIC	
ALLERGIC	**NONANATOMIC**	**ANATOMIC**
Seasonal	Nonallergic, noninfectious (vasomotor) rhinitis	Adenoidal hypertrophy
Perennial	Infectious rhinosinusitis	CSF rhinorrhea
Episodic	Nonallergic rhinitis with eosinophilia	Choanal atresia
	Physical rhinitis	Congenital anomalies
	Rhinitis medicamentosa	Foreign body
		Nasal polyps
		Septal deviation
		Tumors
		Turbinate hypertrophy

CSF, Cerebrospinal fluid.

The hallmarks of allergic rhinitis are clear: thin rhinorrhea; nasal congestion; paroxysms of sneezing; and pruritus of the eyes, nose, ears, and palate. Postnasal drip may result in frequent attempts to clear the throat, nocturnal cough, and hoarseness. It is important to correlate the onset, duration, and severity of symptoms with seasonal or perennial exposures, changes in the home or school environment, and exposure to nonspecific irritants, such as tobacco smoke.

The physical examination includes a thorough nasal examination and an evaluation of the eyes, ears, throat, chest, and skin. Physical findings may be subtle. Classic physical findings include pale pink or bluish gray, swollen, boggy nasal turbinates with clear, watery secretions. Frequent nasal itching and rubbing of the nose with the palm of the hand, the **allergic salute,** can lead to a transverse nasal crease found across the lower bridge of the nose. Children may produce clucking sounds by rubbing the soft palate with their tongue. Oropharyngeal examination may reveal lymphoid hyperplasia of the soft palate and posterior pharynx or visible mucus or both. Orthodontic abnormalities may be seen in children with chronic mouth breathing. **Allergic shiners,** dark periorbital swollen areas caused by venous congestion, along with swollen eyelids or conjunctival injection, are often present in children. Retracted tympanic membranes from eustachian tube dysfunction or serous otitis media also may be present. Other atopic diseases, such as asthma or eczema, may be present, which helps lead the clinician to the correct diagnosis.

LABORATORY AND IMAGING STUDIES
Allergy testing can be performed by in vivo skin tests or by in vitro serum tests (radioallergosorbent test [RAST], fluorescent enzyme immunoassay [FEIA], or enzyme linked immunosorbent assay [ELISA]) to pertinent allergens found in the patient's environment (see Table 77-4). Skin tests (prick/puncture) provide immediate and accurate results. Positive tests correlate strongly with nasal and bronchial allergen provocative challenges. In vitro serum tests are useful for patients with abnormal skin conditions, for those with a tendency for anaphylaxis, or for those taking medications that interfere with skin testing. Disadvantages of serum tests include increased cost, inability to obtain immediate results, and reduced sensitivity compared with skin tests. Widespread screening with

serum testing without regard to symptoms is not recommended. Measurement of total serum IgE or blood eosinophils generally is not helpful. The presence of eosinophils on the nasal smear suggests a diagnosis of allergy, but eosinophils also can be found in patients with nonallergic rhinitis with eosinophilia. Nasal smear eosinophilia is often predictive of a good clinical response to nasal corticosteroid sprays.

DIFFERENTIAL DIAGNOSIS
Rhinitis can be divided into allergic and nonallergic rhinitis (Table 79-1). Nonallergic rhinitis describes a group of nasal diseases in which there is no evidence of allergic etiology. It can be divided further into nonanatomic and anatomic etiologies. The most common form of nonallergic rhinitis in children is infectious rhinitis, which may be acute or chronic. Acute infectious rhinitis (the common cold) is caused by viruses, including rhinoviruses and coronaviruses, and typically resolves within 7 to 10 days (see Chapter 102). An average child has three to six common colds per year, with the most affected being younger children and children attending day care. Infection is suggested by the presence of sore throat, fever, and poor appetite, especially with a history of exposure to others with colds. Chronic infectious **rhinosinusitis,** or sinusitis, should be suspected if there is mucopurulent nasal discharge with symptoms that persist beyond 10 days (see Chapter 104). Classic signs of acute sinusitis in older children include facial tenderness, tooth pain, headache, and fever. Classic signs are usually not present in young children who may present with postnasal drainage with cough, throat clearing, halitosis, and rhinorrhea. The character of the nasal secretions with infectious rhinitis varies from purulent to minimal or absent. Coexistence of middle ear disease, such as otitis media or eustachian tube dysfunction, may be additional clues of infection.

Nonallergic, noninfectious rhinitis (formerly known as *vasomotor rhinitis*) can manifest as rhinorrhea and sneezing in children with profuse clear nasal discharge. Exposure to irritants, such as cigarette smoke and dust, and strong fumes and odors, such as perfumes and chlorine in swimming pools, can trigger these nasal symptoms. Nonallergic rhinitis with eosinophilia syndrome is associated with clear nasal discharge and eosinophils on nasal smear and is seen infrequently in children. Cold air (**skier's nose**), hot/spicy food ingestion (**gustatory rhinitis**), and exposure to bright light (**reflex rhinitis**) are examples of physical rhinitis. Treatment with topical ipratropium before exposure may be helpful.

Rhinitis medicamentosa, which is due primarily to overuse of topical nasal decongestants, such as oxymetazoline, phenylephrine, or cocaine, is not a common condition in younger children. Adolescents or young adults may become dependent on these over-the-counter medications. Treatment requires discontinuation of the offending decongestant spray, topical corticosteroids, and, frequently, a short course of oral corticosteroids.

The most common anatomic problem seen in young children is obstruction secondary to adenoidal hypertrophy, which can be suspected from symptoms such as mouth breathing, snoring, hyponasal speech, and persistent rhinitis with or without chronic otitis media. Infection of the nasopharynx may be secondary to infected hypertrophied adenoid tissue.

Choanal atresia is the most common congenital anomaly of the nose and consists of a bony or membranous septum between the nose and pharynx, either unilateral or bilateral. Bilateral choanal atresia classically presents in neonates as cyclic cyanosis because neonates are preferential nose breathers. Airway obstruction and cyanosis are relieved when the mouth is opened to cry and recurs when the calming infant reattempts to breathe through the nose. Some newborns show respiratory difficulty while feeding only. Nearly half of infants with choanal atresia have other congenital anomalies as a part of the **CHARGE association** (**c**oloboma, congenital **h**eart disease, choanal **a**tresia, **r**etardation, **g**enitourinary defects, **e**ar anomalies). Unilateral choanal atresia may go undiagnosed until later in life and presents with symptoms of unilateral nasal obstruction and discharge.

Nasal polyps typically appear as bilateral, gray, glistening sacs originating from the ethmoid sinuses and may be associated with clear or purulent nasal discharge. Nasal polyps are rare in children younger than 10 years of age but, if present, warrant evaluation for an underlying disease process, such as cystic fibrosis or primary ciliary dyskinesia. **Triad asthma** is asthma, aspirin sensitivity, and nasal polyps with chronic or recurrent sinusitis.

Foreign bodies are seen more commonly in young children who place food, small toys, stones, or other things in their nose. The index of suspicion should be raised by a history of unilateral, purulent nasal discharge, or foul odor. The foreign body can often be seen on examination with a nasal speculum.

TREATMENT

Management of allergic rhinitis is based on disease severity, impact of the disease on the patient, and the ability of the patient to comply with recommendations. Treatment modalities include allergen avoidance, pharmacologic therapy, and immunotherapy. Environmental control and steps to minimize allergen exposure, similar to preventive steps for asthma, should be implemented whenever possible (see Table 78-3).

Pharmacotherapy

Intranasal corticosteroids are the most potent pharmacologic therapy for treatment of allergic and nonallergic rhinitis. These include beclomethasone, budesonide, ciclesonide, flunisolide, fluticasone, mometasone, and triamcinolone. These topical agents work to reduce inflammation, edema, and mucus production. They are effective for symptoms of nasal congestion, rhinorrhea, itching, and sneezing but less helpful for ocular symptoms. Nasal corticosteroid sprays have been used safely in long-term therapy. Deleterious effects on adrenal function or nasal membranes have not been reported when these agents are used appropriately. The most common adverse effects include local irritation, burning, and sneezing, which occur in 10% of patients. Nasal bleeding from improper technique (spraying the nasal septum) can occur. Rare cases of nasal septal perforation have been reported.

Antihistamines are the medications used most frequently to treat allergic rhinitis. They are useful in treating rhinorrhea, sneezing, nasal itching, and ocular itching but are less helpful in treating nasal congestion. **First-generation antihistamines,** such as diphenhydramine and hydroxyzine, easily cross the blood-brain barrier, with sedation as the most common reported adverse effect. Use of first-generation antihistamines in children has an adverse effect on cognitive and academic function. In very young children, a paradoxical stimulatory central nervous system effect, resulting in irritability and restlessness, has been noted. Other adverse effects of first-generation antihistamines include anticholinergic effects, such as blurred vision, urinary retention, dry mouth, tachycardia, and constipation. **Second-generation antihistamines,** such as cetirizine, loratadine, desloratadine, fexofenadine and levocetirizine, are less likely to cross the blood-brain barrier, resulting in less sedation. Cetirizine, fexofenadine, and loratadine are over-the-counter medications. Azelastine and olopatadine, topical nasal antihistamine sprays, are approved for children older than 5 years and older than 6 years, respectively.

Decongestants, taken orally or intranasally, may be used to relieve nasal congestion. Oral medications, such as pseudoephedrine and phenylephrine, are available either alone or in combination with antihistamines. Adverse effects of oral decongestants include insomnia, nervousness, irritability, tachycardia, tremors, and palpitations. For older children participating in sports, oral decongestant use may be restricted. Topical nasal decongestant sprays are effective for immediate relief of nasal obstruction but should be used for less than 5 to 7 days to prevent rebound nasal congestion (rhinitis medicamentosa).

Topical ipratropium bromide, an anticholinergic nasal spray, is used primarily for nonallergic rhinitis and rhinitis associated with viral upper respiratory infection. Leukotriene modifiers have been studied in the treatment of allergic rhinitis. Montelukast is approved for use in seasonal allergic rhinitis.

Immunotherapy

If environmental control measures and medication intervention are only partially effective or produce unacceptable adverse effects, immunotherapy may be recommended. The mechanism of action for allergen immunotherapy is complex but includes increased production of an IgG-blocking antibody, decreased production of specific IgE, and alteration of cytokine expression produced in response to an allergen challenge. Immunotherapy is effective for desensitization to pollens, dust mites, and cat and dog proteins. Use in young children may be limited by the need for frequent injections. Immunotherapy must be administered in a physician's office with 20 to 30 minutes of observation after the allergen injection. Anaphylaxis may occur, and the physician must be experienced in the treatment of these severe adverse allergic reactions.

COMPLICATIONS

Approximately 60% of children with allergic rhinitis have symptoms of reactive airways disease/asthma (see Chapter 78). Chronic allergic inflammation leads to chronic cough from postnasal drip; eustachian tube dysfunction and otitis media; sinusitis; and tonsillar and adenoid hypertrophy, which may lead to obstructive sleep apnea. Children with allergic rhinitis may experience sleep disturbances, limitations of activity, irritability, and mood and cognitive disorders that adversely affect their performance at school and their sense of well-being.

PROGNOSIS AND PREVENTION

Seasonal allergic rhinitis is a common and prominent condition that may not improve as children grow older. Patients become more adept at self-management. Perennial allergic rhinitis improves with allergen control of indoor allergens.

Removal or avoidance of the offending allergen is advised. The only effective measure for minimizing animal allergens from pets is removal of the pet from the home. Avoidance of pollen and outdoor molds can be accomplished by staying indoors in a controlled environment. Air conditioning and keeping windows and doors closed lower exposure to pollen. High-efficiency particle air filters reduce exposure to allergens (e.g., pet dander). Sealing the mattress, pillow, and covers in allergen-proof encasings is the most effective strategy for reduction of mite allergen. Bedding should be washed in hot water (>130 °F) every week.

Chapter 80

ATOPIC DERMATITIS

ETIOLOGY

Atopic dermatitis is a chronic, pruritic, relapsing inflammatory skin condition. The pathogenesis is multifactorial and involves a complex interplay of factors, including genetic predisposition, immunologic abnormalities, disturbances in skin barrier function, environmental interactions, and infectious triggers. Several genes encoding epidermal (filaggrin) or other epithelial structural proteins and genes encoding major elements of the immune system play a major role in atopic dermatitis.

Several immunoregulatory abnormalities have been described in patients with atopic dermatitis. There is an exaggerated cutaneous inflammatory response to environmental triggers, including irritants and allergens. Activated Langerhans cells in the dermis expressing surface-bound IgE stimulate T cells. In acute lesions, activated Th2 lymphocytes infiltrate the

dermis. They initiate and maintain local tissue inflammation primarily through interleukin-4 (IL-4) and IL-13, which promote IgE production, and IL-5, which promotes eosinophil differentiation. As the disease progresses from an acute to a chronic phase, there is a switch from Th2 to Th1/Th0 cellular response. Chronic lesions are characterized by increased IL-12 and IL-18.

Patients with atopic dermatitis have **hyperirritable skin,** and many factors can cause the disease to worsen or relapse. Known triggers include anxiety and stress, climate (extremes of temperature and humidity), irritants, allergens, and infections. Approximately 35% to 40% of infants and young children with moderate to severe atopic dermatitis have coexisting food allergies. The more severe the atopic dermatitis and the younger the patient, the more likely a food allergy will be identified as a contributing factor. Egg allergy is the most common cause of food-induced eczematous reactions.

EPIDEMIOLOGY

The prevalence of atopic dermatitis increased twofold to threefold over the past 30 years. Approximately 15% to 20% of children and 2% to 10% of adults are affected. Atopic dermatitis often starts in early infancy. Approximately 50% of affected children show symptoms in the first year of life, and 80% of these children experience disease onset before 5 years of age. Atopic dermatitis is often the first manifestation of other atopic diseases. Approximately 80% of children with atopic dermatitis develop other allergic diseases, such as asthma or allergic rhinitis. Symptoms of dermatitis often disappear at the onset of respiratory allergy.

CLINICAL MANIFESTATIONS

The clinical manifestations of atopic dermatitis vary with age. In infants, atopic dermatitis involves the face, scalp, cheeks, and extensor surfaces of the extremities (Fig. 80-1). The

Figure 80-1 Atopic dermatitis typical cheek involvement. (*From Eichenfield LF, Frieden IJ, Esterly NB:* Textbook of Neonatal Dermatology, *Philadelphia, 2001, Saunders, p 242.*)

Figure 80-2 Rubbing and scratching the inflamed flexural areas cause thickened (lichenified) skin. *(From Habif T: Clinical Dermatology, ed 4, Philadelphia, 2004, Elsevier.)*

diaper area is spared. In older children, the rash localizes to the antecubital and popliteal flexural surfaces, head, and neck. In adolescents and adults, lichenified plaques are seen in the flexural areas (Fig. 80-2) and the head and neck regions. Itching or pruritus has a significant impact on the child and family's quality of life; it is often worse at night, interrupting sleep. Physical examination may show hyperlinearity of the palms and soles, white dermatographism, pityriasis alba, creases under the lower eyelids (**Dennie–Morgan folds or Dennie lines),** and **keratosis pilaris** (asymptomatic horny follicular papules on the extensor surfaces of the arms).

LABORATORY AND IMAGING STUDIES
The diagnosis of atopic dermatitis is based on clinical features rather than laboratory tests (Table 80-1). Skin biopsy is of little value, but it may be used to exclude other skin diseases that mimic atopic dermatitis. Skin testing or, alternatively, CAP fluorescent immunoassay (also known as *FEIA*) may be helpful in assessing the contribution of food or environmental allergies to disease expression.

DIFFERENTIAL DIAGNOSIS
Many conditions share signs and symptoms of atopic dermatitis (Table 80-2). Infants presenting in the first year of life with failure to thrive, recurrent skin or systemic infections, and scaling, erythematous rash should be evaluated for immunodeficiency disorders. Wiskott-Aldrich syndrome is an X-linked recessive syndrome characterized by atopic

Table 80-1	Criteria for the Diagnosis of Atopic Dermatitis

The diagnosis requires evidence of itchy skin (or parental report of scratching or rubbing) plus three or more of the following:
1. History of involvement of skin creases
2. History of asthma or allergic rhinitis (or history of atopic disease in a first-degree relative if child is <4 years of age)
3. History of generally dry skin in the past year
4. Onset in a child <2 years of age (criterion not used if child is <4 years of age)
5. Visible flexural dermatitis (including dermatitis affecting cheeks, forehead, and outer aspects of limbs in children <4 years of age)

Modified from Williams HC, Burney PG, Hay RJ, et al: Diagnostic criteria for atopic dermatitis. III. Independent hospital validation. Br J Dermatol 131:406–416, 1994.

Table 80-2	Differential Diagnosis of Atopic Dermatitis

CONGENITAL DISORDERS
Netherton syndrome

Familial keratosis pilaris

CHRONIC DERMATOSES
Seborrheic dermatitis

Contact dermatitis (allergic or irritant)

Nummular eczema

Psoriasis

Ichthyoses

INFECTIONS AND INFESTATIONS
Scabies

HIV-associated dermatitis

Dermatophytosis

MALIGNANCIES
Cutaneous T-cell lymphoma (mycosis fungoides/Sezary syndrome)

Langerhans cell histiocytosis

AUTOIMMUNE DISORDERS
Dermatitis herpetiformis

Pemphigus foliaceus

Graft-versus-host disease

Dermatomyositis

IMMUNODEFICIENCIES
Wiskott-Aldrich syndrome

Severe combined immunodeficiency

Hyper-IgE syndromes

IPEX

METABOLIC DISORDERS
Zinc deficiency

Pyridoxine (vitamin B6) and niacin deficiency

Multiple carboxylase deficiency, phenylketonuria

From Leung DYM: Atopic dermatitis. In Leung DYM, Sampson HA, Geha RS, et al, editors: Pediatric allergy: principles and practice, St Louis, 2003, Mosby, p 562.
IPEX, Immunodeficiency polyendocrinopathy X-linked.

dermatitis, thrombocytopenia, small-sized platelets, and recurrent infections. Langerhans cell histiocytosis is characterized by hemorrhagic or petechial lesions. Scabies is an intensely pruritic skin condition caused by the human scabies mite. The presence of a burrow found in the web spaces of the fingers, the flexor surfaces of the wrists, elbows, axilla, or genitals is pathognomonic. Burrows may be few in number or absent, however.

TREATMENT

The goals of therapy are to reduce the number and severity of flares and to increase the number of disease-free periods. Successful management involves skin hydration, pharmacologic therapy to reduce pruritus, and identification and avoidance of triggers. Patients with atopic dermatitis have a decrease in skin barrier function and enhanced transepidermal water loss. Daily, lukewarm baths for 15 to 20 minutes followed immediately by the application of fragrance-free emollients to retain moisture are a major component of therapy. Prevention of xerosis is important for control of pruritus and for maintaining the integrity of the epithelial barrier. Emollients should be ointments or creams, such as petrolatum, Aquaphor, Eucerin, or Cetaphil. Lotions are not as effective because they contain water or alcohol and may have a drying effect owing to evaporation. A mild nonsoap cleanser also is recommended.

Topical anti-inflammatory agents, including corticosteroids and immunomodulators, are the cornerstone of therapy for acute flares and prevention of relapses. Topical corticosteroids are used for reducing inflammation and pruritus; they are effective for the acute and chronic phases of the disease. Ointments generally are preferred over creams and lotions because of enhanced potency and skin penetration. Corticosteroids are ranked by potency into seven classes. The least potent corticosteroid that is effective should be used. Higher potency corticosteroids may be necessary to diminish the dermatitis flare but should be used for limited periods. Low-potency, nonfluorinated corticosteroids should be used on the face, intertriginous areas (groin, axilla), and large areas to reduce the risk of adverse effects. Reduced efficacy of topical corticosteroids may be related to disease severity rather than glucocorticoid resistance. Local adverse effects, such as skin atrophy and striae, and systemic adverse effects, such as hypothalamic-pituitary-adrenal axis and growth suppression and hyperglycemia, are related to the potency, length of use, and extent of medication application. In infants and younger children, the possibility of corticosteroid-induced adverse effects may be greater. When control of inflammatory lesions is achieved, most patients can be managed with emollients and low-potency topical corticosteroids.

The topical immunomodulating drugs, tacrolimus and pimecrolimus, are approved as second-line agents for short-term and intermittent treatment of atopic dermatitis in patients unresponsive to or intolerant of other therapies. They are approved for use in children older than 2 years of age. These agents may be used on all body locations and are especially useful on delicate skin sites, such as the face, neck, and axilla without the adverse effect of cutaneous atrophy seen with topical corticosteroids. These medications have a potential increased cancer risk, and their long-term safety has not been established. Other less serious adverse effects include local burning and the need for sun protection.

COMPLICATIONS

Defective cell-mediated immunity leads to increased susceptibility to many bacterial, viral, and fungal infections of the skin. More than 90% of patients with atopic dermatitis have colonization of lesional skin with *Staphylococcus aureus,* and more than 75% of patients have colonization of uninvolved skin. Colonization and infection by *S. aureus* are associated with disease severity. *S. aureus* secretes exotoxins that act as a superantigen, stimulating T cells and increasing IgE production. Secondarily infected atopic dermatitis often presents as impetiginous, pustular lesions with crusting and honey-colored exudate. Topical antibiotics, such as mupirocin or retapamulin, can be used to treat local areas of infection, or oral antibiotics (such as cephalexin, dicloxacillin, or amoxicillin-clavulanate) can be used for multifocal disease or for infection around the eyes and mouth that is difficult to treat topically. Bacterial cultures may be helpful in patients who do not respond to oral antibiotics or who have infection after multiple antibiotic courses. The incidence of community-acquired methicillin-resistant *S. aureus* is increasing.

Herpes simplex superinfection of affected skin, or **Kaposi varicelliform eruption** or **eczema herpeticum,** results in vesiculopustular lesions that appear in clusters and can become hemorrhagic. Herpes simplex virus infection can be misdiagnosed as bacterial infection and should be considered if skin lesions fail to respond to antibiotics.

In individuals with atopic dermatitis, smallpox vaccination or exposure to a vaccinated individual may lead to **eczema vaccinatum,** a localized vaccinial superinfection of affected skin. Eczema vaccinatum may progress to generalized vaccinia with vaccinial lesions appearing at sites distant from the inoculation. In patients with underlying immunodeficiencies, it may be life threatening.

Widespread infections with human papillomavirus (warts) and molluscum contagiosum are also common in children with atopic dermatitis.

PROGNOSIS

Atopic dermatitis is a chronic, relapsing skin disorder that tends to be more severe and prominent in young children. Symptoms become less severe in two thirds of children, with complete remission for approximately 20%. Early onset disease that is more widespread, concomitant asthma and allergic rhinitis, family history of atopic dermatitis, and elevated serum IgE levels may predict a more persistent course. Patients and families should be taught that a single cause and cure for atopic dermatitis is unlikely but that good control is possible for the majority of affected patients.

PREVENTION

An important step in the management of atopic dermatitis is to identify and avoid allergens and irritants. Common irritants include soaps, detergents, fragrances, chemicals, smoke, and extremes of temperature and humidity. Wool and synthetic fabrics can be irritating to the skin; 100% cotton fabric is preferred. Sweating is a recognized trigger. Fingernails should be trimmed frequently to minimize excoriations from scratching.

In infants and younger children who do not respond to the usual therapies, identifying and removing a food allergen from the diet may lead to clinical improvement. Food allergy is not a common trigger for older patients. Other environmental exposures, such as dust mites, pet dander, or pollens, can also contribute to the disease state.

Chapter 81

URTICARIA, ANGIOEDEMA, AND ANAPHYLAXIS

ETIOLOGY

Urticaria, commonly referred to as **hives,** is swelling of the dermis and one of the most common skin conditions seen in clinical practice. **Angioedema** results from a process similar to urticaria, but the reaction extends below the dermis. Urticaria and angioedema occur in response to the release of inflammatory mediators, including histamine, leukotrienes, platelet-activating factor, prostaglandins, and cytokines from mast cells present in the skin. A variety of stimuli can trigger mast cells and basophils to release their chemical mediators. Typically mast cells degranulate when cross-linking of the membrane-bound IgE occurs. Release of these mediators results in vasodilation, increased vascular leakage, and pruritus. Basophils from the circulatory system also can localize in tissue and release mediators similar to mast cells. Patients with urticaria have elevated histamine content in the skin that is more easily released.

Anaphylaxis is mediated by IgE, whereas **anaphylactoid reactions** result from mechanisms that are due to nonimmunologic mechanisms. Both reactions are acute, severe, and can be life threatening due to a massive release of inflammatory mediators. Urticaria, angioedema, and anaphylaxis are best considered as symptoms because they have a variety of causes.

Not all mast cell activation is IgE-mediated. Immunologic, nonimmunologic, physical, and chemical stimuli can produce degranulation of mast cells and basophils. **Anaphylatoxins,** C3a and C5a, can cause histamine release in a non–IgE-mediated reaction. Anaphylatoxins are generated in serum sickness (reactions to blood transfusions) (see Chapter 82) and in infectious, neoplastic, and rheumatic diseases. In addition mast cell degranulation can occur from a direct pharmacologic effect or physical or mechanical activation, such as urticaria after exposure to opiate medications, and dermatographism.

Urticaria/angioedema can be classified into three subcategories: acute, chronic, and physical. By definition **acute urticaria** and **angioedema** are hives and diffuse swelling that last less than 6 weeks. Often the history is quite helpful in eliciting the cause of the acute reaction (Table 81-1). An IgE mechanism is more commonly found in acute urticaria than in chronic urticaria. **Chronic urticaria** and **angioedema** are characterized by persistence of symptoms beyond 6 weeks (Table 81-2). Some have daily symptoms of hives and swelling, whereas others have intermittent or recurrent episodes. Chronic urticaria can be idiopathic with unknown causal

Table 81-1	Etiology of Acute Urticaria
Foods	Egg, milk, wheat, peanuts, tree nuts, soy, shellfish, fish, strawberries (direct mast cell degranulation)
Medications	Suspect all medications, even over-the-counter or homeopathic medications
Insect stings	Hymenoptera (honeybee, yellow jacket, hornets, wasp, fire ants), biting insects (papular urticaria)
Infections	Bacterial (group A streptococcus pharyngitis, *Mycoplasma*, sinusitis); viral (hepatitis B, mononucleosis [EBV], coxsackieviruses A and B); parasitic (*Ascaris, Ancylostoma, Echinococcus, Fasciola, Filaria, Schistosoma, Strongyloides, Toxocara, Trichinella*); fungal (dermatophytes, *Candida*)
Contact allergy	Latex, pollen, animal saliva, nettle plants, caterpillars
Transfusion reactions	Blood, blood products, or IVIG administration
Idiopathic	

From Lasley MV, Kennedy MS, Altman LC: Urticaria and angioedema. In Altman LC, Becker JW, Williams PV, editors: Allergy in Primary Care, Philadelphia, 2000, Saunders, p 232.
EBV, Epstein-Barr virus; IVIG, intravenous immunoglobulin.

Table 81-2	Etiology of Chronic Urticaria
Idiopathic	75%–90% of cases
	25%–50% of adult patients have IgG, anti-IgE, and anti-FcεR1 (high-affinity IgE receptor alpha chain) autoantibodies
Physical	Dermatographism
	Cholinergic urticaria
	Cold urticaria
	Delayed pressure urticaria
	Solar urticaria
	Vibratory urticaria
	Aquagenic urticaria
Rheumatologic	Systemic lupus erythematosus
	Juvenile idiopathic arthritis
Endocrine	Hyperthyroidism
	Hypothyroidism
Neoplastic	Lymphoma
	Mastocytosis
	Leukemia
Angioedema	Hereditary angioedema (autosomal dominant inherited deficiency of Cl-esterase inhibitor)
	Acquired angioedema
	Angiotensin-converting enzyme inhibitors

From Lasley MV, Kennedy MS, Altman LC: Urticaria and angioedema. In Altman LC, Becker JW, Williams PV, editors: Allergy in Primary Care, Philadelphia, 2000, Saunders, p 234.

factors; 35% to 40% of chronic urticaria cases have an autoimmune process due to IgG autoantibodies binding directly to IgE or to the IgE receptor. **Physical urticaria** and **angioedema** are characterized by known eliciting external factors that may include pressure, cold, heat, exercise, or exposure to sun or water.

The most common physical urticaria is dermatographism, affecting 2% to 5% of persons. **Dermatographism** means "writing on the skin" and is easily diagnosed by firmly scratching the skin with a blunt point, such as the wooden tip of a cotton swab or tongue depressor. It is characterized by an urticarial reaction localized to the site of skin trauma. It has been suggested that trauma induces an IgE-mediated reaction causing histamine to be released from the mast cells.

Cholinergic urticaria, characterized by the appearance of 1- to 3-mm wheals surrounded by large erythematous flares after an increase in core body temperature, occurs commonly in young adults. Lesions may develop during strenuous exercise, after a hot bath, or emotional stress. The lack of airway symptoms differentiates it from exercise-induced anaphylaxis.

Cold urticaria occurs with exposure to cold and may develop within minutes on areas directly exposed to cold or on rewarming of the affected parts. Ingestion of cold drinks may result in lip swelling. Cold urticaria syndromes can be categorized into acquired and familial disorders. Severe reactions resulting in death can occur with swimming or diving into cold water. Patients must never swim alone, avoid total body exposure to cold, and have injectable epinephrine available.

Hereditary angioedema (HAE) is an autosomal dominant disease due to a deficiency of Cl inhibitor. The genetic defect may be caused by spontaneous mutation; approximately 25% of cases occur in patients without any family history. The disease is estimated to affect approximately 10,000 persons in the United States. It is characterized by unpredictable, recurrent attacks of episodic swelling that involves the face, peripheral extremities, genitalia, abdomen, oropharynx, and pharynx. Episodes are often triggered by trauma. Asphyxiation from laryngeal attacks is a significant cause of mortality. Patients with HAE rarely have urticaria associated with angioedema. The majority of patients (85%) have **type I** disease, which is due to decreased production of Cl-esterase inhibitor. A minority of patients (15%) have **type II** disease, which is due to production of dysfunctional Cl esterase inhibitor. A low C4 level serves as an initial screening test. Patients with reduced C4 should have quantitative and functional levels of Cl-esterase inhibitor measured. C2 levels are low during an acute attack. **Type III** HAE patients have normal laboratory evaluation. These patients are more typically females, but some males have been reported in the literature. Three products are approved to treat HAE attacks: Berinert (for acute facial or abdominal attacks in children ≥13 years old), Kalbitor (for acute attacks in children ≥16 years of age), and Cinryze (for prophylaxis in adolescents and adults).

Anaphylactic reactions are type I, IgE-mediated reactions and result from many causes (Table 81-3). Cross-linking of the IgE molecule with the allergen leads to IgE receptor activation on the mast cell and basophil and release of mediators, including histamine, tryptase, tumor necrosis factor, platelet-activating factor, leukotrienes, prostaglandins, and cytokines. Other cell types involved in the reactions include monocytes, macrophages, eosinophils, neutrophils, and platelets. The mediator release results in the clinical picture of anaphylaxis.

Table 81-3	Common Causes of Anaphylaxis in Children*
Foods	Peanuts, tree nuts, milk, eggs, fish, shellfish, seeds, fruits, grains
Drugs	Penicillins, cephalosporins, sulfonamides, nonsteroidal anti-inflammatory drugs, opiates, muscle relaxants, vancomycin, dextran, thiamine, vitamin B_{12}, insulin, thiopental, local anesthetics
Hymenoptera venom	Honeybee, yellow jacket, wasp, hornet, fire ant
Latex	
Allergen immunotherapy	
Exercise	Food-specific exercise, postprandial (nonfood-specific) exercise
Vaccinations	Tetanus, measles, mumps, influenza
Miscellaneous	Radiocontrast media, immunoglobulin, cold temperature, chemotherapeutic agents, blood products, inhalants
Idiopathic	

From Young MC: General treatment of anaphylaxis. In Leung DYM, Sampson HA, Geha RS, et al, editors: Pediatric Allergy: Principles and Practice, *St Louis, 2003, Mosby, p 644.*
*In order of frequency.

Anaphylactoid reactions are due to nonimmunologic mechanisms. Mast cells and basophils can be activated by direct, nonspecific stimulation, although the exact underlying mechanism is unknown. Reactions to agents, such as opiates and radiocontrast material, are classic examples. Complement system activation also can result in mast cell and basophil activation. **Anaphylatoxins,** C3a and C5a, are named because of their ability to trigger mediator release and are generated in serum sickness. The most common cause of this type of reaction is transfusion with blood products. There are other causes of anaphylactoid reactions for which the mechanism has not been clarified.

EPIDEMIOLOGY

Urticaria and angioedema are common skin conditions affecting 15% to 25% of individuals at some point in their lives. Most cases of urticaria are self-limited, but, for some patients, they are chronic. In approximately 50% of patients, urticaria and angioedema occur together. In the remaining 50%, 40% have urticaria alone and 10% have angioedema alone. The incidence of anaphylaxis in children is unknown.

CLINICAL MANIFESTATIONS

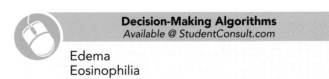

Decision-Making Algorithms
Available @ StudentConsult.com

Edema
Eosinophilia

Raised, erythematous lesions with pale centers that are intensely pruritic characterize **urticaria,** commonly called **hives** (Fig. 81-1). The lesions vary in size and can occur anywhere on

Figure 81-1 Examples of urticaria. *(From Zitelli BJ, Davis HW, editors: Pediatric Physical Diagnosis Electronic Atlas, Philadelphia, 2004, Mosby.)*

the body. Typically urticaria arises suddenly and may resolve within 1 to 2 hours or may persist for 24 hours. **Angioedema** is a similar process that involves the deeper dermis or subcutaneous tissue, with swelling as the principal symptom. Generally angioedema is not pruritic, may be mildly painful, and persists for longer than 24 hours. In rare cases it may become life threatening if swelling affects the upper airway.

The clinical manifestations of **anaphylaxis** and **anaphylactoid** reactions are the same for children and adults. The signs and symptoms vary and can range from mild skin findings to a fatal reaction. Ninety percent of patients present with cutaneous symptoms, including urticaria, angioedema, flushing, and warmth; the absence of dermal symptoms does not exclude the diagnosis of anaphylaxis. Other affected organ systems include the respiratory tract (rhinorrhea, oropharyngeal edema, laryngeal edema, hoarseness, stridor, wheezing, dyspnea, and asphyxiation), cardiovascular system (tachycardia, hypotension, shock, syncope, and arrhythmias), gastrointestinal tract (nausea, abdominal pain, crampy diarrhea, and vomiting), and neurologic system (syncope, seizure, dizziness, and a sense of impending doom). The severity of an anaphylactic reaction is often proportionate to the speed of symptom onset.

LABORATORY AND IMAGING STUDIES

The laboratory evaluation of patients with urticaria and angioedema must be tailored to the clinical situation. Acute urticaria and angioedema do not require specific laboratory evaluation except to document the suspected cause. For patients with chronic urticaria and angioedema, laboratory evaluation should be performed to exclude underlying diseases (Table 81-4). Patients with recurrent angioedema *without* urticaria should be evaluated for HAE (Table 81-5).

Measurement of the mast cell mediators, histamine and tryptase, may be helpful when the diagnosis of anaphylaxis is in question. A tryptase level is a more useful test because histamine is released quickly, has a short half-life, and is often difficult to detect in the serum. Serum tryptase levels peak 1 to 1.5 hours after anaphylaxis. Elevated levels may be helpful in

Table 81-4	Suggested Testing for Chronic Urticaria/Angioedema of Unknown Etiology
BASIC TESTS	**DISCRETIONARY TESTS BASED ON**
Complete blood count with differential	If vasculitis is suspected
Erythrocyte sedimentation rate	Antinuclear antibody
Urinalysis	Skin biopsy
Liver function tests	CH_{50}
Thyroid function and autoantibodies	If liver function tests abnormal
Autoimmune chronic urticaria test-anti-FcεR1 autoantibody	Serology for hepatitis B

From Zuraw B: Urticaria and angioedema. In Leung DYM, Sampson HA, Geha RS, et al, editors: Pediatric Allergy: Principles and Practice, St Louis, 2003, Mosby, p 580.

establishing the diagnosis, but normal tryptase levels do not rule out the diagnosis. It is best to measure a serum tryptase level 1 to 2 hours after the onset of symptoms. It also can be ordered retrospectively on stored serum that is less than 2 days old.

DIFFERENTIAL DIAGNOSIS

The diagnosis of urticaria and angioedema is straightforward; finding the etiology may be more difficult. Other dermatologic conditions can mimic urticaria. **Erythema multiforme** has target-shaped, erythematous, macular or papular lesions that may look similar to urticaria, but the lesions are fixed and last for several days. Other dermatologic diseases include dermatitis herpetiformis and bullous pemphigoid, which are quite pruritic, and early on, the lesions may resemble urticaria. Mastocytosis is characterized by mast cell infiltration of various organs, including the skin. Some patients have skin lesions similar in appearance to urticaria rather than the classic urticaria pigmentosa. Urticaria pigmentosa appears as hyperpigmented, red-brown macules, which may coalesce.

| Table 81-5 | Complement Evaluation of Patients with Recurrent Angioedema |

ASSAY	IDIOPATHIC ANGIOEDEMA	TYPE I HEREDITARY ANGIOEDEMA	TYPE II HEREDITARY ANGIOEDEMA	ACQUIRED C1-ESTERASE INHIBITOR DEFICIENCY	VASCULITIS
C4	Normal	Low	Low	Low	Low or normal
C4d/C4 ratio	Normal	High	High	High	High or normal
C1-esterase inhibitor level	Normal	Low	Normal	Low	Normal
C1-esterase inhibitor function	Normal	Low	Low	Low	Normal
C1q	Normal	Normal	Normal	Low	Low or normal
C3	Normal	Normal	Normal	Normal	Low or normal

From Zuraw B: Urticaria and angioedema. In Leung DYM, Sampson HA, Geha RS, et al, editors: Pediatric Allergy: Principles and Practice, St Louis, 2003, Mosby, p 580.

When these lesions are stroked, they urticate, which is called the **Darier sign.** A rare disorder that should be included in the differential diagnosis of urticaria is **Muckle-Wells syndrome.** It is an autosomal dominant disorder characterized by episodic urticaria presenting in infancy, with sensorineural deafness, amyloidosis, arthralgias, and skeletal abnormalities. Another rare syndrome is **Schnitzler syndrome,** which is characterized by chronic urticaria, macroglobulinemia, bone pain, anemia, fever, fatigue, and weight loss. **Urticarial vasculitis** is a small vessel vasculitis with histologic features of a leukocytoclastic response. The main distinguishing feature is that the lesions last longer than 24 hours, may be tender, and leave behind skin pigmentation. Skin biopsy is required for definitive diagnosis.

The diagnosis of anaphylaxis is usually apparent from the acute and often dramatic onset of multisystem involvement of the skin, respiratory tract, and cardiovascular system. Sudden cardiovascular collapse in the absence of cutaneous symptoms suggests vasovagal collapse, seizure disorder, aspiration, pulmonary embolism, or myocardial infarction. Laryngeal edema, especially with abdominal pain, suggests HAE. Many patients with anaphylaxis are initially thought to have septic shock (see Chapter 40).

TREATMENT

Avoidance of triggering agents is important in the management of urticaria and angioedema. The mainstay of pharmacologic treatment is H_1 antihistamines. Second-generation H_1 antihistamines, such as cetirizine, desloratadine, fexofenadine, levocetirizine, and loratadine, are preferred because they have fewer adverse effects. If a second-generation H_1 antihistamine, by itself, does not provide adequate relief, the next step is to add a sedating H_1 antihistamine at bedtime or H_2 antihistamines, such as cimetidine or ranitidine. Tricyclic antidepressants, such as doxepin, exhibit potent activity at both H_1 and H_2 receptors. Corticosteroids are effective in treating urticaria and angioedema, although adverse effects from long-term use mandate the lowest dose for the shortest time. When urticaria is resistant to treatment, the leukotriene receptor blocker montelukast has been used in several case studies. Other immunomodulating agents, such as cyclosporine, hydroxychloroquine, methotrexate, cyclophosphamide,

and intravenous immunoglobulin, have been used; however, data supporting their use are limited, and they require laboratory monitoring due to potential adverse effects.

Anaphylaxis is a medical emergency; prompt recognition and immediate treatment are crucial (Fig. 81-2). Early administration of intramuscular epinephrine is the mainstay of therapy and should be given at the same time that basic measures of cardiopulmonary resuscitation are being performed. If the child is not in a medical setting, emergency medical services should be called. Supplemental oxygen and intravenous fluid should be administered with the child lying in supine position. An airway must be secured; intubation or tracheotomy may be required. Additional pharmacologic therapies, such as corticosteroids, antihistamines, H_2-receptor antagonists, and bronchodilators, may be given to improve symptoms. Up to 20% of people with anaphylaxis have **biphasic** or **protracted** anaphylaxis.

A person with **biphasic anaphylaxis** has both early- and late-phase reactions. The biphasic reaction is a recurrence of anaphylactic symptoms after an initial remission, occurring within 8 to 72 hours after the initial reaction. A person with **protracted anaphylaxis** has signs and symptoms that persist for hours or even days despite treatment, although this is rare.

PREVENTION

Prevention of urticaria, angioedema, and anaphylaxis focuses on avoidance of known triggers. A referral to an allergy specialist for a thorough history, diagnostic testing, and recommendations for avoidance is suggested for patients following severe reactions or anaphylaxis. Skin testing and serum IgE-specific testing are available for foods, inhalants, insect venoms, drugs (penicillin), vaccines, and latex. Educating the patient and family members about the signs and symptoms of anaphylaxis and using self-administered epinephrine early result in better outcomes. Fatal anaphylaxis has occurred despite timely and appropriate treatment. A **MedicAlert bracelet** with appropriate information should be worn. Medications such as β-blockers, angiotensin-converting enzyme inhibitors, and monoamine oxidase inhibitors should be discontinued because they may exacerbate anaphylaxis or interfere with its treatment.

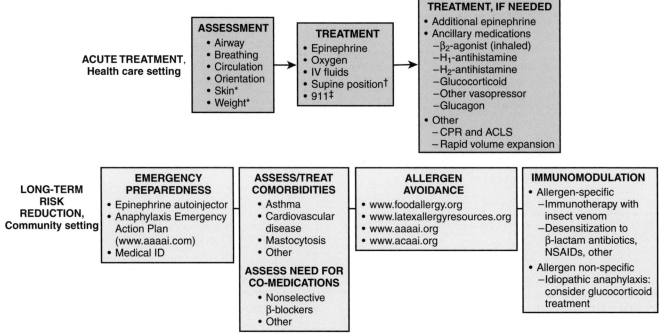

Figure 81-2 Summary of anaphylaxis management. Acute treatment is the same regardless of the mechanism or trigger involved in anaphylaxis. In contrast, for long-term risk reduction, avoidance measures and immunomodulation are trigger-specific; currently immunomodulation is available only for a minority of individuals with anaphylaxis. All at-risk individuals need to have comorbidities and comedications assessed, be taught the importance of emergency preparedness, and be instructed in the use of self-injectable epinephrine. *ACLS,* Advanced cardiac life support; *CPR,* cardiopulmonary resuscitation; *CVS,* cardiovascular; *GI,* gastrointestinal; *ID,* identification (e.g., bracelet, wallet card); *IV,* intravenous. *(From Simon FER: Anaphylaxis, J Allergy Clin Immunol 121:S405, 2008.)*
*The skin should be inspected, and weight estimation is important, especially in infants and children, and also in overweight and obese teens and adults, in order to calculate an optimal dose of epinephrine and other medications needed in treatment and resuscitation.
†Supine position, as tolerated, to prevent empty ventricle syndrome.
‡Call 911/emergency medical services for anaphylaxis occurring in community health care facilities such as medical, dental, or infusion clinics, where optimal backup might not be available for resuscitation.

Chapter 82

SERUM SICKNESS

ETIOLOGY

Serum sickness is a type III hypersensitivity reaction (see Table 77-1). The patient's immune system recognizes the proteins in the drug or antiserum as foreign and produces antibodies against them. The newly formed antibodies bind with the foreign protein to form antigen-antibody or immune complexes, which may enter the circulation and be deposited in blood vessels and in filtering organs. These complexes cause tissue injury by activating the complement cascade and recruiting neutrophils, resulting in increased capillary permeability, toxic mediator release, and tissue damage.

EPIDEMIOLOGY

Immune complexes were first described after administration of heterologous serum, such as horse serum for diphtheria. The availability of human-derived biologics, bioengineered antibodies, and alternative pharmacotherapies has greatly reduced the incidence of serum sickness. Common inciting agents include blood products and foreign proteins, such as antithymocyte globulin and antivenoms. Medications

frequently implicated include penicillin, sulfonamides, minocycline, cefaclor, hydantoins, and thiazides.

CLINICAL MANIFESTATIONS

Decision-Making Algorithm
Available @ StudentConsult.com

Petechiae/Purpura

The symptoms of serum sickness typically occur 7 to 21 days after the administration of drugs, foreign proteins, or infections. Symptom onset may be more rapid (within 1 to 4 days) in previously sensitized individuals. The classic clinical manifestations consist of fever, polyarticular arthralgias, lymphadenopathy, and cutaneous symptoms. Cutaneous lesions vary and may include urticaria, angioedema, erythema multiforme, morbilliform rash, and a palpable purpura or serpiginous rash at the interface of the dorsal and palmar or plantar aspects of the hands and feet.

Carditis, glomerulonephritis, Guillain-Barre syndrome, encephalomyelitis, and peripheral neuritis are rare complications.

LABORATORY AND IMAGING STUDIES

Laboratory tests may show an elevated erythrocyte sedimentation rate, presence of circulating immune complexes, and depressed complement (C3 and C4) levels. Skin biopsy specimens show immune deposits of IgM, IgA, IgE, or C3. Hematuria or proteinuria or both may be present. The diagnosis is established by history of exposure to an inciting cause, characteristic clinical manifestations, and laboratory testing showing circulating immune complexes and depressed complement levels.

TREATMENT AND PREVENTION

Serum sickness is self-limited and resolves within 1 to 2 weeks; therefore, treatment is symptomatic relief. Antihistamines may be administered to relieve pruritus. Nonsteroidal anti-inflammatory drugs are given for fever and joint pain, and, if necessary, prednisone (1 to 2 mg/kg orally daily) is administered with a tapering dose. Allergy skin testing does not predict the likelihood of serum sickness development.

The primary means of prevention is to avoid exposure to the implicated cause.

Chapter 83

INSECT ALLERGIES

ETIOLOGY

Systemic allergic reactions usually result from stinging insects of the order **Hymenoptera,** which include **apids** (honeybee and bumblebee), **vespids** (yellow jacket, wasp, yellow-face, and white-face hornets), and **formicids** (fire and harvester ants). Honeybees have a barbed stinger that remains embedded after a sting. Yellow jackets are responsible for most allergic reactions in most parts of the United States, whereas wasps are the most frequent cause of sting reactions in Texas. Fire ants are found in the southeastern and south central United States.

Biting insects rarely cause anaphylaxis. Anaphylaxis has been described, however, after the bites of a kissing bug (*Triatoma*), bed bug, blackfly, and deerfly. Large local reactions from biting insects, such as mosquitoes, fleas, and flies, are a more common occurrence. The reaction appears urticarial and is caused by the salivary secretions deposited by the biting insect and does not represent an allergic response.

EPIDEMIOLOGY

Insect sting allergy may develop at any age and typically manifests after several uneventful stings. Although children are stung more frequently than adults, systemic allergic reactions occur in only about 1% of children and 3% of adults. Reactions in adults are generally more severe than in children and can result in death. Large local reactions to insect stings are more common in children, with an estimated incidence of 20% for children and 10% for adults.

CLINICAL MANIFESTATIONS

The diagnosis of insect sting allergy is dependent on the history of the reaction and the presence of venom-specific IgE. Normal reactions to insect stings, which are observed in 90%

Table 83-1	Classification of Insect Sting Reactions
REACTION TYPE	**CHARACTERISTICS**
Normal	<2 inches in diameter
	Transient pain and erythema
	Duration <24 hr
Large local reaction	>2 inches in diameter
	Swelling contiguous to the site
	Duration 2–7 days
Systemic	
Nonlife-threatening	Immediate generalized reaction confined to the skin (erythema, urticaria, angioedema)
Life-threatening	Immediate generalized reaction not confined to the skin with respiratory (laryngeal edema, bronchospasm) or cardiovascular (hypotension, shock) symptoms
Toxic	Follows multiple stings, produced by exogenous vasoactive amines in venom
Unusual	Serum sickness, vasculitis, nephrosis, neuritis, encephalitis
	Symptoms start several days to weeks after the insect sting.

of children, include localized pain, swelling, and erythema at the sting site that usually subside within 24 hours. Large local reactions occur in approximately 10% of patients. They are usually late-phase, IgE-mediated reactions, with large swelling, contiguous to the sting site that develops over 24 to 48 hours and resolves within 2 to 7 days. Virtually all individuals with large local reactions have similar reactions with subsequent stings. Systemic reactions are IgE mediated and occur in 1% of children. They can be mild and nonlife-threatening with cutaneous symptoms only or life-threatening with respiratory, cardiovascular, or neurologic symptoms of anaphylaxis (see Chapter 81). Toxic reactions may result if a person receives a large number of stings (50 to 100). Symptoms include malaise, nausea, and emesis resulting from the toxic effects of the venom. Unusual reactions, such as vasculitis, nephrosis, neuritis, serum sickness, and encephalitis, rarely are associated with insect stings (Table 83-1).

LABORATORY AND IMAGING STUDIES

A positive skin test to Hymenoptera venom extract demonstrates the presence of venom-specific IgE in the context of a positive sting reaction history and helps identify specific insects to which an individual is allergic. Venom-specific IgE antibodies also may be measured by in vitro serum tests. Both testing methods should be considered complementary because neither test alone detects all patients with insect sting allergy. Future reactions correlate more with past individual patterns than the level of sensitivity of venom skin testing or serum specific IgE testing.

DIFFERENTIAL DIAGNOSIS

A history of an immediate systemic reaction is necessary before venom testing and immunotherapy should be considered.

Identification of the offending insect is often unreliable. Honeybee stings may be identified by the stinger that remains in place. Vespid stings are usually unprovoked and occur at summer's end when the insects are more aggressive.

TREATMENT

Local reactions should be treated by cleaning the site, applying cold compresses, and administering oral antihistamines and analgesics. Occasionally large local reactions may be mistaken for cellulitis. Infection is unlikely if reaction occurs within 24 to 48 hours after a sting. Treatment is with an oral corticosteroid for 4 to 5 days rather than oral antibiotics.

Treatment of systemic reactions is guided by the severity of the reaction, but epinephrine is the cornerstone of therapy and should be administered without delay. Antihistamines may be administered concurrently with epinephrine. Corticosteroids should be given to prevent recurrent or prolonged symptoms. For severe reactions, intravenous fluids and epinephrine, oxygen, and respiratory support in an intensive care unit may be needed. After acute care of a systemic sting reaction, patients should be provided an epinephrine autoinjector, referral to an allergist/immunologist, and instructions on prevention of insect stings.

COMPLICATIONS

At least 50 to 100 fatalities per year in the United States are attributed to insect sting reactions. Most deaths (80%) occur in adults older than 40 years of age, and only 2% occur in individuals younger than 20 years of age. Approximately one half of deaths occur in persons without any history of a prior sting reaction.

PROGNOSIS

Successfully avoiding the stinging insect is the most important prognostic factor. More than 85% of adults who complete 5 years of immunotherapy tolerate challenge stings without systemic reactions for 5 to 10 years after completion.

PREVENTION

Measures to reduce the chance of accidental sting include exterminating infested areas; not eating or drinking outdoors; wearing long pants and shoes; and avoiding brightly colored clothing, fragrances, or hairspray when outdoors. Common insect repellents are not effective against Hymenoptera.

Current recommendations are to administer **venom immunotherapy** to individuals who have had a systemic life-threatening reaction from an insect sting and have positive venom skin tests or elevated levels of venom-specific IgE. All persons with a history of systemic reactions to insects should be instructed in the use of an epinephrine autoinjector and encouraged to wear a **MedicAlert bracelet.** Children younger than 16 years of age who have had only a cutaneous reaction generally do not require immunotherapy because their prognosis is benign and can be managed with the availability of epinephrine.

Chapter 84

ADVERSE REACTIONS TO FOODS

ETIOLOGY AND EPIDEMIOLOGY

An **adverse reaction to food** is a generic description of any untoward reaction after food ingestion, including toxic reactions such as food poisoning and nontoxic reactions, which can be subdivided further into nonimmune and immune reactions. Lactose intolerance is a nonimmune reaction. Food allergy or hypersensitivity reactions encompass immune reactions to food and can be divided further into IgE-mediated reactions, which are typically rapid in onset, and non-IgE-mediated reactions.

Oral tolerance is the process of suppression of the immune response to the array of dietary elements ingested daily. **Food allergy** or **hypersensitivity reactions** are the result of immune reactions to glycoproteins and develop in genetically predisposed individuals. In children, cow's milk, eggs, peanuts, soybean, wheat, tree nuts, fish, and shellfish cause 90% of IgE-mediated reactions. In older children and adults, peanuts, tree nuts, fish, and shellfish account for most reactions. Exposure to the allergenic food protein results in cross-linking of the IgE receptor found on the mast cells and basophils, which become activated and degranulate, releasing numerous potent mediators and cytokines. Non-IgE-mediated reactions typically occur hours to days after the allergen ingestion and are manifest as gastrointestinal symptoms. A cell-mediated immune mechanism may be responsible.

Approximately 6% to 8% of children are affected with food allergy. In adults this declines to 1% to 2%.

CLINICAL MANIFESTATIONS

Symptoms of hypersensitivity reactions vary from involvement of the skin, gastrointestinal tract, and respiratory tract to anaphylaxis. Non-IgE-mediated food allergy typically presents during infancy as proctitis/proctocolitis, enteropathy, or enterocolitis (Table 84-1).

LABORATORY AND IMAGING STUDIES

In acute IgE reactions, skin prick allergy testing and serum testing to foods may help confirm the suspected food allergy.

DIAGNOSIS

A careful history focuses on symptoms, the time interval from ingestion to onset of symptoms, the quantity of food necessary to evoke the reaction, the most recent reaction, patterns of reactivity, and associated factors such as exercise and medication use. Skin prick testing can be performed to confirm IgE-mediated food allergies. A negative skin test virtually excludes an IgE-mediated reaction (unless the clinical history suggests a severe reaction after an isolated ingestion of the food). A positive skin test indicates sensitization but does not prove clinical reactivity and must be interpreted, based on the history.

Table 84-1	Gastrointestinal Food Allergic Disorders			
DISORDER	**AGE GROUP**	**CHARACTERISTICS**	**DIAGNOSIS**	**PROGNOSIS/COURSE**
IgE-MEDIATED				
Acute gastrointestinal hypersensitivity	Any	Onset: minutes to 2 h Nausea, abdominal pain, emesis, diarrhea Typically in conjunction with cutaneous and/or respiratory symptoms	History, positive PST, and/or serum food-IgE Confirmatory OFC	Variable, food-dependent Milk, soy, egg, and wheat typically outgrown Peanut, tree nuts, seeds, and shellfish typically persist
Pollen-food allergy syndrome (oral allergy syndrome)	Any, most common in young adults (50% of birch pollen adults)	Immediate symptoms on contact of raw fruit with oral mucosa Pruritus, tingling, erythema or angioedema of the lips, tongue, oropharynx, throat pruritus/tightness	History, positive PST with raw fruits or vegetables; OFC-positive with raw fruit, negative with cooked	Severity of symptoms may vary with pollen season Symptoms may improve with pollen immunotherapy in subset of patients
IgE- AND/OR NON-IGE-MEDIATED				
Allergic eosinophilic esophagitis	Any, but especially infants, children, adolescents	Children: chronic/intermittent symptoms of gastroesophageal reflux, emesis, dysphagia, abdominal pain, irritability Adults: abdominal pain, dysphagia, food impaction	History, positive PST, and/or food-IgE in 50%, but poor correlation with clinical symptoms Patch testing may be of value Elimination diet and OFC Endoscopy, biopsy provides conclusive diagnosis and response to treatment information	Variable, not well established, improvement with elimination diet within 6–8 wk Elemental diet may be required Often responds to swallowed topical steroids
Allergic eosinophilic gastroenteritis	Any	Chronic/intermittent abdominal pain, emesis, irritability, poor appetite, failure to thrive, weight loss, anemia, protein-losing gastroenteropathy	History, positive PST, and/or food-IgE in 50%, but poor correlation with clinical symptoms, elimination diet, and OFC Endoscopy, biopsy provides conclusive diagnosis and response to treatment information	Variable, not well established, improvement with elimination diet within 6–8 wk Elemental diet may be required
NON-IgE-MEDIATED				
Allergic proctocolitis	Young infants (<6 mo), frequently breastfed	Blood-streaked or heme-positive stools, otherwise healthy-appearing	History, prompt response (resolution of gross blood in 48 h) to allergen elimination Biopsy conclusive but not necessary in vast majority	Majority able to tolerate milk/soy by 1 yr of age
Food protein-induced enterocolitis syndrome	Young infants	Chronic emesis, diarrhea, failure to thrive on chronic exposure On reexposure following a period of elimination, subacute, repetitive emesis, dehydration (15% shock), diarrhea Breastfeeding protective	History, response to dietary restriction OFC	Most resolve in 1–3 yr
Dietary protein-induced enteropathy	Young infants	Protracted diarrhea, (steatorrhea), emesis, failure to thrive, anemia in 40%	History, endoscopy, and biopsy Response to dietary restriction	Most resolve in 1–2 yr
Celiac disease (gluten-sensitive enteropathy)	Any	Chronic diarrhea, malabsorption, abdominal distention, flatulence, failure to thrive or weight loss May be associated with oral ulcers and/or dermatitis herpetiformis	Biopsy diagnostic: villus atrophy Screening with serum IgA antitissue transglutaminase and antigliadin Resolution of symptoms with gluten elimination and relapse on oral challenge	Lifelong

From Adkinson NF Jr, Bochner BS, Busse WW, et al: Middleton's Allergy: Principles and Practice, ed 7, Philadelphia, 2008, Mosby.
OFC, Oral food challenge; PST, prick skin test.

Table 84-2	Interpretation of Serum IgE Antibody Concentrations	
FOOD	**FOOD-SPECIFIC IgE ANTIBODY CONCENTRATIONS AT OR ABOVE WHICH CLINICAL REACTIONS ARE HIGHLY LIKELY (kUa/L)**	**POSITIVE PREDICTIVE VALUE (%)**
Egg	7	98
≤2 yr of age	2	95
Milk	15	95
≤2 yr of age	5	95
Peanut	14	95–100
Fish	20	100
Soybean	30	73
Wheat	26	74
Tree nuts	≈15	≈5

Adapted from Sampson HA: Food allergy, J Allergy Clin Immunol 111:S544, 2003.

An in vitro serum specific IgE assay can be used to help confirm clinical allergy as well. Many allergists and laboratories regard the ImmunoCAP system as the method of choice. This method uses a quantitative fluorescent immunoassay, which is more sensitive than other assays; this method also has improved specificity and reproducibility compared to other assays. These tests provide supplementary information to skin tests. Researchers have tried to determine concentrations of food-specific IgE at which clinical reactions are highly likely to occur (Table 84-2). Patients with allergen specific IgE levels greater than 95% of the predictive value may be considered allergic, and there is no need for an oral food challenge. Monitoring the allergen specific IgE level may be helpful in predicting whether a child has outgrown the food allergy. Oral food challenges remain the standard of diagnosis and can be performed to determine whether a child can eat the food safely.

TREATMENT

Management of food allergies consists of educating the patient to avoid ingestion of the responsible allergen and to initiate therapy if ingestion occurs. For mild symptoms limited to the skin only, such as mild itching or hives in the area of allergen contact, oral antihistamines such as diphenhydramine or cetirizine can be administered. If symptoms extend beyond skin, including but not limited to difficulty breathing or swallowing, tongue or throat swelling, vomiting, and fainting or symptoms not responding to diphenhydramine within 20 minutes, injectable epinephrine should be administered and immediate medical attention pursued. Types of injectable epinephrine include EpiPen (0.3 mg), EpiPen Jr. (0.15 mg), and Twinject (0.3 or 0.15 mg).

COMPLICATIONS

Anaphylaxis is the most serious complication of allergic food reactions and can result in death (see Chapter 81).

PROGNOSIS AND PREVENTION

Hypersensitivity to egg, milk, wheat, and soy resolves within the first 5 years of life in approximately 80% of children. Sensitivity to certain foods, such as peanuts, tree nuts, fish, and shellfish, tends to be lifelong. However 20% of children who manifested peanut allergy younger than 2 years of age may outgrow it.

Avoidance of the suspect food is crucial. Careful reading of food labels is a priority. A **MedicAlert bracelet** with appropriate information should be worn. The Food Allergy Research & Education organization (www.foodallergy.org) is a useful educational resource for families and physicians.

Recommendations for prevention of allergic diseases aimed at the *high-risk* newborn who has not manifested atopic disease include (1) breastfeeding for the first 4 to 6 months or (2) using a hydrolyzed casein formula (e.g., Alimentum or Nutramigen) or partially hydrolyzed whey formula (e.g., Good Start) (if supplementing) for the first 4 to 6 months and delaying introduction of solid foods until 4 to 6 months of age. Other approaches, such as maternal avoidance diets during pregnancy and during lactation, as well as avoidance of allergenic foods for infants beyond 6 months of age, are unproven.

Chapter 85

ADVERSE REACTIONS TO DRUGS

ETIOLOGY

An **adverse drug reaction** is defined as an unwanted, negative consequence associated with the use of a drug or biologic agent. Drug reactions can be classified as immunologic or nonimmunologic reactions (Table 85-1). Nearly 75% to 80% of adverse drug reactions are caused by a predictable, nonimmunologic mechanism, and between 5% and 10% of all drug reactions are explained by an immune-mediated mechanism. The remaining drug reactions are caused by an unpredictable mechanism, which may or may not be immune-mediated. The **Gell and Coombs classification** can be used to describe some drug-induced allergic reactions (see Table 77-1). Many drug reactions cannot be classified because the exact immune mechanism has not been defined. Most drugs cannot elicit an immune response because of their small size; rather, the drug or a metabolite acts as a hapten and binds to larger molecules, such as tissue or serum proteins, a process called **haptenation.** The multivalent hapten-protein complex forms a new immunogenic epitope that elicits T- and B-lymphocyte responses.

EPIDEMIOLOGY

Drug reactions to penicillins and cephalosporins are the most common allergic drug reactions encountered in the pediatric population. Approximately 6% to 10% of children are labeled as *penicillin allergic*. Risk factors for drug reactions include previous drug exposure, increasing age (>20 years of age), parenteral or topical administration, higher dose, intermittent

Table 85-1	Classification of Adverse Drug Reactions
TYPE	**EXAMPLE**
IMMUNOLOGIC	
Type I reaction (IgE-mediated)	Anaphylaxis from β-lactam antibiotic
Type II reaction (cytotoxic)	Hemolytic anemia from penicillin
Type III reaction (immune complex)	Serum sickness from antithymocyte globulin
Type IV reaction (delayed, cell-mediated)	Contact dermatitis from topical antihistamine
Specific T-cell activation	Morbilliform rash from sulfonamides
Fas/Fas ligand-induced apoptosis	Stevens-Johnson syndrome; toxic epidermal necrolysis
Other	Drug-induced lupus-like syndrome; anticonvulsant hypersensitivity syndrome
NONIMMUNOLOGIC	
Predictable	
Pharmacologic adverse effect	Dry mouth from antihistamines; tremor from albuterol
Secondary pharmacologic adverse effect	Thrush while taking antibiotics; *Clostridium difficile*-associated colitis (pseudomembranous colitis) from clindamycin (and other antibiotics)
Drug toxicity	Hepatotoxicity from methotrexate
Drug-drug interactions	Torsades de pointes arrhythmia from terfenadine with erythromycin
Drug overdose	Hepatic necrosis from acetaminophen
Unpredictable	
Pseudoallergic	Anaphylactoid reaction after radiocontrast media
Idiosyncratic	Hemolytic anemia in a patient with G6PD deficiency after primaquine therapy
Intolerance	Tinnitus after a single, small dose of aspirin

Adapted from Riedl MA, Casillas AM: Adverse drug reactions: types and treatment options, Am Fam Physician 68(9):1781–1790, 2003.
G6PD, Glucose-6-phosphate dehydrogenase.

repeated exposure, and a genetic predisposition of slow drug metabolism. An atopic background does not predispose an individual to the development of drug reactions but may indicate a greater risk of serious reaction.

CLINICAL MANIFESTATIONS

Allergic reactions can be classified as **immediate (anaphylactic) reactions,** which occur within 60 minutes of drug administration; **accelerated reactions**, which begin 1 to 72 hours after drug administration; and **late reactions**, which occur after 72 hours. The most common form of adverse drug reaction is cutaneous. Accelerated reactions are usually dermatologic or serum sickness reactions. Late reactions include desquamating dermatitis, Stevens-Johnson syndrome, toxic epidermal necrolysis, and serum sickness.

LABORATORY AND IMAGING STUDIES

Skin testing protocols are standardized for penicillin and are well described for other agents, such as local anesthetics, muscle relaxants, vaccines, and insulin. Positive skin testing to such reagents confirms the presence of antigen-specific IgE and supports the diagnosis of a type I hypersensitivity reaction in the appropriate clinical setting.

DIFFERENTIAL DIAGNOSIS

The broadest experience with managing adverse drug reactions is with penicillin. Penicillin allergy should be evaluated when the individual is well and not in acute need of treatment. Penicillin skin testing is helpful for IgE-mediated reactions because of its negative predictive value; only 1% to 3% of patients with negative skin tests have a reaction, which is mild, when re-exposed to penicillin. Skin testing for penicillin should be performed using the **major determinant, penicilloyl polylysine** (available as Pre-Pen), and **minor determinants,** which include penicillin G, penicilloate, and penilloate. Skin testing to penicillin does not predict non-IgE-mediated reactions. For patients with a history consistent with serum sickness or desquamative-type reactions, skin testing should not be performed, and penicillin should be avoided indefinitely.

The risk of a child who has reacted positively to penicillin skin testing suffering an allergic reaction to a cephalosporin antibiotic is less than 2%. It is believed that the first-generation cephalosporins (e.g., cephalexin) are more likely than second-generation (e.g., cefuroxime) or third-generation (cefpodoxime) cephalosporins to be cross-reactive. This is due to the chemical similarity of side chains of the β-lactam ring between penicillin and first-generation cephalosporins.

TREATMENT

If penicillin skin testing is positive, penicillin should be avoided, and an alternative antibiotic should be used. If there is a definite need for penicillin, **desensitization** can be accomplished by administration of increasing amounts of drug over a short time in a hospital setting. The exact mechanism of desensitization is unclear; however, it is thought to render mast cells unresponsive to the drug. To maintain desensitization, the drug must be given at least twice daily. If the drug is stopped for longer than 48 hours, the patient is no longer *desensitized,* and the same protocol must be repeated before repeated antibiotic use.

For other antibiotics, the relevant allergenic determinants produced by metabolism or degradation are not well defined. Skin testing to the native antibiotic in nonirritating concentrations can be performed. A negative response does not exclude allergy; however, a positive response suggests the presence of IgE-mediated allergy. In the case of a negative skin test response, a graded challenge or test dose may be administered, depending on the clinical history of the reaction. Patients who have experienced Stevens-Johnson syndrome, toxic epidermal necrolysis, or serum sickness should not be challenged.

COMPLICATIONS

Anaphylaxis is the most serious complication of allergic drug reactions and can result in death (see Chapter 81).

PROGNOSIS

Most drug reactions do not seem to be allergic in nature. Repeated, intermittent exposure during childhood or early adulthood contributes to an increased incidence of adverse drug reactions in adults.

PREVENTION

Avoidance of the suspect drug is paramount. A **MedicAlert bracelet** with appropriate information should be worn. One of the most common concerns in regard to allergic drug reactions is cross-reactivity between penicillin and cephalosporins. In children with a history of penicillin allergy, it is important to determine whether they are truly allergic by skin testing to penicillin, using the major and minor determinants. If the penicillin skin test is negative, there is not an increased risk of an allergic reaction to cephalosporins. A positive penicillin skin test leads to an alternate non-cross-reacting antibiotic, a graded challenge to the required cephalosporin under appropriate monitoring, or desensitization to the required cephalosporin.

For children with a history of a cephalosporin allergy who require another cephalosporin, two approaches may be considered: a graded challenge with a cephalosporin that does not share the same side chain determinant, or skin testing with the same or a different cephalosporin. A positive response suggests the presence of IgE-mediated allergy, and the value of a negative test is unknown. Skin testing with cephalosporins has not been standardized or validated.

Suggested Reading

Bieber T: Atopic dermatitis, *N Engl J Med* 58:483–1494, 2008.

Greenberger P, Grammer L: Northwestern University allergy-immunology syllabus 2012: residents and students, *Allergy Asthma Proc* 33(3), 2012 Suppl 1.

Greer FR, Sicherer SH, Burks AW: Effects of early nutritional interventions on the development of atopic disease in infants and children: the role of maternal dietary restriction, breastfeeding, timing of introduction of complementary foods and hydrolyzed formulas, *Pediatrics* 121:183–191, 2008.

Leung DYM, Sampson HA, Geha RS, et al: *Pediatric Allergy: Principles and Practice*, ed 2, St Louis, 2010, Elsevier.

National Heart, Lung, and Blood Institute and National Asthma Education and Prevention Program: Expert panel report 3: guidelines for the diagnosis and management of asthma. Full report 2007. *NTH Publication No. 08–4051*. Bethesda, MD, 2007, U.S. Department of Health and Human Services. Available at http://www.nhlbi.nih.gov/guidelines/asthma/asthgdln.htm.

National Heart, Lung, and Blood Institute and National Asthma Education and Prevention Program: Expert panel report 3: guidelines for the diagnosis and management of asthma. Summary report 2007. *NTH Publication No. 08–5846*. Bethesda, MD, 2007, U.S. Department of Health and Human Services. Available at http://www.nhlbi.nih.gov/guidelines/asthma/asthsumm.pdf.

Shearer WT, Leung DYM: 2010 primer on allergic and immunologic diseases, *J Allergy Clin Immunol* 125:S1–S2, 2010.

Sicherer SH: *Understanding and Managing Your Child's Food Allergies*, Baltimore, 2006, Johns Hopkins University Press.

Williams HC: Atopic dermatitis, *N Engl J Med* 352:2314–2324, 2005.

Wood RA: *Food Allergies for Dummies*, Hoboken, NJ, 2007, Wiley.

Rheumatic Diseases of Childhood

Hilary M. Haftel

Chapter **86**

ASSESSMENT

The **rheumatic diseases (collagen vascular** or **connective tissue diseases)** of childhood are characterized by autoimmunity and inflammation, which may be localized or generalized. The classic rheumatic diseases of children include juvenile idiopathic arthritis (JIA), formerly called *juvenile rheumatoid arthritis,* systemic lupus erythematosus (SLE), and juvenile dermatomyositis (JDM). Vasculitis is a component of many rheumatic diseases. **Musculoskeletal pain syndromes** are a set of overlapping conditions characterized by poorly localized pain involving the extremities. Scleroderma, Behçet syndrome, and Sjögren syndrome are rare in childhood. The differential diagnosis of rheumatologic disorders typically includes infections, postinfectious processes, and malignancies (Table 86-1).

HISTORY

The history can identify symptoms that reflect the source of the inflammation, including whether it is localized or systemic. Symptoms of systemic inflammation tend to be nonspecific. **Fever,** caused by cytokine release, can take many forms. A hectic fever, without periodicity or pattern, is commonly found in vasculitides such as Kawasaki disease but also occurs in children with underlying infection. Certain illnesses, such as systemic-onset JIA, produce a patterned fever with regular temperature spikes once or twice a day. Other rheumatic illnesses cause low-grade fevers. Charting the child's fever pattern, particularly in the absence of antipyretics, is useful. Rashes occur in many forms (see Table 86-1). Other systemic symptoms (malaise, anorexia, weight loss, and fatigue) can vary from mild to debilitating.

Symptoms of localized inflammation vary depending on the involved site. **Arthritis,** or inflammation of the synovium **(synovitis),** leads to joint pain, swelling, and impaired ability to use the affected joint. Morning stiffness or gelling is described. The child may be slow to arise in the morning and may have a limp. Children may refrain from usual activities and athletics. **Enthesitis** is inflammation at the insertion of a ligament to a bone. **Serositis,** inflammation of serosal lining such as pleuritis, pericarditis, or peritonitis, gives rise to chest pain, shortness of breath, or abdominal pain. **Myositis,** inflammation of the muscle, may lead to symptoms of muscle pain, weakness, or difficulty performing tasks of daily living. **Vasculitis,** inflammation of the blood vessels, leads to nonspecific symptoms of rash (petechiae, purpura) and edema when small vessels deep in the papillary dermis are involved; involvement of medium-sized vessels results in a circumscribed tender nodule.

PHYSICAL EXAMINATION

A thorough history and physical examination is frequently sufficient to narrow the differential diagnosis and elicit the diagnosis. The child's overall appearance, evidence of growth failure, or failure to thrive may point to a significant underlying inflammatory disorder. The head and neck examination may show evidence of mucosal ulceration, seen in diseases such as SLE. The eye examination may show pupillary irregularity and synechiae from uveitis or the conjunctivitis of Kawasaki disease. Diffuse lymphadenopathy may be found and is nonspecific. The respiratory and cardiac examinations may show pericardial or pleural friction rubs, indicating serositis. Splenomegaly or hepatomegaly raises suspicion of activation of the reticuloendothelial system that occurs in systemic-onset JIA or SLE.

The joint examination is crucial for the diagnosis of arthritis and may identify evidence of joint swelling, effusion, tenderness, and erythema from increased blood flow. Joint contractures may be seen. The joint lining, or synovium, may be thickened from chronic inflammation. Activation of epiphyseal growth plates in an area of arthritis can lead to localized bony proliferation and limb length discrepancies. Conversely inflammation at sites of immature growth centers may lead to maldevelopment of bones, such as the carpals or tarsals, resulting in crowding, or the temporomandibular joints, resulting in micrognathia. A rash or evidence of underlying skin disorders, such as skin thickening from scleroderma or sclerodactyly, may be noted. Chronic Raynaud phenomenon may result in nail-fold capillary changes, ulceration, or digital tuft wasting.

COMMON MANIFESTATIONS

The rheumatic diseases of childhood encompass a heterogeneous group of diseases with a shared underlying pathogenesis: disordered functioning of the immune system leading to inflammation directed against native proteins, with secondary increases in numbers of activated lymphocytes, inflammatory

Table 86-1 Differential Diagnosis of Pediatric Arthritis Syndromes

CHARACTERISTIC	SYSTEMIC LUPUS ERYTHEMATOSUS	JUVENILE IDIOPATHIC ARTHRITIS	RHEUMATIC FEVER	LYME DISEASE	LEUKEMIA	GONOCOCCEMIA	KAWASAKI DISEASE
Sex	F > M	Type-dependent	M = F	M = F	M = F	F > M	M = F
Age	10–20 yr	1–16 yr	5–15 yr	>5–20 yr	2–10 yr	>12 yr	<5 yr
Arthralgia	Yes	Yes	Yes	Yes	Yes	Yes	Yes
Morning stiffness	Yes	Yes	No	No	No	No	No
Rash	Butterfly; discoid	Salmon-pink macules (systemic onset)	Erythema marginatum	Erythema migrans	No	Palms/soles, papulopustules	Diffuse maculopapular (nonspecific), desquamation
Monarticular, pauciarticular	Yes	50%	No	Yes	Yes	Yes	—
Polyarticular	Yes	Yes	Yes	No	Yes	No	Yes
Small joints	Yes	Yes	No	Rare	Yes	No	Yes
Temporomandibular joint	No	Rare	No	Rare	No	No	No
Eye disease	Uveitis/retinitis	Iridocyclitis (rare in systemic)	No	Conjunctivitis, keratitis	No	No	Conjunctivitis, uveitis
Total WBC count	Decreased	Increased (decreased in macrophage activation syndrome)	Normal to increased	Normal	Increased or neutropenia ± blasts	Increased	Increased
ANA	Positive (>99%)	Positive (50%)	Negative	Negative	Negative	Negative	Negative
Rheumatoid factor	Positive or negative	Positive (10%) (polyarticular)	Negative	Negative	Negative	Negative	Negative
Other laboratory results	↓Complement, ↑antibodies to double-stranded DNA	Anti-CCP antibody + in adult type RA	↑ASO anti-DNase B	↑Cryoglobulin, ↑immune complexes	+ Bone marrow	+ Culture for *Neisseria gonorrhoeae*	Thrombocytosis, ↑immune complexes
Erosive arthritis	Rare	Yes	Rare	Rare	No	Yes	No
Other clinical manifestations	Proteinuria, serositis	Fever, serositis (systemic onset)	Carditis, nodules, chorea	Carditis, neuropathy, meningitis	Thrombocytopenia	Sexual activity, menses	Fever, lymphadenopathy, swollen hands/feet, mouth lesions
Pathogenesis	Autoimmune	Autoimmune	Group A streptococcus	*Borrelia burgdorferi*	Acute lymphoblastic leukemia	*N. gonorrhoeae*	Unknown
Treatment	NSAIDs, corticosteroids, hydroxychloroquine, immunosuppressive agents	NSAIDs, methotrexate, TNF blockers for resistant disease	Penicillin prophylaxis, aspirin, corticosteroids	Penicillin, doxycycline, ceftriaxone	Corticosteroids, chemotherapy	Ceftriaxone	Intravenous immunoglobulin, aspirin

ANA, Antinuclear antibody; *ASO,* antistreptolysin-O titer; *CCP,* cyclic citrullinated protein; *NSAID,* nonsteroidal anti-inflammatory drug; *TNF,* tumor necrosis factor; *WBC,* white blood cell.

Table 86-2	Manifestations of Autoantibodies

Coombs-positive hemolytic anemia

Immune neutropenia

Immune thrombocytopenia

Thrombosis (anticardiolipin, antiphospholipid, lupus anticoagulant)

Immune lymphopenia

Antimitochondrial (primary biliary cirrhosis, SLE)

Antimicrosomal (chronic active hepatitis, SLE)

Antithyroid (thyroiditis, SLE)

Antineutrophil cytoplasmic antibody (ANCA-cytoplasmic) (granulomatosis with polyangiitis)

ANCA-perinuclear (microscopic polyangiitis)

Anti-CCP (rheumatoid positive JIA)

ANTINUCLEAR ANTIBODIES TO SPECIFIC NUCLEAR ANTIGENS AND ASSOCIATED MANIFESTATIONS

Single-stranded DNA (nonspecific, indicates inflammation)

Double-stranded DNA (SLE, renal disease)

DNA-histone (drug-induced SLE)

Sm (Smith) (SLE, renal, CNS)

RNP (ribonucleoprotein) (SLE, Sjögren syndrome, scleroderma, polymyositis, MCTD)

Ro (Robert: SSA) (SLE, neonatal lupus-congenital heart block, Sjögren syndrome)

La (Lane: SSB) (SLE, neonatal lupus [congenital heart block], Sjögren syndrome)

Jo-1 (polymyositis, dermatomyositis)

Scl-70 (systemic sclerosis)

Centromere (CREST; limited scleroderma)

PM-Scl (scleroderma, UCTD)

Adapted from Condemi J: The autoimmune disease, JAMA 268:2882–2892, 1992.
ANCA, Antineutrophil cytoplasmic antibody; CCP, cyclic citrullinated protein; CNS, central nervous system; CREST syndrome, calcinosis, Raynaud phenomenon, esophageal dysfunction, sclerodactyly, telangiectasia; MCTD, mixed connective tissue disease; SLE, systemic lupus erythematosus; SSA, Sjögren syndrome antigen A; SSB, Sjögren syndrome antigen B; UCTD, undifferentiated connective tissue disease.

cytokines, and circulating antibodies. This antibody production can be nonspecific, or it can be targeted against specific native proteins, leading to subsequent disease manifestations (Table 86-2). Although immune system hyperactivity may be self-limited, the hallmark of most rheumatic diseases of childhood is chronicity, or the perpetuation of the inflammatory process, which can lead to long-term disability.

INITIAL DIAGNOSTIC EVALUATION
Although rheumatic diseases sometimes present with nonspecific symptoms, especially early in the course, over time a characteristic set of symptoms and physical findings can be elicited. In conjunction with carefully chosen confirmatory laboratory tests, an appropriate differential diagnosis is made, and eventually the correct diagnosis and treatment plan is developed.

Most rheumatologic diagnoses are established by clinical findings and fulfillment of classification criteria. Laboratory testing should be judicious and based on a differential diagnosis rather than random screening in search of a diagnosis. Laboratory tests confirm clinical diagnoses rather than develop them.

LABORATORY TESTING
Evidence of an underlying systemic inflammation may be indicated by elevated acute phase reactants, especially the erythrocyte sedimentation rate, but also the white blood cell count, platelet count, and C-reactive protein. The complete blood count may demonstrate a normochromic, normocytic anemia of chronic disease. These laboratory findings are nonspecific for any particular rheumatologic diagnosis. Certain laboratory tests may help confirm a diagnosis, such as autoantibody production in SLE or muscle enzyme elevation in JDM, or identify increased risk for complications, such as uveitis in a patient with JIA with a positive antinuclear antibody.

DIAGNOSTIC IMAGING
Radiologic studies should focus on areas of concern identified by history or physical examination. Radiography of joints in patients with arthritis on examination may be beneficial, but radiographic abnormalities may lag far behind the clinical examination. Tests with greater sensitivity, such as bone scan, computed tomography scan, and magnetic resonance imaging, may be useful when trying to differentiate between synovitis and traumatic soft tissue injury. Magnetic resonance imaging may also be useful to identify evidence of central nervous system involvement with SLE or for evidence of myositis with JDM.

Chapter **87**

HENOCH-SCHÖNLEIN PURPURA

ETIOLOGY
Henoch-Schönlein purpura (HSP) is a vasculitis of unknown etiology characterized by inflammation of small blood vessels with leukocytic infiltration of tissue, hemorrhage, and ischemia. The immune complexes associated with HSP are predominantly composed of IgA.

EPIDEMIOLOGY
HSP is the most common systemic vasculitis of childhood and cause of nonthrombocytopenic purpura, with an incidence of 13 per 100,000 children. It occurs primarily in children 3 to 15 years of age, although it has been described in adults. HSP is slightly more common in boys than girls and occurs more frequently in the winter than in the summer months.

CLINICAL MANIFESTATIONS

Decision-Making Algorithms
Available @ StudentConsult.com

Red Urine and Hematuria
Proteinuria
Scrotal Pain
Fever and Rash
Petechiae/Purpura

HSP is characterized by rash, arthritis, and, less frequently, gastrointestinal or renal vasculitis. The hallmark of HSP is **palpable purpura,** caused by small vessel inflammation in the skin leading to extravasation of blood into the surrounding tissues, frequently with IgA deposition. The rash is classically found in dependent areas: below the waist, on the buttocks, and lower extremities (Fig. 87-1). The rash can begin as small macules or urticarial lesions but rapidly progresses to purpura with areas of ecchymosis. The rash also can be accompanied by edema, particularly of the calves and dorsum of the feet, scalp, and scrotum or labia. HSP occasionally is associated with encephalopathy, pancreatitis, and orchitis.

Arthritis occurs in 80% of patients with HSP and is most common in the lower extremities, particularly the ankles and knees. The arthritis is acute and very painful with refusal to bear weight. Joint swelling can be confused with peripheral edema seen with the rash of HSP.

Gastrointestinal involvement occurs in about one half of affected children and most typically presents as mild to moderate crampy abdominal pain, thought to be due to small vessel involvement of the gastrointestinal tract leading to ischemia. Less commonly, significant abdominal distention, bloody diarrhea, intussusception, or abdominal perforation occurs and requires emergent intervention. Gastrointestinal involvement is typically seen during the acute phase of the illness. It may precede the onset of rash.

One third of children with HSP develop renal involvement, which can be acute or chronic. Although renal involvement is mild in most cases, acute glomerulonephritis manifested by hematuria, hypertension, or acute renal failure can occur. Most cases of glomerulonephritis occur within the first few months of presentation, but rarely patients develop late renal disease, which ultimately can lead to chronic renal disease, including renal failure.

LABORATORY AND IMAGING STUDIES

Erythrocyte sedimentation rate, C-reactive protein, and white blood cell count are elevated in patients with HSP. The platelet count is the most important test, because HSP is characterized by nonthrombocytopenic purpura with a normal, or even high, platelet count, differentiating HSP from other causes of purpura that are associated with thrombocytopenia such as autoimmune thrombocytopenia, systemic lupus erythematosus, or leukemia. A urinalysis screens for evidence of hematuria. A serum blood urea nitrogen and creatinine should be obtained to evaluate renal function. Testing the stool for blood may identify evidence of gut ischemia. Any question of gut perforation requires radiologic investigation.

DIFFERENTIAL DIAGNOSIS

The diagnosis of HSP is based on the presence of two of four criteria (Table 87-1), which provides 87.1% sensitivity and 87.7% specificity for the disease. The differential diagnosis includes other systemic vasculitides (Table 87-2) and diseases associated with thrombocytopenic purpura, such as idiopathic thrombocytopenic purpura and leukemia.

TREATMENT

Therapy for HSP is supportive. A short-term course of nonsteroidal anti-inflammatory drugs can be administered for the acute arthritis. Systemic corticosteroids usually are reserved for children with gastrointestinal disease and provide significant relief of abdominal pain. A typical dosing regimen is prednisone, 1 mg/kg/day for 1 to 2 weeks, followed by a taper schedule. Recurrence of abdominal pain as corticosteroids are weaned may necessitate a longer course of treatment. Acute nephritis typically is treated with corticosteroids but may require more aggressive immunosuppressive therapy.

COMPLICATIONS

Most cases of HSP are monophasic, lasting 3 to 4 weeks and resolving completely. The rash can wax and wane, however, for 1 year after HSP. Parents should be warned regarding possible recurrences. The arthritis of HSP does not leave any permanent joint damage; it does not typically recur. Gastrointestinal involvement can lead to temporary abnormal peristalsis that poses a risk of intussusception, which may be followed by complete obstruction or infarction with bowel perforation. Any child

Figure 87-1 Rash of Henoch-Schönlein purpura on the lower extremities of a child. Note evidence of both purpura and petechiae.

Table 87-1	Criteria for Diagnosis of Henoch-Schönlein Purpura*
CRITERIA	**DEFINITION**
Palpable purpura	Raised, palpable hemorrhagic skin lesions in the absence of thrombocytopenia
Bowel angina	Diffuse abdominal pain or the diagnosis of bowel ischemia
Diagnostic biopsy	Histologic changes showing granulocytes in the walls of arterioles or venules; IgA deposits in vessel wall
Pediatric age group	Age <20 years at onset of symptoms

*The diagnosis of Henoch-Schönlein purpura is based on the presence of two of four criteria.

Table 87-2	Classification of Vasculitides

ANTINEUTROPHIL CYTOPLASMIC ANTIBODY-ASSOCIATED VASCULITIS

Granulomatosis with polyangiitis (formerly known as *Wegener granulomatosis*)

Polyarteritis nodosa

Churg-Strauss syndrome

Microscopic polyangiitis

HYPERSENSITIVITY SYNDROMES

Henoch-Schönlein purpura

Serum sickness (e.g., drug-related)

Vasculitis associated with infections

CONNECTIVE TISSUE DISEASES

Systemic lupus erythematosus

Dermatomyositis

Juvenile idiopathic arthritis

GIANT CELL ARTERITIS

Temporal arteritis

Takayasu arteritis

OTHERS

Behçet syndrome

Kawasaki disease

Hypocomplementemic urticarial vasculitis

with a recent history of HSP who presents with acute abdominal pain, obstipation, or diarrhea should be evaluated for intussusception. Renal involvement rarely may lead to renal failure.

PROGNOSIS

The prognosis of HSP is excellent. Most children have complete resolution of the illness without any significant sequelae. Patients with HSP renal disease (elevated blood urea nitrogen, persistent high-grade proteinuria) are at highest risk for long-term complications, such as hypertension or renal insufficiency, particularly if the initial course was marked by significant nephritis. There is a long-term risk of progression to end-stage renal disease in less than 1% of children with HSP. The rare patients who develop end-stage renal disease may require renal transplantation. HSP may recur in the transplanted kidney.

Chapter 88

KAWASAKI DISEASE

ETIOLOGY

Kawasaki disease (KD) is a vasculitis of unknown etiology that is characterized by multisystem involvement and inflammation of small to medium-sized arteries with resulting aneurysm formation.

EPIDEMIOLOGY

KD is the second most common vasculitis of childhood. It is more common in children of Asian descent. It has been described in variable frequency in all parts of the world; the highest frequency is in Japan. KD most commonly occurs in children younger than 5 years of age, with a peak between 2 to 3 years, and is rare in children older than 7 years. The incidence in the United States is approximately 6 per 100,000 children who are younger than 5 years of age. A seasonal variability has been described with a peak between February and May, but the disease occurs throughout the year.

CLINICAL MANIFESTATIONS

The clinical course of KD can be divided into three phases, each with its own unique manifestations. Aneurysmal involvement of the coronary arteries is the most important manifestation of KD.

Acute Phase

Decision-Making Algorithms
Available @ StudentConsult.com

Lymphadenopathy
Fever Without a Source
Fever of Unknown Origin

The acute phase of KD, which lasts 1 to 2 weeks, is marked by sudden onset of a high, hectic **fever** (>40 °C) without an apparent source. The onset of fever is followed by **conjunctival erythema;** mucosal changes, including dry, **cracked lips** and a **strawberry tongue; cervical lymphadenopathy;** and swelling of the hands and feet (Fig. 88-1). Conjunctivitis is bilateral, bulbar, and nonsuppurative. Cervical lymphadenopathy is found in 70% of children and should be greater than 1.5 cm in diameter for the purposes of diagnosis. A rash, which can vary in appearance, occurs in 80% of children with KD and may be particularly accentuated in the inguinal area and on the chest. Extreme irritability is prominent, especially in infants. Abdominal pain and hydrops of the gallbladder, cerebrospinal fluid pleocytosis, sterile pyuria, and arthritis, particularly of medium-sized to large joints, may occur. Carditis in the acute phase may be manifested by tachycardia, shortness of breath, or overt congestive heart failure. **Giant coronary artery aneurysms,** which are rare but occur most commonly in very young children, can appear during this phase.

Subacute Phase

The subacute phase, which lasts until about the fourth week, is characterized by gradual resolution of fever (if untreated) and other symptoms. **Desquamation** of the skin, particularly of the fingers and toes, appears at this point. The platelet count, previously normal or slightly depressed, increases to a significant degree (often >1 million/mm³). This phase heralds the onset of **coronary artery aneurysms,** which may also appear in the convalescent phase and pose the highest risk of morbidity and mortality. Risk factors for development of coronary artery aneurysms include prolonged fever, prolonged elevation of inflammatory parameters such as the erythrocyte

Figure 88-1 Facial features of Kawasaki disease with (**A**) morbilliform rash and nonsuppurative conjunctivitis and (**B**) red, chapped lips.

sedimentation rate (ESR), age younger than 1 year or older than 6 years, and male gender.

Convalescent Phase
The convalescent phase begins with the disappearance of clinical symptoms and continues until the ESR returns to normal, usually 6 to 8 weeks after the onset of illness. Beau lines of the fingernails may appear during this phase.

LABORATORY AND IMAGING STUDIES
It is particularly important to exclude other causes of fever, notably infection. It is appropriate to obtain blood and urine cultures and to perform a chest x-ray. In the acute phase, inflammatory parameters are elevated, including white blood cell count, C-reactive protein, and the ESR, which can be profoundly elevated (often >80 mm/hr). Platelet counts may be inappropriately low or normal. A lumbar puncture, if performed to exclude infection, may reveal pleocytosis. Tests of hepatobiliary function may be abnormal. Greatly elevated platelet counts develop during the subacute phase. The development of coronary artery aneurysms is monitored by performing two-dimensional echocardiograms, usually during the acute phase, at 2 to 3 weeks, and again at 6 to 8 weeks. More frequent echocardiograms and, potentially, coronary angiography are indicated for patients who develop coronary artery abnormalities.

DIFFERENTIAL DIAGNOSIS
The diagnosis of KD is based on the presence of fever for more than 5 days without an identifiable source and the presence of four of five other clinical criteria (Table 88-1).

The diagnosis of **incomplete (atypical) KD,** which occurs more commonly in infants, is made when fever is present for at least 5 days even if only two or three clinical criteria are present, particularly in the presence of coronary artery aneurysms. The diagnosis of KD should be considered in infants younger than 6 months of age with fever for at least 7 days even if no other criteria are present. Because many of the manifestations of KD are found in other illnesses, many diagnoses must be considered and excluded before the diagnosis of KD can be established (Table 88-2).

TREATMENT
Intravenous immunoglobulin (IVIG) is the mainstay of therapy for KD, although the mechanism of action is unknown.

Table 88-1	Criteria for Diagnosis of Kawasaki Disease
Fever of >5 days' duration associated with at least four* of the following five changes:	
Bilateral nonsuppurative conjunctivitis	
One or more changes of the mucous membranes of the upper respiratory tract, including pharyngeal injection, dry fissured lips, injected lips, and "strawberry" tongue	
One or more changes of the extremities, including peripheral erythema, peripheral edema, periungual desquamation, and generalized desquamation	
Polymorphous rash, primarily truncal	
Cervical lymphadenopathy >1.5 cm in diameter	
Disease cannot be explained by some other known disease process.	

*A diagnosis of Kawasaki disease can be made if fever and only three changes are present in conjunction with coronary artery disease documented by two-dimensional echocardiography or coronary angiography.

Table 88-2	Differential Diagnosis of Kawasaki Disease
INFECTIOUS	
Scarlet fever	
Epstein-Barr virus	
Adenovirus	
Meningococcemia	
Measles	
Rubella	
Roseola infantum	
Staphylococcal toxic shock syndrome	
Scalded skin syndrome	
Toxoplasmosis	
Leptospirosis	
Rocky Mountain spotted fever	
INFLAMMATORY	
Juvenile idiopathic arthritis (systemic onset)	
Polyarteritis nodosa	
Behçet syndrome	
HYPERSENSITIVITY	
Drug reaction	
Stevens-Johnson syndrome (erythema multiforme)	

Table 88-3	Complications of Kawasaki Disease
Coronary artery thrombosis	
Peripheral artery aneurysm	
Coronary artery aneurysms	
Myocardial infarction	
Myopericarditis	
Heart failure	
Hydrops of gallbladder	
Aseptic meningitis	
Irritability	
Arthritis	
Sterile pyuria (urethritis)	
Thrombocytosis (late)	
Diarrhea	
Pancreatitis	
Peripheral gangrene	

A single dose of IVIG (2 g/kg over 12 hours) results in rapid defervescence and resolution of clinical illness in most patients and, more important, reduces the incidence of coronary artery aneurysms. Aspirin is initially given in **anti-inflammatory doses** (80 to 100 mg/kg/day divided every 6 hours) in the acute phase. Once the fever resolves, aspirin is reduced to **antithrombotic doses** (3 to 5 mg/kg/day as a single dose) and given through the subacute and convalescent phases, usually for 6 to 8 weeks, until follow-up echocardiography documents the absence or resolution of coronary artery aneurysms.

Up to 10% of children with KD initially fail to respond satisfactorily to IVIG therapy. Most of these patients respond to retreatment with IVIG, but an alternative preparation of IVIG may be required. Corticosteroids or infliximab are rarely used in KD, as opposed to other vasculitides, but may have a role during the acute phase if active carditis is apparent or for children with persistent fever after two doses of IVIG.

COMPLICATIONS

Most cases resolve without sequelae. Myocardial infarction has been documented, most likely caused by stenosis of a coronary artery at the site of an aneurysm. Coronary artery aneurysms found on autopsy in older children following sudden cardiac death may have been due to past KD. Other complications are listed in Table 88-3.

PROGNOSIS

IVIG reduces the prevalence of coronary artery disease from 20% to 25% in children treated with aspirin alone to 2% to 4% in children treated with IVIG and aspirin. Other than the risk of persistent coronary artery aneurysms, KD has an excellent prognosis.

Chapter 89

JUVENILE IDIOPATHIC ARTHRITIS

ETIOLOGY

The chronic arthritides of childhood include several types, the most common of which is juvenile idiopathic arthritis (JIA), formerly called *juvenile rheumatoid arthritis (JRA)*. The classification of JIA includes several other types of juvenile arthritis, such as enthesitis-related arthritis and psoriatic arthritis. The etiology of this autoimmune disease is unknown. The common underlying manifestation of this group of illnesses is the presence of chronic **synovitis,** or inflammation of the joint synovium. The synovium becomes thickened and hypervascular with infiltration by lymphocytes, which also can be found in the synovial fluid along with inflammatory cytokines. The inflammation leads to production and release of tissue proteases and collagenases. If left untreated, the inflammation can lead to tissue destruction, particularly of the articular cartilage and, eventually, the underlying bony structures.

EPIDEMIOLOGY

JIA is the most common chronic rheumatologic disease of childhood, with a prevalence of 1:1000 children. The disease has two peaks, one at 1 to 3 years and one at 8 to 12 years, but it can occur at any age. Girls are affected more commonly than boys, particularly with the oligoarticular form of the illness.

CLINICAL PRESENTATION

Decision-Making Algorithms
Available @ StudentConsult.com

Red Eye
Limp
Arthritis
Knee Pain
Extremity Pain

JIA can be divided into several subtypes, depending on the number of joints involved (less than five versus five or more), the presence of sacroiliac involvement, and the presence of systemic features, each with particular disease characteristics (Table 89-1). Although the onset of the arthritis is slow, the actual joint swelling is often noticed acutely by the child or parent, such as after an accident or fall, and can be confused with trauma (even though traumatic effusions are rare in children). The child may develop pain and stiffness in the joint that limit use, but rarely refuses to use the joint at all. Morning stiffness and gelling also can occur in the joint and, if present, can be followed in response to therapy.

On physical examination, signs of inflammation are present, including joint tenderness, erythema, and effusion (Fig. 89-1). Joint range of motion may be limited because of pain, swelling, or contractures from lack of use. In children, because of the

Table 89-1	Features of Juvenile Idiopathic Arthritis Subgroups			
FEATURE	**OLIGOARTICULAR**	**POLYARTICULAR**	**SYSTEMIC ONSET**	**SPONDYLOARTHROPATHIES**
No. joints	<5	≥5	Varies, usually ≥5	Varies
Types of joints	Medium to large (also small in extended oligoarthritis)	Small to medium	Small to medium	Medium to large, including sacroiliac joints
Gender predominance	F > M (especially in younger children)	F > M	F = M	M > F
Systemic features	None	Some constitutional	Prominent	Some constitutional
Eye disease	+++ (uveitis)	++ (uveitis)	+ (uveitis)	++ (iritis)
Extra-articular manifestations	None	None	Systemic features	Enthesopathy, psoriasis, bowel disease
ANA positivity	++	+	—	—
RF positivity		+ (in older children with early-onset RA)		
Outcomes	Excellent, >90% complete remission	Good, >50% complete remission, some risk of disability	Variable, depends on extent of arthritis	Variable

ANA, Antinuclear antibody; RA, rheumatoid arthritis; RF, rheumatoid factor.

Figure 89-1 An affected knee in a patient with oligoarticular juvenile idiopathic arthritis. Note sizeable effusion, bony proliferation, and flexion contracture.

presence of an active growth plate, it may be possible to find bony abnormalities of the surrounding bone, causing bony proliferation and localized growth disturbance. In a lower extremity joint, a leg length discrepancy may be appreciable if the arthritis is asymmetric.

All children with chronic arthritis are at risk for chronic **iridocyclitis** or **uveitis**. There is an association between human leukocyte antigens (HLAs) (HLA-DR5, HLA-DR6, and HLA-DR8) and uveitis. The presence of a positive **antinuclear antibody** identifies children with arthritis who are at higher risk for chronic uveitis. Although all children with JIA are at

increased risk, the subgroup of children, particularly young girls, with oligoarticular (less than five affected joints) JIA and a positive antinuclear antibody are at highest risk, with an incidence of uveitis of 80%. The uveitis associated with JIA can be asymptomatic until the point of visual loss, making it a primary treatable cause of blindness in children. It is crucial for children with JIA to undergo regular ophthalmologic screening with a slit-lamp examination to identify anterior chamber inflammation and to initiate prompt treatment of any active disease.

Oligoarticular Juvenile Idiopathic Arthritis
Oligoarticular JIA is defined as the presence of arthritis in fewer than five joints within 6 months of diagnosis. This is the most common form of JIA, accounting for approximately 50% of cases.

Oligoarticular JIA presents in young children, with a peak at 1 to 3 years and another peak at 8 to 12 years. The arthritis is found in medium-sized to large joints; the knee is the most common joint involved, followed by the ankle and the wrist. It is unusual for small joints, such as the fingers or toes, to be involved, although this may occur. Neck and hip involvement also is uncommon. Children with oligoarticular JIA may be otherwise well without any evidence of systemic inflammation (fever, weight loss, or failure to thrive) or any laboratory evidence of systemic inflammation (elevated white blood cell count or erythrocyte sedimentation rate). A subset of these children later develops polyarticular disease (called *extended oligoarthritis*).

Polyarticular Juvenile Idiopathic Arthritis
Polyarticular JIA describes children with arthritis in five or more joints within the first 6 months of diagnosis and accounts for about 40% of cases. Children with polyarticular JIA tend to have symmetric arthritis, which can affect any joint but typically involves the small joints of the hands, feet, ankles, wrists, and knees. The cervical spine can be involved, leading

Table 89-2	Comparison of Juvenile Idiopathic Arthritis and Spondyloarthropathies			
CLINICAL MANIFESTATIONS	**JIA**	**JAS**	**PSA**	**IBD**
Gender predominance	F	M	Equal	Equal
Peripheral arthritis	+++	+	++	+
Back symptoms	–	+++	+	++
Family history	–	++	++	+
ANA positivity	++	–	–	–
HLA-B27 positivity	–	++	–	
RF positivity	+ (in late-onset JIA)	–	–	–
Extra-articular manifestations	Systemic symptoms (systemic-onset JRA)	Enthesopathy	Psoriasis, nail changes	Bowel symptoms
Eye disease	Anterior uveitis iritis		Posterior uveitis	Anterior uveitis

ANA, Antinuclear antibody; *IBD*, inflammatory bowel disease; *JAS*, juvenile ankylosing spondylitis; *JIA*, juvenile idiopathic arthritis; *PSA*, poststreptococcal arthritis; *RF*, rheumatoid factor.

to fusion of the spine over time. In contrast to oligoarticular JIA, children with polyarticular disease can present with evidence of systemic inflammation, including malaise, low-grade fever, growth retardation, anemia of chronic disease, and elevated markers of inflammation. Polyarticular JIA can present at any age, although there is a peak in early childhood. There is a second peak in adolescence, but these children differ by the presence of a positive **rheumatoid factor** (and anti-CCP antibody) and most likely represent a subgroup with true adult rheumatoid arthritis; the clinical course and prognosis are similar to the adult entity.

Systemic-Onset Juvenile Idiopathic Arthritis
A small subgroup of patients (approximately 10%) with juvenile arthritis does not present with onset of arthritis but rather with preceding **systemic inflammation.** This form of JIA, thought to be an autoinflammatory disease, manifests with a typical recurring, spiking fever, usually once or twice per day, which can occur for several weeks to months. This is accompanied by a rash, typically **morbilliform** and **salmon-colored.** The rash may be evanescent and occur at times of high fever only. Rarely the rash can be urticarial in nature. Internal organ involvement also occurs. Serositis, such as pleuritis and pericarditis, occurs in 50% of children. Pericardial tamponade rarely may occur. Hepatosplenomegaly occurs in 70% of children. Children with systemic-onset JIA appear sick; they have significant constitutional symptoms, including malaise and failure to thrive. Laboratory findings show the inflammation, with elevated erythrocyte sedimentation rate, C-reactive protein, white blood cell count, and platelet counts and anemia. The arthritis of JIA follows the systemic inflammation by 6 weeks to 6 months. The arthritis is typically polyarticular in nature and can be extensive and resistant to treatment, placing these children at highest risk for long-term disability.

Spondyloarthropathies
The spondyloarthropathies describe a group of arthritides that include inflammation of the axial skeleton and sacroiliac joints and enthesitis, or inflammation of tendinous insertions. These include juvenile ankylosing spondylitis, psoriatic arthritis, and the arthritis of inflammatory bowel disease. This group

of diseases can also present with peripheral arthritis and can be initially classified in other subgroups. It is only later, when the patient develops evidence of sacroiliac arthritis, psoriasis, or gastrointestinal disease, that the diagnosis becomes clear (Table 89-2). Other important features of this group include the frequent presence of HLA-B27 and the need for earlier treatment with tumor necrosis factor (TNF) blockers.

LABORATORY AND IMAGING STUDIES
Most children with oligoarticular JIA have no laboratory abnormalities. Children with polyarticular and systemic-onset disease commonly show elevated acute phase reactants and anemia of chronic disease. In all pediatric patients with joint or bone pain, a complete blood count should be performed to exclude leukemia, which also can present with limb pain (see Chapter 155). All patients with oligoarticular JIA should have an antinuclear antibody test to help identify those at higher risk for uveitis. Older children and adolescents with polyarticular disease should have a rheumatoid factor performed to identify children with early onset adult rheumatoid arthritis.

Diagnostic arthrocentesis may be necessary to exclude suppurative arthritis in children who present with acute onset of monarticular symptoms. The synovial fluid white blood cell count is typically less than 50,000 to 100,000/mm³ and should be predominantly lymphocytes, rather than neutrophils seen with suppurative arthritis. Gram stain and culture should be negative (see Chapter 118).

The most common radiologic finding in the early stages of JIA is a normal bone x-ray. Over time, periarticular osteopenia, resulting from decreased mineralization, is most commonly found. Growth centers may be slow to develop, whereas there may be accelerated maturation of growth plates or evidence of bony proliferation. Erosions of bony articular surfaces may be a late finding. If the cervical spine is involved, fusion of C1-4 may occur, and atlantoaxial subluxation may be demonstrable.

DIFFERENTIAL DIAGNOSIS
The diagnosis of JIA is established by the presence of arthritis, the duration of the disease for at least 6 weeks, and exclusion of other possible diagnoses. Although a presumptive diagnosis

of systemic-onset JIA can be established for a child during the systemic phase, a definitive diagnosis is not possible until arthritis develops. Children must be younger than 16 years of age at time of onset of disease; the diagnosis of JIA does not change when the child becomes an adult. Because there are so many other causes of arthritis, these disorders need to be excluded before providing a definitive diagnosis of JIA (Table 89-3). The acute arthritides can affect the same joints as JIA but have a shorter time course.

TREATMENT

The treatment of JIA focuses on suppressing inflammation, preserving and maximizing function, preventing deformity, and preventing blindness. Nonsteroidal anti-inflammatory drugs (NSAIDs) are the first choice in the treatment of JIA. Naproxen, sulindac, ibuprofen, indomethacin, and others have been used successfully. Systemic corticosteroid medications, such as prednisone and prednisolone, should be avoided in all but the most extreme circumstances, such as for severe systemic-onset JIA with internal organ involvement or for significant active arthritis leading to the inability to ambulate. In this circumstance, the corticosteroids are used as **bridging therapy** until other medications take effect. For patients with a few isolated inflamed joints, intra-articular corticosteroids may be helpful.

Second-line medications, such as hydroxychloroquine and sulfasalazine, have been used in patients whose arthritis is not completely controlled with NSAIDs alone. **Methotrexate,** given either orally or subcutaneously, has become the drug of choice for polyarticular and systemic-onset JIA, which may not respond to baseline agents alone. Methotrexate can cause bone marrow suppression and hepatotoxicity; regular monitoring can minimize these risks. Leflunomide, with a similar adverse effect profile to methotrexate, has also been used. Biologic agents that inhibit TNF-α and block the inflammatory cascade, including **etanercept, infliximab,** and **adalimumab,** are effective in the treatment of JIA. The risks of these agents are greater, however, and include serious infection and, possibly, increased risk of malignancy. Anakinra, an interleukin-1 receptor antagonist, is very beneficial in the treatment of the systemic features of systemic-onset JIA.

COMPLICATIONS

Complications with JIA result primarily from the loss of function of an involved joint secondary to contractures, bony fusion, or loss of joint space. Physical and occupational therapies, professionally and through home programs, are crucial to preserve and maximize function. More serious complications stem from associated uveitis; if left untreated, it can lead to serious visual loss or blindness.

PROGNOSIS

The prognosis of JIA is excellent, with an overall 85% complete remission rate. Children with oligoarticular JIA uniformly tend to do well, whereas children with polyarticular disease and systemic-onset disease constitute most children with functional disability. Systemic-onset disease, a positive rheumatoid factor, poor response to therapy, and the presence of erosions on x-ray all connote a poorer prognosis. The importance of physical and occupational therapy cannot be overstated because when the disease remits, the physical limitations remain with the patient into adulthood.

Table 89-3 | Differential Diagnosis of Juvenile Arthritis

CONNECTIVE TISSUE DISEASES
Juvenile idiopathic arthritis
Systemic lupus erythematosus
Juvenile dermatomyositis
Scleroderma with arthritis
INFECTIOUS ARTHRITIS
Bacterial arthritis
Viral arthritis
Fungal arthritis
Lyme disease
REACTIVE ARTHRITIS
Poststreptococcal arthritis
Rheumatic fever
Toxic synovitis
Henoch-Schönlein purpura
Reiter syndrome
ORTHOPEDIC DISORDERS
Traumatic arthritis
Legg-Calve-Perthes disease
Slipped capital femoral epiphysis
Osteochondritis dissecans
Chondromalacia patellae
MUSCULOSKELETAL PAIN SYNDROMES
Growing pains
Hypermobility syndromes
Myofascial pain syndromes/fibromyalgia
Reflex sympathetic dystrophy
HEMATOLOGIC/ONCOLOGIC DISORDERS
Leukemia
Lymphoma
Sickle cell disease
Thalassemia
Malignant and benign tumors of bone, cartilage, or synovium
Metastatic bone disease
Hemophilia
MISCELLANEOUS
Rickets/metabolic bone disease
Lysosomal storage diseases
Heritable disorders of collagen

SYSTEMIC LUPUS ERYTHEMATOSUS

ETIOLOGY

Systemic lupus erythematosus (SLE) is a multisystem disorder of unknown etiology characterized by a production of large amounts of **circulating autoantibodies.** This antibody production may be due to loss of T-lymphocyte control on B-lymphocyte activity, leading to hyperactivity of B lymphocytes, which leads to nonspecific and specific antibody and autoantibody production. These antibodies form immune complexes that become trapped in the microvasculature, leading to inflammation and ischemia.

EPIDEMIOLOGY

Although SLE affects primarily women of childbearing age, approximately 5% of cases present in childhood, mainly around puberty. SLE is rare in children younger than 9 years of age. Although there is a female predominance of this disease in adolescence and adulthood, there is an equal gender distribution in children. The overall prevalence of SLE in the pediatric population is 10 to 25 cases per 100,000 children.

CLINICAL MANIFESTATIONS

Patients with SLE can present either in an abrupt fashion with fulminant disease or in an indolent manner (Tables 90-1 and 90-2). Nonspecific symptoms are common but can be quite profound and may include significant fatigue and malaise, low-grade fever, and weight loss.

Skin disease can be a prominent finding, occurring in up to 95% of patients. A raised, erythematous rash on the cheeks, called a *malar butterfly rash,* is common (Fig. 90-1). This rash also can occur across the bridge of the nose, on the forehead, and on the chin. **Photosensitivity** can be problematic, particularly during the summer months. Both of these rashes improve with appropriate therapy. The rash of **discoid lupus,** by contrast, is an inflammatory process that leads to disruption of the dermal-epidermal junction, resulting in permanent scarring and loss of pigmentation in the affected area. If discoid lupus occurs in the scalp, permanent alopecia ensues because of loss of hair follicles. **Raynaud phenomenon,** although not specific for SLE, and livedo reticularis also can occur.

Mouth and nasal sores resulting from mucosal ulceration are a common complaint in patients with SLE and can lead to ulceration and perforation of the nasal septum. Because of reticuloendothelial system stimulation, lymphadenopathy and splenomegaly are common findings in SLE. In particular, axillary lymphadenopathy can be a sensitive indicator of disease activity. Serositis can be seen, with chest pain and pleural or pericardial friction rubs or frank effusion.

Renal involvement is one of the most serious manifestations of SLE and is common in pediatric SLE, occurring in 50% to 70% of children. Renal disease may range from microscopic

Table 90-1	Criteria for Diagnosis of Systemic Lupus Erythematosus*
PHYSICAL SIGNS	
Malar *butterfly* rash	
Discoid lupus	
Photosensitivity	
Oral and nasopharyngeal ulcers	
Nonerosive arthritis (more than two joints with effusion and tenderness)	
Pleuritis or pericarditis (serositis)	
Seizures or psychosis in absence of metabolic toxins or drugs	
LABORATORY DATA	
RENAL DISEASE (NEPHRITIS)	
Proteinuria (>500 mg/24 h) or	
Cellular casts (RBC, granular, or tubular)	
HEMATOLOGIC DISEASE	
Hemolytic anemia with reticulocytosis or	
Leukopenia (<4000 on two occasions) or	
Lymphopenia (<1500 on two occasions) or	
Thrombocytopenia (<100,000/mm^3)	
SEROLOGIC DATA	
Positive anti-dsDNA *or*	
Positive anti-Sm *or*	
Evidence of presence of antiphospholipid antibodies	
IgG or IgM anticardiolipin antibodies *or*	
Lupus anticoagulant *or*	
False-positive VDRL for >6 mo	
Positive ANA in absence of drugs known to induce lupus	

ANA, Antinuclear antibody; *RBC,* red blood cell; *VDRL,* Venereal Disease Research Laboratory.
*These are the 1997 revised criteria for diagnosing systemic lupus erythematosus (SLE). A patient must have 4 of the 11 criteria to establish the diagnosis of SLE. These criteria may be present at the same or at different times during the patient's illness. Additional, less specific diagnostic manifestations are noted in Table 90-2.

proteinuria or hematuria to gross hematuria, nephrotic syndrome, and renal failure. Hypertension or the presence of edema suggests lupus renal disease.

Arthralgias and arthritis are common. The arthritis is rarely deforming and typically involves the small joints of the hands; any joint may be involved. Myalgias or frank myositis, with muscle weakness and muscle fatigability, may occur. SLE can affect the central nervous system (CNS), leading to a myriad of symptoms ranging from poor school performance and difficulty concentrating, to seizures, psychosis, and stroke.

LABORATORY AND IMAGING STUDIES

Testing for SLE is performed to establish the diagnosis, determine prognosis, and monitor response to therapy. Although nonspecific, a positive **antinuclear antibody** is found in more than 97% of patients with SLE, usually at high titers. Because of its high sensitivity, a negative antinuclear antibody has a high negative predictive value for SLE. The presence of

Table 90-2	Additional Manifestations of Systemic Lupus Erythematosus

SYSTEMIC

Fever

Malaise

Weight loss

Fatigue

MUSCULOSKELETAL

Myositis, myalgia

Arthralgia

CUTANEOUS

Raynaud phenomenon

Alopecia

Urticaria-angioedema

Panniculitis

Livedo reticularis

NEUROPSYCHIATRIC

Personality disorders

Stroke

Peripheral neuropathy

Chorea

Transverse myelitis

Migraine headaches

Depression

CARDIOPULMONARY

Endocarditis

Myocarditis

Pneumonitis

OCULAR

Episcleritis

Sicca syndrome

Retinal cytoid bodies

GASTROINTESTINAL

Pancreatitis

Mesenteric arteritis

Serositis

Hepatomegaly

Hepatitis (chronic lupoid)

Splenomegaly

RENAL

Nephritis

Nephrosis

Uremia

Hypertension

REPRODUCTIVE

Repeat spontaneous abortions

Neonatal lupus erythematosus

Congenital heart block

Figure 90-1 Malar *butterfly* rash on teenage boy with systemic lupus erythematosus. Note erythema on cheeks and chin, sparing the nasolabial folds.

antibodies to double-stranded DNA should raise suspicion for SLE because these antibodies are present in most patients with SLE and are found almost exclusively in the disease. Titers of anti-double-stranded DNA antibodies are quantifiable and vary with disease activity. Antibodies directed against Sm (Smith) are specific to SLE but are found in only approximately 30% of persons with SLE, limiting its clinical utility. Antibodies to Ro (SSA) and La (SSB) also can be found in patients with SLE, but they also occur in patients with Sjögren syndrome. Likewise patients with SLE can have antibodies directed against phospholipids, which also can be seen in other rheumatologic diseases and in primary antiphospholipid syndrome.

These antibodies lead to an increased risk of arterial and venous thrombosis and can be detected by the presence of anticardiolipin antibodies, a false-positive Venereal Disease Research Laboratory (VDRL) test, or a prolonged activated partial thromboplastin time.

Hematologic abnormalities also are prevalent in patients with SLE. Leukopenia, primarily manifest as lymphopenia, is common. Thrombocytopenia and anemia of chronic disease may be found. Rarely patients with SLE develop Coombs-positive autoimmune hemolytic anemia. Excessive antibody production can lead to polyclonal hypergammopathy with an elevated globulin fraction in the serum. Excessive circulating antibodies and immune complexes also lead to the consumption of complement proteins, with low levels of C3 and C4 and decreased complement function as measured by CH50. Effective therapy returns the low complement levels to normal. This is one way to monitor therapy except in patients with familial deficiency in complement components, which, itself, predisposes to SLE.

Urinalysis may show hematuria and proteinuria, identifying patients with lupus nephritis. Serum blood urea nitrogen and creatinine evaluate renal function. Hypoalbuminemia and hypoproteinemia may be present. Elevation of muscle enzymes may be a clue for the presence of myositis. Elevated cerebrospinal fluid (CSF) protein and an elevated IgG-to-albumin ratio when comparing CSF with serum (IgG index) can indicate antibody production in the CSF and help diagnose SLE affecting the CNS. CNS lupus has a specific pattern on gadolinium-enhanced magnetic resonance imaging.

DIFFERENTIAL DIAGNOSIS
Because SLE is a multisystem disease, it can be difficult to diagnosis early in the disease course. Suspicion must be high in patients who present with diffuse symptoms, particularly adolescent girls. Many of the clinical manifestations of SLE are found in other inflammatory illnesses and during acute or chronic infection. Criteria have been developed for the diagnosis of SLE (see Table 90-1). The presence of 4 of 11 of these criteria has 98% sensitivity and 97% specificity for SLE.

TREATMENT
Corticosteroids have been the mainstay of treatment for SLE for decades. Initial use of pulse methylprednisolone and high-dose oral prednisone (up to 2 mg/kg) frequently is required, followed by cautious tapering to minimize recurrence of symptoms. Nonsteroidal anti-inflammatory drugs have been used to treat the arthralgias and arthritis associated with SLE. Hydroxychloroquine is used not only for the treatment of lupus skin disease, such as discoid lupus, but as maintenance therapy. Hydroxychloroquine treatment results in longer periods of wellness between flares of disease as well as decreased numbers of flares.

Corticosteroids and hydroxychloroquine frequently are not sufficient therapies for lupus nephritis or cerebritis. Cyclophosphamide is effective for the worst forms of lupus nephritis, with significant improvements in outcome and decreased rates of progression to renal failure. CNS lupus responds to cyclophosphamide. For patients who are not able to tolerate the tapering of corticosteroids, the use of steroid-sparing agents, such as azathioprine, methotrexate, or mycophenolate mofetil, may be indicated.

Patients with SLE should be counseled to wear sun block and avoid sun exposure because exposure to the sun precipitates flares of the disease. Because of this prohibition, patients benefit from calcium and vitamin D supplementation to reduce the risk of osteoporosis that may result from prolonged corticosteroid use. Early treatment of hyperlipidemia to decrease long-term cardiovascular complications is also indicated.

COMPLICATIONS
Long-term complications include avascular necrosis secondary to corticosteroid use, infections, and myocardial infarction. Adult patients with SLE develop accelerated atherosclerosis, not only because of prolonged corticosteroid use but also due to the underlying disease. All patients with SLE should be counseled regarding their weight and maintaining an active lifestyle to reduce other cardiac risk factors.

PROGNOSIS
Outcomes for SLE have improved significantly over the past several decades and depend largely on the organ systems that are involved. Worse prognoses are seen in patients with severe lupus nephritis or cerebritis, with risk of chronic disability or progression to renal failure. With current therapy for the disease and the success of renal transplantation, however, most patients live well into adulthood.

Chapter **91**

JUVENILE DERMATOMYOSITIS

ETIOLOGY
The etiology of juvenile dermatomyositis (JDM) is unknown. It is characterized by activation of T and B lymphocytes, leading to vasculitis affecting small vessels of skeletal muscle, with immune complex deposition and subsequent inflammation of blood vessels and muscle. JDM may follow infections, allergic reactions, or sun exposure, but no causal relationship has been shown.

EPIDEMIOLOGY
JDM is a rare disease, with an incidence of less than 0.1:100,000 children. JDM can occur in all age groups with a peak incidence between 4 to 10 years. The disease is slightly more common in girls than boys.

CLINICAL MANIFESTATIONS
Dermatomyositis tends to present in a slow, progressive fashion, with insidious onset of fatigue, malaise, and progressive muscle weakness, accompanied by low-grade fevers and rash. Some children present in an acute fashion, however, with rapid onset of severe disease.

The muscle disease of JDM primarily affects the proximal muscles, particularly the hip and shoulder girdles, and the abdominal and neck muscles. Children have difficulty climbing steps, getting out of chairs, and getting off the floor. The patient may have a positive **Gower sign.** In severe cases, the patient is not able to sit up from a supine position or even lift the head off the examination table (see Chapter 182). If muscles of the upper airway and pharynx are involved, the patient's voice will sound nasal and the patient may have difficulty swallowing.

A classic **JDM rash** occurs on the face and across the cheeks but also can be found on the shoulders and back **(shawl sign).** Patients may have **heliotrope discoloration** of the eyelids. Scaly, red plaques **(Gottron papules)** classically are found across the knuckles but can be found on the extensor surfaces of any joint. Patients may have periungual erythema and **dilated nail-fold capillaries.** Less commonly, patients develop cutaneous vasculitis, with inflammation, erythema, and skin breakdown.

Table 91-1	Criteria for Diagnosis of Juvenile Dermatomyositis*
Rash typical of dermatomyositis	
Symmetric proximal muscle weakness	
Elevated muscle enzymes (ALT, AST, LDH, CPK, and aldolase)	
EMG abnormalities typical of dermatomyositis (fasciculations, needle insertion irritability, and high-frequency discharges)	
Positive muscle biopsy specimen with chronic inflammation	

ALT, Alanine aminotransferase; *AST*, aspartate aminotransferase; *CPK*, creatine phosphokinase; *EMG*, electromyography; *LDH*, lactate dehydrogenase.
*To make a definitive diagnosis of dermatomyositis, four of five criteria are required.

At some point, 15% of patients with JDM develop arthritis, commonly affecting small joints, but any joint may be involved. Raynaud phenomenon, hepatomegaly, and splenomegaly may also occur.

LABORATORY AND IMAGING STUDIES

Many patients with JDM have no evidence of systemic inflammation (normal blood count and erythrocyte sedimentation rate). Evidence of myositis can be identified in 98% of children with active JDM by elevated serum muscle enzymes, including aspartate aminotransferase, alanine aminotransferase, creatine phosphokinase, aldolase, and lactate dehydrogenase. Electromyography and muscle biopsy can document the myositis. Magnetic resonance imaging is a noninvasive means of showing muscle inflammation.

DIFFERENTIAL DIAGNOSIS

Diagnosis of JDM is based on the presence of documented muscle inflammation in the setting of classic rash (Table 91-1). A small percentage of children have muscle disease without skin manifestations, but polymyositis is sufficiently rare in children that they should have a muscle biopsy to exclude other causes of muscle weakness, such as muscular dystrophy (particularly boys). The differential diagnosis also includes postinfectious myositis and other myopathies (see Chapter 182).

TREATMENT

Methotrexate, supplemented by short-term use of systemic corticosteroids, is the cornerstone of therapy for JDM. Initial treatment with pulse intravenous methylprednisolone is followed by several months of tapering doses of oral prednisone. Early institution of methotrexate significantly decreases the duration of corticosteroid use and its associated toxicities. In severe or refractory cases, it may be necessary to use cyclosporine or cyclophosphamide. Intravenous immunoglobulin is useful as adjunctive therapy. Hydroxychloroquine or dapsone has been used for the skin manifestations. These drugs do not significantly affect the muscle disease. Exposure to the sun worsens the cutaneous manifestations and exacerbates the muscle disease; sunlight may lead to flare. Patients should be advised to wear sun block and refrain from prolonged sun exposure. Accordingly supplementation with calcium and active forms of vitamin D is also indicated.

COMPLICATIONS

The most serious complication of JDM is the development of **calcinosis.** Dystrophic calcification can occur in the skin and soft tissues in any area of the body; it ranges from mild to extensive **(calcinosis universalis).** Although it is difficult to predict who will develop calcinosis, it occurs more commonly in children with cutaneous vasculitis, prolonged disease activity, or delays in onset of therapy. Patients with JDM who develop vasculitis also are at risk for gastrointestinal perforation and gastrointestinal bleeding. JDM has been associated with lipoatrophy and insulin resistance, which can progress to type 2 diabetes. Control of insulin resistance frequently leads to improvement in muscle disease in these patients.

PROGNOSIS

The outcome of JDM depends greatly on the extent of muscle disease and the time between disease onset and initiation of therapy. JDM follows one of three clinical courses: a monophasic course, in which patients are treated and improve without significant sequelae; a chronic recurrent course; and a chronic progressive course marked by poor response to therapy and resulting loss of function. Patients who ultimately develop calcinosis are at risk for chronic loss of mobility, depending on the extent of calcium deposition. The association of dermatomyositis with malignancy seen in adults does not occur in children.

Chapter **92**

MUSCULOSKELETAL PAIN SYNDROMES

GROWING PAINS

Growing pains, or benign musculoskeletal pain syndrome, occur in 10% to 20% of school-age children. The peak age range is 3 to 7 years; the syndrome seems to be more common in boys than girls. There is no known etiology, although there seems to be a familial predisposition.

Children with growing pains complain of deep, crampy pain in the calves and thighs. It most typically occurs in the evening or as nocturnal pain that occasionally can waken the child from sleep. Growing pains tend to be more common in children who are extremely active; bouts are exacerbated by increased physical activity. The physical examination is unremarkable, with no evidence of arthritis or muscular tenderness or weakness. Laboratory studies or x-rays, if performed, are normal.

The **diagnosis** of growing pains is based on a typical history and a normal physical examination. **Hypermobility** excludes the diagnosis. It is important to consider leukemia as a cause of nocturnal leg pain in children of this age group, so it is prudent to document a normal complete blood count.

The **treatment** of growing pains consists of reassurance and a regular bedtime ritual of stretching and relaxation. The pain can be relieved by massage. Some patients may benefit from

Figure 92-1 Hyperextension of the knees, an example of hypermobility.

Table 92-1	Criteria for Diagnosis of Benign Hypermobility*	
Touch thumb to flexor aspect of the forearm	1 point each for right and left	
Extend fifth metacarpophalangeal joint to 90 degrees	1 point each for right and left	
>10 degrees hyperextension of elbow	1 point each for right and left	
>10 degrees hyperextension of knee	1 point each for right and left	
Touch palms to floor with knees straight	1 point	

*>6 points defines hypermobility.

a nighttime dose of acetaminophen or an analgesic dose of a nonsteroidal anti-inflammatory drug (NSAID). Occasionally nocturnal awakening has been of long duration, leading to disruptive behavior patterns. In these cases, intervention must be aimed at decreasing the secondary gain associated with nighttime parental attention and should focus on sleep hygiene. Other than the negative behavioral patterns that can occur, there are no significant complications. Growing pains are not associated with other illnesses and resolve over time.

BENIGN HYPERMOBILITY

Hypermobility syndromes are disorders of unknown etiology that cause musculoskeletal pain secondary to excessive mobility of joints. These disorders most commonly present in children 3 to 10 years of age. Girls are more commonly affected than boys. There is a familial predisposition to hypermobility syndromes.

Hypermobility can be isolated to a specific joint group or can present as a generalized disorder. Symptoms vary depending on the joints involved. The most consistent symptom is pain, which may occur during the day or night. The discomfort may increase after exertion but rarely interferes with regular physical activity. Children with hypermobility of the ankles or feet may complain of chronic leg or back pain.

Joint hypermobility may be quite marked. Range of motion may be exaggerated with excessive flexion or extension at the metacarpophalangeal joints, wrists, elbows, or knees (genu recurvatum) (Fig. 92-1). There may be excessive pronation of the ankles. Hypermobility of the foot (flat foot; pes planus) is shown by the presence of a longitudinal arch of the foot that disappears with weight bearing and may be associated with a shortened Achilles tendon (see Chapter 200). These findings

are rarely associated with tenderness on examination. No laboratory test abnormalities are apparent, and radiographs of affected joints are normal.

The diagnosis of isolated hypermobility is made on the basis of physical examination with demonstration of exaggerated mobility of a joint. Generalized hypermobility is diagnosed by the presence of sufficient criteria (Table 92-1) and the absence of evidence of other underlying disorders. Excessive skin elasticity, easy bruisability, or mitral valve prolapse suggests **Ehlers-Danlos syndrome** or **Marfan syndrome** rather than benign hypermobility.

The **treatment** of hypermobility consists of reassurance and regular stretching, similar to treatment for other benign musculoskeletal disorders. NSAIDs can be administered as needed but do not need to be prescribed on a regular basis. Arch supports can be helpful in children with symptomatic pes planus but are not indicated in the absence of symptoms. Benign hypermobility tends to improve with increasing age and is not associated with long-term complications.

MYOFASCIAL PAIN SYNDROMES AND FIBROMYALGIA

The myofascial pain syndromes are a group of noninflammatory disorders characterized by diffuse musculoskeletal pain, the presence of multiple **tender points,** fatigue, malaise, and poor sleep patterns. The etiology of these disorders is unknown, although there seems to be a familial predisposition. Although these disorders sometimes follow viral infection or trauma, no causal relationship has been shown. The myofascial pain syndromes are most common in adults but can occur in children (particularly >12 years of age). The syndromes are more common in girls than in boys. The prevalence of fibromyalgia in children has been reported to be 6%.

Patients with myofascial pain syndromes complain of long-standing diffuse pain in muscles and in the soft tissues around joints that can occur at any time of day, awaken the patient from sleep, and interfere with regular activities. There is frequently a high degree of school absenteeism, despite maintaining adequate school performance. A significant percentage of patients with myofascial pain syndromes exhibit symptoms consistent with depression. An increased incidence of sexual abuse has been reported in children presenting with fibromyalgia.

Physical examination is typically unremarkable with the exception of the presence of specific points that are painful—not just tender—to digital palpation. These points often are located on the neck, back, lateral epicondyles, greater trochanter, and knees. There is no evidence of arthritis or muscular weakness.

Patients with myofascial pain syndromes frequently undergo extensive medical testing because of the concern for underlying inflammatory disease. These tests are invariably normal. Children may have a false-positive antinuclear antibody, which is found in 20% of the normal pediatric population.

The **diagnosis** of myofascial pain syndrome is based on the presence of multiple tender points in the absence of other illness. To fulfill strict criteria for a diagnosis of fibromyalgia, the patient must have a history of diffuse pain for at least 3 months and the presence of 11 of 18 specific tender points on examination. It is important to exclude underlying inflammatory diseases, such as systemic lupus erythematosus, or the postinfectious fatigue that characteristically follows Epstein-Barr virus and influenza virus infection. Mood and conversion disorders also should be considered.

Treatment consists of pain control, usually using NSAIDs, physical therapy, relaxation techniques, and education regarding sleep hygiene. Patients may require low doses of medications, such as amitriptyline to regulate sleep or gabapentin to reduce pain sensitivity. Education and reassurance are crucial.

Because of the disability associated with myofascial pain syndromes, patients and parents frequently believe that the child has a serious underlying condition and may be resistant to reassurance. It should be emphasized that there is no simple cure, and time and perseverance are required.

The long-term outcomes in the myofascial pain syndromes vary. Patients and families who focus on therapy and are positive in their approach tend to have better outcomes. Patients who demand prolonged evaluations, especially from multiple health care providers, may do more poorly. Overall children with fibromyalgia and myofascial pain syndromes have better prognoses than their adult counterparts.

Suggested Reading

Connelly M, Schanberg L: Latest developments in the assessment and management of chronic musculoskeletal pain syndromes in children, *Curr Opin Rheumatol* 18:496–502, 2006.

Falcini F: Kawasaki disease, *Curr Opin Rheumatol* 18:33–38, 2006.

Feldman BM, Rider LG, Reed AM, et al: Juvenile dermatomyositis and other idiopathic inflammatory myopathies of childhood, *Lancet* 371:2201–2212, 2008.

Gottlieb BS, Ilowite NT: Systemic lupus erythematosus in children and adolescents, *Pediatr Rev* 27:323–330, 2006.

Ravelli A, Martini A: Juvenile idiopathic arthritis, *Lancet* 369:767–778, 2007.

Tizard EJ, Hamilton-Ayres MJJ: Henoch Schonlein purpura, *Arch Dis Child Ed Pract* 93:1–8, 2008.

Infectious Diseases

Matthew P. Kronman and Sherilyn Smith

Chapter 93

ASSESSMENT

Overlapping clinical symptoms caused by infectious and noninfectious illnesses make the diagnosis of some diseases difficult. Clinicians are concerned that an untreated minor infection may progress to a life-threatening illness, if appropriate treatment is not given. However unnecessary treatment with antimicrobial agents may lead to a serious problem— emergence of antimicrobial resistant organisms. Accurate diagnosis of infectious and noninfectious diseases and providing specific treatment only as indicated reduce the unnecessary use of antibiotics.

A thorough assessment of the patient, including a detailed history, complete physical examination, and appropriate diagnostic testing is the cornerstone of optimal care.

INITIAL DIAGNOSTIC EVALUATION

The ability to diagnose specific infections accurately begins with an understanding of the epidemiology; risk factors, including exposures to sick contacts or environmental risks (e.g., zoonosis); and age-related susceptibility reflecting the maturity of the immune system. Obtaining a thorough history and physical examination identifies most of these elements (Tables 93-1 and 93-2) and guides appropriate use of other diagnostic tests.

Unique questions that help identify whether an infection is causing the patient's symptoms include a detailed environmental history (including sick contacts, travel, and animal exposure) (see Table 93-1). Certain infections are more common in specific geographic areas. For instance parasitic infections are more common in tropical climates. Diarrhea may be bacterial, viral, or parasitic in the tropics, but in temperate climates parasitic causes of diarrhea, other than giardiasis, are much less likely. Certain fungal infections have specific geographic distribution (coccidioidomycosis in the southwestern United States, blastomycosis in the upper Midwest, and histoplasmosis in central United States). In other areas, fungal pneumonias are rare except in immunocompromised persons.

An immunization history is critical for determining susceptibility to vaccine preventable diseases. Family history,

especially of unexpected deaths of male infants, may suggest familial immunodeficiency (see Chapters 73 through 76). Localization of symptoms to a specific site may narrow diagnostic possibilities (see Table 93-2).

A complete physical examination is essential to identify signs of infection, which may be systemic, such as fever and shock, or focal, including swelling, erythema, tenderness, and limitation of function. Many infectious diseases are associated with characteristic cutaneous signs (see Table 97-1). Accurate otolaryngologic examination is critical for diagnosing upper respiratory tract infections and otitis media, the most common childhood infectious diseases in the United States.

DIFFERENTIAL DIAGNOSIS

Decision-Making Algorithms
Available @ StudentConsult.com

Fever and Rash
Fever without a Source
Fever of Unknown Origin

Fever does not always represent infection. Rheumatologic disease, inflammatory bowel disease, Kawasaki disease, poisoning, and malignancy also may present with fever. Particularly, children with overwhelming infection may be afebrile or hypothermic. Common symptoms, such as bone pain or lymphadenopathy that suggest infection, may also be due to leukemia, lymphoma, juvenile idiopathic arthritis, or Kawasaki disease (see Chapters 88, 89, and 153). Acute mental status changes or focal neurologic impairment could be manifestations of infections (encephalitis, meningitis, or brain abscess) or noninfectious causes (brain or spinal tumors, inflammatory conditions, postinfectious sequelae, or impairment from toxic ingestions or inhalants). Many manifestations of mucosal allergy (rhinitis, diarrhea) may mimic common infectious diseases (see Chapter 77).

Some infections are prone to recurrence, especially if treatment is suboptimal (inadequate antimicrobial or shorter duration). Recurrent, severe, or unusual (opportunistic) infections suggest the possibility of immunodeficiency (see Chapters 72 and 125).

SCREENING TESTS

Laboratory diagnosis of infection includes examination of bacterial morphology using Gram stain, various culture techniques,

315

Table 93-1	Clues from the History for Risk of Infection

Season of year

Age

General health

Weight change

Fever—presence, duration, and pattern

Previous similar symptoms

Previous infections and other illnesses

Previous surgeries, dental procedures

Preceding trauma

Presence of outbreaks or epidemics in the community

Exposures to infected individuals

Exposures to farm or feral animals and pets

Exposures to ticks and mosquitoes

Sexual history, including possibility of sexual abuse

Illicit drug use

Transfusion of blood or blood products

Travel history

Daycare or school attendance

Sources of water and food (e.g., undercooked meat, unpasteurized dairy products)

Home sanitary facilities and hygiene

Pica

Exposure to soil-borne and waterborne organisms (e.g., swimming in brackish water)

Presence of foreign bodies (e.g., indwelling catheters, shunt, grafts)

Immunization history

Immunodeficiency (chemotherapy, acquired, congenital)

Current medications

molecular microbiologic methods such as polymerase chain reaction, and assessment of the immune response with antibody titers or skin testing. The **acute phase response** is a nonspecific metabolic and inflammatory response to infection, trauma, autoimmune disease, and some malignancies. **Acute phase reactants** such as erythrocyte sedimentation rate and C-reactive protein are commonly elevated during an infection but are not specific for infection and do not identify any specific infection. These tests are often used to monitor response to therapy.

A **complete blood count** is frequently obtained for evidence of infection. The initial response to infection, especially in children, is usually a **leukocytosis** (increased number of circulating leukocytes) with an initial neutrophilic response to both bacterial and viral infections. With most viral infections, this response is transient and is followed quickly by a characteristic mononuclear response. In general, bacterial infections are associated with greater neutrophil counts than viral infections (Table 93-3). A **shift-to-the-left** is an increase in the numbers of circulating immature cells of the neutrophil series, including band forms, metamyelocytes, and myelocytes and indicates the rapid release of cells from the bone marrow. It is characteristic of the early stages of infection and, if sustained, bacterial infections. Transient lymphopenia at the beginning of illness and lasting 24 to 48 hours has been described with many viral infections. **Atypical lymphocytes** are mature T lymphocytes with larger, eccentrically placed, and indented nuclei classically seen with infectious mononucleosis caused by Epstein-Barr virus. Other infections associated with atypical lymphocytosis include cytomegalovirus infection, toxoplasmosis, viral hepatitis, rubella, roseola, mumps, and some drug reactions. **Eosinophilia** is characteristic of allergic diseases but may be seen with tissue-invasive multicellular parasites, such as the migration of the larval stages of parasites through skin, connective tissue, and viscera. High-grade eosinophilia (>30% eosinophils, or a total eosinophil count >3000/μL) frequently occurs during the muscle invasion phase

Table 93-2	Localizing Manifestations of Infection	
SITE	**LOCALIZING SYMPTOMS**	**LOCALIZING SIGNS***
Eye	Eye pain, double vision, photophobia, conjunctival discharge	Periorbital erythema, periorbital edema, drainage, chemosis, limitation of extraocular movements
Ear	Ear pain, drainage	Red bulging tympanic membrane, drainage from ear canal
Upper respiratory tract	Rhinorrhea, sore throat, cough, drooling, stridor, trismus, sinus pain, tooth pain, hoarse voice	Nasal congestion, pharyngeal erythema, enlarged tonsils with exudate, swollen red epiglottis, regional lymphadenopathy
Lower respiratory tract	Cough, chest pain, dyspnea, sputum production, cyanosis	Tachypnea, crackles, wheezing, localized diminished breath sounds, intercostal retractions
Gastrointestinal tract	Nausea, vomiting, diarrhea, abdominal pain (focal or diffuse), anorexia, weight loss	Hypoactive or hyperactive bowel sounds, abdominal tenderness (focal or generalized), hematochezia
Liver	Anorexia, vomiting, dark urine, light stools	Jaundice, hepatomegaly, hepatic tenderness, bleeding diatheses, coma
Genitourinary tract	Dysuria, frequency, urgency, flank or suprapubic pain, vaginal discharge	Costovertebral angle or suprapubic tenderness, cervical motion and adnexal tenderness
Central nervous system	Lethargy, irritability, headache, neck stiffness, seizures	Nuchal rigidity, Kernig sign, Brudzinski sign, bulging fontanelle, focal neurologic deficits, altered mental status, coma
Cardiovascular	Dyspnea, palpitations, fatigue, exercise intolerance, chest pain	Tachycardia, hypotension, cardiomegaly, hepatomegaly, splenomegaly, crackles, petechiae, Osler nodes, Janeway lesions, Roth spots, new or change in murmur, distended neck veins, pericardial friction rub, muffled heart sounds
Musculoskeletal	Limp, bone pain, limited function (pseudoparalysis)	Local swelling, erythema, warmth, limited range of motion, point bone tenderness, joint line tenderness

*Fever usually accompanies infection as a systemic manifestation.

of trichinellosis, the pulmonary phases of ascariasis and hookworm infection (eosinophilic pneumonia), and the hepatic and central nervous system phases of visceral larva migrans.

Other common screening tests include **urinalysis** for urinary tract infections, transaminases for liver function, and **lumbar puncture** for evaluation of the cerebrospinal fluid if there is concern for meningitis or encephalitis (see Chapters 100 and 101). Various tests may help distinguish viral versus bacterial infection, but definitive diagnosis requires identifying the agent by culture or another test, such as polymerase chain reaction.

Cultures are the mainstay of diagnosis of many infections. **Blood cultures** are sensitive and specific for bacteremia, which may be primary or secondary to a focal infection (osteomyelitis, gastroenteritis, urinary tract, and endocarditis). Urine cultures are important to confirm urinary tract infection, which may be occult in young infants. Cultures should be obtained with every lumbar puncture, aspiration, or biopsy of other fluid collections or masses. Specific types of cultures (bacterial, fungal, viral, or mycobacterial) are guided by the clinical problem. Tissue culture techniques are used to identify viruses and intracellular bacterial pathogens.

Antibiotics often are begun before a definitive diagnosis is established, complicating the ability to rely on subsequent cultures for microbiologic diagnosis (see Chapter 95). Although persistent or progressive symptoms, despite antibiotic treatment, may indicate the need to change the regimen, more frequently this indicates the need to stop all antibiotics to facilitate definitive diagnosis by obtaining appropriate cultures. Antibiotics should not be given before obtaining appropriate cultures unless there is a life-threatening situation (e.g., septic shock).

Rapid tests, such as antigen tests, are useful for preliminary diagnosis and are included in numerous bacterial, viral, fungal, and parasitic antigen detection tests. **Serologic tests,** using enzyme-linked immunosorbent assay or Western blotting, showing an IgM response, high IgG titer, or seroconversion between acute and convalescent sera, can be used for diagnosis. **Molecular tests,** such as **polymerase chain reaction** for DNA or RNA, offer the specificity of culture, high sensitivity, and rapid results. When an unusual infection is suspected, a microbiologist should be consulted before samples are obtained.

DIAGNOSTIC IMAGING
The choice of diagnostic imaging mode should be based on the location of the findings. In the absence of localizing signs and during an acute infection, imaging of the entire body is less productive. **Plain x-rays** are useful initial tests for respiratory tract infections. **Ultrasonography** is a noninvasive, nonirradiating technique well suited to infants and children for imaging solid organs. It also is useful to identify soft tissue abscesses with lymphadenitis and to diagnose suppurative arthritis of the hip. **Computed tomography (CT) (with contrast enhancement)** and **magnetic resonance imaging (MRI) (with gadolinium enhancement)** allow characterization of lesions and precise anatomic localization and are the modalities of choice for the brain. CT shows greater bone detail, and MRI shows greater tissue detail. MRI is especially useful for diagnosis of osteomyelitis, myositis, and necrotizing fasciitis. High-resolution CT is useful for complicated chest infections. Judicious use of CT scans is important because of the long-term effects of radiation on children's health. Contrast studies (upper gastrointestinal series, barium enema) are used to identify mucosal lesions of the gastrointestinal tract, whereas CT or MRI is preferred for evaluation of appendicitis and intra-abdominal masses. A voiding cystourethrogram may be used to evaluate for vesicoureteral reflux, a predisposing factor for upper urinary tract infections. **Radionuclide scans,** such as technetium-99m for osteomyelitis and dimercaptosuccinic acid for acute pyelonephritis, are often informative.

Table 93-3	Differentiating Viral from Bacterial Infections	
VARIABLE	**VIRAL**	**BACTERIAL**
Petechiae	Present	Present
Purpura	Rare	If severe
Leukocytosis	Uncommon*	Common
Shift-to-the-left (↑bands)	Uncommon	Common
Neutropenia	Possible	Suggests overwhelming infection
↑ ESR	Unusual*	Common
↑ CRP	Unusual	Common
↑ TNF, IL-1, PAF	Uncommon	Common
Meningitis (pleocytosis)	Lymphocytic†	Neutrophilic
Meningeal signs positive‡	Present	Present

CRP, C-reactive protein; *ESR*, erythrocyte sedimentation rate; *IL*, interleukin; *PAF*, platelet-activating factor; *TNF*, tumor necrosis factor.
*Adenovirus and herpes simplex may cause leukocytosis and increased ESR; Epstein-Barr virus may cause petechiae and increased ESR.
†Early viral (enterovirus, arbovirus) meningitis initially may have a neutrophilic pleocytosis.
‡Nuchal rigidity, bulging fontanelle, Kernig sign, Brudzinski sign.

Chapter **94**

IMMUNIZATION AND PROPHYLAXIS

IMMUNIZATION
Childhood immunization has markedly reduced the impact of major infectious diseases. **Active immunization** induces immunity through the administration of a **vaccine** or **toxoid** (inactivated toxin). **Passive immunization** includes transplacental transfer of maternal antibodies and the administration of antibody, either as immunoglobulin or monoclonal antibody.

Vaccinations may be with live attenuated viruses (measles, mumps, rubella [MMR], varicella, nasal influenza), inactivated or killed viruses (polio, hepatitis A, intramuscular influenza), recombinant products (hepatitis B, human papillomavirus), reassortants (rotavirus), or immunogenic components of bacteria (pertussis, *Haemophilus influenzae* type b, *Neisseria meningitidis,* and *Streptococcus pneumoniae),* including toxoids (diphtheria, tetanus). Many purified polysaccharides are T-independent antigens that initiate B-cell proliferation without involvement of CD4 T lymphocytes and are poor immunogens in children younger than 2 years of age. Conjugation of a polysaccharide to a **protein carrier** induces a T-dependent response in infants and creates immunogenic vaccines for *H. influenzae* type b, *S. pneumoniae, and N. meningitidis.*

Childhood immunization standards and recommendations in the United States (Figs. 94-1 and 94-2) are formulated by the Advisory Committee on Immunization Practices of the Centers for Disease Control and Prevention (ACIP), the American Academy of Pediatrics, and the American Academy of Family Physicians. In the United States, due to state laws requiring immunization for school entry, approximately 95% of children entering kindergarten are vaccinated for the common infectious diseases. The ACIP recommends that children in the United States routinely receive vaccines against 16 diseases (see Fig. 94-1). This schedule includes up to 21 injections in four to five visits by 18 months of age. Children and adolescents who are at increased risk for pneumococcal infections should receive the pneumococcal polysaccharide vaccine, as well. Children who are behind in immunization should receive catch-up immunizations as rapidly as feasible. Infants born prematurely, regardless of birth weight, should be vaccinated at the same chronologic age and according to the same schedule as full-term infants and children (see Fig. 94-2). The single exception to this practice is providing hepatitis B vaccine for infants weighing less than 2000 g if the mother is hepatitis B virus surface antigen (HB$_s$Ag)-negative at 1 month instead of at birth. Vaccines for adolescents should be given at 11 to 12 years of age (see Fig. 94-1), with completion of any vaccine series at 13 to 18 years of age and a booster for *N. meningitidis* at 16 years of age.

Vaccines should be administered after obtaining informed consent. The **National Childhood Vaccine Injury Act** requires that all health care providers provide parents or patients with copies of **Vaccine Information Statements** prepared by the Centers for Disease Control and Prevention (http://www.cdc.gov/vaccines/pubs/vis/default.htm) before administering each vaccine dose.

Most vaccines are administered by intramuscular or subcutaneous injection. The preferred sites for administration are the anterolateral aspect of the thigh in infants and the deltoid region in children and adults. Multiple vaccines can be administered simultaneously at anatomically separate sites (different limbs, or separated by >1 in.) without diminishing the immune response. MMR and varicella vaccines should be administered simultaneously or more than 30 days apart. Administration of blood products and immunoglobulin can diminish response to live virus vaccines if administered before the recommended interval.

General contraindications to vaccination include serious allergic reaction (anaphylaxis) after a previous vaccine dose or to a vaccine component, immunocompromised states or pregnancy (live virus vaccines), and moderate or severe acute illness with or without fever. History of *anaphylactic-like* reactions to eggs is a contraindication to influenza and yellow fever vaccines, which are produced in embryonated chicken eggs. Current preparations of measles and mumps vaccines, which are produced in chick embryo fibroblast tissue culture,

do not contain significant amounts of egg proteins and may be administered without testing children with history of egg allergy. Mild acute illness, with or without fever, convalescent phase of illness, recent exposure to infectious diseases, current antimicrobial therapy, breastfeeding, mild to moderate local reaction or low-grade to moderate fever after previous vaccination, and history of penicillin or other nonvaccine allergy or receiving allergen extract immunotherapy are **not contraindications** to immunization.

Severe immunosuppression resulting from congenital immunodeficiency, human immunodeficiency virus (HIV) infection, leukemia, lymphoma, cancer therapy, or a prolonged course of high-dose corticosteroids (>2 mg/kg/day for >2 weeks) predisposes to complications and is a contraindication for live virus vaccines. For HIV-infected children who do not have evidence of severe immunosuppression, MMR vaccination is recommended at 12 months of age with a second dose 1 month later rather than waiting until 4 to 6 years of age. Varicella vaccine is contraindicated for persons with cellular immunodeficiency but is recommended for persons with impaired humoral immunity (hypogammaglobulinemia or dysgammaglobulinemia) and at 12 months of age for HIV-infected children without evidence of severe immunosuppression, given as two doses 3 months apart.

The National Childhood Vaccine Injury Act requires that clinically significant adverse events after vaccination be reported to the **Vaccine Adverse Event Reporting System (VAERS)** (http://www.vaers.hhs.gov or (800) 822-7967). Suspected cases of vaccine-preventable diseases should be reported to state or local health departments. The act also established the **National Vaccine Injury Compensation Program,** a no-fault system in which persons thought to have suffered an injury or death as a result of administration of a covered vaccine can seek compensation.

PROPHYLAXIS

Prophylaxis may include antibiotics, immunoglobulin or monoclonal antibody, vaccine, alone or in combination; they may be used postexposure, for perinatal exposure, and preexposure for persons at increased risk for infection. **Primary prophylaxis** is used to prevent infection before a first occurrence. **Secondary prophylaxis** is used to prevent recurrence after a first episode.

Meningococcus

Primary prophylaxis to all contacts of index cases of *N. meningitidis* infection should be administered as soon as possible (see Chapter 100). Prophylaxis is recommended for all household contacts, especially young children; child care or nursery school contacts in the previous 7 days; for direct exposure to the index patient's secretions through kissing or sharing of toothbrushes or eating utensils; and for mouth-to-mouth resuscitation or unprotected contact during endotracheal intubation within 7 days before onset of illness. Prophylaxis is also recommended for contacts who frequently sleep or eat in the same dwelling as the index patient or passengers seated directly next to the index case during airline flights lasting longer than 8 hours. Chemoprophylaxis is not recommended for casual contacts with no history of direct exposure to the patient's oral secretions (school or work mate), indirect

Recommended immunization schedule for persons aged 0 through 18 years – 2013.
(FOR THOSE WHO FALL BEHIND OR START LATE, SEE THE CATCH-UP SCHEDULE [FIGURE 94-2]).

These recommendations must be read with the footnotes that follow. For those who fall behind or start late, provide catch-up vaccination at the earliest opportunity as indicated by the green bars in Figure 94-1. To determine minimum intervals between doses, see the catch-up schedule (Fig. 94-2). School entry and adolescent vaccine age groups are in bold.

Vaccines	Birth	1 mo	2 mos	4 mos	6 mos	9 mos	12 mos	15 mos	18 mos	19–23 mos	2-3 yrs	4-6 yrs	7-10 yrs	11-12 yrs	13–15 yrs	16–18 yrs
Hepatitis B[1] (HepB)	1st dose	←2nd dose→			←———————— 3rd dose ————————→											
Rotavirus[2] (RV) RV-1 (2-dose series); RV-5 (3-dose series)			1st dose	2nd dose	See footnote 2											
Diphtheria, tetanus, & acellular pertussis[3] (DTaP: <7 yrs)			1st dose	2nd dose	3rd dose		←———— 4th dose ————→					5th dose				
Tetanus, diphtheria, & acellular pertussis[4] (Tdap: ≥7 yrs)														(Tdap)		
Haemophilus influenzae type b[5] (Hib)			1st dose	2nd dose	See footnote 5		←— 3rd or 4th dose, see footnote 5 —→									
Pneumococcal conjugate[6a,c] (PCV13)			1st dose	2nd dose	3rd dose		←— 4th dose —→									
Pneumococcal polysaccharide[6b,c] (PPSV23)																
Inactivated Poliovirus[7] (IPV) (<18years)			1st dose	2nd dose	←———————— 3rd dose ————————→							4th dose				
Influenza[8] (IIV; LAIV) 2 doses for some : see footnote 8					Annual vaccination (IIV only)						Annual vaccination (IIV or LAIV)					
Measles, mumps, rubella[9] (MMR)						←— 1st dose —→						2nd dose				
Varicella[10] (VAR)						←— 1st dose —→						2nd dose				
Hepatitis A[11] (HepA)						←— 2 dose series, see footnote 11 —→										
Human papillomavirus[12] (HPV2: females only; HPV4: males and females)					see footnote 13									(3-dose series)		
Meningococcal[13] (Hib-MenCY ≥6 weeks; MCV4-D ≥ 9 mos; MCV4-CRM ≥ 2 yrs.)														1st dose		booster

Legend:
- Range of recommended ages for all children
- Range of recommended ages for catch-up immunization
- Range of recommended ages for certain high-risk groups
- Range of recommended ages during which catch-up is encouraged and for certain high-risk groups
- Not routinely recommended

This schedule includes recommendations in effect as of January 1 2013. Any dose not administered at the recommended age should be administered at a subsequent visit, when indicated and feasible. The use of a combination vaccine generally is preferred over separate injections of its equivalent component vaccines. Vaccination providers should consult the relevant Advisory Committee on Immunization Practices (ACIP) statement for detailed recommendations, available online at http://www.cdc.gov/vaccines/pubs/acip-list.htm. Clinically significant adverse events that follow vaccination should be reported to the Vaccine Adverse Event Reporting System (VAERS) online (http://www.vaers.hhs.gov) or by telephone (800-822-7967). Suspected cases of vaccine-preventable diseases should be reported to the state or local health department. Additional information, including precautions and contraindications for vaccination, is available from CDC online (http://www.cdc.gov/vaccines) or by telephone (800-CDC-INFO [800-232-4636]).

This schedule is approved by the Advisory Committee on Immunization Practices (http://www.cdc.gov/vaccines/acip/index.html), the American Academy of Pediatrics (http://www.aap.org), the American Academy of Family Physicians (http://www.aafp.org), and the American College of Obstetricians and Gynecologists (http://www.acog.org).

Figure 94-1 Recommended immunization schedules for persons ages 0 through 18 years—United States, 2013. (Approved by the Advisory Committee on Immunization Practices; American Academy of Pediatrics; American Academy of Family Physicians; and American College of Obstetricians and Gynecologists). (Courtesy of the U.S. Department of Health and Human Services, Centers for Disease Control and Prevention, http://www.cdc.gov/vaccines/schedules/hcp/child-adolescent.html.)

Continued

For further guidance on the use of the vaccines mentioned below, see: http://www.cdc.gov/vaccines/pubs/acip-list.htm.

1. **Hepatitis B (HepB) vaccine. (Minimum age: birth)**
   Routine vaccination:
   At birth
   • Administer monovalent HepB vaccine to all newborns before hospital discharge.
   • For infants born to hepatitis B surface antigen (HBsAg)–positive mothers, administer HepB vaccine and 0.5 mL of hepatitis B immune globulin (HBIG) within 12 hours of birth. These infants should be tested for HBsAg and antibody to HBsAg (anti-HBs) 1 to 2 months after completion of the HepB series, at age 9 through 18 months (preferably at the next well-child visit).
   • If mother's HBsAg status is unknown, within 12 hours of birth administer HepB vaccine to all infants regardless of birth weight. For infants weighing <2,000 grams, administer HBIG in addition to HepB within 12 hours of birth. Determine mother's HBsAg status as soon as possible and, if she is HBsAg-positive, also administer HBIG for infants weighing ≥ 2,000 grams (no later than age 1 week).
   Doses following the birth dose
   • The second dose should be administered at age 1 or 2 months. Monovalent HepB vaccine should be used for doses administered before age 6 weeks.
   • Infants who did not receive a birth dose should receive 3 doses of a HepB-containing vaccine on a schedule of 0, 1 to 2 months, and 6 months starting as soon as feasible. See Figure 2.
   • The minimum interval between dose 1 and dose 2 is 4 weeks and between dose 2 and 3 is 8 weeks. The final (third or fourth) dose in the HepB vaccine series should be administered no earlier than age 24 weeks, and at least 16 weeks after the first dose.
   • Administration of a total of 4 doses of HepB vaccine is recommended when a combination vaccine containing HepB is administered after the birth dose.
   Catch-up vaccination:
   • Unvaccinated persons should complete a 3-dose series.
   • A 2-dose series (doses separated by at least 4 months) of adult formulation Recombivax HB is licensed for use in children aged 11 through 15 years.
   • For other catch-up issues, see Figure 2.

2. **Rotavirus (RV) vaccines. (Minimum age: 6 weeks for both RV-1 [Rotarix] and RV-5 [RotaTeq]).**
   Routine vaccination:
   • Administer a series of RV vaccine to all infants as follows:
      1. If RV-1 is used, administer a 2-dose series at 2 and 4 months of age.
      2. If RV-5 is used, administer a 3-dose series at ages 2, 4, and 6 months.
      3. If any dose in series was RV-5 or vaccine product is unknown for any dose in the series, a total of 3 doses of RV vaccine should be administered.
   Catch-up vaccination:
   • The maximum age for the first dose in the series is 14 weeks, 6 days.
   • Vaccination should not be initiated for infants aged 15 weeks 0 days or older.
   • The maximum age for the final dose in the series is 8 months, 0 days.
   • If RV-1(Rotarix) is administered for the first and second doses, a third dose is not indicated.
   • For other catch-up issues, see Figure 2.

3. **Diphtheria and tetanus toxoids and acellular pertussis (DTaP) vaccine. (Minimum age: 6 weeks)**
   Routine vaccination:
   • Administer a 5-dose series of DTaP vaccine at ages 2, 4, 6, 15–18 months, and 4 through 6 years. The fourth dose may be administered as early as age 12 months, provided at least 6 months have elapsed since the third dose.
   Catch-up vaccination:
   • The fifth (booster) dose of DTaP vaccine is not necessary if the fourth dose was administered at age 4 years or older.
   • For other catch-up issues, see Figure 2.

4. **Tetanus and diphtheria toxoids and acellular pertussis (Tdap) vaccine. (Minimum age: 10 years for Boostrix, 11 years for Adacel).**
   Routine vaccination:
   • Administer 1 dose of Tdap vaccine to all adolescents aged 11 through 12 years.
   • Tdap can be administered regardless of the interval since the last tetanus and diphtheria toxoid-containing vaccine.
   • Administer one dose of Tdap vaccine to pregnant adolescents during each pregnancy (preferred during 27 through 36 weeks gestation) regardless of number of years from prior Td or Tdap vaccination.
   Catch-up vaccination:
   • Persons aged 7 through 10 years who are not fully immunized with the childhood DTaP vaccine series, should receive Tdap vaccine as the first dose in the catch-up series; if additional doses are needed, use Td vaccine. For these children, an adolescent Tdap vaccine should not be given.
   • Persons aged 11 through 18 years who have not received Tdap vaccine should receive a dose followed by tetanus and diphtheria toxoids (Td) booster doses every 10 years thereafter.
   • An inadvertent dose of DTaP vaccine administered to children aged 7 through 10 years can count as part of the catch-up series. This dose can count as the adolescent Tdap dose, or the child can later receive a Tdap booster dose at age 11–12 years.
   • For other catch-up issues, see Figure 2.

5. **Haemophilus influenzae type b (Hib) conjugate vaccine. (Minimum age: 6 weeks)**
   Routine vaccination:
   • Administer a Hib vaccine primary series and a booster dose to all infants. The primary series doses should be administered at 2, 4, and 6 months of age; however, if PRP-OMP (PedvaxHib or Comvax) is administered at 2 and 4 months of age, a dose at age 6 months is not indicated. One booster dose should be administered at age 12 through15 months.
   • Hiberix (PRP-T) should only be used for the booster (final) dose in children aged 12 months through 4 years, who have received at least 1 dose of Hib.
   Catch-up vaccination:
   • If dose 1 was administered at ages 12-14 months, administer booster (as final dose) at least 8 weeks after dose 1.
   • If the first 2 doses were PRP-OMP (PedvaxHIB or Comvax), and were administered at age 11 months or younger, the third (and final) dose should be administered at age 12 through 15 months and at least 8 weeks after the second dose.
   • If the first dose was administered at age 7 through 11 months, administer the second dose at least 4 weeks later and a final dose at age 12 through 15 months, regardless of Hib vaccine (PRP-T or PRP-OMP) used for first dose.
   • For unvaccinated children aged 15 months or older, administer only 1 dose.
   • For other catch-up issues, see Figure 2.
   Vaccination of persons with high-risk conditions:
   • Hib vaccine is not routinely recommended for patients older than 5 years

of age. However one dose of Hib vaccine should be administered to unvaccinated or partially vaccinated persons aged 5 years or older who have leukemia, malignant neoplasms, anatomic or functional asplenia (including sickle cell disease), human immunodeficiency virus (HIV) infection, or other immunocompromising conditions.

6a. **Pneumococcal conjugate vaccine (PCV). (Minimum age: 6 weeks)**
   Routine vaccination:
   • Administer a series of PCV13 vaccine at ages 2, 4, 6 months with a booster at age 12 through 15 months.
   • For children aged 14 through 59 months who have received an age-appropriate series of 7-valent PCV (PCV7), administer a single supplemental dose of 13-valent PCV (PCV13).
   Catch-up vaccination:
   • Administer 1 dose of PCV13 to all healthy children aged 24 through 59 months who are not completely vaccinated for their age.
   • For other catch-up issues, see Figure 2.
   Vaccination of persons with high-risk conditions:
   • For children aged 24 through 71 months with certain underlying medical conditions (see footnote 6c), administer 1 dose of PCV13 if 3 doses of PCV were received previously, or administer 2 doses of PCV13 at least 8 weeks apart if fewer than 3 doses of PCV were received previously.
   • A single dose of PCV13 may be administered to previously unvaccinated children aged 6 through 18 years who have anatomic or functional asplenia (including sickle cell disease), HIV infection or an immunocompromising condition, cochlear implant or cerebrospinal fluid leak. See MMWR 2010;59 (No. RR-11), available at http://www.cdc.gov/mmwr/pdf/rr/rr5911.pdf.
   • Administer PPSV23 at least 8 weeks after the last dose of PCV to children aged 2 years or older with certain underlying medical conditions (see footnotes 6b and 6c).

6b. **Pneumococcal polysaccharide vaccine (PPSV23). (Minimum age: 2 years)**
   Vaccination of persons with high-risk conditions:
   • Administer PPSV23 at least 8 weeks after the last dose of PCV to children aged 2 years or older with certain underlying medical conditions (see footnote 6c). A single revaccination with PPSV should be administered after 5 years to children with anatomic or functional asplenia (including sickle cell disease) or an immunocompromising condition.

6c. **Medical conditions for which PPSV23 is indicated in children 2 years and older and for which use of PCV13 is indicated in children aged 24 through 71 months:**
   • Immunocompetent children with chronic heart disease (particularly cyanotic congenital heart disease and cardiac failure); chronic lung disease (including asthma if treated with high-dose oral corticosteroid therapy), diabetes mellitus; cerebrospinal fluid leaks; or cochlear implant.
   • Children with anatomic or functional asplenia (including sickle cell disease and other hemoglobinopathies, congenital or acquired asplenia, or splenic dysfunction).
   • Children with immunocompromising conditions: HIV infection, chronic renal failure and nephrotic syndrome, diseases associated with treatment with immunosuppressive drugs or radiation therapy, including malignant neoplasms, leukemias, lymphomas and Hodgkin disease; or solid organ transplantation, congenital immunodeficiency.

7. **Inactivated poliovirus vaccine (IPV). (Minimum age: 6 weeks)**
   Routine vaccination:
   • Administer a series of IPV at ages 2, 4, 6–18 months, with a booster at age 4–6 years. The final dose in the series should be administered on or after the fourth birthday and at least 6 months after the previous dose.
   Catch-up vaccination:
   • In the first 6 months of life, minimum age and minimum intervals are only recommended if the person is at risk for imminent exposure to circulating poliovirus (i.e., travel to a polio-endemic region or during an outbreak).
   • If 4 or more doses are administered before age 4 years, an additional dose should be administered at age 4 through 6 years.
   • A fourth dose is not necessary if the third dose was administered at age 4 years or older and at least 6 months after the previous dose.
   • If both OPV and IPV were administered as part of a series, a total of 4 doses should be administered, regardless of the child's current age.
   • IPV is not routinely recommended for U.S. residents aged 18 years or older.
   • For other catch-up issues, see Figure 2.

8. **Influenza vaccines. (Minimum age: 6 months for inactivated influenza vaccine [IIV]; 2 years for live, attenuated influenza vaccine [LAIV])**
   Routine vaccination:
   • Administer influenza vaccine annually to all children beginning at age 6 months. For most healthy, nonpregnant persons aged 2 through 49 years, either LAIV or IIV may be used. However, LAIV should NOT be administered to some persons, including 1) those with asthma, 2) children 2 through 4 years who had wheezing in the past 12 months, or 3) those who have any other underlying medical conditions that predispose them to influenza complications. For all other contraindications to use of LAIV see MMWR 2010; 59 (No. RR-8), available at http://www.cdc.gov/mmwr/pdf/rr/rr5908.pdf.
   • Administer 1 dose to persons aged 9 years and older.
   For children aged 6 months through 8 years:
   • For the 2012-13 season, administer 2 doses (separated by at least 4 weeks) to children who are receiving influenza vaccine for the first time. For additional guidance, follow dosing guidelines in the 2012 ACIP influenza vaccine recommendations, MMWR 2012; 61: 613–618, available at http://www.cdc.gov/mmwr/pdf/wk/mm6132.pdf.
   • For the 2013-14 season, follow dosing guidelines in the 2013 ACIP influenza vaccine recommendations.

9. **Measles, mumps, and rubella (MMR) vaccine. (Minimum age: 12 months for routine vaccination)**
   Routine vaccination:
   • Administer the first dose of MMR vaccine at age 12 through 15 months, and the second dose at age 4 through 6 years. The second dose may be administered before age 4 years, provided at least 4 weeks have elapsed since the first dose.
   • Administer 1 dose of MMR vaccine to infants aged 6 through 11 months before departure from the United States for international travel. These children should be revaccinated with 2 doses of MMR vaccine, the first at age 12 through 15 months (12 months if the child remains in an area where disease risk is high), and the second dose at least 4 weeks later.
   • Administer 2 doses of MMR vaccine to children aged 12 months and older, before departure from the United States for international travel. The first dose should be administered on or after age 12 months and the second dose at least 4 weeks later.
   Catch-up vaccination:
   • Ensure that all school-aged children and adolescents have had 2 doses of MMR vaccine; the minimum interval between the 2 doses is 4 weeks.

10. **Varicella (VAR) vaccine. (Minimum age: 12 months)**
   Routine vaccination:
   • Administer the first dose of VAR vaccine at age 12 through 15 months, and the second dose at age 4 through 6 years. The second dose may be administered before age 4 years, provided at least 3 months have elapsed since the first dose. If the second dose was administered at least 4 weeks after the first dose, it can be accepted as valid.

Catch-up vaccination:
   • Ensure that all persons aged 7 through 18 years without evidence of immunity (see MMWR 2007;56 [No. RR-4], available at http://www.cdc.gov/mmwr/pdf/rr/rr5604.pdf) have 2 doses of varicella vaccine. For children aged 7 through 12 years the recommended minimum interval between doses is 3 months (if the second dose was administered at least 4 weeks after the first dose, it can be accepted as valid); for persons aged 13 years and older, the minimum interval between doses is 4 weeks.

11. **Hepatitis A vaccine (HepA). (Minimum age: 12 months)**
   Routine vaccination:
   • Initiate the 2-dose HepA vaccine series for children aged 12 through 23 months; separate the 2 doses by 6 to 18 months.
   • Children who have received 1 dose of HepA vaccine before age 24 months, should receive a second dose 6 to 18 months after the first dose.
   • For any person aged 2 years and older who has not already received the HepA vaccine series, 2 doses of HepA vaccine separated by 6 to 18 months may be administered if immunity against hepatitis A virus infection is desired.
   Catch-up vaccination:
   • The minimum interval between the two doses is 6 months.
   Special populations:
   • Administer 2 doses of Hep A vaccine at least 6 months apart to previously unvaccinated persons who live in areas where vaccination programs target older children, or who are at increased risk for infection.

12. **Human papillomavirus (HPV) vaccines. (HPV4 [Gardasil] and HPV2 [Cervarix]). (Minimum age: 9 years)**
   Routine vaccination:
   • Administer a 3-dose series of HPV vaccine on a schedule of 0, 1-2, and 6 months to all adolescents aged 11-12 years. Either HPV4 or HPV2 may be used for females, and only HPV4 may be used for males.
   • The vaccine series can be started beginning at age 9 years.
   • Administer the second dose 1 to 2 months after the **first** dose and the third dose 6 months after the **first** dose (at least 24 weeks after the first dose).
   Catch-up vaccination:
   • Administer the vaccine series to females (either HPV2 or HPV4) and males (HPV4) at age 13 through 18 years if not previously vaccinated.
   • Use recommended routine dosing intervals (see above) for vaccine series catch-up.

13. **Meningococcal conjugate vaccine (MCV). (Minimum age: 6 weeks for Hib-MenCY, 9 months for Menactra [MCV4-D], 2 years for Menveo [MCV4-CRM]).**
   Routine vaccination:
   • Administer MCV4 vaccine at age 11–12 years, with a booster dose at age 16 years.
   • Adolescents aged 11 through 18 years with human immunodeficiency virus (HIV) infection should receive a 2-dose primary series of MCV4, with at least 8 weeks between doses. See MMWR 2011; 60:1018–1019 available at: http://www.cdc.gov/mmwr/pdf/wk/mm6030.pdf.
   • For children aged 2 months through 10 years with high-risk conditions, see below.
   Catch-up vaccination:
   • Administer MCV4 vaccine at age 13 through 18 years if not previously vaccinated.
   • If the first dose is administered at age 13 through 15 years, a booster dose should be administered at age 16 through 18 years with a minimum interval of at least 8 weeks between doses.
   • If the first dose is administered at age 16 years or older, a booster dose is not necessary.
   • For other catch-up issues, see Figure 2.
   Vaccination of persons with high-risk conditions:
   • For children younger than 19 months of age with anatomic or functional asplenia (including sickle cell disease), administer an infant series of Hib-MenCY at 2, 4, 6, and 12-15 months.
   • For children aged 2 through 18 months with persistent complement component deficiency, administer either an infant series of Hib-MenCY at 2, 4, 6, and 12 through 15 months or a 2-dose primary series of MCV4-D starting at 9 months, with at least 8 weeks between doses. For children aged 19 through 23 months with persistent complement component deficiency who have not received a complete series of Hib-MenCY or MCV4-D, administer 2 primary doses of MCV4-D at least 8 weeks apart.
   • For children aged 24 months and older with persistent complement component deficiency or anatomic or functional asplenia (including sickle cell disease), who have not received a complete series of Hib-MenCY or MCV4-D, administer 2 primary doses of either MCV4-D or MCV4-CRM. If MCV4-D (Menactra) is administered to a child with asplenia (including sickle cell disease), do not administer MCV4-D until 2 years of age and at least 4 weeks after the completion of all PCV13 doses. See MMWR 2011;60:1391–2, available at http://www.cdc.gov/mmwr/pdf/wk/mm6040.pdf.
   • For children aged 9 months and older who are residents of or travelers to countries in the African meningitis belt or to the Hajj, administer an age appropriate formulation and series of MCV4 for protection against serogroups A and W-135. Prior receipt of Hib-MenCY is not sufficient for children traveling to the meningitis belt or the Hajj. See MMWR 2011;60:1391–2, available at http://www.cdc.gov/mmwr/pdf/wk/mm6040.pdf.
   • For children who are present during outbreaks caused by a vaccine serogroup, administer or complete an age and formulation-appropriate series of Hib-MenCY or MCV4.
   • For booster doses among persons with high-risk conditions refer to http://www.cdc.gov/vaccines/pubs/acip-list.htm#mening.

Additional information
   • For contraindications and precautions to use of a vaccine and for additional information regarding that vaccine, vaccination providers should consult the relevant ACIP statement available online at http://www.cdc.gov/vaccines/pubs/acip-list.htm.
   • For the purposes of calculating intervals between doses, 4 weeks = 28 days. Intervals of 4 months or greater are determined by calendar months.
   • Information on travel vaccine requirements and recommendations is available at http://wwwnc.cdc.gov/travel/page/vaccinations.htm.
   • For vaccination of persons with primary and secondary immunodeficiencies, see Table 13, "Vaccination of persons with primary and secondary immunodeficiencies," in General Recommendations on Immunization (ACIP), available at http://www.cdc.gov/mmwr/preview/mmwrhtml/rr6002a1.htm; and American Academy of Pediatrics. Immunization in Special Clinical Circumstances. In: Pickering LK, Baker CJ, Kimberlin DW, Long SS eds. Red book: 2012 report of the Committee on Infectious Diseases. 29th ed. Elk Grove Village, IL: American Academy of Pediatrics.

Figure 94-1, cont'd

The figure below provides catch-up schedules and minimum intervals between doses for children whose vaccinations have been delayed. A vaccine series does not need to be restarted, regardless of the time that has elapsed between doses. Use the section appropriate for the child's age. Always use this table in conjunction with Figure 94-1 and the footnotes that follow.

Vaccine	Minimum Age for Dose 1	Minimum Interval Between Doses			
		Dose 1 to dose 2	Dose 2 to dose 3	Dose 3 to dose 4	Dose 4 to dose 5
Persons aged 4 months through 6 years					
Hepatitis B[1]	Birth	4 weeks	8 weeks and at least 16 weeks after first dose; minimum age for the final dose is 24 weeks		
Rotavirus[2]	6 weeks	4 weeks	4 weeks[2]		
Diphtheria, tetanus, pertussis[3]	6 weeks	4 weeks	4 weeks	6 months	6 months[3]
Haemophilus influenzae type b[5]	6 weeks	4 weeks if first dose administered at younger than age 12 months 8 weeks (as final dose) if first dose administered at age 12–14 months No further doses needed if first dose administered at age 15 months or older	4 weeks[5] if current age is younger than 12 months 8 weeks (as final dose)[5] if current age is 12 months or older and first dose administered at younger than age 12 months and second dose administered at younger than 15 months No further doses needed if previous dose administered at age 15 months or older	8 weeks (as final dose) This dose only necessary for children aged 12 through 59 months who received 3 doses before age 12 months	
Pneumococcal[6]	6 weeks	4 weeks if first dose administered at younger than age 12 months 8 weeks (as final dose for healthy children) if first dose administered at age 12 months or older or current age 24 through 59 months No further doses needed for healthy children if first dose administered at age 24 months or older	4 weeks if current age is younger than 12 months 8 weeks (as final dose for healthy children) if current age is 12 months or older No further doses needed for healthy children if previous dose administered at age 24 months or older	8 weeks (as final dose) This dose only necessary for children aged 12 through 59 months who received 3 doses before age 12 months or for children at high risk who received 3 doses at any age	
Inactivated poliovirus[7]	6 weeks	4 weeks	4 weeks	6 months[7] minimum age 4 years for final dose	
Meningococcal[13]	6 weeks	8 weeks[13]	see footnote 13	see footnote 13	
Measles, mumps, rubella[9]	12 months	4 weeks			
Varicella[10]	12 months	3 months			
Hepatitis A[11]	12 months	6 months			
Persons aged 7 through 18 years					
Tetanus, diphtheria; tetanus, diphtheria, pertussis[4]	7 years[4]	4 weeks	4 weeks if first dose administered at younger than age 12 months 6 months if first dose administered at 12 months or older	6 months if first dose administered at younger than age 12 months	
Human papillomavirus[12]	9 years	Routine dosing intervals are recommended[12]			
Hepatitis A[11]	12 months	6 months			
Hepatitis B[1]	Birth	4 weeks	8 weeks (and at least 16 weeks after first dose)		
Inactivated poliovirus[7]	6 weeks	4 weeks	4 weeks[7]	6 months[7]	
Meningococcal[13]	6 weeks	8 weeks[13]			
Measles, mumps, rubella[9]	12 months	4 weeks			
Varicella[10]	12 months	3 months if person is younger than age 13 years 4 weeks if person is aged 13 years or older			

Figure 94-2 Catch-up immunization schedule for persons ages 4 months through 18 years who start late or who are more than 1 month behind—United States, 2013. This figure provides catch-up schedules and minimum intervals between doses for children whose vaccinations have been delayed. A vaccine series does not need to be restarted, regardless of the time that has elapsed between doses. Use the section appropriate for the child's age. Always use this table in conjunction with the Recommended Immunization Schedule for 2013 and the footnotes that follow. (Approved by the Advisory Committee on Immunization Practices; American Academy of Pediatrics; American Academy of Family Physicians; and American College of Obstetricians and Gynecologists.) *(Courtesy of the U.S. Department of Health and Human Services, Centers for Disease Control and Prevention,* http://www.cdc.gov/vaccines/schedules/hcp/child-adolescent.html.*)*

Continued

For further guidance on the use of the vaccines mentioned below, see: http://www.cdc.gov/vaccines/pubs/acip-list.htm.

1. **Hepatitis B (HepB) vaccine. (Minimum age: birth)**
   Routine vaccination:
   At birth
   - Administer monovalent HepB vaccine to all newborns before hospital discharge.
   - For infants born to hepatitis B surface antigen (HBsAg)–positive mothers, administer HepB vaccine and 0.5 mL of hepatitis B immune globulin (HBIG) within 12 hours of birth. These infants should be tested for HBsAg and antibody to HBsAg (anti-HBs) 1 to 2 months after completion of the HepB series, at age 9 through 18 months (preferably at the next well-child visit).
   - If mother's HBsAg status is unknown, within 12 hours of birth administer HepB vaccine to all infants regardless of birth weight. For infants weighing <2,000 grams, administer HBIG in addition to HepB vaccine within 12 hours of birth. Determine mother's HBsAg status as soon as possible and, if she is HBsAg-positive, also administer HBIG for infants weighing ≥ 2,000 grams (no later than age 1 week).
   Doses following the birth dose
   - The second dose should be administered at age 1 or 2 months. Monovalent HepB vaccine should be used for doses administered before age 6 weeks.
   - Infants who did not receive a birth dose should receive 3 doses of a HepB-containing vaccine on a schedule of 0, 1 to 2 months, and 6 months starting as soon as feasible. See Figure 2.
   - The minimum interval between dose 1 and dose 2 is 4 weeks and between dose 2 and 3 is 8 weeks. The final (third or fourth) dose in the HepB vaccine series should be administered no earlier than age 24 weeks, and at least 16 weeks after the first dose.
   - Administration of a total of 4 doses of HepB vaccine is recommended when a combination vaccine containing HepB is administered after the birth dose.
   Catch-up vaccination:
   - Unvaccinated persons should complete a 3-dose series.
   - A 2-dose series (doses separated by at least 4 months) of adult formulation Recombivax HB is licensed for use in children aged 11 through 15 years.
   - For other catch-up issues, see Figure 2.

2. **Rotavirus (RV) vaccines. (Minimum age: 6 weeks for both RV-1 [Rotarix] and RV-5 [RotaTeq]).**
   Routine vaccination:
   - Administer a series of RV vaccine to all infants as follows:
     1. If RV-1 is used, administer a 2-dose series at 2 and 4 months of age.
     2. If RV-5 is used, administer a 3-dose series at ages 2, 4, and 6 months.
     3. If any dose in series was RV-5 or vaccine product is unknown for any dose in the series, a total of 3 doses of RV vaccine should be administered.
   Catch-up vaccination:
   - The maximum age for the first dose in the series is 14 weeks, 6 days.
   - Vaccination should not be initiated for infants aged 15 weeks 0 days or older.
   - The maximum age for the final dose in the series is 8 months, 0 days.
   - If RV-1(Rotarix) is administered for the first and second doses, a third dose is not indicated.
   - For other catch-up issues, see Figure 2.

3. **Diphtheria and tetanus toxoids and acellular pertussis (DTaP) vaccine. (Minimum age: 6 weeks)**
   Routine vaccination:
   - Administer a 5-dose series of DTaP vaccine at ages 2, 4, 6, 15–18 months, and 4 through 6 years. The fourth dose may be administered as early as age 12 months, provided at least 6 months have elapsed since the third dose.
   Catch-up vaccination:
   - The fifth (booster) dose of DTaP vaccine is not necessary if the fourth dose was administered at age 4 years or older.
   - For other catch-up issues, see Figure 2.

4. **Tetanus and diphtheria toxoids and acellular pertussis (Tdap) vaccine. (Minimum age: 10 years for Boostrix, 11 years for Adacel).**
   Routine vaccination:
   - Administer 1 dose of Tdap vaccine to all adolescents aged 11 through 12 years.
   - Tdap can be administered regardless of the interval since the last tetanus and diphtheria toxoid-containing vaccine.
   - Administer one dose of Tdap vaccine to pregnant adolescents during each pregnancy (preferred during 27 through 36 weeks gestation) regardless of number of years from prior Td or Tdap vaccination.
   Catch-up vaccination:
   - Persons aged 7 through 10 years who are not fully immunized with the childhood DTaP vaccine series, should receive Tdap vaccine as the first dose in the catch-up series; if additional doses are needed, use Td vaccine. For these children, an adolescent Tdap vaccine should not be given.
   - Persons aged 11 through 18 years who have not received Tdap vaccine should receive a dose followed by tetanus and diphtheria toxoids (Td) booster doses every 10 years thereafter.
   - An inadvertent dose of DTaP vaccine administered to children aged 7 through 10 years can count as part of the catch-up series. This dose can count as the adolescent Tdap dose, or the child can later receive a Tdap booster dose at age 11–12 years.
   - For other catch-up issues, see Figure 2.

5. **Haemophilus influenzae type b (Hib) conjugate vaccine. (Minimum age: 6 weeks)**
   Routine vaccination:
   - Administer a Hib vaccine primary series and a booster dose to all infants. The primary series doses should be administered at 2, 4, and 6 months of age; however, if PRP-OMP (PedvaxHib or Comvax) is administered at 2 and 4 months of age, a dose at age 6 months is not indicated. One booster dose should be administered at age 12 through15 months.
   - Hiberix (PRP-T) should only be used for the booster (final) dose in children aged 12 months through 4 years, who have received at least 1 dose of Hib.
   Catch-up vaccination:
   - If dose 1 was administered at ages 12-14 months, administer booster (as final dose) at least 8 weeks after dose 1.
   - If the first 2 doses were PRP-OMP (PedvaxHIB or Comvax), and were administered at age 11 months or younger, the third (and final) dose should be administered at age 12 through 15 months and at least 8 weeks after the second dose.
   - If the first dose was administered at age 7 through 11 months, administer the second dose at least 4 weeks later and a final dose at age 12 through 15 months, regardless of Hib vaccine (PRP-T or PRP-OMP) used for first dose.
   - For unvaccinated children aged 15 months or older, administer only 1 dose.
   - For other catch-up issues, see Figure 2.
   Vaccination of persons with high-risk conditions:
   - Hib vaccine is not routinely recommended for patients older than 5 years

of age. However one dose of Hib vaccine should be administered to unvaccinated or partially vaccinated persons aged 5 years or older who have leukemia, malignant neoplasms, anatomic or functional asplenia (including sickle cell disease), human immunodeficiency virus (HIV) infection, or other immunocompromising conditions.

6a. **Pneumococcal conjugate vaccine (PCV). (Minimum age: 6 weeks)**
   Routine vaccination:
   - Administer a series of PCV13 vaccine at ages 2, 4, 6 months with a booster at age 12 through 15 months.
   - For children aged 14 through 59 months who have received an age-appropriate series of 7-valent PCV (PCV7), administer a single supplemental dose of 13-valent PCV (PCV13).
   Catch-up vaccination:
   - Administer 1 dose of PCV13 to all healthy children aged 24 through 59 months who are not completely vaccinated for their age.
   - For other catch-up issues, see Figure 2.
   Vaccination of persons with high-risk conditions:
   - For children aged 24 through 71 months with certain underlying medical conditions (see footnote 6c), administer 1 dose of PCV13 if 3 doses of PCV were received previously, or administer 2 doses of PCV13 at least 8 weeks apart if fewer than 3 doses of PCV were received previously.
   - A single dose of PCV13 may be administered to previously unvaccinated children aged 6 through 18 years who have anatomic or functional asplenia (including sickle cell disease), HIV infection or an immunocompromising condition, cochlear implant or cerebrospinal fluid leak. See MMWR 2010;59 (No. RR-11), available at http://www.cdc.gov/mmwr/pdf/rr/rr5911.pdf.
   - Administer PPSV23 at least 8 weeks after the last dose of PCV to children aged 2 years or older with certain underlying medical conditions (see footnotes 6b and 6c).

6b. **Pneumococcal polysaccharide vaccine (PPSV23). (Minimum age: 2 years)**
   Vaccination of persons with high-risk conditions:
   - Administer PPSV23 at least 8 weeks after the last dose of PCV to children aged 2 years or older with certain underlying medical conditions (see footnote 6c). A single revaccination with PPSV should be administered after 5 years to children with anatomic or functional asplenia (including sickle cell disease) or an immunocompromising condition.

6c. **Medical conditions for which PPSV23 is indicated in children aged 2 years and older and for which use of PCV13 is indicated in children aged 24 through 71 months:**
   - Immunocompetent children with chronic heart disease (particularly cyanotic congenital heart disease and cardiac failure); chronic lung disease (including asthma if treated with high-dose oral corticosteroid therapy), diabetes mellitus; cerebrospinal fluid leaks; or cochlear implant.
   - Children with anatomic or functional asplenia (including sickle cell disease and other hemoglobinopathies, congenital or acquired asplenia, or splenic dysfunction);
   - Children with immunocompromising conditions: HIV infection, chronic renal failure and nephrotic syndrome, diseases associated with treatment with immunosuppressive drugs or radiation therapy, including malignant neoplasms, leukemias, lymphomas and Hodgkin disease; or solid organ transplantation, congenital immunodeficiency.

7. **Inactivated poliovirus vaccine (IPV). (Minimum age: 6 weeks)**
   Routine vaccination:
   - Administer a series of IPV at ages 2, 4, 6–18 months, with a booster at age 4–6 years. The final dose in the series should be administered on or after the fourth birthday and at least 6 months after the previous dose.
   Catch-up vaccination:
   - In the first 6 months of life, minimum age and minimum intervals are only recommended if the person is at risk for imminent exposure to circulating poliovirus (i.e., travel to a polio-endemic region or during an outbreak).
   - If 4 or more doses are administered before age 4 years, an additional dose should be administered at age 4 through 6 years.
   - A fourth dose is not necessary if the third dose was administered at age 4 years or older and at least 6 months after the previous dose.
   - If both OPV and IPV were administered as part of a series, a total of 4 doses should be administered, regardless of the child's current age.
   - IPV is not routinely recommended for U.S. residents aged 18 years or older.
   - For other catch-up issues, see Figure 2.

8. **Influenza vaccines. (Minimum age: 6 months for inactivated influenza vaccine [IIV], 2 years for live, attenuated influenza vaccine [LAIV])**
   Routine vaccination:
   - Administer influenza vaccine annually to all children beginning at age 6 months. For most healthy, nonpregnant persons aged 2 through 49 years, either LAIV or IIV may be used. However, LAIV should NOT be administered to some persons, including 1) those with asthma, 2) children 2 through 4 years who had wheezing in the past 12 months, or 3) those who have any other underlying medical conditions that predispose them to influenza complications. For all other contraindications to use of LAIV see MMWR 2010; 59 (No. RR-8), available at http://www.cdc.gov/mmwr/pdf/rr/rr5908.pdf.
   - Administer 1 dose to persons aged 9 years and older.
   For children aged 6 months through 8 years:
   - For the 2012–13 season, administer 2 doses (separated by at least 4 weeks) to children who are receiving influenza vaccine for the first time. For additional guidance, follow dosing guidelines in the 2012 ACIP influenza vaccine recommendations, MMWR 2012; 61: 613–618, available at http://www.cdc.gov/mmwr/pdf/wk/mm6132.pdf.
   - For the 2013–14 season, follow dosing guidelines in the 2013 ACIP influenza vaccine recommendations.

9. **Measles, mumps, and rubella (MMR) vaccine. (Minimum age: 12 months for routine vaccination)**
   Routine vaccination:
   - Administer the first dose of MMR vaccine at age 12 through 15 months, and the second dose at age 4 through 6 years. The second dose may be administered before age 4 years, provided at least 4 weeks have elapsed since the first dose.
   - Administer 1 dose of MMR vaccine to infants aged 6 through 11 months before departure from the United States for international travel. These children should be revaccinated with 2 doses of MMR vaccine, the first at age 12 through 15 months (12 months if the child remains in an area where disease risk is high), and the second dose at least 4 weeks later.
   - Administer 2 doses of MMR vaccine to children aged 12 months and older, before departure from the United States for international travel. The first dose should be administered on or after age 12 months and the second dose at least 4 weeks later.
   Catch-up vaccination:
   - Ensure that all school-aged children and adolescents have had 2 doses of MMR vaccine; the minimum interval between the 2 doses is 4 weeks.

10. **Varicella (VAR) vaccine. (Minimum age: 12 months)**
   Routine vaccination:
   - Administer the first dose of VAR vaccine at age 12 through 15 months, and the second dose at age 4 through 6 years. The second dose may be administered before age 4 years, provided at least 3 months have elapsed since the first dose. If the second dose was administered at least 4 weeks after the first dose, it can be accepted as valid.

Catch-up vaccination:
   - Ensure that all persons aged 7 through 18 years without evidence of immunity (see MMWR 2007;56 [No. RR-4], available at http://www.cdc.gov/mmwr/pdf/rr/rr5604.pdf) have 2 doses of varicella vaccine. For children aged 7 through 12 years the recommended minimum interval between doses is 3 months (if the second dose was administered at least 4 weeks after the first dose, it can be accepted as valid); for persons aged 13 years and older, the minimum interval between doses is 4 weeks.

11. **Hepatitis A vaccine (HepA). (Minimum age: 12 months)**
   Routine vaccination:
   - Initiate the 2-dose HepA vaccine series for children aged 12 through 23 months; separate the 2 doses by 6 to 18 months.
   - Children who have received 1 dose of HepA vaccine before age 24 months, should receive a second dose 6 to 18 months after the first dose.
   - For any person aged 2 years and older who has not already received the HepA vaccine series, 2 doses of HepA vaccine separated by 6 to 18 months may be administered if immunity against hepatitis A virus infection is desired.
   Catch-up vaccination:
   - The minimum interval between the two doses is 6 months.
   Special populations:
   - Administer 2 doses of Hep A vaccine at least 6 months apart to previously unvaccinated persons who live in areas where vaccination programs target older children, or who are at increased risk for infection.

12. **Human papillomavirus (HPV) vaccines. (HPV4 [Gardasil] and HPV2 [Cervarix]). (Minimum age: 9 years)**
   Routine vaccination:
   - Administer a 3-dose series of HPV vaccine on a schedule of 0, 1-2, and 6 months to all adolescents aged 11-12 years. Either HPV4 or HPV2 may be used for females, and only HPV4 may be used for males.
   - The vaccine series can be started beginning at age 9 years.
   - Administer the second dose 1 to 2 months after the **first** dose and the third dose 6 months after the **first** dose (at least 24 weeks after the first dose).
   Catch-up vaccination:
   - Administer the vaccine series to females (either HPV2 or HPV4) and males (HPV4) at age 13 through 18 years if not previously vaccinated.
   - Use recommended routine dosing intervals (see above) for vaccine series catch-up.

13. **Meningococcal conjugate vaccine (MCV). (Minimum age: 6 weeks for Hib-MenCY, 9 months for Menactra [MCV4-D], 2 years for Menveo [MCV4-CRM]).**
   Routine vaccination:
   - Administer MCV4 vaccine at age 11–12 years, with a booster dose at age 16 years.
   - Adolescents aged 11 through 18 years with human immunodeficiency virus (HIV) infection should receive a 2-dose primary series of MCV4, with at least 8 weeks between doses. See MMWR 2011; 60:1018–1019 available at: http://www.cdc.gov/mmwr/pdf/wk/mm6030.pdf.
   - For children aged 2 months through 10 years with high-risk conditions, see below.
   Catch-up vaccination:
   - Administer MCV4 vaccine at age 13 through 18 years if not previously vaccinated.
   - If the first dose is administered at age 13 through 15 years, a booster dose should be administered at age 16 through 18 years with a minimum interval of at least 8 weeks between doses.
   - If the first dose is administered at age 16 years or older, a booster dose is not needed.
   - For other catch-up issues, see Figure 2.
   Vaccination of persons with high-risk conditions:
   - For children younger than 19 months of age with anatomic or functional asplenia (including sickle cell disease), administer an infant series of Hib-MenCY at 2, 4, 6, and 12-15 months.
   - For children aged 2 through 18 months with persistent complement component deficiency, administer either an infant series of Hib-MenCY at 2, 4, 6, and 12 through 15 months or a 2-dose primary series of MCV4-D starting at 9 months, with at least 8 weeks between doses. For children aged 19 through 23 months with persistent complement component deficiency who have not received a complete series of Hib-MenCY or MCV4-D, administer 2 primary doses of MCV4-D at least 8 weeks apart.
   - For children aged 24 months and older with persistent complement component deficiency or anatomic or functional asplenia (including sickle cell disease), who have not received a complete series of Hib-MenCY or MCV4-D, administer 2 primary doses of either MCV4-D or MCV4-CRM. If MCV4-D (Menactra) is administered to a child with asplenia (including sickle cell disease), do not administer MCV4-D until 2 years of age and at least 4 weeks after the completion of all PCV13 doses. See MMWR 2011;60:1391–2, available at http://www.cdc.gov/mmwr/pdf/wk/mm6040.pdf.
   - For children aged 9 months and older who are residents of or travelers to countries in the African meningitis belt or to the Hajj, administer an age appropriate formulation and series of MCV4 for protection against serogroups A and W-135. Prior receipt of Hib-MenCY is not sufficient for children traveling to the meningitis belt or the Hajj. See MMWR 2011;60:1391–2, available at http://www.cdc.gov/mmwr/pdf/wk/mm6040.pdf.
   - For children who are present during outbreaks caused by a vaccine serogroup, administer or complete an age and formulation-appropriate series of Hib-MenCY or MCV4.
   - For booster doses among persons with high-risk conditions refer to http://www.cdc.gov/vaccines/pubs/acip-list.htm#mening.

Additional information
   - For contraindications and precautions to use of a vaccine and for additional information regarding that vaccine, vaccination providers should consult the relevant ACIP statement available online at http://www.cdc.gov/vaccines/pubs/acip-list.htm.
   - For the purposes of calculating intervals between doses, 4 weeks = 28 days. Intervals of 4 months or greater are determined by calendar months.
   - Information on travel vaccine requirements and recommendations is available at http://wwwnc.cdc.gov/travel/page/vaccinations.htm.
   - For vaccination of persons with primary and secondary immunodeficiencies, see Table 13, "Vaccination of persons with primary and secondary immunodeficiencies," in General Recommendations on Immunization (ACIP), available at http://www.cdc.gov/mmwr/preview/mmwrhtml/rr6002a1.htm; and American Academy of Pediatrics. Immunization in Special Clinical Circumstances. In: Pickering LK, Baker CJ, Kimberlin DW, Long SS eds. Red book: 2012 report of the Committee on Infectious Diseases. 29th ed. Elk Grove Village, IL: American Academy of Pediatrics.

Figure 94-2, cont'd

Table 94-1	Guide to Tetanus Prophylaxis in Routine Wound Management				
	CLEAN MINOR WOUNDS		**ALL OTHER WOUNDS***		
Previous Tetanus Immunization (Doses)	**DTap, Tdap, or Td†**	**TIG†,‡**	**DTap, Tdap, or Td**	**TIG‡**
Uncertain or <3 doses	Yes	No	Yes	Yes
≥3 doses	Yes if ≥10 yr since the last tetanus toxoid-containing vaccine dose	No	Yes if ≥5 yr since the last tetanus toxoid-containing vaccine dose	No

Modified from American Academy of Pediatrics. Pickering LK, editor: Red Book: 2012 report of the committee on infectious diseases, ed 29, Elk Grove Village, IL, 2012, American Academy of Pediatrics.

Tdap, tetanus and diphtheria toxoids, adsorbed (for adolescents >11 yr of age and adults); Td, Tetanus-diphtheria toxoid; TIG, tetanus immunoglobulin.

*Such as, but not limited to, wounds contaminated with dirt, feces, soil, or saliva; puncture wounds; avulsions; and wounds resulting from missiles, crushing, burns, and frostbite.

†Tdap is preferred for adolescents who have never received Tdap. Td is preferred to tetanus toxoid for adolescents who received Tdap previously or when Tdap is not available.

‡Immune globulin intravenous should be used if TIG is not available.

contact with the index patient, or medical personnel without direct exposure to the patient's oral secretions. Rifampin twice daily for 2 days, ceftriaxone once, and ciprofloxacin once (>18 years of age) are the recommended regimens. Azithromycin may be used in the case of resistant organisms.

Tetanus

All postexposure wound treatment begins with immediate, thorough cleansing using soap and water, removal of foreign bodies, and debridement of devitalized tissue. Tetanus prophylaxis after wounds and injuries includes vaccination of persons with incomplete immunization and tetanus immunoglobulin for contaminated wounds (soil, feces, saliva), puncture wounds, avulsions, and wounds resulting from missiles, crushing, burns, and frostbite (Table 94-1).

Rabies

Rabies immune globulin (RIG) and rabies vaccine are extremely effective for prophylaxis after exposure to rabies but are of no known benefit after symptoms appear. Because rabies is one of the deadliest infections, recognition of potential exposure and prophylaxis are crucial. Any healthy-appearing domestic animal responsible for an apparently unprovoked bite should be observed for 10 days for signs of rabies, without immediate treatment of the victim. Prophylaxis should be administered if the animal is rabid or suspected to be rabid, or if the animal develops signs of rabies while under observation. A captured wild animal should be euthanized (by animal control officials) without a period of observation and its brain examined for evidence of rabies. If the biting animal is not captured, particularly if it is a wild animal of a species known to harbor the virus in the region, rabies should be presumed and prophylaxis administered to the victim. Skunks, raccoons, foxes, woodchucks, most other carnivores, and bats are regarded as rabid unless proved negative by testing. Prophylaxis also should be provided following exposure to a bat for persons who might be unaware or unable to relate that a bite or direct contact has occurred, such as a mentally disabled person, a sleeping child, or an unattended infant.

All rabies postexposure management begins with immediate thorough cleansing of the bite using soap and water and, if available, irrigation with a virucidal agent such as povidone-iodine. RIG at a dose of 20 U/kg should be administered, with the full dose of RIG infiltrated subcutaneously into the area around the wound, if possible. Any remaining RIG that cannot be infiltrated into the wound should be administered as an intramuscular injection. Inactivated rabies vaccine should be administered simultaneously as soon as possible, with additional vaccine doses at 3, 7, and 14 days.

Chapter 95

ANTI-INFECTIVE THERAPY

The selection of anti-infective therapy depends on a number of factors: the site of infection and clinical syndrome, host immunity, probable causative agents, the pathogen's susceptibility to antimicrobial agents and the local epidemiology of resistance, the pharmacokinetics of the selected agents, and their pharmacodynamics in specific patient populations.

Empirical or presumptive anti infective therapy is based on a clinical diagnosis combined with published evidence and experience of the probable causative pathogens. **Definitive therapy** relies on microbiologic diagnosis by isolation or other direct evidence of a pathogen. Microbiologic diagnosis permits characterization of the pathogen's anti-infective drug **susceptibilities** and delivery of the appropriate anti-infective agent to the site of infection in concentrations sufficient to kill or alter the pathogen and facilitate an effective immune response. Antiviral therapy must include consideration of the intracellular nature of viral replication and, to avoid toxicity to host cells, must be targeted to viral-specific proteins, such as the thymidine kinase of herpesviruses or the reverse transcriptase of human immunodeficiency virus.

Empirical antimicrobial therapy is best initiated after obtaining appropriate cultures of fluids or tissues. In high-risk circumstances, such as neonatal sepsis or bacteremia in immunocompromised persons, empirical therapy includes broad-spectrum antimicrobials (see Chapters 96 and 120).

Empirical antimicrobial therapy may be tailored to specific pathogens based on the clinical diagnosis (e.g., streptococcal pharyngitis) or defined risks (e.g., close exposure to tuberculosis). Definitive therapy can additionally minimize drug toxicity, development of resistant microorganisms, and cost.

Antimicrobial agents are an adjunct to the normal host immune response. Infections associated with foreign bodies, such as an intravascular catheter, are difficult to eradicate with antimicrobials alone because of organism-produced biofilms that impair phagocytosis. Similarly it is difficult for phagocytic cells to eradicate bacteria amid vegetations of fibrin and platelets on infected heart valves. Prolonged, bactericidal therapy is required with these infections, and outcomes are not always satisfactory. Foreign body devices may have to be removed if sterilization does not occur promptly. Infections in closed spaces with limited perfusion (such as abscesses or chronic osteomyelitis with poorly perfused bone) are difficult to cure without surgical drainage, debridement of the infected tissue, and reestablishment of a good vascular supply.

Optimal antimicrobial therapy requires an understanding of both the **pharmacokinetics** (e.g., bioavailability and tissue penetration) of the administered drugs and their **pharmacodynamics** (e.g., metabolism and excretion by the body) in specific patient populations. The bioavailability of orally administered antibiotics varies, depending on the acid stability of the drug; degree of gastric acidity; and whether it is taken with food, antacids, H_2 blockers, or other medications. An ileus or profuse diarrhea may alter intestinal transit time and result in unpredictable absorption.

The **site and nature** of the infection may affect the choice of antimicrobials. Aminoglycosides, active against aerobic organisms only, have significantly reduced activity in abscesses with low pH and oxygen tension. Infections of the central nervous system or the eye necessitate treatment with antimicrobials that penetrate and achieve therapeutic levels in these sites.

Limited renal function (as in premature infants or those with renal failure) requires increasing dosing intervals to allow time for excretion of certain drugs. The larger volume of distribution of certain hydrophilic antimicrobials and increased renal clearance (e.g., in cystic fibrosis) requires higher doses to achieve therapeutic levels. Weight-based dosage regimens may result in overdoses in obese children due to significantly smaller volumes of distribution for hydrophilic drugs. Determining serum drug levels for antibiotics with narrow safety margins (e.g., aminoglycosides and vancomycin) minimizes adverse effects of treatment.

Drug-drug interactions must be considered when multiple antimicrobial agents are used to treat infection. Use of two or more antimicrobial agents may be justified before organism identification or for the benefit of two drugs with different mechanisms of action. Several antimicrobials are administered routinely in combination (e.g., trimethoprim-sulfamethoxazole, amoxicillin-clavulanate) because of **synergism** (significantly greater bacterial killing or spectrum of activity than when either is used alone). The use of a bacteriostatic drug, such as a tetracycline, along with a β-lactam agent, effective against growing organisms only, may result in antibiotic **antagonism,** or less bacterial killing in the presence of both drugs than if either is used alone.

Chapter 96

FEVER WITHOUT A FOCUS

Decision-Making Algorithms
Available @ StudentConsult.com

Fever without a Source
Fever of Unknown Origin

Core body temperature is normally maintained within 1° C to 1.5° C in a range of 37° C to 38° C. Normal body temperature is generally considered to be 37° C (98.6° F; range, 97° F to 99.6° F). There is a normal diurnal variation, with maximum temperature in the late afternoon. Rectal temperatures higher than 38° C (>100.4° F) generally are considered abnormal, especially if associated with symptoms.

Normal body temperature is maintained by a complex regulatory system in the anterior hypothalamus. Development of fever begins with release of endogenous pyrogens into the circulation as the result of infection, inflammatory processes, or malignancy. Microbes and microbial toxins act as **exogenous pyrogens** by stimulating release of **endogenous pyrogens,** including cytokines such as interleukin-1, interleukin-6, tumor necrosis factor, and interferons. These cytokines reach the anterior hypothalamus, liberating arachidonic acid, which is metabolized to prostaglandin E_2. Elevation of the hypothalamic thermostat occurs via a complex interaction of complement and prostaglandin-E_2 production. Antipyretics (acetaminophen, ibuprofen, aspirin) inhibit hypothalamic cyclooxygenase, decreasing production of prostaglandin E2. Aspirin is associated with Reye syndrome in children and is not recommended as an antipyretic. The response to antipyretics does not distinguish bacterial from viral infections.

The **pattern of fever** in children may vary, depending on age and the nature of the illness. Neonates may not have a febrile response and may be hypothermic, despite significant infection, whereas older infants and children younger than 5 years of age may have an exaggerated febrile response with temperatures of up to 105° F (40.6° C) in response to either a serious bacterial infection or an otherwise benign viral infection. Fever to this degree is unusual in older children and adolescents and suggests a serious process. The fever pattern does not reliably distinguish fever caused by infectious microorganisms from that resulting from malignancy, autoimmune diseases, or drugs.

Children with fever without a focus present a diagnostic challenge that includes identifying bacteremia and sepsis. **Bacteremia,** the presence of bacteria in the bloodstream, may be primary or secondary to a focal infection. **Sepsis** is the systemic response to infection that is manifested by hyperthermia or hypothermia, tachycardia, tachypnea, and shock (see Chapter 40). Children with septicemia and signs of central nervous system dysfunction (irritability, lethargy), cardiovascular impairment (cyanosis, poor perfusion), and disseminated intravascular coagulation (petechiae, ecchymosis) are readily recognized as **toxic appearing** or **septic.** Most febrile illnesses in children may be categorized as follows:

- **Fever of short duration** accompanied by localizing signs and symptoms, in which a diagnosis can often be established by clinical history and physical examination
- **Fever without localizing signs (fever without a focus),** frequently occurring in children younger than 3 years of age, in which a history and physical examination fail to establish a cause
- **Fever of unknown origin (FUO),** defined as fever for >14 days without an identified etiology despite history, physical examination, and routine laboratory tests or after 1 week of hospitalization and evaluation

FEVER IN INFANTS YOUNGER THAN 3 MONTHS OF AGE

Fever or **temperature instability** in infants younger than 3 months of age is associated with a higher risk of **serious bacterial infections** than in older infants. These younger infants usually exhibit only fever and poor feeding, without localizing signs of infection. Most febrile illnesses in this age group are caused by common viral pathogens, but serious bacterial infections include **bacteremia** (caused by group B streptococcus [GBS], *Escherichia coli,* and *Listeria monocytogenes* in neonates; and *Streptococcus pneumoniae, Haemophilus influenzae,* nontyphoidal *Salmonella,* and *Neisseria meningitidis* in 1- to 3-month-old infants), **urinary tract infection (UTI)** *(E. coli),* **pneumonia** *(S. pneumoniae,* GBS, or *Staphylococcus aureus),* **meningitis** (S. *pneumoniae, H. influenzae* type b, GBS, *N. meningitidis,* herpes simplex virus [HSV], enteroviruses), **bacterial diarrhea** *(Salmonella, Shigella, E. coli),* and **osteomyelitis** or **septic arthritis** *(S. aureus* or GBS).

Differentiation between viral and bacterial infections in young infants is difficult. Febrile infants <3 months of age who appear ill, especially if follow-up is uncertain, and all febrile infants <4 weeks of age should be admitted to the hospital for empirical antibiotics pending culture results. After blood, urine, and cerebrospinal fluid cultures are obtained, broad-spectrum parenteral antibiotics (typically ampicillin with cefotaxime or gentamicin) are administered. The choice of antibiotics depends on the pathogens suggested by localizing findings. The possibility of neonatal HSV should also be considered in febrile children <4 weeks old, and empirical acyclovir begun in those in whom neonatal HSV is a concern. Well-appearing febrile infants ≥4 weeks of age without an identifiable focus and with certainty of follow-up are at a low risk of developing a serious bacterial infection (0.8% develop bacteremia, and 2% develop a serious localized bacterial infection). Specific criteria identifying these low-risk infants include age older than 1 month, well-appearing without a focus of infection, no history of prematurity or prior antimicrobial therapy, a white blood cell (WBC) count of 5000 to 15,000/μL, and urine with less than 10 WBCs/high-power field. Fecal leukocyte testing and chest radiograph can be considered in infants with diarrhea or respiratory signs. Low-risk infants may be followed as outpatients without empirical antibiotic treatment, or, alternatively, may be treated with intramuscular ceftriaxone. Regardless of antibiotic treatment, close follow-up for at least 72 hours, including re-evaluation in 24 hours or immediately with any clinical change, is essential.

FEVER IN CHILDREN 3 MONTHS TO 3 YEARS OF AGE

A common problem is the evaluation of a febrile but well-appearing child younger than 3 years of age without localizing signs of infection. Although most of these children have self-limited viral infections, some have **occult bacteremia** (bacteremia without identifiable focus) or UTIs, and a few have severe and potentially life-threatening illnesses. It is difficult, even for experienced clinicians, to differentiate patients with bacteremia from those with benign illnesses.

Observational assessment is a key part of the evaluation. Descriptions of normal appearance and **alertness** include *child looking at the observer* and *looking around the room,* with eyes that are *shiny* or *bright.* Descriptions that indicate severe impairment include *glassy eyes* and *stares vacantly into space.* Observations such as *sitting, moving arms and legs on table or lap,* and *sits without support* reflect normal motor ability, whereas *no movement in mother's arms* and *lies limply on table* indicate severe impairment. Normal behaviors, such as *vocalizing spontaneously, playing with objects, reaching for objects,* smiling, and *crying with noxious stimuli,* reflect **playfulness;** abnormal behaviors reflect **irritability.** Normally, crying children are **consolable** and *stop crying when held by the parent,* whereas severe impairment is indicated by *continual cry despite being held and comforted.*

Children between 2 months and 3 years of age are at increased risk for infection with organisms with polysaccharide capsules, including S. *pneumoniae, H. influenzae, N. meningitidis,* and nontyphoidal *Salmonella.* Effective phagocytosis of these organisms requires opsonic antibody. Transplacental maternal IgG initially provides immunity to these organisms, but as the IgG gradually dissipates, risk of infection increases. In the United States, use of conjugate *H. influenzae* type b and S. *pneumoniae* vaccines has dramatically reduced the incidence of these infections. Determining the child's immunization status is essential to evaluate risk of these infections. An approach to evaluation of these children is outlined in Figure 96-1.

Most episodes of fever in children younger than 3 years of age have a demonstrable source of infection elicited by history, physical examination, or a simple laboratory test. In this age group, the most commonly identified serious bacterial infection is a UTI. A blood culture to evaluate for occult bacteremia, and urinalysis and urine culture to evaluate for a UTI, should be considered for all children younger than 3 years of age with fever without localizing signs. Stool culture should be obtained in those with diarrhea marked by blood or mucous. Ill-appearing children should be admitted to the hospital and treated with empirical antibiotics.

Approximately 0.2% of well-appearing febrile children 3 to 36 months of age vaccinated against S. *pneumoniae* and *H. influenzae* and without localizing signs have occult bacteremia. Risk factors for occult bacteremia include temperature of 102.2° F (39° C) or greater, WBC count of 15,000/mm³ or more, and elevated absolute neutrophil count, band count, erythrocyte sedimentation rate, or C-reactive protein. No combination of demographic factors (socioeconomic status, race, gender, and age), clinical parameters, or laboratory tests in these children reliably predicts occult bacteremia. Occult bacteremia in otherwise healthy children is usually transient and self-limited but may progress to serious localizing infections. Well-appearing children usually are followed as

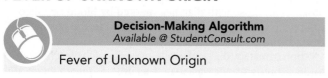

Figure 96-1 Approach to a child younger than 36 months of age with fever without localizing signs. The specific management varies, depending on the age and clinical status of the child.

outpatients without empirical antibiotic treatment or, alternatively, treated with intramuscular ceftriaxone. Regardless of antibiotic treatment, close follow-up for at least 72 hours, including re-evaluation in 24 hours or immediately with any clinical change, is essential. Children with a positive blood culture require immediate re-evaluation, repeat blood culture, consideration for lumbar puncture, and empirical antibiotic treatment.

Children with **sickle cell disease** have impaired splenic function and properdin-dependent opsonization that places them at increased risk for bacteremia, especially during the first 5 years of life. Children with sickle cell disease and fever who appear seriously ill, have a temperature of 104° F (40° C) or greater, or WBC count less than 5000/mm³ or greater than 30,000/mm³ should be hospitalized and treated empirically with antibiotics. Other children with sickle cell disease and fever should have blood culture, empirical treatment with ceftriaxone, and close outpatient follow-up. Osteomyelitis resulting from *Salmonella* or *S. aureus* is more common in children with sickle cell disease; blood culture is not always positive in the presence of osteomyelitis.

FEVER OF UNKNOWN ORIGIN

Decision-Making Algorithm
Available @ StudentConsult.com

Fever of Unknown Origin

FUO is defined as temperature greater than 100.4° F (38° C) lasting for >14 days without an obvious cause despite a complete history, physical examination, and routine screening laboratory evaluation. It is important to distinguish persistent fever from recurrent or periodic fevers, which usually represent serial acute illnesses.

The initial evaluation of FUO requires a thorough history and physical examination supplemented with a few screening laboratory tests (Fig. 96-2). Additional laboratory and imaging tests are guided by abnormalities on initial evaluation.

Important historical elements include the impact the fever has on the child's health and activity; weight loss; the use of drugs, medications, or immunosuppressive therapy; history of unusual, severe, or chronic infection suggesting immunodeficiency (see Chapter 72); immunizations; exposure to unprocessed or raw foods; history of pica and exposure to soil-borne or waterborne organisms; exposure to industrial or hobby-related chemicals; blood transfusions; domestic or foreign travel; exposure to animals; exposure to ticks or mosquitoes; ethnic background; recent surgical procedures or dental work; tattooing and body piercing; and sexual activity.

The etiology of most occult infections causing FUO is an unusual presentation of a common disease. Sinusitis, endocarditis, intra-abdominal abscesses (perinephric, intrahepatic, subdiaphragmatic), and central nervous system lesions (tuberculoma, cysticercosis, abscess, toxoplasmosis) may be relatively asymptomatic. Infections are the most common cause of FUO in children, followed by inflammatory diseases, malignancy, and other etiologies (Table 96-1). **Inflammatory diseases** account for approximately 20% of episodes. **Malignancies** are a less common cause of FUO in children than in adults, accounting for about 10% of all episodes. Approximately 15% of children with FUO have no diagnosis. Fever eventually resolves in many of these cases, usually without sequelae, although some may develop definable signs of rheumatic disease over time. Common infections causing FUO in patients with known or newly diagnosed **immunodeficiency** include viral hepatitis, Epstein-Barr virus, cytomegalovirus, *Bartonella henselae*, ehrlichiosis, *Salmonella*, and tuberculosis.

Factitious fever or fever produced or feigned intentionally by the patient (**Munchausen syndrome**) or the parent of a child (**Munchausen syndrome by proxy**) is an important consideration, particularly if family members are familiar with health care practices (see Chapter 22). Fever should be recorded in the hospital by a reliable individual who remains with the patient when the temperature is taken. Continuous observation over a long period and repetitive evaluation are essential.

Screening tests for FUO include complete blood count with WBC and differential count, platelet count, erythrocyte

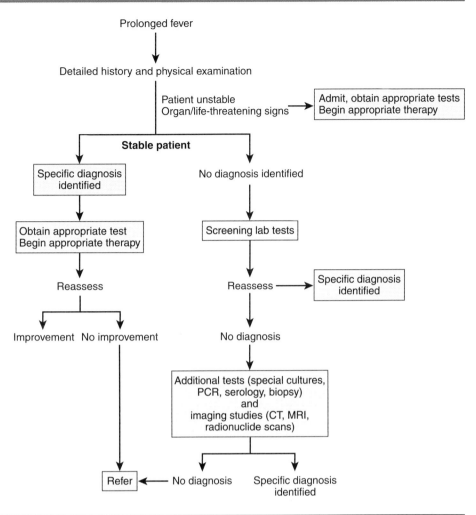

Figure 96-2 Approach to the evaluation of fever of unknown origin (FUO) in children. Screening laboratory tests include a complete blood count and differential white blood cell count, platelet count, erythrocyte sedimentation rate, hepatic transaminase levels, urinalysis, bacterial cultures of urine and blood, chest radiograph, and evaluation for rheumatic disease with antinuclear antibody, rheumatoid factor, and serum complement (C3, C4, CH$_{50}$). *PCR,* polymerase chain reaction.

Table 96-1	Causes of Fever of Unknown Origin in Children

INFECTIONS

LOCALIZED INFECTIONS

Abscesses: abdominal, brain, dental, hepatic, pelvic, perinephric, rectal, subphrenic, splenic, periappendiceal, psoas

Cholangitis

Infective endocarditis

Mastoiditis

Osteomyelitis

Pneumonia

Pyelonephritis

Sinusitis

BACTERIAL DISEASES

Actinomycosis
Bartonella henselae (cat-scratch disease)
Brucellosis

Campylobacter

Francisella tularensis (tularemia)
Gonococcemia (chronic)

Leptospirosis
Listeria monocytogenes (listeriosis)

Lyme disease (*Borrelia burgdorferi*)

Meningococcemia (chronic)

Mycoplasma pneumoniae
Relapsing fever (*Borrelia recurrentis,* other *Borrelia*)

Salmonellosis

Spirillum minus (rat-bite fever)

Streptobacillus moniliformis (rat-bite fever)

Syphilis

Tuberculosis
Whipple disease

Yersiniosis

VIRAL DISEASES

Cytomegalovirus

Hepatitis viruses

HIV (and associated opportunistic infections)

Infectious mononucleosis (Epstein-Barr virus)

CHLAMYDIAL DISEASES

Lymphogranuloma venereum

Psittacosis

RICKETTSIAL DISEASES

Ehrlichiosis

Q fever (*Coxiella burnetii*)

Table 96-1	Causes of Fever of Unknown Origin in Children—cont'd

INFECTIONS	Hodgkin disease
Rocky Mountain spotted fever Tick-borne typhus	Inflammatory pseudotumor
FUNGAL DISEASES	Leukemia
Blastomycosis (extrapulmonary)	Lymphoma
Coccidioidomycosis (disseminated)	Neuroblastoma Pheochromocytoma Wilms tumor
Histoplasmosis (disseminated)	**MISCELLANEOUS**
PARASITIC DISEASES	Addison disease Anhidrotic ectodermal dysplasia
Extraintestinal amebiasis	Castleman disease
Babesiosis	Chronic active hepatitis Cyclic neutropenia
Giardiasis	Deafness, urticaria, amyloidosis syndrome
Malaria	Diabetes insipidus (central and nephrogenic)
Toxoplasmosis Trichinosis	Fabry disease
Trypanosomiasis	Factitious fever Familial dysautonomia
Visceral larva migrans (*Toxocara*)	Familial Mediterranean fever and other autoinflammatory disorders
INFLAMMATORY DISEASES	Granulomatous hepatitis Hemophagocytic syndromes
Behçet syndrome Crohn's disease	Hypertriglyceridemia Hypothalamic-central fever
Drug fever	Ichthyosis Infantile cortical hyperostosis Inflammatory bowel disease
Hypersensitivity pneumonitis Juvenile dermatomyositis	Factitious fever
Juvenile idiopathic arthritis (systemic onset, Still disease)	Kikuchi-Fujimoto disease Metal fume fever Pancreatitis
Inflammatory bowel disease (Crohn's disease, ulcerative colitis)	Periodic fever syndromes Poisoning Postoperative (pericardiotomy, craniectomy)
Kawasaki disease	Pulmonary embolism
Polyarteritis nodosa	Thrombophlebitis Thyrotoxicosis
Rheumatic fever Sarcoidosis	Tumor necrosis factor-α receptor-associated periodic fever syndrome (TRAPS)
Serum sickness	
Systemic lupus erythematosus Weber-Christian disease	
MALIGNANCIES	
Atrial myxoma Cholesterol granuloma	
Ewing sarcoma	
Hepatoma	

Modified from Nield LS, Kamat D: Fever without a focus. In Kliegman RM, Stanton BF, St. Geme III JW, et al: Nelson Textbook of Pediatrics, ed 19, Philadelphia, 2011, Saunders.

sedimentation rate, C-reactive protein, hepatic transaminase levels, urinalysis, cultures of urine and blood, chest radiograph, and evaluation for rheumatic disease with antinuclear antibody, rheumatoid factor, and serum complement (C3, C4, CH$_{50}$). Additional tests for FUO may include throat culture, stool culture, tuberculin skin test or interferon-gamma release assay, HIV antibody, Epstein-Barr virus antibody profile, and *B. henselae* antibody. Consultation with infectious disease, immunology, rheumatic disease, or oncology specialists should be considered. Further tests may include lumbar puncture for cerebrospinal fluid analysis and culture; computed tomography or magnetic resonance imaging of the chest, abdomen, and head; radionuclide scans; and bone marrow biopsy for cytology and culture.

Chapter 97

INFECTIONS CHARACTERIZED BY FEVER AND RASH

Decision-Making Algorithm
Available @ StudentConsult.com

Fever and Rash

Rashes are a common manifestation of many infections; this chapter describes five common childhood viral exanthems characterized by fever and rash. Rash distribution and appearance provide important clues to the differential diagnosis, including other infectious agents (Table 97-1).

MEASLES (RUBEOLA)
Etiology
Measles (rubeola) is highly contagious and is caused by a single-stranded RNA paramyxovirus with one antigenic type. Humans are the only natural host. Measles virus infects the upper respiratory tract and regional lymph nodes and is spread systemically during a brief, low-titer primary viremia. A secondary viremia occurs within 5 to 7 days as virus-infected monocytes spread the virus to the respiratory tract, skin, and other organs. Virus is present in respiratory secretions, blood, and the urine of infected individuals. Measles virus is transmitted by droplets or the airborne route and is highly contagious. Infected persons are contagious from 1 to 2 days before onset of symptoms—from about 5 days before to 4 days after the appearance of rash—and immunocompromised persons can have prolonged excretion of contagious virus.

Epidemiology
Measles remains endemic in regions of the world where measles vaccination is not available and is responsible for about 1 million deaths annually. Since 2000 there typically have been fewer than 100 cases reported annually in the United States, although outbreaks resulting from imported virus after international travel occur. Infections of nonimmigrant children during outbreaks may occur among those too young to be vaccinated or in communities with low immunization rates. Most young infants are protected by transplacental maternal antibody until the end of their first year.

Clinical Manifestations
Measles infection is divided into four phases: incubation, prodromal (catarrhal), exanthematous (rash), and recovery. The incubation period is 8 to 12 days from exposure to symptom onset and a mean of 14 days (range, 7 to 21) from exposure to rash onset. The manifestations of the 3-day prodromal period

Table 97-1	Differential Diagnosis of Fever and Rash
LESION	**PATHOGEN OR DISEASE**
Macular or Maculopapular Rash	
Viruses	Adenovirus
	Measles
	Rubella
	Roseola (HHV-6 or HHV-7)
	Erythema infectiosum (fifth disease, parvovirus B19)
	Epstein-Barr virus
	Echoviruses
	HBV (papular acrodermatitis or Gianotti-Crosti syndrome)
	HIV
Bacteria	Erythema marginatum (rheumatic fever)
	Scarlet fever (group A streptococcus)
	Erysipelas (group A streptococcus)
	Arcanobacterium haemolyticum
	Secondary syphilis
	Leptospirosis
	Pseudomonas aeruginosa
	Meningococcal infection (early)
	Salmonella typhi (typhoid fever, "rose spots")
	Lyme disease (erythema migrans)
	Mycoplasma pneumoniae
Rickettsiae	Rocky Mountain spotted fever (early)
	Typhus (scrub, endemic)
	Ehrlichiosis
Other	Kawasaki disease
	Rheumatoid arthritis
	Drug reaction
Diffuse Erythroderma	
Bacteria	Scarlet fever (group A streptococcus)
	Staphylococcal scalded skin syndrome
	Toxic shock syndrome (*Staphylococcus aureus*, group A streptococcus)
Fungi	*Candida albicans*
Other	Kawasaki disease
Urticarial Rash	
Viruses	Epstein-Barr virus
	HBV
	HIV
Bacteria	*M. pneumoniae*
	Group A streptococcus
Other	Drug reaction Serum sickness
Vesicular, Bullous, Pustular	
Viruses	Herpes simplex viruses
	Varicella-zoster virus

LESION	PATHOGEN OR DISEASE
Table 97-1	Differential Diagnosis of Fever and Rash—cont'd
	Macular or Maculopapular Rash
	Coxsackievirus
Bacteria	Staphylococcal scalded skin syndrome
	Staphylococcal bullous impetigo
	Group A streptococcal crusted impetigo
Rickettsiae	Rickettsialpox
Other	Toxic epidermal necrolysis
	Erythema multiforme (Stevens-Johnson syndrome)
	Petechial-Purpuric
Viruses	Adenovirus
	Atypical measles
	Congenital rubella
	Congenital cytomegalovirus
	Enterovirus
	Papular-purpuric gloves and socks (parvovirus B19)
	HIV
	Hemorrhagic fever viruses
Bacteria	Sepsis (meningococcal, gonococcal, pneumococcal, *Haemophilus influenzae* type b)
	Infective endocarditis
	Ecthyma gangrenosum (*Pseudomonas aeruginosa*) *Vibrio vulnificus*
Rickettsiae	Rocky Mountain spotted fever
	Epidemic typhus
	Ehrlichiosis
Fungi	Necrotic eschar (*Aspergillus, Mucor*)
Other	Vasculitis
	Thrombocytopenia
	Henoch-Schönlein purpura
	Malaria
	Erythema Nodosum
Viruses	Epstein-Barr virus
	HBV
Bacteria	Group A streptococcus
	Mycobacterium tuberculosis
	Yersinia
	Cat-scratch disease (*Bartonella henselae*)
Fungi	Coccidioidomycosis
	Histoplasmosis
Other	Sarcoidosis
	Inflammatory bowel disease
	Estrogen-containing oral contraceptives
	Systemic lupus erythematosus
	Behçet disease

HBV, Hepatitis B virus; *HHV,* human herpesvirus.

are cough, coryza, conjunctivitis, and the pathognomonic **Koplik spots** (gray-white, sand grain-sized dots on the buccal mucosa opposite the lower molars) that last 12 to 24 hours. The conjunctiva may reveal a characteristic transverse line of inflammation along the eyelid margin (**Stimson line**). The classic symptoms of cough, coryza, and conjunctivitis occur during the secondary viremia of the exanthematous phase, which often is accompanied by high fever (40° C to 40.5° C [104° F to 105° F]). The macular rash begins on the head (often above the hairline) and spreads over most of the body in a cephalad to caudal pattern over 24 hours. Areas of the rash often are confluent. The rash fades in the same pattern, and illness severity is related to the extent of the rash. It may be petechial or hemorrhagic (**black measles**). As the rash fades, it undergoes brownish discoloration and desquamation.

Cervical lymphadenitis, splenomegaly, and mesenteric lymphadenopathy with abdominal pain may be noted with the rash. Otitis media, pneumonia, and diarrhea are more common in infants. Liver involvement is more common in adults.

The term **modified measles** describes mild cases of measles occurring in persons with partial protection against measles. Modified measles occurs in persons vaccinated before 12 months of age or with coadministration of immune serum globulin, in infants with disease modified by transplacental antibody, or in persons receiving immunoglobulin.

Laboratory and Imaging Studies

Routine laboratory findings are nonspecific and do not aid in diagnosis. Leukopenia is characteristic. In patients with acute encephalitis, the cerebrospinal fluid reveals an increased protein, a lymphocytic pleocytosis, and normal glucose levels. Measles virus culture is not generally available, though identification of measles RNA via reverse transcriptase-polymerase chain reaction (PCR) may be available through state public health departments or the Centers for Disease Control and Prevention (CDC). Serologic testing for IgM antibodies that appear within 1 to 2 days of the rash and persist for 1 to 2 months in unimmunized persons confirms the clinical diagnosis, though IgM antibodies may be present only transiently in immunized people. Suspected cases should be reported immediately to the local or state health department.

Differential Diagnosis

The constellation of fever, rash, cough, and conjunctivitis is diagnostic for measles. Koplik spots are pathognomonic but are not always present at the time the rash is most pronounced. Confirmation is by diagnostic antibody increases in acute and convalescent sera. The rash must be differentiated from rubella, roseola, enteroviral or adenoviral infection, infectious mononucleosis, toxoplasmosis, meningococcemia, scarlet fever, rickettsial disease, Kawasaki disease, serum sickness, and drug rash.

Treatment

Routine supportive care includes maintaining adequate hydration and antipyretics. High-dose vitamin A supplementation has been shown to improve the outcome of infants with measles in developing countries. The World Health Organization recommends routine administration of vitamin A for 2 days to all children with acute measles.

Complications and Prognosis

Otitis media is the most common complication of measles infection. Interstitial (measles) pneumonia can occur, or pneumonia may result from secondary bacterial infection with *Streptococcus pneumoniae, Staphylococcus aureus,* or group A streptococcus. Persons with impaired cell-mediated immunity may develop **giant cell (Hecht) pneumonia,** which is usually fatal. Myocarditis and mesenteric lymphadenitis are infrequent complications.

Encephalomyelitis occurs in 1 to 2 per 1000 cases and usually occurs 2 to 5 days after the onset of the rash. Early encephalitis probably is caused by direct viral infection of brain tissue, whereas later onset encephalitis is a demyelinating and probably an immunopathologic phenomenon. **Subacute sclerosing panencephalitis** is a late neurologic complication of slow measles infection that is characterized by progressive behavioral and intellectual deterioration and eventual death. It occurs in approximately 1 in every 1 million cases of measles, an average of 8 to 10 years after measles. There is no effective treatment.

Deaths most frequently result from bronchopneumonia or encephalitis, with much higher risk in persons with malignancy, severe malnutrition, age under 5 years, or immunocompromise (such as HIV infection). Late deaths in adolescents and adults usually result from subacute sclerosing panencephalitis. Other forms of measles encephalitis in immunocompetent persons are associated with a mortality rate of approximately 15%, with 20% to 30% of survivors having serious neurologic sequelae.

Prevention

Live measles vaccine prevents infection and is recommended as measles, mumps, and rubella (MMR) for children at 12 to 15 months and 4 to 6 years of age. The MMRV (MMR combined with varicella vaccine) is an alternative vaccine for children 12 months to 12 years of age, provided there are no contraindications, but is associated with a higher rate of febrile seizures following administration. The second dose of MMR is not a booster dose but significantly reduces the primary vaccine failure rate, from <5% to <1%. Contraindications to measles vaccine include immunocompromised states or an immunosuppressive course of corticosteroids (>2 mg/kg/day for >14 days); pregnancy; or recent administration of immunoglobulin (3 to 11 months, depending on dose). MMR vaccination is recommended for all HIV-infected persons without evidence of severe immunosuppression (low age-specific total CD4 T-lymphocyte count or a low CD4 T-lymphocyte count as a percentage of total lymphocytes), children with cancer in remission who have not received chemotherapy in the previous 3 months, and children who have not received immunosuppressive corticosteroids in the previous month. Susceptible household contacts with a chronic disease or who are immunocompromised should receive **postexposure prophylaxis** with measles vaccine within 72 hours of measles exposure or immunoglobulin within 6 days of exposure.

RUBELLA (GERMAN OR 3-DAY MEASLES)
Etiology

Rubella, also known as **German measles** or **3-day measles,** is caused by a single-stranded RNA virus with a glycolipid envelope and is a member of the togavirus family. Humans are the only natural host. Rubella virus invades the respiratory epithelium and disseminates via a primary viremia. After replication in the reticuloendothelial system, a secondary viremia ensues, and the virus can be isolated from peripheral blood monocytes, cerebrospinal fluid, and urine. Rubella virus is most contagious through direct or droplet contact with nasopharyngeal secretions from 2 days before until 5 to 7 days after rash onset, although virus may be present in nasopharyngeal secretions from 7 days before until 14 days after the rash.

Infection **in utero** results in significant morbidity from **congenital rubella syndrome (CRS)** with associated ophthalmologic, cardiac, and neurologic manifestations (see Chapter 66). Maternal infection during the first trimester results in fetal infection with generalized vasculitis in more than 90% of cases. Infants with congenital rubella may shed the virus in nasopharyngeal secretions and urine for longer than 12 months after birth and may transmit the virus to susceptible contacts.

Epidemiology

In unvaccinated populations, rubella usually occurs in the spring, with epidemics occurring in cycles of every 6 to 9 years. Approximately 25% to 50% of cases are subclinical. Fewer than 20 cases of rubella now occur annually in the United States. Outbreaks of rubella occasionally occur in nonvaccinated groups from internationally imported cases. Transplacental antibody is protective during the first 6 months of life.

Clinical Manifestations

Decision-Making Algorithm
Available @ StudentConsult.com

Fever and Rash

The incubation period for postnatal rubella is typically 16 to 18 days (range, 14 to 21 days). The mild catarrhal symptoms of the prodromal phase of rubella may go unnoticed. The characteristic signs of rubella are retroauricular, posterior cervical, and posterior occipital lymphadenopathy accompanied by an erythematous, maculopapular, discrete rash. The rash begins on the face and spreads to the body, lasting for 3 days and less prominent than that of measles. Rose-colored spots on the soft palate, known as **Forchheimer spots,** develop in 20% of patients and may appear before the rash. Other manifestations of rubella include mild pharyngitis, conjunctivitis, anorexia, headache, malaise, and low-grade fever. Polyarthritis, usually of the hands, may occur, especially among adult females, but usually resolves without sequelae. Paresthesias and tendinitis may occur.

Laboratory and Imaging Studies

Routine laboratory findings are nonspecific and generally do not aid in diagnosis. The white blood cell count usually is normal or low, and thrombocytopenia rarely occurs. Diagnosis is confirmed by serologic testing for IgM antibodies (typically positive 5 days after symptom onset) or by a fourfold or greater increase in specific IgG antibodies in paired acute and convalescent sera. **CRS** cases can have detectable IgM until

3 months of age, and stable or rising IgG titers over the first 7 to 11 months of age. False-positive IgM results can occur. Cases of suspected congenital rubella syndrome and postnatal rubella infection should be reported to the local and state health department.

Differential Diagnosis
The rash must be differentiated from measles, roseola, enteroviral or adenoviral infection, infectious mononucleosis, toxoplasmosis, scarlet fever, rickettsial disease, Kawasaki disease, serum sickness, and drug rash.

Treatment
There is no specific therapy for rubella. Routine supportive care includes maintaining adequate hydration and antipyretics.

Complications and Prognosis
Other than **congenital rubella syndrome** (see Chapter 66) arising from rubella infection during pregnancy, complications are rare. Deaths rarely occur with rubella encephalitis.

Prevention
Live rubella vaccine prevents infection and is recommended as MMR for children at 12 to 15 months and at 4 to 6 years of age. After vaccination, rubella virus is shed from the nasopharynx for several weeks, but it is not communicable. In children, rubella vaccine rarely is associated with adverse effects, but in postpubertal females, it causes arthralgias in 25% of vaccinated individuals and acute arthritis-like symptoms in 10% of vaccinated individuals. These symptoms typically develop 1 to 3 weeks after vaccination and last 1 to 3 days.

Contraindications to rubella vaccine include immunocompromised states or an immunosuppressive course of corticosteroids (>2 mg/kg/day for >14 days); pregnancy; or recent administration of immunoglobulin (3 to 11 months, depending on dose). Vaccine virus has been recovered from fetal tissues, although no cases of **CRS** have been identified among infants born to women inadvertently vaccinated against rubella during pregnancy. Nevertheless women are cautioned to avoid pregnancy after receipt of rubella-containing vaccine for 28 days. All pregnant women should have prenatal serologic testing to determine their immune status to rubella, and susceptible mothers should be vaccinated after delivery and before hospital discharge.

Susceptible, nonpregnant persons exposed to rubella should receive rubella vaccination. Immunoglobulin is not recommended for postexposure prophylaxis of susceptible, pregnant women exposed to rubella.

ROSEOLA INFANTUM (EXANTHEM SUBITUM)
Etiology
Roseola infantum (exanthem subitum, sixth disease) is caused primarily by human herpesvirus type 6 (HHV-6), and by HHV-7 in 10% to 30% of cases. HHV-6 and HHV-7 are large, enveloped double-stranded DNA viruses that are members of the herpesvirus family. They infect mature mononuclear cells and cause a relatively prolonged (3 to 5 day) viremia during primary infection. They can be detected in the saliva of healthy adults, which suggests, as with other herpesviruses, the development of lifelong latent infection and intermittent viral shedding.

Epidemiology
Transplacental antibody protects most infants until 6 months of age. The incidence of infection increases as maternally derived antibody levels decline. By 12 months of age, approximately 60% to 90% of children have antibodies to HHV-6, and essentially all children are seropositive by 2 to 3 years of age. The virus is likely acquired from asymptomatic adults who periodically shed these viruses. HHV-6 is a major cause of acute febrile illnesses in infants and may be responsible for 20% of visits to the emergency department for children 6 to 18 months of age.

Clinical Manifestations
Roseola is characterized by high fever (often >40° C) with an abrupt onset that lasts 3 to 5 days. A maculopapular, rose-colored rash erupts coincidentally with defervescence, although it may be present earlier. The rash usually lasts 1 to 3 days but may fade rapidly and is not present in all infants with HHV-6 infection. Upper respiratory symptoms, nasal congestion, erythematous tympanic membranes, and cough may occur. Gastrointestinal symptoms are described. Most children with roseola are irritable and appear toxic. Roseola is associated with approximately one third of febrile seizures. Roseola caused by HHV-6 and HHV-7 is clinically indistinguishable, although HHV-6-associated roseola typically occurs in younger infants. Reactivation of HHV-6 following bone marrow transplantation may result in bone marrow suppression, hepatitis, rash, and encephalitis.

Laboratory and Imaging Studies
Routine laboratory findings are nonspecific and do not aid in diagnosis. Encephalitis with roseola is characterized by pleocytosis (30 to 200 cells/mm^3) with mononuclear cell predominance, elevated protein concentration, and normal glucose concentration. Serologic testing showing a fourfold rise in acute and convalescent sera or documentation of HHV-6 DNA by PCR in the cerebrospinal fluid is diagnostic.

Differential Diagnosis
The pattern of high fever for 3 to 5 days without significant physical findings followed by onset of rash with defervescence of fever is characteristic. Many febrile illnesses may be easily confused with roseola during the preeruptive stage. Serious infections must be excluded, although most children are alert, behave normally, and continue with their usual daily activities.

Treatment
There is no specific therapy for roseola. Routine supportive care includes maintaining adequate hydration and antipyretics. In immunocompromised hosts, use of ganciclovir or foscarnet can be considered.

Complications and Prognosis

The prognosis for roseola is excellent. A few deaths have been attributed to HHV-6, usually in cases complicated by encephalitis or virus-associated **hemophagocytosis syndrome.**

Prevention

There are no guidelines for prevention of roseola.

ERYTHEMA INFECTIOSUM (FIFTH DISEASE)
Etiology

Erythema infectiosum (fifth disease) is caused by the human parvovirus B19, a single-stranded DNA virus producing a benign viral exanthem in healthy children. The viral affinity for red blood cell progenitor cells makes it an important cause of aplastic crisis in patients with hemolytic anemias, including sickle cell disease, spherocytosis, and thalassemia. Parvovirus B19 also causes fetal anemia and hydrops fetalis after primary infection during pregnancy. The cell receptor for parvovirus B19 is the **erythrocyte P antigen,** a glycolipid present on erythroid cells. The virus replicates in actively dividing erythroid stem cells, leading to cell death that results in erythroid aplasia and anemia.

Epidemiology

Erythema infectiosum is common. Parvovirus B19 seroprevalence is only 2% to 9% in children younger than 5 years of age but increases to 15% to 35% in children 5 to 18 years and 30% to 60% in adults. Community epidemics usually occur in the spring. The virus is transmitted by respiratory secretions and by blood product transfusions.

Clinical Manifestations

The incubation period is typically 4 to 14 days and rarely may last 21 days. Parvovirus B19 infections usually begin with a mild, nonspecific illness characterized by fever, malaise, myalgias, and headache. In some cases, the characteristic rash appears 7 to 10 days later. Erythema infectiosum is manifested by rash, low-grade or no fever, and occasionally pharyngitis and mild conjunctivitis. The rash appears in three stages. The initial stage is typically a **"slapped cheek" rash** with circumoral pallor. An erythematous symmetric, maculopapular, truncal rash appears 1 to 4 days later, then fades as central clearing takes place, giving a distinctive **lacy, reticulated rash** that lasts 2 to 40 days (mean, 11 days). This rash may be pruritic, does not desquamate, and may recur with exercise, bathing, rubbing, or stress. Adolescents and adults may experience myalgia, significant arthralgias or arthritis, headache, pharyngitis, coryza, and gastrointestinal upset.

Children with shortened erythrocyte life span (e.g., sickle cell disease) may develop a **transient aplastic crisis** characterized by ineffective erythroid production typically lasting 7 to 10 days (see Chapter 150). Most children with parvovirus B19-induced transient aplastic crisis have multiple symptoms, including fever, lethargy, malaise, pallor, headache, gastrointestinal symptoms, and respiratory symptoms. The reticulocyte count is extremely low, and the hemoglobin level is lower than usual for the patient. Transient neutropenia and thrombocytopenia also commonly occur.

Persistent parvovirus B19 infection may develop in children with immunodeficiency, causing severe anemia resulting from pure red blood cell aplasia. These children do not display the typical manifestations of erythema infectiosum.

Laboratory and Imaging Studies

Hematologic abnormalities occur with parvovirus infection, including reticulocytopenia lasting 7 to 10 days, mild anemia, thrombocytopenia, lymphopenia, and neutropenia. Parvovirus B19 can be detected by PCR and by electron microscopy of erythroid precursors in the bone marrow. Serologic tests showing specific IgM antibody to parvovirus are diagnostic, demonstrating infection that probably occurred in the prior 2 to 4 months.

Differential Diagnosis

The diagnosis of erythema infectiosum in children is established on the basis of the clinical findings of typical facial rash with absent or mild prodromal symptoms, followed by a reticulated rash over the body that waxes and wanes. The differential diagnosis includes measles, rubella, scarlet fever, enteroviral or adenoviral infection, infectious mononucleosis, scarlet fever, Kawasaki disease, systemic lupus erythematosus, serum sickness, and drug reaction.

Treatment

There is no specific therapy. Routine supportive care includes maintaining adequate hydration and antipyretics. Transfusions may be required for transient aplastic crisis. Intrauterine transfusion has been performed for hydrops fetalis associated with fetal parvovirus B19 infection. Intravenous immunoglobulin may be used for immunocompromised persons with severe anemia or chronic infection.

Complications and Prognosis

The prognosis for erythema infectiosum is excellent. Fatalities associated with transient aplastic crisis are rare. Parvovirus B19 is not teratogenic, but in utero infection of fetal erythroid cells may result in fetal heart failure, hydrops fetalis, and fetal death. Of the approximately 50% of women of childbearing age susceptible to parvovirus B19 infection, 30% of exposed women develop infection, with 25% of exposed fetuses becoming infected and 10% of these culminating in fetal death.

Prevention

The greatest risk is to pregnant women. Effective control measures are limited. Exclusion of affected children from school is not recommended, because children generally are not infectious by the time the rash is present. Good handwashing and hygiene are practical measures that should help reduce transmission.

VARICELLA-ZOSTER VIRUS INFECTION (CHICKENPOX AND ZOSTER)
Etiology

Chickenpox and zoster are caused by varicella-zoster virus (VZV), an enveloped, icosahedral, double-stranded DNA virus that is a member of the herpesvirus family. Humans are the only natural host. **Chickenpox (varicella)** is the manifestation of primary infection. VZV infects susceptible individuals via the conjunctivae or respiratory tract and replicates in the nasopharynx and upper respiratory tract. It disseminates by a primary viremia and infects regional lymph nodes, the liver, the spleen, and other organs. A secondary viremia follows, resulting in a cutaneous infection with the typical vesicular rash. After resolution of chickenpox, the virus persists in latent infection in the dorsal root ganglia cells. **Zoster (shingles)** is the manifestation of reactivated latent infection of endogenous VZV. Chickenpox is highly communicable in susceptible individuals, with a secondary attack rate of more than 90%. The period of communicability ranges from 2 days before to 7 days after the onset of the rash, when all lesions are crusted.

Epidemiology

In the prevaccine era, the peak age of occurrence was 5 to 10 years, with peak seasonal infection in late winter and spring. In the postvaccine era, the incidence of varicella has declined in all age groups, with the peak incidence now in 10 to 14 year olds. Transmission is by direct contact, droplet, and air. **Zoster** is a recurrence of latent VZV and is transmitted by direct contact. Only 5% of cases of zoster occur in children younger than 15 years of age. The overall incidence of zoster (215 cases per 100,000 person-years) results in a cumulative lifetime incidence of approximately 10% to 20%, with 75% of cases occurring after 45 years of age. The incidence of zoster is increased in immunocompromised persons.

Clinical Manifestations

Decision-Making Algorithms
Available @ StudentConsult.com
Ataxia
Alopecia
Vesicles and Bullae
Fever and Rash
Petechiae/Purpura

The incubation period of varicella is generally 14 to 16 days, with a range of 10 to 21 days after exposure. Prodromal symptoms of fever, malaise, and anorexia may precede the rash by 1 day. The characteristic rash appears initially as small red papules that rapidly progress to nonumbilicated, oval, "teardrop" vesicles on an erythematous base. The fluid progresses from clear to cloudy, and the vesicles ulcerate, crust, and heal. New crops appear for 3 to 4 days, usually beginning on the trunk followed by the head, the face, and, less commonly, the extremities. There may be a total of 100 to 500 lesions, with all forms of lesions being present at the same time. Pruritus is universal and marked. Lesions may be present on mucous membranes. Lymphadenopathy may be generalized. The severity of the rash varies, as do systemic signs and fever, which generally abate after 3 to 4 days.

The preeruption phase of **zoster** includes intense localized and constant pain and tenderness **(acute neuritis)** along a dermatome, accompanied by malaise and fever. In several days, the eruption of papules, which quickly vesiculate, occurs in the dermatome or in two adjacent dermatomes. Groups of lesions

occur for 1 to 7 days and then progress to crusting and healing. Thoracic and lumbar regions are typically involved. Lesions generally are unilateral and are accompanied by regional lymphadenopathy. In one third of patients, a few vesicles occur outside of the primary dermatome. Any branch of cranial nerve V may be involved, which also may cause corneal and intraoral lesions. Involvement of cranial nerve VII may result in facial paralysis and ear canal vesicles **(Ramsay Hunt syndrome).** Ophthalmic zoster may be associated with ipsilateral cerebral angiitis and stroke. Immunocompromised persons may have unusually severe, painful herpes zoster that involves cutaneous and, rarely, visceral dissemination (to liver, lungs, and central nervous system). **Postherpetic neuralgia,** defined as pain persisting longer than 1 month, is uncommon in children.

Laboratory and Imaging Studies

Laboratory testing confirmation for diagnosis is usually unnecessary. PCR is the current diagnostic method of choice, and genotyping to distinguish vaccine and wild-type strains is available through the CDC. Detection of varicella-specific antigen in vesicular fluid by immunofluorescence using monoclonal antibodies or demonstration of a fourfold antibody increase of acute and convalescent sera is also diagnostic but not as sensitive as PCR.

Differential Diagnosis

The diagnosis of varicella and zoster is based on the distinctive characteristics of the rash. **Eczema herpeticum,** or **Kaposi varicelliform eruption,** is a localized, vesicular eruption caused by HSV that develops on skin affected by underlying eczema or trauma. The differentiation between zoster and HSV infection may be difficult because HSV may cause eruption that appears to be in a dermatomal distribution. Coxsackievirus A infection has a vesiculopustular appearance, but lesions are usually localized to the extremities and oropharynx. A previously healthy patient with more than one recurrence probably has HSV infection, which can be confirmed by viral culture.

Treatment

Symptomatic therapy of varicella includes nonaspirin antipyretics, cool baths, and careful hygiene. Routine oral administration of acyclovir is not recommended in otherwise healthy children with varicella. The decision to use antiviral medications, the route, and duration of treatment depend on host factors and the risk for severe infection or complications. Early therapy with antivirals (especially within 24 hours of rash onset) in immunocompromised persons is effective in preventing severe complications, including pneumonia, encephalitis, and death from varicella. Acyclovir or valacyclovir may be considered in those at risk of severe varicella, such as unvaccinated persons older than 12 years; those with chronic cutaneous or pulmonary disease; receiving short-course, intermittent, or aerosolized corticosteroids; or receiving long-term salicylate therapy. The dose of acyclovir used for VZV infections is much higher than that for HSV.

Antiviral treatment of zoster accelerates cutaneous healing, hastens the resolution of acute neuritis, and reduces the risk of postherpetic neuralgia. Oral famciclovir and valacyclovir have much greater oral bioavailability than acyclovir and are recommended for treatment of zoster in adults. Acyclovir is recommended for children and is an alternative therapy for adults. The necessity of concomitant oral corticosteroids for zoster is controversial.

Complications and Prognosis

Secondary infection of skin lesions by streptococci or staphylococci is the most common complication. These infections may be mild, resembling impetigo, or life-threatening with toxic shock syndrome or necrotizing fasciitis. Pneumonia is uncommon in healthy children but occurs in 15% to 20% of healthy adults and immunocompromised persons. Myocarditis, pericarditis, orchitis, hepatitis, ulcerative gastritis, glomerulonephritis, and arthritis may complicate varicella. Reye syndrome may follow varicella; thus, salicylate use is contraindicated during varicella infection.

Neurologic complications frequently include postinfectious encephalitis, cerebellar ataxia, nystagmus, and tremor. Less common neurologic complications include Guillain-Barre syndrome, transverse myelitis, cranial nerve palsies, optic neuritis, and hypothalamic syndrome.

Primary varicella can be a fatal disease in immunocompromised persons as a result of visceral dissemination, encephalitis, hepatitis, and pneumonitis. The mortality rate approaches 15% in children with leukemia who do not receive prophylaxis or therapy for varicella (see Chapter 66).

A severe form of neonatal varicella may develop in newborns of mothers with varicella (but not shingles) occurring 5 days before to 2 days after delivery. The fetus is exposed to a large inoculum of virus but is born before the maternal antibody response develops and can cross the placenta. These infants should be treated as soon as possible with varicella-zoster immunoglobulin (VZIG) or intravenous immunoglobulin if VZIG is unavailable, to attempt to prevent or ameliorate the infection.

Primary varicella usually resolves spontaneously. The mortality rate is much higher for persons older than 20 years of age and for immunocompromised persons. Zoster usually is self-limited, especially in children. Advanced age and severity of pain at presentation and at 1 month are predictors of prolonged pain. Scarring is more common with zoster because of involvement of the deeper layers of the skin.

Prevention

Children with chickenpox should not return to school until all vesicles have crusted. A hospitalized child with chickenpox should be isolated in a negative-pressure room to prevent transmission.

A live attenuated varicella vaccine—two doses for all children—is recommended. The first dose should be administered at age 12 to 15 months and the second dose at 4 to 6 years. Varicella vaccine is 85% effective in preventing any disease and 97% effective in preventing moderately severe and severe disease. Transmission of vaccine virus from a healthy vaccinated individual is rare but possible.

Passive immunity can be provided by VZIG, which is indicated within 96 hours of exposure for susceptible individuals at increased risk for severe illness. Administration of VZIG does not eliminate the possibility of disease in recipients and prolongs the incubation period up to 28 days.

Chapter 98

CUTANEOUS INFECTIONS

SUPERFICIAL BACTERIAL INFECTIONS
Impetigo

Decision-Making Algorithms
Available @ StudentConsult.com

Vesicles and Bullae
Fever and Rash

Nonbullous or crusted impetigo is caused most often by *Staphylococcus aureus* and occasionally by group A streptococcus. It begins as a single erythematous papulovesicle that progresses to one or many **honey-colored, crusted lesions** weeping serous drainage. **Bullous impetigo** accounts for approximately 10% of all impetigo. The skin lesions are thin-walled (0.5 to 3 cm) bullae with erythematous margins resembling second-degree burns and are associated with *S. aureus* phage type 71. Impetigo most frequently occurs on the face, around the nares and mouth, and on the extremities. Fever is uncommon. The diagnosis usually is established by the clinical appearance alone.

Recommended treatment for nonbullous impetigo is topical 2% mupirocin or oral antistaphylococcal antibiotics. Extensive or disseminated lesions, bullous impetigo, lesions around the eyes, or lesions otherwise not amenable to topical therapy are best treated with oral antibiotics. Streptococcal impetigo is associated with increased risk of postinfectious glomerulonephritis but not acute rheumatic fever (see Chapter 163). Antibiotic treatment does not decrease the risk of postinfectious glomerulonephritis but decreases possible spread of nephritogenic strains to close contacts. Children with impetigo should remain out of school or day care until 24 hours of antibiotic therapy have been completed.

Cellulitis

Decision-Making Algorithms
Available @ StudentConsult.com

Red Eye
Extremity Pain

Cellulitis is infection involving the subcutaneous tissues and the dermis and is usually caused by *S. aureus* or group A streptococci. Cellulitis typically presents with indurated, warm, and erythematous macules with indistinct borders that expand rapidly. Additional manifestations commonly include fever, lymphangitis, and regional lymphadenitis. **Erysipelas** is a superficial variant of cellulitis usually caused by group A streptococcus that involves the dermis only. The rapidly advancing lesions are tender, bright red in appearance, and have sharp margins. The patients may appear toxic. Blood cultures are recommended for erysipelas. Empirical antibiotic treatment for cellulitis is recommended with a first-generation cephalosporin unless the local *S. aureus* methicillin-resistance rate is high, in which case alternatives include clindamycin or trimethoprim-sulfamethoxazole (although this agent has poor group A streptococcal activity). Many patients may be managed with oral antibiotics and close follow-up; hospitalization and intravenous antibiotics are recommended for erysipelas and cellulitis of the face, hands, feet, or perineum; those with lymphangitis; and those not responding to outpatient therapy.

Ecthyma usually is caused by group A streptococcus and may complicate impetigo. Initially it is characterized by a lesion with a rim of erythematous induration surrounding an eschar, which, if removed, reveals a shallow ulcer. **Ecthyma gangrenosum** is a serious skin infection occurring in immunocompromised persons due to hematogenous spread of septic emboli to the skin, classically caused by *Pseudomonas aeruginosa,* other gram-negative organisms, or occasionally *Aspergillus.* The lesions begin as purple macules that undergo central necrosis to become exquisitely tender, deep, punched-out ulcers 2 to 3 cm in diameter with a dark necrotic base, raised red edges, and sometimes a yellowish green exudate. Fever usually is present.

Necrotizing fasciitis is the most extensive form of cellulitis and involves deeper subcutaneous tissues and fascial planes. It may progress to **myonecrosis** of the underlying muscle. Common causes include *S. aureus* and group A streptococcus alone or in combination with anaerobic organisms, such as *Clostridium perfringens.* Risk factors include underlying immunodeficiency, recent surgery or trauma, and varicella infection. Lesions progress rapidly with raised or sharply demarcated margins, although disease typically extends on a deeper plane beyond superficially evident lesions. Warning signs of necrotizing fasciitis include pain out of proportion to evident skin lesions, shock or toxic appearance, or crepitus due to subcutaneous gas formation by anaerobes. Necrotizing fasciitis is a surgical emergency, and early consultation with an experienced surgeon is recommended. Adjunctive tests such as magnetic resonance imaging can confirm the presence of gas in tissues, but obtaining imaging should not delay surgical consultation. Treatment includes rapid surgical debridement of all necrotic tissues and broad-spectrum intravenous antibiotics, such as clindamycin plus cefotaxime or ceftriaxone, with or without an aminoglycoside or vancomycin.

Folliculitis

Folliculitis refers to small, dome-shaped pustules or erythematous papules predominantly caused by *S. aureus* and located in hair follicles, with superficial, limited inflammatory reaction in the surrounding tissue. **Furuncles (boils)** are deeper hair follicle infections that manifest as nodules with intense surrounding inflammatory reaction. These occur most frequently on the neck, trunk, axillae, and buttocks. A **carbuncle** represents the deepest of hair follicle infections and is characterized by multiseptate, loculated abscesses. Boils and carbuncles frequently require incisional drainage. Superficial folliculitis can be treated with topical therapy, such as an antibacterial chlorhexidine wash or an antibacterial lotion or solution such as clindamycin 1%, applied twice a day for 7 to 10 days. Oral antibiotics are necessary for unresponsive cases, or for furuncles and carbuncles.

P. aeruginosa folliculitis (**hot tub folliculitis**) presents as pruritic papules; pustules; or deeper, purple-red nodules predominantly on skin areas covered by a swimsuit after bathing in hot tubs. Folliculitis develops 8 to 48 hours after exposure, usually without associated systemic symptoms, and resolves in 1 to 2 weeks without treatment.

Perianal Dermatitis

Perianal dermatitis (perianal streptococcal disease) is caused by group A streptococcus and is characterized by well-demarcated, tender, marked perianal erythema extending 2 cm from the anus. Manifestations include anal pruritus and painful defecation, sometimes with blood-streaked stools. The differential diagnosis includes diaper dermatitis, candidiasis, pinworm infection, and anal fissures. Treatment is oral penicillin or cefuroxime.

SUPERFICIAL FUNGAL INFECTIONS

Decision-Making Algorithms
Available @ StudentConsult.com

Alopecia
Lymphadenopathy

Cutaneous fungal infections are common in children (Table 98-1). The estimated lifetime risk of developing a **dermatophytosis** is 10% to 20%. Diagnosis is usually established by visual inspection and may be confirmed by potassium hydroxide (KOH) examination or fungal culture of skin scrapings from the margins of the lesion. **Recommended tinea treatment** is usually for 4 to 6 weeks and 2 weeks after resolution; topical antifungal creams (e.g., miconazole, clotrimazole, ketoconazole, tolnaftate) are appropriate for tinea corporis, tinea pedis, and tinea cruris, whereas tinea capitis requires oral treatment. The diagnosis of **onychomycosis** should be confirmed by KOH examination and fungal culture. Recommended treatment is terbinafine or itraconazole for at least 12 weeks.

SUPERFICIAL VIRAL INFECTIONS
Herpes Simplex Virus

Decision-Making Algorithms
Available @ StudentConsult.com

Sore Throat
Vaginal Discharge
Seizures and Other Paroxysmal Disorders
Vesicles and Bullae
Fever and Rash
Lymphadenopathy

Primary herpetic infections can occur after inoculation of the virus at any mucocutaneous site. Herpes simplex virus type 1 (HSV-1) is common in children and classically causes gingivostomatitis, whereas HSV-2 classically infects the genitalia as a sexually transmitted infection (see Chapter 116), though HSV-1 may cause approximately 30% of genital herpes, and

Table 98-1	Superficial Fungal Infections			
NAME	**ETIOLOGY**	**MANIFESTATIONS**	**DIAGNOSIS**	**THERAPY**
		DERMATOPHYTES		
Tinea capitis (ringworm)	*Microsporum audouinii, Trichophyton tonsurans, Microsporum canis*	Prepubertal infection of scalp, hair-shafts; *black dot* alopecia; *T. tonsurans* common in African Americans	*M. audouinii* fluorescence: blue-green with Wood lamp*; +KOH, culture	Griseofulvin; terbinafine, itraconazole
Kerion	Inflammatory reaction to tinea capitis	Swollen, boggy, crusted, purulent, tender mass with lymphadenopathy; secondary distal *id* reaction common	As above	As above, plus steroids for *id* reactions
Tinea corporis (ringworm)	*M. canis, Trichophyton rubrum,* others	Slightly pruritic ringlike, erythematous papules, plaques with scaling and slow outward expansion of the border; check cat or dog for *M. canis*	+KOH, culture; *M. canis* fluorescence: blue-green with Wood lamp; differential diagnosis: granuloma annulare, pityriasis rosea, nummular eczema, psoriasis	Topical miconazole, clotrimazole, terbinafine, tolnaftate, ciclopirox, oxiconazole, or butenafine
Tinea cruris (jock itch)	*Epidermophyton floccosum, Trichophyton mentagrophytes, T. rubrum*	Symmetric, pruritic, scrotal sparing, scaling plaques	+KOH, culture; differential diagnosis: erythrasma (*Corynebacterium minutissimum*)	See Tinea corporis, Therapy; wear loose cotton underwear
Tinea pedis (athlete's foot)	*T. rubrum, T. mentagrophytes*	Moccasin or interdigital distribution, dry scales, interdigital maceration with secondary bacterial infection	+KOH, culture; differential diagnosis: *C. minutissimum* erythrasma	Medications as above; wear cotton socks
Tinea unguium (onychomycosis)	*T. mentagrophytes, T. rubrum, Candida albicans*	Uncommon before puberty; peeling of distal nail plate; thickening, splitting of nails	+KOH, culture	Oral terbinafine or itraconazole
Tinea versicolor	*Malassezia furfur*	Tropical climates, steroids or immunosuppressive drugs; uncommon before puberty; chest, back, arms; oval hypopigmented or hyperpigmented in African Americans, red-brown in Caucasians; scaling patches	+KOH; orange-gold fluorescence with Wood lamp; differential diagnosis: pityriasis alba	Topical selenium sulfide, oral ketoconazole
YEAST				
Candidiasis	*Candida albicans*	Diaper area, intense erythematous plaques or pustules, isolated or confluent	+KOH, culture	Topical nystatin; oral nystatin treats concomitant oral thrush

KOH, Potassium hydroxide.
*Wood lamp examination uses an ultraviolet source in a completely darkened room. *Trichophyton* usually has no fluorescence.

HSV-2 can cause gingivostomatitis. For the cutaneous manifestations of neonatal HSV infection, see Chapter 65.

Herpes gingivostomatitis involves the gingivae and the vermilion border of the lips. Herpes labialis (**cold sores or fever blisters**) is limited to the vermilion border involving skin and mucous membranes. Clinical manifestations of primary HSV gingivostomatitis include typical oropharyngeal vesicular lesions with high fever, malaise, stinging mouth pain, drooling, fetid breath, and cervical lymphadenopathy.

Herpetic skin lesions are quite painful and characteristically begin as erythematous papules that quickly progress to the characteristically grouped, 2- to 4-mm, fluid-filled vesicles on an erythematous base. Removal of the vesicle roof reveals a small, sharply demarcated ulcer with a punched-out appearance. The characteristic grouped vesicles distinguish HSV from chickenpox (see Chapter 97). Within several days, the vesicles become pustular, rupture, and encrust. Diagnosis is made clinically, or with viral culture, fluorescent antibody staining, or polymerase chain reaction. Scarring is uncommon, but there may be residual hyperpigmentation. After primary infection, the virus remains latent in nerve dorsal root ganglia. About 20% to 40% of adults experience recurrent oral episodes of HSV labialis throughout life. Recurrences occur in roughly the same location and may be preceded by prodromal symptoms of tingling or burning without fever or lymphadenopathy.

Viral paronychia (**herpetic whitlow**) is a painful, localized infection of a digit, usually of the distal pulp space, with erythematous and occasionally vesiculopustular eruption. It occurs in children who suck their thumbs, bite their nails, and those with herpetic gingivostomatitis. **Herpes gladiatorum** occurs in wrestlers and rugby players who acquire cutaneous herpes from close body contact with other players' cutaneous infections. Cutaneous HSV infection in persons with an underlying skin disorder (e.g., atopic dermatitis) can result in **eczema herpeticum (Kaposi varicelliform eruption)**, a disseminated cutaneous infection. There may be hundreds of herpetic vesicles over the body, usually concentrated in the areas of skin affected by the underlying disorder.

Treatment with oral valacyclovir or famciclovir may shorten duration of disease for primary and recurrent infection. Prophylactic antiviral therapy may be warranted in those with frequent recurrences. Infants, persons with eczema, and persons with immunodeficiency are at increased risk for disseminated and severe HSV disease and should receive intravenous acyclovir therapy.

Human Papillomaviruses (Warts)

Decision-Making Algorithms
Available @ StudentConsult.com

Hoarseness
Vaginal Discharge

Warts are caused by the human papillomaviruses (HPVs), nonenveloped, double-stranded DNA viruses that infect skin and mucous membrane keratinocytes. More than 100 HPV serotypes have been identified, with different serotypes accounting for the variation in location and clinical presentations. There are 15 to 20 **oncogenic (high-risk)** types, including 16, 18, 31, 33, 35, 39, 45, 51, 52, and 58. HPV types 16 and 18 are associated with 70% of cases of cervical cancer as well as vulvar and vaginal cancers. Common **nononcogenic (low-risk)** types include 1, 2, 3, 6, 10, 11, 40, 42, 43, 44, and 54. Regardless of the infecting serotype, all warts are associated with hyperplasia of the epidermal cells.

Warts occur at all ages. **Common warts (verruca vulgaris),** associated with HPV types 1 and 2, are the most common form (71%). They occur frequently in school-age children, with a prevalence of 4% to 20%. They are transmitted by direct contact or by fomites and have an incubation period of approximately 1 month before clinical presentation. The common wart is a painless, well-circumscribed, small (2- to 5-mm) papule with a papillated or verrucous surface typically distributed on the fingers, toes, elbows, and knees. They also may be found on the nose, ears, and lips. **Filiform warts** are verrucous, exophytic, 2-mm papules that have a narrow or pedunculated base. **Flat warts (verruca plana)** are associated with HPV types 3 and 10 and are multiple, flat-topped 2- to 4-mm papules clustered on the dorsal surface of the hands, on the soles of the feet (**plantar warts**), or on the face. Plantar warts may be painful because of the effect of pressure and friction on the lesions. **Genital warts (condylomata acuminata)** are associated with the HPV types 6 and 11 (90%). They are flesh-colored, hyperpigmented, or erythematous lesions that are filiform, fungating, or plaquelike in appearance and involve multiple sites on the vulva, vagina, penis, or perineum. Genital warts are the most common sexually transmitted infection, with 1 million new cases annually.

Warts typically are self-limited and resolve spontaneously over years without specific treatment. Treatment options are available for common and flat warts as well as condylomata acuminata. Topical preparations for common and flat warts disrupt infected epithelium (using salicylic acid, liquid nitrogen, or laser therapy) and result in the cure of approximately 75% of patients. Treatment of anogenital warts is complex, and specific treatments (www.cdc.gov/std/hpv/default.htm) may include topical podophyllotoxin or imiquimod. Additional treatment methods include laser ablation and immunotherapy with intralesional interferon; immunotherapy may result in significant toxicities.

The most serious consequence of HPV infection is cervical cancer (more than 12,000 new cases annually), vulvar, vaginal, penile, and anal cancers. A quadrivalent, recombinant HPV vaccine against serotypes 6, 11, 31, and 33 is recommended for all children at 11 to 12 years of age but may be given to children between 9 and 26 years of age. The three-dose regimen has 98% to 100% efficacy in preventing the precancerous dysplasia that precedes cervical cancer.

Molluscum Contagiosum

Molluscum contagiosum virus, a poxvirus that replicates in host epithelial cells, produces discrete, small (2 to 4 mm), pearly flesh-colored or pink, nontender, dome-shaped papules with central umbilication. Papules occur most commonly in intertriginous regions, such as the axillae, groin, and neck. They rarely occur on the face or in the periocular region. The infection typically affects toddlers and young children and is acquired through direct contact with infected individuals. Spread occurs by autoinoculation. Infection with molluscum contagiosum may be complicated by a surrounding dermatitis. Severely immunocompromised persons or persons with extensive atopic dermatitis often have widespread lesions.

Diagnosis is made clinically. Lesions are self-limited, resolving over months to years, and usually no specific treatment is recommended. Available treatment options are limited to destructive modalities, such as cryotherapy with topical liquid nitrogen, vesicant therapy with topical 0.9% cantharidin, or removal by curettage, and should be reserved for extensive disease.

Chapter **99**

LYMPHADENOPATHY

ETIOLOGY

Decision-Making Algorithm
Available @ StudentConsult.com

Lymphadenopathy

Lymphoid tissue steadily enlarges until puberty and subsequently undergoes progressive atrophy. Lymph nodes are most prominent in children 4 to 8 years of age. Normal lymph node size is 10 mm in diameter, with the exceptions of 15 mm for inguinal nodes, 5 mm for epitrochlear nodes, and 2 mm for supraclavicular nodes, which are usually undetectable. **Lymphadenopathy** is enlargement of lymph nodes and occurs in response to a wide variety of infectious, inflammatory, and malignant processes. **Generalized lymphadenopathy** is enlargement of two or more noncontiguous lymph node groups, whereas **regional lymphadenopathy** involves one lymph node group only.

Table 99-1	Infectious Causes of Generalized Lymphadenopathy

VIRAL

Epstein-Barr virus (infectious mononucleosis)

Cytomegalovirus (infectious mononucleosis-like syndrome)

HIV (acute retroviral syndrome)

Hepatitis B virus

Hepatitis C virus

Varicella

Adenoviruses

Rubeola (measles)

Rubella

BACTERIAL

Endocarditis

Brucella (brucellosis)

Leptospira interrogans (leptospirosis)

Streptobacillus moniliformis (bacillary rat-bite fever)

Mycobacterium tuberculosis (tuberculosis)

Treponema pallidum (secondary syphilis)

FUNGAL

Coccidioides immitis (coccidioidomycosis)

Histoplasma capsulatum (histoplasmosis)

PROTOZOAL

Toxoplasma gondii (toxoplasmosis)
Trypanosoma cruzi (Chagas disease)

Table 99-2	Infectious Causes of Regional Lymphadenopathy

NONVENEREAL ORIGIN

Staphylococcus aureus

Group A streptococcus

Group B streptococcus (in infants)

Bartonella henselae (cat-scratch disease)

Yersinia pestis (plague)

Francisella tularensis (glandular tularemia)

Mycobacterium tuberculosis

Nontuberculous mycobacteria

Sporothrix schenckii (sporotrichosis)

Epstein-Barr virus

Toxoplasma gondii

SEXUALLY TRANSMITTED INFECTIONS (PRIMARILY INGUINAL LYMPHADENOPATHY)

Neisseria gonorrhoeae (gonorrhea)

Treponema pallidum (syphilis)

Herpes simplex virus

Haemophilus ducreyi (chancroid)

Chlamydia trachomatis serovars L$_{1-3}$ (lymphogranuloma venereum)

LYMPHOCUTANEOUS SYNDROMES

Bacillus anthracis (anthrax)

F. tularensis (ulceroglandular tularemia)

B. henselae (cat-scratch disease)

Pasteurella multocida (dog or cat bite)
Rickettsialpox

Spirillum minus (spirillary rat-bite fever)

Y. pestis (plague)

Nocardia (nocardiosis)

Cutaneous diphtheria (*Corynebacterium diphtherial*)

Cutaneous coccidioidomycosis (*Coccidioides immitis*)

Cutaneous histoplasmosis (*Histoplasma capsulatum*)
Cutaneous leishmaniasis

Cutaneous sporotrichosis (*S. schenckii*)

Lymphadenitis is acute or chronic inflammation of lymph nodes. Acute lymphadenitis usually results when bacteria and toxins from a site of acute inflammation are carried via lymph to regional nodes. Numerous infections cause lymphadenopathy and lymphadenitis (Tables 99-1 and 99-2). Causes of inguinal regional lymphadenopathy also include sexually transmitted infections (see Chapter 116). Regional lymphadenitis associated with a characteristic skin lesion at the site of inoculation defines various **lymphocutaneous syndromes**. **Lymphangitis** is an inflammation of subcutaneous lymphatic channels that presents as an acute bacterial infection, usually caused by *Staphylococcus aureus* and group A streptococci.

Cervical lymphadenitis is the most common regional lymphadenitis among children and is associated most commonly with pharyngitis caused by group A streptococcus (see Chapter 103), respiratory viruses, and Epstein-Barr virus (EBV). Other common infectious causes of cervical lymphadenitis include *Bartonella henselae* (cat-scratch disease) and nontuberculous mycobacteria.

EBV is the primary cause of **infectious mononucleosis,** a clinical syndrome characterized by fever, fatigue and malaise, cervical or generalized lymphadenopathy, tonsillitis, and pharyngitis. EBV, a member of the herpesvirus family, infects B lymphocytes and is spread by salivary secretions. After primary infection, EBV is maintained latently in multiple episomes in the cell nucleus of resting B lymphocytes and establishes lifelong infection that remains clinically inapparent. Most persons shed EBV intermittently, with approximately 20% of healthy individuals shedding EBV at any given time. Cytomegalovirus (CMV), *Toxoplasma gondii,* adenoviruses, hepatitis B virus, hepatitis C virus, and initial human immunodeficiency virus (HIV) infection, known as **acute retroviral syndrome,** can cause an infectious mononucleosis-like syndrome with lymphadenopathy.

The cause of **cat-scratch disease** is *B. henselae,* a small, pleomorphic, gram-negative bacillus that stains with Warthin-Starry silver stain. *B. henselae* causes apparently asymptomatic bacteremia in cats, and kittens under 1 year of age are more likely to harbor the organism. *B. henselae* is transmitted to humans by bites and scratches, which may be minor. *B. henselae* also causes bacillary angiomatosis and peliosis hepatis in persons with HIV infection (see Chapter 125).

Nontuberculous mycobacteria are ubiquitous in soil, vegetation, dust, and water. *Mycobacterium* species commonly causing lymphadenitis in children includes *M. avium* complex, *M. scrofulaceum,* and *M. kansasii. M. tuberculosis* uncommonly causes cervical lymphadenitis.

EPIDEMIOLOGY

Acute cervical lymphadenitis as a complication of group A streptococcal infection parallels the incidence of streptococcal pharyngitis (see Chapter 103). Many cases are caused by *S. aureus.* EBV and CMV are ubiquitous, with most infections occurring in young children, who may often be asymptomatic or only mildly symptomatic. Risk factors for other specific causes of lymphadenopathy may be indicated by past medical and surgical history; preceding trauma; exposure to animals; contact with persons infected with tuberculosis; sexual history; travel history; food and ingestion history, especially of undercooked meat or unpasteurized dairy products; and current medications.

CLINICAL MANIFESTATIONS

The exact location and detailed measurement of the size, shape, characteristics, and number of involved nodes should be noted, including their consistency, mobility, tenderness, warmth, fluctuance, firmness, and adherence to adjacent tissues. Important findings include presence or absence of dental disease, oropharyngeal or skin lesions, ocular disease, other nodal enlargement, and any other signs of systemic illness, including hepatosplenomegaly and skin lesions.

Acute cervical lymphadenopathy associated with pharyngitis is characterized by small and rubbery lymph nodes in the anterior cervical chain with minimal to moderate tenderness. Suppurative cervical lymphadenitis, frequently caused by *S. aureus* or group A streptococcus, shows erythema and warmth of the overlying skin with moderate to exquisite tenderness.

The characteristic triad of EBV infectious mononucleosis is fever, pharyngitis, and lymphadenopathy. The pharynx shows enlarged tonsils and exudate and, sometimes, an enanthem with pharyngeal petechiae. Lymphadenopathy is most prominent in the anterior and posterior cervical and submandibular lymph nodes and less commonly involves axillary and inguinal lymph nodes. Other findings include splenomegaly in 50% of cases, hepatomegaly in 10% to 20%, and maculopapular or urticarial rash in 5% to 15%. A diffuse, erythematous rash develops in approximately 80% of mononucleosis patients treated with amoxicillin. Compared with EBV infection, infectious mononucleosis-like illness caused by CMV has minimal pharyngitis and often more prominent splenomegaly; it often presents with fever only. The most common manifestation of toxoplasmosis is asymptomatic cervical lymphadenopathy, but approximately 10% of cases of acquired toxoplasmosis develop chronic posterior cervical lymphadenopathy and fatigue, usually without significant fever.

Cat-scratch disease typically presents with a cutaneous papule or conjunctival granuloma at the site of bacterial inoculation, followed by lymphadenopathy of the draining regional nodes. The nodes are tender, with suppuration in approximately 10% of cases. Lymphadenopathy may persist 1 to 4 months. Less common features of cat-scratch disease include erythema nodosum, osteolytic lesions, encephalitis, oculoglandular (Parinaud) syndrome, hepatic or splenic granulomas, endocarditis, polyneuritis, and transverse myelitis.

Lymphadenitis caused by **nontuberculous mycobacteria** usually is unilateral in the cervical, submandibular, or preauricular nodes and is more common in toddlers. The nodes are relatively painless and firm initially, but gradually soften, rupture, and drain over time. The local reaction is circumscribed, and overlying skin may develop a violaceous discoloration without warmth. Fever and systemic symptoms are minimal or absent.

LABORATORY AND IMAGING STUDIES

Initial laboratory tests of regional lymphadenopathy include a complete blood count and inflammatory markers. Infectious mononucleosis is characterized by lymphocytosis with **atypical lymphocytes**; thrombocytopenia and elevated hepatic enzymes are common.

Cultures of infected skin lesions and tonsillar exudates should be obtained. Isolation of group A streptococci from the oropharynx suggests, but does not confirm, streptococcal cervical lymphadenitis. A blood culture should be obtained from children with systemic signs and symptoms of bacteremia.

Serologic testing for EBV and for *B. henselae* should be obtained if there are appropriate findings. The most reliable test for diagnosis of acute EBV infection is the IgM antiviral capsid antigen (Fig. 99-1). Heterophil antibody is also diagnostic but is not reliably positive in children younger than 4 years with infectious mononucleosis.

Extended diagnostic workup for lymphadenopathy is guided by the specific risk factors in the history and physical examination findings. Chest radiograph, throat culture, antistreptolysin O titer, and serologic tests for CMV, toxoplasmosis, syphilis, tularemia, *Brucella,* histoplasmosis, and coccidioidomycosis may be indicated. Genital tract evaluation and specimens should be obtained with regional inguinal lymphadenopathy (see Chapter 116). Screening for tuberculosis can be performed using the standard tuberculin skin test or an interferon gamma release assay; both may be positive with atypical mycobacterial infection.

Aspiration is indicated for acutely inflamed, fluctuant cervical lymph nodes, especially those larger than 3 cm in diameter or not responding to antibiotic treatment. Ultrasound or computed tomography may help in establishing the extent of lymphadenopathy and defining whether the mass is solid, cystic, or suppurative with abscess formation. Pus from fluctuant lesions should be examined by Gram and acid-fast stains and cultured for aerobic and anaerobic bacteria and mycobacteria. Biopsy should be performed if lymphoma is suspected because of firm, matted, nontender nodes and other systemic findings.

If the diagnosis remains uncertain and lymphadenopathy persists despite empirical antibiotic therapy for presumed *S. aureus* and group A streptococcus, excisional biopsy of the entire node should be performed, if possible. This is curative for nontuberculous mycobacterial lymphadenitis. Biopsy material should be submitted for histopathology as well as Gram, acid-fast, Giemsa, periodic acid-Schiff, Warthin-Starry silver *(B. henselae),* and methenamine silver stains. Cultures for aerobic and anaerobic bacteria, mycobacteria, and fungi should be performed.

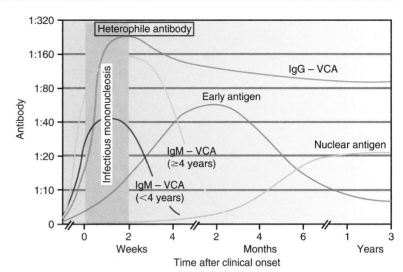

Figure 99-1 The development of antibodies to various Epstein-Barr virus antigens in patients with infectious mononucleosis. The titers are geometric mean values expressed as reciprocals of the serum dilution. The IgM response to viral capsid antigen (VCA) is divided because of the significant differences noted according to the age of the patient. *(From Jenson HB, Ench Y: Epstein-Barr virus. In Rose NR, Hamilton RG, Detrick B: Manual of Clinical Laboratory Immunology, ed 7, Washington DC, 2006, American Society for Microbiology Press, p 640.)*

DIFFERENTIAL DIAGNOSIS

Noninfectious causes of cervical swelling and/or lymphadenopathy include congenital and acquired cysts, Kawasaki disease, sarcoidosis, benign neoplasms, and malignancies. The differential diagnosis for generalized lymphadenopathy includes juvenile idiopathic arthritis; systemic lupus erythematosus; and serum sickness and other adverse drug reactions, especially with phenytoin and other antiepileptic medications, allopurinol, isoniazid, antithyroid medications, and pyrimethamine. Leukemia, lymphoma, and occasionally neuroblastoma may have lymph nodes that are usually painless, uninflamed, matted, and firm (see Chapters 155 and 156). A syndrome of **periodic fever, aphthous stomatitis, pharyngitis, and adenitis** is an occasional cause of recurrent fever and cervical lymphadenitis (see Chapter 103).

TREATMENT

Management of lymphadenopathy and lymphadenitis depends on patient age, associated findings, node size and location, and severity of the acute systemic symptoms. In children most cases of cervical lymphadenopathy, without other signs of acute inflammation, require no specific therapy and usually regress within 2 to 3 weeks. Progression to lymphadenitis or development of generalized lymphadenopathy requires further evaluation.

The specific treatment of cervical lymphadenitis depends on the underlying etiology. Empirical treatment targeting *S. aureus* and group A streptococcus includes a penicillinase-resistant penicillin (e.g., oxacillin) or first-generation cephalosporin (e.g., cefazolin). For patients with hypersensitivity to β-lactam antibiotics, or if community-acquired methicillin-resistant *S. aureus* is suspected, clindamycin is appropriate. Response to empirical antibiotic therapy for suppurative cervical lymphadenitis obviates the need for further evaluation. Absence of a clinical response within 48 to 72 hours is an indication for further laboratory evaluation and possible excisional biopsy and culture.

There is no specific treatment for infectious mononucleosis. Cat-scratch disease usually does not require treatment because the lymphadenopathy resolves in 2 to 4 months without sequelae. Azithromycin may hasten resolution and reduces

node size at 30 days but no benefit is evident at 90 days. Aspiration is indicated for suppurative nodes. The recommended treatment of cervical lymphadenitis caused by nontuberculous mycobacteria is complete surgical excision. Antimycobacterial drugs are necessary only if there is recurrence or inability to excise infected nodes completely, or if *M. tuberculosis* is identified, which requires 6 months of antituberculous chemotherapy (see Chapter 124).

COMPLICATIONS AND PROGNOSIS

Most acute infections caused by *S. aureus* and group A streptococcus respond to treatment and have an excellent prognosis. Complications such as abscess formation, cellulitis, and bacteremia may occur. Abscess formation is treated with incision and drainage in conjunction with appropriate antibiotic therapy.

Infectious mononucleosis usually resolves in 2 to 4 weeks, but fatigue and malaise may wax and wane for several weeks to months. EBV also is associated with numerous complications during the acute illness. Neurologic complications include seizures, aseptic meningitis syndrome, Bell palsy, transverse myelitis, encephalitis, and Guillain-Barre syndrome. Hematologic complications include Coombs-positive hemolytic anemia, antibody-mediated thrombocytopenia, hemophagocytic syndrome, and, rarely, aplastic anemia. Corticosteroids have been used for respiratory compromise resulting from tonsillar hypertrophy, which responds rapidly, and for thrombocytopenia, hemolytic anemia, and neurologic complications. Splenic rupture is very rare. **X-linked lymphoproliferative disease,** which results from a mutation of the *SH2D1A* gene located in the Xq25 region, manifests as fulminant infectious mononucleosis with primary EBV infection and progresses to malignant lymphoproliferative disease or dysgammaglobulinemia.

EBV infection, as with other herpesviruses, persists for life, but no symptoms are attributed to intermittent reactivation in immunocompetent hosts. EBV is causally associated with nasopharyngeal carcinoma; Burkitt lymphoma; Hodgkin disease; leiomyosarcoma in immunocompromised persons; and EBV lymphoproliferative disease, especially in posttransplant patients and in those with acquired immunodeficiency syndrome (AIDS).

Lymphadenitis caused by nontuberculous mycobacteria has an excellent prognosis. Surgical excision of cervical lymphadenitis caused by nontuberculous mycobacteria is curative in >97% of cases.

PREVENTION

The incidence of suppurative regional lymphadenitis reflects the incidence of predisposing conditions, such as dental disease, streptococcal pharyngitis, otitis media, impetigo, and other infections involving the face and scalp. There are no guidelines to prevent lymphadenitis caused by nontuberculous mycobacteria.

Chapter 100

MENINGITIS

ETIOLOGY

Meningitis, inflammation of the leptomeninges, can be caused by bacteria, viruses, or, rarely, fungi. The term **aseptic meningitis** refers principally to viral meningitis, but meningitis with negative cerebrospinal fluid (CSF) bacterial cultures may be seen with other infectious organisms (Lyme disease, syphilis, tuberculosis), parameningeal infections (brain abscess, epidural abscess, venous sinus empyema), chemical exposure (nonsteroidal anti-inflammatory drugs, intravenous immunoglobulin), autoimmune disorders, and other diseases.

The organisms commonly causing bacterial meningitis (Table 100-1) before the availability of current conjugate vaccines were *Haemophilus influenzae, Streptococcus pneumoniae,* and *Neisseria meningitidis.* In the United States, the rates of *H. influenzae* type b and *S. pneumoniae* meningitis have declined substantially after the introduction of targeted vaccines. The bacteria causing neonatal meningitis are the same as those causing neonatal sepsis (see Chapter 65). Staphylococcal meningitis occurs primarily after neurosurgery or penetrating head trauma.

Partially treated meningitis refers to bacterial meningitis complicated by antibiotic treatment before the lumbar puncture, which may result in negative CSF cultures, although other CSF findings suggestive of bacterial infection persist. The etiology can sometimes be confirmed by polymerase chain reaction of the CSF.

Viral meningitis is caused principally by enteroviruses and parechoviruses. Fecal excretion and transmission are continuous and persist for several weeks. Enteroviruses, parechoviruses, and arboviruses (St. Louis, LaCrosse, West Nile, California encephalitis viruses) are the principal causes of meningoencephalitis (see Chapter 101). Other viruses that cause meningitis include herpes simplex virus, Epstein-Barr virus, cytomegalovirus, lymphocytic choriomeningitis virus, and human immunodeficiency virus (HIV). Mumps virus is a common cause of viral meningitis in unvaccinated children. Less frequent causes of meningitis include *Borrelia burgdorferi* (Lyme disease), *Bartonella henselae* (cat-scratch disease), *Mycobacterium tuberculosis, Toxoplasma,* fungi (*Cryptococcus,*

Table 100-1	Bacterial Causes of Meningitis	
AGE	**MOST COMMON**	**LESS COMMON**
Neonatal	Group B streptococcus *Escherichia coli* *Klebsiella* *Enterobacter*	*Listeria monocytogenes* Coagulase-negative staphylococci *Enterococcus faecalis* *Citrobacter diversus* *Salmonella* *Pseudomonas aeruginosa* *Haemophilus influenzae* types a, b, c, d, e, f, and nontypable
>1 mo	*Streptococcus pneumoniae* *Neisseria meningitidis*	*H. influenzae* type b Group A streptococcus Gram-negative bacilli *L. monocytogenes*

Histoplasma, Blastomycosis, and *Coccidioides*), and parasites (*Angiostrongylus cantonensis, Naegleria fowleri,* and *Acanthamoeba*).

EPIDEMIOLOGY

The incidence of bacterial meningitis is highest among children under 1 year of age. Extremely high rates are found in Native Americans, Alaskan Natives, and Australian aboriginals, suggesting that genetic factors play a role in susceptibility. Other risk factors include acquired or congenital immunodeficiencies, hemoglobinopathies such as sickle cell disease, functional or anatomic asplenia, and crowding such as occurs in some households, day care centers, or college and military dormitories. A CSF leak (fistula), resulting from congenital anomaly or following a basilar skull fracture, increases the risk of meningitis, especially that caused by *S. pneumoniae.*

Enteroviruses and parechoviruses cause meningitis with peaks during summer and fall in temperate climates. These infections are more prevalent among low socioeconomic groups, young children, and immunocompromised persons. The prevalence of arboviral meningitis is determined by geographic distribution and seasonal activity of the arthropod (mosquito) vectors. In the United States, most arboviral infections occur during the summer and fall.

CLINICAL MANIFESTATIONS

Decision-Making Algorithms
Available @ StudentConsult.com

Apnea
Stiff or Painful Neck
Headaches
Hearing Loss
Fever without a Source
Irritable Infant

Preceding upper respiratory tract symptoms are common. Rapid onset is typical of *S. pneumoniae* and *N. meningitidis.* Indications of meningeal inflammation include headache, irritability, nausea, nuchal rigidity, lethargy, photophobia, and vomiting. Fever usually is present. Kernig and Brudzinski

Table 100-2	Cerebrospinal Fluid (CSF) Findings in Various Central Nervous System Disorders				
CONDITION	**PRESSURE**	**LEUKOCYTES (/μL)**	**PROTEIN (mg/dL)**	**GLUCOSE (mg/dL)**	**COMMENTS**
Normal	50–180 mm H_2O	<4; 60%–70% lymphocytes, 30%–40% monocytes, 1%–3% neutrophils	20–45	>50% of serum glucose	
Acute bacterial meningitis	Usually elevated	100–60,000+; usually a few thousand; PMNs predominate	100–500	Usually <40 or <40% of serum glucose	Organisms may be seen on Gram stain and recovered by culture
Partially treated bacterial meningitis	Normal or elevated	1–10,000; PMNs usual but mononuclear cells may predominate if pretreated for extended period	>100	Depressed or normal	Organisms may be seen; pretreatment may render CSF sterile in pneumococcal and meningococcal disease, but these may be detected by PCR
Tuberculous meningitis	Usually elevated; may be low because of CSF block in advanced stages	10–500; PMNs early but lymphocytes and monocytes predominate later	100–500; may be higher in presence of CSF block	Usually <50; decreases with time if treatment not provided	Acid-fast organisms may be seen on smear; organisms can be recovered in culture or by PCR; consider TST or IGRA and chest x-ray to confirm or support diagnosis
Fungal	Usually elevated	25–500; PMNs early; mononuclear cells predominate later	20–500	Usually <50; decreases with time if treatment not provided	Budding yeast may be seen; organisms may be recovered in culture; India ink preparation may be positive and antigen usually positive in cryptococcal disease
Viral meningitis or meningoen-cephalitis	Normal or slightly elevated	PMNs early; mononuclear cells predominate later; rarely more than 1000 cells except in eastern equine encephalitis	<200	Generally normal; may be depressed to 40 in some viral diseases (in 15%–20% of mumps)	Enteroviruses may be recovered from CSF by appropriate viral cultures or detected by PCR; HSV detected by PCR
Abscess (parameningeal infection)	Normal or elevated	0–100 PMNs unless rupture into CSF	20–200	Normal	Profile may be completely normal

HSV, Herpes simplex virus; *IGRA*, interferon gamma release assay for tuberculosis; *PCR*, polymerase chain reaction; *PMNs*, polymorphonuclear leukocytes; *TST*, tuberculin skin test.

signs of meningeal irritation are often positive in children older than 12 months. In young infants, signs of meningeal inflammation may be minimal with only irritability, restlessness, depressed mental status, and poor feeding present. Focal neurologic signs, seizures, arthralgia, myalgia, petechial or purpuric lesions, sepsis, shock, and coma may occur. Symptoms of increased intracranial pressure include headache, diplopia, and vomiting; a bulging fontanelle may be present in infants. Ptosis, sixth nerve palsy, anisocoria, bradycardia with hypertension, and apnea are signs of increased intracranial pressure with brain herniation. Papilledema is uncommon, unless there is occlusion of the venous sinuses, subdural empyema, or brain abscess.

LABORATORY AND IMAGING STUDIES

If bacterial meningitis is suspected, a lumbar puncture should be performed unless there is evidence of cardiovascular instability or of increased intracranial pressure (because of the risk of herniation), other than a bulging fontanelle. Routine CSF examination includes a white blood cell count, differential, protein and glucose levels, and Gram stain (Table 100-2). CSF should be

cultured for bacteria and, when appropriate, fungi, viruses, and mycobacteria. The polymerase chain reaction is used to diagnose enteroviruses, parechoviruses, and herpes simplex virus; it is more sensitive and rapid than viral culture. Peripheral leukocytosis is common, and blood cultures are positive in 90% of cases of bacterial meningitis. An electroencephalogram may confirm an encephalitis component (see Chapter 101).

DIFFERENTIAL DIAGNOSIS

Many disorders may show signs of meningeal irritation and increased intracranial pressure, including the infectious causes of meningitis or encephalitis, hemorrhage, rheumatic diseases, and malignancies. Seizures are associated with meningitis, encephalitis, and intracranial abscess or can be the sequelae of brain edema, cerebral infarction or hemorrhage, or vasculitis.

TREATMENT

Treatment of bacterial meningitis focuses on sterilization of the CSF by antibiotics (Table 100–3) and maintenance of

Table 100-3	Initial Antimicrobial Therapy by Age for Presumed Bacterial Meningitis	
AGE	**RECOMMENDED TREATMENT**	**ALTERNATIVE TREATMENTS**
Newborns (0–28 days)	Cefotaxime or ceftriaxone plus ampicillin with or without gentamicin	Ampicillin plus gentamicin Ceftazidime plus ampicillin
Infants and toddlers (1 mo–4 yr)	Ceftriaxone or cefotaxime plus vancomycin	Cefotaxime or ceftriaxone plus rifampin
Children and adolescents (5–13 yr) and adults	Ceftriaxone or cefotaxime plus vancomycin	Cefepime or ceftazidime plus vancomycin

adequate cerebral and systemic perfusion. Due to increasing *S. pneumoniae* resistance to penicillin and cephalosporins, empirical cefotaxime (or ceftriaxone) *plus* vancomycin should be administered until antibiotic susceptibility testing is available. Cefotaxime or ceftriaxone are also adequate to treat *N. meningitidis* and *H. influenzae*. For infants younger than 2 months of age, ampicillin is added to cover the possibility of *Listeria monocytogenes*. Duration of treatment is 5 to 7 days for *N. meningitidis*, 7 to 10 days for *H. influenzae*, and 10 to 14 days for *S. pneumoniae*.

Dexamethasone (0.6 to 0.8 mg/kg daily in two to three divided doses for 2 days), as **adjunctive therapy** initiated just before or concurrently with the first dose of antibiotics, significantly diminishes the incidence of hearing loss and neurologic deficits resulting from *H. influenzae* meningitis. Adjuvant steroids do not appear to decrease mortality or hospital stay in studies in the developed world.

Supportive therapy involves treatment of dehydration, shock, disseminated intravascular coagulation, syndrome of inappropriate antidiuretic hormone (SIADH), seizures, increased intracranial pressure, apnea, arrhythmias, and coma. Adequate cerebral perfusion must be maintained in the presence of cerebral edema.

COMPLICATIONS AND PROGNOSIS

Decision-Making Algorithm
Available @ StudentConsult.com

Hearing Loss

SIADH may complicate meningitis and necessitates monitoring of urine output and fluid administration. Computed tomography or magnetic resonance imaging commonly detects subdural effusions with *S. pneumoniae* and *H. influenzae* meningitis. Most effusions are sterile and asymptomatic and do not necessitate drainage unless associated with increased intracranial pressure or focal neurologic signs. Persistent fever is common during treatment but also may be related to infective treatment or immune complex-mediated pericardial or joint effusions, thrombophlebitis, drug fever, or nosocomial infection. A repeat lumbar puncture after 48 hours of therapy should be considered for those whose condition

has not improved or has worsened and for those who received adjunct steroids, which can interfere with the ability to monitor clinical response.

Even with appropriate antibiotic therapy, the mortality rate for bacterial meningitis in children is significant: 25% for *S. pneumoniae,* 15% for *N. meningitidis,* and 8% for *H. influenzae*. Of survivors, 35% have sequelae, particularly after pneumococcal infection, including deafness, seizures, learning disabilities, blindness, paresis, ataxia, or hydrocephalus. All patients with meningitis should have a hearing evaluation before discharge and at follow-up. Poor prognosis is associated with young age, long duration of illness before effective antibiotic therapy, seizures, coma at presentation, shock, low or absent CSF white blood cell count in the presence of visible bacteria on CSF Gram stain, and immunocompromised status.

Rarely **relapse** may occur 3 to 14 days after treatment, possibly from parameningeal foci or resistant organisms. **Recurrence** may indicate an underlying immunologic or anatomic defect that predisposes the patient to meningitis.

PREVENTION

Routine **immunizations** against *H. influenzae* and *S. pneumoniae* are recommended for children beginning at 2 months of age. Quadrivalent vaccines against *N. meningitidis* (serotypes A, C, Y, and W-135) are recommended for adolescents, college freshmen, military personnel, and travelers to highly endemic areas (see Chapter 94), and are licensed down to 2 years of age. **Chemoprophylaxis** with rifampin, ciprofloxacin, or ceftriaxone to eradicate the carrier state and decrease transmission is recommended both for index cases with *N. meningitidis* or *H. influenzae* and for their close contacts.

Chapter **101**

ENCEPHALITIS

ETIOLOGY

Encephalitis is an inflammatory process of the brain parenchyma leading to cerebral dysfunction. It is usually an acute process but may be a postinfectious encephalomyelitis, a chronic degenerative disease, or a slow viral infection. Encephalitis may be diffuse or localized. Organisms cause encephalitis by one of two mechanisms: (1) direct infection of the brain parenchyma or (2) an apparent immune-mediated response in the central nervous system that usually begins several days after the appearance of extraneural manifestations of the infection.

Viruses are the principal causes of acute infectious encephalitis (Table 101-1). The most common viral causes of encephalitis in the United States are the enteroviruses, arboviruses, and herpesviruses. Human immunodeficiency virus (HIV) is an important cause of subacute encephalitis in children and adolescents and may present as an acute febrile illness but, more commonly, is insidious in onset (see Chapter 125).

Table 101-1	Causes of Acute Encephalitis
AGENT	**FREQUENCY**
Enterovirus and parechovirus	+++
Herpes simplex viruses (HSV 1, 6, 7)	++
Arthropod-borne viruses (especially West Nile virus, St. Louis, California, LaCrosse, and equine encephalitis viruses)	++
Epstein-Barr virus	+
Adenovirus	+
Human immunodeficiency virus	+
Borrelia burgdorferi (Lyme disease)	+
Bartonella henselae (cat-scratch disease)	+
Mycoplasma pneumoniae	+
Rickettsia rickettsii	+

Adapted from Willoughby RE Jr, Long SS: Encephalitis, meningoencephalitis, acute disseminated encephalomyelitis, and acute necrotizing encephalopathy. In Long SS, Pickering LK, Prober CG : Principles and Practice of Pediatric Infectious Diseases, revised reprint, ed 3, Philadelphia, 2008, Saunders.

Other causes of subacute encephalitis include measles, slow viruses (e.g., JC virus), and prion-associated diseases (e.g., Creutzfeldt-Jakob disease). Encephalitis also may result from metabolic, toxic, and neoplastic disorders.

Acute disseminated encephalomyelitis (ADEM) is the abrupt development of multiple neurologic signs related to an inflammatory, demyelinating disorder of the brain and spinal cord. ADEM follows childhood viral infections (such as measles and chickenpox) or vaccinations and resembles multiple sclerosis clinically.

EPIDEMIOLOGY
Arboviral and enteroviral encephalitides characteristically appear in clusters or epidemics that occur from midsummer to early fall, although sporadic cases of enteroviral encephalitis occur throughout the year. Herpesviruses and other infectious agents account for additional sporadic cases throughout the year.

Arboviruses tend to be limited to certain geographic areas, reflecting the reservoir and mosquito vector. St. Louis encephalitis virus is present throughout the United States in birds. California encephalitis virus, common in the Midwest, is carried by rodents and spread by mosquitoes. Eastern equine encephalitis virus is limited to the East Coast in birds. Western equine encephalitis virus is present throughout the Midwest and West in birds. West Nile virus infection occurs worldwide and causes outbreaks of summer encephalitis in North America. The principal vector for West Nile virus is the *Culex pipiens* mosquito, but the organism can be isolated in nature from a wide variety of *Culex* and *Aedes* species. A broad range of birds serves as the major reservoir for West Nile virus.

CLINICAL MANIFESTATIONS
Acute infectious encephalitis usually is preceded by a prodrome of several days of nonspecific symptoms such as sore throat, fever, headache, and abdominal complaints followed by the characteristic symptoms of progressive lethargy, behavioral changes, and neurologic deficits. Seizures are common at presentation. Children with encephalitis also may have a maculopapular rash and severe complications such as fulminant coma, transverse myelitis, anterior horn cell disease, or peripheral neuropathy.

West Nile encephalitis produces a broad spectrum of illness from asymptomatic infection to death. Severity of disease increases with advancing age. Most children are asymptomatic. Typical symptoms include mild, nonspecific extraneurologic illness characterized by fever, rash, arthralgias, lymphadenopathy, gastrointestinal complaints, and conjunctivitis.

DIFFERENTIAL DIAGNOSIS
The diagnosis is established presumptively by the presence of characteristic neurologic signs, typical epidemiology findings, and evidence of infection by cerebrospinal fluid (CSF) analysis, electroencephalogram (EEG), and brain imaging techniques. Encephalitis may result from infections with bacteria, *Mycoplasma*, *Rickettsia*, fungi, and parasites and from many noninfectious diseases, including metabolic diseases (encephalopathy), such as Reye syndrome, hypoglycemia, collagen vascular disorders, drugs, hypertension, and malignancies.

LABORATORY AND IMAGING STUDIES
The diagnosis of viral encephalitis is supported by examination of the CSF, which typically shows a lymphocytic pleocytosis, slight elevation in protein content, and normal glucose level. The CSF occasionally may be normal. Extreme elevations of protein and reductions of glucose suggest tuberculosis, cryptococcal infection, or meningeal carcinomatosis. The EEG is the definitive test and shows diffuse, slow wave activity, although focal changes may be present. Neuroimaging studies may be normal or may show diffuse cerebral swelling of the parenchyma or focal abnormalities. A temporal lobe focus on EEG or brain imaging is the characteristic feature of herpes simplex virus (HSV) infection.

Serologic studies should be obtained for arboviruses (including West Nile virus, if indicated by the patient risk factors), Epstein-Barr virus, *Mycoplasma pneumoniae*, cat-scratch disease, and Lyme disease. Additional serologic testing for less common pathogens should be performed as indicated by the travel, social, or medical history. In most cases of viral encephalitis, the virus is difficult to isolate from the CSF. Polymerase chain reaction tests for HSV, enteroviruses, West Nile virus, and other viruses are available and should be sent. Viral cultures of stool and a nasopharyngeal swab may also be obtained. Even with extensive testing and the use of

Decision-Making Algorithms
Available @ StudentConsult.com

Stiff or Painful Neck
Headaches
Ataxia
Altered Mental Status
Hearing Loss Query
Polyuria

polymerase chain reaction assays, the cause of encephalitis remains undetermined in one third of cases.

Brain biopsy is seldom performed but may be useful in patients with focal neurologic findings. It may be appropriate for patients with severe encephalopathy who show no clinical improvement if the diagnosis remains obscure. Rabies encephalitis and prion-related diseases (Creutzfeldt-Jakob disease and kuru) may be routinely diagnosed by culture or pathologic examination of brain biopsy tissue. Brain biopsy may be helpful to identify arbovirus and enterovirus infections, tuberculosis, fungal infections, and noninfectious illnesses, particularly primary central nervous system vasculopathies and malignancies.

TREATMENT

With the exception of HSV, varicella-zoster virus, cytomegalovirus, and HIV, there is no specific therapy for viral encephalitis. Management is supportive and frequently requires intensive care unit admission to facilitate aggressive therapy for seizures, timely detection of electrolyte abnormalities, and, when necessary, airway monitoring and protection or reduction of increased intracranial pressure and maintenance of adequate cerebral perfusion pressure.

Intravenous acyclovir is the treatment of choice for HSV and varicella-zoster virus infections. Cytomegalovirus infection is treated with ganciclovir. HIV infections may be treated with a combination of antiretroviral agents. *M. pneumoniae* infections may be treated with doxycycline, erythromycin, azithromycin, or clarithromycin, although the clinical value of treating encephalitis associated with mycoplasmal disease is uncertain.

ADEM has been treated with high-dose intravenous corticosteroids, but it is unclear whether the improved outcome with corticosteroids reflects milder cases recognized by magnetic resonance imaging, fewer cases of ADEM caused by measles (which causes severe ADEM), or improved supportive care.

COMPLICATIONS AND PROGNOSIS

Among survivors, symptoms usually resolve over several days to 2 to 3 weeks. Although most patients with epidemic forms of infectious encephalitis (St. Louis, California, West Nile, and enterovirus infections) in the United States recover without sequelae, severe cases leading to death or substantial neurologic sequelae can occur with virtually any of these neurotropic viruses. About two thirds of patients recover fully before being discharged from the hospital. The remainder show clinically significant residua, including paresis or spasticity, cognitive impairment, weakness, ataxia, and recurrent seizures. Most patients with neurologic sequelae of infectious encephalitis at the time of hospital discharge gradually recover some or all of their function. The overall mortality for infectious encephalitis is approximately 5%.

Disease caused by HSV, Eastern equine encephalitis, or *M. pneumoniae* is associated with a worse prognosis. The prognosis may be worse for encephalitis in children younger than 1 year of age or with coma. Rabies, with very rare exceptions, is fatal.

Relapses of ADEM occur in 14%, usually within 1 year with the same or new clinical signs. Recurrences of ADEM may represent onset of multiple sclerosis in childhood.

PREVENTION

The best prevention for arboviral encephalitis is to avoid mosquito-borne or tick-borne exposures and to remove ticks carefully (see Chapter 122). There are no vaccines in use in the United States for the prevention of arboviral infection or for enteroviruses except for poliomyelitis. There are no specific preventive measures for HSV encephalitis except for cesarean section for mothers with active genital lesions (see Chapter 65). Rabies can be prevented by preexposure or postexposure vaccination. Influenza encephalitis can be prevented by use of influenza vaccination. Reye syndrome can be prevented by avoiding use of aspirin or aspirin-containing compounds for children with fever as well as use of varicella and influenza vaccines.

Chapter **102**

THE COMMON COLD

ETIOLOGY

The common cold is a viral infection with prominent symptoms of rhinorrhea and nasal obstruction, absent or mild fever, and no systemic manifestations. It is often referred to as **rhinitis** but usually involves the sinus mucosa and is more correctly termed **rhinosinusitis.**

The viruses primarily associated with colds are rhinoviruses and, less commonly, coronaviruses. Other viruses that cause common cold symptoms include respiratory syncytial virus and, less commonly, influenza, parainfluenza, and adenoviruses. Viral infection of nasal epithelium causes an acute inflammatory response with mucosal infiltration by inflammatory cells and release of cytokines. The inflammatory response is partly responsible for many of the symptoms.

EPIDEMIOLOGY

Colds occur throughout the year with peak incidence from early fall through late spring, reflecting the seasonal prevalence of viral pathogens and confined habitation during colder months. Young children have an average of 6 to 7 colds each year, and 10% to 15% of children have at least 12 colds each year. The annual number of colds decreases with age, to two to three colds each year by adulthood. Children in out-of-home day care during the first year of life have 50% more colds than children cared for at home only. This difference diminishes during subsequent years in day care.

CLINICAL MANIFESTATIONS

Decision-Making Algorithms
Available @ StudentConsult.com

Rhinorrhea
Sore Throat

Common cold symptoms typically develop 1 to 3 days after viral infection and include nasal obstruction, rhinorrhea, sore or *scratchy* throat, and occasional nonproductive cough. Colds usually persist about 1 week, although 10% last 2 weeks. There is often a change in the color or consistency of nasal secretions, which is not indicative of sinusitis or bacterial superinfection. Examination of the nasal mucosa may reveal swollen, erythematous nasal turbinates.

LABORATORY AND IMAGING STUDIES

Laboratory studies often are not helpful. A **nasal smear** for eosinophils may be useful in the evaluation for allergic rhinitis (see Chapter 79).

DIFFERENTIAL DIAGNOSIS

The differential diagnosis of the common cold includes allergic rhinitis, foreign body (especially with unilateral nasal discharge), sinusitis, pertussis, and streptococcal nasopharyngitis. Allergic rhinitis is characterized by absence of fever, eosinophils in the nasal discharge, and other manifestations, such as allergic shiners, nasal polyps, a transverse crease on the nasal bridge, and pale, edematous, nasal turbinate mucosa. Rare causes of rhinorrhea are choanal atresia or stenosis, cerebrospinal fluid fistula, diphtheria, tumor, congenital syphilis (with *snuffles),* nasopharyngeal malignancy, and Wegener granulomatosis.

TREATMENT

There is no specific therapy for the common cold. Antibacterial therapy is not beneficial. Management consists of symptomatic therapies. Antihistamines, decongestants, and combination antihistamine-decongestants are not recommended for children younger than 6 years of age because of adverse effects and lack of benefits. Low-grade fever is seen with colds, particularly in the first few days of illness and can be treated with antipyretic medications. Cough suppressants and expectorants have not been shown to be beneficial. Vitamin C and inhalation of warm, humidified air are no more effective than placebo. The benefit of zinc lozenges or sprays has been inconsistent.

COMPLICATIONS AND PROGNOSIS

Otitis media is the most common complication and occurs in 5% to 20% of children with a cold (see Chapter 105). Other complications include bacterial sinusitis, which should be considered if rhinorrhea or daytime cough persists without improvement for at least 10 to 14 days or if severe signs of sinus involvement develop, such as fever, facial pain, or facial swelling (see Chapter 104). Colds may lead to exacerbation of asthma and may result in inappropriate antibiotic treatment.

PREVENTION

There are no proven methods for prevention of colds other than good hand washing and avoiding contact with infected persons. No significant effect of vitamin C or Echinacea for prevention of the common cold has been confirmed.

Chapter 103

PHARYNGITIS

ETIOLOGY

Many infectious agents can cause pharyngitis (Table 103-1). **Group A streptococci** (*Streptococcus pyogenes*) are gram-positive, nonmotile cocci that are facultative anaerobes. On sheep blood agar, the colonies are small (1 to 2 mm in diameter) and have a surrounding zone of β (clear) hemolysis. Other bacterial organisms less often associated with pharyngitis include group C streptococcus (also β-hemolytic), *Arcanobacterium haemolyticum* (β-hemolytic, gram-positive rod), and *Francisella tularensis* (gram-negative coccobacillus and cause of tularemia). *Chlamydophila pneumoniae,* strain TWAR, is associated with lower respiratory disease but also causes sore throat. *Mycoplasma pneumoniae* is associated with atypical pneumonia and may cause mild pharyngitis without distinguishing clinical manifestations. Other bacteria, including *Staphylococcus aureus, Haemophilus influenzae,* and *Streptococcus pneumoniae,* are cultured frequently from the throats of children with pharyngitis, but their role in causing pharyngitis is unclear.

Many viruses cause acute pharyngitis. Some viruses, such as adenoviruses, are more likely than others to cause pharyngitis as a prominent symptom, whereas other viruses, such as rhinoviruses, are more likely to cause pharyngitis as a minor part of an illness that primarily features other symptoms, such as rhinorrhea or cough. Epstein-Barr virus, enteroviruses (herpangina), herpes simplex virus, and primary human immunodeficiency virus (HIV) infection also produce pharyngitis.

EPIDEMIOLOGY

Sore throat is the primary symptom in approximately one third of upper respiratory tract illnesses. Streptococcal pharyngitis is relatively uncommon before 2 to 3 years of age, but the incidence increases in young school-age children and then declines in late adolescence and adulthood. Streptococcal pharyngitis occurs throughout the year in temperate climates, with a peak during the winter and early spring. The illness often spreads to siblings and classmates. Viral infections generally spread via close contact with an infected person and peak during winter and spring.

CLINICAL MANIFESTATIONS

Decision-Making Algorithms
Available @ StudentConsult.com

Sore Throat
Fever and Rash
Lymphadenopathy

Pharyngeal inflammation causes cough, sore throat, dysphagia, and fever. If involvement of the tonsils is prominent, the term **tonsillitis** or **tonsillopharyngitis** is often used.

Table 103-1	Major Microbial Causes of Acute Pharyngitis	
AGENT	**SYNDROME OR DISEASE**	**ESTIMATED PROPORTION OF ALL PHARYNGITIS (%)**
BACTERIAL		
Group A streptococcus (*Streptococcus pyogenes*)	Pharyngitis, tonsillitis	15–30
Group C streptococcus	Pharyngitis, tonsillitis	1–5
Arcanobacterium haemolyticum	Pharyngitis (Scarlet fever-like syndrome)	0.5–3
Fusobacterium necrophorum	Lemierre syndrome	Unknown
Other (e.g., *Corynebacterium diphtheriae*)	Pharyngitis, laryngitis	<5
VIRAL		
Rhinoviruses (>100 types)	Common cold	20
Coronaviruses (>4 types)	Common cold	>5
Adenoviruses (types 3, 4, 7, 14, 21)	Pharyngoconjunctival fever, acute respiratory disease	5
Herpes simplex viruses (types 1 and 2)	Gingivitis, stomatitis, pharyngitis	4
Parainfluenza viruses (types 1–4)	Common cold, croup	2
Influenza viruses (types A and B)	Influenza	2
Epstein-Barr virus	Mononucleosis	Unknown
Coxsackie virus	Herpangina	Unknown
UNKNOWN		40

Adapted from Hayden GF, Hendley JO, Gwaltney JM Jr: Management of the ambulatory patient with a sore throat, Curr Clin Top Infect Dis 9:62–75, 1988.

The onset of streptococcal pharyngitis is often rapid and associated with prominent sore throat and moderate to high fever. Headache, nausea, vomiting, and abdominal pain are frequent. In a typical, florid case, the pharynx is distinctly red. The tonsils are enlarged and covered with a yellow, blood-tinged exudate. There may be petechiae or *doughnut-shaped* lesions on the soft palate and posterior pharynx. The uvula may be red, stippled, and swollen. Anterior cervical lymph nodes are enlarged and tender to touch. Many children, however, present with only mild pharyngeal erythema without tonsillar exudate or cervical lymphadenitis. Conjunctivitis, cough, coryza, hoarseness, or ulcerations suggest a viral etiology. The diagnosis of streptococcal pharyngitis cannot be made on clinical features alone.

In addition to sore throat and fever, some patients exhibit the stigmata of **scarlet fever**: circumoral pallor, strawberry tongue, and a fine diffuse erythematous macular-papular rash that has the feeling of goose flesh. The tongue initially has a white coating, but red and edematous lingual papillae later project through this coating, producing a **white strawberry tongue.** When the white coating peels off, the resulting **red strawberry tongue** is beefy red with prominent papillae. Patients infected with *A. haemoyticum* may present with similar findings.

Compared with classic streptococcal pharyngitis, the onset of viral pharyngitis is typically more gradual, and symptoms more often include rhinorrhea, cough, and diarrhea. Many upper respiratory tract infections present with symptoms of rhinorrhea and nasal obstruction, whereas systemic symptoms and signs, such as myalgia and fever, are absent or mild.

Gingivostomatitis is characteristic of herpes simplex virus-1 (see Chapter 65). **Herpangina** is an enteroviral infection with sudden onset of high fever, vomiting, headache, malaise, myalgia, backache, conjunctivitis, poor intake, drooling, sore throat, and dysphagia. The oral lesions of herpangina may be nonspecific, but classically there are one or more small, tender, papular, or pinpoint vesicular lesions on an erythematous base scattered over the soft palate, uvula, and tongue. These vesicles enlarge from 1 to 2 mm to 3 to 4 mm over 3 to 4 days, rupture, and produce small, punched-out ulcers that persist for several days.

Mononucleosis
SEE CHAPTER 99

LABORATORY EVALUATION

The principal challenge is to distinguish pharyngitis caused by group A streptococcus from pharyngitis caused by nonstreptococcal (usually viral) organisms. A rapid streptococcal antigen test, a throat culture, or both are often performed to improve diagnostic precision and to identify children most likely to benefit from antibiotic therapy of streptococcal disease.

Many rapid diagnostic techniques for streptococcal pharyngitis are available with excellent specificity of 95% to 99%. The sensitivity of these rapid tests varies, however, and negative rapid tests should be confirmed by a throat culture.

Throat culture is the diagnostic *gold standard* for establishing the presence of streptococcal pharyngitis. False-positive cultures can occur if other organisms are incorrectly identified as group A streptococcus. As many as 20% of positive cultures in children during winter months reflect **streptococcal carriers** and not acute pharyngitis.

The predictive values of white blood cell count and differential, erythrocyte sedimentation rate, and C-reactive protein are not sufficient to distinguish streptococcal from nonstreptococcal pharyngitis, and these tests are not routinely recommended. The white blood cell count in patients with infectious mononucleosis usually shows a predominance of atypical lymphocytes.

DIFFERENTIAL DIAGNOSIS

Decision-Making Algorithm
Available @ StudentConsult.com

Lymphadenopathy

The differential diagnosis of infectious pharyngitis includes other local infections of the oral cavity, retropharyngeal abscesses (*S. aureus,* streptococci, anaerobes), diphtheria (if unimmunized), peritonsillar abscesses (with quinsy sore throat or unilateral tonsil swelling caused by streptococci, anaerobes, or, rarely, *S. aureus*), and epiglottitis. In addition neutropenic mucositis (leukemia, aplastic anemia), thrush (candidiasis secondary to T-cell immune deficiency), autoimmune ulceration (systemic lupus erythematosus, Behçet disease), and Kawasaki disease may cause pharyngitis. Pharyngitis is often a prominent feature of Epstein-Barr virus-associated mononucleosis (see Chapter 99).

Vincent infection or **trench mouth** is a fulminant form of **acute necrotizing ulcerative gingivitis** with synergistic infection with certain spirochetal organisms, notably *Treponema vincentii*, with anaerobic *Selenomonas* and *Fusobacterium*. **Vincent angina** refers to a virulent form of anaerobic pharyngitis; gray pseudomembranes are found on the tonsils. **Lemierre syndrome** is acute pharyngitis complicated by thrombosis of the internal jugular vein and septic emboli (most often to the lungs). It occurs primarily in adolescents and is caused by *Fusobacterium necrophorum*.

Ludwig angina is a mixed anaerobic bacterial cellulitis of the submandibular and sublingual regions. Although often applied to any infection of the sublingual or submandibular region, the term originally was reserved for a rapidly spreading bilateral cellulitis of the sublingual and submandibular spaces. It typically is due to spreading from a periapical abscess of the second or third mandibular molar. It also has been associated with tongue piercing. A propensity for rapid spread, glottic and lingual swelling, and consequent airway obstruction makes prompt intervention imperative.

A syndrome of **periodic fever, aphthous stomatitis, pharyngitis, and cervical adenitis** is a rare cause of recurrent fever in children. Recurring nonspecific pharyngitis is accompanied by fever and painful solitary vesicular lesions in the mouth. The fevers begin at a young age (usually <5 years). Episodes last approximately 5 days, with a mean of 28 days between episodes. Episodes are shorter with oral prednisone and unresponsive to nonsteroidal anti-inflammatory drugs or antibiotics. The syndrome resolves in some but persists in other children. Long-term sequelae do not develop.

TREATMENT

Even if untreated, most episodes of streptococcal pharyngitis resolve uneventfully over a few days. Early antimicrobial therapy accelerates clinical recovery by 12 to 24 hours. The major benefit of antimicrobial therapy is prevention of acute rheumatic fever (see Chapter 146). Because the latent (incubation) period of acute rheumatic fever is relatively long (1 to 3 weeks), treatment instituted within 9 days of illness is virtually 100% successful in preventing rheumatic fever. Treatment begun more than 9 days after the onset of illness, although less than 100% successful, has some preventive value. Antibiotic therapy should be started promptly in children with a positive rapid test for group A streptococcus, scarlet fever, symptomatic pharyngitis whose sibling has documented streptococcal pharyngitis, a past history of rheumatic fever or a recent family history of rheumatic fever, or symptomatic pharyngitis and living in an area experiencing an epidemic of acute rheumatic fever or poststreptococcal glomerulonephritis.

A variety of antimicrobial agents can be used to treat streptococcal pharyngitis (Table 103-2). Cephalosporins have superior pharyngeal bacterial eradication rates compared to

Table 103-2	Antimicrobial Treatment of Group A Streptococcal Pharyngitis

Penicillin

Oral penicillin V (2–3 times daily for 10 days) 10 mg/kg/dose, maximum dose 250 mg/dose

Intramuscular benzathine penicillin G (single dose)

For children ≤27 kg: 600,000 U

For larger children and adults: 1.2 million U

For persons allergic to penicillin

Cephalexin 20 mg/kg/dose BID, maximum dose 500 mg/dose × 10 days

Cefadroxil 30 mg/kg OD maximum, maximum dose 1 g × 10 days

Clindamycin 7 mg/kg/dose TID, maximum dose 300 mg/dose × 10 days

For persons allergic to β-lactams

Erythromycin

Erythromycin ethyl succinate: 40–50 mg/kg/day (max 1 g/day) in 3–4 doses for 10 days

Erythromycin estolate: 20–40 mg/kg/day in 2–4 doses (max 1 g/day) for 10 days

Azithromycin, children: 12 mg/kg orally once daily for 5 days (to maximum adult dose); adults: 500 mg orally on day 1, then 250 mg orally on days 2–5

BID, Twice daily; *OD*, once daily; *TID*, three times daily.

penicillin. One proposed explanation is that staphylococci or anaerobes in the pharynx produce β-lactamase, which inactivates penicillin and reduces its efficacy. Another possible explanation is that cephalosporins are more effective in eradicating streptococcal carriage.

Children with recurrent throat culture episodes of group A streptococcal pharyngitis pose a particular problem. An alternative antibiotic may be chosen to treat β-lactamase producing flora, which may be responsible for the recurrences. Either amoxicillin-clavulanate or clindamycin is an effective regimen for eliminating streptococcal carriage.

Specific antiviral therapy is unavailable for most cases of viral pharyngitis. Patients with primary herpetic gingivostomatitis benefit from early treatment with oral acyclovir.

COMPLICATIONS AND PROGNOSIS

Pharyngitis caused by streptococci or respiratory viruses usually resolves completely. The complications of group A streptococcal pharyngitis include local suppurative complications, such as parapharyngeal abscess and other infections of the deep fascial spaces of the neck, and nonsuppurative complications, such as acute rheumatic fever and acute postinfectious glomerulonephritis. Viral respiratory tract infections, including infections caused by influenza A, adenoviruses, parainfluenza type 3, and rhinoviruses, may predispose to bacterial middle ear infections.

PREVENTION

Antimicrobial prophylaxis with daily oral penicillin V prevents recurrent streptococcal infections and is recommended only to prevent recurrences of rheumatic fever.

Chapter 104

SINUSITIS

ETIOLOGY

Sinusitis is a suppurative infection of the paranasal sinuses and often complicates the common cold and allergic rhinitis. The maxillary and ethmoid sinuses are present at birth, but only the ethmoidal sinuses are pneumatized. The maxillary sinuses become pneumatized at 4 years of age. Frontal sinuses begin to develop at 7 years of age and are not completely developed until adolescence. The sphenoid sinuses are present by 5 years of age. The ostia draining the sinuses are narrow (1 to 3 mm) and drain into the middle meatus in the **ostiomeatal complex.** The mucociliary system maintains the sinuses as normally sterile.

Obstruction to mucociliary flow, such as mucosal edema resulting from the common cold, impedes sinus drainage and predisposes to bacterial proliferation. In 90% of children with acute sinusitis, the bacterial causes are *Streptococcus pneumoniae,* nontypable *Haemophilus influenzae, Moraxella catarrhalis, Staphylococcus aureus,* and group A streptococcus. Anaerobes emerge as important pathogens in subacute and chronic sinusitis. Indwelling nasogastric and nasotracheal tubes predispose to nosocomial sinusitis, which may be caused by gram-negative bacteria *(Klebsiella* or *Pseudomonas).* Antibiotic therapy predisposes to infection with antibiotic-resistant organisms. Sinusitis in neutropenic and immunocompromised persons may be caused by *Aspergillus* or the Zygomycetes (e.g., *Mucor, Rhizopus).*

EPIDEMIOLOGY

The true incidence of sinusitis is unknown. The common cold is the major predisposing factor for developing sinusitis at all ages. Other risk factors include allergy, cystic fibrosis, immunodeficiency, human immunodeficiency virus (HIV) infection, nasogastric or nasotracheal intubation, immotile cilia syndrome, nasal polyps, and nasal foreign body. Sinusitis also is a frequent problem in immunocompromised children after organ transplantation.

CLINICAL MANIFESTATIONS

Decision-Making Algorithms
Available @ StudentConsult.com

Rhinorrhea
Cough
Vomiting
Headaches

Clinical manifestations most commonly include persistent, mucopurulent, unilateral or bilateral rhinorrhea, nasal stuffiness, and cough, especially at night. Less common symptoms include a nasal quality to the voice, halitosis, facial swelling, facial tenderness and pain, and headache. Sinusitis may exacerbate asthma.

LABORATORY AND IMAGING STUDIES

Culture of the nasal mucosa is not useful. Sinus aspirate culture is the most accurate diagnostic method but is not practical or necessary in immunocompetent patients.

Plain x-ray and computed tomography may reveal sinus clouding, mucosal thickening, or an air-fluid level. Abnormal radiographic findings do not differentiate infection from allergic disease; computed tomography and magnetic resonance imaging often show abnormalities, including air-fluid levels, in the sinuses of asymptomatic persons. Conversely normal radiographs have high negative predictive value for bacterial sinusitis.

DIFFERENTIAL DIAGNOSIS

The diagnosis usually is based on history and physical findings for longer than 10 to 14 days without improvement or increased severity of symptoms compared to the common cold.

TREATMENT

Amoxicillin-clavulanate for 10 to 14 days is recommended as first-line therapy of sinusitis in children. High-dose therapy is recommended for children at increased risk for resistant bacteria (antibiotic treatment in the preceding 1 to 3 months, day care attendance, age <2 years, high rates of antimicrobial resistance locally). Levofloxacin is recommended for children with type I hypersensitivity to penicillins. Clindamycin plus a third generation cephalosporin (cefixime, cefpodoxime) is recommended for children with non-type I hypersensitivity.

COMPLICATIONS AND PROGNOSIS

Complications include orbital cellulitis, epidural or subdural empyema, brain abscess, dural sinus thrombosis, osteomyelitis of the outer or inner table of the frontal sinus (**Pott puffy tumor),** and meningitis. These all should be managed with sinus drainage and broad-spectrum parenteral antibiotics. Sinusitis also may exacerbate bronchoconstriction in asthmatic patients.

Orbital cellulitis is a serious complication of sinusitis that follows bacterial spread into the orbit through the wall of the infected sinus. It typically begins as ethmoid sinusitis and spreads through the lamina papyracea, a thin, bony plate that separates the medial orbit and the ethmoid sinus. Orbital involvement can lead to subperiosteal abscess, ophthalmoplegia, cavernous sinus thrombosis, and vision loss. Manifestations of orbital cellulitis include orbital pain, proptosis, chemosis, ophthalmoplegia and limited extraocular muscle motion, diplopia, and reduced visual acuity. Infection of the orbit must be differentiated from that of the preseptal (anterior to the palpebral fascia) or periorbital space. **Preseptal (periorbital) cellulitis** usually occurs in children younger than 3 years of age; these children do not have proptosis or ophthalmoplegia. Periorbital cellulitis may be associated with a skin lesion or trauma and usually is caused by *S. aureus* or group A streptococcus.

The diagnosis of orbital cellulitis is confirmed by a computed tomography scan of the orbit, which determines the extent of orbital infection and the need for surgical drainage. Disorders to be considered in the differential diagnosis are zygomycosis (mucormycosis), aspergillosis, rhabdomyosarcoma, neuroblastoma, Wegener granulomatosis, inflammatory pseudotumor of the orbit, and trichinosis. Therapy for orbital cellulitis involves broad-spectrum parenteral antibiotics, such as vancomycin and ceftriaxone.

More than half of children with acute bacterial sinusitis recover without any antimicrobial therapy. Fever and nasal discharge should improve dramatically within 48 hours of initiating treatment. Persistent symptoms suggest another etiology.

PREVENTION

The best means of prevention are good hand washing to minimize acquisition of colds and management of allergic rhinitis.

Chapter 105

OTITIS MEDIA

ETIOLOGY

Otitis media (OM) is a suppurative infection of the middle ear cavity. Bacteria gain access to the middle ear when the normal patency of the eustachian tube is blocked by upper airway infection or hypertrophied adenoids. Air trapped in the middle ear is resorbed, creating negative pressure in this cavity and facilitating reflux of nasopharyngeal bacteria. Obstructed flow of secretions from the middle ear to the pharynx combined with bacterial reflux leads to infected middle ear effusion.

Both bacteria and viruses can cause OM. The common bacterial pathogens are *Streptococcus pneumoniae,* nontypable *Haemophilus influenzae, Moraxella catarrhalis,* and, less frequently, group A streptococcus. *S. pneumoniae* that is **relatively resistant** to penicillin (minimal inhibitory concentration 0.1 to 1 μg/mL) or **highly resistant** to penicillin (minimal inhibitory concentration ≥2 μg/mL) is isolated with increasing frequency from young children, particularly those who attend day care or have received antibiotics recently. Viruses, including rhinoviruses, influenza, and respiratory syncytial virus, are recovered alone or as co-pathogens in 20% to 25% of patients.

EPIDEMIOLOGY

Diseases of the middle ear account for approximately one third of office visits to pediatricians. The peak incidence of acute OM is between 6 and 15 months of life. By the first birthday, 62% of children experience at least one episode. Few first episodes occur after 18 months of age. OM is more common in boys and in patients of lower socioeconomic status. There is increased incidence of OM in Native Americans and Alaskan Natives and in certain high-risk populations, such as children with human immunodeficiency virus (HIV), cleft palate, and trisomy 21. In most of the United States, OM is a seasonal disease with a distinct peak in January and February, which corresponds to the rhinovirus, respiratory syncytial virus, and

influenza seasons. The major risk factors for acute OM are young age, lack of breastfeeding, passive exposure to tobacco smoke, and increased exposure to infectious agents (day care).

As defined by the presence of six or more acute OM episodes in the first 6 years of life, at least 12% of children in the general population have **recurrent OM** and would be considered **otitis-prone.** Craniofacial anomalies and immunodeficiencies often are associated with recurrent OM; most children with recurrent acute OM are otherwise healthy.

CLINICAL MANIFESTATIONS

Decision-Making Algorithms
Available @ StudentConsult.com

Ear Pain
Strabismus
Abnormal Eye Movements
Diarrhea
Hearing Loss
Fever without a Source

In infants, the most frequent symptoms of acute OM are nonspecific and include fever, irritability, and poor feeding. In older children and adolescents, acute OM usually is associated with fever and **otalgia** (acute ear pain). Acute OM also may present with **otorrhea** (ear drainage) after spontaneous rupture of the tympanic membrane. Signs of a common cold, which predisposes to acute OM, are often present (see Chapter 102). A bulging tympanic membrane, air fluid level, or visualization of purulent material by otoscopy are reliable signs of infection (Table 105-1).

Examination of the ears is essential for diagnosis and should be part of the physical examination of any child with fever. The hallmark of OM is the presence of effusion in the middle ear cavity (see Table 105-1). The presence of an effusion does not define its nature or potentially infectious etiology, but it does define the need for appropriate diagnosis and therapy.

Pneumatic otoscopy, using an attachment to a hermetically sealed otoscope, allows evaluation of ventilation of the middle ear and is a standard for clinical diagnosis. The tympanic membrane of the normal, air-filled middle ear has much greater compliance than if the middle ear is fluid-filled. With acute OM, the tympanic membrane is characterized by **hyperemia,** or red color rather than the normal pearly gray color, but it can be pink, white, or yellow with a full to bulging position and with poor or absent mobility to negative and positive pressure. The light reflex is lost, and the middle ear structures are obscured and difficult to distinguish. A hole in the tympanic membrane or purulent drainage confirms perforation. Occasionally bullae are present on the lateral aspect of the tympanic membrane, which characteristically are associated with severe ear pain.

LABORATORY AND IMAGING STUDIES

Routine laboratory studies, including complete blood count and erythrocyte sedimentation rate, are not useful in the evaluation of OM. **Tympanometry** provides objective acoustic measurements of the tympanic membrane–middle ear system by reflection or absorption of sound energy from the external

Table 105-1	Definition of Acute Otitis Media (AOM)

A diagnosis of AOM requires:

   History of acute onset of signs and symptoms

   Presence of middle ear effusion

   Signs and symptoms of middle ear inflammation

The definition of AOM includes all of the following:

   Recent, usually abrupt, onset of signs and symptoms of middle ear inflammation and middle ear effusion

The presence of middle ear effusion that is indicated by any of the following:

   Bulging of the tympanic membrane

   Limited or absent mobility of the tympanic membrane

   Air-fluid level behind the tympanic membrane

   Otorrhea

Signs or symptoms of middle ear inflammation as indicated by either:

   Distinct erythema of the tympanic membrane

   Distinct otalgia (discomfort clearly referable to the ear that results in interference with or precludes normal activity or sleep)

ear duct as pressure in the duct is varied. Measurements of the resulting **tympanogram** correlate well with the presence or absence of middle ear effusion.

Instruments using **acoustic reflectometry** are available for office and home use. Use of reflectometry as a screening test for acute OM should be followed by examination with pneumatic otoscopy when abnormal reflectometry is identified.

Bacteria recovered from the nasopharynx do not correlate with bacteria isolated by tympanocentesis. Tympanocentesis and middle ear exudate culture are not always necessary, but they are required for accurate identification of bacterial pathogens and may be useful in neonates, immunocompromised patients, and patients not responding to therapy.

DIFFERENTIAL DIAGNOSIS

The major difficulty is differentiation of acute OM from **OM with effusion,** which also is referred to as **chronic OM.** Acute OM is accompanied by signs of acute illness, such as fever, pain, and upper respiratory tract inflammation. OM with effusion is the presence of effusion without any of the other signs and symptoms.

TREATMENT

Recommendations for treatment are based on certainty of diagnosis and severity of illness. A certain diagnosis can be made if there is rapid onset, signs of middle ear effusion, and signs and symptoms of middle ear inflammation. The recommended first-line therapy for most children with a certain diagnosis of acute OM or those with an uncertain diagnosis but who are younger than 2 years of age or have fever greater than 39° C or otalgia is amoxicillin (80 to 90 mg/kg/day in two divided doses). Children with an uncertain diagnosis who are older than 2 years of age may be observed if appropriate follow-up can be arranged. Failure of initial therapy with amoxicillin at 3 days suggests infection with β-lactamase-producing

H. influenza, M. *catarrhalis* or resistant *S. pneumoniae.* Recommended next-step treatments include high-dose amoxicillin-clavulanate (amoxicillin 80 to 90 mg/kg/day), cefuroxime axetil, cefdinir, or ceftriaxone (50 mg/kg intramuscularly in daily doses for 1 to 3 days). Intramuscular ceftriaxone is especially appropriate for children younger than 3 years of age with vomiting that precludes oral treatment. Tympanocentesis may be required for patients who are difficult to treat or who do not respond to therapy. Acetaminophen and ibuprofen are recommended for fever. Decongestants or antihistamines are not effective.

COMPLICATIONS AND PROGNOSIS

        Decision-Making Algorithms
        Available @ StudentConsult.com

      Ear Pain
      Strabismus
      Hearing Loss

The complications of OM are chronic effusion, hearing loss, cholesteatoma (mass-like keratinized epithelial growth), petrositis, intracranial extension (brain abscess, subdural empyema, or venous thrombosis), and mastoiditis. **Acute mastoiditis** is a suppurative complication of OM with inflammation and potential destruction of the mastoid air spaces. The disease progresses from a periostitis to an osteitis with mastoid abscess formation. Posterior auricular tenderness, swelling, and erythema, in addition to the signs of OM, are present. The pinna is displaced downward and outward. Radiographs or computed tomography scan of the mastoid reveals clouding of the air cells, demineralization, or bone destruction. Treatment includes systemic antibiotics and drainage if the disease has progressed to abscess formation.

OM with effusion is the most frequent sequela of acute OM and occurs most frequently in the first 2 years of life. **Persistent middle ear effusion** may last for many weeks or months in some children but usually resolves by 3 months following infection. Evaluating young children for this condition is part of all well-child examinations.

Conductive hearing loss should be assumed to be present with persistent middle ear effusion; the loss is mild to moderate and often is transient or fluctuating. Normal tympanograms after 1 month of treatment obviate the need for further follow-up. In children at developmental risk or with frequent episodes of recurrent acute OM, 3 months of persistent effusion with significant bilateral hearing loss is a reasonable indicator of need for intervention with insertion of pressure equalization tubes.

PREVENTION

Parents should be encouraged to continue exclusive breastfeeding as long as possible and should be cautioned about the risks of *bottle-propping* and of children taking a bottle to bed. The home should be a smoke-free environment.

Children identified at high-risk for recurrent acute OM are candidates for prolonged courses of antimicrobial prophylaxis, which can reduce recurrences significantly. Amoxicillin (20 to 30 mg/kg/day) or sulfisoxazole (50 mg/kg/day) given once daily at bedtime for 3 to 6 months or longer is used for prophylaxis.

The conjugate *S. pneumoniae* vaccine reduces pneumococcal OM caused by vaccine serotypes by 50%, all pneumococcal OM by 33%, and all OM by 6%. Annual immunization against influenza virus may be helpful in high-risk children.

Chapter 106

OTITIS EXTERNA

ETIOLOGY

Otitis externa, also known as **swimmer's ear,** is defined by inflammation and exudation in the external auditory canal in the absence of other disorders, such as otitis media or mastoiditis. The most common bacterial pathogens are *Pseudomonas aeruginosa,* especially in association with swimming in pools or lakes, and *Staphylococcus aureus.* Otitis externa develops in approximately 20% of children with **tympanostomy tubes,** associated with *S. aureus, Streptococcus pneumoniae, Moraxella catarrhalis, Proteus, Klebsiella,* and occasionally anaerobes. Coagulase-negative staphylococci and *Corynebacterium* are isolated frequently from cultures of the external canal but represent normal flora. **Malignant otitis externa** is caused by *P. aeruginosa* in immunocompromised persons and adults with diabetes.

EPIDEMIOLOGY

Otitis externa cases peak in summer, in contrast to otitis media, which occurs primarily in colder seasons in association with viral upper respiratory tract infections. Cleaning of the auditory canal, swimming, and, in particular, diving disrupt the integrity of the cutaneous lining of the ear canal and local defenses such as cerumen, predisposing to otitis externa.

CLINICAL MANIFESTATIONS

Decision-Making Algorithm
Available @ StudentConsult.com

Ear Pain

Pain, tenderness, and aural discharge are the characteristic clinical findings of otitis externa. Fever is notably absent, and hearing is unaffected. Tenderness with movement of the pinna, especially the tragus, and with chewing is particularly characteristic, symptoms notably absent in otitis media. Inspection usually reveals that the lining of the auditory canal is inflamed with mild to severe erythema and edema. Scant to copious discharge from the auditory canal may obscure the tympanic membrane. The most common symptoms of **malignant otitis externa** are similar, but facial nerve palsy occasionally occurs. The most common physical findings are swelling and granulation tissue in the canal, usually with a discharge from the external auditory canal.

LABORATORY AND IMAGING STUDIES

The diagnosis of uncomplicated otitis externa usually is established solely on the basis of the clinical symptoms and physical examination findings without the need for additional laboratory or microbiologic evaluation. In malignant otitis externa, an elevated erythrocyte sedimentation rate is a constant finding. Cultures are required to identify the etiologic agent, which is usually *P. aeruginosa,* and the antimicrobial susceptibility.

DIFFERENTIAL DIAGNOSIS

Otitis media with tympanic perforation and discharge into the auditory canal may be confused with otitis externa. Pain on movement of the pinnae or tragus, typical of otitis externa, is not present. Local and systemic signs of mastoiditis indicate a process more extensive than otitis externa. **Malignancies** or cholesteatoma presenting in the auditory canal are rare in children but may present with discharge, unusual pain, or hearing loss.

TREATMENT

Topical antimicrobial/corticosteroid otic preparations (such as ofloxacin, ciprofloxacin with hydrocortisone or dexamethasone, and polymyxin B-neosporin-hydrocortisone) are sufficient in most cases of otitis externa. These preparations are equally effective and are active against *S. aureus* and most gram-negative bacteria, including *P. aeruginosa.* None of these antibiotics has any antifungal activity. Use of aminoglycosides such as neomycin should be avoided in cases of tympanic membrane rupture due to their ototoxicity. **Tympanostomy tube otorrhea** is best treated with quinolone otic drugs, which is considered less likely to be ototoxic.

Treatment with topical otic analgesics and cerumenolytics is usually unnecessary. It is important with any topical therapy to remove purulent discharge from the external auditory canal with a swab or with suction to permit instillation of the solution. Excess water should be removed after bathing and the ear canal dried using a hairdryer. The predisposing activity, such as swimming or diving, should be avoided until the inflammation has resolved.

Fungi such as *Aspergillus, Candida,* and dermatophytes occasionally are isolated from the external ear. It may be difficult to determine whether they represent normal flora or are the cause of inflammation. In most cases, local therapy and restoration of normal pH as recommended for bacterial otitis externa are sufficient.

Malignant otitis externa is treated by parenteral antimicrobials with activity against *P. aeruginosa,* such as an expanded-spectrum penicillin (mezlocillin, piperacillin-tazobactam) or a cephalosporin with activity against *P. aeruginosa* (ceftazidime, cefepime) plus an aminoglycoside.

COMPLICATIONS AND PROGNOSIS

Acute otitis externa usually resolves promptly without complications within 1 to 2 days of initiating treatment. Persistent pain, especially if severe or if accompanied by other symptoms such as fever, should prompt re-evaluation for other conditions.

Complications of malignant otitis externa include invasion of the bones of the base of the skull, which may cause cranial nerve palsies. A mortality of 15% to 20% occurs in adults with malignant otitis media. Relapses within the first year after treatment are common.

PREVENTION

Overvigorous cleaning of an asymptomatic auditory canal should be avoided. Drying the auditory canals with acetic acid (2%), Burow solution, or diluted isopropyl alcohol (rubbing alcohol) after swimming may be used prophylactically to help prevent the maceration that facilitates bacterial invasion. Often underwater gear, such as earplugs or diving equipment, must be avoided to prevent recurrent disease. There is no role for prophylactic otic antibiotics.

Chapter **107**

CROUP (LARYNGOTRACHEOBRONCHITIS)

ETIOLOGY AND EPIDEMIOLOGY

Croup, or laryngotracheobronchitis, is the most common infection of the middle respiratory tract (Table 107-1). The most common causes of croup are parainfluenza viruses (types 1, 2, 3, and 4) and respiratory syncytial virus. Laryngotracheal airway inflammation disproportionately affects children because a small decrease in diameter secondary to mucosal edema and inflammation exponentially increases airway resistance and the work of breathing. During inspiration, the walls of the subglottic space are drawn together, aggravating the obstruction and producing the stridor characteristic of croup. Croup is most common in children 6 months to 3 years of age, with a peak in fall and early winter. It typically follows a common cold. Symptomatic reinfection is common, yet reinfections are usually mild. In adolescents, it manifests as laryngitis.

CLINICAL MANIFESTATIONS

Decision-Making Algorithms
Available @ StudentConsult.com

Cough
Hoarseness
Stridor
Apnea

The manifestations of croup are a harsh cough described as **barking** or **brassy**, hoarseness, inspiratory stridor, low-grade fever, and respiratory distress that may develop slowly or quickly. **Stridor** is a harsh, high-pitched respiratory sound produced by turbulent airflow. It is usually inspiratory, but it may be biphasic and is a sign of upper airway obstruction. Signs of upper airway obstruction, such as labored breathing

and marked suprasternal, intercostal, and subcostal retractions, may be evident on examination (see Chapter 135). Wheezing may be present if there is associated lower airway involvement.

LABORATORY AND IMAGING STUDIES

Anteroposterior radiographs of the neck often show the diagnostic subglottic narrowing of croup known as the **steeple sign** (Fig. 107-1). Routine laboratory studies are not useful in establishing the diagnosis. Leukocytosis is uncommon and suggests epiglottitis or bacterial tracheitis. Many rapid tests (using polymerase chain reaction or fluorescent antibodies) are available for parainfluenza viruses, respiratory syncytial virus, and other less common viral causes of croup, such as influenza and adenoviruses.

DIFFERENTIAL DIAGNOSIS

The diagnosis of croup usually is established by clinical manifestations. The infectious differential diagnosis includes epiglottitis, bacterial tracheitis, and parapharyngeal abscess. Noninfectious causes of stridor include mechanical and anatomic causes (foreign body aspiration, laryngomalacia, subglottic stenosis, hemangioma, vascular ring, vocal cord paralysis). Stridor in infants younger than 4 months of age or persistence of symptoms for longer than 1 week indicates an increased probability of another lesion and the need for imaging and direct laryngoscopy (see Chapter 135).

Epiglottitis is a medical emergency because of the risk of sudden airway obstruction. This illness is now rare and usually caused by group A streptococcus or *Staphylococcus aureus* or *Haemophilus influenza* type b in unimmunized patients. Patients typically prefer sitting, often with the head held forward, the mouth open, and the jaw thrust forward (**sniffing position**). Lateral radiograph reveals thickened and bulging epiglottis (**thumb sign**) and swelling of the aryepiglottic folds. The diagnosis is confirmed by direct observation of the inflamed and swollen supraglottic structures and swollen, cherry-red epiglottitis, which should be performed only in the operating room with an anesthesiologist and a competent surgeon prepared to place an endotracheal tube or perform a tracheostomy if needed. Epiglottitis requires antibiotic therapy and endotracheal intubation to maintain the airway. Clinical recovery is rapid, and most children can be extubated safely within 48 to 72 hours.

Bacterial tracheitis is a rare but serious superinfection of the trachea that may follow viral croup and is most commonly caused by *S. aureus*. **Spasmodic croup** describes sudden onset of croup symptoms, usually at night, but without a significant upper respiratory tract prodrome. These episodes may be recurrent and severe but usually are of short duration. Spasmodic croup has a milder course than viral croup and responds to relatively simple therapies, such as exposure to cool or humidified air. The etiology is not well understood and may be allergic.

TREATMENT

Oral or intramuscular dexamethasone for children with mild, moderate, or severe croup reduces symptoms, the need for hospitalization, and shortens hospital stays. Dexamethasone

	VIRAL LARYNGOTRA-CHEOBRONCHITIS	EPIGLOTTITIS	BACTERIAL TRACHEITIS	SPASMODIC CROUP
Table 107-1	**Clinical Features of Laryngotracheal Respiratory Tract Infections**			

FEATURE	VIRAL LARYNGOTRA-CHEOBRONCHITIS	EPIGLOTTITIS	BACTERIAL TRACHEITIS	SPASMODIC CROUP
Viral prodromal illness	++	−	+	+
Mean age	6–36 mo (60% <24 mo)	3–4 yr (25% <2 yr)	4–5 yr	6–36 mo (60% <24 mo)
Onset of illness	Gradual (2–3 days)	Acute (6–24 hr)	Acute (1–2 days)	Sudden (at night)
Fever	±	+	+	−
Toxicity	−	++	++	−
Quality of stridor	Harsh	Mild	Harsh	Harsh
Drooling, neck hyperextension	−	++	+	−
Cough	++	−	++	++
Sore throat	±	++	±	−
Positive blood culture	−	+	±	−
Leukocytosis	−	+	+	−
Recurrence	+	−	−	++
Hospitalization and endotracheal intubation	Rare	Frequent	Frequent	Rare

From Bell LM: Middle respiratory tract infections. In Jenson HB, Baltimore RS: Pediatric Infectious Diseases: Principles and Practice, ed 2, Philadelphia, 2002, Saunders, p 772.
+, frequently present; −, absent; ±, may or may not be present; ++, present and usually pronounced.

Figure 107-1 Croup (laryngotracheo-bronchitis). **A,** Posteroanterior view of the upper airway shows the so-called steeple sign, the tapered narrowing of the immediate subglottic airway (arrows). **B,** Lateral view of the upper airway shows good delineation of the supraglottic anatomy. The subglottic trachea is hazy and poorly defined (arrow) because of the inflammatory edema that has obliterated the sharp undersurface of the vocal cords and extends down the trachea in a diminishing manner. (From Bell LM: Middle respiratory tract infections. In Jenson HB, Baltimore RS: Pediatric Infectious Diseases: Principles and Practice, ed 2, Philadelphia, 2002, Saunders, p 774.)

phosphate (0.6 to 1 mg/kg) may be given once intramuscularly or dexamethasone (0.6 to 1 mg/kg) once orally. Alternatively prednisolone (2 mg/kg per day) may be given orally in two to three divided doses. For significant airway compromise, administration of aerosolized racemic (D- and L-) epinephrine reduces subglottic edema by adrenergic vasoconstriction, temporarily producing marked clinical improvement. The peak effect is within 10 to 30 minutes and fades within 60 to 90 minutes. A rebound effect may occur, with worsening of symptoms as the effect of the drug dissipates. Aerosol treatment may need to be repeated every 20 minutes (for no more than 1 to 2 hours) in severe cases.

Children should be kept as calm as possible to minimize forceful inspiration. One useful calming method is for a child with croup to sit on the parent's lap. Sedatives should be used cautiously and in the intensive care unit only. Cool mist administered by face mask may help prevent drying of the secretions around the larynx.

Hospitalization is often required for children with stridor at rest. Children receiving aerosol treatment should be hospitalized or observed for at least 2 to 3 hours because of the risk of rebound airway obstruction. Decreased symptoms may indicate improvement or fatigue and impending respiratory failure.

COMPLICATIONS AND PROGNOSIS

The most common complication of croup is viral pneumonia, which occurs in 1% to 2% of children. Parainfluenza virus pneumonia and secondary bacterial pneumonia are more common in immunocompromised persons. Bacterial tracheitis may also be a complication of croup.

The prognosis for croup is excellent. Illness usually lasts approximately 5 days. As children grow, they become less susceptible to the airway effects of viral infections of the middle respiratory tract.

PREVENTION

There is no vaccine for parainfluenza.

Chapter 108

PERTUSSIS

ETIOLOGY

Classic pertussis (**whooping cough**) is caused by *B. pertussis*, a gram-negative pleomorphic bacillus with fastidious growth requirements. *B. pertussis* infects only humans and is transmitted person to person by coughing.

EPIDEMIOLOGY

The incubation period is 7 to 10 days. Patients are most contagious during the first 2 weeks of cough. The peak incidence of pertussis in the United States is among those less than 4 months of age—infants too young to be completely immunized and most likely to have severe complications. The annual rate of pertussis was approximately 100 to 200 cases per 100,000 population in the prevaccination era; worldwide there are an estimated 30 to 50 million cases of pertussis and 300,000 deaths annually. In the United States, the incidence of pertussis decreased after the introduction of vaccine but has increased steadily since the 1980s with more than 27,000 cases reported in 2010. Infections in adolescents have also been rising, likely due to waning immunity from previous vaccines. Likewise when vaccination rates are low, pertussis rates increase: there was a steady decline in the incidence of pertussis until the late 1970s in the United Kingdom, when the incidence increased dramatically as the vaccination rate declined. Epidemics also occur in fully immunized patients, as vaccine-induced immunity wanes.

CLINICAL MANIFESTATIONS

Decision-Making Algorithms
Available @ StudentConsult.com

Cough
Cyanosis
Apnea

Classic pertussis is seen in children between 1 and 10 years old. The progression of the disease is divided into catarrhal, paroxysmal, and convalescent stages. The **catarrhal stage** is marked by nonspecific signs (increased nasal secretions and low-grade fever) lasting 1 to 2 weeks. The **paroxysmal stage** is the most distinctive stage of pertussis and lasts 2 to 4 weeks. Coughing occurs in **paroxysms** during expiration, causing young children to lose their breath. This pattern of coughing is needed to dislodge plugs of necrotic bronchial epithelial tissues and thick mucus. The forceful inhalation against a narrowed glottis that follows this paroxysm of cough produces the characteristic **whoop**. Posttussive emesis is common. The **convalescent stage** is marked by gradual resolution of symptoms over 1 to 2 weeks. Coughing becomes less severe, and the paroxysms and whoops slowly disappear. Although the disease typically lasts 6 to 8 weeks, residual cough may persist for months, especially with physical stress or respiratory irritants.

Infants may not display the classic findings, and the first sign in the neonate may be apnea. Young infants are unlikely to have the classic whoop, more likely to have central nervous system damage as a result of hypoxia, and more likely to have secondary bacterial pneumonia. Adolescents and adults with pertussis usually present with a prolonged bronchitic illness with persistent, nonproductive cough that often begins as a nonspecific upper respiratory tract infection. Generally adolescents and adults do not have a whoop with the cough, although they may have severe paroxysms. The cough may persist many weeks to months.

LABORATORY AND IMAGING STUDIES

The diagnosis depends on isolation of *B. pertussis* or detection of its nucleic acids. Culture on specialized media is usually accomplished during the early phases of illness on specimens from nasopharyngeal swabs or aspirates but can be difficult to accomplish given the organism's fastidious nature. Polymerase chain reaction, although potentially lacking sensitivity in previously immunized individuals, is likely as sensitive as culture and is available in many clinical laboratories. False positive results can occur. Direct fluorescent antibody staining is not recommended. Serologic tests are not useful for diagnosing acute infection but can be confirmatory in the convalescent phase of illness, though there are no commercial kits approved by the U.S. Food and Drug Administration.

Lymphocytosis is present in 75% to 85% of infants and young children but is not diagnostic. The white blood cell count may increase from 20,000 cells/mm³ to more than 50,000 cells/mm³, consisting primarily of mature lymphocytes. Physical examination and radiographic signs of segmental lung atelectasis may develop during pertussis, especially during the paroxysmal stage. Perihilar infiltrates are common and are similar to those seen in viral pneumonia.

DIFFERENTIAL DIAGNOSIS

For a young child with classic pertussis, the diagnosis based on the pattern of illness is quite accurate. The paroxysmal stage is the most distinctive part of the syndrome. Other causes of pertussis-like prolonged cough illnesses include *Bordetella parapertussis,* which causes a similar but milder illness and is not prevented by *B. pertussis* vaccination, *Mycoplasma pneumoniae, Chlamydia pneumoniae* and *Chlamydophila pneumoniae,* adenoviruses, and respiratory syncytial virus.

TREATMENT

Azithromycin, clarithromycin, or erythromycin are recommended for children under 1 month of age. Azithromycin should be used in neonates due to the association between erythromycin treatment and the development of pyloric stenosis. Treatment during the catarrhal phase eradicates nasopharyngeal carriage of organisms within 3 to 4 days and may lessen symptom severity. Treatment in the paroxysmal stage does not alter the course of illness but decreases the potential for spread to others. Trimethoprim-sulfamethoxazole is an alternative therapy among children older than 2 months, though studies of its use for this indication are limited.

COMPLICATIONS AND PROGNOSIS

Major complications are most common among infants and young children and include hypoxia, apnea, pneumonia, seizures, encephalopathy, malnutrition, and death. The most frequent complication is pneumonia caused by *B. pertussis* itself or resulting from secondary bacterial infection with *Streptococcus pneumoniae, Haemophilus influenzae,* and *Staphylococcus aureus.* Atelectasis may develop secondary to mucous plugs. The force of the paroxysm may produce pneumomediastinum, pneumothorax, or interstitial or subcutaneous emphysema; epistaxis; hernias; and retinal and subconjunctival hemorrhages. Otitis media and sinusitis may occur.

Most children recover normal pulmonary function with complete healing of the respiratory epithelium. Most permanent disability is a result of encephalopathy.

PREVENTION

Active immunity is induced with acellular pertussis components given as a vaccine in combination with the tetanus and diphtheria toxoids (DTaP). The acellular pertussis vaccines contain two to five antigens of *B. pertussis,* including pertussis toxin, pertactin, filamentous hemagglutinin, and fimbrial agglutinogens, FIM-2 and FIM-3. DTaP vaccine is recommended at 2, 4, 6, and 15 to 18 months, with a booster at 4 to 6 years, and has an efficacy of 70% to 90%. A single booster dose of Tdap vaccine is recommended at 11 to 12 years or once for all adults.

Macrolides are effective in preventing secondary cases in contacts exposed to pertussis. Underimmunized close contacts under 7 years of age should receive a booster dose of DTaP (unless a booster dose has been given within the preceding 3 years), whereas those 7 to 10 years of age should receive Tdap. All close contacts should receive prophylactic antibiotics for 5 days (azithromycin) or 7 to 14 days (clarithromycin or erythromycin, duration based on age).

Chapter 109

BRONCHIOLITIS

ETIOLOGY

Bronchiolitis is a disease of small bronchioles with increased mucus production and occasional bronchospasm, sometimes leading to airway obstruction. It is most commonly caused by a viral lower respiratory tract infection. Bronchiolitis is most commonly seen in infants and young children, with most severe cases occurring among infants. Bronchiolitis is potentially life-threatening.

Respiratory syncytial virus (RSV) is a primary cause of bronchiolitis, followed in frequency by human metapneumovirus, parainfluenza viruses, influenza viruses, adenoviruses, rhinoviruses, coronaviruses, and, infrequently, *Mycoplasma pneumoniae.* Viral bronchiolitis is extremely contagious and is spread by contact with infected respiratory secretions. Although coughing produces aerosols, hand carriage of contaminated secretions is the most frequent mode of transmission.

EPIDEMIOLOGY

Bronchiolitis is a leading cause of hospitalization of infants. Bronchiolitis occurs almost exclusively during the first 2 years of life, with a peak age at 2 to 6 months. Many healthy children with bronchiolitis can be managed as outpatients; however, premature infants and children with chronic lung disease of prematurity, hemodynamically significant congenital heart disease, neuromuscular weakness, or immunodeficiency are at increased risk of severe, potentially fatal disease. Children acquire infection after exposure to infected family members, who typically have symptoms of an upper respiratory tract infection, or from infected children in day care. In the United States, annual peaks are usually in the late winter months from December through March.

CLINICAL MANIFESTATIONS

Decision-Making Algorithms
Available @ StudentConsult.com

Wheezing
Apnea

Bronchiolitis caused by RSV has an incubation period of 4 to 6 days. Bronchiolitis classically presents as a progressive respiratory illness similar to the common cold in its early phase with cough and rhinorrhea. It progresses over 3 to 7 days to noisy, raspy breathing and audible wheezing. There is usually a low-grade fever accompanied by irritability, which may reflect the increased work of breathing. In contrast to the classic progression of disease, young infants infected with RSV may not have a prodrome and may have apnea as the first sign of infection.

Physical signs of bronchiolar obstruction include prolongation of the expiratory phase of breathing, nasal flaring, intercostal retractions, suprasternal retractions, and air trapping with hyperexpansion of the lungs. During the wheezing phase, percussion of the chest usually reveals only hyperresonance, but auscultation usually reveals diffuse wheezes and crackles throughout the breathing cycle. With more severe disease, grunting and cyanosis may be present.

LABORATORY AND IMAGING STUDIES

Routine laboratory tests are not required to confirm the diagnosis. It is important to assess oxygenation in severe cases of bronchiolitis. **Pulse oximetry** is adequate for monitoring oxygen saturation. Frequent, regular assessments and cardiorespiratory monitoring of infants are necessary because respiratory failure may develop precipitously in very tired infants even though blood gas values taken before rapid decompensation are reassuring.

Antigen tests (usually by immunofluorescence or enzyme-linked immunosorbent assay [also referred to as *ELISA*]) of nasopharyngeal secretions for RSV, parainfluenza viruses, influenza viruses, and adenoviruses are sensitive tests to confirm the infection. Rapid viral diagnosis also is performed by polymerase chain reaction. Identifying the viral agent is helpful for cohorting children with the same infection but is not necessary to make the diagnosis of bronchiolitis.

Chest radiographs frequently show signs of lung hyperinflation, including increased lung lucency and flattened or depressed diaphragms. Areas of increased density may represent either viral pneumonia or localized atelectasis.

DIFFERENTIAL DIAGNOSIS

The major difficulty in the diagnosis of bronchiolitis is to differentiate other diseases associated with wheezing. It may be difficult to differentiate asthma from bronchiolitis by physical examination, but age of presentation, presence of fever, and absence of personal or family history of asthma are the major differential factors. Bronchiolitis occurs primarily in the first year of life and is accompanied by fever, whereas asthma usually presents in older children with previous wheezing episodes typically unaccompanied by fever unless a respiratory tract infection is the trigger for the asthma exacerbation.

Wheezing also may be due to an airway foreign body, congenital airway obstructive lesion, cystic fibrosis, exacerbation of chronic lung disease, viral or bacterial pneumonia, and other lower respiratory tract diseases (see Chapter 78). **Cardiogenic asthma**, which can be confused with bronchiolitis in infants, is wheezing associated with pulmonary congestion secondary to left-sided heart failure.

Wheezing associated with gastroesophageal reflux is likely to be chronic or recurrent, and the patient may have a history of frequent emesis. Cystic fibrosis is associated with poor growth, chronic diarrhea, and a positive family history. A focal area on radiography that does not inflate or deflate suggests **foreign body aspiration.**

TREATMENT

Bronchiolitis treatment consists of supportive therapy, including respiratory monitoring, control of fever, hydration, upper airway suctioning, and, if needed, oxygen administration. Indications for hospitalization include moderate to marked respiratory distress, hypoxemia, apnea, inability to tolerate oral feeding, and lack of appropriate care available at home. Hospitalization of high-risk children with bronchiolitis should be considered. Among hospitalized infants, supplemental oxygen by nasal cannula is often necessary, but intubation and ventilatory assistance for respiratory failure or apnea are required in fewer than 10% of these infants. Bronchodilators and corticosteroids are seldom effective and are not generally recommended.

COMPLICATIONS AND PROGNOSIS

Most hospitalized children show marked improvement in 2 to 5 days with supportive treatment alone. The course of the wheezing phase varies, however. Tachypnea and hypoxia may progress to respiratory failure requiring assisted ventilation. Apnea is a major concern for very young infants with bronchiolitis.

Most cases of bronchiolitis resolve completely, although minor abnormalities of pulmonary function and bronchial hyperreactivity may persist for several years. Recurrence is common but tends to be mild and should be assessed and treated similarly to the first episode. The incidence of asthma seems to be higher for children hospitalized for bronchiolitis as infants, but it is unclear whether this is causal or whether children prone to asthma are more likely to be hospitalized with bronchiolitis. There is a 1% to 2% mortality rate, highest among infants with preexisting cardiopulmonary or immunologic impairment.

PREVENTION

Monthly injections of **palivizumab,** an RSV-specific monoclonal antibody, initiated just before the onset of the RSV season confers some protection from severe RSV disease. Palivizumab is indicated for some infants under 2 years old with chronic lung disease, very low birth weight, and those with hemodynamically significant cyanotic and acyanotic congenital heart disease. Immunization with influenza vaccine is recommended for all children older than 6 months and may prevent influenza-associated disease.

Chapter 110

PNEUMONIA

ETIOLOGY

Pneumonia is an infection of the lower respiratory tract that involves the airways and parenchyma with consolidation of the alveolar spaces. The term **lower respiratory tract infection** is often used to encompass bronchitis, bronchiolitis (see Chapter 109), pneumonia, or any combination of the three. **Pneumonitis** is a general term for lung inflammation that may or may not be associated with consolidation. **Lobar pneumonia** describes pneumonia localized to one or more lobes of the lung. **Atypical pneumonia** describes patterns typically more diffuse or interstitial than lobar pneumonia. **Bronchopneumonia** refers to inflammation of the lung that is centered in the bronchioles and leads to the production of a mucopurulent exudate that obstructs some of these small airways and causes patchy consolidation of the adjacent lobules. **Interstitial pneumonitis** refers to inflammation of the interstitium, which is composed of the walls of the alveoli, the alveolar sacs and ducts, and the bronchioles. Interstitial pneumonitis is characteristic of acute viral infections but also may be a chronic inflammatory or fibrosing process.

Defects in host defenses increase the risk of pneumonia. Lower airways and secretions are sterile as a result of a multifactorial system. Airway contaminants are caught in the mucus secreted by the goblet cells. Cilia on epithelial surfaces, composing the **ciliary elevator system,** beat synchronously to move particles upward toward central airways and into the throat, where they are swallowed or expectorated. Polymorphonuclear neutrophils from the blood and tissue macrophages ingest and kill microorganisms. IgA secreted into the upper airway fluid protects against invasive infections and facilitates viral neutralization.

Infectious agents that commonly cause community-acquired pneumonia vary by age (Table 110-1). Most common causes are respiratory syncytial virus (RSV) in infants (see Chapter 109), other respiratory viruses (parainfluenza viruses, influenza viruses, human metapneumovirus, adenoviruses) in children younger than 5 years old, and *Mycoplasma pneumoniae* in children older than age 5 years. *Streptococcus pneumoniae* is the most common bacterial cause of **lobar** pneumonia, and occurs in children of any age outside the neonatal period. *M. pneumoniae* and *Chlamydophila pneumoniae* are principal causes of **atypical pneumonia.**

Chlamydia trachomatis and less commonly *Mycoplasma hominis, Ureaplasma urealyticum,* and cytomegalovirus (CMV) cause a similar respiratory syndrome in infants 1 to 3 months of age with subacute onset of an **afebrile pneumonia;** cough and hyperinflation are the predominant signs. These infections are difficult to diagnose and to distinguish from each other. In adults these organisms are carried primarily as part of the genital mucosal flora. Women who harbor these agents may transmit them perinatally to newborns.

Additional agents occasionally cause pneumonia. **Severe acute respiratory syndrome (SARS)** is due to SARS-associated coronavirus (SARS-CoV). **Avian influenza (bird flu)** is a highly contagious viral disease of poultry and other birds caused by **influenza A (H5N1).** There were outbreaks among humans in South East Asia in 1997 and 2003 to 2004 with high mortality rates. A novel influenza A (H1N1) of swine origin began circulating in 2009. Other etiologic agents to consider, based on specific exposure history, include *Mycobacterium tuberculosis, Francisella tularensis, Brucella* spp., *Coxiella burnetii, Chlamydophila psittaci, Legionella pneumophila,* hantavirus, *Histoplasma capsulatum, Coccidioides immitis,* and *Blastomyces dermatitidis.*

Causes of pneumonia in immunocompromised persons include gram-negative enteric bacteria, mycobacteria (*M. avium* complex), fungi (aspergillosis), viruses (CMV), and *Pneumocystis jiroveci (carinii).* Pneumonia in patients with cystic fibrosis usually is caused by *Staphylococcus aureus* in infancy and *Pseudomonas aeruginosa* or *Burkholderia cepacia* in older patients.

EPIDEMIOLOGY

Immunizations have had a great impact on the incidence of pneumonia caused by pertussis, diphtheria, measles, *Haemophilus influenza* type b, and *S. pneumoniae.* Where used, bacille Calmette-Guerin (BCG) for tuberculosis also has had an impact. An estimated 2 million deaths in developing countries are due to acute respiratory tract infections annually. Risk factors for lower respiratory tract infections include gastroesophageal reflux, neurologic impairment (aspiration), immunocompromised states, anatomic abnormalities of the respiratory tract, residence in residential care facilities, and hospitalization, especially in an intensive care unit.

CLINICAL MANIFESTATIONS

Decision-Making Algorithms
Available @ StudentConsult.com

Cough
Wheezing
Hemoptysis
Chest Pain
Abdominal Pain
Failure to Thrive
Acidemia

Age is a determinant in the clinical manifestations of pneumonia. Neonates may have fever or hypoxia only, with subtle or absent physical examination findings (see Chapter 65). With a young infant, apnea may be the first sign of pneumonia. Fever, chills, tachypnea, cough, malaise, pleuritic chest pain, retractions, and apprehension, because of difficulty breathing or shortness of breath, are common in older infants and children. Physical examination findings cannot reliably distinguish viral and bacterial pneumonias, but complete physical examination may help identify other foci of disease or associated findings to suggest an etiology.

In general viral pneumonias are associated more often with cough, wheezing, or stridor; fever is less prominent than with bacterial pneumonia. Mucosal congestion and upper airway inflammation suggest a viral infection. Bacterial pneumonias typically are associated with higher fever, chills, cough, dyspnea, and auscultatory findings of lung consolidation. Atypical pneumonia in young infants is characterized by tachypnea, cough, crackles on auscultation, and concomitant (chlamydial) conjunctivitis (infants) may be present. Other signs of respiratory distress include nasal flaring, intercostal and subcostal retractions, and grunting.

Asymmetry or shallow breathing may be due to splinting from pain. Hyperexpansion, common in asthma but also frequently accompanying viral lower respiratory infections, may cause a low diaphragm or liver. Poor diaphragmatic excursion may indicate hyperexpanded lungs or an inability for expansion due to a large consolidation or effusion. Dullness to percussion may be due to lobar or segmental infiltrates or pleural fluid. Auscultation may be normal in early or very focal pneumonia, but the presence of localized crackles, rhonchi, and wheezes may help one detect and locate pneumonia. Distant breath sounds may indicate a large, poorly ventilated area of consolidation or pleural fluid.

Table 110-1	Etiologic Agents and Empirical Antimicrobial Therapy for Pneumonia in Patients without History of Recent Antibiotic Therapy				
AGE GROUP	COMMON PATHOGENS* (IN APPROXIMATE ORDER OF FREQUENCY)	LESS COMMON PATHOGENS	OUTPATIENTS† (7–10 DAYS TOTAL DURATION OF TREATMENT)	PATIENTS REQUIRING HOSPITALIZATION‡ (10–14 DAYS TOTAL DURATION OF TREATMENT)	PATIENTS REQUIRING INTENSIVE CARE‡ (10–14 DAYS TOTAL DURATION OF TREATMENT)
Neonates (up to 1 month of age)	Group B streptococcus, Escherichia coli, other gram-negative bacilli, Streptococcus pneumoniae	Cytomegalovirus, Herpes simplex virus, Listeria monocytogenes, Treponema pallidum, Haemophilus influenzae (type b,§ nontypable)	Outpatient management not recommended	Ampicillin plus cefotaxime or an aminoglycoside plus an antistaphylococcal agent if Staphylococcus aureus is suspected	Ampicillin plus cefotaxime or an aminoglycoside plus antistaphylococcal agent if S. aureus is suspected
1 to 3 months					
Febrile pneumonia	Respiratory syncytial virus, other respiratory viruses (parainfluenza viruses, influenza viruses, adenoviruses), S. pneumoniae, H. influenzae (type b,§ nontypable)		Initial outpatient management not recommended	Amoxicillin or ampicillin if fully immunized for age for S. pneumoniae and H. influenzae type b. Alternatives: cefotaxime or ceftriaxone if not fully immunized or local S. pneumoniae penicillin resistance is significant, with clindamycin if MRSA suspected	Cefotaxime or ceftriaxone plus nafcillin, oxacillin, clindamycin, or vancomycin
Afebrile pneumonia	Chlamydia trachomatis, Mycoplasma hominis, Ureaplasma urealyticum, cytomegalovirus, Bordetella pertussis		Erythromycin, azithromycin, or clarithromycin with close follow-up	Erythromycin, azithromycin, or clarithromycin	Erythromycin, azithromycin, or clarithromycin plus cefotaxime or ceftriaxone plus nafcillin, oxacillin, clindamycin, or vancomycin
3 months to 5 years	Respiratory syncytial virus, other respiratory viruses (parainfluenza viruses, influenza viruses, human metapneumovirus adenoviruses), S. pneumoniae, H. influenzae (type b,§ nontypable)	C. trachomatis, Mycoplasma pneumoniae, Chlamydophila pneumoniae, group A streptococcus, Staphylococcus aureus, Mycobacterium tuberculosis	Amoxicillin plus erythromycin, azithromycin, or clarithromycin if atypical pneumonia suspected	Ampicillin Alternatives: cefotaxime or ceftriaxone if not fully immunized or local S. pneumoniae penicillin resistance is significant, with clindamycin if MRSA suspected; Add erythromycin, azithromycin, or clarithromycin if atypical pneumonia suspected	Cefuroxime or ceftriaxone plus azithromycin, erythromycin or clarithromycin with or without clindamycin or vancomycin
5 to 18 years	M. pneumoniae, S. pneumoniae, C. pneumoniae,	H. influenzae (type b,§ nontypable), influenza viruses, adenoviruses, other respiratory viruses	Amoxicillin or erythromycin, azithromycin, or clarithromycin if atypical pneumonia suspected	Ampicillin plus erythromycin, azithromycin, or clarithromycin if atypical pneumonia suspected	Cefuroxime or ceftriaxone plus azithromycin, erythromycin or clarithromycin with or without clindamycin or vancomycin
≥18 years§	M. pneumoniae, S. pneumoniae, C. pneumoniae, H. influenzae (type b,§ nontypable), influenza viruses, adenoviruses,	Legionella pneumophila, M. tuberculosis	Amoxicillin, or erythromycin, azithromycin, clarithromycin, doxycycline, moxifloxacin, gatifloxacin, levofloxacin, or gemifloxacin‖ if atypical pneumonia suspected	Ampicillin plus erythromycin, azithromycin, or clarithromycin if atypical pneumonia suspected or moxifloxacin, gatifloxacin, levofloxacin, or gemifloxacin	Cefotaxime or ceftriaxone, plus either azithromycin or clarithromycin with or without clindamycin or vancomycin or moxifloxacin, gatifloxacin, levofloxacin, or gemifloxacin with or without clindamycin or vancomycin

MRSA, Methicillin-resistant Staphylococcus aureus.

*Severe pneumonia, from S. pneumoniae, S. aureus, group A streptococcus, H. influenzae, or M. pneumoniae requiring admission to an intensive care unit. Antipseudomonal agents should be added if Pseudomonas is suspected.

†Oral administration.

‡Intravenous administration for inpatients except for the macrolides (erythromycin, azithromycin, and clarithromycin), which are given orally.

§H. influenzae type b infection is uncommon with universal H. influenzae type b immunization.

‖Fluoroquinolones are contraindicated for children younger than 18 years of age and pregnant or lactating women. Tetracyclines are not recommended for children younger than 9 years.

LABORATORY AND IMAGING STUDIES

Bacterial flora of the upper respiratory tract do not accurately reflect flora present in lower respiratory tract infections, and high-quality sputum is rarely obtainable from children. In otherwise healthy children without life-threatening disease, invasive procedures to obtain lower respiratory tissue or secretions usually are not indicated. Serologic tests are not useful for the most common causes of bacterial pneumonia.

The white blood cell (WBC) count with viral pneumonias is often normal or mildly elevated, with a predominance of lymphocytes, whereas with bacterial pneumonias the WBC count is elevated (>20,000/mm³) with a predominance of neutrophils. Mild eosinophilia is characteristic of infant *C. trachomatis* pneumonia. Blood cultures should be performed on hospitalized children to attempt to diagnose a bacterial cause of pneumonia. Blood cultures are positive in 10% to 20% of bacterial pneumonia and are considered to be confirmatory of the cause of pneumonia if positive for a recognized respiratory pathogen. Urinary antigen tests are especially useful for *L. pneumophila* (legionnaires' disease).

Viral respiratory pathogens can be diagnosed using polymerase chain reaction (PCR) or rapid viral antigen detection, but neither rules out concomitant bacterial pneumonia. *M. pneumoniae* should be suspected if cold agglutinins are present in peripheral blood samples and can be confirmed by *Mycoplasma* PCR. CMV and enterovirus can be cultured from the nasopharynx, urine, or bronchoalveolar lavage fluid. The diagnosis of *M. tuberculosis* is established by tuberculin skin test, serum interferon-gamma release assay, or analysis of sputum or gastric aspirates by culture, antigen detection, or PCR.

The need to establish an etiologic diagnosis of pneumonia is greater for patients who are ill enough to require hospitalization, immunocompromised patients, patients with recurrent pneumonia, or patients with pneumonia unresponsive to empirical therapy. For these patients, bronchoscopy with bronchoalveolar lavage and brush mucosal biopsy, needle aspiration of the lung, and open lung biopsy are methods of obtaining material for microbiologic diagnosis.

When there is a pleural **effusion or empyema**, a thoracentesis to obtain pleural fluid can be diagnostic and therapeutic. Evaluation differentiates between empyema and a sterile parapneumonic effusion caused by irritation of the pleura contiguous with the pneumonia. Gram stain, culture, or broad-range bacterial PCR may lead to microbiologic diagnosis. The pleural fluid should be cultured for bacteria, mycobacteria, fungi, and viruses. If the fluid is grossly purulent, removal reduces the patient's toxicity and associated discomfort and may facilitate more rapid recovery. If the accumulation is large and impairs the ability of the lung to expand, removal of the fluid improves pulmonary mechanics and gas exchange.

Frontal and lateral radiographs are required to localize disease and adequately visualize retrocardiac infiltrates and are recommended for diagnosis among hospitalized children, but they are not necessary to confirm the diagnosis in well-appearing outpatients. Although there are characteristic radiographic findings of pneumonia, radiography alone cannot provide a definitive microbiologic diagnosis. Bacterial pneumonia characteristically shows lobar consolidation, or a round pneumonia, with pleural effusion in 10% to 30% of cases (Fig. 110-1). Viral pneumonia characteristically shows diffuse, streaky infiltrates of bronchopneumonia (Fig. 110-2) and hyperinflation. Atypical pneumonia, such as with *M. pneumoniae* and

Figure 110-1 Acute lobar pneumonia of the lingula in a 6-year-old child with high fever, cough, and chest pain. Frontal chest radiograph shows airspace consolidation, which obliterates the silhouette of the heart border on the left. The left hemidiaphragm is mildly elevated as a result of splinting. *(From Markowitz RI: Diagnostic imaging. In Jenson HB, Baltimore RS, editors:* Pediatric Infectious Diseases: Principles and Practice, *ed 2, Philadelphia, Saunders, 2002, p 133.)*

Figure 110-2 Diffuse viral bronchopneumonia in a 12-year-old boy with cough, fever, and wheezing. Frontal chest radiograph shows bilateral, perihilar, peribronchial thickening, and shaggy infiltrate. Focal airspace disease representing consolidation or atelectasis is present in the medial portion of the right upper lobe. The findings are typical of bronchopneumonia. *(From Markowitz RI: Diagnostic imaging. In Jenson HB, Baltimore RS, editors:* Pediatric Infectious Diseases: Principles and Practice, *ed 2, Philadelphia, Saunders, 2002, p 132.)*

C. pneumoniae, shows increased interstitial markings or bronchopneumonia (Fig. 110-3). Chest radiographs may be normal in early pneumonia, with infiltrates appearing during treatment as hydration is restored. Hilar lymphadenopathy is uncommon with bacterial pneumonia but may be a sign of tuberculosis, histoplasmosis, or an underlying malignant neoplasm. Decubitus views or ultrasound should be used to assess size of pleural effusions and whether they are freely mobile.

Figure 110-3 *Mycoplasma pneumoniae* infection (atypical pneumonia) in a 14-year-old boy with malaise, dry cough, and mild shortness of breath for 1 week. Frontal chest radiograph shows a diffuse pattern of increased interstitial markings, including Kerley lines. The heart is normal, and there are no focal infiltrates. Cold agglutinins were markedly elevated, and the patient responded to erythromycin. This radiographic pattern of reticulonodular interstitial disease is observed in 25% to 30% of patients with pneumonia caused by *Mycoplasma pneumoniae*. (*From Baltimore RS: Pneumonia. In Jenson HB, Baltimore RS, editors: Pediatric Infectious Diseases: Principles and Practice, ed 2, Philadelphia, Saunders, 2002, p 808.*)

Table 110-2	Differential Diagnosis of Recurrent Pneumonia
HEREDITARY DISORDERS	
Cystic fibrosis	
Sickle cell disease	
DISORDERS OF IMMUNITY	
AIDS	
Bruton agammaglobulinemia	
Selective IgG subclass deficiencies	
Common variable immunodeficiency syndrome	
Severe combined immunodeficiency syndrome	
DISORDERS OF LEUKOCYTES	
Chronic granulomatous disease	
Hyperimmunoglobulin E syndrome (Job syndrome)	
Leukocyte adhesion defect	
DISORDERS OF CILIA	
Immotile cilia syndrome	
Kartagener syndrome	
ANATOMIC DISORDERS	
Sequestration	
Lobar emphysema	
Esophageal reflux	
Foreign body	
Tracheoesophageal fistula (H type)	
Cystic adenomatoid malformation	
Gastroesophageal reflux	
Bronchiectasis	
Aspiration (oropharyngeal incoordination)	

Computed tomography (CT) is used to evaluate serious disease, pleural abscesses, bronchiectasis, and effusion characteristics. Unusual etiologies or recurrent pneumonias require special considerations (Table 110-2). Lung abscesses, pneumatoceles, and empyema all require special management.

DIFFERENTIAL DIAGNOSIS

Pneumonia must be differentiated from other acute pulmonary diseases, including allergic pneumonitis, asthma, and cystic fibrosis; cardiac diseases, such as pulmonary edema caused by heart failure; and autoimmune diseases, such as certain vasculitides and systemic lupus erythematosus. Radiographically pneumonia must be differentiated from lung trauma and contusion, hemorrhage, foreign body aspiration, and sympathetic effusion due to subdiaphragmatic inflammation.

TREATMENT

Decision-Making Algorithm
Available @ StudentConsult.com

Fever without a Source

Therapy for pneumonia includes supportive and specific treatment and depends on the degree of illness, complications, and knowledge of the infectious agent likely causing the pneumonia. Most cases of pneumonia in healthy children can be managed on an outpatient basis. However children with hypoxemia, inability to maintain adequate hydration, or moderate to severe respiratory distress should be hospitalized. Hospitalization should be considered in infants under 6 months with suspected bacterial pneumonia, those in whom there is a concern for a pathogen with increased virulence (e.g., methicillin-resistant *Staphylococcus aureus*), or when concern exists about a family's ability to care for the child and to assess symptom progression.

Because viruses cause most community-acquired pneumonias in young children, not all children require empirical antibiotic treatment for pneumonia. Recommended therapies in those without recent antibiotic exposure are listed in Table 110-1. Exceptional situations include lack of response to empirical therapy, unusually severe presentations, nosocomial pneumonia, and immunocompromised children susceptible to infections with opportunistic pathogens (Table 110-3). In contrast to pneumococcal meningitis, presumed pneumococcal pneumonia can be treated with high-dose cephalosporin therapy even with high-level penicillin resistance. Vancomycin can be used if the isolate shows high-level resistance and the patient is severely ill. For infants 4 to 18 weeks old with afebrile pneumonia most likely caused by *C. trachomatis*, a macrolide is the recommended treatment. Oseltamivir or zanamivir should be used if influenza is identified or suspected, ideally within 48 hours of symptom onset.

Table 110-3	Antimicrobial Therapy for Pneumonia Caused by Specific Pathogens*	
PATHOGEN	**RECOMMENDED TREATMENT**	**ALTERNATIVE TREATMENT**
Streptococcus pneumoniae with MIC for penicillin ≤2.0 µg/mL	Ampicillin or penicillin IV; amoxicillin PO	Ceftriaxone, cefotaxime, clindamycin or vancomycin IV; Cefuroxime, cefpodoxime, levofloxacin[†], or linezolid PO
Streptococcus pneumoniae with MIC for penicillin ≥4.0 µg/mL	Ceftriaxone IV; levofloxacin[†] or linezolid PO	Ampicillin, levofloxacin[†], clindamycin or vancomycin IV; clindamycin PO
Group A streptococcus	Penicillin or ampicillin IV; amoxicillin or penicillin PO	Ceftriaxone, cefotaxime, clindamycin or vancomycin IV; clindamycin PO
Group B streptococcus	Penicillin or ampicillin IV; amoxicillin or penicillin PO	Ceftriaxone, cefotaxime, clindamycin or vancomycin IV; clindamycin PO
Haemophilus influenzae	Ampicillin IV or amoxicillin PO if β-lactamase negative; ceftriaxone or cefotaxime IV or amoxicillin-clavulanate PO if β-lactamase positive	Ciprofloxacin[†] or levofloxacin[†] IV; cefdinir, cefixime, or cefpodoxime PO
Mycoplasma pneumoniae, Chlamydophila pneumoniae, or *Chlamydia trachomatis*	Azithromycin IV or PO	Erythromycin or levofloxacin IV; clarithromycin, erythromycin, doxycycline[†], or a fluoroquinolone[†] PO
Staphylococcus aureus, methicillin susceptible (MSSA)	Cefazolin, oxacillin, or nafcillin IV; cephalexin PO	Clindamycin or vancomycin IV; clindamycin PO
Staphylococcus aureus, methicillin resistant (MRSA)	Clindamycin or vancomycin IV; clindamycin PO	Linezolid IV or PO
Gram-negative aerobic bacilli (except *P. aeruginosa*)	Cefotaxime or ceftriaxone with or without an aminoglycoside IV; amoxicillin-clavulanate, cefdinir, or cefixime PO	Piperacillin-tazobactam plus an aminoglycoside[‡]; fluoroquinolone[†] PO
P. aeruginosa	Ceftazidime IV with or without an aminoglycoside[‡]; ciprofloxacin[†] if susceptible PO	Piperacillin-tazobactam IV plus an aminoglycoside[‡]
Herpes simplex virus	Acyclovir IV	

IV, Intravenous; *MIC,* minimum inhibitory concentration; *PO, per os* (orally); *TMP-SMX,* trimethoprim-sulfamethoxazole.

*Oral outpatient therapy may be used for mild illness. Intravenous inpatient therapy should be used for moderate to severe illness.

[†]Appropriate fluoroquinolones include moxifloxacin, gatifloxacin, levofloxacin, and gemifloxacin. Fluoroquinolones are contraindicated for children younger than 18 years of age and pregnant or lactating women. Tetracyclines are not recommended for children younger than 9 years.

[‡]Aminoglycoside dosing should be guided by serum antibiotic concentrations after a steady state has been reached.

COMPLICATIONS AND PROGNOSIS

Bacterial pneumonias frequently cause inflammatory fluid to collect in the adjacent pleural space, causing a **parapneumonic effusion** or, if grossly purulent, an **empyema.** Small effusions may not require any special therapy. Large effusions may restrict breathing and require drainage. Air dissection within lung tissue results in a **pneumatocele.** Scarring of the airways and lung tissue may leave dilated bronchi, resulting in **bronchiectasis** and increased risk for recurrent infection.

Pneumonia that causes necrosis of lung tissue may evolve into a **lung abscess.** Lung abscess is an uncommon problem in children and usually is caused by aspiration, infection behind an obstructed bronchus, or certain virulent organisms. Anaerobic bacteria usually predominate, along with various streptococci, *Escherichia coli, Klebsiella pneumoniae, Pseudomonas aeruginosa,* and *Staphylococcus aureus.* Chest radiograph or CT scan reveals a cavitary lesion, often with an air-fluid level, surrounded by parenchymal inflammation. If the cavity communicates with the bronchi, organisms may be isolated from sputum. Diagnostic bronchoscopy may be indicated to exclude a foreign body and obtain microbiologic specimens. Lung abscesses usually respond to appropriate antimicrobial therapy with clindamycin, penicillin G, or ampicillin-sulbactam.

Most children recover from pneumonia rapidly and completely, although radiographic abnormalities may take 6 to 8 weeks to return to normal. In a few children, pneumonia may persist longer than 1 month or may be recurrent. In such cases, the possibility of underlying disease must be investigated further, such as with tuberculin skin test, sweat chloride determination for cystic fibrosis, serum immunoglobulin and IgG subclass determinations, bronchoscopy to identify anatomic abnormalities or foreign body, and barium swallow for gastroesophageal reflux.

Severe adenovirus pneumonia may result in **bronchiolitis obliterans,** a subacute inflammatory process in which the small airways are replaced by scar tissue, resulting in a reduction in lung volume and lung compliance. **Unilateral hyperlucent lung,** or **Swyer-James syndrome,** is a focal sequela of severe necrotizing pneumonia in which all or part of a lung has increased translucency radiographically; it has been linked to adenovirus type 21.

PREVENTION

Annual influenza vaccine is recommended for all children over 6 months of age (see Chapter 94). Trivalent, inactivated influenza vaccine is licensed for use beginning at 6 months of age; live, attenuated vaccine can be used for persons 2 to 49 years of age. Universal childhood vaccination with conjugate vaccines for *H. influenzae* type b and *S. pneumoniae* has greatly diminished the incidence of these pneumonias. The severity of RSV infections can be reduced by use of palivizumab in high-risk patients (see Chapter 109).

Reducing the duration of mechanical ventilation and administering antibiotics judiciously reduces the incidence of ventilator-associated pneumonias. The head of the bed should be raised to 30 to 45 degrees for intubated patients to minimize risk of aspiration, and all suctioning equipment and saline should be sterile. Hand washing before and after every patient contact and use of gloves for invasive procedures are important measures to prevent nosocomial transmission of infections. Hospital staff with respiratory illnesses or who are carriers of certain organisms, such as methicillin-resistant *S. aureus,* should comply with infection control policies to prevent transfer of organisms to patients. Treating sources of aerosols, such as air coolers, can prevent *Legionella* pneumonia.

Table 111-1	Pathogens Causing Infective Endocarditis in Children
BACTERIA	
Viridans streptococci (the most common causative organism at all ages)*	
*Staphylococcus aureus**	
*Enterococcus**	
Coagulase-negative staphylococci	
Hemolytic streptococci: groups A, B (in neonates and elderly), C, G, D	
Streptococcus pneumoniae	
Gram-negative enteric bacilli	
HACEK organisms (i.e., *Haemophilus aphrophilus, Actinobacillus actinomycetemcomitans, Cardiobacterium hominis, Eikenella corrodens,* and *Kingella kingae*)	
FUNGI	
Candida albicans	
Non-albicans Candida	
Aspergillus	
Cryptococcus neoformans	
OTHERS	
Coxiella burnetii (Q fever)	
Chlamydia	
Agents of culture-negative endocarditis	

*Most common causes of infective endocarditis in children.

Chapter 111

INFECTIVE ENDOCARDITIS

ETIOLOGY

Infective endocarditis is an infection on the endothelial surface of the heart, including the heart valves. The management of infections on the endothelial surfaces of blood vessels is very similar. Infectious endothelial lesions, called **vegetations,** usually occur on the valve leaflets and are composed of microorganisms trapped in a fibrin mesh that extends into the bloodstream.

Many microorganisms have been reported to cause endocarditis, although there are only a few principal causes in children (Table 111-1). Viridans streptococci are the principal causes in children with congenital heart diseases without previous surgery. *Staphylococcus aureus* and coagulase-negative staphylococci are important causes of endocarditis, especially following cardiac surgery and in the presence of prosthetic cardiac and endovascular materials.

EPIDEMIOLOGY

Infective endocarditis among children is primarily a complication of congenital heart disease and cardiac surgery, although it can occur in a previously normal native valve. Patients at high risk for infective endocarditis include those with prosthetic cardiac valves or prior infective endocarditis; children who have unrepaired cyanotic congenital heart disease, are within 6 months of repair using prosthetic material, or have residual defects at or near a site of prosthetic material; or transplant patients who develop valvular lesions. The risk is increased after dental and oral procedures or instrumentation or surgical procedures of the respiratory tract, genitourinary tract, or gastrointestinal tract. Rheumatic heart disease is a risk factor but is uncommon. Neonatal endocarditis is associated with the use of central vascular catheters and surgery

in neonates. Endocarditis is a sporadic disease with no geographic predisposition and little gender or socioeconomic predisposition in children.

CLINICAL MANIFESTATIONS

Decision-Making Algorithms
Available @ StudentConsult.com

Heart Murmurs
Fever and Rash

The most common early symptoms of infective endocarditis are nonspecific and include fever, malaise, and weight loss. Tachycardia and a new or changed heart murmur are common findings. The subtle and nonspecific findings underscore the need to obtain blood cultures if endocarditis is suspected, especially for children with congenital heart disease and for unexplained illness after dental or surgical procedures. Endocarditis is usually a **subacute,** slowly progressive process, but **acute endocarditis** is often due to *S. aureus* and may resemble sepsis. Heart failure, splenomegaly, petechiae, and embolic phenomena (Osler nodes, Roth spots, Janeway lesions, and splinter hemorrhages) may be present.

LABORATORY STUDIES AND IMAGING

The key to diagnosis is confirming continuous bacteremia or fungemia by culturing the blood. Multiple blood cultures are performed before initiating antibiotic therapy. Three separate venipunctures for blood culture achieve near-maximal sensitivity (about 95%) among patients who have not been treated recently with antibiotics. Patients who have been treated with antibiotics recently or who are currently receiving antibiotics should have additional serial cultures performed. Despite adequate blood culture techniques, the microbiologic diagnosis is not confirmed in 10% to 15% of cases, known as **culture-negative endocarditis.**

Erythrocyte sedimentation rate and C-reactive protein are often elevated. Leukocytosis, anemia, and hematuria are common laboratory findings. A positive rheumatoid factor or antinuclear antibody may also be seen.

Echocardiography visualizes endocardial and valvular vegetations measuring 2 mm or greater. Transesophageal echocardiography is more sensitive than transthoracic echocardiography for adolescents and adults and for patients with prosthetic valves but is often unnecessary in children.

DIFFERENTIAL DIAGNOSIS

Infective endocarditis must be differentiated from other causes of bacteremia or other cardiac conditions using the **Modified Duke Criteria** for categorizing the strength of the endocarditis diagnosis (Table 111-2). Noninfectious causes of endocardial vegetations must be excluded, such as sterile clots and vegetations associated with rheumatoid disease and lupus erythematosus. Prolonged bacteremia can be caused by infectious endothelial foci outside of the heart, often associated with congenital malformations, vascular trauma, an infected venous thrombosis, and previous vascular surgery.

TREATMENT

Severely ill patients must be stabilized with supportive therapies for cardiac failure, pulmonary edema, and low cardiac output (see Chapter 145). Empirical antibiotic therapy may be started for acutely ill persons after blood cultures are obtained. With subacute disease, awaiting results of blood cultures to confirm the diagnosis is recommended to direct therapy according to the susceptibility of the isolate. Because antibiotics must reach the organisms by passive diffusion through the fibrin mesh, high doses of bactericidal antibiotics are required for an extended period of treatment (4 to 8 weeks). Infective carditis from susceptible viridans streptococci can be treated with monotherapy penicillin G for 4 weeks. A 2-week regimen of penicillin G plus an aminoglycoside is effective in adults. Surgery is indicated if medical treatment is unsuccessful, with persistent bacteremia, an unusual or difficult to treat pathogen (fungal endocarditis), valve annulus or myocardial abscess, rupture of a valve leaflet, valvular insufficiency with acute or refractory heart failure, recurrent serious embolic complications, or refractory prosthetic valve disease.

COMPLICATIONS AND PROGNOSIS

The major complications of infective endocarditis are direct damage to the heart and heart valves and distant complications secondary to sterile and **septic emboli** from vegetations. Damage to the heart and heart valves may include regurgitation with vegetations or actual defects in the leaflets resulting from embolization of the leaflet tissue, abscess of the valve

Table 111-2	Modified Duke Clinical Criteria for Diagnosis of Infective Endocarditis

DEFINITE INFECTIVE ENDOCARDITIS

Histopathologic Criteria

Microorganisms shown by culture or histopathologic examination in a vegetation, emboli, intracardiac abscess *or*

Active endocardial lesions on pathologic examination

Clinical Criteria

Two major criteria or one major and three minor criteria or five minor criteria)

Major Criteria

Positive blood cultures

Two or more separate cultures positive with typical organisms for infective endocarditis

Two or more positive cultures of blood drawn more than 12 hours apart or 4 positive blood cultures irrespective of timing of obtaining specimen

A positive blood culture for *Coxiella burnetii* or positive IgG titer >1:800

Evidence of endocardial involvement

Positive findings on echocardiogram (vegetation on valve or supporting structure, abscess, new valvular regurgitation)

Minor Criteria

Predisposition—predisposing heart condition or injection drug use

Fever—temperature >38° C (>100.4° F)

Vascular phenomena (major arterial emboli, septic pulmonary infarcts, mycotic aneurysm, intracranial hemorrhage, conjunctival hemorrhages, Janeway lesions)

Immunologic phenomena (glomerulonephritis, Osler nodes, Roth spots, rheumatoid factor)

Microbiologic evidence (positive blood culture result, but not meeting major criteria, or serologic evidence of active infection with organism consistent with infective endocarditis)

POSSIBLE INFECTIVE ENDOCARDITIS

Clinical Criteria

One major and one minor criteria or three minor criteria

REJECTED

Firm alternative diagnosis for manifestations of endocarditis *or*

Resolution of manifestations of endocarditis with antibiotic therapy for <4 days *or*

No pathologic evidence of endocarditis at surgery or autopsy after antibiotic therapy of >4 days *or* does not meet criteria for possible endocarditis

Adapted from Tissieres P, Gervaix A, Beghetti M, et al: Value and limitations of the van Reyn, Duke, and modified Duke criteria for the diagnosis of infective endocarditis in children, Pediatrics 112: e467–e471, 2003.

ring, or myocardial abscess. These complications should be monitored by physical examination and echocardiography. Cerebral abscesses or aneurysms can cause a stroke-like picture. Splenic abscesses can cause fatal bleeding.

The outcome of infective endocarditis caused by the most common organisms is often good. The cure rate is greater than 90% in uncomplicated endocarditis caused by viridans streptococci on a natural valve, 75% to 90% for *Enterococcus* endocarditis treated by a synergistic combination of antibiotics, and 60% to 75% for *S. aureus* endocarditis with an acute, severe presentation. The prognosis for endocarditis caused by gram-negative bacilli and rarer organisms is poor. Fungal endocarditis has the poorest prognosis, with a cure rate of about 50% even with valve replacement.

PREVENTION

In high-risk patients, prophylactic antibiotics are required before and during all dental procedures that involve manipulation of gingival tissue or the periapical region as well as invasive procedures of the respiratory tract, infected skin, or muscle. In most cases, oral amoxicillin 50 mg/kg (maximum dose, 2 g) taken 30 to 60 minutes before the procedure is the recommended regimen. Clindamycin or azithromycin are alternative regimens indicated for most patients allergic to β-lactams. Prolonged or continuous antibiotic prophylaxis is not recommended.

Chapter 112

ACUTE GASTROENTERITIS

ETIOLOGY AND EPIDEMIOLOGY

Acute enteritis or **acute gastroenteritis** refers to **diarrhea**, which is abnormally frequent, and liquidity of fecal discharges. Diarrhea is caused by different infectious or inflammatory processes in the intestine that directly affect enterocyte secretory and absorptive functions. Enteritis has many viral, bacterial, and parasitic causes (Table 112-1). Some of these processes act by increasing cyclic adenosine monophosphate levels (*Vibrio cholerae, Escherichia coli* heat-labile toxin). Other processes (*Shigella* toxin) cause secretory diarrhea by affecting ion channels or by unknown mechanisms (Table 112-2).

Diarrhea is a leading cause of morbidity and a common disease in children in the United States. In the developing world, it is a major cause of childhood fatality. The epidemiology of gastroenteritis depends on the specific organisms. Some organisms are spread person to person, others are spread via contaminated food or water, and some are spread from animal to human. Many organisms spread by multiple routes. The ability of an organism to infect relates to the mode of spread, ability to colonize the gastrointestinal tract, and minimum number of organisms required to cause disease.

Viral causes of gastroenteritis in children include rotaviruses, caliciviruses (including the noroviruses), astroviruses, and enteric adenoviruses (serotypes 40 and 41). **Rotavirus** is the most frequent cause of diarrhea during the winter months. Vomiting may last 3 to 4 days, and diarrhea may last 7 to 10 days. Dehydration is common in younger children. Primary infection with rotavirus may cause moderate to severe disease in infancy but is less severe later in life. This illness is much less common in areas where infants receive the rotavirus vaccine.

Table 112-1	Common Pathogenic Organisms Causing Diarrhea and Their Virulence Mechanisms
ORGANISMS	**PATHOGENIC MECHANISM(S)**
VIRUSES	
Rotaviruses	Damage to microvilli
Caliciviruses (noroviruses)	Mucosal lesion
Astroviruses	Mucosal lesion
Enteric adenoviruses (serotypes 40 and 41)	Mucosal lesion
Bacteria	
Campylobacter jejuni	Invasion, enterotoxin
Clostridium difficile	Cytotoxin, enterotoxin
Escherichia coli	
Enteropathogenic (EPEC)	Adherence, effacement
Enterotoxigenic (ETEC) (traveler's diarrhea)	Enterotoxins (heat-stable or heat-labile)
Enteroinvasive (EIEC)	Invasion of mucosa
Enterohemorrhagic (EHEC) (includes O157: H7 causing HUS)	Adherence, effacement, cytotoxin
Enteroaggregative (EAEC)	Adherence, mucosal damage
Salmonella	Invasion, enterotoxin
Shigella	Invasion, enterotoxin, cytotoxin
Vibrio cholerae	Enterotoxin
Vibrio parahaemolyticus	Invasion, cytotoxin
Yersinia enterocolitica	Invasion, enterotoxin
Parasites	
Entamoeba histolytica	Invasion, enzyme and cytotoxin production; cyst resistant to physical destruction
Giardia lamblia	Adheres to mucosa; cyst resistant to physical destruction
Spore-forming intestinal protozoa *Cryptosporidium parvum Isospora belli Cyclospora cayetanensis*	Adherence, inflammation
Microsporidia (*Enterocytozoon bieneusi, Encephalitozoon intestinalis*)	

HUS, Hemolytic uremic syndrome.

Typhoid fever is caused by *Salmonella typhi* and, occasionally, *Salmonella paratyphi*. Worldwide, there are an estimated 16 million cases of typhoid fever annually, resulting in 600,000 deaths. The typhoid bacillus infects humans only. These infections are distinguished by prolonged fever and extraintestinal manifestations, despite inconsistent presence of diarrhea. In the United States, approximately 400 cases of typhoid fever occur each year. Most occur in travelers returning from other countries. The incubation period of typhoid fever is usually 7 to 14 days (range 3 to 60 days). Infected persons without symptoms, or **chronic carriers,** serve as reservoirs and sources of continuous spread. Carriers often have cholelithiasis.

Nontyphoidal *Salmonella* produces diarrhea by invading the intestinal mucosa. The organisms are transmitted through

Table 112-2	Mechanisms of Infectious Diarrhea			
PRIMARY MECHANISM	**DEFECT**	**STOOL EXAMINATION**	**EXAMPLES**	**COMMENTS**
Secretory	Decreased absorption, increased secretion: electrolyte transport	Watery, normal osmolality; osmoles = 2 × (Na+ + K+)	Cholera, toxigenic *Escherichia coli* (EPEC, ETEC); carcinoid, *Clostridium difficile*, cryptosporidiosis (in AIDS)	Persists during fasting; bile salt malabsorption also may increase intestinal water secretion; no stool leukocytes
Mucosal invasion	Inflammation, decreased mucosal surface area and/or colonic reabsorption, increased motility	Blood and increased WBCs in stool	Celiac disease, *Salmonella* infection, shigellosis, amebiasis, yersiniosis, *Campylobacter* infection, rotavirus enteritis	Dysentery (blood, mucus, and WBCs)

From Wyllie R: Major symptoms and signs of digestive tract disorders. In Kliegman RM, Behrman RE, Jenson HB, editors: Nelson Textbook of Pediatrics, ed 18, Philadelphia, 2007, Saunders, Table 303-7, p 152.
WBCs, White blood cells; infection may also contribute to increased motility.

contact with infected animals (chickens, pet iguanas, other reptiles, turtles) or from contaminated food products, such as dairy products, eggs, and poultry. A large inoculum, of 1000 to 10 billion organisms, is required because *Salmonella* is killed by gastric acidity. The incubation period for gastroenteritis ranges from 6 to 72 hours but usually is less than 24 hours.

Shigella dysenteriae may cause disease by producing **Shiga toxin**, either alone or combined with tissue invasion. The incubation period is 1 to 7 days. Infected adults may shed organisms for 1 month. Infection is spread by person-to-person contact or by the ingestion of contaminated food with 10 to 100 organisms. The colon is selectively affected. High fever and febrile seizures may occur in addition to diarrhea.

Only certain strains of *E. coli* produce diarrhea. *E. coli* strains associated with enteritis are classified by the mechanism of diarrhea: enterotoxigenic (ETEC), enterohemorrhagic (EHEC), enteroinvasive (EIEC), enteropathogenic (EPEC), or enteroaggregative (EAEC). ETEC strains produce **heat-labile (cholera-like) enterotoxin, heat-stable enterotoxin**, or both. ETEC causes 40% to 60% of cases of **traveler's diarrhea.** ETEC adhere to the epithelial cells in the upper small intestine and produce disease by liberating toxins that induce intestinal secretion and limit absorption. EHEC, especially the *E. coli* O157:H7 strain, produce a **Shiga-like toxin** that is responsible for a hemorrhagic colitis and most cases of diarrhea associated with **hemolytic uremic syndrome (HUS),** which is a syndrome of microangiopathic hemolytic anemia, thrombocytopenia, and renal failure (see Chapter 164). EHEC is associated with contaminated food, including unpasteurized fruit juices and, especially, undercooked beef. EHEC is associated with a self-limited form of gastroenteritis, usually with bloody diarrhea, but production of this toxin blocks host cell protein synthesis and affects vascular endothelial cells and glomeruli, resulting in the clinical manifestations of HUS. EIEC invades the colonic mucosa, producing widespread mucosal damage with acute inflammation, similar to *Shigella*. EPEC is responsible for many of the epidemics of diarrhea in newborn nurseries and in day care centers.

Campylobacter jejuni is spread by person-to-person contact and by contaminated water and food, especially poultry, raw milk, and cheese. The organism invades the mucosa of the jejunum, ileum, and colon. *Yersinia enterocolitica* is transmitted by pets and contaminated food, especially chitterlings. Infants and young children characteristically have a diarrheal disease, whereas older children usually have acute lesions of the terminal ileum or acute mesenteric lymphadenitis mimicking appendicitis or Crohn's disease. Postinfectious arthritis, rash, and spondylopathy may develop.

Clostridium difficile causes **C. difficile-associated diarrhea** or **antibiotic-associated diarrhea,** secondary to its toxin. The organism produces spores that spread from person to person. *C. difficile-associated* diarrhea may follow exposure to any antibiotic.

Important enteric parasites found in North America include *Entamoeba histolytica* (amebiasis), *Giardia lamblia*, and *Cryptosporidium parvum*. **Amebiasis** occurs in warmer climates, whereas giardiasis is endemic throughout the United States and is common among infants in day care centers. *E. histolytica* infects the colon; amebae may pass through the bowel wall and invade the liver, lung, and brain. Diarrhea is of acute onset, is bloody, and contains leukocytes. **G. lamblia** is transmitted through ingestion of cysts, either from contact with an infected individual or from food or freshwater or well water contaminated with infected feces. The organism adheres to the microvilli of the duodenal and jejunal epithelium. Insidious onset of progressive anorexia, nausea, gaseousness, abdominal distention, watery diarrhea, secondary lactose intolerance, and weight loss is characteristic of giardiasis. *Cryptosporidium* causes mild, watery diarrhea in immunocompetent persons that resolves without treatment. It produces severe, prolonged diarrhea in persons with acquired immunodeficiency syndrome (AIDS) (see Chapter 125).

CLINICAL MANIFESTATIONS

Decision-Making Algorithms
Available @ StudentConsult.com

Vomiting
Diarrhea
Edema
Eosinophilia

Gastroenteritis may be accompanied by systemic findings, such as fever, lethargy, and abdominal pain. Patients often present with clinical syndromes. **Viral diarrhea** is characterized by watery stools, with no blood or mucus. Vomiting may be present, and dehydration may be prominent, especially in infants and younger children. Fever, when present, is low grade.

Typhoid fever is characterized by bacteremia and fever that usually precede the final enteric phase. Fever, headache, and abdominal pain worsen over 48 to 72 hours with nausea, decreased appetite, and constipation over the first week. If untreated, the disease persists for 2 to 3 weeks marked by significant weight loss and, occasionally, hematochezia or melena. Bowel perforation is a common complication in adults but is rare in children. Infected persons without symptoms, or **chronic carriers,** serve as reservoirs and sources of continuous spread.

Dysentery is enteritis involving the colon and rectum, with blood and mucus, possibly foul smelling stools, and fever. *Shigella* is the prototype cause of dysentery, which must be differentiated from infection with EIEC, EHEC, *E. histolytica* **(amebic dysentery),** *C. jejuni, Y. enterocolitica,* and nontyphoidal *Salmonella.* Gastrointestinal bleeding and blood loss may be significant.

Enterotoxigenic disease is caused by agents that produce enterotoxins, such as *V. cholerae* and ETEC. Fever is absent or low grade. Diarrhea usually involves the ileum with watery stools without blood or mucus and usually lasts 3 to 4 days with four to five loose stools per day.

A chief consideration in management of a child with diarrhea is to assess the degree of dehydration as evident from clinical signs and symptoms, ongoing losses, and daily requirements (see Chapter 33). The degree of dehydration dictates the urgency of the situation and the volume of fluid needed for rehydration. Mild to moderate dehydration usually can be treated with oral rehydration; severe dehydration usually requires intravenous (IV) rehydration and may require ICU admission.

LABORATORY AND IMAGING STUDIES

Initial laboratory evaluation of moderate to severe diarrhea includes electrolytes, blood urea nitrogen, creatinine, and urinalysis for specific gravity as an indicator of hydration. Stool specimens should be examined for mucus, blood, and leukocytes, which indicate colitis in response to bacteria that diffusely invade the colonic mucosa, such as *Shigella, Salmonella, C. jejuni,* and invasive *E. coli.* Patients infected with Shiga toxin-producing *E. coli* and *E. histolytica* generally have minimal fecal leukocytes.

A rapid diagnostic test for rotavirus in stool should be performed, especially during the winter. Bacterial stool cultures are recommended for patients with fever, profuse diarrhea, and dehydration or if HUS or pseudomembranous colitis is suspected. If the stool test result is negative for blood and leukocytes, and there is no history to suggest contaminated food ingestion, a viral etiology is most likely. Stool evaluation for parasitic agents should be considered for acute dysenteric illness, especially in returning travelers, and in protracted cases of diarrhea in which no bacterial agent is identified. The diagnosis of *E. histolytica* is based on identification of the organism in the stool. Serologic tests are useful for diagnosis of extraintestinal amebiasis, including amebic hepatic abscess. Giardiasis can be diagnosed by identifying trophozoites or cysts in stool but require three specimens. More specific and sensitive fecal immunoassays are the diagnostic tests of choice.

Positive blood cultures are uncommon with bacterial enteritis except for *S. typhi* (typhoid fever), nontyphoidal *Salmonella,* and *E. coli* enteritis in very young infants. In typhoid fever, blood cultures are positive early in the disease, whereas stool cultures become positive only after the secondary bacteremia.

DIFFERENTIAL DIAGNOSIS

Decision-Making Algorithms
Available @ StudentConsult.com

Abdominal Pain
Vomiting
Diarrhea
Failure to Thrive

Diarrhea can be caused by infection, toxins, gastrointestinal allergy (including allergy to milk or soy proteins), malabsorption defects, inflammatory bowel disease, celiac disease, or any injury to enterocytes. Specific infections are differentiated from each other by the use of stool cultures and enzyme-linked immunosorbent assay or polymerase chain reaction tests, when necessary. Acute enteritis may mimic other acute diseases, such as intussusception and acute appendicitis, which are best identified by diagnostic imaging. Many noninfectious causes of diarrhea produce chronic diarrhea, with persistence for more than 14 days. Persistent or chronic diarrhea may require tests for malabsorption or invasive studies, including endoscopy and small bowel biopsy (see Chapter 129).

Common-source diarrhea usually is associated with ingestion of contaminated food. In the United States, the most common bacterial food-borne causes (in order of frequency) are nontyphoidal *Salmonella, Campylobacter, Shigella, E. coli* O157:H7, *Yersinia, Listeria monocytogenes,* and *V. cholerae.* The most common parasitic food-borne causes are *Cryptosporidium parvum* and *Cyclospora cayetanensis.*

Common-source diarrhea also includes ingestion of preformed enterotoxins produced by bacteria, such as *S. aureus* and *Bacillus cereus,* which multiply in contaminated foods, and nonbacterial toxins such as from fish, shellfish, and mushrooms. After a short incubation period, vomiting and cramps are prominent symptoms, and diarrhea may or may not be present. Heavy metals that leach into canned food or drinks causing gastric irritation and emetic syndromes may mimic symptoms of acute infectious enteritis.

TREATMENT

Most infectious causes of diarrhea in children are self-limited. Management of viral and most bacterial causes of diarrhea is primarily supportive and consists of correcting dehydration and ongoing fluid and electrolyte deficits and managing secondary complications resulting from mucosal injury.

Hyponatremia is common; hypernatremia is less common. Metabolic acidosis results from losses of bicarbonate in stool, lactic acidosis results from shock, and phosphate retention results from transient prerenal-renal insufficiency. Traditionally therapy for 24 hours with oral rehydration solutions alone is effective for viral diarrhea. Therapy for severe fluid and electrolyte losses involves IV hydration. Less severe degrees of dehydration (<10%) in the absence of excessive vomiting or shock may be managed with oral rehydration solutions containing glucose and electrolytes. Ondansetron may be administered to reduce emesis when persistent.

Antibiotic therapy is necessary only for patients with *S. typhi* (typhoid fever) and sepsis or bacteremia with signs of systemic toxicity, those with metastatic foci, or infants younger than 3 months with nontyphoidal salmonella. Antibiotic treatment of *Shigella* produces a bacteriologic cure in 80% of patients after 48 hours, reducing the spread of the disease. Many *Shigella sonnei* isolates, the predominant strain affecting children, are resistant to amoxicillin and trimethoprim-sulfamethoxazole. Recommended treatment for children is an oral third-generation cephalosporin or a fluoroquinolone for patients 18 years and older.

Treatment of *C. difficile* (pseudomembranous colitis) includes discontinuation of the antibiotic and, if diarrhea is severe, oral metronidazole or vancomycin. *E. histolytica* dysentery is treated with metronidazole followed by a luminal agent, such as iodoquinol. The treatment of *G. lamblia* is with albendazole, metronidazole, furazolidone, or quinacrine. Nitazoxanide can be used in children younger than 12 months of age for the treatment of *Cryptosporidium.*

COMPLICATIONS AND PROGNOSIS

The major complication of gastroenteritis is dehydration and hypovolemic shock. Seizures may occur with high fever, especially with *Shigella*. Intestinal abscesses can form with *Shigella* and *Salmonella* infections, especially typhoid fever, leading to intestinal perforation, a life-threatening complication. Severe vomiting associated with gastroenteritis can cause esophageal tears or aspiration pneumonia.

Deaths resulting from diarrhea reflect the principal problem of disruption of fluid and electrolyte homeostasis, which leads to dehydration, electrolyte imbalance, vascular instability, and shock. In the United States, approximately 75 to 150 deaths occur annually from diarrheal disease, primarily in children under 1 year of age. These deaths occur in a seasonal pattern between October and February, concurrent with the rotavirus season.

At least 10% of patients who have typhoid fever shed *S. typhi* for about 3 months, and 4% become chronic carriers. The risk of becoming a chronic carrier is low in children. Ciprofloxacin is recommended for adult carriers with persistent *Salmonella* excretion.

PREVENTION

The most important means of preventing childhood diarrhea is the provision of clean, uncontaminated water and proper hygiene in growing, collecting, and preparing foods. Good hygienic measures, especially good hand washing with soap and water, are the best means of controlling person-to-person spread of most organisms causing gastroenteritis. Similarly poultry products should be considered potentially contaminated with *Salmonella* and should be handled and cooked appropriately.

Immunization against rotavirus infection is recommended for all children beginning at 6 weeks of age, with the first dose by 14 weeks 6 days and the last dose by 8 months (see Chapter 94). Two typhoid vaccines are licensed in the United States: an oral live attenuated vaccine (Ty21a) for children 6 years and older, and a capsular polysaccharide vaccine (ViCPS) for intramuscular administration for persons 2 years and older. These are recommended for travelers to endemic areas of developing countries or for household contacts of *S. typhi* chronic carriers.

Families should be aware of the risk of acquiring salmonellosis from household reptile pets. Transmission of *Salmonella* from reptiles can be prevented by thorough hand washing with soap and water after handling reptiles or reptile cages. Children under 5 years of age and immunocompromised persons should avoid contact with reptiles.

The risk for traveler's diarrhea, caused primarily by ETEC, may be minimized by avoiding uncooked food and untreated drinking water. Prophylaxis with bismuth subsalicylate (Pepto-Bismol) for adults (2 oz or two tablets orally four times a day) may be effective for prevention but is not recommended for children. Symptomatic self-treatment for mild diarrhea with loperamide (Imodium) and WHO **oral rehydration solution** is recommended for children at least 6 years of age and adults. Self-treatment of moderate diarrhea and fever with a fluoroquinolone is recommended in adults of at least 18 years old. Prompt medical evaluation is indicated for disease persisting more than 3 days, bloody stools, fever above 102° F (38.9° C) or chills, persistent vomiting, or moderate to severe dehydration, especially in children.

Lactobacillus acidophilus is a **probiotic** and reduces the incidence of community-acquired and antibiotic-associated diarrhea in children treated with oral antibiotics for other infectious diseases.

Chapter 113

VIRAL HEPATITIS

ETIOLOGY

There are six primary hepatotropic viruses:
Hepatitis A virus (HAV)
Hepatitis B virus (HBV)
Hepatitis C virus (HCV)
Hepatitis D virus (HDV)
Hepatitis E virus (HEV)
Hepatitis G virus (HGV)

They differ in their virologic characteristics, transmission, severity, likelihood of persistence, and subsequent risk of hepatocellular carcinoma (Table 113-1). HDV, also known as the **delta agent,** is a defective virus that requires HBV for spread and causes either coinfection with HBV or superinfection in chronic HBsAg (hepatitis B surface antigen) carriers. HBV, HCV, and HDV infections can result in chronic hepatitis, or a chronic carrier state, which facilitates spread. The cause of 10% to 15% of cases of acute hepatitis is unknown.

EPIDEMIOLOGY

HAV causes approximately half of all cases of viral hepatitis in the United States. Among U.S. children, approximately 70% to 80% of all new cases of viral hepatitis are caused by HAV, 5% to 30% by HBV, and 5% to 15% by HCV. The major risk factors for HBV and HCV are injectable drug use, frequent exposure

Table 113-1	Characteristics of Agents Causing Acute Viral Hepatitis						
	HEPATITIS VIRUSES						
FEATURE	**HAV***	**HBV**	**HCV†**	**HDV**	**HEV‡**	**HGV**	**TTV, SEN-V**
Viral structure	27-nm ssRNA virus	42-nm dsDNA virus	30- to 60-nm ssRNA virus	36-nm circular ssRNA hybrid particle with HB$_s$Ag coat	27–34 nm ssRNA virus	50- to 100-nm ssRNA virus	30- to 50- nm ssDNA virus
Family	Picornavirus	Hepadnavirus	Flavivirus	Satellite	Flavivirus	Flavivirus	Circovirus
Transmission	Fecal-oral, rarely parenteral	Transfusion, sexual, inoculation, perinatal	Parenteral, transfusion, perinatal	Similar to HBV	Fecal-oral (endemic and epidemic)	Parenteral, transfusion	Parenteral, perinatal
Incubation period	15–30 days	60–180 days	30–60 days	Coinfection with HBV	35–60 days	Unknown	Unknown
Serum markers	Anti-HAV	HBsAg, HBcAg, HB$_e$Ag, anti-HB$_s$, anti-HBc	Anti-HCV (IgG, IgM), RIBA, PCR assay for HCV RNA	Anti-HDV, RNA	Anti-HEV	RNA by RT-PCR assay	
Fulminant liver failure	Rare	<1% unless coinfection with HDV	Uncommon	2%–20%	20%	Probably no	
Persistent infection	No	5%–10% (90% with perinatal infection)	85%	2%–70%	No	Persistent infection common; chronic disease rare	
Increased risk of hepatocellular carcinoma	No	Yes	Yes	No	No	Unknown	
Prophylaxis	Vaccine: immune serum globulin	Vaccine: hepatitis B immunoglobulin (HBIG)					

dsDNA, Double-stranded DNA; *HAV*, hepatitis A virus; *HBV*, hepatitis B virus; *HCV*, hepatitis C virus; *HDV*, hepatitis D virus; *HEV*, hepatitis E virus; *HGV*, hepatitis G virus; *PCR*, polymerase chain reaction; *RIBA*, recombinant immunoblot assay; *RT-PCR*, reverse transcriptase-polymerase chain reaction; *ssDNA/ssRNA*, single-stranded DNA/RNA; *TTV*, transfusion-transmitted virus.
*I.e., enterovirus 72.
†Formerly posttransfusion non-A, non-B virus.
‡Formerly enteral non-A, non-B virus.

to blood products, and prenatal transmission from maternal infection. HEV occurs following travel to endemic areas outside of the United States. HGV is prevalent in HIV-infected persons. HBV and HCV cause chronic infection, which may lead to cirrhosis and is a significant risk factor for hepatocellular carcinoma and represents a persistent risk of transmission.

CLINICAL MANIFESTATIONS

Decision-Making Algorithms
Available @ StudentConsult.com

Jaundice
Hepatomegaly
Fever without a Source

There is considerable overlap in the characteristic clinical courses of HAV, HBV, and HCV (Fig. 113-1). The **preicteric phase,** which lasts approximately 1 week, is characterized by headache, anorexia, malaise, abdominal discomfort, nausea, and vomiting and usually precedes the onset of clinically detectable disease. Infants with perinatal acquired HBV may have immune complexes accompanied by urticaria and arthritis before the onset of icterus. Jaundice and tender hepatomegaly are the most common physical findings and are characteristic of the **icteric phase.** Prodromal symptoms, particularly in children, may abate during the icteric phase. Asymptomatic or mild, nonspecific illness without icterus is common with HAV, HBV, and HCV, especially in young children. Hepatic enzymes may increase 15- to 20-fold. Resolution of the hyperbilirubinemia and normalization of the transaminases may take 6 to 8 weeks.

LABORATORY AND IMAGING STUDIES

Alanine aminotransferase and aspartate aminotransferase levels are elevated and generally reflect the degree of parenchymal inflammation. Alkaline phosphatase, 5α-nucleotidase, and total and direct (conjugated) bilirubin levels indicate the degree of cholestasis, which results from hepatocellular and bile duct damage. The **prothrombin time** is a good predictor

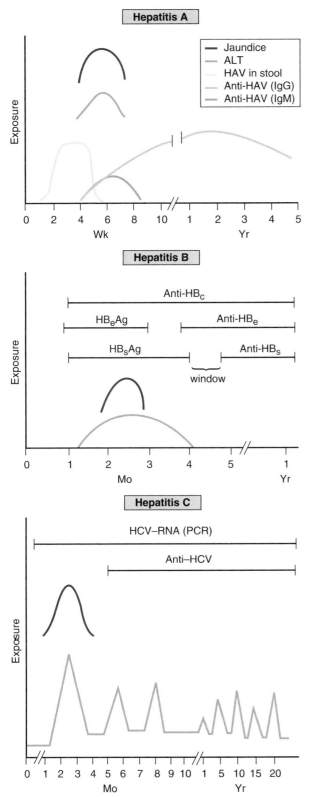

Figure 113-1 Clinical course and laboratory findings associated with hepatitis A, hepatitis B, and hepatitis C. *ALT*, Alanine aminotransferase; *HAV*, hepatitis A virus; *anti-HBc*, antibody to hepatitis B core antigen; *HBeAg*, hepatitis B early antigen; *anti-HBe*, antibody to hepatitis B early antigen; *HBsAg*, hepatitis B surface antigen; anti-HBs, antibody to hepatitis B surface antigen; *HCV*, hepatitis C virus; *PCR*, polymerase chain reaction.

of severe hepatocellular injury and progression to fulminant hepatic failure (see Chapter 130).

The diagnosis of viral hepatitis is confirmed by serologic testing (see Table 113-1 and Fig. 113-1). The presence of IgM-specific antibody to HAV with low or absent IgG antibody to HAV is presumptive evidence of HAV. There is no chronic carrier state of HAV. The presence of HBsAg signifies acute or chronic infection with HBV. Antigenemia appears early in the illness and is usually transient but is characteristic of chronic infection. Maternal HBsAg status should always be determined when HBV infection is diagnosed in children younger than 1 year of age because of the likelihood of vertical transmission. Hepatitis B early antigen (HBeAg) appears in the serum with acute HBV. The continued presence of HBsAg and HBeAg in the absence of antibody to e antigen (anti-HBe) indicates high risk of transmissibility that is associated with ongoing viral replication. Clearance of HBsAg from the serum precedes a variable **window period** followed by the emergence of the antibody to surface antigen (anti-HBs), which indicates development of lifelong immunity and is also a marker of immunization. Antibody to core antigen (anti-HBc) is a useful marker for recognizing HBV infection during the window phase (when HBsAg has disappeared but before the appearance of anti-HBs). Anti-HBe is useful in predicting a low degree of infectivity during the carrier state. Seroconversion after HCV infection may occur 6 months after infection. A positive result of HCV enzyme-linked immunosorbent assay should be confirmed with the more specific recombinant immunoblot assay, which detects antibodies to multiple HCV antigens. Detection of HCV RNA by polymerase chain reaction (PCR) is a sensitive marker for active infection, and results of this test may be positive 3 days after inoculation.

DIFFERENTIAL DIAGNOSIS

Many other viruses may cause hepatitis as part of systemic infection, including Epstein-Barr virus, cytomegalovirus, varicella zoster virus (chickenpox), herpes simplex virus, and adenoviruses. Bacterial infections that may cause hepatitis include *Escherichia coli* sepsis and leptospirosis. Patients with cholecystitis, cholangitis, and choledocholithiasis may present with acute symptoms and jaundice. Other causes of acute liver disease in childhood include drugs (isoniazid, phenytoin, valproic acid, carbamazepine, oral contraceptives, acetaminophen), toxins (ethanol, poisonous mushroom), Wilson disease, metabolic disease (galactosemia, tyrosinemia), α_1-antitrypsin deficiency, tumor, shock, anoxia, and graft-versus-host disease (see Chapter 130).

TREATMENT

The treatment of acute hepatitis is largely supportive and involves rest, hydration, and adequate nutrition. Hospitalization is indicated for persons with severe vomiting and dehydration, a prolonged prothrombin time, or signs of hepatic encephalopathy. When the diagnosis of viral hepatitis is established, attention should be directed toward preventing its spread to close contacts. For HAV, hygienic measures include hand washing and careful disposal of excreta, contaminated diapers or clothing, needles, and other blood-contaminated items.

Chronic HBV infection may be treated with interferon alfa-2b or lamivudine, and HCV may be treated with interferon alfa alone or usually in combination with ribavirin. Mostly adults experience these treatment regimens. The decision to treat is based on the patient's current age, age at HBV acquisition, development of viral mutations during therapy, and stage of viral infection. Transmission of HBV by vertical transmission or infection early in life often results in chronic HBV infection in an immune tolerant phase, in which interferon usually is not effective.

COMPLICATIONS AND PROGNOSIS

A protracted or relapsing course may develop in 10% to 15% of cases of HAV in adults, lasting up to 6 months with an undulating course before eventual clinical resolution. **Fulminant hepatitis** with encephalopathy, gastrointestinal bleeding from esophageal varices or coagulopathy, and profound jaundice is uncommon but is associated with a high mortality rate.

Most cases of acute viral hepatitis resolve without specific therapy, with less than 0.1% of cases progressing to fulminant hepatic necrosis. HAV and HEV cause acute infection only. HBV, HCV, and HDV may persist as chronic infection with chronic inflammation, fibrosis, and cirrhosis and the associated risk of hepatocellular carcinoma.

From 5% to 10% of adults with HBV develop persistent infection, defined by persistence of HBsAg in the blood for more than 6 months, compared with 90% of children who acquire HBV by perinatal transmission. Chronic HBsAg carriers are usually HBeAg-negative and have no clinical, biochemical, or serologic evidence of active hepatitis, unless there is superinfection with HDV. Approximately 10% to 15% of HBsAg carriers eventually clear HBsAg.

Approximately 85% of persons infected with HCV remain chronically infected, which is characterized by fluctuating transaminase levels (see Fig. 113-1). There is poor correlation of symptoms with ongoing liver damage. Approximately 20% of persons with chronic infection develop cirrhosis, and approximately 25% of those develop hepatocellular carcinoma. HIV infection and ethanol use increase the risk of HCV progression.

PREVENTION

Good hygienic practices significantly reduce the risk of fecal-oral transmission of HAV. Screening blood donors for evidence of hepatitis significantly reduces the risk of blood-borne transmission. Specific postexposure measures are recommended to prevent secondary cases in susceptible persons.

HAV vaccine is recommended for routine immunization of all children beginning at 12 months and for unvaccinated older children in areas with targeted vaccination programs. Unvaccinated household and sexual contacts of persons with HAV should receive postexposure prophylaxis as soon as possible and within 2 weeks of the last exposure. A single dose of HAV vaccine at the age-appropriate dose is preferred for persons 12 months to 40 years of age. Immunoglobulin (0.02 mL/kg) given intramuscularly is preferred for children under 12 months of age, persons over 40 years of age, and immunocompromised persons. Unvaccinated travelers to endemic regions should receive a single dose of HAV vaccine administered at any time before departure.

HBV vaccine is recommended for routine immunization of all infants beginning at birth and for all children and adolescents through 18 years of age who have not been immunized previously (see Fig. 94-1). It also is recommended as a preexposure vaccination for older children and adults at increased risk of exposure to HBV, including persons undergoing hemodialysis, recipients of clotting factor concentrates, residents and staff of institutions for developmentally disabled persons, men who have sex with men, injectable drug users, inmates of juvenile detention and other correctional facilities, and health care workers. HBV vaccine already has shown effectiveness in reducing the incidence of hepatocellular carcinoma in high-risk populations. Routine prenatal screening for HBsAg is recommended for all pregnant women in the United States. Infants born to HBsAg-positive mothers should receive HBV vaccine and hepatitis B immunoglobulin (HBIG) (0.5 mL) within 12 hours of birth, with subsequent vaccine doses at 1 month and 6 months of age followed by testing for HBsAg and anti-HBs at 9 to 15 months of age. Infants born to mothers whose HBsAg status is unknown should receive vaccine within 12 hours of birth. If maternal testing is positive for HBsAg, the infant should receive HBIG as soon as possible (no later than 1 week of age). The combination of HBIG and vaccination is 99% effective in preventing vertical transmission of HBV. Vaccination alone without HBIG may prevent 75% of cases of perinatal HBV transmission and approximately 95% of cases of symptomatic childhood HBV infection.

Postexposure prophylaxis of unvaccinated persons using HBIG and vaccine is recommended following needle stick injuries with blood from an HBsAg-positive patient and for household members with intimate contact, including sex partners.

Chapter **114**

URINARY TRACT INFECTION

ETIOLOGY

Urinary tract infections (UTIs) include **cystitis** (infection localized to the bladder), **pyelonephritis** (infection of the renal parenchyma, calyces, and renal pelvis), and **renal abscess,** which may be intrarenal or perinephric. The urinary tract and urine are normally sterile. *Escherichia coli,* ascending from bowel flora, accounts for 90% of first infections and 75% of recurrent infections. Over 90% of nephritogenic *E. coli* possess P fimbriae that binds to uroepithelial cells and P blood group antigens. Individuals with high-level expression of P1 blood group antigen are predisposed to pyelonephritis and bacteremia, as well as recurrent UTIs. Other bacteria commonly causing infection include *Klebsiella, Proteus, Enterococcus,* and *Pseudomonas. Staphylococcus saprophyticus* is associated with UTI in some children and in sexually active adolescent girls. *S. saprophyticus, Chlamydia trachomatis,* and *E. coli* are the chief causes of the **acute urethral syndrome**, or **postcoital urethritis,** which typically occur 12 to 72 hours after sexual intercourse.

EPIDEMIOLOGY

Approximately 8% of girls and 2% of boys have a UTI by 11 years of age. The lifetime incidence of UTI in females is about 30% compared to only 1% in males. Approximately 75% of infants younger than 3 months of age with bacteriuria are male compared with only 10% between 3 and 8 months of age. After 12 months of age, UTI in healthy children usually is seen in girls.

A short urethra predisposes girls to UTI. Uncircumcised male infants are at 5- to 12-fold increased risk for UTI compared with circumcised male infants. Obstruction to urine flow and urinary stasis is the major risk factor and may result from anatomic abnormalities, nephrolithiasis, renal tumor, indwelling urinary catheter, ureteropelvic junction obstruction, megaureter, extrinsic compression, and pregnancy. Vesicoureteral reflux, whether primary (70% of cases) or secondary to urinary tract obstruction, predisposes to chronic infection and renal scarring. Scarring also may develop in the absence of reflux.

CLINICAL MANIFESTATIONS

Decision-Making Algorithms
Available @ StudentConsult.com

Dysuria
Enuresis
Red Urine and Hematuria

The symptoms and signs of UTI vary markedly with age. Few have high positive predictive values in neonates, with failure to thrive, feeding problems, and fever as the most consistent symptoms. Direct hyperbilirubinemia may develop secondary to gram-negative endotoxin. Infants 1 month to 2 years old may present with feeding problems, failure to thrive, diarrhea, vomiting, or unexplained fever. The symptoms may masquerade as gastrointestinal illness with colic, irritability, and screaming periods. At 2 years of age, children begin to show the classic signs of UTI such as urgency, dysuria, frequency, and abdominal or back pain. The presence of UTI should be suspected in all infants and young children with unexplained fever and in patients of all ages with fever and congenital anomalies of the urinary tract.

LABORATORY AND IMAGING STUDIES

The diagnosis of UTI in infants and young children requires the presence of both pyuria and at least 50,000 CFU/mL of a single pathogenic organism. For older children and adolescents, >100,000 CFU/mL indicates infection. Urine samples for urinalysis should be examined promptly (within 20 minutes) or refrigerated until cultured. Urine obtained by midstream, clean-catch technique for older children and adolescents is an appropriate collection method, whereas transurethral catheterization is the appropriate method for younger children and infants in which antibiotics are being started. Perineal bags for urine collection are prone to contamination and are not recommended for urine collection for culture. If there is uncertainty about diagnosis of UTI in a younger child or infant, urine can be collected by the most convenient method for urinalysis and if suggestive of infection, collect urine by catheterization prior to starting antibiotics.

Urinalysis showing **pyuria** (leukocyturia of >10 white blood cells [WBCs]/mm^3) suggests infection, but also is consistent with urethritis, vaginitis, nephrolithiasis, glomerulonephritis, and interstitial nephritis. Urinary dipstick tests that combine both the leukocyte esterase and nitrite (or positive leukocyte esterase and positive microscopy for bacteria) have sensitivity of 70% and specificity of 99% for detecting a UTI. Either test used alone has poor sensitivity.

Ultrasonography of the bladder and kidneys is recommended for infants with febrile UTIs to exclude structural abnormalities or detect hydronephrosis. Voiding cystourethrogram (VCUG) is indicated if the ultrasound is abnormal (hydronephrosis, scarring, or other findings to suggest obstruction or congenital abnormality). Vesicoureteral reflux is the most common abnormality found and is ranked from grade I (ureter only) to grade V (complete gross dilation of the ureter and obliteration of caliceal and pelvic anatomy) (see Chapter 167). A technetium-99m DMSA scan can identify acute pyelonephritis and is most useful to define renal scarring as a late effect of UTI.

DIFFERENTIAL DIAGNOSIS

The diagnosis of a UTI is confirmed by a positive urine culture, but this does not distinguish between upper tract and lower tract infection. Localization of a UTI is important because upper UTI is associated more frequently with bacteremia and with anatomic abnormalities than is uncomplicated cystitis. The clinical manifestations of UTI do not reliably distinguish the site of infection in neonates, infants, and toddlers. Fever and abdominal pain may occur with either lower or upper UTI, although high fever, costovertebral tenderness, high erythrocyte sedimentation rate, leukocytosis, and bacteremia each suggest upper tract involvement. DMSA scan is sensitive for detecting acute pyelonephritis but not commonly used.

The manifestations of UTI overlap with signs of sepsis seen in young children and with enteritis, appendicitis, mesenteric lymphadenitis, and pneumonia in older children. Dysuria may indicate pinworm infection, hypersensitivity to soaps or detergents, vaginitis, or sexual abuse and infection.

TREATMENT

Decision-Making Algorithm
Available @ StudentConsult.com

Fever without a Source

Empirical therapy should be initiated for symptomatic children and for all children with a urine culture confirming UTI. For an older child who does not appear ill but has a positive urine culture, oral antibiotic therapy should be initiated. For a child with suspected UTI who appears toxic, appears dehydrated, or is unable to retain oral fluids, initial antibiotic therapy should be administered parenterally, and hospitalization should be considered.

Neonates with UTI are treated for 10 to 14 days with parenteral antibiotics because of the higher rate of bacteremia. Older children with UTI are treated for 7 to 14 days. Initial treatment with parenteral antibiotics is determined by clinical status. Parenteral antibiotics should be continued until there is clinical improvement (typically 24 to 48 hours). Specific antibiotic therapy should be guided by the local antimicrobial susceptibility patterns and the results of the patient's urine cultures because of increasing problems related to antimicrobial resistance. Commonly used parenteral antibiotics include ceftriaxone or gentamicin. Oral regimens include a cephalosporin, amoxicillin plus clavulanic acid, or trimethoprim sulfamethoxazole. Infants and children who do not show the expected clinical response within 2 days of starting antimicrobial therapy should be re-evaluated, have another urine specimen obtained for culture, and undergo imaging promptly.

The degree of toxicity, dehydration, and ability to retain oral intake of fluids should be assessed carefully. Restoring or maintaining adequate hydration, including correction of electrolyte abnormalities that are often associated with vomiting or poor oral intake, is important.

COMPLICATIONS AND PROGNOSIS

Bacteremia occurs in 2% to 5% of episodes of pyelonephritis and is more likely in infants than in older children. Focal renal abscesses are an uncommon complication.

The relapse rate of UTI is approximately 25% to 40%. Most relapses occur within 2 to 3 weeks of treatment. Parents should be counseled to follow up for evaluation for subsequent fevers to evaluate for the possibility of a recurrence of UTI. If a recurrent UTI is diagnosed, further imaging studies (VCUG) are indicated to evaluate the possibility of vesicoureteral reflux (see Chapter 167).

PREVENTION

Primary prevention is achieved by promoting good perineal hygiene and managing underlying risk factors for UTI, such as chronic constipation, encopresis, and daytime and nighttime urinary incontinence. There is evidence that antibiotic prophylaxis may prevent more severe symptomatic recurrent infections, although the effect is small. The impact of secondary prophylaxis to prevent renal scarring is unknown. Acidification of the urine with cranberry juice is not recommended as the sole means of preventing UTI in children at high risk.

Chapter 115

VULVOVAGINITIS

ETIOLOGY

Vulvovaginitis, which is inflammation of the vulva or the vagina or both, is the most common gynecologic problem in children. Low prepubertal levels of estrogen result in thin, atrophic vaginal epithelium that is susceptible to bacterial invasion. At puberty estrogen increases, and the pH of the

vagina becomes more acidic. There are several specific causes of vulvovaginitis (Table 115-1), including sexually transmitted infections such as *Trichomonas vaginalis* and herpes simplex virus (see Chapter 116). **Nonspecific vaginitis** results from overgrowth of normal aerobic vaginal flora that is associated with poor hygiene. **Bacterial vaginosis** is caused by *Gardnerella vaginalis,* which interacts synergistically with vaginal anaerobes, including *Bacteroides, Mobiluncus,* and *Peptostreptococcus.*

EPIDEMIOLOGY

Nonspecific vaginitis is the most common cause of vulvovaginitis in young girls. *G. vaginalis* is often present as part of the normal vaginal flora in preadolescent girls but is more common in girls who are sexually active. *Candida* is much less common in preadolescent girls than in women.

CLINICAL MANIFESTATIONS

Decision-Making Algorithms
Available @ StudentConsult.com

Abnormal Vaginal Bleeding
Vaginal Discharge

The primary symptoms of vulvovaginitis are vaginal discharge, erythema, and pruritus. Characteristics of specific etiologies are outlined in Table 115-1.

LABORATORY AND IMAGING STUDIES

Wet mount microscopic examination, prepared by mixing vaginal secretions with normal saline solution, and culture may be used to confirm a specific diagnosis (see Table 115-1). **Clue cells** are vaginal epithelial cells that are covered with *G. vaginalis* and have a granular appearance. Vaginal cultures for *G. vaginalis* are not useful. *Candida* may be identified by saline wet mount or by culture.

DIFFERENTIAL DIAGNOSIS

Noninfectious causes of vulvovaginitis include physical agents (foreign body, sand), chemical agents (bubble bath, soap, detergent), and vulvar skin disease (atopic dermatitis, seborrhea, psoriasis). Physiologic vaginal discharge or **physiologic leukorrhea** of desquamated vaginal cells and mucus occurs normally in girls soon after birth, with discharge lasting for about 1 week, and appears again at 6 to 12 months before menarche. The discharge is minimal, clear, and thin without pruritus or inflammation. No treatment is necessary.

TREATMENT

The treatment of vulvovaginitis depends on the etiology (see Table 115-1). Treatment of nonspecific vaginitis focuses on improving perineal hygiene. The recommended treatment for bacterial vaginosis is oral metronidazole or clindamycin. Imidazole creams and vaginal tablets and suppositories all are effective for the treatment of acute

Table 115-1	Characteristics of Vulvovaginitis		
ETIOLOGY CONDITION/ DISORDER	**PRESENTATION**	**DIAGNOSIS**	**TREATMENT**
Physiologic vaginal discharge (physiologic leukorrhea)	Minimal, clear, thin discharge without pruritus or inflammation; occurs soon after birth and again at 6–12 months before menarche	No pathogenic organisms on culture	Reassurance
Nonspecific vaginitis	Vaginal discharge, dysuria, itching; fecal soiling of underwear	Evidence of poor hygiene; no pathogenic organisms on culture	Improved hygiene, sitz baths 2–3 times/day
Bacterial vaginosis	Often asymptomatic; possible thin vaginal discharge with a "fishy" odor	At least three of the following four criteria: (1) thin, homogeneous vaginal discharge; (2) vaginal pH ≥4.5; (3) a fishy odor of volatile amines on the addition of a drop of 10% potassium hydroxide to a drop of vaginal discharge (the whiff test); and (4) the presence of clue cells on a saline wet mount of vaginal discharge (*Gardnerella vaginalis* and anaerobes)	Metronidazole, clindamycin
Candidiasis	Itching, dysuria, white "cottage cheese" vaginal discharge	*Candida* on saline wet mount of vaginal discharge	Topical antifungal (e.g., butoconazole, clotrimazole, miconazole, nystatin)
Enterobiasis (pinworms)	Perineal pruritus (nocturnal); gastrointestinal symptoms; variable vulvovaginal contamination from feces	Adult worms in stool or eggs on perianal skin	Mebendazole or albendazole
Giardiasis	Asymptomatic fecal contaminant, vaginal discharge, diarrhea, malabsorption syndrome	Protozoal flagellate (cyst or trophozoites) in feces	Metronidazole or albendazole
Molluscum contagiosum	Vulvar lesions, nodules with papule; white core of curd-like material	Isolation of poxvirus	Dermal curettage of umbilicated area
Phthirus pubis infection (pediculosis pubis)	Pruritus, excoriation, sky-blue macules; inner thigh or lower abdomen	Nits on hair shafts, lice on skin or clothing	1% permethrin
Sarcoptes scabiei infection (scabies)	Nocturnal pruritus, pruritic vesicles, pustules in runs	Mites; ova black, dots of feces (microscopic)	5% permethrin
Shigella infection	Bloody vaginal discharge; fever, malaise, fecal contamination, diarrhea; blood and mucus in stool, abdominal cramps	Stools: white blood cells and red blood cells, positive for *Shigella*	Oral third-generation cephalosporin
Staphylococcus, Streptococcus infection	Vaginal discharge, possibly bloody; spread from primary lesion		First-generation cephalosporin or dicloxacillin
Foreign body	Foul-smelling vaginal discharge, sometimes bloody	Foreign body on physical examination	Removal of foreign body

vulvovaginal candidiasis. Douching or vaginal irrigation is not beneficial and is not recommended.

COMPLICATIONS AND PROGNOSIS
Complications are rare. The prognosis is excellent.

PREVENTION
There are no recognized prophylactic measures for bacterial vaginosis or nonspecific vaginitis. Douching is not protective and reduces normal vaginal flora, which are protective against pathogenic organisms.

Chapter **116**

SEXUALLY TRANSMITTED INFECTIONS

Decision-Making Algorithms
Available @ StudentConsult.com

Dysmenorrhea
Abnormal Vaginal Bleeding
Vaginal Discharge

Adolescents have the highest rates of sexually transmitted infections (STIs). Compared with adults, sexually active adolescents are more likely to believe they will not contract an STI, more likely to come into contact with an infected sexual partner, less likely to receive health care when an STI develops, and less likely to be compliant with treatment for an STI.

Although numerous organisms cause STIs, the diseases can be grouped by the characteristic clinical presentation. **Urethritis** and **endocervicitis** (Table 116-1) are characteristic of *Neisseria gonorrhoeae* and *C. trachomatis* and are the most common STIs. Note that more than 70% of genital chlamydial infections in women are asymptomatic. **Genital ulcers** (Table 116-2) are characteristic of syphilis (*Treponema pallidum*), genital herpes simplex virus (HSV) infections, chancroid (*Haemophilus ducreyi*), and granuloma inguinale, also known as *donovanosis* (*Klebsiella granulomatis*). **Vaginal discharge** (Table 116-3) is a symptom of trichomoniasis (*Trichomonas vaginalis*) and is part of the spectrum of vulvovaginitis (see Chapter 115), which is not always associated with sexual activity. Human papillomavirus (HPV) causes **condylomata acuminata,** or **genital warts** (Table 116-4), and is the major risk factor for cervical, vulvar, and vaginal cancers.

STIs are associated with significant physiologic and psychological morbidity. Early diagnosis and treatment are important

Table 116-1	Features of Sexually Transmitted Infections Caused by *Chlamydia trachomatis* and *Neisseria gonorrhoeae**	
FEATURE	**C. TRACHOMATIS**	**N. GONORRHOEAE**
Incubation period	5–12 days	3–14 days
Possible presentations	Pharyngitis, conjunctivitis (including neonatal conjunctivitis), disseminated disease (arthritis, dermatitis, endocarditis, meningitis)	
	Female	*Male*
	Asymptomatic	Asymptomatic
	Urethritis	Urethritis
	Skenitis/bartholinitis	Epididymo-orchitis
	PID	Proctitis
Signs/symptoms of common syndromes		
Urethritis	*Female* Dysuria, frequency >10 PMNs/hpf	*Male* Penile discharge >10 PMNs/hpf
Mucopurulent cervicitis	Cervical erythema, friability, with thick creamy discharge >10 PMNs/hpf Mild cervical tenderness Gram-negative intracellular diplococci	
Pelvic inflammatory disease	Onset of symptoms day 3–10 of menstrual cycle	
	Lower abdominal pain (95%)	
	Adnexal tenderness, mass (95%)	
	Pain on cervical motion (95%)	
	Fever (35%)	
	Mucopurulent cervical discharge (variable)	
	Menstrual irregularities (variable)	
	Nausea, vomiting (variable)	
	Weakness, syncope, dizziness (variable)	
	Perihepatitis (5%)	
Diagnostic tests	NAAT, culture (using Thayer-Martin selective media)	NAAT
Treatment	Ceftriaxone *plus* doxycycline *or* azithromycin	

hpf, High-powered field; *NAAT,* nucleic acid amplification test; *PID,* pelvic inflammatory disease; *PMN,* polymorphonuclear cells.
*Coinfection is common, and clinical presentations have significant overlap.

Table 116-2	Features of Sexually Transmitted Infections Characterized by Genital Ulcers

	SYPHILIS	GENITAL HERPES	CHANCROID	GRANULOMA INGUINALE (DONOVANOSIS)
Agent	*Treponema pallidum*	HSV-1, HSV-2	*Haemophilus ducreyi*	*Klebsiella granulomatis*
Incubation	10–90 days	4–14 days	3–10 days	8–80 days
Systemic findings	Fever, rash, malaise, anorexia, arthralgia, lymphadenopathy	Headache, fever, malaise, myalgia in one third of cases	None	Local spread only
Inguinal lymphadenopathy	Late, bilateral, nontender, no suppuration	Early, bilateral, tender, no suppuration	Early, rapid, tender, and unilateral; suppuration likely	Lymphatic obstruction
Primary lesion	Papule	Vesicle	Papule to pustule	Papule
Ulcer characteristics				
Number	>1	Multiple	<3	>1, may coalesce
Edges	Distinct	Reddened, ragged	Ragged, undermined	Rolled, distinct
Depth	Shallow	Shallow	Deep	Raised
Base	Red, smooth	Red, smooth	Necrotic	Beefy red, clean
Secretion	Serous	Serous	Pus, blood	None
Induration	Firm	None	None	Firm
Pain	None	Usual	Often	None
Diagnosis				
Serology	VDRL or RPR MHA-TP or FTA-ABS	Seroconversion (primary infection only)	None	None
Isolation	No in vitro test; rabbit inoculation	Culture	Aspirate of node, swab of ulcer on selective medium	None
Microscopic	Dark-field examination	PCR or fluorescent antibody staining	Gram-negative pleomorphic rods	Staining of ulcer biopsy material for Donovan bodies
Treatment	*Early:* Benzathine penicillin G (2.4 million U IM) once *Late (>1 yr duration):* Benzathine penicillin G (2.4 million U IM) weekly × 3 doses	Acyclovir *or* famciclovir *or* valacyclovir	Aspirate fluctuant nodes Incision and drainage of buboes >5 cm Azithromycin *or* ceftriaxone *or* ciprofloxacin *or* erythromycin	Doxycycline *or* TMP-SMX

FTA-ABS, Fluorescent treponemal antibody-absorption; *HSV,* herpes simplex virus; *MHA-TP,* microhemagglutination assay-*Treponema pallidum; PCR,* polymerase chain reaction; *RPR,* rapid plasma reagin; *TMP-SMX,* trimethoprim-sulfamethoxazole; *VDRL,* Venereal Disease Research Laboratory.

Table 116-3	Features of Sexually Transmitted Infections Characterized by Vaginal Discharge

FEATURE	PHYSIOLOGIC LEUKORRHEA (NORMAL)	TRICHOMONIASIS	BACTERIAL VAGINOSIS (GARDNERELLA VAGINALIS-ASSOCIATED VAGINITIS)
Agent	Normal flora	*Trichomonas vaginalis*	*G. vaginalis* and anaerobes
Incubation	—	5–28 days	Not necessarily sexually transmitted
Predominant symptoms			
Pruritus	None	Mild to moderate	None to mild
Discharge	Minimal	Moderate to severe	Mild to moderate
Pain	None	Mild	Uncommon

Continued

| Table 116-3 | Features of Sexually Transmitted Infections Characterized by Vaginal Discharge—cont'd |

FEATURE	PHYSIOLOGIC LEUKORRHEA (NORMAL)	TRICHOMONIASIS	BACTERIAL VAGINOSIS (*GARDNERELLA VAGINALIS*-ASSOCIATED VAGINITIS)
Vulvar inflammation	None	Common	Uncommon
Characteristics of discharge			
Amount	Small	Profuse	Moderate
Color	Clear, milky	Yellow-green or grey	Grey
Consistency	Flocculent	Frothy	Homogeneous
Viscosity	Thin	Thin	Thin
Foul odor	None	Possible	Yes
Odor with KOH	None	Possible	Characteristic fishy odor (amine)
pH	<4.5	>5.0	>4.5
Diagnosis			
Saline drop	Squamous and few WBCs	WBC; Motile flagellates, slightly larger than WBCs	Squamous cells studded with bacteria ("clue cells") and WBCs
Gram stain	Gram-positive and gram-negative rods and cocci	*Trichomonas*	Predominance of gram-negative rods and cocci with paucity of gram-positive rods
Culture	Mixed flora with *Lactobacillus* predominant	Culture generally not indicated; antibody and nucleic acid tests available	Culture not useful
Treatment	Reassurance	Metronidazole or tinidazole	Metronidazole, tinidazole, or clindamycin

KOH, Potassium hydroxide; *WBCs*, white blood cells.

| Table 116-4 | Features of Sexually Transmitted Infections Characterized by Nonulcerative External Genital Symptoms |

FEATURE	GENITAL WARTS	VULVOVAGINAL CANDIDIASIS	PEDICULOSIS PUBIS (CRABS)
Agent	Human papillomavirus	*Candida albicans*	*Phthirus pubis*
Incubation/transmission	30–90 days	Uncommon sexual transmission	5–10 days
Presenting complaints	Genital warts are seen or felt	Vulvar itching or discharge	Pubic itching; live organisms may be seen; sexual partner has "crabs"
Signs	Firm, gray-to-pink, single or multiple, fimbriated, painless excrescences on vulva, introitus, vagina cervix, penis, perineum, anus	Inflammation of vulva, with thick, white, "cottage cheese" discharge, pH <5; friable mucosa that easily bleeds	Eggs (nits) at base of pubic hairs, lice may be visible; excoriated, red skin secondary to infestation
Clinical associations	Cervical neoplasia, dysplasia	Oral contraceptives, diabetes, antibiotics	—
Diagnosis	Clinical appearance; most infections asymptomatic; acetowhite changes on colposcopy; enlarged cells with perinuclear halo and hyperchromatic nuclei	KOH (10%): pseudohyphae; Gram stain: gram-positive pseudohyphae; Nickerson or Sabouraud medium for culture	History and clinical appearance
Treatment	*Patient-applied therapies:* Podofilox solution or gel *or* Imiquimod cream	*Intravaginal agents:* butoconazole *or* clotrimazole *or* miconazole	Permethrin 1% cream
	Provider-applied therapies: cryotherapy with liquid nitrogen or cryoprobe *or* topical podophyllin resin *or* trichloroacetic acid or dichloroacetic acid *or* surgical removal	*or* nystatin *or* tioconazole *or* terconazole *Oral agent:* fluconazole	*or* pyrethrin with piperonyl butoxide

KOH, Potassium hydroxide.

for preventing medical complications and infertility. All STIs are preventable; primary prevention of STIs should be a goal for all health care providers for adolescents. Diagnosis of an STI necessitates evaluation or treatment for concomitant STIs, notification and treatment of sexual partners, and some are reportable to state health departments.

Many infections that are not traditionally considered STIs are sexually transmissible, including those caused by human immunodeficiency virus (HIV), human T cell leukemia viruses types I and II, cytomegalovirus, Epstein-Barr virus, human herpes virus (HHV-6, HHV-7), hepatitis B virus, molluscum contagiosum virus, and *Sarcoptes scabiei*. The presence of any STI suggests behavior that increases risk for HIV (see Chapter 125), and HIV counseling and testing should be provided to all adolescents with STIs. Acquisition of gonorrhea, syphilis, HSV-2, and trichomoniasis in prepubertal children beyond the neonatal period indicates sexual contact and signifies the need to investigate for possible sexual abuse (see Chapter 22); diagnosis of STIs in infants can represent abuse or perinatal acquisition. The association of sexual abuse with vulvovaginitis and genital HPV infection, which may result from skin or genital HPV types, is less certain.

PELVIC INFLAMMATORY DISEASE

Direct extension of *N. gonorrhoeae*, often in combination with *C. trachomatis*, to the endometrium, fallopian tubes, and peritoneum causes **pelvic inflammatory disease (PID).** PID complications include tubo-ovarian abscess, perihepatitis **(Fitz-Hugh-Curtis syndrome,** an inflammation of the liver capsule), and infertility. The differential diagnosis of PID includes ectopic pregnancy, septic abortion, ovarian cyst torsion or rupture, urinary tract infection, appendicitis, mesenteric lymphadenitis, and inflammatory bowel disease. Pelvic ultrasound may detect thickened adnexal structures and is the imaging study of choice to exclude other possible diagnoses. Minimum clinical criteria for diagnosis of PID are lower abdominal tenderness with uterine, adnexal, or cervical motion tenderness. Additional criteria that support the diagnosis are fever, mucopurulent cervix discharge, elevated white blood cell (WBC) count, elevated inflammatory markers, and documented infection with *N. gonorrhoeae* or *C. trachomatis*. Adolescents should be hospitalized for treatment if there is uncertainty about the diagnosis, pregnancy; no clinical response to oral therapy within 72 hours; inability to adhere to or tolerate oral therapy; a tubo-ovarian abscess; or severe illness with high fever, nausea, and vomiting. The recommended parenteral treatment for hospitalized patients is cefotetan or cefoxitin, plus doxycycline orally. The recommended ambulatory treatment of PID for younger persons is ceftriaxone (250 mg) in a single intramuscular (IM) dose, plus doxycycline orally for 14 days, with or without metronidazole for 14 days. Follow-up examination should be performed within 72 hours.

GONORRHEA (*NEISSERIA GONORRHOEAE*)

N. gonorrhoeae, a gram-negative coccus, is often seen microscopically as diplococci. Gonorrhea is a common STI among adolescents. The highest incidence in the United States is in 15- to 24-year-old females and 20- to 24-year-old males, and incidence rates differ by race. The organism causes infection at the site of acquisition, which commonly results in mucopurulent cervicitis and urethritis (see Table 116-1), but infection of the rectum and pharynx can also occur. **Disseminated gonococcal infections** can occur with hematogenous spread and results in petechial or pustular acral skin lesions, asymmetric arthralgia, tenosynovitis or septic arthritis, and, occasionally, endocarditis or meningitis. Perinatal transmission of maternal infection can lead to neonatal sepsis and meningitis (see Chapter 65) and ophthalmia neonatorum (see Chapter 119).

Treatment regimens should be effective against *N. gonorrhoeae* and *C. trachomatis* because of the high frequency of coinfection. Increasing rates of resistance to fluoroquinolones limit treatment options. A single IM dose of ceftriaxone (250 mg) is recommended for uncomplicated gonococcal infections of the cervix, urethra, and rectum. Hospitalization and treatment with ceftriaxone are recommended for disseminated gonococcal infections. For all gonococcal infections, azithromycin or doxycycline also should be administered unless chlamydial infection is excluded.

CHLAMYDIA (*CHLAMYDIA TRACHOMATIS*)

Decision-Making Algorithms
Available @ StudentConsult.com

Dysuria
Scrotal Pain
Abnormal Vaginal Bleeding
Vaginal Discharge

Chlamydiae are obligate intracellular bacteria with a biphasic life cycle, existing as relatively inert elementary bodies in their extracellular form and as **reticulate bodies** when phagocytosed and replicating within a phagosome. Reticulate bodies divide by binary fission and, after 48 to 72 hours, reorganize into elementary bodies that are released from the cell. *Chlamydia* infects nonciliated squamocolumnar cells and the transitional epithelial cells that line the mucosa of the urethra, cervix, rectum, and conjunctiva.

C. trachomatis serovars D through K cause urethritis, cervicitis, PID, inclusion conjunctivitis in newborns, and infant pneumonia. *C. trachomatis* serovars L1–3 cause lymphogranuloma venereum, an infrequent STI characterized by unilateral, painful inguinal lymphadenitis. *C. trachomatis* serovars A, B, Ba, and C produce trachoma (hyperendemic blinding), which eventually leads to blindness from extensive local scarring.

Chlamydia is the most frequently diagnosed bacterial STI in adolescents and accounts for most cases of **nongonococcal urethritis and cervicitis** (see Table 116-1). There is a 5:1 female-to-male ratio. Males often have dysuria and a mucopurulent discharge, although approximately 25% may be asymptomatic. Women are more often asymptomatic (approximately 70%) or may have minimal symptoms including dysuria, mild abdominal pain, or vaginal discharge. Prepubertal girls may have vaginitis. At least 30% of persons with gonococcal cervicitis, urethritis, proctitis, or epididymitis have *C. trachomatis* coinfection.

Chlamydia infection usually is diagnosed by the detection of bacterial nucleic acids (polymerase chain reaction [PCR] tests, using ligase chain reaction and transcription-mediated amplification) of cervical, urethral, and early morning first-voided urine specimens. Amplification tests have supplanted less sensitive culture and enzyme-linked immunosorbent assay tests. Because of false positive results, only culture should be used for medicolegal purposes to confirm *C. trachomatis* infection in cases of suspected sexual abuse.

Treatment regimens should be effective against *C. trachomatis* and *N. gonorrhoeae* because of the high frequency of coinfection. A single oral dose of azithromycin (1 g) or doxycycline for 7 days is recommended, which can be combined with a single dose of ceftriaxone (250 mg) to treat concomitant gonorrhea infection.

SYPHILIS (*TREPONEMA PALLIDUM*)

Decision-Making Algorithms
Available @ StudentConsult.com

Vaginal Discharge
Fever and Rash
Lymphadenopathy
Petechiae/Purpura

Syphilis is caused by *T. pallidum*, a long, slender, coiled spirochete. It cannot be cultivated routinely in vitro but can be observed by dark-field microscopy. Untreated infection progresses through several clinical stages (see Table 116-2). **Primary syphilis** is manifested as a single, painless genital ulcer, or **chancre**, usually on the genitalia, that appears 3 to 6 weeks after inoculation. **Secondary syphilis** follows 6 to 8 weeks later and is manifested as fever, generalized lymphadenopathy, and a disseminated maculopapular rash that also is present on the palms and soles. Plaquelike skin lesions, **condylomata lata,** and mucous membrane lesions occur and are infectious. **Tertiary syphilis** is a slowly progressive disease that involves the cardiovascular, neurologic, and musculoskeletal systems and is not seen in children. **Latent syphilis** is an asymptomatic infection detected by serologic testing. Early latent syphilis indicates acquisition within the preceding year; all other cases of latent syphilis are designated either late latent syphilis or latent syphilis of unknown duration. Infection can be passed from pregnant women and infect their infants resulting in **congenital syphilis** (see Chapter 66).

The diagnosis of syphilis is based on serologic testing. **Nontreponemal antibody tests**, the **Venereal Disease Research Laboratory (VDRL)** test, and the **rapid plasma reagin (RPR)** test are screening tests and can be quantified as titers that increase with increasing duration of infection and decrease in response to therapy. A nonquantitative VDRL test can be performed on cerebrospinal fluid but is insensitive. Rheumatic disease and other infectious diseases may cause false positive results. Confirmatory, specific **treponemal antibody tests**, the **microhemagglutination assay-*T. pallidum*** (MHA-TP) and **fluorescent treponemal antibody-absorption** (FTA-ABS) are more specific and are used to confirm the diagnosis of syphilis. These tests usually remain positive lifelong even if the infection is treated and cured. Dark-field examination of chancres, mucous membranes, or cutaneous lesions may reveal motile organisms.

The treatment of choice for all stages of syphilis is parenteral penicillin G. Primary syphilis, secondary syphilis, and early latent syphilis are treated with a single IM dose of benzathine penicillin G. Tertiary, late latent, and latent syphilis of unknown duration are treated with three doses at 1-week intervals. Neurosyphilis is treated with intravenous aqueous crystalline penicillin G for 10 to 14 days. A systemic, febrile **Jarisch-Herxheimer reaction** occurs in 15% to 20% of syphilitic patients treated with penicillin.

HERPES SIMPLEX VIRUS (HSV) INFECTION

Decision-Making Algorithms
Available @ StudentConsult.com

Sore Throat
Dysuria
Vaginal Discharge
Vesicles and Bullae
Fever and Rash
Lymphadenopathy

HSV-1 and HSV-2 are large, double-stranded DNA viruses of the herpesvirus family with a linear genome contained within an icosahedral capsid. There is significant DNA homology between types 1 and 2. The virus initially infects mucosal surfaces and enters cutaneous neurons where it migrates along the axons to sensory ganglia. As viral replication occurs in the ganglia, infectious virus moves along the axon to infect and destroy epithelial cells. Infection may disseminate to other organs in immunocompromised patients. Virus latency is maintained in the ganglia where it undergoes periodic reactivation and replication triggered by undefined events. Although either virus can be found in any site, HSV-1 more commonly occurs in the central nervous system, eyes, and mouth, whereas HSV-2 more commonly involves the genitalia. Reinfection can occur with exposure to the other type or even a second strain of the same type.

Primary genital herpes is characterized by multiple painful, grouped vesicles or ulcerative and crusted external genital lesions on an erythematous base (see Table 116-2). In females the cervix is also involved. Symptoms may include regional lymphadenopathy, discharge, and dysuria. Primary illness lasts 10 to 20 days with recurrences in 50% to 80% of patients. **Secondary, recurrent,** or **reactivation eruptions** are not as dramatic and are not associated with systemic symptoms. In primary infection, viral shedding lasts 1 to 2 weeks, and the entire course from vesicle and ulcer onset resolves over 16 to 20 days. In recurrent disease, virus shedding lasts for less than 7 days, and the course resolves over 8 to 10 days. Many persons experience five to eight recurrences per year. Some primary and many recurrent episodes are asymptomatic.

Viral cultures and PCR are the preferred methods of diagnosis; culture typically shows cytopathic effect in 1 to 3 days and seldom takes longer than 5 days. PCR assays have increased sensitivity over culture. Viral shedding is intermittent after primary infection, so both culture and PCR can fail to detect latent infection. Serologic testing is useful for primary infection only (to show seroconversion between acute and convalescent sera), and positive serologies persist lifelong. Titers are not helpful in guiding management of recurrences.

Oral famciclovir and valacyclovir are effective treatments in reducing the severity and duration of symptoms in primary cases and may reduce recurrences. Once-daily suppressive therapy reduces the frequency of genital herpes recurrences by 70% to 80% among patients who have frequent recurrences (more than six recurrences per year). Local hygiene and sitz baths may relieve discomfort. The use of condoms provides some protection against sexual transmission of HSV.

TRICHOMONIASIS (*TRICHOMONAS VAGINALIS*)

Decision-Making Algorithms
Available @ StudentConsult.com

Abnormal Vaginal Bleeding
Vaginal Discharge

Trichomoniasis is caused by the protozoan *T. vaginalis* and often is associated with other STIs such as gonorrhea and *Chlamydia*. Infection is asymptomatic in as many as 90% of men and 85% of women. Symptomatic males can have urethritis. Symptomatic females have vaginitis with thin, malodorous, frothy yellow-green discharge, vulvar irritation, and cervical "strawberry hemorrhages" (see Table 116-3). Diagnosis is based on visualization of motile, flagellated protozoans in the urine or in a saline wet mount, which has a sensitivity of only 60% to 70% among symptomatic women. Culture is the most sensitive method of diagnosis. Treatment of both sexual partners with oral metronidazole or tinidazole in a single dose is recommended.

GENITAL WARTS (HUMAN PAPILLOMAVIRUSES)

Decision-Making Algorithms
Available @ StudentConsult.com

Hoarseness
Vaginal Discharge

HPV, the cause of genital warts **(condylomata acuminata),** is the most common STI in the United States with the highest prevalence rates among 15- to 24-year-olds. Most HPV infections are asymptomatic or subclinical. HPV types 6 and 11 cause 90% of genital warts and are nononcogenic. HPV types 16 and 18 are associated with 70% of cases of cervical cancer. HPV types 31, 33, and 35 are also oncogenic.

Genital warts can occur on the squamous epithelium or mucous membranes of the genital and perineal structures of females and males (see Table 116-4). Genital warts are usually multiple, firm, gray-to-pink excrescences. Untreated genital warts may remain unchanged, increase in size or number, or resolve spontaneously. They can become tender if macerated or secondarily infected. The diagnosis usually is established by appearance without biopsy. The differential diagnosis includes condylomata lata (secondary syphilis) and tumors.

The goal of treatment is removal of symptomatic warts to induce wart-free periods. Treatment modalities involve destruction of infected epithelium; patient-applied therapies include podofilox or imiquimod, and provider-applied therapies include cryotherapy with liquid nitrogen or cryoprobe, topical podophyllin resin, and trichloroacetic acid or bichloracetic acid. An alternative is surgical removal.

Intralesional interferon and laser surgery also have been effective. Factors that may influence selection of treatment include wart number, size, anatomic sites, wart morphology, patient preference, treatment cost, convenience, adverse effects, and provider experience. Recurrences after treatment are common and are frequently asymptomatic.

PUBIC LICE (*PHTHIRUS PUBIS*)

Pubic lice, or pediculosis pubis, are caused by infestation with *Phthirus pubis,* the **pubic crab louse.** The louse is predominantly sexually transmitted and lives out its life cycle on pubic hair, where it causes characteristic, intense pruritus (see Table 116-4). Diagnosis can be made clinically; lice are visible to the naked eye. Erythematous papules and **egg cases (nits)** are not seen before puberty. Treatment consists of education regarding personal and environmental hygiene and the application of an appropriate pediculicide, such as permethrin 1% cream or pyrethrins with piperonyl butoxide. Bedding and clothing should be decontaminated (machine washed and machine dried using the heat cycle or dry cleaned) or removed from body contact for at least 72 hours.

Chapter **117**

OSTEOMYELITIS

ETIOLOGY

Acute hematogenous osteomyelitis is the most common manifestation of osteomyelitis in children and evolves secondary to bacteremia. **Subacute osteomyelitis** usually follows local inoculation by penetrating trauma and is not associated with systemic symptoms, and **chronic osteomyelitis** results from an untreated or inadequately treated (usually subacute) osteomyelitis.

In children beyond the newborn period and without hemoglobinopathies, bone infections occur almost exclusively in the metaphysis of long bones due to sluggish blood flow through tortuous vascular loops unique to this site. Preceding nonpenetrating trauma is often reported and may lead to local bone injury that predisposes to infection. Bone infections in children with sickle cell disease occur in the diaphyseal portion of the long bones, probably as a consequence of antecedent focal infarction. In children younger than 12 to 18 months of age, capillaries perforate the epiphyseal growth plate, permitting spread of infection across the epiphysis leading to suppurative arthritis, whereas in older children, infection is contained in the metaphysis because these vessels no longer cross the epiphyseal plate (Figs. 117-1AB).

Staphylococcus aureus is responsible for more than 80% of acute skeletal infections. Other common causes include Group A streptococcus and *Streptococcus pneumoniae*. *Neisseria meningitidis, Mycobacterium tuberculosis, Bartonella henselae, Actinomyces* spp., and anaerobes are less common causes. Group B streptococcus and enteric gram-negatives are other major causes in neonates. Sickle cell disease and other hemoglobinopathies predispose to osteomyelitis caused by *Salmonella* and *S. aureus*. *Pasteurella multocida* osteomyelitis may

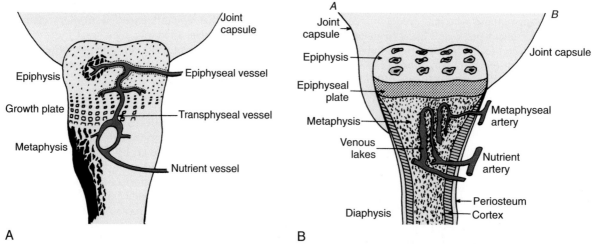

Figure 117-1 A, Major structures of the bone of an infant before maturation of the epiphyseal growth plate. Note the transphyseal vessel, which connects the vascular supply of the epiphysis and metaphysis, facilitating spread of infection between these two areas. B, Major structures of the bone of a child. Joint capsule *A* inserts below the epiphyseal growth plate, as in the hip, elbow, ankle, and shoulder. Rupture of a metaphyseal abscess in these bones is likely to produce pyarthrosis. Joint capsule *B* inserts at the epiphyseal growth plate, as in other tubular bones. Rupture of a metaphyseal abscess in these bones is likely to lead to a subperiosteal abscess but seldom to an associated pyarthrosis. *(From Gutman LT: Acute, subacute, and chronic osteomyelitis and pyogenic arthritis in children,* Curr Probl Pediatr *15:1–72, 1985.)*

follow cat or dog bites. The use of polymerase chain reaction testing reveals that a significant proportion of **culture negative osteomyelitis** is due to *Kingella kingae*. Conjugate vaccine has reduced greatly the incidence of *Haemophilus influenzae* type b infections.

Subacute focal bone infections caused by *Pseudomonas aeruginosa* and *S. aureus* usually occur in ambulatory persons who sustain **puncture wounds** of the foot. *Pseudomonas* **chondritis** is strongly associated with puncture wounds through sneakers, which harbor *Pseudomonas* in the foam insole. *S. aureus* is the most common cause of chronic osteomyelitis. **Chronic recurrent multifocal osteomyelitis** is an autoinflammatory syndrome characterized by recurrent episodes of fever, bone pain, and radiographic findings of osteomyelitis. Bones uncommonly involved in acute hematogenous osteomyelitis such as the clavicle, scapula, or small bones of the hands or feet are often affected, pathogens are not identified on culture, and histopathology demonstrates plasmacytic infiltrates.

EPIDEMIOLOGY

Osteomyelitis may occur at any age but is most common in children 3 to 12 years of age and affects boys twice as frequently as girls. Osteomyelitis from penetrating trauma or peripheral vascular disease is more common in adults.

CLINICAL MANIFESTATIONS

Decision-Making Algorithms
Available @ StudentConsult.com

Limp
Knee Pain
Extremity Pain
Stiff or Painful Neck
Fever without a Source
Fever of Unknown Origin

The most common presenting complaints are focal pain, exquisite point tenderness over the bone, warmth, erythema, and swelling. Fever, anorexia, irritability, and lethargy may accompany the focal findings. Weight bearing and active and passive motion of the affected extremity are decreased, mimicking paralysis (**pseudoparalysis**). Muscle spasm may make the extremity difficult to examine. The adjacent joint space may be involved in young children, suggested by pain with minimal joint range of motion (see Chapter 118).

Usually only one bone is involved. The femur, tibia, or humerus is affected in approximately two thirds of patients. Approximately 15% of cases involve the bones of the hands or feet, and 10% involve the pelvis. Vertebral osteomyelitis is notable for an insidious onset, vague symptoms, backache, occasional spinal cord compression, and, usually, little associated fever or systemic toxicity. Patients with osteomyelitis of the pelvis may present with fever, limp, and vague abdominal, hip, groin, or thigh pain. Pyomyositis of pelvic muscles may mimic osteomyelitis.

LABORATORY AND IMAGING STUDIES

The presence of leukocytosis is inconsistent. Blood cultures are important but are negative in many cases. Elevated acute phase reactants, erythrocyte sedimentation rate (ESR) and C-reactive protein (CRP), are sensitive but nonspecific findings. Serial determinations of ESR and CRP are helpful in monitoring the course of the illness and response to treatment. Direct subperiosteal or metaphyseal needle aspiration definitively establishes the diagnosis. Identification of bacteria in aspirated material by Gram stain can establish the diagnosis within hours of clinical presentation.

Plain radiographs can demonstrate soft tissue swelling such as the **loss of the periosteal fat line** within the first 3 days of symptoms, but bony lesions such as **periosteal elevation** and **bone destruction** are absent until after 10 to 14 days of symptoms (Fig. 117-2). **Brodie abscess** is a subacute intraosseous abscess that does not drain into the subperiosteal space and is classically located in the distal tibia. **Sequestra,** portions of

Figure 117-2 Multifocal acute osteomyelitis in a 3-week-old infant with multiple joint swelling and generalized malaise. Frontal (**A**) and lateral (**B**) radiographs of the left knee show focal destruction of the distal femoral metaphysis with periosteal reaction and generalized soft tissue swelling. Frontal (**C**) and lateral (**D**) views of the right knee show an area of focal bone destruction at the distal femoral metaphysis with periosteal reaction and medial soft tissue swelling. Needle aspiration of multiple sites revealed *Staphylococcus aureus*. *(From Moffett KS, Aronoff SC: Osteomyelitis. In Jenson HB, Baltimore RS, editors: Pediatric Infectious Diseases: Principles and Practice, ed 2, Philadelphia, 2002, Saunders, p 1038.)*

avascular bone that have separated from adjacent bone, frequently are covered with a thickened sheath, or **involucrum**, both of which are hallmarks of chronic osteomyelitis.

Radionuclide scanning for osteomyelitis has largely been supplanted by magnetic resonance imaging, which is sensitive to the inflammatory marrow changes even during the earliest stages of osteomyelitis. Technetium-99m bone scans are useful for identifying multifocal disease. Gallium-67 scans are often positive if the technetium-99m bone scan is negative.

DIFFERENTIAL DIAGNOSIS

Osteomyelitis must be differentiated from infectious arthritis (see Chapter 118), cellulitis, pyomyositis, fasciitis, diskitis, trauma, juvenile idiopathic arthritis, bone cysts, histiocytosis, and malignancy.

TREATMENT

Decision-Making Algorithm
Available @ StudentConsult.com

Fever without a Source

Initial antibiotic therapy for osteomyelitis is based on the likely organism for the age of the child, Gram stain of bone aspirate, and associated diseases (Table 117-1). Initial therapy includes an antibiotic that targets *S. aureus* and *Kingella*, such as oxacillin or nafcillin. Clindamycin or vancomycin should be used if methicillin-resistant *S. aureus* is suspected based on patient factors or local *S. aureus* epidemiology. For patients with sickle cell disease, initial therapy should include an antibiotic with activity against *Salmonella*.

Table 117-1	Recommended Antibiotic Therapy for Osteomyelitis in Children
COMMON PATHOGEN	**RECOMMENDED TREATMENT***
ACUTE HEMATOGENOUS OSTEOMYELITIS	
Staphylococcus aureus	
Methicillin-sensitive	Nafcillin (or oxacillin) or cefazolin
Methicillin-resistant	Clindamycin or vancomycin or linezolid
Streptococcus pyogenes (group A streptococci)	Penicillin G
Streptococcus pneumoniae	Penicillin G or ceftriaxone/cefotaxime or vancomycin
Subacute Focal Osteomyelitis	
Pseudomonas aeruginosa	Ceftazidime or piperacillin-tazobactam plus an aminoglycoside
Kingella kingae	Penicillin G, oxacillin, or cefotaxime

*Optimal specific therapy is based on susceptibilities of the organism that is isolated.

Response to intravenous (IV) antibiotics usually occurs within 48 hours. Lack of improvement after 48 hours indicates that surgical drainage may be necessary or that an unusual pathogen may be present. Surgical drainage is indicated for extensive or severe disease, if the disease is chronic or atypical, if the hip joint is involved, or **sequestrum** or spinal cord compression is present. Antibiotics are administered for a minimum of 4 to 6 weeks. After initial inpatient treatment and adequate clinical response, including decreases in CRP or ESR, transition to home therapy with oral or IV antibiotics may be considered if adherence is ensured.

COMPLICATIONS AND PROGNOSIS

Complications of acute osteomyelitis are uncommon and usually arise because of inadequate or delayed therapy or concomitant bacteremia. Vascular insufficiency, which affects delivery of antibiotics, and trauma are associated with higher rates of complications.

Hematogenous osteomyelitis has an excellent prognosis if treated promptly and if surgical drainage is performed when appropriate. The poorest outcomes are in neonates and in infants with involvement of the hip or shoulder joints (see Chapter 118). Approximately 2% to 4% of acute infections recur despite adequate therapy, and approximately 25% of these fail to respond to extensive surgical debridement and prolonged antimicrobial therapy, ultimately resulting in bone loss, sinus tract formation, or amputation (although rare). Sequelae related to skeletal growth disturbance are most common with neonatal osteomyelitis.

PREVENTION

There are no effective means to prevent hematogenous *S. aureus* osteomyelitis. Universal immunization of infants with conjugate *Haemophilus influenzae* type b vaccine has practically eliminated serious bacterial infections from this organism, including bone and joint infections.

Children with puncture wounds to the foot should receive prompt irrigation, cleansing, debridement, removal of any visible foreign body or debris, and tetanus prophylaxis. The value of oral prophylactic antibiotics for preventing osteomyelitis after penetrating injury is uncertain.

Chapter 118

INFECTIOUS ARTHRITIS

ETIOLOGY

Infectious arthritis (**suppurative** or **septic arthritis**) is a serious bacterial infection of the joint space resulting from hematogenous dissemination of bacteria. Infectious arthritis less often results from contiguous spread of infection from surrounding soft tissues or direct inoculation into the joint (penetrating trauma). Spread of osteomyelitis into the joint space is more common in children under 18 months of age and occurs via organisms passing through transphyseal vessels to the epiphysis (see Fig. 117-1A). The bacteria causing infectious arthritis are similar to bacteria causing osteomyelitis (Table 118-1). Lyme disease also may cause arthritis (see Chapter 122).

The arthritis of **disseminated gonococcal infections** includes both reactive and suppurative forms in early and late gonococcal disease, respectively. With untreated genital infection, gonococcemia may occur with fever and a polyarticular, symmetric arthritis and rash, known as the **arthritis-dermatitis syndrome.** Bacterial cultures of the synovium are sterile at this stage, despite a relatively high prevalence of bacteremia. Monarticular arthritis of large, weight-bearing joints develops

Table 118-1	Pathogenic Organisms Causing Arthritis in Children	
COMMON		**UNCOMMON**
YOUNG INFANT (<2 MONTHS)		
Group B streptococci		Neisseria gonorrhoeae
Staphylococcus aureus		Candida
Escherichia coli		
Klebsiella pneumoniae		
Older Infants and Children (2 Months to Maturity)		
S. aureus		Anaerobic bacteria
Streptococcus pneumoniae		Pseudomonas aeruginosa
Group A streptococci		Enterobacteriaceae
Kingella kingae		Haemophilus influenzae type b*
N. gonorrhoeae		Mycobacterium tuberculosis
Borrelia burgdorferi (Lyme disease)		
Reactive Arthritis		
Yersinia enterocolitica		
Campylobacter jejuni		
Shigella flexneri		
Salmonella Group A streptococci		
Neisseria meningitidis		
Coccidioides immitis		
Rubella virus		

*The incidence of invasive infections caused by *H. influenzae* type b has diminished greatly with universal childhood Hib vaccination.

days to weeks later. Cultures of affected synovial fluid at this stage often yield the pathogen.

Reactive arthritis is immune-mediated synovial inflammation that follows a bacterial or viral infection, especially *Yersinia* and other enteric infections. Reactive arthritis of the hip joints in children 3 to 6 years of age is known as **toxic** or **transient synovitis** (see Chapter 200).

EPIDEMIOLOGY

Infectious arthritis occurs most commonly in children younger than 5 years of age and adolescents.

CLINICAL MANIFESTATIONS

Decision-Making Algorithms
Available @ StudentConsult.com

Limp
Arthritis
Knee Pain
Extremity Pain

The typical features of suppurative arthritis include monarticular involvement with erythema, warmth, swelling, and tenderness over the affected joint with a palpable effusion

Table 118-2	Synovial Fluid Findings in Various Joint Diseases

CONDITION	APPEARANCE	WBC COUNT (mm³/L)	PMNs (%)	MUCIN CLOT	SYNOVIAL FLUID–BLOOD GLUCOSE DIFFERENCE (mg/dL)	COMMENTS
Normal	Clear, yellow	0–200 (200)*	<10	Good	No difference	—
Trauma	Clear, turbid, or hemorrhagic	50–4000 (600)	<30	Good	No difference	Common in hemophilia
Systemic lupus erythematosus	Clear or slightly turbid	0–9000 (3,000)	<20	Good to fair	No difference	LE cell positive, complement decreased
Rheumatoid arthritis, reactive arthritis (Reiter syndrome, inflammatory bowel disease)	Turbid	250–80,000 (19,000)	>70	Poor	30	Decreased complement
Infectious pyogenic infection	Turbid	10,000–250,000 (80,000)	>90	Poor	50–90	Positive culture result, positive Gram stain
Tuberculosis	Turbid	2500–100,000 (20,000)	>60	Poor	40–70	Positive results on culture, PPD testing, and acid-fast stain
Lyme arthritis	Turbid	500–100,000 (20,000)	>60	Poor	70	History of tick bite or erythema migrans

LE, Lupus erythematosus; *PMN*, polymorphonuclear cell; *PPD*, purified protein derivative of tuberculin; *WBC*, white blood cell.
*Average in parentheses.

and markedly decreased range of movement. The onset may be sudden or insidious with symptoms noted when the joint is moved only, such as during a diaper change, or if parents become aware of decreased voluntary movement of a joint or limb. Toddlers may exhibit a limp or refuse to walk. In septic arthritis of the hip, the lower limb may be preferentially held in external rotation and flexion to minimize pain from pressure on the joint capsule. Similarly the knee and elbow joints usually are held in flexion. The joints of the lower extremity are most often involved: the knees (40%), the hips (20%), and the ankles (14%). Small joints, such as those of the hand, usually are involved after penetrating trauma or closed fist injuries.

Minor genital tract symptoms that have been ignored may precede development of the early arthritis-dermatitis syndrome associated with disseminated gonococcal infection. A history of febrile illness antedating the development of monarticular arthritis characterizes late gonococcal arthritis.

Reactive arthritis is typically symmetric, polyarticular, and usually involves the large joints, especially the hips. Patients may have had a preceding episode of gastroenteritis or urethritis. Urethritis may appear with the arthritis.

LABORATORY AND IMAGING STUDIES
Leukocytosis and an elevated erythrocyte sedimentation rate (ESR) and C-reactive protein (CRP) are common. Arthrocentesis is important to distinguish among the causes of arthritis (Table 118-2). Adolescents with acute infectious arthritis should have urethral, cervical, rectal, and pharyngeal examinations and cultures or nucleic acid amplification tests performed for *Neisseria gonorrhoeae*.

Blood or joint cultures are positive in approximately 50% of cases. Joint fluid that exhibits the characteristics of pyogenic infection may not reveal bacterial pathogens, even in the absence of preceding antibiotic therapy, because of the bacteriostatic effects of synovial fluid. Gram stain, acid-fast stain, and potassium hydroxide preparation for fungi should be performed and are often informative even if the cultures are negative.

Plain radiographs typically add little information to the physical findings. Radiographs may show swelling of the joint capsule, a widened joint space, and displacement of adjacent normal fat lines. Radionuclide scans are of limited use, although magnetic resonance imaging or technetium-99m bone scans may be helpful to exclude concurrent bone infection or deep abscesses. Ultrasound is especially useful for identifying joint effusions and is the initial diagnostic procedure of choice for evaluation of suppurative infections of the hip.

DIFFERENTIAL DIAGNOSIS
The differential diagnosis of infectious arthritis in infants, children, and adolescents includes other infectious diseases, autoimmune disorders, rheumatic fever, and trauma.

Suppurative arthritis must be distinguished from Lyme disease, osteomyelitis, suppurative bursitis, fasciitis, myositis, cellulitis, and soft tissue abscesses. Psoas muscle abscess often presents with fever and pain on hip flexion and rotation. Juvenile idiopathic arthritis, Kawasaki disease, Henoch-Schönlein purpura, other rheumatic disorders, and Crohn's disease must be differentiated from infectious arthritis. In most of these diseases, the presence of symmetric or multiple joint involvement

Table 118-3	Recommended Antibiotic Therapy for Infectious Arthritis in Children	
AGE GROUP	**COMMON PATHOGENS**	**RECOMMENDED TREATMENT**
Infants (younger than 2 months of age)	Group B streptococci	Ampicillin *plus* aminoglycoside
	Escherichia coli	Cefotaxime (*or* ceftriaxone) *plus* aminoglycoside
	Klebsiella pneumoniae	Cefotaxime (*or* ceftriaxone) *plus* aminoglycoside
	Staphylococcus aureus	Nafcillin (*or* oxacillin), vancomycin
Older infants and children	*S. aureus*	Nafcillin (*or* oxacillin), vancomycin
	Streptococcus pneumoniae	Cefotaxime (*or* ceftriaxone) *or* vancomycin (based on susceptibilities)
	Group A streptococci	Penicillin G
	Kingella kingae	Penicillin G, nafcillin (*or* oxacillin) or cefotaxime
	Haemophilus influenzae type b*	Cefotaxime *or* ceftriaxone
	Neisseria gonorrhoeae: disseminated gonococcal infection	Ceftriaxone

*The incidence of invasive infections caused by *H. influenzae* type b has diminished greatly with universal childhood Hib vaccination.

often excludes infectious arthritis. **Suppurative bursitis** with *Staphylococcus aureus* occurs most often in older boys and men and is usually a consequence of trauma or, less commonly, a complication of bacteremia.

TREATMENT

Initial antibiotic therapy for infectious arthritis is based on the likely organism for the age of the child and the Gram stain of joint fluid. Suppurative arthritis of the hip joint, especially, or shoulder joint necessitates prompt surgical drainage. With insertion of the joint capsule below the epiphysis in these ball-and-socket joints, increased pressure in the joint space can adversely affect the vascular supply to the head of the femur or humerus, leading to avascular necrosis. Infections of the knee may be treated with repeated arthrocenteses, in addition to appropriate parenteral antibiotics.

Several antimicrobial agents provide adequate antibiotic levels in joint spaces (Table 118-3). Initial therapy for neonates should include antibiotics with activity against *S. aureus*, group B streptococcus, and aerobic gram-negative rods, such as nafcillin and cefotaxime. Initial therapy for children 3 months to 5 years old should include antibiotics with activity against *S. aureus*. Addition of appropriate antibiotics should be considered if the child is unimmunized against *Haemophilus influenzae* type b (Hib). Confirmed methicillin-susceptible

S. aureus infections are best treated with nafcillin or oxacillin, and methicillin-resistant *S. aureus* infections are best treated with clindamycin, if susceptible, or vancomycin otherwise.

The duration of therapy depends on clinical resolution of fever and pain and decline of the ESR and CRP. Infection with virulent organisms, such as *S. aureus*, usually necessitates treatment for at least 21 days. Treatment may be changed to oral antibiotics if adherence can be ensured. Oral agents with excellent activity against *S. aureus* that are often used to complete therapy include cephalexin, clindamycin, amoxicillin-clavulanate, dicloxacillin, and ciprofloxacin (for patients >18 years).

COMPLICATIONS AND PROGNOSIS

The prognosis for the common forms of infectious arthritis encountered in infants and children is excellent. The major complications of neonatal, childhood, and gonococcal arthritis are loss of joint function resulting from damage to the articular surface. The highest incidence of these complications occurs with hip and shoulder infections, presumably resulting from avascular necrosis. The high incidence of concurrent suppurative arthritis with adjacent osteomyelitis in neonates places the epiphyseal growth plate at high risk for growth abnormalities. Neonates with osteomyelitis have an approximately 40% to 50% likelihood of growth disturbances with loss of longitudinal bone growth and ultimate limb shortening.

PREVENTION

There are no effective means to prevent hematogenous *S. aureus* arthritis. Universal immunization of infants with conjugate Hib vaccine has practically eliminated serious bacterial infections from this organism, including bone and joint infections.

Chapter **119**

OCULAR INFECTIONS

ETIOLOGY

Acute conjunctivitis is usually a bacterial or viral infection of the eye characterized by a rapid onset of symptoms that persist for a few days. Nontypable *Haemophilus influenzae*, *Streptococcus pneumoniae*, and *Moraxella catarrhalis* account for approximately two thirds of bacterial causes (Table 119-1). Other causes include *Neisseria gonorrhoeae* and *Pseudomonas aeruginosa*, which is associated with extended-wear soft contact lenses. Viral conjunctivitis most commonly is caused by adenoviruses, which cause **epidemic keratoconjunctivitis,** and less frequently by coxsackieviruses and other enteroviruses. **Keratitis,** or inflammation of the cornea, is not commonly associated with conjunctivitis but occurs with *N. gonorrhoeae*, herpes simplex virus (HSV), and adenovirus infections.

Neonatal conjunctivitis, or **ophthalmia neonatorum,** is purulent conjunctivitis during the first month of life, usually

Table 119-1	Manifestations of Acute Conjunctivitis in Children	
	CLINICAL CHARACTERISTICS	
FEATURE	**BACTERIAL**	**VIRAL**
Common pathogens	*Haemophilus influenzae* (usually nontypable)	Adenoviruses types 8, 19
	Streptococcus pneumoniae	Enteroviruses
	Moraxella catarrhalis	Herpes simplex virus
Incubation	24–72 hours	1–14 days
Symptoms		
Photophobia	Mild	Moderate to severe
Blurred vision	Common with discharge	If keratitis is present
Foreign body sensation	Unusual	Yes
Signs		
Discharge	Purulent discharge	Mucoid/serous discharge
Palpebral reaction	Papillary response	Follicular response
Preauricular lymph node	Unusual for acute (<10%)	More common (20%)
Chemosis	Moderate	Mild
Hemorrhagic conjunctivae	Occasionally with *Streptococcus* or *Haemophilus*	Frequent with enteroviruses
Treatment (topical)	Polymyxin B-trimethoprim *or* sulfacetamide 5% *or* erythromycin	Adenovirus: self-limited Herpes simplex virus: trifluridine 1% solution *or* vidarabine 3% ointment; ophthalmologic consultation
End of contagious period	24 hours after start of effective treatment	7 days after onset of symptoms

acquired during birth. The common causes of neonatal conjunctivitis, in order of decreasing prevalence, are chemical conjunctivitis secondary to silver nitrate gonococcal prophylaxis, *Chlamydia trachomatis,* common bacterial causes of conjunctivitis, *Escherichia coli,* other gram-negative enteric bacilli, HSV, and *N. gonorrhoeae.*

EPIDEMIOLOGY

Conjunctivitis is common in young children, especially if they come in contact with other children with conjunctivitis. Predisposing factors for bacterial infection include nasolacrimal duct obstruction, sinus disease, ear infection, and allergic disease when children rub their eyes frequently. Conjunctivitis occurs in 1% to 12% of neonates. A mild to moderate chemical conjunctivitis commonly is present from 24 to 48 hours of age in most newborns who receive ophthalmic silver nitrate as gonococcal prophylaxis. Approximately 50% of infants born vaginally to infected mothers have neonatal acquisition of *C. trachomatis,* in which the risk of chlamydial conjunctivitis (**inclusion conjunctivitis**) is 25% to 50%.

CLINICAL MANIFESTATIONS

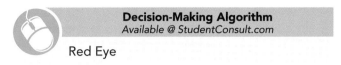

Decision-Making Algorithm
Available @ StudentConsult.com
Red Eye

Symptoms include redness, discharge, matted eyelids, and mild photophobia. Physical examination findings include chemosis, injection of the conjunctiva, and edema of the eyelids. Corneal involvement suggests gonococcal or herpetic infection. Herpetic corneal lesions appear as dendritic or ameboid ulcers or, more commonly, in recurrent infection, as a deep keratitis. Unilateral conjunctivitis with ipsilateral otitis media is often caused by nontypable *H. influenzae.*

The timing and manifestations of neonatal conjunctivitis are helpful in identifying the cause (Table 119-2). *N. gonorrhoeae* causes severe conjunctivitis with profuse purulent discharge. Chlamydial conjunctivitis usually occurs in the second week of life but may appear 3 days to 6 weeks after delivery. There is mild to moderate inflammation with purulent discharge issuing from one or both eyes.

LABORATORY AND IMAGING STUDIES

Cultures are not routinely obtained because bacterial conjunctivitis is usually self-limited or responds quickly to topical antibiotic treatment. If gonococcal conjunctivitis is suspected, especially in neonates, Gram stain and culture must be obtained. In these infants, blood and other sites of infection (such as cerebrospinal fluid) should be cultured. Additional testing for *Chlamydia,* human immunodeficiency virus (HIV), and syphilis should be performed on the mother and infant as necessary as well.

DIFFERENTIAL DIAGNOSIS

Distinguishing bacterial from viral conjunctivitis by presentation and appearance is difficult (see Table 119-1). Vesicular lid lesions, if present, suggest HSV. **Hyperpurulent conjunctivitis** characterized by reaccumulation of purulent discharge within minutes is characteristic of *N. gonorrhea* infection. The differential diagnosis is delineated in Table 119-3.

Blepharitis is associated with staphylococcal infections, seborrhea, and meibomian gland dysfunction. The child complains of photophobia, burning, irritation, and a foreign body sensation that causes the child to rub the eyes. Eyelid hygiene with an **eyelid scrub** routine is the initial step in treatment.

Hordeola are acute suppurative nodular inflammatory lesions of the eyelids associated with pain and redness. **External hordeola** or **styes** occur on the anterior eyelid, in the Zeis glands, or in the lash follicles and usually are caused by staphylococci. **Internal hordeola** occur in the meibomian glands and may be infected with staphylococci or may be sterile. If the meibomian gland becomes obstructed, the gland secretions accumulate, and a **chalazion** develops. Hordeola usually respond spontaneously to local treatment measures but may recur.

Dacryocystitis is an infection or inflammation of the lacrimal sac, which is usually obstructed, and is most commonly caused by *Staphylococcus aureus* or coagulase-negative staphylococci. A mucopurulent discharge can be expressed with

Table 119-2 | Clinical Manifestations and Treatment of Neonatal Conjunctivitis

ETIOLOGIC AGENT	CASES (%)	DISCHARGE AND EXTERNAL EXAMINATION	TYPICAL AGE AT ONSET	DIAGNOSIS	ASSOCIATED MANIFESTATIONS	TREATMENT
Chemical: silver nitrate	Variable (1%), depending on use of silver nitrate	Watery discharge	1–3 days	No organisms on smear or culture	None	None
Chlamydia trachomatis (inclusion conjunctivitis)	2–40	Scant discharge; mild swelling; hyperemia; follicular response; late corneal staining	4–19 days	Test of discharge with a DIF test or PCR assay	May presage *C. trachomatis* pneumonia (at 3 weeks–3 months of age)	Erythromycin (oral)
Bacterial: *Staphylococcus, Streptococcus, Pseudomonas, E. coli*	30–50	Purulent moderate discharge; mild lid and conjunctival swelling; corneal involvement with risk for perforation	2–7 days	Gram stain; culture on blood agar		Topical therapy
Neisseria gonorrhoeae	<1	Copious, purulent discharge; swelling of lids and conjunctivae; corneal involvement common; risk for perforation and corneal scar	1–7 days	Gram stain (gram-negative intracellular diplococci); culture on chocolate agar Culture other sites including blood and CSF	May be associated with severe disseminated gonococcal infection	Ceftriaxone Hospitalize patient
HSV	<1	Clear or serosanguineous discharge; lid swelling; keratitis with cloudy cornea; dendrite formation	3 days–3 weeks	Viral culture; DIF test, PCR assay	May be associated with disseminated perinatal HSV infection	Acyclovir (intravenous) for systemic involvement

CSF, Cerebrospinal fluid; *DIF,* direct immunofluorescence; *HSV,* herpes simplex virus; *PCR,* polymerase chain reaction.

Table 119-3 | Differential Diagnosis of Ocular Infections

CONDITION	ETIOLOGIC AGENTS	SIGNS AND SYMPTOMS	TREATMENT
Bacterial conjunctivitis	*Haemophilus influenzae, Haemophilus aegyptius, Streptococcus pneumoniae, Neisseria gonorrhoeae*	Mucopurulent unilateral or bilateral discharge, normal vision, photophobia, conjunctival injection and edema (chemosis); gritty sensation	Topical antibiotics, parenteral ceftriaxone for gonococcus
Viral conjunctivitis	Adenovirus, echovirus, coxsackievirus	Same as for bacterial infection; may be hemorrhagic, unilateral	Self-limited
Neonatal conjunctivitis	*Chlamydia trachomatis,* gonococcus, chemical (silver nitrate), *Staphylococcus aureus*	Palpebral conjunctival follicle or papillae; same as for bacterial infection	Ceftriaxone for gonococcus and oral erythromycin for *C. trachomatis*
Allergic conjunctivitis	Seasonal pollens or allergen exposure	Itching, incidence of bilateral chemosis (edema) greater than that of erythema, tarsal papillae	Antihistamines, steroids, cromolyn
Keratitis	Herpes simplex, adenovirus, *S. pneumoniae, S. aureus, Pseudomonas, Acanthamoeba,* chemicals	Severe pain, corneal swelling, clouding, limbus erythema, hypopyon, cataracts; contact lens history with amebic infection	Specific antibiotics for bacterial/fungal infections; keratoplasty, acyclovir for herpes
Endophthalmitis	*S. aureus, S. pneumoniae, Candida albicans,* associated surgery or trauma	Acute onset, pain, loss of vision, swelling, chemosis, redness; hypopyon and vitreous haze	Antibiotics
Anterior uveitis (iridocyclitis)	JIA, reactive arthritis, sarcoidosis, Behçet disease, inflammatory bowel disease	Unilateral/bilateral; erythema, ciliary flush, irregular pupil, iris adhesions; pain, photophobia, small pupil, poor vision	Topical steroids, plus therapy for primary disease
Posterior uveitis (choroiditis)	Toxoplasmosis, histoplasmosis, *Toxocara canis*	No signs of erythema, decreased vision	Specific therapy for pathogen

Table 119-3	Differential Diagnosis of Ocular Infections—cont'd		
CONDITION	**ETIOLOGIC AGENTS**	**SIGNS AND SYMPTOMS**	**TREATMENT**
Episcleritis/scleritis	Idiopathic autoimmune disease (e.g., SLE, Henoch-Schönlein purpura)	Localized pain, intense erythema, unilateral; blood vessels bigger than in conjunctivitis; scleritis may cause globe perforation	Episcleritis is self-limiting; topical steroids for fast relief
Foreign body	Occupational or other exposure	Unilateral, red, gritty feeling; visible or microscopic size	Irrigation, removal; check for ulceration
Blepharitis	*S. aureus, Staphylococcus epidermidis*, seborrheic, blocked lacrimal duct; rarely molluscum contagiosum, *Phthirus pubis, Pediculus capitis*	Bilateral, irritation, itching, hyperemia, crusting, affecting lid margins	Topical antibiotics, warm compresses
Dacryocystitis	Obstructed lacrimal sac: *S. aureus, H. influenzae, S. pneumoniae*	Pain, tenderness, erythema and exudate in areas of lacrimal sac (inferomedial to inner canthus); tearing (epiphora); possible orbital cellulitis	Systemic, topical antibiotics; surgical drainage
Dacryoadenitis	*S. aureus, S. pneumoniae*, CMV, measles, EBV, enteroviruses; trauma, sarcoidosis, leukemia	Pain, tenderness, edema, erythema over gland area (upper temporal lid); fever, leukocytosis	Systemic antibiotics; drainage of orbital abscesses
Orbital cellulitis (postseptal cellulitis)	Paranasal sinusitis: *H. influenzae, S. aureus, S. pneumoniae*, other streptococci Trauma: *S. aureus* Fungi: *Aspergillus, Mucor* if immunodeficient	Rhinorrhea, chemosis, vision loss, painful extraocular motion, proptosis, ophthalmoplegia, fever, lid edema, leukocytosis	Systemic antibiotics, drainage of orbital abscesses
Periorbital cellulitis (preseptal cellulitis)	Trauma: *S. aureus*, other streptococci Bacteremia: pneumococcus, streptococci, *H. influenzae*	Cutaneous erythema, warmth, normal vision, minimal involvement of orbit; fever, leukocytosis, toxic appearance	Systemic antibiotics

CMV, Cytomegalovirus; *EBV*, Epstein-Barr virus; *JIA*, juvenile idiopathic arthritis; *SLE*, systemic lupus erythematosus.

gentle pressure on the nasolacrimal sac. Treatment usually requires probing of the nasolacrimal system to establish communication.

Endophthalmitis is an emergent, sight-threatening infection that usually follows trauma, surgery, or hematogenous spread from a distant focus. Causative organisms include coagulase-negative staphylococci, *S. aureus, S. pneumoniae, Bacillus cereus*, and *Candida albicans*. Examination is difficult because of severe blepharospasm and extreme photophobia. A **hypopyon** and haze may be visible on examination.

TREATMENT

The lids should be treated as needed with warm compresses to remove accumulated discharge. Acute bacterial conjunctivitis is frequently self-limited, but topical antibiotics hasten resolution. Antibiotics are instilled between the eyelids four times a day until the discharge and chemosis subside. Recommended treatment includes topical trimethoprim-polymyxin B solution, sulfacetamide 5% solution, or erythromycin ointment. Ciprofloxacin solution should be restricted to corneal infections and resistant gram-negative infections in hospitalized patients. Gonococcal conjunctivitis in adults is treated with a single intramuscular (IM) dose of ceftriaxone (1 g) plus azithromycin (to treat possible concomitant chlamydial infection).

The treatment of ophthalmia neonatorum depends on the cause (see Table 119-2). Gonococcal ophthalmia neonatorum is treated with a single dose of ceftriaxone (25 to 50 mg/kg intravenous [IV] or IM; maximum dose 125 mg). These infants

should be hospitalized. Antibiotic treatment also is recommended for newborns to mothers with untreated gonorrhea. Chlamydial conjunctivitis is treated with oral erythromycin for 14 days, partly to reduce the risk of subsequent chlamydial pneumonia.

COMPLICATIONS AND PROGNOSIS

The prognosis for bacterial and viral conjunctivitis is excellent. The major complication is keratitis, which can lead to ulcerations and perforation, and is uncommon except with *N. gonorrhoeae* and HSV infections. Chlamydial conjunctivitis may progress in infants to chlamydial pneumonia, which typically develops from 4 to 12 weeks of age (see Chapter 110).

PREVENTION

Careful hand washing is important to prevent spread of conjunctivitis. Bacterial conjunctivitis is considered contagious for 24 hours after initiating effective treatment. Children may return to school, but treatment measures must be continued until there is complete clinical resolution.

All newborns, whether delivered vaginally or by cesarean section, should receive prophylaxis for gonococcal ophthalmia neonatorum as soon as possible after delivery. Silver nitrate 1% is used frequently but usually causes a chemical conjunctivitis. Alternative methods are equally effective and less irritating and include a single application of erythromycin 0.5% ointment or tetracycline 1% ointment.

Chapter **120**

INFECTION IN THE IMMUNOCOMPROMISED PERSON

ETIOLOGY

Many diseases or their treatments adversely affect the immune system, including genetic immunodeficiencies, human immunodeficiency virus (HIV) infection and acquired immunodeficiency syndrome (AIDS), cancer, stem cell and organ transplantation, and immunosuppressive drugs used to treat cancer, autoimmune diseases, and transplant patients. These patients are at significant risk of life-threatening infections from invasive **endogenous infection** from bacterial or fungal flora of the oropharynx, skin, and gastrointestinal tract, acquisition of **exogenous infection** from infected persons, and reactivation of latent infections until immune function recovers (Table 120-1).

The infections seen in immunocompromised persons can often be predicted by which component of the immune system is abnormal, and the evaluation of fever in immunocompromised hosts differs. Episodes of fever and **neutropenia,** defined as an **absolute neutrophil count** of less than 500/mm³ neutrophils and bands, are especially common in cancer and transplant patients and increase risk for bacterial and fungal infections. The use of corticosteroids and potent immunosuppressive drugs that impair the activation of T lymphocytes increases the risk for pathogens normally controlled by T cell–mediated responses, such as *Pneumocystis jiroveci* and *Toxoplasma gondii,* and intracellular pathogens, such as *Salmonella, Listeria,* and *Mycobacterium.*

Staphylococcus aureus, Escherichia coli, Pseudomonas aeruginosa, Klebsiella pneumoniae, and coagulase-negative staphylococci are the most commonly identified bacterial pathogens in immunocompromised persons. Central indwelling catheters often are associated with infections caused by coagulase-negative staphylococci, *S. aureus,* gram-negative bacteria, *Enterococcus,* and *Candida.*

Fungal pathogens account for approximately 10% of all infections associated with childhood cancer. *Candida* causes 60% of all fungal infections, with *Aspergillus* as the second most common pathogen. Other risk factors for fungal infections include oropharyngeal and gastrointestinal mucositis

Table 120-1	Pathogens of Importance in Patients with Cancer (listed alphabetically)		
BACTERIA	**FUNGI**	**PROTOZOA**	**VIRUSES**
Bacteroides fragilis	*Aspergillus*	*Cryptosporidium parvum*	Adenoviruses
Campylobacter	*Blastoschizomyces capitatus*	*Cyclospora cayetanensis*	Cytomegalovirus
Clostridium difficile	*Candida* spp.	*Cystoisospora belli*	Echoviruses
Clostridium septicum	*Chrysosporium*	*Enterocytozoon bieneusi*	Epstein-Barr virus
Clostridium perfringens	*Cryptococcus neoformans*	*Giardia lamblia*	Hepatitis A virus
Comamonas acidovorans	*Cunninghamella bertholletiae*	*Leishmania donovani*	Herpes simplex viruses
Enterobacter cloacae	*Fusarium* spp.	*Septata intestinalis*	Human herpes virus 6
Enterococcus	*Geotrichum candidum*		Human metapneumovirus
Escherichia coli	*Malassezia furfur*		Influenza viruses
Haemophilus influenzae	*Mucor*		Norovirus
Klebsiella pneumoniae	*Pseudallescheria boydii*		Parainfluenza viruses
Listeria monocytogenes	*Rhizopus*		Parvovirus B19
Moraxella catarrhalis	*Scopulariopsis*		Respiratory syncytial virus
Mycobacterium avium complex	*Trichosporon beigelii*		Varicella-zoster virus
Mycobacterium chelonae			
Mycobacterium haemophilum			
Nocardia asteroides			
Pediococcus acidilactici			
Propionibacterium granulosum			
Pseudomonas aeruginosa			
Pseudomonas pseudomallei			
Coagulase-negative staphylococci			
Staphylococcus aureus			
Vibrio vulnificus			

facilitating systemic fungal invasion, presence of long-term indwelling intravascular catheters, extreme prematurity, and broad-spectrum antibacterial therapy that promotes fungal colonization as a precursor to infection.

Infection with *T. gondii* represents reactivation of quiescent infection facilitated by cancer-associated or therapy-associated cellular immunodeficiency. *P. jirovecii* primarily causes pneumonitis in patients with leukemia, lymphoma, HIV or those on long-term corticosteroids, but can also cause extrapulmonary disease (sinusitis, otitis media).

Viral opportunistic infections in patients with cancer usually represent symptomatic reactivation from latency facilitated by cancer-associated or therapy-associated cellular immunodeficiency. Herpes simplex virus (HSV) can cause severe and prolonged mucocutaneous infection or disseminated disease. Cytomegalovirus (CMV) can cause focal disease in immunocompromised persons, especially in stem cell transplant patients. Manifestations of CMV disease include hepatitis, pneumonitis, esophagitis, encephalitis, and enteritis with gastrointestinal ulcerations. Reactivation of Epstein-Barr virus (EBV) is associated with posttransplant lymphoproliferative disorder. Varicella zoster virus (VZV) can cause serious primary infection in susceptible persons, often with accompanying encephalitis, hepatitis, or, most ominously, pneumonitis. Zoster also can reactivate during chemotherapy and may be disseminated.

EPIDEMIOLOGY

Chemotherapeutic agents target rapidly dividing cells, especially myeloproliferative cells, which cause myelosuppression. Children receiving allogeneic transplants are at greater risk for infection than children receiving autologous transplants. Prolonged time to hematologic engraftment is a significant risk factor for infection in these patients. Children receiving stem cell or organ transplants have significantly greater immunosuppression as a consequence of the myeloablative conditioning regimens. Foreign bodies (shunts, central venous catheters) interfere with cutaneous barriers against infection and together with neutropenia or immunosuppression increase the risk of bacterial or fungal infections (see Chapter 121).

The relative rate of infection in patients with cancer at admission or during hospitalization is 10% to 15%. The most frequently infected sites, in descending order, are the respiratory tract, the bloodstream, surgical wounds, and the urinary tract.

CLINICAL MANIFESTATIONS

Decision-Making Algorithms
Available @ StudentConsult.com

Neutropenia
Pancytopenia
Fever without a Source
Recurrent Infections

Fever is the most common, and sometimes the only, presenting symptom of serious infection in cancer and transplant patients. The presence of fever with neutropenia, even in the absence of other signs or symptoms, demands prompt evaluation because of the potential for life-threatening infection. Despite being immunocompromised, these patients develop fever and some typical signs and symptoms associated with infections. All symptoms and signs should be evaluated thoroughly. However, some symptoms may be absent based on the underlying immunodeficiency. For example, in the absence of neutrophils to contain and induce localized signs of inflammation, determination of the source of infection by physical examination is often difficult. Chest findings may be absent, despite pneumonia, and revealed only by chest radiograph at presentation or when the neutrophil count recovers.

LABORATORY TESTS AND IMAGING

Assessing fever and neutropenia in immunocompromised persons requires blood cultures for bacterial and fungal pathogens obtained by peripheral venipuncture and from all lumens of any indwelling vascular catheters. A complete blood count with differential, C-reactive protein, complete chemistry panel, culture of urine and Gram staining/culture of potential sites of specific infection found during history and physical should be performed. Antigen tests, especially for serum cryptococcal antigen, should be considered. Chest radiographs are important to assess for the presence of pulmonary infiltrates. Specialized imaging studies, such as the CT or MRI, can be useful in selected cases, such as with suspected sinusitis or intra-abdominal infection, or to further delineate the location and extent of abnormalities seen on plain radiographs. Sinus infection with bacteria, *Aspergillus*, or Zygomycetes is common in neutropenic hosts and may be detected only on the CT scan.

DIFFERENTIAL DIAGNOSIS

Initially the patient should have a complete physical examination, including careful scrutiny of the oropharynx, nares, external auditory canals, skin and axilla, groin, perineum, and rectal area. The exit site and subcutaneous tunnel of any indwelling vascular catheter should be examined closely for erythema and palpated for tenderness and expression of purulent material. Perirectal abscess is a potentially serious infection in neutropenic hosts, with tenderness and erythema that may be the only clues to infection. Any presumptive infection identified during the evaluation should direct appropriate cultures and tailor anti-infective therapy.

TREATMENT

Treatment should be provided as appropriate for focal infections identified by physical examination or diagnostic imaging. Select *low-risk* patients may be managed as outpatients. Empirical treatment of fever and neutropenia without an identified source should include an extended-spectrum penicillin or cephalosporin with activity against gram-negative bacilli, including *P. aeruginosa*, sometimes in combination with an aminoglycoside (Fig. 120-1). If the patient has an indwelling vascular catheter, vancomycin should be added because of the increasing prevalence of methicillin-resistant *S. aureus* but can be discontinued if *S. aureus* is not cultured after 48 to 72 hours. Specific antibiotic regimens should be guided by local antibiotic resistance patterns at each institution.

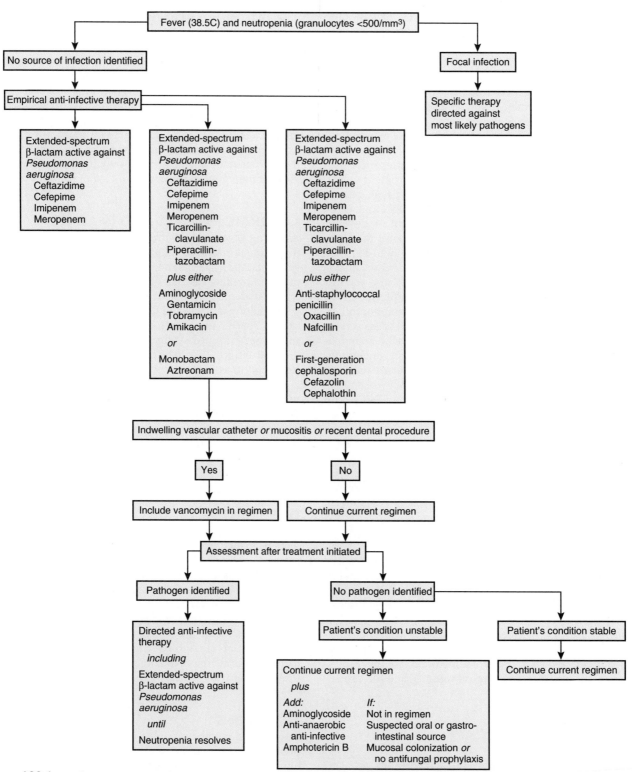

Figure 120-1 Initial management of fever and neutropenia without an identified source in cancer and transplant patients. *(From Conrad DA: Patients with cancer. In Jenson HB, Baltimore RS, editors: Pediatric Infectious Diseases: Principles and Practice, ed 2, Philadelphia, 2002, Saunders, p 1161.)*

If no microbiologic cause is isolated, empirical broad-spectrum antibiotics are continued as long as the patient remains neutropenic, regardless of whether the fever resolves (Fig. 120-2). Antibiotic therapy should be modified as indicated by new findings or if the patient's clinical status deteriorates. Further investigation for fungal infection and empirical

treatment with amphotericin B or another antifungal agent is instituted in patients who have neutropenia and persistent fever without a focus, despite broad-spectrum antibacterial therapy for approximately 5 days (see Fig. 120-2).

The use of recombinant granulocyte colony-stimulating factor or granulocyte-macrophage colony-stimulating factor

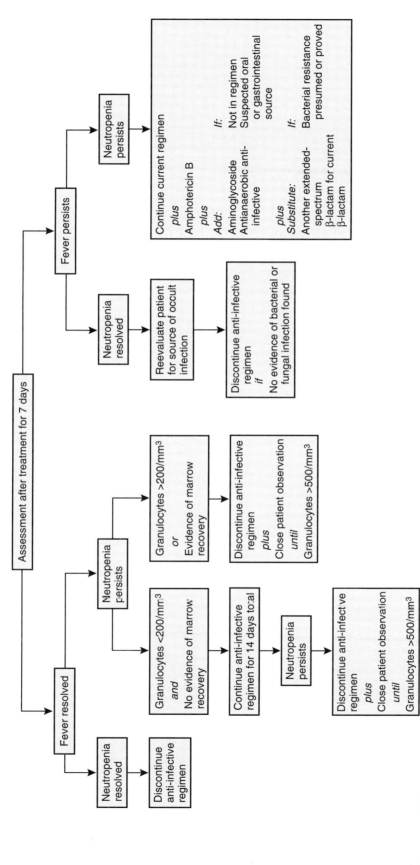

Figure 120-2 Continuing management of possible infection after 7 days of fever without an identified source in cancer and transplant patients. *(From Conrad DA: Patients with cancer. In Jenson HB, Baltimore RS editors: Pediatric Infectious Diseases: Principles and Practice, ed 2, Philadelphia, 2002, Saunders, p 1165.)*

stimulates neutrophil production by the bone marrow, reduces the duration and severity of neutropenia, and decreases the risk of infection. Some chemotherapeutic protocols for the treatment of solid tumors that result in prolonged neutropenia incorporate hematopoietic cytokine therapy as part of the treatment protocol.

PREVENTION

Current guidelines discourage the use of broad-spectrum prophylactic antibiotics to prevent fever and neutropenia because of lack of efficacy and concerns about development of antibiotic resistance. Administration of trimethoprim-sulfamethoxazole to prevent *P. jiroveci* infection is routine for patients undergoing intensive chemotherapy or immunosuppression for transplantation. Prophylaxis generally is begun with initiation of anticancer therapy and continued until 6 months after chemotherapy has been completed. In select populations, such as patients undergoing hematopoietic stem cell transplantation, prophylactic antifungals such as fluconazole are beneficial.

Immunocompromised susceptible persons exposed to chickenpox within 2 days before the onset of rash until 5 days after the onset of rash in the index case should receive varicella zoster immune globulin (VZIG). Modified infection after VZIG may not result in protective immunity, and persons who receive VZIG prophylaxis should be considered still at risk with any subsequent exposures.

Chapter 121

INFECTIONS ASSOCIATED WITH MEDICAL DEVICES

Infections are a common and important complication of medical devices and are a major part of **health care–associated infections** (formerly known as **nosocomial infections**).

VASCULAR DEVICE INFECTIONS

Vascular catheters are inserted in most inpatients and used in many outpatients. The use of catheters for long-term access to the bloodstream has been an important advance for the care of persons who require parenteral nutrition, chemotherapy, or extended parenteral antibiotic therapy. The major complication of catheters is infection.

Short, peripheral intravenous (IV) catheters used for short-term access in stable patients are associated with a low rate of infection, especially in children. **Peripherally inserted central catheters** are commonly used for short-term venous access. **Central catheters** are commonly placed for extended venous access, such as for chemotherapy, using tunneled silicone elastomer catheters **(Broviac** or **Hickman catheters)** that are surgically inserted into a central vein, passed through a

Table 121-1	Organisms Causing Catheter-Related Infections	
CLASSIFICATION OF PATHOGEN	**COMMON**	**UNCOMMON**
Gram-positive organisms	Coagulase-negative staphylococci, *Staphylococcus aureus, Enterococcus*	Diphtheroids, *Bacillus,* Micrococcus
Gram-negative organisms	*Escherichia coli, Klebsiella, Pseudomonas aeruginosa*	*Acinetobacter, Enterobacter, Neisseria*
Fungi	*Candida albicans*	*Malassezia furfur, Candida parapsilosis, Candida glabrata, Candida tropicalis*
Miscellaneous		Nontuberculous mycobacteria

subcutaneous tunnel before exiting the skin, and anchored by a subcutaneous cuff. Contamination of the catheter hub or any connection of the IV tubing is common and is a major predisposition to catheter-associated infection. Totally implanted venous access systems (Port-a-Cath, Infuse-a-Port) have a silicone elastomer catheter tunneled beneath the skin to a reservoir implanted in a subcutaneous pocket. Implanted catheters or ports decrease, but do not eliminate, the opportunity for microbial entry at the skin site.

Catheter-related thrombosis and catheter-related infection can develop separately or together. Ultrasound or radiographs can identify thrombi, but infection can be identified by culture only. **Thrombophlebitis** is inflammation with thrombosis. **Septic thrombophlebitis** is thrombosis with organisms embedded in the clot. **Catheter-related bloodstream infection** implies isolation of the same organism from a catheter and from peripheral blood of a patient with clinical symptoms of bacteremia and no other apparent source of infection. Confirmation requires quantitative colony counts of both samples, which is not routinely performed. Possible sources of the bacteremia include the infusate, contamination via tubing and catheter connections, or established infection, which may or may not be clinically apparent. Infection may appear as an **exit site infection** limited to the insertion site or may extend along the catheter tunnel of buried catheters to cause a **tunnel infection.**

Many microorganisms cause catheter-related infections, most commonly *Staphylococcus aureus,* coagulase-negative staphylococci, *Enterococcus,* and *Candida* (Table 121-1). Gram-positive cocci, primarily staphylococci, cause more than 50% of central venous catheter associated bacteremias and exit site infections. Other skin flora, diphtheroids, and *Bacillus* are often involved. Gram-negative organisms cause 25% to 40% of infections. Polymicrobial infections of central venous catheters are common. Fungal catheter infections, usually *Candida albicans,* are most common among persons receiving broad-spectrum antibiotics or parenteral nutrition.

The rates of bloodstream infection of peripheral venous catheters are from 0 to 2 per 1000 catheter-days and for central catheters from less than 2 to 30 per 1000 catheter-days. Risk factors for infection include prematurity, burns and skin disorders that adversely affect the skin integrity, neutropenia, and

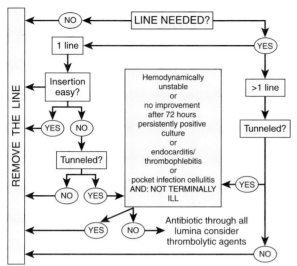

Figure 121-1 Management of central venous catheter infection. *(From De Paw BE, Verweij PE: Infections in patients with hematologic malignancies. In Mandell GL, Bennett JE, Dolin R, editors: Principles and Practice of Infectious Diseases, ed 6, Philadelphia, 2005, Churchill Livingstone, Fig. 307-1, p 3434.)*

other immunodeficiencies (see Chapter 120). Infection rates are lower for tunneled and implanted catheters. Catheters inserted in emergency settings are more likely to be infected than catheters placed electively.

Clinical signs of catheter-associated bacteremia or fungemia range from mild fever to overwhelming sepsis. Infection at the site of the central catheter entrance is manifested as a localized cellulitis with warmth, tenderness, swelling, erythema, and discharge. Tunnel infection is manifested by similar findings along the tunnel route. Peripheral phlebitis or catheter-related infection is classically manifested as a warm, erythematous, tender palpable cord originating at the IV catheter site but may be subclinical or manifested only by fever without signs of local inflammation.

Decision-Making Algorithm
Available @ StudentConsult.com

Fever and Rash

The treatment of catheter-related infection depends on the site of the infection and the pathogen involved. Catheters that are no longer necessary should be removed if infection is suspected. Catheter-associated bacteremia can be treated with simple catheter removal, removal plus antibiotics, or, in a stable patient, an attempt of antibiotic therapy alone (Fig. 121-1). Infection with organisms of low virulence may be manifested by fever alone, and removal of the catheter frequently is followed by prompt defervescence and complete resolution of infection. Empirical initial therapy for suspected infection should include antibiotics active against gram-negative organisms such as a broad-spectrum cephalosporin, and against *S. aureus* and coagulase-negative staphylococci such as oxacillin, nafcillin, or vancomycin. Antibiotic regimens should be tailored to the specific organism identified. Eradication of infection can be accomplished without removal of the central line in 89% of uncomplicated bacteremic infections, 94% of exit site infections, and 25% of tunnel infections. If the patient

is not critically ill and the pathogen is likely to be susceptible to antibiotic therapy, a trial of antibiotics is given through the infected catheter. The total duration of therapy depends on the pathogen and the duration of positive cultures and is usually 10 to 14 days after sterilization of the bloodstream. Catheter removal is indicated with sepsis, septic thrombophlebitis, clinical deterioration (despite appropriate therapy), persistently positive blood culture results after 48 to 72 hours of appropriate antimicrobial therapy, embolic lesions, or fungal infection because of poor response to antifungal therapy alone (see Fig. 121-1). Infection of the pocket around an implanted port is unlikely to respond to antibiotics, and removal of the foreign body is usually necessary.

Antibiotic-lock is a method of sterilizing intravascular catheters by using high concentrations of antibiotics infused into the portion of the catheter between the hub and the vessel entry. The solution is allowed to dwell within the catheter segment for several hours. It also may be useful for treatment of catheter-associated infections and for prevention of infection.

Aseptic technique is essential during catheter insertion. Catheters that are placed during emergency situations should be replaced as soon as medically feasible. Care of indwelling catheters involves meticulous attention to sterile technique whenever the system is entered. Care of the catheter entry site commonly involves a topical antibiotic or disinfectant. Catheters that are no longer necessary should be removed.

VENTILATOR-ASSOCIATED PNEUMONIA

Intubation of the airway provides direct access to the lungs and bypasses normal host defenses. Organisms enter the lungs directly through the lumen of the tube or by descending around the tube, which may result in ventilator-associated pneumonia. Contaminated respiratory equipment, humidification systems, or condensate introduces bacteria directly into lower airways. The continuously open upper airway increases the risk of aspiration of oropharyngeal flora and reflux of gastric contents and interferes with clearance of the airway by coughing because an effective cough requires a closed glottis. Suctioning of the upper respiratory tract or mouth requires clean technique but does not require aseptic technique. Suction catheters that reach the lower airways must be sterile and usually are designed for single use.

URINARY CATHETERS

The most important risk factors for urinary tract infections (UTIs) are the presence of catheters, instrumentation, and anatomic abnormalities (see Chapter 114). Organisms enter the bladder through the catheter by instillation of contaminated irrigation fluids, backflow of contaminated urine from the drainage bag, or ascent of bacteria around the meatus along the outside of the catheter. Indwelling catheters facilitate direct access to the bladder and should have a closed drainage system. After simple, straight catheterization, the incidence of UTI is 1% to 2%. Organisms that cause catheter-associated UTIs include fecal flora, such as gram-negative enteric bacilli, most commonly *Escherichia coli,* and *Enterococcus.* With concomitant antibiotic treatment, resistant organisms predominate, and fungi emerge as pathogens.

The most important aspect of prevention is to minimize the duration and use of catheterization. Intermittent catheterization is preferred over indwelling catheter drainage whenever feasible. Insertion of catheters must be performed with aseptic technique, and the drainage system must remain closed at all times, with sterile technique used whenever the system is entered. Drainage bags always should be dependent to avoid backflow of urine into the bladder.

PERITONEAL DIALYSIS–ASSOCIATED INFECTIONS

Indwelling catheters used for peritoneal dialysis may develop exit site infections, tunnel infections, or lead to peritonitis. The usual route of infection is from the skin surface along the tunnel and into the peritoneum. The most common pathogens are skin flora, including *Staphylococcus;* organisms that contaminate water, such as *Pseudomonas* and *Acinetobacter;* enteric flora, such as *E. coli* and *Klebsiella;* and fungi, such as *C. albicans.* Peritonitis may present with fever, vague abdominal pain, and cloudy dialysate. The diagnosis is established on clinical manifestations and confirmed by culture of the dialysate. Prevention of infection requires careful planning of the location of the exit site to minimize contamination, aseptic insertion of the catheter, meticulous care of the catheter site, securing of the catheter to avoid tension and motion, and aseptic technique during dialysis.

CENTRAL NERVOUS SYSTEM SHUNTS

Important risk factors of health care–associated central nervous system infections are surgery, ventriculoperitoneal shunts, and cerebrospinal fluid (CSF) leaks. Infection of ventriculoperitoneal shunts results from contamination of the system at the time of placement or from hematogenous seeding. Externalized ventricular drains and subdural bolts allow direct access of skin flora to the CSF. For these devices, the rates of infection increase with the duration of catheterization, especially beyond 5 days.

The most common pathogens causing shunt infections are coagulase-negative staphylococci and *S. aureus.* After skull fracture or cranial surgery, a CSF fistula leak may facilitate ascending infection from the nasopharynx, especially with *Streptococcus pneumoniae,* which frequently colonizes the nasopharynx. Patients with shunt infections may present with only fever and headache, or may present with typical signs and symptoms of meningitis (see Chapter 100). Infections caused by coagulase-negative staphylococci typically present with insidious onset of fever, malaise, headache, and vomiting. Empirical therapy is with vancomycin, with additional antibiotics if gram-negative bacteria are suspected.

Antibiotics frequently are used perioperatively during placement of shunts and other neurosurgical procedures. There is no proof that antibiotics decrease infection rates in these clean procedures. External ventricular drains should be maintained as closed systems with aseptic technique and removed as soon as possible. Drainage bags always should be dependent to avoid backflow.

Chapter 122

ZOONOSES

Zoonoses are infections that are transmitted in nature between vertebrate animals and humans. Many zoonotic pathogens are maintained in nature by means of an **enzootic cycle,** in which mammalian hosts and arthropod vectors reinfect each other. Humans frequently are only incidentally infected. Of the more than 150 different human zoonotic diseases that have been described (Table 122-1), Lyme disease (*Borrelia burgdorferi*) accounts for 90% of reported vector-borne infections in the United States. Other common pathogens include *Rickettsia rickettsii* (Rocky Mountain spotted fever), ehrlichiosis (*Ehrlichia chaffeensis*), West Nile virus, and anaplasmosis (*Anaplasma phagocytophilum*). The epidemiology of zoonoses is related to the geographic distribution of the hosts and, if vector-borne, the distribution and seasonal life cycle of the vector.

Many zoonoses are spread by ticks including Lyme disease, Rocky Mountain spotted fever, ehrlichiosis, tularemia, tick typhus, and babesiosis. Mosquitoes transmit the arboviral encephalitides (see Chapter 101), dengue fever, malaria, and yellow fever. Preventive measures to avoid tick-borne and mosquito-borne diseases include using insect repellants that contain **DEET** (N,N-diethyl-*m*-toluamide) on skin and insect repellants that contain **permethrin** on clothing; avoiding tick-infested habitats (thick scrub oak, briar, poison ivy sites); avoiding excretory products of wild animals; wearing appropriate protective clothing (closed-toe shoes, long pants, etc.); and promptly removing ticks.

Ticks are best removed using blunt forceps or tweezers to grasp the tick as close to the skin as possible to pull the tick steadily outward. Squeezing, twisting, or crushing the tick should be avoided because the tick's bloated abdomen can act like a syringe if squeezed. Transmission of infection seems to be most efficient after 30 to 36 hours of nymphal tick attachment for human granulocytic ehrlichiosis, after 36 to 48 hours for *B. burgdorferi,* and after 56 to 60 hours for *Babesia.* Prophylactic antimicrobial therapy after a tick bite or exposure is not recommended.

LYME DISEASE (*BORRELIA BURGDORFERI*)
Etiology

Lyme disease is a tick-borne infection caused by the spirochete, *B. burgdorferi.* The vector in the eastern and midwestern United States is *Ixodes scapularis,* the **black-legged tick** that is commonly known as the **deer tick.** The vector on the Pacific Coast is *Ixodes pacificus,* the **western black-legged tick.** Ticks usually become infected by feeding on the white-footed mouse (*Peromyscus leucopus*), which is a natural reservoir for *B. burgdorferi.* The larvae are dormant over winter and emerge the following spring in the nymphal stage, the stage of the tick that is most likely to transmit the infection to humans.

Epidemiology

Over 20,000 cases are reported annually in the United States, with 96% of cases reported from New England, the eastern parts of the Middle Atlantic states, and the upper Midwest

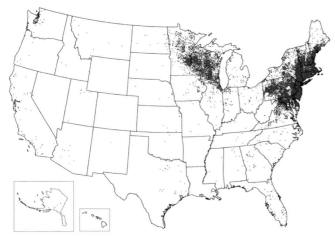

Figure 122-1 The geographic distribution of 24,364 confirmed cases of Lyme disease in the United States in 2011. The risk for acquiring Lyme disease varies by the distribution of *Ixodes scapularis* and *Ixodes pacificas,* the proportion of infected ticks for each species at each stage of the tick's life cycle, and the presence of grassy or wooded locations favored by white-tailed deer. *(From Centers for Disease Control and Prevention: Lyme Disease—United States, 2011, available from the CDC website: http://www.cdc.gov/lyme/stats/maps/map2011.html.)*

(Fig. 122-1). In Europe most cases occur in Scandinavian countries and central Europe. Because exposure to ticks is more common in warm months, Lyme disease is noted predominantly in summer. The incidence is highest among children 5 to 10 years old, at almost twice the incidence among adolescents and adults.

Clinical Manifestations

Decision-Making Algorithms
Available @ StudentConsult.com

Arthritis
Fever and Rash

The clinical manifestations are divided into early and late stages. Early infection may be localized or disseminated. **Early localized disease** develops 7 to 14 days after a tick bite as the site forms an erythematous papule that expands to form a red, raised border, often with central clearing. The lesion, **erythema migrans,** harbors *B. burgdorferi* and may be 15 cm wide, pruritic, or painful. Systemic manifestations may include malaise, lethargy, fever, headache, arthralgias, stiff neck, myalgias, and lymphadenopathy. The skin lesions and early manifestations resolve without treatment over 2 to 4 weeks. Not all patients with Lyme disease recall a tick bite or develop erythema migrans.

Approximately 20% of patients develop **early disseminated disease** with multiple secondary skin lesions, aseptic meningitis, pseudotumor, papilledema, cranioneuropathies including Bell palsy, polyradiculitis, peripheral neuropathy, mononeuritis multiplex, or transverse myelitis. Carditis with various degrees of heart block rarely may develop during this stage. Neurologic manifestations usually resolve by 3 months but may recur or become chronic.

Late disease begins weeks to months after infection. Arthritis is the usual manifestation and may develop in 50% to 60% of untreated patients. The male to female ratio is 7:1. The knee is involved in greater than 90% of cases, but any joint may be affected. Symptoms may resolve over 1 to 2 weeks but often recur in other joints. If untreated most cases resolve, but chronic erosive arthritis persists in 10% of patients as the episodes increase in duration and severity. Cardiac abnormalities occur in approximately 10% of untreated patients. **Neuroborreliosis,** the late manifestations of Lyme disease involving the central nervous system (CNS), is rarely reported in children.

Laboratory and Imaging Studies

Antibody tests during early, localized Lyme disease may be negative and are not useful. The diagnosis of late disease is confirmed by serologic tests specific for *B. burgdorferi.* The sensitivity and specificity of serologic tests for Lyme disease vary substantially. A positive enzyme-linked immunosorbent assay or immunofluorescence assay result must be confirmed by immunoblot showing antibodies against at least either two to three (for IgM) or five (for IgG) proteins of *B. burgdorferi* (at least one of which is one of the more specific, low-molecular-weight, outer-surface proteins).

In late disease, the erythrocyte sedimentation rate is elevated and complement may be reduced. The joint fluid shows an inflammatory response with total white blood cell count of 25,000 to 125,000 cells/mm^3, often with a polymorphonuclear predominance (see Table 118-2). The rheumatoid factor and antinuclear antibody are negative, but the Venereal Disease Research Laboratory test may be falsely positive. With CNS involvement, the cerebrospinal fluid shows a lymphocytic pleocytosis with normal glucose and slightly elevated protein.

Differential Diagnosis

A history of a tick bite and the classic rash is helpful but is not always present. Erythema migrans of early, localized disease may be confused with nummular eczema, tinea corporis, granuloma annulare, an insect bite, or cellulitis. **Southern tick-associated rash illness,** which is similar to erythema migrans, occurs in southeastern and south central states and is associated with the bite of *Amblyomma americanum,* the lone star tick, and infection with *Borrelia lonestari.*

During early, disseminated Lyme disease, multiple lesions may appear as erythema multiforme or urticaria. The aseptic meningitis is similar to viral meningitis, and the seventh nerve palsy is indistinguishable from herpetic or idiopathic Bell palsy. Lyme carditis is similar to viral myocarditis. Monarticular or pauciarticular arthritis of late Lyme disease may mimic suppurative arthritis, juvenile idiopathic arthritis, or rheumatic fever (see Chapter 89). The differential diagnosis of neuroborreliosis includes degenerative neurologic illness, encephalitis, and depression.

Treatment

Early localized disease and early disseminated disease, including facial nerve palsy (or other cranial nerve palsy) and carditis with first-degree or second-degree heart block, is treated with doxycycline or amoxicillin for 14 to 21 days. Early disease with carditis with third-degree heart block or meningitis and

Table 122-1	Major Zoonotic and Vector-Borne Infections*

DISEASE	CAUSATIVE AGENT	COMMON ANIMAL RESERVOIRS	VECTORS/MODES OF TRANSMISSION	GEOGRAPHIC DISTRIBUTION
BACTERIAL DISEASES				
Anthrax	*Bacillus anthracis*	Cattle, goats, sheep, swine, cats, wild animals	Aerosol inhalation of spores in hides and other animal by-products, direct contact	Worldwide; rare in United States
Brucellosis	*Brucella*	Cattle, sheep, goats, swine, horses, dogs	Aerosol inhalation, direct contact, ingestion of contaminated goat cheese and milk	Worldwide
Campylobacteriosis	*Campylobacter jejuni*	Rodents, dogs (puppies), cats, fowl (chickens), swine	Direct contact, ingestion of contaminated food or water	Worldwide
Cat-scratch disease	*Bartonella henselae*	Cats, dogs	Bites and scratches	United States
Erysipeloid	*Erysipelothrix rhusiopathiae*	Sheep, swine, turkeys, ducks, fish	Direct contact	Worldwide
Listeriosis	*Listeria monocytogenes*	Cattle, fowl, goats, sheep	Ingestion of contaminated food, unpasteurized cheese and dairy products	Worldwide
Plague	*Yersinia pestis*	Wild and domestic rodents, cats, dogs	Direct contact, flea bite	New Mexico, Arizona, Utah, Colorado, California
Rat-bite fever (bacillary fever)	*Streptobacillus moniliformis*	Mice, rats, hamsters	Bites, ingestion of contaminated food or water	Japan, Asia; rare in United States
Salmonellosis	Nontyphoidal *Salmonella*	Fowl, dogs, cats, reptiles, amphibians	Direct contact, ingestion of contaminated food or water	Worldwide
Tularemia	*Francisella tularensis*	Rabbits, squirrels, dogs, cats	Aerosol inhalation, direct contact, ingestion of contaminated meat, tick bite, deerfly bite	California, Utah, Arkansas, Oklahoma
Yersiniosis	*Yersinia enterocolitica, Yersinia pseudotuberculosis*	Rodents, cattle, goats, sheep, swine, fowl, dogs	Direct contact, ingestion of contaminated food or water	Worldwide
Wound infection, bacteremia	*Pasteurella multocida, Capnocytophaga canimorsus*	Cats, dogs, rodents	Direct contact, bites and scratches	Worldwide
Mycobacterial Diseases				
Wound infection	*Mycobacterium marinum, Mycobacterium fortuitum, Mycobacterium kansasii*	Fish, aquarium	Direct contact, scratches	Worldwide
Spirochetal Diseases				
Leptospirosis	*Leptospira interrogans*	Dogs, rodents, livestock	Direct contact, contact with water or soil contaminated by urine of infected animals	Worldwide
Lyme disease	*Borrelia burgdorferi*	Deer, rodents	Tick bite (*Ixodes scapularis, Ixodes pacificus*)	Northeast and Midwest United States, California
Rat-bite fever (Haverhill fever)	*Spirillum minus*	Mice, rats, hamsters	Bites, ingestion of contaminated food or water	Japan, Asia; rare in United States
Relapsing fever	*Borrelia*	Rodents, fleas	Louse bite, flea bite, transplacental transmission	Western and southern United States
Southern tick-associated rash illness	*Borrelia lonestari*	Deer, rodents	Tick bite (*I. scapularis*)	Southeastern and south-central U.S.

Table 122-1	Major Zoonotic and Vector-Borne Infections*—cont'd			
DISEASE	**CAUSATIVE AGENT**	**COMMON ANIMAL RESERVOIRS**	**VECTORS/MODES OF TRANSMISSION**	**GEOGRAPHIC DISTRIBUTION**
Rickettsial Diseases				
Spotted Fever Group				
Rocky Mountain spotted fever	*Rickettsia rickettsii*	Dogs, rodents	Tick bite (*Dermacentor variabilis*, the American dog tick; *Dermacentor andersoni*, the wood tick; *Rhipicephalus sanguineus*, the brown dog tick; *Amblyomma cajennense*)	Western hemisphere
Mediterranean spotted fever (boutonneuse fever)	*Rickettsia conorii*	Dogs, rodents	Tick bite	Africa, Mediterranean region, India, Middle East
African tick-bite fever	*Rickettsia africae*	Cattle, goats (?)	Tick bite	Sub-Saharan Africa, Caribbean
Rickettsialpox	*Rickettsia akari*	Mice	Mite bite	North America, Russia, Ukraine, Adriatic region, Korea, South Africa
Murine typhus–like illness	*Rickettsia felis*	Opossums, cats, dogs	Flea bite	Western hemisphere, Europe
Typhus Group				
Murine typhus	*Rickettsia typhi*	Rats	Rat flea or cat flea feces	Worldwide
Epidemic typhus	*Rickettsia prowazekii*	Humans	Louse feces	Africa, South America, Central America, Mexico, Asia
Brill-Zinsser disease (recrudescent typhus)	*R. prowazekii*	Humans	Reactivation of latent infection	Potentially worldwide; United States, Canada, Eastern Europe
Flying squirrel (sylvatic) typhus	*R. prowazekii*	Flying squirrels	Lice or fleas of flying squirrel	United States
Scrub Typhus				
Scrub typhus	*Orientia tsutsugamushi*	Rodents (?)	Chigger bite	Southern Asia, Japan, Indonesia, Australia, Korea, Asiatic Russia, India, China
Ehrlichiosis and Anaplasmosis				
Human monocytic ehrlichiosis	*Ehrlichia chaffeensis*	Deer, dogs	Tick bite (*Amblyomma americanum*)	United States, Europe, Africa
Anaplasmosis (human granulocytic ehrlichiosis)	*Anaplasma phagocytophilum*	Rodents, deer, ruminants	Tick bite (*I. scapularis*)	United States, Europe
Ehrlichiosis ewingii	*Ehrlichia ewingii*	Dogs	Tick bite	United States
Sennetsu ehrlichiosis	*Neorickettsia sennetsu*	Unknown	Ingestion of helminth-contaminated fish (?)	Japan, Malaysia
Q Fever				
Q fever	*Coxiella burnetii*	Cattle, sheep, goats, cats, rabbits	Inhalation of infected aerosols, ingestion of contaminated dairy products, ticks (?)	Worldwide
Viral Diseases				
Colorado tick fever	Orbivirus	Rodents, ticks	Aerosol inhalation, tick bite, blood transfusion, ingestion of contaminated food	Rocky Mountains, Pacific Northwest, western Canada
Dengue fever	Dengue viruses (types 1-4)	Humans	Mosquito bite (*Aedes aegypti, Aedes albopictus*)	Tropical areas of the Caribbean, the Americas, and Asia

Continued

Table 122-1	Major Zoonotic and Vector-Borne Infections*—cont'd			
DISEASE	**CAUSATIVE AGENT**	**COMMON ANIMAL RESERVOIRS**	**VECTORS/MODES OF TRANSMISSION**	**GEOGRAPHIC DISTRIBUTION**
Hantavirus cardiopulmonary syndrome	Hantavirus	Rodents, mice, cats	Aerosol inhalation	Southwestern United States
Herpesvirus B infection	Herpesvirus B	Old World primates (rhesus, *Macaca cynomolgus*)	Animal bite	Africa, Asia (and primate centers worldwide)
Lymphocytic choriomeningitis	Lymphocytic choriomeningitis virus	Rodents, hamsters, mice	Aerosol inhalation, direct contact, bite	Worldwide
Rabies	Rabies virus	Dogs, skunks, bats, raccoons, foxes, cats	Bites and scratches	Worldwide
Vesicular stomatitis	Vesicular stomatitis virus	Horses, cattle, swine	Direct contact	Americas
Protozoan Diseases				
African trypanosomiasis				
East African sleeping sickness	*Trypanosoma brucei rhodesiense*	Wild and domestic animals	Insect bite (tsetse fly)	East Africa
West African sleeping sickness	*Trypanosoma brucei gambiense*	Wild and domestic animals	Insect bite (tsetse fly)	West Africa
American trypanosomiasis (Chagas disease)	*Trypanosoma cruzi*	Wild and domestic animals	Insect bite (reduviid bug); contact with fecal material of reduviid bug	South America, Central America, South Texas
Babesiosis	*Babesia*	Cattle, wild and domestic rodents	Tick bite (*I. scapularis*), blood transfusion	Worldwide
Leishmaniasis, mucocutaneous and cutaneous	*Leishmania*	Domestic and wild dogs	Sandfly bite	Tropics
Leishmaniasis, visceral	*Leishmania donovani* complex	Domestic and wild dogs	Sandfly bite	Tropics
Malaria	*Plasmodium*	Humans	Mosquito bite (*Anopheles*)	Usually imported to the United States, Southern California
Toxoplasmosis	*Toxoplasma gondii*	Cats, livestock, pigs	Ingestion of oocysts in fecally contaminated material or ingestion of tissue cysts in undercooked meat	Worldwide

Adapted from Christenson JC: Epidemiology of infectious diseases. In Jenson HB, Baltimore RS, editors: Pediatric Infectious Diseases: Principles and Practice, ed 2, Philadelphia, 2002, Saunders, pp 18–20.
*Many helminths are also zoonotic (see Tables 123-4 and 123-5).

late neurologic disease (other than facial nerve or other cranial nerve palsy) are treated with intravenous or intramuscular ceftriaxone or intravenous penicillin G for 14 to 28 days. Arthritis is treated with doxycycline (for children >9 years of age) or amoxicillin for 28 days. If there is recurrence, treatment should be with a repeated oral regimen or with the regimen for late neurologic disease.

Complications and Prognosis
Carditis, especially conduction disturbances, and arthritis are the major complications of Lyme disease. Even untreated, most cases eventually resolve without sequelae.

Lyme disease is readily treatable and curable. The long-term prognosis is excellent for early and late disease. Early treatment may prevent progression to carditis and meningitis. Recurrences of arthritis are rare after recommended treatment.

A community-based study of children with Lyme disease found no evidence of impairment 4 to 11 years later.

Prevention
Measures to minimize exposure to tick-borne diseases are the most reasonable means of preventing Lyme disease. Postexposure prophylaxis is not routinely recommended because the overall risk of acquiring Lyme disease after a tick bite is only 1% to 2% even in endemic areas, and treatment of the infection, if it develops, is highly effective. Nymphal stage ticks must feed for 36 to 48 hours, and adult ticks must feed for 48 to 72 hours before the risk of transmission of *B. burgdorferi* from infected ticks becomes substantial. In hyperendemic regions, prophylaxis of adults with doxycycline, 200 mg as a single dose, within 72 hours of a nymphal tick bite is effective in preventing Lyme disease.

ROCKY MOUNTAIN SPOTTED FEVER (*RICKETTSIA RICKETTSII*)
Etiology

The cause of Rocky Mountain spotted fever is *R. rickettsii,* gram-negative coccobacillary organisms that resemble bacteria but have incomplete cell walls and require an intracellular site for replication. The organism invades and proliferates within the endothelial cells of blood vessels, causing vasculitis and resulting in increased vascular permeability, edema, and, eventually, decreased vascular volume, altered tissue perfusion, and widespread organ failure. Many tick species are capable of transmitting *R. rickettsii*. The principal ticks are the **American dog tick** (*Dermacentor variabilis*) in the eastern United States and Canada, the **wood tick** (*Dermacentor andersoni*) in the western United States and Canada, the **brown dog tick** (*Rhipicephalus sanguineus*) in Mexico, and *Amblyomma cajennense* in Central and South America.

Epidemiology

Rocky Mountain spotted fever is the most common rickettsial illness in the United States, occurring primarily in the eastern coastal, southeastern, and western states. Most cases occur from May to October after outdoor activity in wooded areas, with peak incidence among children 1 to 14 years of age. Approximately 40% of infected persons are unable to recall a tick bite.

Clinical Manifestations

Decision-Making Algorithms
Available @ StudentConsult.com

Hepatomegaly
Fever and Rash
Petechiae/Purpura
Fever without a Source

The incubation period of Rocky Mountain spotted fever is 2 to 14 days, with an average of 7 days. The onset is nonspecific with headache, malaise, and fever. A pale, rose-red macular or maculopapular rash appears in 90% of cases. The rash begins peripherally and spreads to involve the entire body, including palms and soles. The early rash blanches on pressure and is accentuated by warmth. It progresses over hours or days to a petechial and purpuric eruption that appears first on the feet and ankles, then the wrists and hands, and progresses centripetally to the trunk and head. Myalgias, especially of the lower extremities, and intractable headaches are common. Severe cases progress with splenomegaly, myocarditis, renal impairment, pneumonitis, and shock.

Laboratory and Imaging Studies

Thrombocytopenia (usually <100,000 cells/mm^3), anemia, hyponatremia, and elevated hepatic transaminase levels are common laboratory findings. Organisms can be detected in skin biopsy specimens by fluorescent antibodies or polymerase chain reaction, although this test is not widely available. Serologic testing is used to confirm the diagnosis, although treatment is begun before confirmation.

Differential Diagnosis

The differential diagnosis includes meningococcemia, bacterial sepsis, toxic shock syndrome, leptospirosis, ehrlichiosis, measles, enteroviruses, infectious mononucleosis, collagen vascular diseases, Henoch-Schönlein purpura, and idiopathic thrombocytopenic purpura. The diagnosis of Rocky Mountain spotted fever should be suspected with fever and petechial rash, especially with a history of a tick bite or outdoor activities during spring and summer in endemic regions. Fever, headache, and myalgias lasting more than 1 week in patients in endemic areas indicate Rocky Mountain spotted fever. Delayed diagnosis and late treatment usually result from atypical initial symptoms and late appearance of the rash.

Treatment

Therapy for suspected Rocky Mountain spotted fever should not be postponed pending results of diagnostic tests. Doxycycline is the drug of choice, even for young children, despite the theoretical risk of dental staining in children younger than 9 years of age. Fluoroquinolones also are active against *R. rickettsii* and may be an alternative treatment.

Complications and Prognosis

In severe infections, capillary leakage results in noncardiogenic pulmonary edema (acute respiratory distress syndrome), hypotension, disseminated intravascular coagulation, circulatory collapse, and multiple organ failure, including encephalitis, myocarditis, hepatitis, and renal failure.

Untreated illness may persist for 3 weeks before progressing to multisystem involvement. The mortality rate is 25% without treatment, which is reduced to 3.4% with treatment. Permanent sequelae are common after severe disease.

Prevention

Preventive measures to avoid tick-borne infections and careful removal of ticks are recommended.

EHRLICHIOSIS (*EHRLICHIA CHAFFEENSIS*) AND ANAPLASMOSIS (*ANAPLASMA PHAGOCYTOPHILUM*)
Etiology

The term **ehrlichiosis** often is used to refer to all forms of infection with *Ehrlichia*. **Human monocytic ehrlichiosis** is caused by *E. chaffeensis,* which infects predominantly monocytic cells and is transmitted by the tick *A. americanum.* Disease may also be caused by *Ehrlichia ewingii*. **Human anaplasmosis** is caused by *A. phagocytophilum* and is transmitted by the tick *I. scapularis.*

Epidemiology

Ehrlichiosis occurs commonly in the United States. Human monocytic ehrlichiosis occurs in broad areas across the southeastern, south central, and Mid-Atlantic United States in a distribution that parallels that of Rocky Mountain spotted fever. Anaplasmosis is found mostly in the northeastern and upper midwestern United States, but infections have now been identified in northern California, the Mid-Atlantic states, and broadly across Europe.

Clinical Manifestations

Human monocytic ehrlichiosis, anaplasmosis, and *Ehrlichiosis ewingii* cause similar acute febrile illness characterized by fever, malaise, headache, myalgias, anorexia, and nausea, but often without a rash. In contrast to adult patients, nearly two thirds of children with human monocytic ehrlichiosis present with a macular or maculopapular rash, although petechial lesions may occur. Symptoms usually last for 4 to 12 days.

Laboratory and Imaging Studies

Characteristic laboratory findings include leukopenia, lymphocytopenia, thrombocytopenia, anemia, and elevated hepatic transaminases. Morulae are found infrequently in circulating monocytes of persons with human monocytic ehrlichiosis but are found in 40% of circulating neutrophils in 20% to 60% of persons with anaplasmosis (Fig. 122-2). Seroconversion or fourfold rise in antibody titer confirms the diagnosis.

Differential Diagnosis

Ehrlichiosis is clinically similar to other arthropod-borne infections, including Rocky Mountain spotted fever, tularemia, babesiosis, early Lyme disease, murine typhus, relapsing fever, and Colorado tick fever. The differential diagnosis also includes infectious mononucleosis, Kawasaki disease, endocarditis, viral infections, hepatitis, leptospirosis, Q fever, collagen vascular diseases, and leukemia.

Treatment

As with Rocky Mountain spotted fever, therapy for suspected ehrlichiosis should not be postponed pending results of diagnostic tests. Ehrlichiosis and anaplasmosis are treated with doxycycline.

Figure 122-2 A morula (*arrowhead*) containing *Anaplasma phagocytophilum* in a neutrophil. *Ehrlichia chaffeensis* and *A. phagocytophilum* have similar morphologies but are serologically and genetically distinct. (Wright stain, original magnification X 1200.) (*From Walker DH, Dumler JS: Ehrlichia chaffeensis (human monocytotropic ehrlichiosis), Anaplasma phagocytophilum (human granulocytotropic anaplasmosis), and other ehrlichieae. In Mandell GL, Bennett JE, Dolin R, editors: Principles and Practice of Infectious Diseases, ed 6, Philadelphia, 2005, Churchill Livingstone, Fig. 190-2, p 2315.*)

Complications and Prognosis

Severe pulmonary involvement with acute respiratory distress syndrome has been reported in several cases. Other reported severe complications include meningoencephalitis and myocarditis. Most patients improve within 48 hours.

Prevention

Preventive measures to avoid tick-borne infections and careful removal of ticks are recommended.

Chapter 123

PARASITIC DISEASES

PROTOZOAL DISEASES

Protozoa are the simplest organisms of the animal kingdom. They are unicellular. Most are free living, but some have a commensal or parasitic existence. Protozoal diseases include malaria, toxoplasmosis, babesiosis, and the intestinal protozoal diseases, amebiasis, cryptosporidiosis, and giardiasis.

Malaria
Etiology

Malaria is caused by obligate intracellular protozoa of the genus *Plasmodium*, including *P. falciparum, P. malariae, P. ovale, P. vivax,* and *P. knowlesi. Plasmodium* has a complex life cycle that enables survival in different cellular environments in the human host and in the mosquito vector. There are two major phases in the life cycle, an **asexual phase (schizogony)** in humans and a **sexual phase (sporogony)** in mosquitoes. The **erythrocytic phase** of *Plasmodium* asexual development begins when the merozoites released from exoerythrocytic schizonts in the liver penetrate erythrocytes. When inside the erythrocyte, the parasite transforms into the **ring form,** which enlarges to become a **trophozoite.** These latter two forms can be identified with Giemsa stain on blood smear, which is the primary means of confirming the diagnosis of malaria.

The parasites usually are transmitted to humans by female *Anopheles* mosquitoes. Malaria also can be transmitted through blood transfusion via contaminated needles and transplacentally to a fetus.

Epidemiology

Malaria is a worldwide problem with transmission in more than 100 countries with a combined population of more than 1.6 billion people. Malaria is an important cause of fever and morbidity in the tropical world. The principal areas of transmission are sub-Saharan Africa, southern Asia, Southeast Asia, Mexico, Haiti, the Dominican Republic, Central and South America, Papua New Guinea, and the Solomon Islands. Approximately 1000 to 2000 imported cases are recognized annually in the United States, with most cases occurring among infected foreign civilians from endemic areas who travel to the United States and among U.S. citizens who travel to endemic areas without appropriate chemoprophylaxis.

Clinical Manifestations

Decision-Making Algorithm
Available @ StudentConsult.com

Fever of Unknown Origin

The clinical manifestations of malaria range from asymptomatic infection to fulminant illness and death, depending on the virulence of the infecting malaria species and the host immune response. The incubation period ranges from 6 to 30 days, depending on the *Plasmodium* species (Table 123-1). The most characteristic clinical feature of malaria, which is seldom noted with other infectious diseases, is **febrile paroxysms** alternating with periods of fatigue but otherwise relative wellness. The classic symptoms of the febrile paroxysms of malaria include high fever, rigors, sweats, and headache. Paroxysms coincide with the rupture of schizonts that occur every 48 hours with *P. vivax* and *P. ovale* (**tertian periodicity**) and every 72 hours with *P. malariae* (**quartan periodicity**).

Short-term relapse describes the recurrence of symptoms after a primary attack that is due to the survival of erythrocyte forms in the bloodstream. **Long-term relapse** describes the renewal of symptoms long after the primary attack, usually due to the release of merozoites from an exoerythrocytic source in the liver. Long-term relapse occurs with *P. vivax* and *P. ovale* because of persistence in the liver and with *P. malariae* because of persistence in the erythrocyte.

Laboratory and Imaging Studies

The diagnosis of malaria is established by the identification of organisms on stained smears of peripheral blood. In nonimmune persons, symptoms typically occur 1 to 2 days before parasites are detectable on blood smear. Although *P. falciparum* is most likely to be identified from blood during a febrile paroxysm, the timing of the smears is less important than obtaining smears several times each day over 3 successive days. Both thick and thin blood smears should be examined. The concentration of erythrocytes on a **thick smear** is approximately 20 to 40 times greater than that on a **thin smear**. Thick smears are used to scan large numbers of erythrocytes quickly. Thin smears allow for positive identification of the malaria species and determination of the percentage of infected erythrocytes, which also is useful in following the response to therapy. Rapid diagnostic tests may emerge as point of care tests in the near future.

Differential Diagnosis

The most important aspect of diagnosing malaria in children is to consider the possibility of malaria in any child who has fever, chills, splenomegaly, anemia, or decreased level of consciousness with a history of recent travel or residence in an endemic area, regardless of the use of chemoprophylaxis. The differential diagnosis is broad and includes many infectious diseases, such as typhoid fever, tuberculosis, brucellosis, relapsing fever, infective endocarditis, influenza, poliomyelitis, yellow fever, trypanosomiasis, kala-azar, and amebic liver abscess.

Table 123-1	Characteristics of *Plasmodium* Species Causing Malaria				
CHARACTERISTIC	**P. FALCIPARUM**	**P. VIVAX**	**P. OVALE**	**P. MALARIAE**	**P. KNOWLESI**
Exoerythrocytic cycle	5.5–7 days	6–8 days	9 days	12–16 days	8-9 days
Erythrocytic cycle	48 hours	42–48 hours	49–50 hours	72 hours	24 hours
Usual incubation period (range)	12 days (9–14 days)	13 days (12–17 days; may be longer)	17 days (16–18 days; may be longer)	28 days (18–40 days; may be longer)	~12 days
Erythrocyte preference	Young erythrocytes, but can infect all	Reticulocytes	Reticulocytes	Older erythrocytes	Older erythrocytes
Usual parasite load (% erythrocytes infected)	≥1–5	1–2	1–2	1–2	Variable
Secondary exoerythrocytic cycle (hypnozoites) and relapses	Absent	Present	Present	Absent	Absent
Duration of untreated infection	1–2 years	1.5–4 years (includes liver stage)	1.5–4 years (includes liver stage)	3–50 years	Unknown
Severity of primary attack	Severe in nonimmune forms; subpatent patients—**a medical emergency**—failure to recognize and treat can lead to death	Mild to severe—danger of splenic rupture, relapse related to persistence of latent exoerythrocytic forms	Mild—danger of splenic rupture, relapse related to persistence of latent exoerythrocytic forms	Can be chronic in subclinical and subpatent forms; can cause nephritis in children	Variable, can be fatal
Usual periodicity of febrile attacks	None	48 hours	48 hours	72 hours	24 hours
Duration of febrile paroxysm	16–36 hours (may be longer)	8–12 hours	8–12 hours	8–10 hours	Unknown

Adapted from Strickland GT: Malaria. In Strickland GT, editor: Hunter's Tropical Medicine, ed 7, Philadelphia, 1991, WB Saunders, p 589.

Treatment

Oral chloroquine is the recommended treatment except for chloroquine-resistant *P. falciparum*. Either atovaquone-proguanil (Malarone) or artemether-lumefantrine (Coartem) is an appropriate first-line therapy for malaria acquired in areas of chloroquine resistance. Specific treatment should be guided by where the patient acquired the infection and the local resistance patterns. Patients with malaria usually require hospitalization and may require intensive care unit admission. Quinidine gluconate is the only drug available in the United States that is used for parenteral treatment.

Complications and Prognosis

Cerebral malaria is a complication of *P. falciparum* infection and a frequent cause of death (20% to 40% of cases), especially among children and nonimmune adults. Similar to other complications, cerebral malaria is more likely to occur among patients with intense parasitemia (>5%). Other complications include splenic rupture, renal failure, severe hemolysis (**blackwater fever),** pulmonary edema, hypoglycemia, thrombocytopenia, and **algid malaria** (sepsis syndrome with vascular collapse).

Death may occur with any of the malarial species but is most frequent with complicated *P. falciparum* malaria. The likelihood of death is increased in children with preexisting health problems, such as measles, intestinal parasites, schistosomiasis, anemia, and malnutrition. Death is much more common in developing countries.

Prevention

There are two components of malaria prevention: reduction of exposure to infected mosquitoes and chemoprophylaxis. Mosquito protection is necessary because no prophylactic regimen can guarantee protection in every instance due to the widespread development of resistant organisms.

Chemoprophylaxis is necessary for all visitors to and residents of the tropics who have not lived there since infancy. Children of nonimmune women should have chemoprophylaxis from birth. Children of women from endemic areas have passive immunity until 3 to 6 months of age, after which they are increasingly likely to acquire malaria. Specific chemoprophylaxis should be guided by the distribution of resistance pattern and determined before making specific recommendations (http://www.cdc.gov/malaria/travelers/country_table/a.html). Mefloquine, doxycycline, chloroquine, and Malarone are commonly prescribed medications.

Toxoplasmosis

Decision-Making Algorithms
Available @ StudentConsult.com

Splenomegaly
Lymphadenopathy
Petechiae/Purpura
Fever of Unknown Origin

Toxoplasmosis is a zoonosis caused by *Toxoplasma gondii,* an intracellular protozoan parasite. Infection is acquired by infectious oocysts, such as those excreted by newly infected cats, which play an important role in amplifying the organism in nature, or from ingesting cysts in contaminated, undercooked meat. Less commonly, transmission occurs transplacentally during acute infection of pregnant women. In the United States, the incidence of congenital infection is 1 to 2 per 1000 live births.

Acquired toxoplasmosis is usually asymptomatic. Symptomatic infection is typically a heterophile-negative mononucleosis syndrome that includes lymphadenopathy, fever, and hepatosplenomegaly. Disseminated infection, including myocarditis, pneumonia, and central nervous system (CNS) toxoplasmosis, is more common among immunocompromised persons, especially persons with acquired immunodeficiency syndrome (AIDS). Among women infected during pregnancy, 40% to 60% give birth to an infected infant. The later in pregnancy that infection occurs, the more likely it is that the fetus will be infected, but the less severe the illness (see Chapter 66). Serologic diagnosis can be established by a fourfold increase in antibody titer or seroconversion, a positive IgM antibody titer, or positive polymerase chain reaction for *T. gondii* in peripheral white blood cells, cerebrospinal fluid (CSF), serum, or amniotic fluid.

Treatment includes pyrimethamine and sulfadiazine, which act synergistically against *Toxoplasma*. Because these compounds are folic acid inhibitors, they are used in conjunction with folinic acid. Spiramycin, which is not licensed in the United States, also is used in therapy of pregnant women with toxoplasmosis. Corticosteroids are reserved for patients with acute CNS or ocular infection.

Ingesting only well-cooked meat and avoiding cats or soil in areas where cats defecate are prudent measures for pregnant or immunocompromised persons. Administration of spiramycin to infected pregnant women has been associated with lower risks of congenital infection in their offspring.

HELMINTHIASES

Helminths are divided into three groups: roundworms, or nematodes, and two groups of flatworms, the trematodes (flukes) and the cestodes (tapeworms).

Hookworm Infections

Hookworm infection is caused by several species of hookworms, with *Ancylostoma duodenale* and *Necator americanus* being the most important (Table 123-2). There are more than 9 million humans worldwide infected with hookworms. *Ancylostoma duodenale* is the predominant species in Europe, the Mediterranean region, northern Asia, and the west coast of South America. *N. americanus* predominates in the Western hemisphere, sub-Saharan Africa, Southeast Asia, and the Pacific Islands. Optimal soil conditions and fecal contamination are found in many agrarian tropical countries and in the southeastern United States. Infection typically occurs in young children, especially during the first decade of life. The larvae are found in warm, damp soil and infect humans by penetrating the skin. They migrate to the lungs, ascend the trachea, are swallowed, and reside in the intestine. The worms mature and attach to the intestinal wall, where they suck blood and shed eggs.

Table 123-2	Major Pediatric Syndromes Caused by Parasitic Nematodes		
SYNDROME	**ETIOLOGIC AGENT**	**TRANSMISSION**	**TREATMENT**
Hookworm iron deficiency	*Ancylostoma duodenale*	Larval ingestion and penetration	Albendazole *or* mebendazole *or* pyrantel pamoate
	Necator americanus	Larval penetration	
Cutaneous larva migrans	*Ancylostoma braziliense* (azoonotic hookworm)	Larval penetration (and failure to migrate)	Albendazole *or* ivermectin *or* thiabendazole topically
Infant ancylostomiasis	*A. duodenale*	Perinatal (?)	Albendazole *or* mebendazole *or* pyrantel pamoate
Trichuris dysentery or colitis	*Trichuris trichiura*	Egg ingestion	Mebendazole *or* albendazole *or* pyrantel pamoate and oxantel pamoate
Intestinal ascariasis	*Ascaris lumbricoides*	Ingestion of *Ascaris* eggs	Albendazole *or* mebendazole *or* pyrantel pamoate
Visceral larva migrans	*Toxocara canis*	Egg ingestion	Albendazole *or* mebendazole
Ocular larva migrans	*Toxocara cati* *Baylisascaris procyonis*		
Diarrhea, malabsorption (celiac-like)	*Strongyloides stercoralis*	Larval penetration	Ivermectin *or* thiabendazole
Swollen belly syndrome	*Strongyloides fuelleborni*	Perinatal	Ivermectin *or* thiabendazole
Pinworm	*Enterobius vermicularis*	Ingestion of embryonated eggs	Albendazole *or* mebendazole *or* pyrantel pamoate
Trichinellosis	*Trichinella spiralis*	Ingestion of infected undercooked meat	Mebendazole *or* albendazole *plus* corticosteroids for severe symptoms
Abdominal angiostrongyliasis	*Angiostrongylus costaricensis*	Ingestion of contaminated food	Mebendazole *or* thiabendazole
Eosinophilic meningitis	*Angiostrongylus cantonensis* (rat lungworm)	Ingestion of undercooked contaminated seafood	Mebendazole

Infections are usually asymptomatic. Intense pruritus (*ground itch*) occurs at the site of larval penetration, usually the soles of the feet or between the toes, and may include papules and vesicles. Migration of larvae through the lungs usually is asymptomatic. Symptoms of abdominal pain, anorexia, indigestion, fullness, and diarrhea occur with hookworm infestation. The major manifestation of infection is anemia. Examination of fresh stool for hookworm eggs is diagnostic. Therapy includes anthelmintic treatment with albendazole, mebendazole, or pyrantel pamoate and treatment for anemia. Eradication depends on sanitation of the patient's environment and chemotherapy.

Ascariasis

Ascariasis is caused by *Ascaris lumbricoides,* a large nematode. It is the most prevalent helminthiasis, affecting 1 billion people (see Table 123-2). After humans ingest the eggs, larvae are released and penetrate the intestine, migrate to the lungs, ascend the trachea, and are swallowed. On entering the intestines again, they mature and produce eggs that are excreted in the stool and are deposited in the soil, where they survive for prolonged periods.

Manifestations may be the result of migration of the larvae to other sites of the body or the presence of adult worms in the intestine. **Pulmonary ascariasis** occurs as the larvae migrate through the lung, producing cough, blood-stained sputum, eosinophilia, and transient infiltrates on chest x-ray films.

Adult larvae in the small intestine may cause abdominal pain and distention. Intestinal obstruction from adult worms rarely occurs. Migration of worms into the bile duct may rarely cause acute biliary obstruction. Examination of fresh stool for characteristic eggs is diagnostic. Effective control depends on adequate sanitary treatment and disposal of infected human feces.

Visceral Larva Migrans

Visceral larva migrans is a systemic nematodiasis caused by ingestion of the eggs of the dog tapeworm, *Toxocara canis,* or, less commonly, the cat tapeworm, *Toxocara cati,* or the raccoon tapeworm, *Baylisascaris procyonis* (see Table 123-2). These organisms also cause **ocular larva migrans.**

Visceral larva migrans is most common in young children with pica who have dogs or cats as pets. Ocular toxocariasis occurs in older children. The eggs of these roundworms are produced by adult worms residing in the dog and cat intestine. Ingested eggs hatch into larvae that penetrate the gastrointestinal tract and migrate to the liver, lung, eye, CNS, and heart, where they die and calcify.

Symptoms of visceral larva migrans are the result of the number of migrating worms and the associated immune response. Light infections are often asymptomatic. Symptoms include fever, cough, wheezing, and seizures. Physical findings may include hepatomegaly, crackles, rash, and lymphadenopathy. Visual symptoms may include decreased acuity, strabismus, periorbital edema, or blindness. Eye examination

Table 123-3	Major Pediatric Syndromes Caused by Parasitic Trematodes		
SYNDROME	**ETIOLOGIC AGENT**	**TRANSMISSION**	**TREATMENT**
Schistosomiases		Freshwater contact with penetration through the skin	
Intestinal or hepatic schistosomiasis	Schistosoma mansoni		Praziquantel or oxamniquine
	Schistosoma japonicum		Praziquantel
	Schistosoma mekongi		Praziquantel Praziquantel
	Schistosoma haematobium		
Urinary schistosomiasis			
Parasitoses due to other trematodes		Ingestion of raw or inadequately cooked foods	
Clonorchiasis	Clonorchis sinensis (Chinese liver fluke)		Praziquantel or albendazole
Fascioliasis	Fasciola hepatica (sheep liver fluke)		Triclabendazole or bithionol
Fasciolopsiasis	Fasciolopsis buski		Praziquantel
Heterophyiasis	Heterophyes heterophyes		Praziquantel
Metagonimiasis	Metagonimus yokogawai		Praziquantel
Metorchiasis	Metorchis conjunctus (North American liver fluke)		Praziquantel
Nanophyetiasis	Nanophyetus salmincola (salmon fluke)		Praziquantel
Opisthorchiasis	Opisthorchis viverrini (Southeast Asian liver fluke)		Praziquantel
Paragonimiasis	Paragonimus westermani, P. miyazaki, P. mexicanus, P. kellicotti, P. uterobilateralis, P. skjabini, P. hueitungensis, P. heterotrema, P. africanus (lung flukes)		Praziquantel or bithionol

may reveal granulomatous lesions near the macula or disc. Ocular larva migrans is characterized by isolated, unilateral ocular disease and no systemic findings. Larvae probably enter the anterior vitreous of the eye from a peripheral branch of the retinal artery and elicit granulomas in the posterior and peripheral poles that cause vision loss.

Eosinophilia and hypergammaglobulinemia associated with elevated isohemagglutinin levels suggest the diagnosis, which is confirmed by serology (enzyme-linked immunosorbent assay) or, less commonly, by biopsy. This is usually a self-limited illness. In severe disease, albendazole or mebendazole is used. Deworming puppies and kittens, major excreters of eggs, decreases the risk of infection.

Enterobiasis (Pinworm)

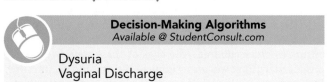

Decision-Making Algorithms
Available @ StudentConsult.com

Dysuria
Vaginal Discharge

Pinworm is caused by *Enterobius vermicularis,* a nematode that is distributed worldwide. Enterobiasis affects individuals at all socioeconomic levels, especially children. Crowded living conditions predispose to infection. Humans ingest the eggs carried on hands, present in house dust or on bedclothes. The eggs hatch in the stomach, and the larvae migrate to the cecum and mature. At night the females migrate to the perianal area to lay their eggs, which are viable for 2 days.

The most common symptoms are nocturnal anal pruritus **(pruritus ani)** and sleeplessness, presumably resulting from the migratory female worms. Vaginitis and salpingitis may develop secondary to aberrant worm migration. The eggs are detected by microscopically examining adhesive cellophane tape pressed against the anus in the morning to collect eggs. Less commonly, a worm may be seen in the perianal region. Treatment is with albendazole (400 mg), mebendazole (100 mg), or pyrantel pamoate (11 mg/kg, maximum 1 g) each given as a single oral dose and repeated in 2 weeks.

Schistosomiasis

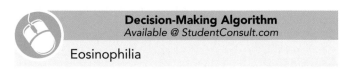

Decision-Making Algorithm
Available @ StudentConsult.com

Eosinophilia

Schistosomiasis (bilharziasis) is caused by flukes that parasitize the bloodstream, including *Schistosoma haematobium, Schistosoma mansoni, Schistosoma japonicum,* and, rarely, *Schistosoma intercalatum* and *Schistosoma mekongi* (Table 123-3). Schistosomiasis affects more than 2 million people, mainly children and young adults with a peak age range of 10 to 20 years. Humans are infected by cercariae in contaminated water that emerge in an infectious form from snails and penetrate intact skin. Each adult worm migrates to specific sites: *S. haematobium* to the **bladder plexus** and *S. intercalatum* and *S. mekongi* to the **mesenteric vessels.** The eggs are deposited by the adult flukes in urine (*S. haematobium*) or stool (*S. mansoni*

Table 123-4	Major Pediatric Syndromes Caused by Parasitic Cestodes		
SYNDROME	**ETIOLOGIC AGENT**	**TRANSMISSION**	**TREATMENT**
Echinococcosis		Ingestion of *Echinococcus* eggs	
Unilocular	*Echinococcus granulosus*		Surgical resection *plus* albendazole
Echinococcosis	*Echinococcus granulosus* var. *canadensis*		Expectant observation
Alveolar echinococcosis	*Echinococcus multilocularis*		Surgical resection is only reliable means of treatment; some reports suggest adjunct use of albendazole or mebendazole
Neurocysticercosis	Larval stage of *Taenia solium* (cysticerci)	Ingestion of infected raw/undercooked pork	Albendazole *or* praziquantel
Adult tapeworm infections	*T. solium* (pork tapeworm)	Ingestion of contaminated raw/undercooked pork	Praziquantel
	Hymenolepis diminuta	Fecal-oral transmission	Praziquantel
	Hymenolepis nana	Fecal-oral	Praziquantel

and *S. japonicum*). *S. haematobium* is prevalent in Africa and the Middle East; *S. mansoni* in Africa, the Middle East, the Caribbean, and South America; *S. japonicum* in China, the Philippines, and Indonesia; *S. mekongi* in the Far East; and *S. intercalatum* in West Africa.

The manifestations of schistosomiasis result from eggs that are trapped at the site of deposition or at metastatic locations. Within 3 to 12 weeks of infection, while the worms are maturing, a syndrome of fever, malaise, cough, abdominal pain, and rash can occur. This syndrome is followed by a resultant inflammatory response that leads to further symptoms. **Katayama fever** is an acute condition, with fever, weight loss, hepatosplenomegaly, and eosinophilia. Eggs may be found in the urine (*S. haematobium*) or stool (*S. mansoni* and *S. japonicum*) of infected individuals. Sanitary measures, molluscacides, and therapy for infected individuals may help control the illness.

Echinococcosis

Echinococcosis includes **hydatid or unilocular cyst disease,** caused by *Echinococcus granulosus* (the **minute dog tapeworm**) or *Echinococcus vogeli,* and **alveolar cyst disease,** caused by *Echinococcus multilocularis* (Table 123-4). Dogs become infected with tapeworms by eating infected sheep or cattle viscera and excrete eggs in their stools. Humans acquire echinococcosis by ingesting eggs and become an intermediate host. The eggs hatch in the intestinal tract, and the larva **(oncospheres)** penetrate the mucosa and enter the circulation to pass to the liver and other visceral organs, forming cysts 2 cm in diameter.

E. granulosus has a worldwide distribution and is endemic in sheep-raising and cattle-raising areas of Australia, South America, South Africa, the former Soviet Union, and the Mediterranean region. The prevalence is highest in children. Symptoms caused by *E. granulosus* result from space-occupying cysts. Pulmonary cysts may cause hemoptysis, cough, dyspnea, and respiratory distress. Brain cysts appear as tumors; liver cysts cause problems as they compress and obstruct blood flow. Ultrasonography identifies cystic lesions, and the diagnosis is confirmed by serologic testing. Large or asymptomatic granulosa cysts are removed surgically. Treatment with albendazole has shown some benefit.

Neurocysticercosis

Neurocysticercosis is caused by infection with the larval stages **(cysticerci)** of the **pork tapeworm,** *Taenia solium,* and is the most frequent helminthic infection of the CNS (see Table 123-4). Humans are infected after consuming cysticerci in raw or undercooked larva-containing pork. *T. solium* is endemic in Asia, Africa, and Central and South Americas.

Cysts typically enlarge slowly, causing no or minimal symptoms for years or decades until the organism begins to die. The cyst then begins to swell, and leakage of antigen incites an inflammatory response, resulting in the presenting signs of focal or generalized seizures and calcified cerebral cysts identified by computed tomography or magnetic resonance imaging. The CSF shows lymphocytic or eosinophilic pleocytosis. The diagnosis is confirmed by serologic testing. Neurocysticercosis is treated with albendazole or praziquantel, corticosteroids for concomitant cerebral inflammation from cyst death, and anticonvulsant drugs.

Chapter **124**

TUBERCULOSIS

ETIOLOGY

Mycobacterium tuberculosis are pleomorphic, weakly gram-positive curved rods. Mycobacteria are **acid fast,** which is the capacity to form stable mycolate complexes with arylmethane dyes. Mycobacteria grow slowly; culture from clinical specimens on solid synthetic media usually takes 3 to 6 weeks. Drug-susceptibility testing requires an additional 4 weeks. Growth can be detected in 1 to 3 weeks in selective liquid media using radiolabeled nutrients. Polymerase chain reaction (PCR) of clinical specimens allows rapid diagnosis in many laboratories.

EPIDEMIOLOGY

An estimated 10 to 15 million persons in the United States have latent tuberculosis infection (infection with *M. tuberculosis* and no disease). Without treatment, tuberculosis *disease* develops in 5% to 10% of immunologically normal adults with tuberculosis *infection* at some time during their lives; the risk is higher in infants. An estimated 8 million new cases of tuberculosis occur each year among adults worldwide. Three million deaths are attributed to the disease annually. In developing countries, 1.3 million new cases of the disease occur in children under 15 years of age, and 450,000 children die each year of tuberculosis. Most children with tuberculosis infection and disease acquire *M. tuberculosis* from an infectious adult.

Transmission of *M. tuberculosis* is from person to person, usually by **respiratory droplets** that become airborne when the ill individual coughs, sneezes, laughs, sighs, or breathes. Infected droplets dry and become **droplet nuclei,** which may remain suspended in the air for hours, long after the infectious person has left the environment.

Several patient-related factors are associated with an increased chance of transmission. Of these a positive acid-fast smear of the sputum most closely correlates with infectivity. Children with primary pulmonary tuberculosis disease rarely, if ever, infect other children or adults. Tubercle bacilli are relatively sparse in the endobronchial secretions of children with primary pulmonary tuberculosis, and a significant cough is usually lacking. When young children cough, they rarely produce sputum, lacking the tussive force necessary to project and suspend infectious particles of the requisite size. Hospitalized children with suspected pulmonary tuberculosis are placed initially in respiratory isolation. Most infectious patients become noninfectious within 2 weeks of starting effective treatment, and many become noninfectious within several days.

In North America, tuberculosis rates are highest in foreign-born persons from high-prevalence countries, residents of prisons, residents of nursing homes, homeless persons, users of illegal drugs, persons who are poor and medically indigent, health care workers, and children exposed to adults in high-risk groups. Among U.S. urban dwellers with tuberculosis, persons with acquired immunodeficiency syndrome (AIDS) and racial minorities are overrepresented. Most children are infected with *M. tuberculosis* from household contacts, but outbreaks of childhood tuberculosis centered in elementary and high schools, nursery schools, family day care homes, churches, school buses, and stores still occur. A high-risk adult working in the area has been the source of the outbreak in most cases.

CLINICAL MANIFESTATIONS

Decision-Making Algorithms
Available @ StudentConsult.com

Cough
Hemoptysis
Back Pain
Fever and Rash
Lymphadenopathy
Fever of Unknown Origin

Latent tuberculosis describes the asymptomatic stage of infection with *M. tuberculosis.* The tuberculin skin test (TST) is positive, but the chest radiograph is normal, and there are no signs or symptoms of illness. **Tuberculosis disease** occurs when there are clinical signs and symptoms or an abnormal chest radiograph. The term *tuberculosis* usually refers to the disease. The interval between latent tuberculosis and the onset of disease may be several weeks or many decades in adults. In young children, tuberculosis usually develops as an immediate complication of the primary infection, and the distinction between infection and disease may be less obvious.

Primary pulmonary tuberculosis in older infants and children is usually an asymptomatic infection. Often the disease is manifested by a positive TST with minimal abnormalities on the chest radiograph, such as an infiltrate with hilar lymphadenopathy or **Ghon complex.** Hilar lymphadenopathy may compress the bronchi or trachea malaise, low-grade fever, erythema nodosum, or symptoms resulting from lymph node enlargement may occur after the development of delayed hypersensitivity.

Lymphadenopathy is common in primary pulmonary disease. Hilar lymphadenopathy may compress the bronchi or trachea. The most common extrathoracic sites of lymphadenitis are the cervical, supraclavicular, and submandibular areas **(scrofula).**

Progressive primary disease is characterized by a primary pneumonia that develops shortly after initial infection. Progression to pulmonary disease, disseminated miliary disease, or progression of central nervous system (CNS) granulomas to meningitis occurs most commonly in the first year of life.

Tuberculous pleural effusion, which may accompany primary infection, generally represents the immune response to the organisms and most commonly occurs in older children or adolescents. Pleurocentesis reveals lymphocytes and an increased protein level, but the pleural fluid usually does not contain bacilli.

Reactivation pulmonary tuberculosis, common in adolescents and typical in adults, usually is confined to apical segments of upper lobes or superior segments of lower lobes. There is usually little lymphadenopathy and no extrathoracic infection because of established hypersensitivity. This is a manifestation of a secondary expansion of infection at a site seeded years previously during primary infection. Advanced disease is associated with cavitation and endobronchial spread of bacilli. Symptoms include fever, night sweats, malaise, and weight loss. A productive cough and hemoptysis often herald cavitation and bronchial erosion.

Miliary tuberculosis refers to widespread hematogenous dissemination to multiple organs. The lesions are of roughly the same size as a millet seed, from which the name *miliary* is derived. Miliary tuberculosis is characterized by fever, general malaise, weight loss, lymphadenopathy, night sweats, and hepatosplenomegaly. Diffuse bilateral pneumonitis is common, and meningitis may be present. The chest radiograph reveals bilateral miliary infiltrates, showing overwhelming infection. The TST may be nonreactive as a result of **anergy.** Liver or bone marrow biopsy is useful for the diagnosis.

Tuberculous meningitis most commonly occurs in children under 5 years old and often within 6 months of primary infection. Tubercle bacilli that seed the meninges during the primary infection replicate, triggering an inflammatory response. This condition may have an insidious onset, initially characterized by low-grade fever, headache, and subtle personality change. Progression of the infection results in basilar meningitis with impingement of the cranial nerves and is manifested by meningeal irritation and, eventually, increased intracranial pressure, deterioration of mental status, and coma. Computed tomography (CT) scans show hydrocephalus, edema, periventricular lucencies, and infarctions. Cerebrospinal fluid (CSF) analysis reveals pleocytosis (50 to 500 leukocytes/mm³), which early in the course of disease may be either lymphocytes or polymorphonuclear leukocytes. Glucose is low, and protein is significantly elevated. Acid-fast bacilli are not detected frequently in the CSF by either routine or fluorescent staining procedures. Although culture is the standard for diagnosis, PCR for *M. tuberculosis* is useful to confirm meningitis.

Skeletal tuberculosis results from either hematogenous seeding or direct extension from a **caseous lymph node.** This is usually a chronic disease with an insidious onset that may be mistaken for chronic osteomyelitis caused by *Staphylococcus aureus*. Radiographs reveal cortical destruction. Biopsy and culture are essential for proper diagnosis. Tuberculosis of the spine, **Pott's disease,** is the most common skeletal site followed by the hip as well as fingers and toes **(dactylitis).**

Other forms of tuberculosis include **abdominal tuberculosis** that occurs from swallowing infected material. This is a relatively uncommon complication in developed nations where dairy herds are inspected for bovine tuberculosis. **Tuberculous peritonitis** is associated with abdominal tuberculosis and presents as fever, anorexia, ascites, and abdominal pain. **Urogenital tuberculosis** is a late reactivation complication and is rare in children. Symptomatic illness presents as dysuria, frequency, urgency, hematuria, and *sterile* pyuria.

LABORATORY AND IMAGING STUDIES
Tuberculin Skin Test

Two types of tests are used to detect the immune response to *M. tuberculosis* and are used to screen patients for latent tuberculosis and investigation of active tuberculosis. The TST response to tuberculin antigen is a manifestation of a T cell–mediated delayed hypersensitivity. The **Mantoux test,** an intradermal injection of 5 TU (tuberculin units) of **purified protein derivative standard (PPD-S),** usually on the volar surface of the forearm, is the standard TST. It is usually positive 2 to 6 weeks after onset of infection (occasionally 3 months) and at the time of symptomatic illness. This test is preferred in children less than 5 years of age. It may also be used in other settings such as contact investigations or in older patients. Only persons at high risk should be offered a Mantoux test (Table 124-1). False-negative responses may occur early in the illness, with use of inactivated antigen (as a result of poor storage practice or inadequate administration), or as a result of immunosuppression (secondary to underlying illness, AIDS, malnutrition, or overwhelming tuberculosis). Tests with questionable results should be repeated after several weeks of therapy and adequate nutrition. Because of poor nutrition, a high proportion of internationally adopted children arriving in the United States have an initial false-positive TST. All internationally adopted children with an initially negative TST should have a repeat TST after 3 months in the United States. The TST is interpreted based on the host status and size of induration (Table 124-2).

Table 124-1 | Tuberculin Skin Test (TST) Recommendations for Infants, Children, and Adolescents*

CHILDREN FOR WHOM IMMEDIATE TST OR IGRA IS INDICATED:†

- Contacts of people with confirmed or suspected contagious tuberculosis (contact investigation)
- Children with radiographic or clinical findings suggesting tuberculosis disease
- Children immigrating from countries with endemic infection (e.g., Asia, Middle East, Africa, Latin America, countries of the former Soviet Union), including international adoptees
- Children with travel histories to countries with endemic infection and substantial contact with indigenous people from such countries

CHILDREN WHO SHOULD HAVE ANNUAL TST OR IGRA:‡

- Children infected with HIV infection (TST only)

CHILDREN AT INCREASED RISK OF PROGRESSION OF LTBI TO TUBERCULOSIS DISEASE:

Children with other medical conditions, including diabetes mellitus, chronic renal failure, malnutrition, and congenital or acquired immunodeficiencies deserve special consideration. Without recent exposure, these people are not at increased risk of acquiring tuberculosis infection. Underlying immune deficiencies associated with these conditions theoretically would enhance the possibility for progression to severe disease. Initial histories of potential exposure to tuberculosis should be included for all of these patients. If these histories or local epidemiologic factors suggest a possibility of exposure, immediate and periodic TST or IGRA should be considered. **An initial TST or IGRA should be performed before initiation of immunosuppressive therapy, including prolonged steroid administration, use of tumor necrosis factor-alpha antagonists, or other immunosuppressive therapy in any child requiring these treatments.**

Recommendations from American Academy of Pediatrics: Tuberculosis. In Pickering LK, Baker CJ, Kimberlin DW, et al, editors. Red Book: 2012 Report of the Committee on Infectious Diseases, ed 29, Elk Grove Village, IL, 2012, American Academy of Pediatrics.
HIV, Human immunodeficiency virus; IGRA, interferon-gamma release assay; LTBI, latent tuberculosis infection.
*Bacille Calmette-Guérin immunization is not a contraindication to a TST.
†Beginning as early as 3 months of age.
‡If the child is well, the TST or IGRA should be delayed for up to 10 weeks after return.

A whole blood test of interferon-gamma (INF-γ) release assay (IGRA), a cytokine elaborated by lymphocytes in response to tuberculosis antigens, is the recommended diagnostic test for persons older than 5 years of age in the United States. It has similar sensitivity as the TST but improved specificity because it is unaffected by prior bacille Calmette-Guérin vaccination.

Culture

The ultimate diagnostic confirmation relies on culture of the organism, a process that usually is more successful with tissue, such as pleura or pericardial membrane from biopsy, rather than pleural or pericardial fluid. Sputum is an excellent source for diagnosis in adults but is difficult to obtain in young children. Induced sputum or gastric fluid obtained via an indwelling nasogastric tube with samples taken before or immediately on waking contains swallowed sputum and provides appropriate samples in young children. Large volumes of fluid (CSF, pericardial fluid) yield a higher rate of recovery of organisms,

Table 124-2	Criteria for Positive Tuberculin Skin Test Results in Clinically Defined Pediatric Populations*
POSITIVE RESULT	**POPULATION(S)**
Induration ≥5 mm	Children in close contact with persons with known or suspected contagious tuberculosis disease
	Children suspected to have tuberculosis disease Findings on chest radiograph consistent with active or previously active tuberculosis Clinical evidence of tuberculosis disease†
	Children receiving immunosuppressive therapy‡ or with immunosuppressive conditions, including HIV infection
Induration ≥10 mm	Children at increased risk for disseminated disease
	Children <4 years of age Children with other medical conditions, including Hodgkin disease, lymphoma, diabetes mellitus, chronic renal failure, and malnutrition
	Children with increased exposure to tuberculosis disease Children born, or whose parents were born, in high-prevalence regions of the world Children frequently exposed to adults who are HIV-infected, homeless, users of illicit drugs, residents of nursing homes, incarcerated or institutionalized, or migrant farm workers Children who travel to high-prevalence regions of the world
Induration ≥15 mm	Children ≥4 years of age without any risk factors

*These criteria apply regardless of previous bacille Calmette-Guérin immunization. Erythema at tuberculin skin test site does not indicate a positive test result. Tuberculin reactions should be read at 48 to 72 hours after placement.
†Evidence by physical examination or laboratory assessment that would include tuberculosis in the working differential diagnosis (e.g., meningitis).
‡Including immunosuppressive doses of corticosteroids.

but slow growth of the mycobacteria makes culture less helpful in very ill children. When the organism is grown, drug susceptibilities should be determined because of the increasing incidence of resistant organisms.

Antigen detection and DNA probes have expedited diagnosis, especially with CNS disease.

Diagnostic Imaging

Because many cases of pulmonary tuberculosis in children are clinically relatively silent, radiography is a cornerstone for the diagnosis of disease. All lobar segments of the lung are at equal risk of being the focus of the initial infection. In 25% of cases, two or more lobes of the lungs are involved, although disease usually occurs at one site only. Spread of infection to regional lymph nodes occurs early.

The hallmark of childhood pulmonary tuberculosis is the relatively large size and importance of the hilar lymphadenitis compared with the less significant size of the initial parenchymal focus, together historically referred to as the **Ghon complex** (with or without calcification of the lymph nodes). Hilar lymphadenopathy is inevitably present with childhood tuberculosis. Partial bronchial obstruction caused by external compression from the enlarging nodes can cause air trapping, hyperinflation, and lobar emphysema. Occasionally children have a picture of lobar pneumonia without impressive hilar lymphadenopathy. If the infection is progressively destructive, liquefaction of the lung parenchyma leads to formation of a thin-walled primary tuberculous cavity. Adolescents with pulmonary tuberculosis may develop segmental lesions with hilar lymphadenopathy or the apical infiltrates, with or without cavitation, that are typical of adult reactivation tuberculosis.

Radiographic studies aid greatly in the diagnosis of **extrapulmonary tuberculosis** in children. Plain radiographs, CT, and magnetic resonance imaging (MRI) of the tuberculous spine usually show collapse and destruction of the vertebral body with narrowing of the involved disk spaces. Radiographic findings in bone and joint tuberculosis range from mild joint effusions and small lytic lesions to massive destruction of the bone.

In tuberculosis of the CNS, CT or MRI of the brains of patients with tuberculous meningitis may be normal during early stages of the infection. As disease progresses, basilar enhancement and communicating hydrocephalus with signs of cerebral edema or early focal ischemia are the most common findings.

DIFFERENTIAL DIAGNOSIS

The differential diagnosis of tuberculosis includes a multitude of diagnoses because tuberculosis may affect any organ, and in early disease the symptoms and signs may be nonspecific. In pulmonary disease, tuberculosis may appear similar to pneumonia, malignancy, and any systemic disease in which generalized lymphadenopathy occurs. The diagnosis of tuberculosis should be suspected if the TST or IGRA is positive or if there is history of tuberculosis in a close contact.

The differential diagnosis of tuberculous lymphadenopathy includes infections caused by atypical mycobacteria, catscratch disease, fungal infection, viral or bacterial disease, toxoplasmosis, sarcoidosis, drug reactions, and malignancy. The diagnosis may be confirmed by fine-needle aspiration but may necessitate excisional biopsy accompanied by appropriate histologic and microbiologic studies.

TREATMENT

The treatment of tuberculosis is affected by the presence of naturally occurring drug-resistant organisms in large bacterial populations, even before therapy is initiated, and the fact that mycobacteria replicate slowly and can remain dormant in the body for prolonged periods. Although a population of bacilli as a whole may be considered drug susceptible, a subpopulation of drug-resistant organisms occurs at fairly predictable frequencies of 10^5 to 10^7, depending on the drug. Cavities may contain 10^9 tubercle bacilli with thousands of organisms resistant to any one drug, but only rare organisms are resistant to multiple drugs.

Patients with latent tuberculosis infection have small bacterial populations and a single drug, such as isoniazid, can be

Table 124-3	Recommended Treatment Regimens for Drug-Susceptible Tuberculosis in Infants, Children, and Adolescents	
INFECTION OR DISEASE CATEGORY	**REGIMEN**	**COMMENTS**
LATENT TUBERCULOSIS INFECTION (POSITIVE TST RESULT, NO DISEASE)		
Isoniazid-susceptible	9 months of isoniazid, once a day	If daily therapy is not possible, DOT twice a week can be used for 9 months.
Isoniazid-resistant	6 months of rifampin, once a day	
Isoniazid-rifampin–resistant	Consult a tuberculosis specialist.	
Pulmonary and extrapulmonary (except meningitis)	2 months of isoniazid, rifampin, and pyrazinamide daily, followed by 4 months of isoniazid and rifampin twice weekly under DOT	If possible drug resistance is a concern, another drug (ethambutol or an aminoglycoside) is added to the initial three-drug therapy until drug susceptibilities are determined. DOT is highly desirable.
		If hilar lymphadenopathy only, a 6-month course of isoniazid and rifampin is sufficient.
		Drugs can be given 2 or 3 times per week under DOT in the initial phase if nonadherence is likely.
Meningitis	2 months of isoniazid, rifampin, pyrazinamide, and an aminoglycoside or ethionamide, once a day, followed by 7–10 months of isoniazid and	A fourth drug, usually an aminoglycoside, is given with initial therapy until drug susceptibility is known.
	rifampin, once a day or twice a week (9–12 months total)	For patients who may have acquired tuberculosis in geographic areas where resistance to streptomycin is common, capreomycin, kanamycin, or amikacin may be used instead of streptomycin.

Recommendations from Pickering LK, Baker CJ, Long SS, et al: Red Book: 2012 Report of the Committee on Infectious Diseases, ed 27, Elk Grove Village, IL, 2012, American Academy of Pediatrics.
DOT, Directly observed therapy; TST, tuberculin skin test.

given. Therapy for latent infection is aimed at eradicating the presumably small inoculum of organisms sequestered within macrophages and suppressed by normal T cell activity. To prevent reactivation of these latent bacilli, therapy with a single agent (usually isoniazid for 9 months) is suggested. Children with primary pulmonary tuberculosis and patients with extrapulmonary tuberculosis have medium-sized populations in which significant numbers of drug-resistant organisms may or may not be present. In general these patients are treated with at least two drugs (Table 124-3) for a prolonged course, typically 6 to 9, depending on the type of disease. Isoniazid and rifampin are bactericidal for *M. tuberculosis* and are effective against all populations of mycobacteria. Along with pyrazinamide, they form the backbone of the antimicrobial treatment of tuberculosis. Other drugs are used in special circumstances, such as tuberculous meningitis and antibiotic-resistant tuberculosis.

A 9-month regimen of isoniazid and rifampin cures greater than 98% of cases of drug-susceptible pulmonary tuberculosis. After daily administration for the first 1 to 2 months, both drugs can be given daily or twice weekly for the remaining 7 to 8 months, with equivalent results and low rates of adverse reactions. The addition of pyrazinamide for the first 2 months of the regimen reduces the total duration of treatment to 6 months and has similar efficacy. **Noncompliance**, or **nonadherence**, is a major problem in tuberculosis control because of the long-term nature of treatment and the sometimes difficult social circumstances of the patients. As treatment regimens become shorter, adherence assumes an even greater importance. Improvement in compliance occurs with **directly observed therapy**, which means that the health care worker is physically present when the medications are administered, and is the standard of care in most settings.

COMPLICATIONS AND PROGNOSIS

The prognosis of tuberculosis in infants, children, and adolescents is excellent with early recognition and effective chemotherapy. In most children with pulmonary tuberculosis, the disease completely resolves, and ultimately radiographic findings are normal. The prognosis for children with bone and joint tuberculosis and tuberculous meningitis depends directly on the stage of disease at the time antituberculosis medications are started. Tuberculosis of the spine may result in angulation or **gibbus** formation that requires surgical correction after the infection is cured. Most childhood tuberculous meningitis occurs in developing countries, where the prognosis is poor.

PREVENTION

Tuberculosis control programs involve case finding and treatment, which interrupts secondary transmission of infection from close contacts. Infected close contacts are identified by positive TST reactions and can be started on appropriate treatment to prevent transmission.

Prevention of transmission in health care settings involves appropriate physical ventilation of the air around the source case. Offices, clinics, and hospital rooms used by adults with possible tuberculosis should have adequate ventilation, with air exhausted to the outside (**negative-pressure ventilation**). Health care providers should have annual TSTs.

The only available vaccine against tuberculosis is the **bacille Calmette-Guérin vaccine.** The original vaccine organism was a strain of *Mycobacterium bovis* attenuated by subculture every 3 weeks for 13 years. The preferred route of administration is intradermal injection with a syringe and needle because this is the only method that permits accurate measurement of an individual dose. The official recommendation of the World Health Organization is a single dose administered during infancy. This vaccine is not routinely used in the United States. Some studies show bacille Calmette-Guérin to provide 80% to 90% protection from tuberculosis, and other studies show no protective efficacy at all. Many infants who receive bacille Calmette-Guérin vaccine never have a positive TST reaction. When a reaction does occur, the induration size is usually less than 10 mm, and the reaction wanes after several years.

Chapter 125

HIV AND AIDS

ETIOLOGY

The cause of acquired immunodeficiency syndrome (AIDS) is the human immunodeficiency virus (HIV), a single-stranded RNA virus of the retrovirus family that produces a **reverse transcriptase** enabling the viral RNA to act as a template for DNA transcription and integration into the host genome. HIV-1 causes 99% of all human cases. HIV-2, which is less virulent, causes 1% to 9% of cases in parts of Africa and is very rare in the United States.

HIV infects **helper T cells (CD4 cells)** and cells of monocyte-macrophage lineage via interaction of viral protein gp120 with the CD4 molecule and chemokines (CXCR4 on T cells and CCR5 on dendritic cells and macrophages) that serve as coreceptors. Interaction with these molecules facilitates membrane fusion and cell entry by the virus. HIV infection directly and indirectly depletes CD4 T cells. Because helper T cells are important for delayed hypersensitivity, T cell–dependent B cell antibody production, and T cell–mediated lymphokine activation of macrophages, their destruction produces a profound combined (B and T cell) immunodeficiency. A lack of T cell regulation and unrestrained antigenic stimulation result in polyclonal hypergammaglobulinemia with nonspecific and ineffective globulins. Other cells bearing CD4, such as microglia, astrocytes, oligodendroglia, and placental tissues also may be infected with HIV.

HIV infection is a continuously progressive process with a variable period of clinical latency before development of AIDS-defining conditions. All untreated patients have evidence of ongoing viral replication and progressive CD4 lymphocyte depletion. There are no overt manifestations of immunodeficiency until CD4 cell numbers decline to critical threshold levels. *Quantitation of the viral load has become an important parameter in management.*

Horizontal transmission of HIV is by sexual contact (vaginal, anal, or orogenital), percutaneous contact (from contaminated needles or other sharp objects), or mucous membrane exposure to contaminated blood or body fluid. Transmission by contaminated blood and blood products has been eliminated in developed countries but still occurs in developing countries. **Vertical transmission** of HIV from mother to infant may occur transplacentally in utero, during birth, or by breastfeeding. Risk factors for perinatal transmission include prematurity, rupture of membranes more than 4 hours, and high maternal circulating levels of HIV at delivery. Perinatal transmission can be decreased from approximately 25% to less than 8% with antiretroviral treatment of the mother before and during delivery and postnatal treatment of the infant. Breastfeeding by HIV-infected mothers increases the risk of vertical transmission by 30% to 50%. In untreated infants, the mean incubation interval for development of an AIDS-defining condition after vertical transmission is 5 months (range, 1 to 24 months) compared with a longer incubation period after horizontal transmission of 7 to 10 years.

EPIDEMIOLOGY

Worldwide, as of 2010, approximately 34 million persons are living with HIV and 3.4 million of them are children. There were 2.7 million new infections in 2010 with approximately 390,000 new infections in children. Roughly 70% of all people living with HIV reside in sub-Saharan Africa. Worldwide, 1.8 million people died from HIV-related illnesses in 2010. In 2010 the estimated number of people over the age of 13 years and living with HIV in the United States was 1.1 million, and approximately 9800 children are infected. Vertical transmission is much less common than previously, and approximately 50 infants are born with HIV infection each year in the United States. Most pediatric cases now occur in adolescents who engage in unprotected sexual activities. Worldwide the number of deaths related to HIV and the number of children infected with HIV have steadily decreased in large part due to treatment with antiretroviral therapy.

CLINICAL MANIFESTATIONS

Decision-Making Algorithms
Available @ StudentConsult.com

Neck Masses
Hoarseness
Diarrhea
Arthritis
Fever and Rash
Lymphadenopathy
Anemia
Petechiae/Purpura
Failure to Thrive

In adolescents and adults, primary infection results in the **acute retroviral syndrome** that develops after an incubation period of 2 to 6 weeks and consists of fever, malaise, weight loss, pharyngitis, lymphadenopathy, and often a maculopapular rash. The risk of opportunistic infections and other AIDS-defining conditions is related to the depletion of CD4 T cells. A combination of CD4 cell count and percentage and clinical manifestations is used to classify HIV infection in children (Tables 125-1 and 125-2).

Initial symptoms with vertical transmission vary and may include failure to thrive, neurodevelopmental delay, lymphadenopathy, hepatosplenomegaly, chronic or recurrent diarrhea, interstitial pneumonia, or oral thrush. These findings may be subtle and remarkable only by their persistence.

Table 125-1	1994 Revised HIV Pediatric Classification System: Immune Categories					
	LABORATORY CRITERIA					
	<12 MONTHS		**1–5 YEARS**		**6–12 YEARS**	
IMMUNE CATEGORY	**CD4+ CELLS/ mm³**	**% TOTAL LYMPHOCYTES**	**CD4+ CELLS/ mm³**	**% TOTAL LYMPHOCYTES**	**CD4+ CELLS/ mm³**	**% TOTAL LYMPHOCYTES**
Category 1 (no suppression)	≥1500	≥25	≥1000	≥25	≥500	≥25
Category 2 (moderate suppression)	750–1499	15–24	500–999	15–24	200–499	15–24
Category 3 (severe suppression)	<750	<15	<500	<15	<200	<15

From Centers for Disease Control and Prevention: 1994 revised classification system for human immunodeficiency virus infection in children less than 13 years of age, MMWR 43(RR-12):1–10, 1994.

Manifestations that are more common in children than adults with HIV infection include recurrent bacterial infections, lymphoid hyperplasia, chronic parotid swelling, lymphocytic interstitial pneumonitis, and earlier onset of progressive neurologic deterioration. Pulmonary manifestations of HIV infection are common and include *Pneumocystis jiroveci* pneumonia, which can present early in infancy as a primary pneumonia characterized by hypoxia, tachypnea, retractions, elevated serum lactate dehydrogenase, and fever.

In the United States, most pregnant women are screened and, if indicated, treated for HIV infection. Infants born to HIV-infected mothers receive prophylaxis and are prospectively tested for infection. The diagnosis of HIV infection in most infants born in the United States is confirmed before development of clinical signs of infection.

LABORATORY AND IMAGING STUDIES
HIV infection can be diagnosed definitively by 1 month of age and in virtually all infected infants by 6 months of age using viral diagnostic assays (RNA polymerase chain reaction [PCR], DNA PCR, or virus culture). Maternal antibodies may be detectable until 12 to 15 months of age, and a positive serologic test is not considered diagnostic until 18 months of age.

HIV DNA PCR is the preferred virologic method for diagnosing HIV infection during infancy and identifies 38% of infected infants at 48 hours and 96% at 28 days. Diagnostic viral testing should be performed by 48 hours of age, at 1 to 2 months of age, and at 3 to 6 months of age. An additional test at 14 days of age is often performed because the diagnostic sensitivity increases rapidly by 2 weeks of age. HIV RNA PCR has 25% to 40% sensitivity during the first weeks of life, increasing to 90% to 100% by 2 to 3 months of age. However a negative HIV RNA PCR cannot be used to exclude infection and, thus, is not recommended as first-line testing.

HIV infection of an exposed infant is confirmed if virologic tests are positive on two separate occasions. HIV infection can be reasonably excluded in nonbreastfed infants with at least two virologic tests performed at older than 1 month of age, with one test being performed after 4 months of age, or at least two negative antibody tests performed after 6 months of age, with an interval of at least 1 month between the tests. Loss of HIV antibody combined with negative HIV DNA

PCR confirms absence of HIV infection. Persistence of a positive HIV antibody test after 18 months of age indicates HIV infection.

DIFFERENTIAL DIAGNOSIS
The differential diagnosis of AIDS in infants includes primary immunodeficiency syndromes and intrauterine infections with cytomegalovirus (CMV) and syphilis. Prominence of individual symptoms, such as diarrhea, may suggest other etiologies.

TREATMENT
Management of HIV infection in children and adolescents is rapidly evolving and becoming increasingly complex. It should be directed by a specialist in the treatment of HIV infection. Therapy is initiated based on the severity of HIV disease, as indicated by AIDS-defining conditions, and the risk of disease progression, as indicated by CD4 cell count and plasma HIV RNA level (Table 125-3). Initiation of antiretroviral therapy while the patient is still asymptomatic may preserve immune function and prevent clinical progression but incurs the adverse effects of therapy and may facilitate emergence of drug-resistant virus. Because the risk of HIV progression is fourfold to sixfold greater in infants and very young children, treatment recommendations for children are more aggressive than for adults. All age groups show rapid increases in risk as CD4 cell percentage declines to less than 15%.

Initiation of therapy (see Table 125-3) is recommended for infants less than 12 months of age regardless of symptoms of HIV disease or HIV RNA level. Initiation of therapy is recommended for all children 1 to 5 years of age with AIDS or significant HIV-related symptoms or CD4 below 25% (clinical category C or most clinical category B) regardless of symptoms or HIV RNA level. For children older than 5 years with AIDS or significant HIV-related symptoms, CD4 count below 350/mm³ should be treated. Indications for treatment of adolescents and adults include CD4 cell count less than 200 to 350/mm³ or plasma HIV RNA levels above 55,000 copies/mL.

Combination therapy with **highly active antiretroviral therapy (HAART)** is recommended based on the risk of disease progression as determined by CD4 percentage or count and plasma HIV RNA copy number; the potential benefits

Table 125-2	1994 Revised HIV Pediatric Classification System: Clinical Categories

CATEGORY N: NOT SYMPTOMATIC

Children who have no signs or symptoms considered to be the result of HIV infection or who have only one of the conditions listed in category A

CATEGORY A: MILDLY SYMPTOMATIC

Children with two or more of the following conditions, but none of the conditions listed in categories B and C:

Lymphadenopathy (nodal tissue enlargement of ≥0.5 cm palpable at more than two sites; bilateral = one site)

Hepatomegaly

Splenomegaly

Dermatitis

Parotitis

Recurrent or persistent upper respiratory infection, sinusitis, or otitis media

CATEGORY B: MODERATELY SYMPTOMATIC

Children who have symptomatic conditions, other than those listed for category A or category C, that are attributed to HIV infection. Examples of conditions in clinical category B include, but are not limited to, the following:

Anemia (<8 g/dL), neutropenia (<1000/mm^3), or thrombocytopenia (<100,000/mm^3) persisting ≥30 days

Bacterial meningitis, pneumonia, or sepsis (single episode)

Candidiasis, oropharyngeal (i.e., thrush) persisting for >2 months in children younger than 6 months of age

Cardiomyopathy

Cytomegalovirus infection with onset before the age of 1 month

Diarrhea, recurrent or chronic

Hepatitis

HSV stomatitis, recurrent (i.e., more than two episodes within 1 year)

HSV bronchitis, pneumonitis, or esophagitis with onset before the age of 1 month

Herpes zoster (i.e., shingles) involving at least two distinct episodes or more than one dermatome

Leiomyosarcoma

LIP or pulmonary lymphoid hyperplasia complex

Nephropathy

Nocardiosis

Fever lasting >1 month

Varicella, disseminated (i.e., complicated chickenpox)

CATEGORY C: SEVERELY SYMPTOMATIC

Serious bacterial infections, multiple or recurrent (i.e., any combination of at least two culture-confirmed infections within a 2-year period), of the following types: septicemia, pneumonia, meningitis, bone or joint infection, or abscess of an internal organ or body cavity (excluding otitis media, superficial skin or mucosal abscesses, and indwelling catheter-related infections)

Candidiasis, esophageal or pulmonary (bronchi, trachea, lungs)

Coccidioidomycosis, disseminated (at site other than or in addition to lungs or cervical or hilar lymph nodes)

Cryptococcosis, extrapulmonary

Cryptosporidiosis or isosporiasis with diarrhea persisting >1 month

Cytomegalovirus disease with onset of symptoms before the age of 1 month (other than liver, spleen, or lymph nodes)

Encephalopathy (at least one progressive deficit present for at least 2 months in the absence of a concurrent illness): (a) failure to attain or loss of developmental milestones/intellectual ability, verified by standard scale or tests; (b) impaired brain growth or acquired microcephaly; (c) acquired symmetric motor deficit manifested by two or more of the following: paresis, pathologic reflexes, ataxia, or gait disturbance

Herpes simplex virus infection (mucocutaneous ulcer persisting for >1 month; bronchitis, pneumonitis, or esophagitis affecting a child younger than 1 month of age

Histoplasmosis, disseminated (other than or in addition to lungs or cervical or hilar lymph nodes)
Kaposi sarcoma

Lymphoma (primary tumor, in brain; Burkitt lymphoma; immunoblastic or large cell lymphoma of B cell or unknown immunologic phenotype)

Mycobacterium tuberculosis, disseminated or extrapulmonary

Mycobacterium, other species or unidentified species, disseminated (other than or in addition to lungs, skin, or cervical or hilar lymph nodes)

Mycobacterium avium complex or *Mycobacterium kansasii,* disseminated (other than or in addition to lungs, skin, or cervical or hilar lymph nodes)

Pneumocystis jiroveci (carinii) pneumonia

Progressive multifocal leukoencephalopathy

Salmonella (nontyphoid) septicemia, recurrent

Toxoplasmosis of the brain with onset before the age of 1 month

Wasting syndrome in the absence of a concurrent illness could explain the following findings: (a) persistent weight loss >10% of baseline *or* (b) downward crossing of at least two percentile lines on the weight-for-age chart *or* (c) below the 5th percentile on the weight-for-height chart on two consecutive measurements, ≥30 days apart, *plus* (1) chronic diarrhea (i.e., two or more loose stools per day for >30 days) *or* (2) documented fever (for ≥30 days, intermittent or constant)

From the Working Group on Antiretroviral Therapy and Medical Management of HIV-infected Children: Guidelines for the Use of Antiretroviral Agents in Pediatric HIV Infection. Department of Health and Human Services. February 23, 2009. Available at http://aidsinfo.nih.gov/contentfiles/PediatricGuidelines.pdf. Updated from Centers for Disease Control and Prevention: 1994 revised classification system for human immunodeficiency virus infection in children less than 13 years of age, MMWR 43(RR-12):1–10, 1994.
HIV, Human immunodeficiency virus infection; *HSV,* herpes simplex virus; *LIP,* lymphoid interstitial pneumonia.

Table 125-3	Indications for Initiation of Antiretroviral Therapy in Children Infected with HIV	
AGE	**CRITERIA**	**RECOMMENDATION**
<12 months	• Regardless of clinical symptoms, immune status, or viral load	Treat
1<5 years	• AIDS or significant HIV-related symptoms*	Treat
	• CD4 <25%, regardless of symptoms or HIV RNA level†	Treat
	• Asymptomatic or mild symptoms‡ and	Consider
	○ CD4 ≥25% and	
	○ HIV RNA ≥100,000 copies/mL	
	• Asymptomatic or mild symptoms‡ and	Defer§
	○ CD4 ≥25% and	
	○ HIV RNA < 100,000 copies/mL	
≥5 years	• AIDS or significant HIV-related symptoms*	Treat
	• CD4 <350 cells/mm³ ‖	Treat
	• Asymptomatic or mild symptoms‡ and	Consider
	○ CD4 ≥350 cells/mm³ and	
	○ HIV RNA < 100,000 copies/mL	
	• Asymptomatic or mild symptoms‡ and	Defer§
	○ CD4 >350 cells/mm³ and	
	○ HIV RNA < 100,000 copies/mL	

*CDC clinical categories C and B (except for the following category B conditions: single episode of serious bacterial infection or lymphoid interstitial pneumonitis).
†The data supporting this recommendation are stronger for those with CD4 percentage <20% than for those with CD4 percentage of 20% to 24%.
‡CDC clinical category A or N or the following category B conditions: single episode of serious bacterial infection or lymphoid interstitial pneumonitis.
§Clinical and laboratory data should be re-evaluated every 3 to 4 months.
‖The data supporting this recommendation are stronger for those with CD4 count <200 than for those with CD4 counts of 200 to 350 cells/mm³.

and risks of therapy; and the ability of the caregiver to adhere to administration of the therapeutic regimen. Effective combination therapy significantly reduces viral loads and leads to the amelioration of clinical symptoms and opportunistic infections. Combination therapy that includes either a non-nucleoside reverse transcriptase inhibitor or a protease inhibitor (PI) plus a dual–nucleoside/nucleotide reverse transcriptase inhibitor backbone is recommended for initial treatment of all HIV infected children. The goal of therapy is to reduce the plasma HIV RNA to below the level of detection and normalize or preserve the patient's immune status. The most recent specific recommendations for treatment regimens (http://aidsinfo.nih.gov/guidelines/) should be consulted before initiating therapy for any patient.

The ability of HIV to develop resistance to antiretroviral agents rapidly and the development of cross-resistance to several classes of agents simultaneously are major problems. Determination of HIV RNA, CD4 cell count, and HIV phenotype and genotype is essential for monitoring and modifying antiretroviral treatment.

Routine immunizations are recommended to prevent vaccine-preventable infections but may result in suboptimal immune responses. In addition to heptavalent pneumococcal conjugate vaccine, 23-valent pneumococcal polysaccharide vaccine is recommended for HIV-infected children at 2 years of age and adolescents and adults with CD4 counts at or above 200/mm³. Because of the risk of fatal measles in children with AIDS, children without severe immunosuppression should receive their first dose of MMR at 12 months of age and may receive the booster as soon as 4 weeks later. Varicella zoster virus (VZV) vaccine should be given only to asymptomatic, nonimmunosuppressed children beginning at 12 months of age as two doses of vaccine at least 3 months apart. Inactivated split influenza virus vaccine should be administered annually to all HIV-infected children at or after 6 months of age. HIV-infected children exposed to varicella or measles should receive varicella zoster immune globulin or immunoglobulin prophylaxis.

COMPLICATIONS

The approach to the numerous opportunistic infections in HIV-infected patients involves treatment and prophylaxis for infections likely to occur as CD4 cells are depleted. With potent antiretroviral therapy and immune reconstitution, routine prophylaxis for common opportunistic infections depends on the child's age and CD4 count. Infants born to HIV-infected mothers receive prophylaxis for *P. jiroveci* pneumonia with trimethoprim-sulfamethoxazole (TMP-SMZ) beginning at 4 to 6 weeks of age and continued for the first year of life or discontinued if HIV infection is subsequently excluded. TMP-SMZ prophylaxis for *P. jiroveci* pneumonia for older children and adolescents is provided if CD4 cell counts are less than 200/mm³ or there is history of oropharyngeal candidiasis. Clarithromycin prophylaxis for *Mycobacterium avium-complex* infection is provided if CD4 cell counts are below 50/mm³.

P. jiroveci pneumonia is treated with high-dose TMP-SMZ and corticosteroids. Oral and gastrointestinal candidiasis is common in children and usually responds to imidazole therapy. VZV infection may be severe and should be treated with acyclovir or other antivirals. Recurrent herpes simplex virus (HSV) infections also may require long-term antiviral prophylaxis. Other common infections in HIV-infected patients include toxoplasmosis, CMV, Epstein-Barr virus infection, salmonellosis, and tuberculosis.

Children and adults with HIV are prone to malignancies, especially non-Hodgkin lymphomas, with the gastrointestinal tract being the most common site. Leiomyosarcomas are the second most common tumors among HIV-infected children. Kaposi sarcoma, caused by HHV-8, is distinctly rare in children with HIV. It was once common among adults with AIDS and is now infrequent with HAART.

PROGNOSIS

The availability of HAART has improved the prognosis for HIV and AIDS dramatically. Risk of death is directly related to the degree of immunosuppression, viral load, and young age.

Children less than 1 year of age with very low CD4 percentiles and high viral loads have the poorest prognosis.

PREVENTION

Identification of HIV-infected women before or during pregnancy is crucial to providing optimal therapy for infected women and their infants and to preventing perinatal transmission. Prenatal HIV counseling and testing with consent should be provided for all pregnant women in the United States.

The rate of vertical transmission is reduced to less than 8% by chemoprophylaxis with a regimen of zidovudine to the mother (100 mg five times/24 hours orally) started by 4 weeks gestation, continued during delivery (2 mg/kg loading dose intravenously followed by 1 mg/kg/hour intravenously), and then administered to the newborn for the first 6 weeks of life (2 mg/kg every 6 hours orally). Other regimens incorporating single-dose nevirapine for infants have been shown to be similarly effective and are used in developing countries. The current recommendations for the United States include a 6-week prophylactic with zidovudine for the infant in combination with maternal intrapartum therapy. The maternal regimen includes continuation of antiretroviral therapy (if appropriate) and intravenous zidovudine if the mother's viral load is >400 copies/mL or is unknown (http://aidsinfo.nih.gov/contentfiles/lvguidelines/peri_recommendations.pdf). Scheduled cesarean section at 38 weeks to prevent vertical transmission is recommended for women with HIV RNA levels greater than 1000 copies/mL, but it is unclear whether cesarean section is beneficial when viral load is less than 1000 copies/mL or when membranes have already ruptured.

Preventing HIV infection in adults decreases the incidence of infection in children. Adult prevention results from behavior changes such as safe-sex practices, decrease in intravenous drug use, and needle exchange programs. Prevention of pediatric AIDS includes avoidance of pregnancy and breastfeeding (in developed countries) in high-risk women. Screening of blood donors has almost eliminated the risk of HIV transmission from blood products. HIV infection almost never is transmitted in a casual or nonsexual household setting.

Suggested Reading

Feigin RD, Cherry J, Demmler GJ, et al: *Textbook of Pediatric Infectious Diseases*, ed 6, Philadelphia, 2009, Saunders.

Isaacs D: *Evidence-based Pediatric Infectious Disease*, Malden, MA, 2007, Blackwell Publishing.

Kliegman RM, Stanton BF, Behrman RE, et al: *Nelson Textbook of Pediatrics*, ed 19, Philadelphia, 2007, Saunders.

Long SS, Pickering LK, Prober CG: *Principles and Practice of Pediatric Infectious Diseases*, ed 4, Philadelphia, 2012, Churchill Livingstone.

Pickering LK, Baker CJ, Long SS, et al: *Red Book: 2012 Report of the Committee on Infectious Diseases*, ed 27, Elk Grove Village, IL, 2012, American Academy of Pediatrics.

Plotkin SA, Orenstein WA, Offit PA: *Vaccines*, ed 5, Philadelphia, 2008, WB Saunders.

The Digestive System

Warren P. Bishop and Dawn R. Ebach

Chapter 126

ASSESSMENT

HISTORY

After identifying the major gastrointestinal (GI) symptom, onset and progression should be determined (improved, unchanged, worsening). Characterization of signs and symptoms should identify factors such as triggers; actions that alleviate the symptom; timing, frequency and duration of symptoms; relationship to meals and defecation; and associated symptoms (e.g., fever or weight loss). Other key history includes exposures to others (family, school contacts), travel, environmental exposure, and impact of illness on the child (school absences).

PHYSICAL EXAMINATION

The history may suggest a diagnosis and direct the evaluation, which should include a full examination as well as a thorough abdominal examination. Extraintestinal disorders may produce GI manifestations (e.g., emesis with group A streptococcal pharyngitis, abdominal pain with lower lobe pneumonia). The examination should begin with a careful external inspection for abdominal distention, bruising or discoloration, abnormal veins, jaundice, surgical scars, and ostomies. Abnormalities of intensity and pitch of bowel sounds can occur with bowel obstruction. When palpating for tenderness, the examiner should note location, facial expression, guarding, and rebound tenderness. Palpation can also detect enlargement of the liver or spleen as well as feces and masses. If detected, organomegaly should be measured (with a tape measure), noting abnormal firmness or contour. A rectal examination, including inspection for fissures, skin tags, abscesses, and fistulous openings, should be performed for children with history suggesting constipation, GI bleeding, abdominal pain, chronic diarrhea, and suspicion of inflammatory bowel disease (IBD). Digital rectal examination should include assessment of anal sphincter tone, anal canal size and elasticity, tenderness, extrinsic masses, presence of fecal impaction, and caliber of the rectum. Stool should be tested for occult blood.

SCREENING TESTS

A **complete blood count** may provide evidence for inflammation (white blood cell [WBC] and platelet count), poor nutrition or bleeding (hemoglobin, red blood cell volume, reticulocyte count), and infection (WBC number and differential, presence of toxic granulation). Serum electrolytes, blood urea nitrogen (BUN), and creatinine help define hydration status. Tests of liver dysfunction include total and direct bilirubin, alanine aminotransferase, aspartate aminotransferase for evidence of hepatocellular injury, and γ-glutamyltransferase or alkaline phosphatase for evidence of bile duct injury. **Hepatic synthetic function** can be assessed by coagulation factor levels, prothrombin time, and albumin level. Pancreatic enzyme tests (amylase, lipase) provide evidence of pancreatic injury or inflammation. Urinalysis can gauge dehydration and identify a possible source of protein loss.

DIAGNOSTIC IMAGING
Radiology

Consultation with a radiologist is often advisable to discuss appropriate imaging, decide what variants of the technique to use, and learn how to prepare the patient for the study.

A plain abdominal x-ray to document excessive retained stool when history is consistent with constipation and encopresis is not necessary, as examination alone can confirm the diagnosis.

Endoscopy

Endoscopy permits the direct visualization of the interior of the gut. **Video endoscopes** may be used even in very small infants by pediatric gastroenterologists. **Wireless capsule endoscopy** (Fig. 126-1) enables visualization of lesions beyond the reach of conventional endoscopes.

Consultation with a pediatric gastroenterologist for endoscopy is recommended for further evaluation of suspected esophageal or gastric inflammation unresponsive to medications and to confirm the diagnosis of eosinophilic esophagitis or celiac disease, evaluate gastrointestinal bleeding, evaluate suspected inflammatory bowel disease, and screen for polyp disorders. In addition, a trained endoscopist can remove esophageal and gastric foreign bodies and place feeding tubes.

COMMON MANIFESTATIONS OF GASTROINTESTINAL DISORDERS
Abdominal Pain

Decision-Making Algorithm
Available @ StudentConsult.com

Abdominal Pain

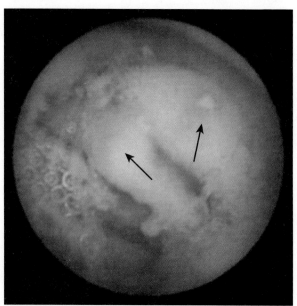

Figure 126-1 Wireless capsule endoscopy: Aphthous ulcers *(arrows)* in jejunum diagnostic of Crohn's disease in patient with negative findings on upper endoscopy and colonoscopy.

General Considerations

Abdominal pain can result from injury to the intra-abdominal organs or overlying somatic structures in the abdominal wall, or from extra-abdominal diseases. **Visceral pain** results when autonomic nerves within the gut detect injury, transmitting sensation by nonmyelinated fibers. The pain is vague, dull, slow in onset, and poorly localized. A variety of stimuli, including normal peristalsis and various intraluminal chemical and osmotic states, activate these fibers to some degree. Regardless of the stimulus, visceral pain is perceived when a threshold of intensity or duration is crossed. Lower degrees of activation may result in perception of nonpainful or perhaps vaguely uncomfortable sensations, whereas more intensive stimulation of these fibers results in pain. Overactive sensation may be the basis of some kinds of abdominal pain, such as **functional abdominal pain** and **irritable bowel syndrome**.

In contrast to visceral pain, **somatic pain** results when overlying body structures are injured. Somatic structures include the parietal peritoneum, fascia, muscles, and skin of the abdominal wall. In contrast to pain emanating from visceral injury, somatic nociceptive fibers are myelinated and are capable of rapid transmission of well-localized painful stimuli. When intra-abdominal processes cause inflammation or injury to the parietal peritoneum or abdominal wall structures, poorly localized visceral pain becomes well-localized somatic pain. For example, in acute appendicitis, the initial activation of visceral nociceptive fibers yields poorly localized discomfort in the mid-abdomen. When the inflammatory process extends to the overlying parietal peritoneum, the pain becomes severe and localizes to the right lower quadrant. This is called **somatoparietal pain**.

Referred pain is a painful sensation in a body region distant from the true source of pain. The location of referred pain is predictable based on the locus of visceral injury. Stomach pain is referred to the epigastric and retrosternal regions, and liver and pancreas pain is referred to the epigastric region. Gallbladder pain often is referred to the region below the right

scapula. Somatic pathways stimulated by small bowel visceral afferents affect the periumbilical area, and colonic injury results in infraumbilical referred pain.

Acute Abdominal Pain
Distinguishing Features

Acute abdominal pain can signal the presence of a dangerous intra-abdominal process (e.g., appendicitis or bowel obstruction) or may originate from extraintestinal sources (e.g., lower lobe pneumonia or urinary tract stone). Not all episodes of acute abdominal pain require emergency intervention. Appendicitis and volvulus, for example, must be ruled out as quickly as possible. Few patients presenting with acute abdominal pain actually have a surgical emergency, but they must be separated from cases that can be managed conservatively.

Initial Diagnostic Evaluation

Table 126-1 lists a diagnostic approach to acute abdominal pain in children. Events that occur with a discrete, abrupt onset, such as passage of a stone, perforation of a viscus, or infarction, result in a sudden **onset of pain**. Gradual onset of pain is common with infectious or inflammatory causes, such as appendicitis and IBD.

A standard group of laboratory tests usually is performed for acute abdominal pain (see Table 126-1). An abdominal x-ray series evaluates for bowel obstruction or nephrolithiasis. Ultrasound or computed tomography (CT) can visualize the appendix if appendicitis is suspected but the diagnosis remains in doubt. If the initial evaluation suggests intussusception, a barium or pneumatic (air) enema may be used to diagnose and treat this condition (see Chapter 129).

Differential Diagnosis

Table 126-2 lists the differential diagnosis of acute abdominal pain in children. The urgent task of the clinician is to rule out surgical emergencies. In young children, malrotation with volvulus, incarcerated hernia, congenital anomalies, and intussusception are common concerns. In older children and teenagers, appendicitis is more common. An acute surgical abdomen is characterized by signs of peritonitis, including tenderness, abdominal wall rigidity, guarding, and absent or diminished bowel sounds. Helpful characteristics of onset, location, referral, and quality of pain are noted in Table 126-3.

Functional Abdominal Pain and Irritable Bowel Syndrome

Decision-Making Algorithms
Available @ StudentConsult.com

Abdominal Pain
Vomiting

Recurrent abdominal pain is a common problem, affecting more than 10% of all children. The peak incidence occurs between ages 7 and 12 years. Although the differential diagnosis of recurrent abdominal pain is fairly extensive (Table 126-4), most children do not have a serious (or even identifiable) underlying illness causing the pain.

Table 126-1	Diagnostic Approach to Acute Abdominal Pain

HISTORY

Onset	Sudden or gradual, prior episodes, association with meals, history of injury
Nature	Sharp versus dull, colicky or constant, burning
Location	Epigastric, periumbilical, generalized, right or left lower quadrant, change in location over time
Associated symptoms	Fever, vomiting (bilious?), diarrhea (bloody?), abdominal distention
Extraintestinal symptoms	Cough, dyspnea, dysuria, urinary frequency, flank pain
Course of symptoms	Worsening or improving, change in nature or location of pain, aggravating and alleviating factors

PHYSICAL EXAMINATION

General position	Growth and nutrition, general appearance, hydration, degree of discomfort, body position
Abdominal	Tenderness, distention, bowel sounds, rigidity, guarding, mass
Genitalia	Testicular torsion, hernia, pelvic inflammatory disease, ectopic pregnancy
Surrounding structures	Breath sounds, rales, rhonchi, wheezing, flank tenderness, tenderness of abdominal wall structures, ribs, costochondral joints
Rectal examination	Perianal lesions, stricture, tenderness, fecal impaction, blood

LABORATORY

CBC, C-reactive protein, ESR	Evidence of infection or inflammation
AST, ALT, GGT, bilirubin	Biliary or liver disease
Amylase, lipase	Pancreatitis
Urinalysis	Urinary tract infection; bleeding due to stone, trauma, or obstruction
Pregnancy test (older females)	Ectopic pregnancy

RADIOLOGY

Plain flat and upright abdominal films	Bowel obstruction, appendiceal fecalith, free intraperitoneal air, kidney stones
CT scan	Intra-abdominal or pelvic abscess, appendicitis, Crohn's disease, pancreatitis, gallstones, kidney stones
Barium enema	Intussusception, malrotation
Ultrasound	Gallstones, appendicitis, intussusception, pancreatitis, kidney stones
Endoscopy	
Upper endoscopy	Suspected peptic ulcer or esophagitis

ALT, Alanine aminotransferase; *AST*, aspartate aminotransferase; *CBC*, complete blood count; *CT*, computed tomography; *ESR*, erythrocyte sedimentation rate; *GGT*, γ-glutamyltransferase.

Table 126-2	Differential Diagnosis of Acute Abdominal Pain

TRAUMATIC

Duodenal hematoma

Ruptured spleen

Perforated viscus

Traumatic pancreatitis

FUNCTIONAL

Constipation*

Irritable bowel syndrome*

Dysmenorrhea*

Mittelschmerz (ovulation)*

Infantile colic*

Abdominal migraine

INFECTIOUS

Appendicitis*

Viral or bacterial gastroenteritis/adenitis*

Abscess

Spontaneous bacterial peritonitis

Pelvic inflammatory disease

Cholecystitis

Urinary tract infection*

Pneumonia

Bacterial typhlitis

Hepatitis

GENITAL

Testicular torsion

Ovarian torsion

Ruptured ovarian cyst

Ectopic pregnancy

GENETIC

Sickle cell crisis*

Familial Mediterranean fever

Porphyria

METABOLIC

Diabetic ketoacidosis

INFLAMMATORY

Inflammatory bowel disease

Vasculitis

Henoch-Schönlein purpura*

Pancreatitis

OBSTRUCTIVE

Intussusception*

Malrotation with volvulus

Ileus*

Incarcerated hernia

Postoperative adhesion

Continued

Table 126-2	Differential Diagnosis of Acute Abdominal Pain—cont'd

Meconium ileus equivalent (cystic fibrosis)

Duplication cyst

Congenital stricture

BILIARY

Gallstone

Gallbladder hydrops

Biliary dyskinesia

PEPTIC

Gastric or duodenal ulcer

Gastritis*

Esophagitis

RENAL

Kidney stone

Hydronephrosis/ureteropelvic junction obstruction

*Common.

Differential Diagnosis

Children with **functional abdominal pain** characteristically have pain almost daily. The pain is not associated with meals or relieved by defecation and is often associated with a tendency toward anxiety and perfectionism. Symptoms often result from stress at school or in novel social situations. The pain often is worst in the morning and often prevents or delays children from attending school. **Irritable bowel syndrome (IBS)** is a subset of functional abdominal pain, characterized by onset of pain at the time of a change in stool frequency or consistency, a stool pattern fluctuating between diarrhea and constipation, and relief of pain with defecation. Symptoms in IBS are linked to gut motility. Pain is commonly accompanied in both groups of children by school avoidance, secondary gains, anxiety about imagined causes, lack of coping skills, and disordered peer relationships (Table 126-5).

Distinguishing Features

One needs to distinguish between functional pain/IBS and more serious underlying disorders. **Warning signs** for underlying illness are listed in Table 126-6. If present, further investigation is necessary. Some laboratory evaluation is warranted

Table 126-3	Distinguishing Features of Abdominal Pain in Children

DISEASE	ONSET	LOCATION	REFERRAL	QUALITY	COMMENTS
Functional: irritable bowel syndrome	Recurrent	Periumbilical, splenic and hepatic flexures	None	Dull, crampy, intermittent; duration 2 h	Family stress, school phobia, diarrhea and constipation; hypersensitive to pain from distention
Esophageal reflux	Recurrent, after meals, at bedtime	Substernal	Chest	Burning	Sour taste in mouth; Sandifer syndrome
Duodenal ulcer	Recurrent, before meals, at night	Epigastric	Back	Severe burning, gnawing	Relieved by food, milk, antacids; family history important; GI bleeding
Pancreatitis	Acute	Epigastric-hypogastric	Back	Constant, sharp, boring	Nausea, emesis, marked tenderness
Intestinal obstruction	Acute or gradual	Periumbilical–lower abdomen	Back	Alternating cramping (colic) and painless periods	Distention, obstipation, bilious emesis, increased bowel sounds
Appendicitis	Acute	Periumbilical or epigastric; localizes to right lower quadrant	Back or pelvis if retrocecal	Sharp, steady	Nausea, emesis, local tenderness, ± fever, avoids motion
Meckel diverticulum	Recurrent	Periumbilical–lower abdomen	None	Sharp	Hematochezia; painless unless intussusception, diverticulitis, or perforation
Inflammatory bowel disease	Recurrent	Depends on site of involvement		Dull cramping, tenesmus	Fever, weight loss, ± hematochezia
Intussusception	Acute	Periumbilical–lower abdomen	None	Cramping, with painless periods	Guarded position with knees pulled up, currant jelly stools, lethargy
Lactose intolerance	Recurrent with milk products	Lower abdomen	None	Cramping	Distention, gaseousness, diarrhea
Urolithiasis	Acute, sudden	Back	Groin	Severe, colicky pain	Hematuria
Pyelonephritis	Acute, sudden	Back	None	Dull to sharp	Fever, costochondral tenderness, dysuria, urinary frequency, emesis
Cholecystitis and cholelithiasis	Acute	Right upper quadrant	Right shoulder	Severe, colicky pain	Hemolysis ± jaundice, nausea, emesis

Adapted from Andreoli TE, Carpenter CJ, Plum F, et al: Cecil Essentials of Medicine, Philadelphia, 1986, WB Saunders.

Table 126-4	Differential Diagnosis of Recurrent Abdominal Pain

Functional abdominal pain*

Irritable bowel syndrome*

Chronic pancreatitis

Gallstones

Peptic disease

    Duodenal ulcer

    Gastric ulcer

    Esophagitis

Lactose intolerance*

Fructose malabsorption

Inflammatory bowel disease*

    Crohn's disease

    Ulcerative colitis

Constipation*

Obstructive uropathy

Congenital intestinal malformation

    Malrotation

    Duplication cyst

    Stricture or web

Celiac disease*

Abdominal migraine

Eosinophilic esophagitis*

*Common.

even in the absence of warning signs. The initial evaluation recommended in Table 126-7 is a sensible approach, avoiding unnecessary testing and providing ample sensitivity for most serious underlying disorders. While waiting for laboratory and ultrasound results, a 3-day trial of a lactose-free diet can evaluate for lactose intolerance. If tests are normal and no warning signs are present, testing should be stopped. If there are warning signs, progression of symptoms, or laboratory abnormalities that suggest a specific diagnosis, additional investigation may be warranted.

Treatment of Recurrent Abdominal Pain

A child who is repeatedly kept home from school because of pain receives reinforcement in the form of being excused from responsibilities and withdraws from full social functioning. This tends to both increase anxiety and prolong the course. To break the cycle of pain and disability, the child with functional pain must be assisted in **returning to normal activities** immediately. Instead of being sent home from school with stomachaches, a child may be allowed to take a short break from class until symptoms abate. The child and parents should be informed that pain is likely to be worse on the day the child returns to school as anxiety worsens dysmotility and enhances pain perception. Medications may be helpful. **Fiber supplements** may help to manage symptoms of IBS. Probiotics and peppermint oil can be beneficial in treating IBS. In difficult and persistent cases, cognitive behavioral

Table 126-5	Rome III Criteria for Pediatric Functional Gastrointestinal Syndromes

A. Diagnostic Criteria for Childhood Functional Abdominal Pain

Must include all of the following:
1. Episodic or continuous abdominal pain
2. Insufficient criteria for other functional gastrointestinal diseases
3. No evidence of an inflammatory, anatomic, metabolic, or neoplastic process that explains the subject's symptoms.

*Criteria fulfilled at least once per week for at least 2 months before diagnosis

B. Diagnostic Criteria for Childhood Functional Abdominal Pain Syndrome

Must include functional abdominal pain at least 25% of the time and 1 or more of the following:
1. Some loss of daily functioning
2. Additional somatic symptoms such as headache, limb pain, or difficulty sleeping

*Criteria fulfilled at least once per week for at least 2 months before diagnosis

C. Diagnostic Criteria for Irritable Bowel Syndrome

Must include all of the following:
1. Abdominal discomfort (an uncomfortable sensation not described as pain) or pain associated with 2 or more of the following at least 25% of the time:
   a. improved with defecation
   b. onset associated with change in frequency of stool
   c. onset associated with a change in form (appearance) of stool
2. No evidence of an inflammatory, anatomic, metabolic, or neoplastic process that explains the subject's symptoms.

*Criteria fulfilled at least once per week for at least 2 months before diagnosis

D. Diagnostic Criteria for Abdominal Migraine

Must include all of the following:
1. Paroxysmal episodes of intense, acute periumbilical pain that lasts for 1 hour or more.
2. Intervening periods of usual health lasting weeks to months.
3. The pain interferes with normal activities.
4. The pain is associated with 2 or more of the following:
   a. anorexia
   b. nausea
   c. vomiting
   d. headache
   e. photophobia
   f. pallor
5. No evidence of an inflammatory, anatomic, metabolic, or neoplastic process considered that explains the subject's symptoms.

*Criteria fulfilled 2 or more times in the preceding 12 months.

E. Diagnostic Criteria for Cyclic Vomiting Syndrome

Must include all of the following:
1. Two or more periods of intense nausea and unremitting vomiting or retching lasting hours to days.
2. Return to usual state of health lasting weeks to months.

F. Functional Diarrhea

Must include all of the following
1. Daily painless, recurrent passage of three or more large, unformed stools.
2. Symptoms lasting more than 4 weeks.
3. Onset of symptoms that begins between 6 and 36 months of age.
4. Passage of stools that occur during waking hours.
5. There is no failure to thrive if caloric intake is adequate.

Courtesy of the Rome Foundation.

Table 126-6	Warning Signs of Underlying Illness in Recurrent Abdominal Pain

Vomiting

Abnormal screening laboratory study (anemia, hypoalbuminemia, inflammatory markers)

Fever

Bilious emesis

Growth failure

Pain awakening child from sleep

Weight loss

Location away from periumbilical region

Blood in stools or emesis

Delayed puberty

Nocturnal diarrhea

Dysphagia

Arthritis

Perianal disease

Family history of inflammatory bowel disease, celiac disease, or peptic ulcer disease

Table 126-7	Suggested Evaluation of Recurrent Abdominal Pain

INITIAL EVALUATION	FOLLOW-UP EVALUATION*
Complete history and physical examination	CT scan of the abdomen and pelvis with oral, rectal, and intravenous contrast
Ask about "warning signs" (see Table 126-6)	Celiac disease serology—endomysial antibody or tissue transglutaminase antibody
Determine degree of functional impairment (e.g., missing school)	
CBC	Barium upper GI series with small bowel follow-through
ESR	
Amylase, lipase	Endoscopy of the esophagus, stomach, and duodenum
Urinalysis	
Abdominal ultrasound—examine liver, bile ducts, gallbladder, pancreas, kidneys, ureters (move to follow up)	Colonoscopy
Trial of 3-day lactose-free diet	

CBC, Complete blood count; *CT*, computed tomography; *ESR*, erythrocyte sedimentation rate; *GI*, gastrointestinal.

Consider using one or more of these to investigate warning signs, abnormal laboratory tests, or specific or persistent symptoms.

therapy, amitriptyline, or a selective serotonin reuptake inhibitor may be helpful. When significant anxiety or social dysfunction persists, a mental health professional should be consulted.

Decision-Making Algorithm
Available @ StudentConsult.com

Vomiting

Vomiting

Vomiting is a coordinated, sequential series of events that leads to forceful oral emptying of gastric contents. It is a common problem in children and has many causes. Vomiting should be distinguished from **regurgitation** of stomach contents, also known as gastroesophageal reflux (GER), chalasia, or "spitting up." Although the end result of vomiting and regurgitation is similar, they have completely different characteristics. Vomiting is usually preceded by nausea and is accompanied by forceful gagging and retching. Regurgitation, on the other hand, is effortless and not preceded by nausea.

Differential Diagnosis

In neonates with true vomiting, congenital obstructive lesions should be considered. Allergic reactions to formula in the first 2 months of life may present with vomiting. **Infantile GER** ("spitting up") occurs in most infants and can be large in volume, but is effortless and these infants do not appear ill. **Pyloric stenosis** occurs in the first months of life and is characterized by steadily worsening, forceful vomiting that occurs immediately after feedings. A visibly distended stomach, often with visible peristaltic waves, is often seen before vomiting. Pyloric stenosis is more common in male infants; the family history may be positive. Other obstructive lesions, such as intestinal duplication cysts, atresias, webs, and midgut

malrotation, should be considered. Metabolic disorders (e.g., organic acidemias, galactosemia, urea cycle defects, adrenogenital syndromes) may present with vomiting in infants. In older children with acute vomiting, viruses and food poisoning are common. Other infections, especially streptococcal pharyngitis, urinary tract infections, and otitis media, commonly result in vomiting. When vomiting is chronic, central nervous system (CNS) causes (increased intracranial pressure, migraine) must be considered. **Cyclic vomiting syndrome** or migraine may be the etiology of recurrent vomiting. When abdominal pain or bilious emesis accompanies vomiting, evaluation for bowel obstruction, peptic disorders, and appendicitis must be immediately initiated.

Distinguishing Features

Table 126-8 lists common diagnoses that must be considered and their important historical features. Given the frequency of viral gastroenteritis as the etiology, it is important to be alert for unusual features that suggest another diagnosis. Viral gastroenteritis usually is not associated with severe abdominal pain or headache and does not recur at frequent intervals.

Physical examination should include assessment of the child's hydration status, including examination of capillary refill, moistness of mucous membranes, and skin turgor (see Chapter 38). The chest should be auscultated for evidence of rales or other signs of pulmonary involvement. The abdomen must be examined carefully for distention, organomegaly, bowel sounds, tenderness, and guarding. A rectal examination and testing stool for occult blood should be considered.

Laboratory evaluation of vomiting should include serum electrolytes, tests of renal function, complete blood count, amylase, lipase, and liver function tests. Additional testing may be required immediately when history and examination suggest a specific etiology. Ultrasound is useful to look for pyloric stenosis, gallstones, renal stones, hydronephrosis, biliary obstruction, pancreatitis, malrotation, intussusception, and other anatomic

Table 126-8	Differential Diagnosis and Historical Features of Vomiting

DIFFERENTIAL DIAGNOSIS	HISTORICAL CLUES
Viral gastroenteritis	Fever, diarrhea, sudden onset, absence of pain
Gastroesophageal reflux	Effortless, not preceded by nausea, chronic
Hepatitis	Jaundice, history of exposure
Extra-gastrointestinal infections	
Otitis media	Fever, ear pain
Urinary tract infection	Dysuria, unusual urine odor, frequency, incontinence
Pneumonia	Cough, fever, chest discomfort
Allergic	
Milk or soy protein intolerance (infants)	Associated with particular formula or food, blood in stools
Other food allergy (older children)	
Peptic ulcer or gastritis	Epigastric pain, blood or coffee-ground material in emesis, pain relieved by acid blockade
Appendicitis	Fever, abdominal pain migrating to the right lower quadrant, tenderness
Pancreatitis	Severe epigastric abdominal pain
Anatomic obstruction	
Intestinal atresia	Neonate, usually bilious, polyhydramnios
Midgut malrotation	Pain, bilious vomiting, GI bleeding, shock
Intussusception	Colicky pain, lethargy, vomiting, currant jelly stools, mass occasionally
Duplication cysts	Colic, mass
Pyloric stenosis	Nonbilious vomiting, postprandial, <4 mo old, hunger, progressive weight loss
Bacterial gastroenteritis	Fever, often with bloody diarrhea
CNS	
Hydrocephalus	Large head, altered mental status, bulging fontanelles
Meningitis	Fever, stiff neck
Migraine syndrome	Attacks scattered in time, relieved by sleep; headache
Cyclic vomiting syndrome	Similar to migraine, usually no headache
Brain tumor	Morning vomiting, accelerating over time, headache, diplopia
Motion sickness	Associated with travel in vehicle
Labyrinthitis	Vertigo
Metabolic disease	Presentation early in life, worsens when catabolic or exposure to substrate
Pregnancy	Morning, sexually active, cessation of menses
Drug reaction or side effect	Associated with increased dose or new medication
Cancer chemotherapy	Temporarily related to administration of chemotherapeutic drugs
Eosinophilic esophagitis	May have dysphagia or abdominal pain

abnormalities. CT may be indicated to rule out appendicitis or to observe structures that cannot be visualized well by ultrasound. Barium studies can show obstructive or inflammatory lesions of the gut and can be therapeutic, as in the use of contrast enemas for intussusception (see Chapter 129).

Treatment needs to address the consequences and the causes of the vomiting. Dehydration must be treated with fluid resuscitation. This can be accomplished in most cases with oral fluid-electrolyte solutions, but intravenous (IV) fluids may be required. Electrolyte imbalances should be corrected by appropriate choice of fluids. Underlying causes should be treated when possible.

The use of **antiemetic medications** is controversial. These drugs should not be prescribed until the etiology of the vomiting is known, and then only for severe symptoms. Phenothiazines,

such as prochlorperazine, may be useful for reducing symptoms in food poisoning and motion sickness. Their side-effect profile must be considered carefully, however, and the dose prescribed should be conservative. Anticholinergics (e.g., scopolamine) and antihistamines (e.g., dimenhydrinate) are useful for the prophylaxis and treatment of motion sickness. Drugs that block serotonin 5-HT$_3$ receptors, such as ondansetron and granisetron, are frequently used for viral gastroenteritis and can improve tolerance of oral rehydration therapy. They are helpful for chemotherapy-induced vomiting, often combined with dexamethasone. No antiemetic should be used in patients with surgical emergencies or when a specific treatment of the underlying condition is possible. Correction of dehydration, ketosis, and acidosis is helpful to reduce vomiting in most patients with viral gastroenteritis.

Decision-Making Algorithm
Available @ StudentConsult.com

Diarrhea

Acute and Chronic Diarrhea

Diarrhea is a major cause of childhood morbidity and mortality worldwide. Deaths from diarrhea are rare in industrialized countries, but are common elsewhere. **Acute diarrhea** is a major problem when it occurs with malnutrition or in the absence of basic medical care (see Chapter 30). In North America, most acute diarrhea is viral and is self-limited, requiring no diagnostic testing or specific intervention. Bacterial agents tend to cause much more severe illness and typically are seen in food-associated outbreaks or in regions with poor public sanitation. Bacterial enteritis should be suspected when there is **dysentery** (bloody diarrhea with fever) and whenever severe symptoms are present. These infections can be diagnosed by stool culture or other assays for specific pathogens. **Chronic diarrhea** lasts more than 2 weeks and has a wide range of possible causes, including serious and benign conditions that are more difficult to diagnose.

Parents use the word *diarrhea* to describe loose or watery stools, excessively frequent stools, or stools that are large in volume. Constipation with overflow incontinence can be mislabeled as diarrhea. A more exact definition of diarrhea is excessive daily stool liquid volume (>10 mL stool/kg body weight/day). Stool texture, volume, and frequency help to characterize the episode of diarrhea.

Differential Diagnosis

Diarrhea may be classified by etiology or by physiologic mechanisms (secretory or osmotic). Etiologic agents include viruses, bacteria or their toxins, chemicals, parasites, malabsorbed substances, and inflammation. Table 126-9 lists common causes of diarrhea in childhood. **Secretory diarrhea** occurs when the intestinal mucosa directly secretes fluid and electrolytes into the stool and is the result of inflammation (e.g., inflammatory bowel disease, chemical stimulus). Secretion also is stimulated by mediators of inflammation and by various hormones, such as vasoactive intestinal peptide secreted by a neuroendocrine tumor. Cholera is a secretory diarrhea stimulated by the enterotoxin of *Vibrio cholerae*, which causes increased levels of cAMP within enterocytes and leads to secretion into the small-bowel lumen.

Osmotic diarrhea occurs after malabsorption of an ingested substance, which "pulls" water into the bowel lumen. A classic example is the diarrhea of lactose intolerance. Osmotic diarrhea also can result from generalized maldigestion, such as that seen with pancreatic insufficiency or with intestinal injury. Certain nonabsorbable laxatives, such as polyethylene glycol and milk of magnesia, also cause osmotic diarrhea. Fermentation of malabsorbed substances (e.g., lactose) often occurs, resulting in gas, cramps, and acidic stools. A common cause of chronic loose stools in early childhood is **functional diarrhea**, commonly known as **toddler's diarrhea**. This condition is defined by frequent watery stools in the setting of normal growth and

Table 126-9	Differential Diagnosis of Diarrhea		
	INFANT	**CHILD**	**ADOLESCENT**
ACUTE			
Common	Gastroenteritis* Systemic infection Antibiotic associated (?)	Gastroenteritis* Food poisoning Systemic infection Antibiotic associated	Gastroenteritis* Food poisoning Antibiotic associated
Rare	Primary disaccharidase deficiency Hirschsprung toxic colitis Adrenogenital syndrome		Hyperthyroidism
CHRONIC			
Common	Postinfectious secondary lactase deficiency Cow's milk/soy protein intolerance Chronic nonspecific diarrhea of infancy (toddler's diarrhea) Celiac disease Cystic fibrosis AIDS enteropathy	Postinfectious secondary lactase deficiency Irritable bowel syndrome Celiac disease Lactose intolerance Giardiasis Inflammatory bowel disease	Irritable bowel syndrome Inflammatory bowel disease Lactose intolerance Giardiasis Laxative abuse (anorexia nervosa) Celiac disease
Rare	Primary immune defects Familial villous atrophy (?) Secretory tumors Congenital chloridorrhea Acrodermatitis enteropathica Lymphangiectasia Abetalipoproteinemia Eosinophilic gastroenteritis Short bowel syndrome Intractable diarrhea syndrome Autoimmune enteropathy Factitious	Acquired immune defects Secretory tumor Pseudo-obstruction Factitious AIDS enteropathy	Secretory tumors Primary bowel tumor AIDS enteropathy

AIDS, Acquired immunodeficiency syndrome.

*Gastroenteritis includes viral (rotavirus, norovirus, astrovirus) and bacterial (*Salmonella, Shigella, Escherichia coli, Clostridium difficile, Yersinia, Campylobacter,* other) agents.

weight gain and is caused by excessive intake of sweetened liquids, overwhelming the disaccharide absorptive capacity of the intestine. Diarrhea typically improves tremendously when the child's beverage intake is reduced or changed.

Distinguishing Features

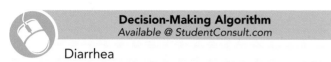

Decision-Making Algorithm
Available @ StudentConsult.com

Diarrhea

Stools are isosmotic, even in osmotic diarrhea, because of the relatively free exchange of water across the intestinal mucosa. Osmoles present in the stool are a mixture of electrolytes and other osmotically active solutes. To determine whether the diarrhea is osmotic or secretory, the **osmotic gap** is calculated:

$$\text{Osmotic gap} = 290 - 2\left([Na^+] + [K^+]\right)$$

Assuming the stool is isosmotic (an osmolarity of 290 mOsm/L), the measured stool sodium and potassium (and their associated anions, accounting for an equal amount) accounts for much of the osmolality. Secretory diarrhea is characterized by an osmotic gap of less than 50. A number significantly higher than 50 defines osmotic diarrhea and indicates that malabsorbed substances other than electrolytes account for fecal osmolarity.

Another way to differentiate between osmotic and secretory diarrhea is to stop all feedings (in hospitalized patients receiving intravenous fluids). If the diarrhea stops completely while the child is NPO (nothing by mouth), the patient has osmotic diarrhea. A child with a pure secretory diarrhea would continue to have massive stool output. Neither method for classifying diarrhea works perfectly, because most diarrheal illnesses are a mixture of secretory and osmotic components. Viral enteritis damages the intestinal lining, causing malabsorption and osmotic diarrhea. The associated inflammation results in release of mediators that cause excessive secretion. A child with viral enteritis may have decreased stool volume while NPO, but the secretory component of the diarrhea persists until the inflammation resolves.

The **history** should include the onset of diarrhea, number and character of stools, estimates of stool volume, and presence of other symptoms, such as blood in the stool, fever, and weight loss. Recent travel and exposures should be documented, dietary factors should be investigated, and a list of medications recently used should be obtained. Factors that seem to worsen or improve the diarrhea should be determined. **Physical examination** should be thorough, evaluating for abdominal distention, tenderness, quality of bowel sounds, presence of blood in the stool or a large fecal mass on rectal examination, and anal sphincter tone.

Laboratory testing should include stool culture and complete blood count if bacterial enteritis is suspected. If diarrhea occurs after a course of antibiotics, a *Clostridium difficile* toxin assay should be ordered; if stools are reported to be oily or fatty, fecal fat content or fecal elastase to test for pancreatic

insufficiency should be measured. Tests for specific diagnoses should be sent when appropriate (e.g., serum antibody tests for celiac disease; colonoscopy for suspected ulcerative colitis). A trial of lactose restriction for several days or lactose breath hydrogen testing is helpful in the evaluation of lactose intolerance.

Constipation and Encopresis

Decision-Making Algorithm
Available @ StudentConsult.com

Constipation

Constipation is a common problem in childhood. When a child is thought to be constipated, his parents may be concerned about straining with defecation, hard stool consistency, large stool size, decreased stool frequency, fear of passing stools, or any combination of these. Physicians define **constipation** as *two or fewer stools per week or passage of hard, pellet-like stools for at least 2 weeks*. A common pattern of constipation is **functional constipation**, which is characterized by two or fewer stools per week, voluntary withholding of stool, and infrequent passage of large-diameter, often painful stools. Children with functional fecal retention often exhibit "retentive posturing" (standing or sitting with legs extended and stiff or crossed legs) and have associated fecal incontinence caused by leakage of retained stool (**encopresis**).

Differential Diagnosis

The differential diagnosis is listed in Table 126-10. **Functional constipation** commonly occurs during toilet training, when the child is unwilling to defecate on the toilet. Retained stool becomes harder and larger over time, leading to painful defecation. This aggravates voluntary withholding of stool, with perpetuation of the constipation.

Hirschsprung disease is characterized by delayed meconium passage in newborns, abdominal distention, vomiting, occasional fever, and foul-smelling stools. This condition is caused by failure of ganglion cells to migrate into the distal bowel, resulting in spasm and functional obstruction of the aganglionic segment. Only about 6% of infants with Hirschsprung disease pass meconium in the first 24 hours of life, compared with 95% of normal infants. Most affected babies rapidly become ill with symptoms of enterocolitis or obstruction. Affected older children do not pass large-caliber stools because of rectal spasm, and they do not have encopresis. Other causes of constipation include spinal cord abnormalities, hypothyroidism, drugs, cystic fibrosis, and anorectal malformations (see Table 126-10). A variety of systemic disorders affecting metabolism or muscle function can result in constipation. Children with **developmental disabilities** have a great propensity for constipation because of diminished capacity to cooperate with toileting, reduced effort or control of pelvic floor muscles during defecation, and diminished perception of the need to pass stool.

Distinguishing Features

Table 126-10 includes typical characteristics of the common causes of constipation. Congenital malformations usually cause

Table 126-10	Common Causes of Constipation and Characteristic Features
CAUSES OF CONSTIPATION	**CLINICAL FEATURES**
Hirschsprung disease	*History:* Failure to pass stool in first 24 h, abdominal distention, vomiting, symptoms of enterocolitis (fever, foul-smelling diarrhea, megacolon). Not associated with large-caliber stools or encopresis *Examination:* Snug anal sphincter, empty, contracted rectum. May have explosive release of stool as examiner's finger is withdrawn *Laboratory:* Absence of ganglion cells on rectal suction biopsy specimen, absent relaxation of the internal sphincter, "transition zone" from narrow distal bowel to dilated proximal bowel on barium enema
Functional constipation	*History:* No history of significant neonatal constipation, onset at potty training, large-caliber stools, retentive posturing, may have encopresis *Examination:* Normal or reduced sphincter tone, dilated rectal vault, fecal impaction, soiled underwear, palpable fecal mass in left lower quadrant *Laboratory:* No abnormalities, barium enema would show dilated distal bowel

Anorectal and colonic malformations
  Anal stenosis
  Anteriorly displaced anus
  Imperforate anus
  Colonic stricture
	History: Constipation from birth due to abnormal anatomy
	Examination: Anorectal abnormalities are shown easily on physical examination
	Anteriorly displaced anus is found chiefly in females, with a normal-appearing anus located close to the posterior fourchette of the vagina
	Laboratory: Barium enema shows the anomaly

Multisystem disease
  Muscular dystrophy
  Cystic fibrosis
  Diabetes mellitus
  Developmental delay
  Celiac disease
	History: Presence of other symptoms or prior diagnosis
	Examination: Specific abnormalities may be present that directly relate to the underlying diagnosis
	Laboratory: Tests directed at suspected disorder confirm the diagnosis

Spinal cord abnormalities
  Meningomyelocele
  Tethered cord
  Sacral teratoma or lipoma
	History: History of swelling or exposed neural tissue in the lower back, history of urinary incontinence
	Examination: Lax sphincter tone due to impaired innervation, visible or palpable abnormality of lower back usually (but not always) present
	Laboratory: Bony abnormalities often present on plain x-ray. Magnetic resonance imaging (MRI) of spinal cord reveals characteristic abnormalities

Drugs Narcotics Psychotropics	*History:* Recent use of drugs known to cause constipation *Examination:* Features suggest functional constipation *Laboratory:* No specific tests available

symptoms from birth. Functional constipation is overwhelmingly the most common diagnosis in older patients. Constipation in older children often begins after starting school, when free and private access to toilets may be restricted. Use of some drugs, especially opiates and some psychotropic medications, also is associated with constipation.

For a few specific causes of constipation, directed diagnostic testing can make the diagnosis. A narrowed, aganglionic distal bowel and dilated proximal bowel on barium enema suggests Hirschsprung disease. Rectal suction biopsy confirms the absence of ganglion cells in the rectal submucosal plexus, with hypertrophy of nerve fibers. Lack of internal anal sphincter relaxation can be shown by anorectal manometry in Hirschsprung's disease. Hypothyroidism is diagnosed by examination and by thyroid function testing. Anorectal malformations are easily detected by rectal examination. Cystic fibrosis (meconium ileus) is diagnosed by sweat chloride determination or *CFTR* gene mutation analysis (see Chapter 137). Most children with constipation have functional constipation and do not have any laboratory abnormality. Examination reveals normal or reduced anal sphincter tone (owing to stretching by passage of large stools). Fecal impaction is usually present, but a large-caliber, empty rectum may be found if a stool has just been passed.

Evaluation and Treatment of Functional Constipation

In most cases of constipation, the history is consistent with functional constipation—absence of neonatal constipation,

active fecal retention, and infrequent, large stools with soiling. In these patients, no testing other than a good physical examination is necessary. Young children with painful defecation must have a prolonged course of stool softener therapy to alleviate fear of defecation. The child should be asked to sit on the toilet for a few minutes on awakening in the morning and immediately after meals, when the colon is most active and it is easiest to pass a stool. Use of a positive reinforcement system for taking medication and sitting on the toilet is helpful for younger children. The stool softener chosen should be non–habit forming, safe, and palatable. Polyethylene glycol and milk of magnesia are the most commonly used agents.

Gastrointestinal Bleeding

Decision-Making Algorithm
Available @ StudentConsult.com

Gastrointestinal Bleeding

GI tract bleeding can be an emergency when large-volume bleeding is present, but even the presence of small amounts of blood in stool or emesis is sufficient to cause concern. Evaluation of bleeding should include confirmation that blood truly is present, estimation of the amount of bleeding, stabilization of the patient's intravascular blood volume, localization of the source of bleeding, and appropriate treatment of the underlying cause. When bleeding is massive, it is crucial that the

| Table 126-11 | Causes and Distinguishing Characteristics of Gastrointestinal Bleeding |

AGE	TYPE OF BLEEDING	CHARACTERISTICS
NEWBORN		
Ingested maternal blood*	Hematemesis or rectal, large	Apt test indicates adult hemoglobin is present, cracked maternal nipples, amount
Peptic disease	Hematemesis, amount varies	Blood found in stomach on lavage
Coagulopathy	Hematemesis or rectal, bruising, other sites	History of home birth (no vitamin K)
Allergic colitis*	Streaks of bloody mucus in stool	Eosinophils in feces and in rectal mucosa
Necrotizing enterocolitis	Rectal	Sick infant with tender and distended abdomen
Duplication cyst	Hematemesis	Cystic mass in abdomen on imaging study
Volvulus	Hematemesis, hematochezia	Acute tender distended abdomen
INFANCY TO 2 YEARS OLD		
Peptic disease	Usually hematemesis, rectal possible	Epigastric pain, coffee-ground emesis
Esophageal varices	Hematemesis	History or evidence of liver disease
Intussusception*	Rectal bleeding	Crampy pain, distention, mass
Meckel diverticulum*	Rectal	Massive, bright red bleeding; no pain
Bacterial enteritis*	Rectal	Bloody diarrhea, fever
NSAID injury	Usually hematemesis, rectal possible	Epigastric pain, coffee-ground emesis
>2 YEARS OLD		
Peptic disease	See above	See above
Esophageal varices	See above	See above
NSAID injury*	See above	See above
Inflammatory bowel disease	Usually rectal	Crampy pain, poor weight gain, diarrhea
Bacterial enteritis*	See above	See above
Pseudomembranous colitis	Rectal	History of antibiotic use, bloody diarrhea
Juvenile polyp	Rectal	Painless, bright red blood in stool; not massive
Meckel diverticulum*	See above	See above
Nodular lymphoid hyperplasia	Rectal	Streaks of blood in stool, no other symptoms
Mallory-Weiss syndrome*	Hematemesis	Bright red or coffee-ground, follows retching
Hemolytic uremic syndrome	Rectal	Thrombocytopenia, anemia, uremia
Hemorrhoids	Rectal	Dilated external veins, blood with wiping

NSAID, Nonsteroidal anti-inflammatory drug.
*Common

patient receive adequate resuscitation with fluid and blood products before moving ahead with diagnostic testing.

Differential Diagnosis
GI bleeding has different causes at different ages (Table 126-11).

Distinguishing Features
Red substances in foods, beverages, or medications (such as cefdinir) occasionally can be mistaken for blood. A test for occult blood is worth performing whenever the diagnosis is in doubt.

The GI tract may not be the source of the observed fecal blood. A history of cough and examination of the mouth, nostrils, and lungs is needed to exclude these as a source of hematemesis. Blood in the toilet or diaper may be coming from the urinary tract, vagina, or even a severe diaper rash. If the bleeding is GI, it is important to determine the source as high in the GI tract or distal to the ligament of Treitz. Vomited blood is always proximal. Rectal bleeding may be coming from anywhere in the gut. When dark clots or melena are seen mixed with stool, a higher location is suspected, whereas bright red blood on the surface of stool probably is coming from lower in the colon. When upper GI tract bleeding is suspected, a nasogastric tube may be placed and gastric contents aspirated for evidence of recent bleeding.

The location and hemodynamic significance of the bleeding can also be assessed by history and examination. The parents should be asked to quantify the bleeding. Details of associated symptoms should be sought. Assessment of the vital signs including orthostatic changes when bleeding volume is large, pulses, capillary refill and assessment of pallor of the mucous membranes provides valuable information. Laboratory assessment and imaging studies should be ordered as indicated (Table 126-12).

Table 126-12	Evaluation of Gastrointestinal Bleeding

LABORATORY INVESTIGATION	Sigmoidoscopy or colonoscopy
All Patients	Meckel scan
CBC and platelet count	Mesenteric arteriogram
Coagulation tests: prothrombin time, partial thromboplastin time	Video capsule endoscopy
	INITIAL RADIOLOGIC EVALUATION
Tests of liver dysfunction: AST, ALT, GGT, bilirubin	*All Patients*
Occult blood test of stool or vomitus	Abdominal x-ray series
Blood type and crossmatch	*Evaluation of Hematemesis*
Evaluation of Bloody Diarrhea	Barium upper GI series if endoscopy not available
Stool culture, *Clostridium difficile* toxin	*Evaluation of Bleeding with Pain and Vomiting (Bowel Obstruction)*
Sigmoidoscopy or colonoscopy	
CT with contrast	Abdominal x-ray series
Evaluation of Rectal Bleeding with Formed Stools	Pneumatic or contrast enema
External and digital rectal examination	Upper GI series

ALT, Alanine aminotransferase; *AST,* aspartate aminotransferase; *CBC,* complete blood count; *CT,* computed tomography; *GGT,* γ-glutamyltransferase; *GI,* gastrointestinal.

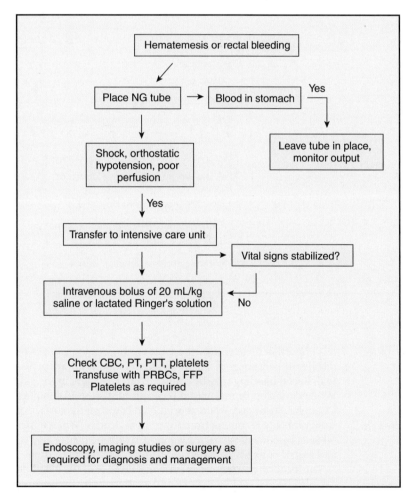

Figure 126-2 Initial management of gastrointestinal bleeding. *CBC,* Complete blood count; *FFP,* fresh frozen plasma; *NG,* nasogastric; *PRBCs,* packed red blood cells; *PT,* prothrombin time; *PTT,* partial thromboplastin time.

Treatment

Treatment of GI bleeding should begin with an initial assessment, rapid stabilization, and a logical sequence of diagnostic tests. When a treatable cause is identified, specific therapy should be started. In many cases, the amount of blood is small, and no resuscitation is required. For children with large-volume bleeds, the **ABCs** of resuscitation (airway, breathing, circulation) should be addressed first (see Chapters 38 and 40). Oxygen should be administered and the airway protected with an endotracheal tube if massive hematemesis is present.

Fluid boluses and transfusion with packed red blood cells as required should be administered through two large-bore IVs. Frequent reassessment should continue to ensure maintenance of physiological stability (Fig. 126-2).

Chapter 127

ORAL CAVITY

EFFECTS OF SYSTEMIC DISEASE ON THE ORAL CAVITY

Medications taken for a variety of conditions may cause oral abnormalities. Drugs with anticholinergic properties diminish saliva production and increase the risk of dental caries and parotitis. Tetracyclines taken before the eruption of the permanent teeth stain the enamel. Excessive fluoride in vitamin preparations or in drinking water can result in mottled teeth. Gingival hypertrophy may be caused by cyclosporine, phenytoin, and calcium channel blockers.

Gastroesophageal reflux disease (GER) can lead to substantial enamel erosion and caries. Neonatal hyperbilirubinemia can result in bluish discoloration of the deciduous teeth. Renal failure is associated with mottled enamel of the permanent teeth. Congenital syphilis causes marked abnormalities in the shape of teeth, especially incisors and molars. Celiac disease can result in enamel defects. Crohn's disease is associated with oral aphthous ulcers. Abnormal pigmentation of the lips and buccal mucosa is seen with Peutz-Jeghers syndrome and Addison disease. Candidiasis is seen commonly with immunodeficiency disorders and diabetes. Leukemic infiltrates result in gum hyperplasia and bleeding; treatment of neoplastic conditions can cause severe mucositis. Some tumors, including lymphoma, may present as mass lesions of the buccal cavity.

Osteogenesis imperfecta is associated with abnormal dentin and risk of caries. Children with *ectodermal dysplasias* commonly have malformed or missing teeth. Pierre Robin syndrome is associated with micrognathia and cleft palate. Disorders resulting in facial dysmorphism can have a profound effect on dental occlusion and mandibular function. Examples include mandibulofacial dysostosis, Crouzon syndrome, conditions associated with dwarfism, and others.

DECIDUOUS AND PRIMARY TEETH

Most infants are born without teeth. *Natal teeth* are present at birth, are usually supernumerary, and may be poorly attached. Usually, no treatment is necessary, but removal by a dentist may be needed if they are causing difficulties with feeding or injuries to the tongue. Table 127-1 presents the ages when normal **deciduous teeth** are acquired. The lower central incisors are typically the first to erupt, followed by the upper central incisors, lateral incisors, first molars, and bicuspids. **Delayed eruption** may occur in association with hypopituitarism, hypothyroidism, osteopetrosis, Gaucher disease, Down syndrome, cleidocranial dysplasia, and rickets. Deciduous teeth begin to be replaced by the permanent teeth at around age 6

Table 127-1	Time of Eruption of the Primary and Permanent Teeth			
	PRIMARY, AGE (mo)		PERMANENT, AGE (yr)	
Tooth type	Upper	Lower	Upper	Lower
Central incisor	6 ± 2	7 ± 2	7–8	6–7
Lateral incisor	9 ± 2	7 ± 2	8–9	7–8
Cuspids	18 ± 2	16 ± 2	11–12	9–10
First bicuspids	—	—	10–11	10–12
Second bicuspids	—	—	10–12	11–12
First molars	14 ± 2	12 ± 2	6–7	6–7
Second molars	24 ± 2	20 ± 2	12–13	11–13
Third molars	—	—	17–21	17–21

years. The sequence of replacement is similar to that of the appearance of deciduous teeth.

DENTAL CARIES
Etiology

Dental caries, commonly referred to as "cavities," occurs as a result of interactions between the tooth enamel, dietary carbohydrates, and oral flora. There is increased susceptibility if the enamel is abnormal or hypoplastic. Bacteria (*Streptococcus mutans*) that can adhere to and colonize the teeth, survive at low pH, and produce acids during fermentation of carbohydrates cause dental caries. The diet has a significant role. A classic example is "bottle mouth," or **baby bottle caries**. This condition results when infants are allowed to have a bottle in the mouth for prolonged periods, especially during sleep, and with sweet beverages or milk in the bottle. Bacteria then have continuous substrate for acid production and can destroy multiple teeth, especially the upper incisors. Sticky sweet foods, such as candy, have the same effect.

Epidemiology and Treatment

Risk of caries is associated with lack of dental care and poor socioeconomic status and, predictably, is greatest in developing countries. Baby bottle caries is seen in 50% to 70% of low-income infants. Treatment of caries is with dental restorative surgery. The carious portion is removed and filled with silver amalgam or plastic. If the damage is severe, a protective crown may be required; extraction of the tooth may be necessary when not salvageable. If not properly treated, dental decay results in inflammation and infection of the dental pulp and surrounding alveolar bone, which can lead to abscess and facial space infections.

Prevention

Avoiding inappropriate use of bottles and excessive sweets is a commonsense remedy for baby bottle caries. Oral hygiene offers some protection, but young children (<8 years old) do not have the ability to brush their own teeth adequately; brushing should be done by the parents. Fluoride supplementation of community water supplies to a concentration of 1 ppm is highly effective in reducing dental caries. Home water supplies, such as from a well, should have the fluoride content tested before supplements are prescribed. If the child spends part of the day at another location, the total fluoride concentration from all sources must be considered before prescribing any oral supplements. Excessive fluoride supplementation causes fluorosis, a largely cosmetic defect of chalky white marks and brown staining of the teeth.

CLEFT LIP AND PALATE
Epidemiology
Cleft lip and palate occur separately or together and affect approximately 1 in 700 infants. It is more common in Asians (1:500) and least common in Africans (1:2500). Clefting occurs with two possible patterns: isolated soft tissue cleft palate or cleft lip with or without associated clefts of the hard palate. Isolated cleft palate is associated with a higher risk of other congenital malformations. The combined cleft lip/palate type has a male predominance.

Etiology
Cleft lip is due to hypoplasia of the mesenchymal tissues with subsequent failure of fusion. There is a strong genetic component; the risk is highest in children with affected first-degree relatives. Monozygotic twins are affected with only 60% concordance, suggesting other nongenomic factors. Environmental factors during gestation also increase risk, including drugs (phenytoin, valproic acid, thalidomide), maternal alcohol and tobacco use, dioxins and other herbicides, and possibly high altitude. Chromosomal and nonchromosomal syndromes are associated with clefting, as are specific genes in some families.

Clinical Manifestations and Treatment
Cleft lip can be unilateral or bilateral and associated with cleft palate and defects of the alveolar ridge and dentition. When present, palatal defects allow direct communication between the nasal and oral cavities, creating problems with speech and feeding. Management includes squeeze-bottle feedings, special nipples, nipples with attached shields to seal the palate, and gastrostomy in severe cases. Surgical closure of the cleft lip is usually done by 3 months of age. Closure of the palate follows, usually before 1 year of age. Missing teeth are replaced by prostheses. Cosmetic results are often good, but depend on the severity of the defect.

Complications
Speech is nasal as a result of the cleft palate. Surgical treatment is effective, but sometimes does not restore palatal function completely. Speech therapy or, occasionally, the use of a speech-assisting appliance may help. Frequent episodes of otitis media are common, as are defects of teeth and the alveolar ridge.

THRUSH
Epidemiology
Oropharyngeal *Candida albicans* infection, or thrush, is common in healthy neonates. The organism may be acquired in the birth canal or from the environment. Persistent infection is common in breastfed infants as a result of colonization or infection of the mother's nipples. Thrush in healthy older patients can occur, but should suggest the possibility of an immunodeficiency, broad-spectrum antibiotic use, or diabetes.

Clinical Manifestations
Thrush is easily visible as white plaques, often with a "fuzzy" appearance, on oral mucous membranes. When scraped with a tongue depressor, the plaques are difficult to remove, and the underlying mucosa is inflamed and friable. Clinical diagnosis is usually adequate, but may be confirmed by fungal culture or potassium hydroxide smear. Oropharyngeal candidiasis is sometimes painful (especially if associated with esophagitis) and can interfere with feeding.

Treatment
Thrush is treated with topical nystatin or an azole antifungal agent such as fluconazole. When the mother's breasts are infected and painful, consideration should be given to treating her at the same time. Because thrush is commonly self-limited in newborns, withholding therapy in asymptomatic infants and treating only persistent or severe cases is a reasonable approach.

Chapter **128**

ESOPHAGUS AND STOMACH

GASTROESOPHAGEAL REFLUX
Etiology and Epidemiology

Decision-Making Algorithms
Available @ StudentConsult.com

Cough
Wheezing
Abdominal Pain
Vomiting
Gastrointestinal Bleeding

Gastroesophageal reflux (GER) is defined as the effortless retrograde movement of gastric contents upward into the esophagus or oropharynx. In infancy, GER is not always an abnormality. **Physiologic GER** ("spitting up") is normal in infants younger than 8 to 12 months old. Nearly half of all infants are reported to spit up at 2 months of age. Infants who regurgitate meet the criteria for physiologic GER so long as they maintain adequate nutrition and have no signs of respiratory complications or esophagitis. Factors involved in causing infantile GER include liquid diet; horizontal body position; short, narrow esophagus; small, noncompliant stomach; frequent, relatively large-volume feedings; and an immature lower esophageal sphincter (LES). As infants grow, they spend more time upright, eat more solid foods, develop a longer and larger diameter esophagus, have a larger and more compliant stomach, and experience lower caloric needs per unit of body weight. As a result, most infants stop spitting up by 9 to 12 months of age.

Gastroesophageal reflux *disease* (GERD) occurs when GER leads to troublesome symptoms or complications such as poor growth, pain, or breathing difficulties. GERD occurs in a minority of infants but is often implicated as the cause of fussiness. GERD is seen in fewer than 5% of older children. In older children, normal protective mechanisms against GER include antegrade esophageal motility, tonic contraction of the LES, and the geometry of the gastroesophageal junction. Abnormalities that cause GER in older children and adults include reduced tone of the LES, transient relaxations of the LES, esophagitis (which impairs esophageal motility), increased intra-abdominal pressure, cough, respiratory difficulty (asthma or cystic fibrosis), and hiatal hernia.

Clinical Manifestations

Decision-Making Algorithms
Available @ StudentConsult.com

Cough
Hoarseness
Wheezing
Abdominal Pain
Failure to Thrive

The presence of GER is easy to observe in an infant who spits up. In older children, the refluxate is usually kept down by reswallowing, but GER may be suspected by associated symptoms, such as heartburn, cough, epigastric abdominal pain, dysphagia, wheezing, aspiration pneumonia, hoarse voice, failure to thrive, and recurrent otitis media or sinusitis. In severe cases of esophagitis, there may be laboratory evidence of anemia and hypoalbuminemia secondary to esophageal bleeding and inflammation.

When esophagitis develops as a result of acid reflux, esophageal motility and LES function are impaired further, creating a cycle of reflux and esophageal injury.

Laboratory and Imaging Studies
A clinical diagnosis is often sufficient in children with classic effortless regurgitation and no complications. Diagnostic studies are indicated if there are persistent symptoms or complications or if other symptoms suggest the possibility of GER in the absence of regurgitation. A child with recurrent pneumonia, chronic cough, or apneic spells without overt emesis may have occult GER. A **barium upper GI series** helps to rule out gastric outlet obstruction, malrotation, or other anatomic contributors to GER. Because of the brief nature of the examination, a negative barium study does *not* rule out GER. Another study, **24-hour esophageal pH probe monitoring**, uses a pH

electrode placed transnasally into the distal esophagus, with continuous recording of esophageal pH. Data typically are gathered for 24 hours and analyzed for the number and temporal pattern of acid reflux events. **Esophageal impedance monitoring** records the migration of electrolyte-rich gastric fluid in the esophagus. **Endoscopy** is useful to evaluate for esophagitis, esophageal stricture, and anatomic abnormalities.

Treatment
In otherwise healthy young infants, no treatment is necessary. For infants with complications of GER, an H_2 blocker or proton-pump inhibitor may be offered (Table 128-1), but these have shown little benefit in infants with uncomplicated GER and/or fussiness. Prokinetic drugs, such as metoclopramide, occasionally are helpful by enhancing gastric emptying and increasing LES tone, but they are seldom very effective and may lead to complications. When severe symptoms persist despite medication, or if life-threatening aspiration is present, surgical intervention may be required. Fundoplication procedures, such as the Nissen operation, are designed to enhance the antireflux anatomy of the LES. In children with a severe neurologic defect who cannot tolerate oral or gastric tube feedings, placement of a feeding jejunostomy may be considered as an alternative to fundoplication. In older children, lifestyle changes should be discussed, including cessation of smoking, weight loss, not eating before bed or exercise, and limiting intake of caffeine, carbonation, and high-fat foods. However, proton pump inhibitor therapy is more effective in reducing symptoms and healing.

EOSINOPHILIC ESOPHAGITIS (EOE)
Etiology and Epidemiology
This chronic immune-mediated disorder is characterized by infiltration of eosinophils into mucosa of the esophagus. It is thought to be triggered by non–IgE-mediated allergic reactions to ingested foods or aeroallergens. EoE may have a familial connection; no specific gene has yet been identified. Incidence appears to be increasing with estimated prevalence of more than 4 per 10,000 children. It may be more common in males than females.

Clinical Manifestations
The presentation of EoE often varies with age. In young children, it may present with oral aversion, vomiting, and failure to thrive. In school-age children, it may present with vague abdominal pain or vomiting. In adolescents and adults, it presents with dysphagia and food impactions. These symptoms are attributed to the inflammatory response in the esophagus leading to edema and poor esophageal motility.

Laboratory and Imaging Studies
Diagnosis requires multilevel esophageal biopsies via flexible endoscopy with the finding of more than 15 eosinophils per high-power field (Fig. 128-1). Treatment with high-dose proton pump inhibitor therapy is recommended to exclude the possibility that findings are secondary to severe acidic esophageal injury. Gross findings at endoscopy include normal appearance, esophageal furrowing, trachealization, and eosinophilic abscesses (Fig. 128-2). A barium study may reveal

Table 128-1	Treatment of Gastroesophageal Reflux	
THERAPIES		**COMMENTS**
CONSERVATIVE THERAPIES		
Towel on caregiver's shoulder		Cheap, effective. Useful only for physiologic reflux
Thickened feedings		Reduces number of episodes, enhances nutrition
Smaller, more frequent feedings		Can help some. Be careful not to *underfeed* child
Avoidance of tobacco smoke and alcohol		Always a good idea. May help reflux symptoms
Abstaining from caffeine		Inexpensive, offers some benefit
Positional therapy—upright in seat, elevate		Prone positioning with head of crib or bed up is helpful, but *not* for young infants because of risk of SIDS
Weight loss when indicated		Increased weight (especially abdominal) increases intra-abdominal pressure, leading to reflux
MEDICAL THERAPY		
Proton-pump inhibitor		Effective medical therapy for heartburn and esophagitis
H₂ receptor antagonist		Reduces heartburn, less effective for healing esophagitis
Metoclopramide		Enhances stomach emptying and LES tone. Real benefit is often minimal
SURGICAL THERAPY		
Nissen or other fundoplication procedure		For life-threatening or medically unresponsive cases
Feeding jejunostomy		Useful in child requiring tube feeds. Delivering feeds downstream eliminates GERD

GERD, Gastroesophageal reflux disease; *LES,* lower esophageal sphincter; *SIDS,* sudden infant death syndrome.

Figure 128-1 Histologic image of eosinophilic esophagitis. Note the large number of eosinophils within the lamina propria.

Figure 128-2 Endoscopic picture of eosinophilic esophagitis. White plaques on the surface are collections of eosinophils (eosinophilic abscesses). Linear furrowing is also seen.

a food impaction in an acutely symptomatic patient or esophageal stricture in someone with chronic disease.

Treatment and Prognosis

Exposure to identified causative antigens needs to be eliminated. Identification can be difficult, as typical allergy testing (skin prick, RAST, and immunocap assays) only identifies IgE-mediated antigens. Atopic patch testing may be more reliable but is not standardized and can be difficult to perform. One approach is to eliminate cow's milk, soy, wheat, eggs, peanuts, and fish/shellfish from the diet, as these are the most common causative dietary antigens. Repeat endoscopies are often necessary to document efficacy of these eliminations. An elemental diet can also be used and is very effective, but often requires either nasogastric or gastrotomy administration because of its poor palatability.

Systemic glucocorticoids can decrease symptoms, but long-term use is discouraged secondary to complications. Swallowed "topical" glucocorticoids administered via a metered dose inhaler (fluticasone) or mixed as a slurry (budesonide)

Esophageal atresia
with distal TEF
(85%)

Esophageal atresia
with no TEF
(8%)

H-type TEF
(4%)

Esophageal atresia
with proximal TEF
(2%)

Esophageal atresia with
proximal and distal TEF
(1%)

Figure 128-3 Various types of tracheoesophageal fistulas (TEF) with relative frequency (%).

have shown benefit. *Candida* esophagitis or oral thrush are the most common side effects.

Endoscopy can be used to relieve food impactions and to dilate esophageal strictures secondary to EoE. The prognosis for EoE is largely unknown. Symptoms tend to wax and wane over time.

Complications
Failure to thrive or weight loss may be seen due to difficulty in eating. Food impactions are a common complication in the older child and may require endoscopic removal. Chronic inflammation of the esophagus can predispose to esophageal strictures and possibly dysplasia.

ESOPHAGEAL ATRESIA AND TRACHEOESOPHAGEAL FISTULA
Etiology and Epidemiology
The esophagus and trachea develop in close proximity to each other during weeks 4 to 6 of fetal life. Defects in the mesenchyme separating these two structures result in a tracheoesophageal fistula (TEF), often in association with other anomalies (renal, heart, spine, limbs). This defect occurs in about 1 in 3000 live births. TEF is not thought to be a genetic defect.

Clinical Manifestations
The most common forms of TEF occur with esophageal atresia; the "H-type" TEF without atresia is uncommon, as is esophageal atresia without TEF (Fig. 128-3). Associated defects include the **VACTERL** association—**v**ertebral anomalies (70%), **a**nal atresia (imperforate anus) (50%), **c**ardiac anomalies (30%), **TEF** (70%), **r**enal anomalies (50%), and **l**imb anomalies (polydactyly, forearm defects, absent thumbs,

syndactyly) (70%). A single-artery umbilical cord is often present. Infants with esophageal atresia have a history of polyhydramnios, exhibit drooling, and have mucus and saliva bubbling from the nose and mouth. Patients with a TEF are vulnerable to aspiration pneumonia. When TEF is suspected, the first feeding should be delayed until a diagnostic study is performed.

Laboratory and Imaging Studies
The simplest test for TEF is to gently attempt to place a 10F or larger tube via the mouth into the stomach. The passage of the tube is blocked at the level of the atresia. A chest x-ray reveals the tube coiled in the esophageal pouch. Air can be injected through the tube to outline the atretic pouch. Barium should not be used because of extreme risk of aspiration, but a tiny amount of dilute water-soluble contrast agent can be given carefully, then aspirated when the defect is clearly shown.

Treatment and Prognosis
The treatment of TEF is surgical. The fistula is divided and ligated. The esophageal ends are approximated and anastomosed. In some cases, primary anastomosis cannot be performed because of a long gap between the proximal and distal esophagus. Various techniques have been described to treat this problem, including pulling up the stomach, elongating the esophagus by myotomy, and simply delaying esophageal anastomosis and providing continuous suction to the upper pouch while allowing for growth.

Complications
The surgically reconstructed esophagus is not normal and is prone to poor motility, GER, anastomotic stricture, recurrent fistula,

and leakage. The trachea also is malformed; tracheomalacia and wheezing are common.

ESOPHAGEAL FOREIGN BODIES
Etiology and Epidemiology

Young children often place nonfood items in their mouths. When these items are swallowed, they may become lodged in the esophagus at the thoracic inlet or at the LES. The most common objects are coins. Smaller coins may pass harmlessly into the stomach, where they rarely cause symptoms. Other common esophageal foreign bodies include food items, small toys or toy parts, disk batteries, and other small household items. Children with a prior history of esophageal atresia or with poor motility secondary to GER or eosinophilic esophagitis are more prone to food impactions, which seldom occur in the normal esophagus.

Clinical Manifestations

Some children are asymptomatic, but most exhibit some degree of drooling, food refusal, or chest discomfort. Older children usually can point to the region of the chest where they feel the object to be lodged. Respiratory symptoms tend to be minimal, but cough or wheezing may be present, especially when the esophagus is completely blocked by a large object, such as a piece of meat, which presses on the trachea.

Diagnosis

Plain chest and abdominal radiographs should be taken when foreign body ingestion is suspected. Metallic objects are easily visualized. A plastic object often can be seen if the child is given a small amount of dilute x-ray contrast material to drink, although endoscopy is probably safer and more definitive.

Treatment

Endoscopy is ultimately necessary in most cases to remove an esophageal foreign body. Various devices can be used to remove the object, depending on its size, shape, and location. Coins usually are grasped with special-purpose forceps and removed. Nets, baskets, and snares also are available. Whenever objects that may threaten the airway are being recovered, endoscopy should be performed with endotracheal intubation and under general anesthesia. Removal is usually not necessary if the object is small and in the stomach as it will most likely pass without complication. Endoscopy is emergent for removal of any esophageal foreign body if symptomatic or if the ingested foreign body is a suspected disc battery in the esophagus or multiple magnets located in the upper tract.

Complications

Sharp objects may lacerate or perforate the esophagus; smooth objects present for a long time also may result in perforation due to ulceration. Corrosive objects, such as zinc-containing pennies and disc batteries, can cause considerable local tissue injury and esophageal perforation. Magnets can lead to perforation and fistula formation when they connect between adjacent loops of bowel.

CAUSTIC INJURIES AND PILL ULCERS
Etiology and Epidemiology

In adolescents, caustic ingestion injuries are usually the result of suicide attempts. In toddlers, ingestion of household cleaning products typically is accidental. Injurious agents include drain cleaners, toilet bowl cleaners, dishwasher detergents, and powerful bleaching agents. Childproof lids for commercial products offer some protection, but have not eliminated the problem. Lye-based drain cleaners, especially liquid products, cause the worst injuries because they are swallowed easily and liquefy tissue rapidly. Full-thickness burns can occur in seconds. Granular products are less likely to cause esophageal injury during accidental exposures because they burn the tongue and lips and often are expelled before swallowing. Less caustic agents, such as bleach and detergents, cause less serious injury. **Pill ulcers** occur when certain medications (tetracyclines and nonsteroidal anti-inflammatory drugs [NSAIDs]) are swallowed without sufficient liquids, allowing prolonged direct contact of the pill with the esophageal mucosa.

Clinical Manifestations

Caustic burns cause immediate and severe mouth pain. The child cries out, drools, spits, and usually drops the container immediately. Burns of the lips and tongue are visible almost immediately. These burns clearly indicate the possibility of esophageal involvement, although esophageal injury can occur in the absence of oral burns. Symptoms may not be present; further evaluation by endoscopy usually is indicated with any significant history of caustic ingestion. Pill injury causes severe chest pain and often prominent odynophagia (painful swallowing) and dysphagia.

Laboratory and Imaging Studies

A chest x-ray should be obtained to rule out aspiration and to inspect for mediastinal air. The child should be admitted to the hospital and given intravenous (IV) fluids until endoscopy. The true extent of burns may not be endoscopically apparent immediately, but delayed endoscopy can increase the risk of perforation. Most endoscopists perform the initial endoscopy soon after injury, when the patient has been stabilized. The extent of injury and severity of the burn should be carefully determined. Risk of subsequent esophageal strictures is related to the degree of burn and whether the injury is circumferential.

Treatment

A nasogastric tube can be placed over a guidewire at the time of the initial endoscopy to provide a route for feeding and to stent the esophagus. Systemic steroid use has not been found to be beneficial in reducing stricture formation. Broad-spectrum antibiotics should be prescribed if infection is suspected.

Complications

Esophageal strictures, if they occur, usually develop within 1 to 2 months and can be treated with endoscopic dilation. There is a risk of perforation during dilation. When esophageal destruction is severe, surgical reconstruction of the esophagus using stomach or intestine may be necessary.

PYLORIC STENOSIS
Etiology and Epidemiology

Decision-Making Algorithm
Available @ StudentConsult.com

Vomiting

Pyloric stenosis is an acquired condition caused by hypertrophy and spasm of the pyloric muscle, resulting in gastric outlet obstruction. It occurs in 6 to 8 per 1000 live births, has a 5-to-1 male predominance, and is more common in first-born children. Its cause is unknown.

Clinical Manifestations

Infants with pyloric stenosis typically begin vomiting during the first weeks of life, but onset may be delayed. The emesis becomes increasingly frequent and forceful as time passes. Vomiting differs from spitting up because of its extremely forceful and often projectile nature. The vomited material never contains bile, because the gastric outlet obstruction is proximal to the duodenum. This feature differentiates pyloric stenosis from most other obstructive lesions of early childhood. Affected infants are ravenously hungry early in the course of the illness, but become more lethargic with increasing malnutrition and dehydration. The stomach becomes massively enlarged with retained food and secretions, and gastric **peristaltic waves** are often visible in the left upper quadrant. A hypertrophied pylorus (the "olive") may be palpated. As the illness progresses, very little of each feeding is able to pass through the pylorus, and the child becomes progressively thinner and more dehydrated.

Laboratory and Imaging Studies

Decision-Making Algorithm
Available @ StudentConsult.com

Alkalemia

Repetitive vomiting of purely gastric contents results in loss of hydrochloric acid; the classic laboratory finding is a **hypochloremic, hypokalemic metabolic alkalosis** with elevated blood urea nitrogen (BUN) secondary to dehydration. Jaundice with unconjugated hyperbilirubinemia may also occur. Plain abdominal x-rays typically show a huge stomach and diminished or absent gas in the intestine (Fig. 128-4). Ultrasound examination shows marked elongation and thickening of the pylorus (Fig. 128-5). A barium upper GI series also may be obtained whenever doubt about the diagnosis exists; this shows a "string sign" caused by barium moving through an elongated, constricted pyloric channel.

Figure 128-4 Pyloric stenosis. Note the huge, gas-filled stomach extending across the midline, with minimal air in the intestine downstream. *(Courtesy Warren Bishop, MD.)*

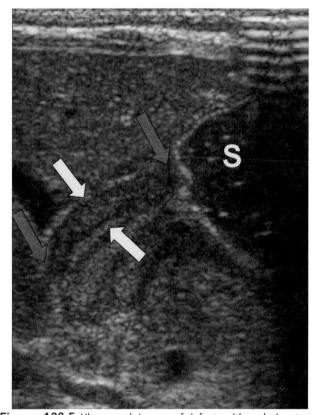

Figure 128-5 Ultrasound image of infant with pyloric stenosis. Large, fluid-filled stomach (*S*) is seen at right, with an elongated, thickened pylorus. The length of the pylorus is marked by the *red arrows*; the wall thickness is marked by the *yellow arrows.*

Table 128-2	Risk Factors for Peptic Ulcer Disease

Helicobacter pylori infection

Drugs

    NSAIDs, including aspirin

    Tobacco use

    Bisphosphonates

    Potassium supplements

Family history

Sepsis

Head trauma

Burn injury

Hypotension

NSAIDs, Nonsteroidal anti-inflammatory drugs.

Table 128-3	Peptic Disorders, Symptoms, and Clinical Investigation

SYNDROME AND ASSOCIATED SYMPTOMS	CLINICAL INVESTIGATION
ESOPHAGITIS	
Retrosternal and epigastric location Burning pain Sensation of regurgitation Dysphagia, odynophagia	Endoscopy Therapeutic trial of acid-blocker therapy pH probe study
NONULCER DYSPEPSIA	
Upper abdominal location Fullness Bloating Nausea	Endoscopy Therapeutic trial of acid-blocker therapy Upper GI series to ligament of Treitz—rule out malrotation CBC, ESR, amylase, lipase, abdominal ultrasound
PEPTIC ULCER DISEASE	
"Alarm" symptoms Weight loss Hematemesis Melena, heme-positive stools Chronic vomiting Microcytic anemia Nocturnal pain Other symptoms—same as for esophagitis and nonulcer dyspepsia	Endoscopy—mandatory with alarm symptoms Test for *Helicobacter pylori* CBC, ESR, amylase, lipase, abdominal ultrasound

CBC, Complete blood count; *ESR,* erythrocyte sedimentation rate; *GI,* gastrointestinal.

Treatment

Treatment of pyloric stenosis includes IV fluid and electrolyte resuscitation followed by surgical pyloromyotomy. Before surgery, dehydration and hypochloremic alkalosis must be corrected, generally with an initial normal saline fluid bolus followed by infusions of half-normal saline containing 5% dextrose and potassium chloride when urine output is observed. In pyloromyotomy (often by laparoscope), the pyloric muscle is incised longitudinally to release the constriction. Care is taken not to cut into the mucosa itself.

PEPTIC DISEASE
Etiology and Epidemiology

Acid-related injury can occur in the esophagus, stomach, or duodenum. Table 128-2 lists risk factors for **peptic ulcer disease** in children. ***Helicobacter pylori*** is responsible for more than half of ulcers in the stomach and duodenum in adults. *H. pylori* plays a significant but lesser role in childhood ulcer disease. Risk factors for acquisition of *H. pylori* are low socioeconomic status and poor sanitation, with the highest incidence in developing countries. **Nonulcer dyspepsia** includes upper abdominal symptoms (pain, bloating, nausea, early satiety) in the absence of gastric or duodenal ulceration. Nonulcer dyspepsia is *not* associated with *H. pylori* infection. GER (see Chapter 128) allows acidic gastric contents to injure the esophagus, resulting in **esophagitis**. Esophagitis is characterized by retrosternal and epigastric burning pain and is best diagnosed by endoscopy. It can range from minimal, with only erythema and microscopic inflammation on biopsy, to superficial erosions and finally to frank ulceration.

Clinical Manifestations

Typical symptoms are listed in Table 128-3. The presence of recurrent burning epigastric and retrosternal pain is a risk factor for esophagitis. With duodenal ulcers, pain typically occurs several hours after meals and often awakens patients at night. Eating tends to relieve the pain. Gastric ulcers differ in that pain is commonly aggravated by eating, resulting in weight loss. GI bleeding from either can occur. Many patients report symptom relief with antacids or acid blockers.

Laboratory and Imaging Studies

Endoscopy can be used to diagnose the underlying condition. Empiric therapy with H_2 blockers or proton pump inhibitors can be used but may delay diagnosis of conditions such as *H. pylori*. For patients with chronic epigastric pain, the possibilities of inflammatory bowel disease, anatomic abnormality such as malrotation, pancreatitis, and biliary disease should be ruled out by appropriate testing when suspected (see Chapter 126 and Table 128-3 for recommended studies). Testing for *H. pylori* can be performed by biopsy during endoscopy with use of a urease test or presence histologically on tissue. If endoscopy is not done, noninvasive tests for infection can be done with reasonable accuracy with *H. pylori* fecal antigen and ^{13}C urea breath tests (urea is metabolized into $^{13}CO_2$ by the organism).

Treatment

If *H. pylori* is present in association with ulcers, it should be treated with a multidrug regimen, such as omeprazole-clarithromycin-metronidazole, omeprazole-amoxicillin-clarithromycin, or omeprazole-amoxicillin-metronidazole, given twice daily for 1 to 2 weeks. Other proton-pump inhibitors may be substituted when necessary. Bismuth compounds are effective against *H. pylori* and can be considered. In North America, only the subsalicylate salt is available, the use of which raises some concerns about Reye syndrome and potential salicylate toxicity. Tetracycline is useful in adults, but should be avoided in children less than 8 years of age. In the absence of *H. pylori*, esophagitis and peptic ulcer disease are treated with a proton-pump inhibitor, which yields higher rates of healing than H_2 receptor antagonists. Gastric and duodenal ulcers heal in 4 to 8 weeks in at least 80% of patients. Esophagitis requires 4 to 5 months of proton-pump inhibitor treatment for optimal healing.

CYCLIC VOMITING SYNDROME
Etiology and Epidemiology

Decision-Making Algorithm
Available @ StudentConsult.com

Vomiting

Cyclic vomiting syndrome (CVS) presents with intermittent episodes of prolonged nausea and vomiting with periods of health in between. It can occur at any age but is diagnosed most frequently in preschool to school-age children. It is thought to be a migraine variant; many patients have a positive family history of migraines, and some with CVS will eventually develop migraine headaches. Triggers to an episode often include viral illnesses, stressful or exciting events (holidays, birthdays, vacations), physical exhaustion, and menses.

Clinical Manifestations
Episodes can start at any time, but will often start in the early morning hours. Episodes are similar to each other in timing and duration. Repetitive vomiting can last hours to days. Patients can also have abdominal pain, diarrhea, and headaches. Those affected are typically pale, listless, and prefer to be left alone. They may have photo- or phonophobia.

Laboratory and Imaging Studies
There are no specific tests for CVS, which is diagnosed based on the history and the exclusion of other disorders. Diagnoses that should be considered include malrotation with intermittent volvulus, UPJ obstruction, eosinophilic esophagitis, and intracranial mass lesions, and metabolic disorders. Rome III criteria for diagnosis are outlined in Table 126-5.

Treatment
For the acute episode, supportive treatment includes hydration; dark, quiet environment; and antiemetics such as ondansetron. In addition, abortive therapy using antimigraine medications such as NSAIDs and triptans can be used. For those with frequent or prolonged episodes, prophylactic therapy can be used, such as cyproheptadine, tricyclic antidepressants, beta blockers, or topiramate.

Chapter 129

INTESTINAL TRACT

MIDGUT MALROTATION
Etiology and Epidemiology
During early fetal life, the midgut is attached to the yolk sac and loops outward into the umbilical cord. Beginning at around 10 weeks' gestation, the bowel reenters the abdomen and rotates counterclockwise around the superior mesenteric artery until the cecum arrives in the right lower quadrant. The duodenum rotates behind the artery and terminates at the **ligament of Treitz** in the left upper quadrant. The base of the mesentery becomes fixed along a broad attachment posteriorly, running from the cecum to the ligament of Treitz (Fig. 129-1A). When rotation is incomplete or otherwise abnormal, "malrotation" is present. Incomplete rotation occurs when the cecum stops near the right upper quadrant, and the duodenum fails to move behind the mesenteric artery; this results in an extremely narrow mesenteric root (see Fig. 129-1B) that makes the child susceptible to midgut **volvulus**, causing intestinal obstruction or mesenteric artery occlusion and intestinal infarction (Fig. 129-2). It is also common for abnormal mesenteric attachments (Ladd bands) to extend from the cecum across the duodenum, causing partial obstruction.

Clinical Manifestations

Decision-Making Algorithms
Available @ StudentConsult.com

Abdominal Pain
Vomiting
Gastrointestinal Bleeding

About 60% of children with malrotation present with symptoms of bilious vomiting during the first month of life. The remaining 40% present later in infancy or childhood. The emesis initially may be due to obstruction by Ladd bands without volvulus. When midgut volvulus occurs, the venous drainage of the gut is impaired; congestion results in ischemia, pain, tenderness, and often bloody emesis and stools. The bowel undergoes ischemic necrosis, and the child may appear septic. Physicians must be alert to the possibility of volvulus in patients with vomiting and fussiness or abdominal pain.

Laboratory and Imaging Studies
Plain abdominal x-rays generally show evidence of obstruction. Abdominal ultrasound may show evidence of malrotation. An upper gastrointestinal (GI) series shows the absence of a typical duodenal "C-loop," with the duodenum instead remaining on the right side of the abdomen. Abnormal placement of the cecum on follow-through (or by contrast enema) confirms the diagnosis. Laboratory studies are nonspecific, showing evidence of dehydration, electrolyte loss, or evidence

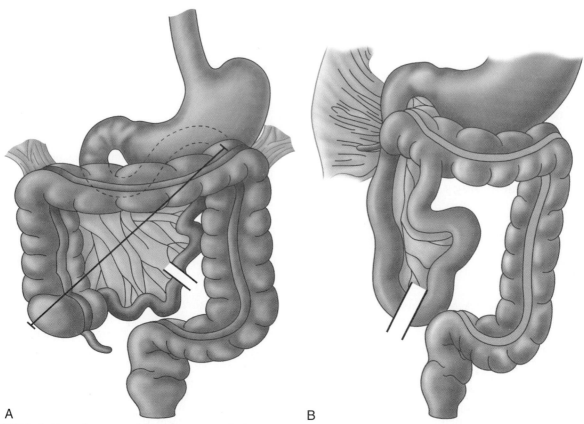

A   B

Figure 129-1 **A,** Normal rotation of the midgut. Note the long axis of mesenteric attachment *(line).* **B,** Midgut malrotation. Note the narrow mesentery, which predisposes to volvulus, and the presence of Ladd bands extending across the duodenum from the abnormally elevated cecum. *(From Donellan WJ, editor: Abdominal Surgery of Infancy and Childhood, Luxembourg, 1996, Harwood Academic, pp 43/6, 43/8.)*

Figure 129-2 Malrotation with volvulus. Midgut is twisted around the mesentery, with an area of darker, ischemic intestine visible. *(Courtesy Robert Soper, MD.)*

of sepsis. A decreasing platelet count is a common indicator of bowel ischemia.

Treatment

Treatment is surgical. The bowel is untwisted, and Ladd bands and other abnormal membranous attachments are divided. The mesentery is spread out and flattened against the posterior wall of the abdomen by moving the cecum to the left side of the abdomen. Sutures may be used to hold the bowel

in position, but postoperative adhesions tend to hold the mesentery in place, resulting in a broad attachment and eliminating the risk of recurrent volvulus. Necrotic bowel is resected and, at times, results in short gut syndrome.

INTESTINAL ATRESIA
Etiology and Epidemiology

Decision-Making Algorithms
Available @ StudentConsult.com

Abdominal Pain
Vomiting

Congenital partial or complete blockage of the intestine is a developmental defect that occurs in about 1 in 1500 live births. Atresia occurs in several forms (Fig. 129-3). One or more segments of bowel may be missing completely, there may be varying degrees of obstruction caused by webs or stenosis, or there may be obliteration of the lumen in cord-like bowel remnants. The end result is obstruction with upstream dilation of the bowel and small, disused intestine distally. When obstruction is complete or high grade, bilious vomiting and abdominal distention are present in the newborn period. In lesser cases, as in "windsock" types of intestinal webs, the obstruction is partial, and symptoms are more subtle.

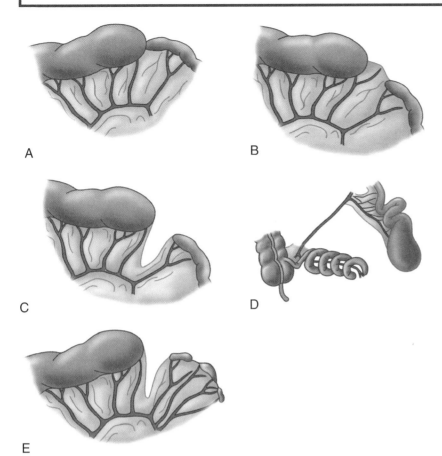

Figure 129-3 Types of intestinal atresia. **A**, Internal web; **B**, Cordlike remnant connecting proximal and distal bowel; **C**, Interrupted bowel with V-shaped mesenteric defect; **D**, "Apple peel" atresia with surviving bowel spiraling around a marginal artery; **E**, Multiple atresias. *(From Grosfeld JL, Ballantine TVN, Shoemaker R: Operative management of intestinal atresia based on pathologic findings, J Pediatr Surg 14:368–375, 1979.)*

Clinical Manifestations

Intestinal atresia presents with a history of polyhydramnios, abdominal distention and bilious vomiting in the neonatal period. If intestinal perforation is present, peritonitis and sepsis may develop.

Laboratory and Imaging Studies

Plain abdominal x-rays may localize the area of atresia and identify evidence of perforation, such as free air or calcifications typical of meconium peritonitis. Duodenal atresia appears as a double-bubble sign (gas in the stomach and enlarged proximal duodenum), with no gas distally. Atresias of the distal intestine are characterized by longer segments of dilated, air-filled bowel. Contrast studies are helpful if plain films are not sufficient. Atresia may be a complication of **meconium ileus** associated with cystic fibrosis. Laboratory evaluation for **cystic fibrosis** (see Chapter 137) is indicated in cases of small bowel atresia. A complete blood count, serum electrolytes, liver functions, and amylase should be measured to identify dehydration, pancreatitis, and other complications.

Treatment

The treatment of intestinal atresia is surgical, but surgery must be preceded by adequate hemodynamic stabilization of the patient. Intravenous (IV) fluids, nasogastric suction, and broad-spectrum antibiotics should be given.

OTHER CONGENITAL DISORDERS

Gastroschisis is an abdominal wall defect, not involving the umbilicus, through which intestinal contents have herniated. In contrast to omphalocele, the bowel is not covered by peritoneum or amniotic membrane. As a result, prolonged contact with the amniotic fluid typically causes a thick, exudative covering (a "peel") on the exposed bowel. Gastroschisis is not associated with extraintestinal anomalies, but segments of intestinal atresia are common. After surgical reduction of the defect, return of normal bowel function may be slow and requires prolonged parenteral nutrition for infants with long atretic segments (short bowel syndrome) and infants with a thick peel.

Omphalocele is an abdominal wall defect through the umbilicus caused by failure of the intestine to return to the abdomen during fetal life. The bowel remains within the umbilical cord and is covered by peritoneum and amniotic membranes. This defect is associated with other congenital anomalies, especially cardiac defects, **Beckwith-Wiedemann syndrome**, and intestinal complications. Treatment is surgical closure, which sometimes must be performed in stages to fit the bowel into a congenitally small abdominal cavity.

Anorectal malformations, including imperforate anus and its variants, are embryologic defects recognized at birth by the absence of a normal anal opening. Evaluation of these infants should include observation for emergence of meconium from the urethra or fistulas on the perineum. A urinary catheter should be placed if urinary distention is present. In low lesions, a fistulous opening that drains meconium is present on the perineum. Low lesions commonly are associated with fistulization between the bowel and bladder, vagina, or urethra. Lateral plain x-rays show the level of the defect and show gas in the bladder caused by a fistula. Initial treatment is a colostomy to divert the fecal flow, with subsequent anogenital reconstruction. The internal sphincter muscle is functionally absent in high lesions, and continence after repair is difficult to achieve. All children with imperforate anus require magnetic resonance imaging (MRI) of the lumbosacral spinal cord because of high incidence of tethered spinal cord. Urologic dysfunction is common and should be evaluated.

Hirschsprung disease is a motility defect caused by failure of ganglion cell precursors to migrate into the distal bowel during fetal life. The aganglionic distal segment does not exhibit normal motility and is functionally obstructed secondary to spasm. In 75% of cases, the involved segment is limited to the rectosigmoid; total colonic involvement is seen in 8%. Rarely, long segments of small bowel also are aganglionic. "Ultrashort" segment involves only a few centimeters of distal rectum. About 95% of normal infants pass stool spontaneously by 24 hours of age; 95% of infants with Hirschsprung disease do not. Symptoms of distal bowel obstruction occur with distention and bilious vomiting. If the diagnosis is not made quickly, **enterocolitis** can result, associated with a high rate of mortality. Diagnosis is based on examination and one or more diagnostic studies. Abdominal distention is present in most cases. Digital rectal examination reveals an empty rectum that clenches around the examiner's finger, giving the impression of an elongated sphincter. When the finger is withdrawn, a powerful gush of retained stool is often expelled. A deep **rectal biopsy** specimen obtained surgically or by using a suction biopsy instrument is required for diagnosis. When no ganglion cells are shown in the submucosal plexus, accompanied by nerve trunk hyperplasia, the diagnosis is certain. **Barium enema** and **anorectal manometry** may be used before biopsy, but false-negative and false-positive results can occur. Therapy is surgical. When the bowel is markedly distended or inflamed, an initial colostomy usually is performed above the aganglionic segment, followed weeks later by one of several definitive repair procedures. The transanal pull-through excises the aganglionic bowel and creates a primary colorectal anastomosis without laparotomy. This procedure can be considered in patients with uncomplicated involvement limited to the rectosigmoid region.

Meckel diverticulum is a remnant of the fetal omphalomesenteric duct and is an outpouching of the distal ileum present in 1% to 2% of the population. Although most diverticula are asymptomatic throughout life, some cause massive, painless GI bleeding. Ectopic gastric tissue within the diverticulum causes ulceration of mucosa in the adjacent ileum. Meckel diverticulum may be a lead point for intussusception or may enable twisting (volvulus) of neighboring bowel around its vascular supply. Diverticulitis mimics appendicitis. Diagnosis may be made in most cases by technetium scan (Meckel scan), which labels the acid-producing mucosa. Because not all diverticula are seen, ultrasound, barium enteroclysis, or video capsule endoscopy may be useful. When the level of suspicion is high, surgical or laparoscopic investigation is warranted. The treatment is surgical excision.

INFLAMMATORY BOWEL DISEASE (IBD)
Epidemiology and Etiology

Decision-Making Algorithms
Available @ StudentConsult.com

Abdominal Pain
Diarrhea
Fever and Rash
Pubertal Delay

The peak incidence of IBD in children is in the second decade of life. IBD includes Crohn's disease (CD), which can involve any part of the gut, and ulcerative colitis (UC), which affects only the colon. The incidence of IBD is increasing, especially in industrialized countries, for reasons that are unclear. IBD is uncommon in tropical and Third World countries. It is more common in Jewish than in other ethnic populations. Genetic factors play a role in susceptibility, with significantly higher risk if there is a family history of IBD. Having a first-degree relative with IBD increases the risk about 30-fold. Susceptibility has been linked to some HLA subtypes, and linkage analysis has identified multiple other susceptibility loci on several chromosomes. Environmental factors (not yet identified) also seem to play a role because there is often nonconcordance among monozygotic twins. It is possible that viral infections can initiate the inflammatory process. Dietary triggers are unproven. Smoking doubles the risk of CD and halves the risk for UC.

Clinical manifestations depend on the region of involvement. UC involves only the colon, whereas CD can include the entire gut from mouth to anus. **Colitis** from either condition results in diarrhea, blood, and mucus in the stool; urgency; and *tenesmus,* a sensation of incomplete emptying after defecation. When colitis is severe, the child often awakens from sleep to pass stool. **Toxic megacolon** is a life-threatening complication characterized by fever, abdominal distention and pain, massively dilated colon, anemia, and low serum albumin owing to fecal protein losses. Symptoms of colitis always are present in UC and usually suggest the diagnosis early in its course. Extraintestinal manifestations of UC occur in a few patients and may include primary sclerosing cholangitis, arthritis, uveitis, and pyoderma gangrenosum (Table 129-1).

Symptoms can be subtle in CD. **Small bowel involvement** in CD is associated with loss of appetite, crampy postprandial pain, poor growth, delayed puberty, fever, anemia, and lethargy. Some symptoms may be present for some time before the diagnosis is made. Severe CD with fibrosis may cause partial or complete small bowel obstruction. Perineal abnormalities, including skin tags and fistulas, are another feature distinguishing CD from UC. Other extraintestinal manifestations of CD include arthritis, erythema nodosum, and uveitis or iritis.

Laboratory and Imaging Studies
Blood tests should include complete blood count, albumin, erythrocyte sedimentation rate, and C-reactive protein (Table 129-2). Anemia and elevated platelet counts are typical. Testing for abnormal serum antibodies can be helpful in diagnosing IBD and in discriminating between the colitis of CD and UC. **Antineutrophil cytoplasmic antibody** is found in about 66% of UC patients and in only a few CD

Table 129-1	Comparison of Crohn's Disease and Ulcerative Colitis	
FEATURE	**CROHN'S DISEASE**	**ULCERATIVE COLITIS**
Malaise, fever, weight loss	Common	Common
Rectal bleeding	Sometimes	Usual
Abdominal mass	Common	Rare
Abdominal pain	Common	Common
Perianal disease	Common	Rare
Ileal involvement	Common	None (backwash ileitis)
Strictures	Common	Unusual
Fistula	Common	Very rare
Skip lesions	Common	Not present
Transmural Involvement	Usual	Not present
Crypt abscesses	Variable	Usual
Intestinal granulomas	Common	Rarely present
Risk of cancer*	Increased	Greatly increased
Erythema nodosum	Common	Less common
Mouth ulceration	Common	Rare
Osteopenia at onset	Yes	No
Autoimmune hepatitis	Rare	Yes
Sclerosing cholangitis	Rare	Yes

*Colonic cancer, cholangiocarcinoma, lymphoma in Crohn's disease.

Table 129-2	Diagnostic Studies for Inflammatory Bowel Disease	
STUDIES	**INTERPRETATION**	
BLOOD TESTS		
CBC with WBC differential	Anemia, elevated platelets suggest IBD	
ESR	Elevated in many, but not all, IBD patients	
C-reactive protein	Elevated in many, but not all, IBD patients	
Albumin	May be low in IBD due to fecal loss	
ASCA	Found in about 50% of CD patients and few UC patients	
Atypical p-ANCA	Found in most UC patients and few CD patients	
Anti-OmpC	Found in some UC and CD patients, rare in non-IBD	
Anti-C Bir1	Found in about 50% of CD patients	
IMAGING STUDIES		
Upper GI series with SBFT	Evaluate for ileal and jejunal CD	
CT scan	Used to detect abscess, small bowel involvement	
Tagged WBC scan	Sometimes helpful in determining extent of disease	
Magnetic Resonance Enterography	Used to detect bowel thickening, inflammation, and strictures as well as abscesses and fistulas	
ENDOSCOPY		
Upper endoscopy	Evaluate for CD of esophagus, stomach, and duodenum; obtain tissue for histologic diagnosis	
Colonoscopy	Show presence or absence of colitis and terminal ileal CD; obtain tissue for histology	
Video Capsule endoscopy	Emerging role in diagnosis of small bowel CD, more sensitive than upper GI series with SBFT	

Anti-OmpC, Antibody to outer membrane protein C; *ASCA*, anti–*Saccharomyces cerevisiae* antibody; *atypical p-ANCA*, atypical perinuclear staining by antineutrophil cytoplasmic antibody; *CBC*, complete blood count; *CD*, Crohn's disease; *ESR*, erythrocyte sedimentation rate; *GI*, gastrointestinal; *IBD*, inflammatory bowel disease; *SBFT*, small bowel follow-through; *WBC*, white blood cell.

cases. **Anti–*Saccharomyces cerevisiae* antibody** is present in about 50% of CD patients and is uncommon in UC. More IBD-specific antibodies are being developed and include anti-OmpC, directed against an *Escherichia coli* membrane protein, and anti-CBir1, directed against bacterial flagellin, among others. Because there is overlap between CD and UC, none of these tests can discriminate absolutely between the two conditions.

In patients with suspected IBD, an **upper GI series with small bowel follow-through** is often used to detect small bowel involvement. **Colonoscopy** is preferred over contrast enema because biopsy specimens can be obtained and because visual features can be diagnostic. Findings in UC include diffuse carpeting of the distal or entire colon with tiny ulcers and loss of haustral folds. Within the involved segment, no skip areas are present. In CD, ulcerations tend to be much larger with a linear, branching, or aphthous appearance; skip areas are usually present. **Upper endoscopy** cannot evaluate the jejunum and ileum, but is more sensitive than contrast studies in identifying proximal CD involvement. Other methods to detect small bowel involvement include **video capsule endoscopy**; computed tomography (CT) scanning, which can detect small bowel disease as well as abscesses; and **MR enterography**, which has the advantage of no radiation and good sensitivity for finding active bowel disease.

Treatment
Ulcerative Colitis
UC is treated with the aminosalicylate drugs, which deliver **5-aminosalicylic acid** (5-ASA) to the distal gut. Because it is rapidly absorbed, pure 5-ASA (mesalamine) must be specially packaged in coated capsules or pills or taken as a suppository to be effective in the colon. Other aminosalicylates (sulfasalazine, olsalazine, and balsalazide) use 5-ASA covalently linked to a carrier molecule. Sulfasalazine is the least expensive, but side effects resulting from its sulfapyridine component are common. When aminosalicylates alone cannot control the disease, steroid therapy may be required to induce remission. Whenever possible, steroids should not be used for long-term therapy. An immunosuppressive drug, such as **6-mercaptopurine** or **azathioprine**, is useful to spare excessive steroid use in difficult cases. More potent immunosuppressives, such as cyclosporine or anti–tumor necrosis factor (TNF) agents such as infliximab may be used as rescue therapy when other treatments fail. Surgical colectomy with ileoanal anastomosis is an option for unresponsive severe disease or

electively to end chronic symptoms and to reduce the risk of colon cancer, which is increased in patients with UC.

Crohn's Disease

Inflammation in CD typically responds less well to aminosalicylates; oral or IV steroids are more important in inducing remission. To avoid the need for repetitive steroid therapy, immunosuppressive drugs, usually either azathioprine or 6-mercaptopurine, are often started soon after diagnosis. CD that is difficult to control also may be treated with subcutaneous methotrexate or with agents that block the action of TNF-α. **Infliximab** is the most effective such drug and is given intravenously. Other antibodies that inhibit white blood cell (WBC) migration or action, such as natalizumab, also show promise. As with UC, surgery is sometimes necessary, usually because of obstructive symptoms, abscess, or severe, unremitting symptoms. Because surgery is not curative in CD, its use must be limited, and the length of bowel resection must be minimized.

CELIAC DISEASE
Etiology and Epidemiology

Celiac disease is an injury to the mucosa of the small intestine caused by the ingestion of **gluten** (a protein component) from wheat, rye, barley, and related grains. Rice does not contain gluten and can be eaten freely, as can special pure preparations of oats not contaminated by other grains. In its severe form, celiac disease causes malabsorption and malnutrition. Diagnosis was based on the presence of typical symptoms, followed by small bowel biopsy. The availability of more sensitive and specific serologic testing has revealed many patients with few or no gastrointestinal symptoms who have early, attenuated, or latent disease. Approximately 1 in 110 persons in the United States have celiac disease, but only a small proportion have been diagnosed. The disease is seen in association with type 1 diabetes, thyroiditis, Turner syndrome, and trisomy 21.

Clinical Manifestations

Decision-Making Algorithms
Available @ StudentConsult.com

Diarrhea
Pubertal Delay
Failure to Thrive

Symptoms can begin at any age when gluten-containing foods are given. Diarrhea, abdominal bloating, failure to thrive, irritability, decreased appetite, and ascites caused by hypoproteinemia are classic. Children may be minimally symptomatic or may be severely malnourished. Constipation is found in a few patients, probably because of reduced intake. A careful inspection of the child's growth curve and evaluation for reduced subcutaneous fat and abdominal distention are crucial. Celiac disease should be considered in any child with chronic abdominal complaints. Extraintestinal manifestations include osteoporosis, pulmonary hemorrhage, seizures/encephalopathy, dermatitis herpetiformis, and erythema nodosum.

Laboratory and Imaging Studies

Serologic markers include IgA antiendomysial antibody and IgA tissue transglutaminase antibody. Because IgA deficiency is common in celiac disease, total serum IgA also must be measured to document the accuracy of these tests. In the absence of IgA deficiency, either test yields a sensitivity and specificity of 95%. An endoscopic **small bowel biopsy** is essential to confirm the diagnosis and should be performed while the patient is still taking gluten. The biopsy specimen shows various degrees of villous atrophy (short or absent villi), mucosal inflammation, crypt hyperplasia, and increased numbers of intraepithelial lymphocytes. When there is any question about response to treatment, a repeat biopsy specimen may be obtained several months later. Other laboratory studies should be performed to rule out complications, including complete blood count, calcium, phosphate, vitamin D, iron, total protein and albumin, and liver function tests. Mild elevations of the transaminases are common and should normalize with dietary therapy.

Treatment

Treatment consists of complete elimination of gluten from the diet. Consultation with a dietitian experienced in celiac disease is helpful, as is membership in a celiac disease support group. Lists of prepared foods that contain hidden gluten are particularly important for patients to use. Starchy foods that are safe include rice, soy, tapioca, buckwheat, potatoes, and (pure) oats. Many resources also are available via the Internet to help families cope with the large changes in diet that are required. Most patients respond clinically within a few weeks with weight gain, improved appetite, and improved sense of well-being. Histologic improvement lags behind clinical response, requiring several months to normalize.

MILK AND SOY PROTEIN INTOLERANCE (ALLERGIC COLITIS)

SEE CHAPTER 34.

INTUSSUSCEPTION
Etiology and Epidemiology

Intussusception is the "telescoping" of a segment of proximal bowel (the intussusceptum) into downstream bowel (the intussuscipiens). Most cases occur in infants 1 to 2 years old; in this age group, nearly all cases are idiopathic. Viral-induced lymphoid hyperplasia may produce a lead point in these children. In older children, the proportion of cases caused by a pathologic lead point increases. In young children, **ileocolonic** intussusception is common; the ileum invaginates into the colon, beginning at or near the ileocecal valve. When pathologic lead points are present, the intussusception may be ileoileal, jejunoileal, or jejunojejunal.

Clinical Manifestations

Decision-Making Algorithms
Available @ StudentConsult.com

Abdominal Pain
Gastrointestinal Bleeding
Irritable Infant

An infant with intussusception has sudden onset of crampy abdominal pain; the infant's knees draw up, and the infant cries out and exhibits pallor with a colicky pattern occurring every 15 to 20 minutes. Feedings are refused. As the intussusception progresses, and obstruction becomes prolonged, bilious vomiting becomes prominent, and the dilated, fatigued intestine generates less pressure and less pain. As the intussuscepted bowel is pulled further and further into the downstream intestine by motility, the mesentery is pulled with it and becomes stretched and compressed. The venous outflow from the intussusceptum is obstructed, leading to edema, weeping of fluid, and congestion with bleeding. Third space fluid losses and "currant jelly" stools result. Another unexpected feature of intussusception is **lethargy**. Between episodes of pain, the infant is glassy-eyed and groggy and appears to have been sedated. A sausage-shaped mass caused by the swollen, intussuscepted bowel may be palpable in the right upper quadrant or epigastrium.

Laboratory and Imaging Studies

The diagnosis depends on the direct demonstration of bowel-within-bowel. A simple way of showing this is by abdominal ultrasound. If the ultrasound is positive, or if good visualization has not been achieved, a pneumatic or contrast enema under fluoroscopy is indicated. This is a potentially useful way to both identify and **treat** intussusception. Air and barium can show the intussusception quickly and, when administered with controlled pressure, usually can reduce it completely. The success rate for pneumatic reduction is probably a bit higher than hydrostatic reduction with barium and approaches 90% if done when symptoms have been present for less than 24 hours. The pneumatic enema has the additional advantages over barium of not preventing subsequent radiologic studies and having no risk of causing barium peritonitis if perforation occurs. Nonoperative reduction should not be attempted if the patient is unstable or has evidence of pre-existing perforation or peritonitis.

Treatment

Therapy must begin with placement of an IV catheter and a nasogastric tube. Before radiologic intervention is attempted, the child must have adequate **fluid resuscitation** to correct the often severe dehydration caused by vomiting and third space losses. Ultrasound may be performed before the fluid resuscitation is complete. Surgical consultation should be obtained early as the surgeon may prefer to be present during nonoperative reduction. If pneumatic or hydrostatic reduction is successful, the child should be admitted to the hospital for overnight observation of possible recurrence (risk is 5% to 10%). If reduction is not complete, emergency surgery is required. The surgeon attempts gentle manual reduction but may need to resect the involved bowel after failed radiologic reduction because of severe edema, perforation, a pathologic lead point (polyp, Meckel diverticulum), or necrosis.

APPENDICITIS
Etiology and Epidemiology

Appendicitis is the most common surgical emergency in childhood. The prevalence of appendicitis varies by age with the peak between the ages of 10 and 12 years. It is much less common in children under the age of 5. Appendicitis begins with obstruction of the lumen, most commonly by fecal matter (fecalith), but appendiceal obstruction also can occur, secondary to hyperplasia of lymphoid tissue associated with viral infections or rarely the presence of neoplastic tissue, such as an appendiceal carcinoid tumor. Trapped bacteria proliferate and begin to invade the appendiceal wall, inducing inflammation and secretion. The obstructed appendix becomes engorged, its blood supply is compromised, and it finally ruptures. The entire process is rapid, with appendiceal rupture usually occurring within 48 hours of the onset of symptoms.

Clinical Manifestations

Decision-Making Algorithms
Available @ StudentConsult.com

Abdominal Pain
Vomiting

Classic appendicitis begins with **visceral pain**, localized to the periumbilical region. Nausea and vomiting occur soon after, triggered by the appendiceal distention. As the inflammation begins to irritate the parietal peritoneum adjacent to the appendix, **somatic pain** fibers are activated, and the pain localizes to the right lower quadrant. Examination of the patient reveals a tender right lower quadrant. Voluntary guarding is present initially, progressing to rigidity, then to rebound tenderness with rupture and peritonitis. These classic findings may not be present, especially in young children or if the appendix is retrocecal, covered by omentum, or in another unusual location. Clinical prediction rules have been developed for the diagnosis of appendicitis. The Alvarado/MANTRELS rule is scored by 1 point for each of the following: migration of pain to the right lower quadrant, anorexia, nausea/vomiting, rebound pain, temperature of at least 37.3°C, and WBC shift to greater than 75% neutrophils; 2 points are given for each of tenderness in the right lower quadrant and leukocytosis greater than 10,000/μL. Children with a score of 4 or less are unlikely to have appendicitis; a score of 7 or greater increases the likelihood that the patient has appendicitis. When classic history and physical examination findings are present, the patient is taken to the operating room. When doubt exists, imaging is helpful to rule out complications (right lower quadrant abscess, liver disease) and other disorders, such as mesenteric adenitis and ovarian or fallopian tube disorders. If the evaluation is negative and some doubt remains, the child should be admitted to the hospital for close observation and serial examinations.

Laboratory and Imaging Studies

The history and examination are often enough to make the diagnosis, but laboratory and imaging studies are helpful when the diagnosis is uncertain (Table 129-3). A WBC count greater than 10,000/mm3 is found in 89% of patients with appendicitis and 93% with perforated appendicitis. This criterion is met by 62% of abdominal pain patients without appendicitis. Urinalysis is done to rule out urinary tract infection, and x-rays of the chest or the kidney, ureter, and bladder (KUB) rule

Table 129-3	Diagnostic Studies in Suspected Appendicitis
INITIAL LABORATORY TESTING	
CBC with differential	
Urinalysis	
Amylase and lipase	
ALT, AST, GGT	
Flat and upright abdominal radiographs (KUB)	
FOLLOW-UP STUDIES*	
Abdominal ultrasound	
CT scan of abdomen	

ALT, Alanine aminotransferase; *AST*, aspartate aminotransferase; *CBC*, complete blood count; *CT*, computed tomography; *GGT*, γ-glutamyltransferase; *KUB*, kidney, ureter, bladder.
*Perform when diagnosis remains in doubt.

out lower lobe pneumonia masquerading as abdominal pain. Amylase, lipase, and liver enzymes are done to look for pancreatic or liver and gallbladder disease. The plain abdominal x-ray may reveal a calcified fecalith, which strongly suggests the diagnosis. When these studies are inconclusive, imaging is indicated with an abdominal ultrasound or CT scan, which may reveal the presence of an enlarged, thick-walled appendix with surrounding fluid. A diameter of more than 6 mm is considered diagnostic.

Treatment

Treatment of appendicitis is surgical. Simple appendectomy is curative if performed before perforation. With perforation, a course of postoperative IV antibiotics is required. Broad-spectrum coverage is necessary to cover the mixed bowel flora.

Chapter **130**

LIVER DISEASE

CHOLESTASIS
Etiology and Epidemiology

Cholestasis is defined as reduced bile flow and is characterized by elevation of the conjugated, or direct, bilirubin fraction. This condition must be distinguished from ordinary neonatal jaundice, in which the direct bilirubin is never elevated (see Chapter 62). Neonatal jaundice that is secondary to unconjugated hyperbilirubinemia is the result of immature hepatocellular excretory function or hemolysis, which increases the production of bilirubin. When direct bilirubin is elevated, many potentially serious disorders must be considered (Fig. 130-1). Emphasis must be placed on the rapid diagnosis of treatable and potentially imminently lethal disorders, especially biliary atresia and metabolic disorders, such as galactosemia or tyrosinemia.

Clinical Manifestations

Decision-Making Algorithm
Available @ StudentConsult.com

Jaundice

The jaundice of **extrahepatic biliary atresia** (biliary atresia) usually is not evident immediately at birth, but develops in the first week or two of life. The reason is that extrahepatic bile ducts are usually present at birth, but are then destroyed by an idiopathic inflammatory process. Aside from jaundice, these infants do not initially appear ill. The liver injury progresses rapidly to cirrhosis; symptoms of portal hypertension with splenomegaly, ascites, muscle wasting, and poor weight gain are evident by a few months of age. If surgical drainage is not performed successfully early in the course (ideally by 2 months), progression to liver failure is inevitable.

Neonatal hepatitis is characterized by an ill-appearing infant with an enlarged liver and jaundice. There is no specific diagnostic test. If liver biopsy is performed, the presence of hepatocyte giant cells is characteristic. Cytomegalovirus, herpes simplex virus, and syphilis must be ruled out. Hepatobiliary scintigraphy typically shows slow hepatic uptake with eventual excretion of isotope into the intestine. These infants have a good prognosis overall, with spontaneous resolution occurring in most.

α_1-**Antitrypsin deficiency** presents with clinical findings indistinguishable from neonatal hepatitis. Only about 10% to 20% of all infants with the genetic defect exhibit neonatal cholestasis. Of these affected infants, about 20% to 30% develop chronic liver disease, which may result in cirrhosis and liver failure. Life-threatening α_1-antitrypsin deficiency occurs in only 3% to 5% of affected pediatric patients. α_1-Antitrypsin deficiency is the leading metabolic disorder requiring liver transplantation.

Alagille syndrome is characterized by chronic cholestasis with the unique liver biopsy finding of paucity of bile ducts in the portal triads. Associated abnormalities in some (syndromic) types include peripheral pulmonic stenosis or other cardiac anomalies; hypertelorism; unusual facies with deep-set eyes, prominent forehead, and a pointed chin; butterfly vertebrae; and a defect of the ocular limbus (*posterior embryotoxon*). Cholestasis is variable but is usually lifelong and associated with hypercholesterolemia and severe pruritus. Progression to end-stage liver disease is uncommon. Liver transplantation sometimes is performed electively to relieve severe and uncontrollable pruritus.

Laboratory and Imaging Studies

The laboratory approach to diagnosis of a neonate with cholestatic jaundice is presented in Table 130-1. Noninvasive studies may aid a rapid diagnosis. Early imaging studies are performed to evaluate for biliary obstruction and other anatomic lesions that may be surgically treatable. When necessary to rule out biliary atresia or to obtain prognostic information, liver biopsy is a final option (Fig. 130-2).

Treatment

Treatment of extrahepatic biliary atresia is the surgical **Kasai procedure**, in which the fibrotic extrahepatic bile duct remnant

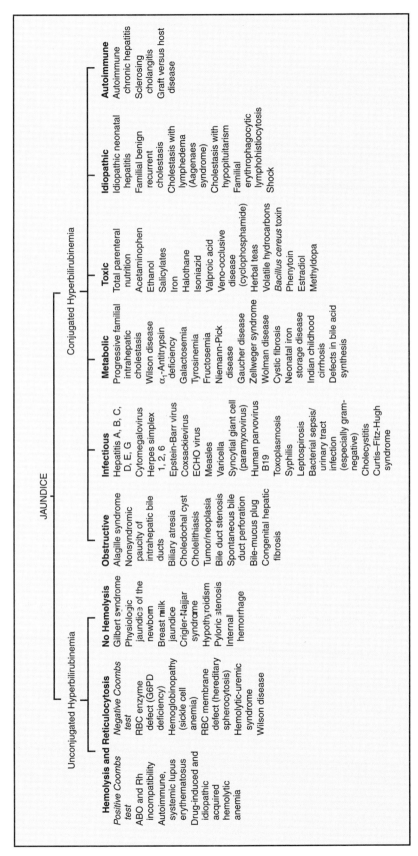

JAUNDICE

Unconjugated Hyperbilirubinemia

Hemolysis and Reticulocytosis
Positive Coombs test
ABO and Rh incompatibility
Autoimmune, systemic lupus erythematosus
Drug-induced and idiopathic acquired hemolytic anemia

Negative Coombs test
RBC enzyme defect (G6PD deficiency)
Hemoglobinopathy (sickle cell anemia)
RBC membrane defect (hereditary spherocytosis)
Hemolytic-uremic syndrome
Wilson disease

No Hemolysis
Gilbert syndrome
Physiologic jaundice of the newborn
Breast milk jaundice
Crigler-Najjar syndrome
Hypothyroidism
Pyloric stenosis
Internal hemorrhage

Conjugated Hyperbilirubinemia

Obstructive
Alagille syndrome
Nonsyndromic paucity of intrahepatic bile ducts
Biliary atresia
Choledochal cyst
Cholelithiasis
Tumor/neoplasia
Bile duct stenosis
Spontaneous bile duct perforation
Bile-mucus plug
Congenital hepatic fibrosis

Infectious
Hepatitis A, B, C, D, E, G
Cytomegalovirus
Herpes simplex 1, 2, 6
Epstein-Barr virus
Coxsackievirus
ECHO virus
Measles
Varicella
Syncytial giant cell (paramyxovirus)
Human parvovirus B19
Toxoplasmosis
Syphilis
Leptospirosis
Bacterial sepsis/urinary tract infection (especially gram-negative)
Cholecystitis
Curtis–Fitz-Hugh syndrome

Metabolic
Progressive familial intrahepatic cholestasis
Wilson disease
α_1-Antitrypsin deficiency
Galactosemia
Tyrosinemia
Fructosemia
Niemann-Pick disease
Gaucher disease
Zellweger syndrome
Wolman disease
Cystic fibrosis
Neonatal iron storage disease
Indian childhood cirrhosis
Defects in bile acid synthesis

Toxic
Total parenteral nutrition
Acetaminophen
Ethanol
Salicylates
Iron
Halothane
Isoniazid
Valproic acid
Veno-occlusive disease (cyclophosphamide)
Herbal teas
Volatile hydrocarbons
Bacillus cereus toxin
Phenytoin
Estradiol
Methyldopa

Idiopathic
Idiopathic neonatal hepatitis
Familial benign recurrent cholestasis
Cholestasis with lymphedema (Aagenaes syndrome)
Cholestasis with hypopituitarism
Familial erythrophagocytic lymphohistiocytosis
Shock

Autoimmune
Autoimmune chronic hepatitis
Sclerosing cholangitis
Graft versus host disease

Figure 130-1 Differential diagnosis of jaundice in childhood. *G6PD*, Glucose-6-phosphate dehydrogenase; *RBC*, red blood cell.

Table 130-1	Laboratory and Imaging Evaluation of Neonatal Cholestasis
EVALUATION	**RATIONALE**
INITIAL TESTS	
Total and direct bilirubin	Elevated direct fraction confirms cholestasis
AST, ALT	Hepatocellular injury
GGT	Biliary obstruction/injury
RBC galactose-1-phosphate uridyltransferase	Galactosemia
α_1-Antitrypsin level	α_1-Antitrypsin deficiency
Urinalysis and urine culture	Urinary tract infection can cause cholestasis in neonates
Blood culture	Sepsis can cause cholestasis
Serum amino acids	Aminoacidopathies
Urine organic acids	Organic acidurias
Very long chain fatty acids	Zellweger syndrome, peroxisomal disorders
Carnitine profile	Mitochondrial and fatty acid oxidation disorders
Sweat chloride or CF mutation analysis	Cystic fibrosis
Urine culture for cytomegalovirus	Congenital cytomegalovirus infection
INITIAL IMAGING STUDY	
Abdominal ultrasound	Choledochal cyst, gallstones, mass lesion, Caroli disease
SECONDARY IMAGING STUDY	
Hepatobiliary scintigraphy	Evaluate for biliary atresia
Pathology	
Percutaneous liver biopsy	Biliary atresia, idiopathic giant cell hepatitis, α_1-antitrypsin deficiency

ALT, Alanine aminotransferase; *AST,* aspartate aminotransferase; *CF,* cystic fibrosis; *GGT,* γ-glutamyltransferase; *RBC,* red blood cell.

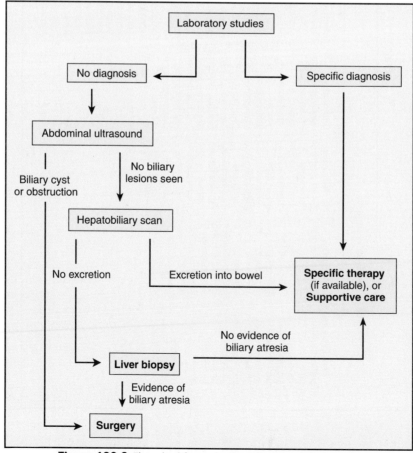

Figure 130-2 Flow chart for evaluation of neonatal cholestasis.

is removed and replaced with a roux-en-Y loop of jejunum. This operation must be performed before 3 months of age to have the best chance of success. Even so, the success rate is low; many children require liver transplantation. Some metabolic causes of neonatal cholestasis are treatable by dietary manipulation (galactosemia) or medication (tyrosinemia); all affected patients require supportive care. This includes fat-soluble vitamin supplements (vitamins A, D, E, and K) and formula containing medium-chain triglycerides, which can be absorbed without bile salt–induced micelles. Choleretic agents, such as ursodeoxycholic acid, may improve bile flow in some conditions.

VIRAL HEPATITIS
SEE CHAPTER 113.

FULMINANT LIVER FAILURE
Etiology and Epidemiology
Fulminant liver failure is defined as severe liver disease with onset of hepatic encephalopathy within 8 weeks after initial symptoms, in the absence of chronic liver disease. Etiology includes viral hepatitis, metabolic disorders, autoimmune hepatitis, ischemia, neoplastic disease, and toxins (Table 130-2).

Clinical Manifestations

Decision-Making Algorithm
Available @ StudentConsult.com

Hepatomegaly

Liver failure is a multisystem disorder with complex interactions among the liver, kidneys, vascular structures, gut, central nervous system (CNS), and immune function. Hepatic encephalopathy is characterized by varying degrees of impairment (Table 130-3). Respiratory compromise occurs as severity of the failure increases and requires early institution of ventilatory support. Hypoglycemia resulting from impaired glycogenolysis and gluconeogenesis must be prevented. Renal function is impaired, and frank renal failure, or **hepatorenal syndrome**, may occur. This syndrome is characterized by low urine output, azotemia, and low urine sodium content. Ascites develops secondary to hypoalbuminemia and disordered regulation of fluid and electrolyte homeostasis. Increased risk of infection occurs and may cause death. Esophageal varices may cause significant hemorrhage, whereas hypersplenism from portal hypertension may produce thrombocytopenia.

Laboratory and Imaging Studies
Coagulation tests and serum albumin are used to follow hepatic synthetic function. These tests are confounded by administration of blood products and clotting factors. Vitamin K should be administered to maximize the liver's ability to synthesize factors II, VII, IX, and X. In addition to monitoring prothrombin time and partial thromboplastin time, many centers measure factor V serially as a sensitive index of synthetic function. Renal function tests, electrolytes, serum

Table 130-2	Causes of Fulminant Liver Failure in Childhood

METABOLIC
Neonatal hemochromatosis
Electron chain transport defects
Disorders of fatty acid oxidation
Galactosemia
Tyrosinemia
Hereditary fructose intolerance
Bile acid synthesis disorders
Wilson disease
CARDIOVASCULAR
Shock, hypotension
Congestive heart failure
Budd-Chiari syndrome
INFECTIOUS
Hepatitis virus A, B
Echovirus
Coxsackievirus
Adenovirus
Parvovirus
Cytomegalovirus
Sepsis
Herpes simplex
NEOPLASTIC
Acute leukemia
Lymphoproliferative disease
TOXIC
Acetaminophen
Valproic acid
Phenytoin
Isoniazid
Halothane
Amanita mushrooms
IMMUNOLOGIC
Autoimmune hepatitis

ammonia, blood counts, and urinalysis also should be followed. In the setting of acute liver failure, liver biopsy may be indicated to ascertain the nature and degree of injury and estimate the likelihood of recovery. In the presence of coagulopathy, biopsy must be done using a transjugular or surgical approach.

Treatment
Because of the life-threatening and complex nature of this condition, management must be carried out in an intensive care unit at a liver transplant center. Treatment of acute liver failure is supportive; the definitive lifesaving therapy is liver transplantation. Supportive measures are listed in Table 130-4.

Table 130-3	Stages of Hepatic Encephalopathy

STAGE I

Alert and awake

Agitated and distractible

Infants and young children—irritable and fussy

Normal reflexes

Tremor, poor handwriting

Obeys age-appropriate commands

STAGE II

Confused and lethargic

Combative or inappropriate euphoria

Hyperactive reflexes

Asterixis present

Purposeful movements, but may not obey commands

STAGE III

Stuporous but arousable

Sleepy

Incoherent speech

Motor response to pain

Hyperreflexic

Hyperventilation

Asterixis present

STAGE IV

Unconscious, not arousable

Unresponsive or responds nonpurposefully to pain

Reflexes hyperactive

Irregular respirations

Pupil response sluggish

STAGE V

Unconscious

Hypoactive reflexes

Flaccid muscle tone

Apneic

Pupils fixed

Table 130-4	Treatment of Fulminant Liver Failure
Hepatic encephalopathy	Avoid sedatives Lactulose via nasogastric tube—start with 1-2 mL/kg/day, adjust dose to yield several loose stools per day Rifaximin or neomycin Enemas if constipated Mechanical ventilation if stage III or IV
Coagulopathy	Fresh frozen plasma only if active bleeding, monitor coagulation studies frequently Platelet transfusions as required
Hypoglycemia	IV glucose supplied with ≥10% dextrose solution, electrolytes as appropriate
Ascites	Restrict fluid intake to 50%-60% maintenance Restrict sodium intake to 0.5-1 mEq/kg/day Monitor central venous pressure to maintain adequate intravascular volume (avoid renal failure)
Renal failure	Maintain adequate intravascular volume, give albumin if low Diuretics Vasoconstrictors Dialysis or hemofiltration Exchange transfusion Liver transplantation

fibrosis, and biliary obstruction secondary to choledochal cyst are leading causes.

Clinical Manifestations

Decision-Making Algorithms
Available @ StudentConsult.com

Gastrointestinal Bleeding
Jaundice
Abdominal Masses
Bleeding

Chronic liver disease is characterized by the consequences of portal hypertension, impaired hepatocellular function, and cholestasis. **Portal hypertension** caused by cirrhosis results in risk of gastrointestinal bleeding, ascites, and reduced hepatic blood flow. Blood entering the portal vein from the splenic and mesenteric veins is diverted to collateral circulation that bypasses the liver, enlarging these previously tiny vessels in the esophagus, stomach, and abdomen. **Esophageal varices** are particularly prone to bleed, but bleeding also can occur from hemorrhoidal veins, engorged gastric mucosa, and gastric varices. **Ascites** develops as a result of weeping of a high-pressure ultrafiltrate from the surfaces of the viscera and is at risk of becoming infected (spontaneous bacterial peritonitis); ascites can often be massive and interfere with patient comfort and respiration. The spleen enlarges secondary to impaired splenic vein outflow, causing excessive scavenging of platelets and white blood cells; this increases the patient's susceptibility to bleeding and infection.

Impaired hepatocellular function is associated with coagulopathy unresponsive to vitamin K, low serum albumin, elevated ammonia, and **hepatic encephalopathy**. The diversion

Efforts are made to treat metabolic derangements, avoid hypoglycemia, support respiration, minimize hepatic encephalopathy, and support renal function.

CHRONIC LIVER DISEASE
Etiology and Epidemiology
Chronic liver disease in childhood is characterized by the development of cirrhosis and its complications, and by progressive hepatic failure. Causative conditions may be congenital or acquired. Major congenital disorders leading to chronic disease include biliary atresia, tyrosinemia, untreated galactosemia, and α_1-antitrypsin deficiency. In older children, hepatitis B or C virus, autoimmune hepatitis, Wilson disease, primary sclerosing cholangitis, cystic

Table 130-5	Laboratory and Imaging Investigation of Chronic Liver Disease

METABOLIC TESTING	Serum albumin
Serum α₁-antitrypsin level	AST, ALT, GGT, alkaline phosphatase
α₁-Antitrypsin phenotype if low serum level	Total and direct bilirubin
Serum ceruloplasmin	Serum cholylglycine or bile acids
Sweat chloride, CF gene tests if CF suspected	Serum cholesterol
Testing for other specific conditions as indicated by clinical/laboratory findings	Ultrasound examination of liver and bile ducts
	Doppler ultrasound of hepatic vessels*
VIRAL HEPATITIS	Magnetic resonance cholangiography*
HBsAg	Magnetic resonance angiography of hepatic vessels*
Hepatitis B viral DNA, HBeAg if HBsAg positive	Percutaneous or endoscopic cholangiography*
Hepatitis C antibody	Liver biopsy*
Hepatitis C antibody confirmatory test if positive	**ANATOMIC EVALUATION**
Hepatitis C viral RNA, genotype if antibody confirmed	Ultrasound of liver, pancreas, and biliary tree
AUTOIMMUNE HEPATITIS	Consider magnetic resonance cholangiography or ERCP if evidence of biliary process
Antinuclear antibody	Liver biopsy—as required for diagnosis or prognosis
Liver-kidney microsomal antibody	**TESTS TO EVALUATE NUTRITIONAL STATUS**
Anti–smooth muscle antibody	Height, weight, skinfold thickness
Antineutrophil cytoplasmic antibody	25-Hydroxyvitamin D level
Total serum IgG (usually elevated)	Vitamin A level
TESTS TO EVALUATE LIVER FUNCTION AND INJURY	Vitamin E level
Prothrombin time and partial thromboplastin time	Prothrombin time and partial thromboplastin time before and after vitamin K administration
Serum ammonia	Serum albumin and prealbumin
CBC with platelet count	

ALT, Alanine aminotransferase; *AST*, aspartate aminotransferase; *CBC*, complete blood count; *CF*, cystic fibrosis; *ERCP*, endoscopic retrograde cholangiopancreatography; *GGT*, γ-glutamyltransferase; *HBeAg*, hepatitis B early antigen; *HBsAg*, hepatitis B surface antigen.
*Perform when indicated to obtain specific anatomic information.

of portal blood away from the liver via collateral circulation worsens this process. Malaise develops and contributes to poor nutrition, leading to muscle wasting and other consequences.

Chronic cholestasis causes debilitating pruritus and deepening jaundice. The reduced excretion of bile acids impairs absorption of fat calories and fat-soluble vitamins, which contributes to the poor nutritional state. Deficiency of vitamin K impairs production of clotting factors II, VII, IX, and X and increases the risk of bleeding. Vitamin E deficiency leads to hematologic and neurologic consequences unless corrected.

Laboratory and Imaging Studies

Laboratory studies include specific tests for diagnosis of the underlying illness and testing to monitor the status of the patient. Children presenting for the first time with evidence of chronic liver disease should have a standard investigation (Table 130-5). Monitoring should include coagulation tests, electrolytes and renal function testing, complete blood count with platelet count, transaminases, alkaline phosphatase, and γ-glutamyltransferase at appropriate intervals. Frequency of testing should be tailored to the pace of the patient's illness. Ascites fluid can be tested for infection by culture and cell count and generally is found to have an albumin concentration lower than that of serum.

Treatment

Treatment of chronic liver disease is complex. Supportive care for each of the many problems encountered in these patients is outlined in Table 130-6. Ultimately, survival depends on the availability of a donor liver and the patient's candidacy for transplantation. When transplantation is not possible or is delayed, palliative procedures, such as portosystemic shunts, can be considered. The transjugular intrahepatic portosystemic shunt is an expandable stent placed between the hepatic vein and a branch of the portal vein within the hepatic parenchyma. This procedure is performed using catheters inserted via the jugular vein and is entirely nonsurgical. All portosystemic shunts carry increased risk of hepatic encephalopathy.

SELECTED CHRONIC HEPATIC DISORDERS
Wilson Disease

Decision-Making Algorithms
Available @ StudentConsult.com

Jaundice
Hepatomegaly
Involuntary Movements
Hypocalcemia

Table 130-6	Management of Chronic Liver Disease		
PROBLEM	**CLINICAL MANIFESTATIONS**	**DIAGNOSTIC TESTING**	**TREATMENT**
Gastrointestinal variceal bleeding*	Hematemesis, rectal bleeding, melena, anemia	CBC, coagulation tests, Doppler ultrasound, magnetic resonance angiography, endoscopy	Somatostatin (octreotide) infusion, variceal band ligation or sclerotherapy, propranolol to reduce portal pressure, acid-blocker therapy, TIPSS or surgical portosystemic shunt if transplant not possible
Ascites	Abdominal distention, shifting dullness and fluid wave, respiratory compromise, spontaneous bacterial peritonitis	Abdominal ultrasound, diagnostic paracentesis; measure ascites fluid albumin (and serum albumin), cell count, WBC differential, culture fluid in blood culture bottles	Restrict sodium intake to 0.5-1 mEq/kg/day, restrict fluids, monitor renal function, treat peritonitis and portal hypertension. Central portosystemic shunt may be required
Nutritional compromise	Muscle wasting, fat-soluble vitamin deficiencies, poor or absent weight gain, fatigue	Coagulation studies, serum albumin, 25-hydroxyvitamin D level, vitamin E level, vitamin A level	Fat-soluble vitamin supplements: vitamins A, D, E, and K; use water-soluble form of vitamins. Supplemental feedings—nasogastric or parenteral if necessary
Hepatic encephalopathy	Irritability, confusion, lethargy, somnolence, coma	Serum ammonia	Lactulose orally or via nasogastric tube, avoid narcotics and sedatives, liver transplantation

CBC, Complete blood count; *TIPSS*, transjugular intrahepatic portosystemic shunt; *WBC*, white blood cell.
*May also have peptic ulcerations.

Wilson disease is characterized by abnormal storage of copper in the liver, leading to hepatocellular injury, CNS dysfunction, and hemolytic anemia. It is an autosomal recessive trait caused by mutations in the *ATP7B* gene. The encoded protein of this gene functions as an ATP-driven copper pump. The **diagnosis** is made by identifying depressed serum levels of ceruloplasmin, elevated 24-hour urine copper excretion, the presence of Kayser-Fleischer rings in the iris, evidence of hemolysis, and elevated hepatic copper content. In any single patient, one or more of these measures may be normal. **Clinical presentation** also varies, but seldom occurs before age 3 years. Neurologic abnormalities may predominate, including tremor, decline in school performance, worsening handwriting, and psychiatric disturbances. Anemia may be the first noted symptom. Hepatic presentations include appearance of jaundice, spider hemangiomas, portal hypertension and its consequences, and fulminant hepatic failure. **Treatment** consists of administration of copper-chelating drugs (penicillimine or trientine), with monitoring of urine copper excretion at intervals. Zinc salts often replace chelating agents after chelation therapy has successfully reduced excessive body copper stores. Adequate therapy must be continued for life to prevent liver and CNS deterioration.

Autoimmune Hepatitis
Immune-mediated liver injury may be primary or occur in association with other autoimmune disorders, such as inflammatory bowel disease or systemic lupus erythematosus. **Diagnosis** is made on the basis of elevated serum total IgG and the presence of an autoantibody, most commonly antinuclear, anti–smooth muscle, or anti–liver-kidney microsomal antibody. Liver biopsy specimen shows the presence of a plasma cell–rich portal infiltrate with piecemeal necrosis. **Treatment** consists of corticosteroids initially, usually with the addition of an immunosuppressive drug after remission is achieved. Steroids are tapered gradually as tolerated to minimize glucocorticoid side effects. Many patients require

lifelong immunosuppressive therapy, but some may be able to stop medications after several years under careful monitoring for recurrence.

Nonalcoholic Steatohepatitis
Steatohepatitis, also known as *nonalcoholic fatty liver disease* or *nonalcoholic fatty hepatitis,* is characterized by the presence of macrovesicular fatty change in hepatocytes on biopsy. Varying degrees of inflammation and portal fibrosis may be present. This disorder occurs in obese children, sometimes in association with insulin-resistant (type 2) diabetes and hyperlipidemia. Children with marked obesity, with or without type 2 diabetes, who have elevated liver enzymes and no other identifiable liver disease are likely to have this condition. Nonalcoholic fatty liver disease can progress to significant fibrosis. Treatment is with diet and exercise. Vitamin E may have some benefit. Efforts should be made to control blood glucose and hyperlipidemia and promote weight loss. In general, the rate of progression to end-stage liver disease is slow.

Chapter 131

PANCREATIC DISEASE

PANCREATIC INSUFFICIENCY
Etiology and Epidemiology
The cause of inadequate pancreatic digestive function in 95% of cases is **cystic fibrosis** (see Chapter 137). The defect in *CFTR* chloride channel function results in thick secretions in the lungs, intestines, pancreas, and bile ducts. In the

pancreas, there is destruction of pancreatic function, often before birth. Some mutations result in less severe defects in *CFTR* function and later onset of lung disease and pancreatic insufficiency. Less common causes of pancreatic insufficiency are Shwachman-Diamond syndrome and Pearson syndrome in developed countries and severe malnutrition in developing countries.

Clinical Manifestations

Decision-Making Algorithm
Available @ StudentConsult.com

Failure to Thrive

Children with pancreatic exocrine insufficiency have many bulky, foul-smelling stools each day, usually with visible oil or fat. They typically have voracious appetites because of massive malabsorption of calories from fat, complex carbohydrates, and proteins. Failure to thrive is uniformly present if diagnosis and treatment are not accomplished rapidly. It is important to distinguish children with malabsorption due to pancreatic disease from children with intestinal disorders that interfere with digestion or absorption. Appropriate testing should be performed to rule out conditions such as celiac disease and inflammatory bowel disease if any doubt about the state of pancreatic sufficiency exists.

Laboratory and Imaging Studies

Testing of pancreatic function is difficult. Direct measurement of enzyme concentrations in aspirated pancreatic juice is not routine and is technically difficult. Stools can be tested for the presence of maldigested fat, which usually indicates poor fat digestion. Measuring fecal fat can give either a qualitative assessment of fat absorption (fecal Sudan stain) or a semi-quantitative measurement (72-hour fecal fat determination) of fat maldigestion. Another way to assess pancreatic function is to test for the presence of pancreatic enzymes in the stool. Of these, measuring **fecal elastase-1** by immunoassay seems to be the most accurate method of assessment. Depressed fecal elastase-1 concentration correlates well with the presence of pancreatic insufficiency.

Treatment

Replacement of missing pancreatic enzymes is the best available therapy. Pancreatic enzymes are available as capsules containing enteric-coated microspheres. The coating on these spheres is designed to protect the enzymes from gastric acid degradation. For children unable to swallow capsules, the contents may be sprinkled on a spoonful of soft food, such as applesauce. Excessive use of enzymes must be avoided because high doses (usually >6000 U/kg/meal) can cause colonic fibrosis. In infants, typical dosing is 2000 to 4000 U of lipase/120 mL of formula. In children younger than 4 years old, 1000 U/kg/meal is given. For older children, 500 U/kg/meal is usual. This dose may be adjusted upward as required to control steatorrhea, but a dose of 2500 U/kg/meal should not be exceeded. Use of H_2 receptor antagonists or proton-pump inhibitors can increase the efficacy of pancreatic enzymes by enhancing their release from the microspheres and reducing inactivation by acid.

ACUTE PANCREATITIS
Etiology and Epidemiology

The exocrine pancreas produces numerous proteolytic enzymes, including trypsin, chymotrypsin, and carboxypeptidase. These are produced as inactive proenzymes to protect the pancreas from autodigestion. Trypsin is activated after leaving the pancreas by enterokinase, an intestinal brush border enzyme. After activation, trypsin cleaves other proteolytic proenzymes into their active states. Protease inhibitors found in pancreatic juice inhibit early activation of trypsin; the presence of self-digestion sites on the trypsin molecule allows for feedback inactivation. Pancreatitis occurs when digestive enzymes are activated inside the pancreas, causing injury. Triggers for acute pancreatitis differ between adults and children. In the adult patient, most episodes are related to alcohol abuse or gallstones. In children, most cases are idiopathic or due to medications. Some cases are caused by pancreatic sufficient cystic fibrosis, hypertriglyceridemia, biliary microlithiasis, trauma, or viral infection. Collagen vascular disorders and parasite infestations are responsible for the remainder (Table 131-1).

Clinical Manifestations

Decision-Making Algorithms
Available @ StudentConsult.com

Abdominal Pain
Vomiting
Hyponatremia
Hypocalcemia

Acute pancreatitis presents with relatively rapid onset of pain, usually in the epigastric region. The pain may radiate to the back and is nearly always aggravated by eating. The patient moves frequently to find a position of comfort. Nausea and vomiting occur in most cases. Pain is typically continuous and quite severe, usually requiring narcotics. Severe pancreatitis can lead to hemorrhage, visible as ecchymoses in the flanks (Grey Turner sign) or periumbilical region (Cullen sign). Rupture of a minor pancreatic duct can lead to development of a pancreatic pseudocyst, characterized by persistent severe pain and tenderness and a palpable mass. With necrosis and fluid collections, patients experiencing severe pancreatitis are prone to infectious complications, and the clinician must be alert for fever and signs of sepsis.

Laboratory and Imaging Studies

Acute pancreatitis can be difficult to diagnose. Elevations in total serum amylase or lipase support the diagnosis. These pancreatic enzymes are released into the blood during pancreatic injury. Nonspecific elevations of the enzymes are common, however. As acute pancreatitis progresses, the amylase level tends to decline faster than lipase, making the latter a

Table 131-1	Causes of Acute Pancreatitis in Children

OBSTRUCTIVE

Cholelithiasis and biliary sludge

Choledochal cyst

Pancreas divisum

Anomalous junction of biliary and pancreatic ducts

Annular pancreas

Ampullary obstruction (mass, inflammation from Crohn's disease)

Ascaris infection

MEDICATIONS AND TOXINS

L-Asparaginase

Valproic acid

Azathioprine and 6-mercaptopurine

Didanosine

Pentamidine

Tetracycline

Opiates

Mesalamine

Sulfasalazine

Alcohol

Cannabis

SYSTEMIC DISEASES

Inflammatory bowel disease

Hemolytic uremic syndrome

Diabetic ketoacidosis

Collagen vascular disease

Kawasaki disease

Shock

Sickle cell disease

INFECTIOUS

Sepsis

Mumps

Coxsackievirus

Cytomegalovirus

Varicella zoster

Herpes simplex

Mycoplasma

Ascaris

GENETIC

Cystic fibrosis—*CFTR* mutations

Hereditary pancreatitis—*SPINK* and *PRSS1* mutations

OTHER

Trauma

Hyperlipidemia

Hypercalcemia

Autoimmune

good choice for diagnostic testing late in the course of the disease.

Serial measurement of laboratory studies is important to monitor for severe complications. At diagnosis, baseline complete blood count, C-reactive protein, electrolytes, blood urea nitrogen, creatinine, glucose, calcium, and phosphorus should be obtained. These should be measured at least daily, along with amylase and lipase, until the patient has recovered.

Because enzyme levels are not 100% sensitive or specific, imaging studies are important for the diagnosis of pancreatitis. In acute pancreatitis, edema is present in all but the mildest cases. Ultrasound is capable of detecting this edema and should be performed as part of the overall diagnostic approach. If overlying bowel gas obscures the pancreas, a computed tomography (CT) scan allows complete visualization of the gland. CT scans should be done with oral and intravenous (IV) contrast agents to facilitate interpretation. Ultrasound and CT also can be used to monitor for the development of **pseudocysts** and for evidence of ductal dilation secondary to obstruction. The other important reason to perform imaging studies early in the course of pancreatitis is to rule out gallstones; the liver, gallbladder, and common bile duct all should be visualized. Magnetic resonance cholangiopancreatography may be used to detect anatomic variants causing pancreatitis.

Treatment

There are no proven specific therapies for acute pancreatitis. If a predisposing etiology is found, such as a drug reaction or a gallstone obstructing the sphincter of Oddi, this should be specifically treated. Initially, oral intake is prohibited, an acid-blocking drug is prescribed, and (except in mild cases) nasogastric suction is begun. Fluid resuscitation is necessary because of vomiting and third space losses. Pain relief should be provided. Meperidine, fentanyl, and hydromorphone are most commonly used. Nutritional support should be provided early in the course if the patient will be nothing by mouth (NPO) for extended periods. Feedings can begin once pain subsides or can be administered downstream from the duodenum. If this is not possible, parenteral nutrition is an option. Fewer complications and more rapid recovery occur with jejunal feedings compared with parenteral nutrition. Antibiotics should be considered if the patient is febrile, has extensive pancreatic necrosis, or has laboratory evidence of infection. A broad-spectrum antibiotic, such as imipenem, is considered the best choice.

CHRONIC PANCREATITIS
Etiology and Epidemiology

Chronic pancreatitis is defined as recurrent or persistent attacks of pancreatitis, which have resulted in irreversible morphologic changes in pancreatic structure. These include scarring of the ducts with irregular areas of narrowing and dilation (beading), fibrosis of parenchyma, and loss of acinar and islet tissue. Pancreatic exocrine insufficiency and diabetes mellitus may result from unremitting chronic pancreatitis. Most patients have discrete attacks of acute symptoms occurring repeatedly, but chronic pain may be present. The causes of chronic pancreatitis include hereditary pancreatitis and milder phenotypes of cystic fibrosis associated with pancreatic sufficiency. Familial disease is caused by one of several known mutations in the trypsinogen gene. These mutations obliterate autodigestion sites on the trypsin molecule, inhibiting feedback inhibition of trypsin digestion. Genetic testing is readily available for these mutations. Genetic testing for cystic fibrosis can be performed, but must include screening for the less common mutations associated with pancreatic sufficiency. Sweat chloride testing is less expensive and is abnormal in most. Less commonly, mutations in the *SPINK1* gene, which codes for pancreatic trypsin inhibitor, and PRSS1, a mutation of cationic trypsinogen, are found.

Clinical Manifestations

Children with chronic pancreatitis initially present with recurring attacks of acute pancreatitis. Injury to the pancreatic ducts predisposes these children to continued attacks owing to scarring of small and large pancreatic ducts, stasis of pancreatic secretions, stone formation, and inflammation. Loss of pancreatic exocrine and endocrine tissue over time can lead to exocrine and endocrine deficiency. More than 90% of the pancreatic mass must be destroyed before exocrine deficiency becomes clinically apparent; this is a late complication that does not occur in all cases. Chronic pain is a serious problem in most affected individuals. These patients have many episodes; many do not require hospitalization.

Laboratory and Imaging Studies

Laboratory diagnosis of chronic pancreatitis is similar to acute pancreatitis but with more severe loss of pancreatic tissue it becomes less likely that the patient with elevation of amylase or lipase. Monitoring also should include looking for consequences of chronic injury, including diabetes mellitus and compromise of the pancreatic and biliary ducts. Pancreatic and biliary imaging has been accomplished by endoscopic retrograde cholangiopancreatography (ERCP). ERCP offers the possibility of therapeutic intervention to remove gallstones, dilate strictures, and place stents to enhance flow of pancreatic juice. Magnetic resonance cholangiopancreatography is an alternative to ERCP. Plain abdominal x-rays may show pancreatic calcifications. Diagnostic testing for the etiology of chronic pancreatitis should include genetic testing for hereditary pancreatitis and cystic fibrosis and sweat chloride determination.

Treatment

Treatment is largely supportive. Potential but unproven therapies include the use of daily pancreatic enzyme supplements, octreotide (somatostatin) to abort early attacks, low-fat diets, and daily antioxidant therapy. Care must be taken that extreme diets do not result in nutritional deprivation. Interventional ERCP to dilate large strictures and remove stones and surgical pancreatic drainage procedures to decompress dilated pancreatic ducts by creating a side-to-side pancreaticojejunostomy may have some value.

PERITONITIS

Etiology and Epidemiology

The peritoneum consists of a single layer of mesothelial cells that covers all intra-abdominal organs. The portion that covers the abdominal wall is derived from the underlying somatic structures and is innervated by somatic nerves. The portion covering the viscera is derived from visceral mesoderm and is innervated by nonmyelinated visceral afferents. Inflammation of the peritoneum, or peritonitis, usually is caused by infection but may result from exogenous irritants introduced by penetrating injuries or surgical procedures, radiation, and endogenous irritants such as meconium. Infectious peritonitis can be an acute complication of intestinal inflammation and perforation, as in appendicitis, or it can occur secondary to contamination of preexisting ascites associated with renal, cardiac, or hepatic disease. In this setting, when there is no other intra-abdominal source, it is referred to as **spontaneous bacterial peritonitis**. Spontaneous bacterial peritonitis is usually due to pneumococcus and less often to *Escherichia coli*.

Clinical Manifestations

Decision-Making Algorithm
Available @ StudentConsult.com

Abdominal Pain

Peritonitis is characterized on examination by marked abdominal tenderness. Rebound tenderness also generally is quite pronounced. The patient tends to move very little owing to intense peritoneal irritation and pain. Fever is not always present, and absence of fever should not be regarded as contradictory to the diagnosis. Patients who are taking corticosteroids for an underlying condition, such as nephrotic syndrome, are likely to have little fever and reduced tenderness.

Laboratory and Imaging Studies

Blood tests should focus on identifying the nature of the inflammation and its underlying cause. An elevated white blood cell count, erythrocyte sedimentation rate, and C-reactive protein suggest infection. In children older than 5 years, appendicitis is the leading cause. Total serum protein, albumin, and urinalysis should be ordered to rule out nephrotic syndrome. Liver function tests should be performed to rule out chronic liver disease causing ascites. The best way to diagnose suspected peritonitis is to sample the peritoneal fluid with a needle or catheter (paracentesis). Peritoneal fluid in spontaneous bacterial peritonitis has a high neutrophil count of greater than 250 cells/mm³. Other tests that should be run on the peritoneal fluid include amylase (to rule out pancreatic ascites), culture, albumin, and lactate dehydrogenase concentration. For culture, a large sample of fluid should be placed into aerobic and anaerobic blood culture bottles immediately on obtaining the sample.

Appendicitis may be identified by ultrasound or computed tomography (CT) scan. When other intra-abdominal emergencies are suspected, such as midgut volvulus, meconium ileus, peptic disease, or any other condition predisposing to intestinal perforation, specific testing should be performed.

Treatment

Peritonitis caused by an intra-abdominal surgical process, such as appendicitis or a penetrating wound, must be managed surgically. Spontaneous bacterial peritonitis should be treated with a broad-spectrum antibiotic with good coverage of resistant pneumococcus and enteric bacteria. Cefotaxime is generally effective as initial therapy while awaiting culture and sensitivity results. Anaerobic coverage with metronidazole should be added whenever a perforated viscus is suspected.

Suggested Reading

Bishop W, editor: *Pediatric Practice: Gastroenterology*, New York, 2010, McGraw-Hill Medical.

Feldman M, Friedman LS, Brandt LJ, editors: *Gastrointestinal and Liver Disease: Pathophysiology/Diagnosis/Management*, Philadelphia, 2010, Saunders.

Kleinman R, Goulet OJ, Mieli-Vergani G, et al: *Walker's Pediatric Gastrointestinal Disease*, Hamilton, Ontario, 2008, BC Decker.

Kliegman RM, Stanton BF, St. Jeme JW, et al: *Nelson Textbook of Pediatrics*, ed 19, Philadelphia, 2011, Saunders.

Wyllie R, Hyams JS, Kay M, editors: *Pediatric Gastrointestinal and Liver Disease*, Philadelphia, 2011, Saunders.

The Respiratory System

Thida Ong, Amanda Striegl, and Susan G. Marshall

Acute and chronic respiratory diseases are common in pediatrics. Children with respiratory problems typically present with symptoms, although abnormal imaging may sometimes precede physical findings. The underlying etiology of childhood respiratory diseases includes the following: genetic (e.g., cystic fibrosis); anatomic (e.g., laryngomalacia); incomplete maturation (e.g., premature birth); iatrogenic (e.g., oxygen toxicity); immunologic (e.g., immune deficiency); infectious (e.g., croup or pneumonia); environmental (e.g., toxins or pollutants); and extrapulmonary (e.g., congenital heart disease). The optimal functioning of the entire respiratory tract allows children not only to survive, but thrive.

Chapter 133

RESPIRATORY SYSTEM ASSESSMENT

ANATOMY OF THE RESPIRATORY SYSTEM

Air enters the **nose** and passes over the large surface area of the **nasal turbinates**, which warm, humidify, and filter the inspired air. Secretions draining from the paranasal sinuses are carried to the **pharynx** by the mucociliary action of the ciliated respiratory epithelium. Lymphoid tissue can obstruct airflow through the nasopharynx (adenoids) or the posterior pharynx (tonsils).

The **epiglottis** protects the larynx during swallowing by deflecting material toward the esophagus. The **arytenoid cartilages**, which assist in opening and closing the glottis, are less prominent in children than in adults. The opening formed by the vocal cords (the **glottis**) is V-shaped, with the apex of the V being anterior. Below the vocal cords, the walls of the **subglottic space** converge toward the **cricoid** portion of the trachea. In children under 3 years of age, the cricoid ring is the narrowest portion of the airway, whereas in older children and adults it is the glottis. C-shaped cartilage, extending approximately 320° around the airway circumference, supports the **trachea** and mainstem **bronchi**. The posterior wall of the trachea is membranous. Beyond the lobar bronchi, the cartilaginous support for the airways becomes discontinuous.

The right lung has three lobes (upper, middle, lower) and comprises approximately 55% of the total lung volume. The left lung has two lobes (upper, lower). The inferior division of the left upper lobe, the lingula, is analogous to the right middle lobe.

The pediatric lung has tremendous capacity for growth. A full-term infant has approximately 25 million alveoli; an adult nearly 300 million alveoli. The growth of new alveoli occurs during the first 2 years of life and is complete by 8 years of age. After this time, lung volume increases primarily by increase in alveolar dimensions, with new alveoli rarely formed.

PULMONARY PHYSIOLOGY
Pulmonary Mechanics

The major function of the lungs is to **exchange oxygen** (O_2) and **carbon dioxide** (CO_2) between the atmosphere and the blood. The anatomy of the airways, mechanics of the respiratory muscles and rib cage, nature of the alveolar-capillary interface, pulmonary circulation, tissue metabolism, and neuromuscular control of ventilation all influence gas exchange.

Air enters the lungs when intrathoracic pressure is less than atmospheric pressure. During inspiration, negative intrathoracic pressure is generated by contraction and lowering of the **diaphragm**. The accessory muscles of inspiration (**external intercostal**, **scalene**, and **sternocleidomastoid muscles**) are not used during quiet breathing but are recruited during exercise or in disease states to raise and enlarge the rib cage. Exhalation is normally passive, but with active exhalation, the **abdominal** and **internal intercostal muscles** are recruited.

During normal breathing at rest, lung volumes are usually in the mid-range of inflation (Fig. 133-1). **Tidal volume (TV)** is the amount of air inspired with each *relaxed* breath. The volume of gas retained in the lung at the end of a *relaxed* exhalation is

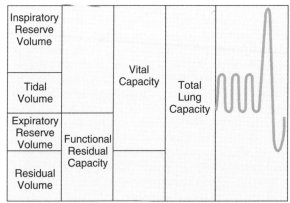

Figure 133-1 Lung volumes and capacities. Vital capacity and its subdivisions can be measured by spirometry, but calculation of residual volume requires measurement of functional residual capacity by body plethysmography, helium dilution, or nitrogen washout. *(From Andreoli TE, Bennett JC, Carpenter CJ, et al, editors:* Cecil Essentials of Medicine, *ed 4, Philadelphia, 1997, WB Saunders, p 127.)*

Table 133-1	Causes of Hypoxemia				
CAUSE	**EXAMPLE(S)**	**Pao₂**	**Paco₂**		**Pao₂ IMPROVES WITH SUPPLEMENTAL OXYGEN**
Ventilation-perfusion mismatch	Asthma Bronchopulmonary dysplasia Pneumonia Atelectasis	↓	Normal, ↓, or ↑		Yes
Hypoventilation	Apnea Narcotic overdose Neuromuscular disease	↓	↑		Yes
Extrapulmonary shunt	Cyanotic heart disease	↓	Normal or ↑		No
Intrapulmonary shunt	Pulmonary arteriovenous malformation Pulmonary edema	↓	Normal or ↑		No
Low FIO₂	High altitude	↓	↓		Yes
Diffusion defect	Scleroderma Hepatopulmonary syndrome Pulmonary fibrosis	↓	Normal		Yes

FIO₂, Fraction of inspired oxygen; *Paco₂*, arterial partial pressure of carbon dioxide; *Pao₂*, arterial partial pressure of oxygen.

the **functional residual capacity (FRC)**. This gas volume maintains exchange of O₂ during exhalation. **Total lung capacity (TLC)** is the volume of gas in the lungs at the end of *maximal* inhalation and **residual volume (RV)** is the volume of gas left in the lungs at the end of a *maximal* exhalation. **Vital capacity (VC)** is the maximal amount of air that can be expelled from the lungs and is the difference between TLC and RV.

Airway resistance is influenced by the diameter and length of the conducting airways, the viscosity of gas, and the nature of the airflow. During quiet breathing, airflow in the smaller airways may be laminar (streamlined), and resistance is inversely proportional to the fourth power of the radius of the airway. At higher flow rates, turbulent flow, especially in the larger airways, increases resistance. Relatively small changes in airway diameter can result in large changes in airway resistance. Excessive airway secretions, bronchospasm, mucosal edema and inflammation, airway stenosis, foreign bodies, loss of airway wall integrity (as with bronchiectasis), and airway compression may all produce symptomatic increases in airway resistance. In pediatrics, laryngomalacia and croup are very common causes of increased upper airway resistance; whereas asthma, bronchiolitis and cystic fibrosis (CF) are among the most common causes of increased lower airway resistance.

Lung compliance (change in volume for a given change in pressure) is a measure of the ease with which the lung can be inflated. Processes that decrease lung compliance (surfactant deficiency, pulmonary fibrosis, pulmonary edema) may lead to decreases in measured lung volumes. Restrictive lung diseases are characterized by normal to low FRC and RV, low TLC and VC, decreased lung compliance, and relatively normal flow rates. Restrictive lung disease can result from neuromuscular weakness, an alveolar filling process (lobar pneumonia, pulmonary edema), pleural disease (pleural effusion, inflammation, or mass), thoracic narrowing/stiffness (scoliosis, severe pectus excavatum), and abdominal distention.

Respiratory Gas Exchange

Alveolar ventilation is defined as the exchange of carbon dioxide between the alveoli and external environment.

Normally, about 30% of each tidal breath fills the conducting (non–gas-exchanging) airways (**anatomic dead space**). Because the anatomic dead space is relatively constant, increasing the tidal volume may increase the efficacy of ventilation. Conversely, if tidal volume decreases, then the dead space/tidal volume ratio increases, and alveolar ventilation decreases.

Gas exchange depends on **alveolar ventilation**, **pulmonary capillary blood flow**, and the **diffusion** of gases across the alveolar-capillary membrane. Exchange of CO₂ is determined by alveolar ventilation, whereas the exchange of O₂ is influenced primarily by the regional matching of ventilation (V) with pulmonary blood flow (Q) (V/Q matching). V/Q matching is maintained, in part, by **hypoxic pulmonary vasoconstriction** (local constriction of the pulmonary vessels in areas that are hypoventilated). There are five causes of **hypoxemia** (Table 133-1). Disorders resulting in **V/Q mismatching** (such as pneumonia and atelectasis) are the most common causes of hypoxemia.

Lung Defense Mechanisms

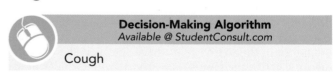

Decision-Making Algorithm
Available @ StudentConsult.com

Cough

The lungs are constantly exposed to particles and infectious agents. The **nose** is the primary filter for large particles. The **ciliated epithelium** of the paranasal sinuses and nasal turbinates move filtered particles toward the pharynx. Particles less than 10 μm in diameter may reach the trachea and bronchi and deposit on the mucosa. Particles less than 1 μm may reach the alveoli. Ciliated cells lining the airways from the larynx to the bronchioles continuously propel a thin layer of mucus toward the mouth. **Alveolar macrophages** and **polymorphonuclear cells** engulf particles and pathogens that have been opsonized by locally secreted IgA antibodies or transudated serum antibodies.

Cough, important in protecting the lungs, is a forceful expiration that can clear the airways of debris and secretions. Cough may be voluntary or generated by reflex irritation of the nose, sinus, pharynx, larynx, trachea, bronchi, or bronchioles. Effective cough requires the ability to (1) inhale to near total lung capacity, (2) close and open the glottis, and (3) contract abdominal muscles to forcibly exhale. Loss of the ability to cough, as with neuromuscular weakness, results in poor secretion clearance and predisposes to atelectasis and pneumonia.

HISTORY

Decision-Making Algorithm
Available @ StudentConsult.com

Cough

The complete respiratory history includes **onset, duration, and frequency** of respiratory symptoms (cough, noisy breathing, work of breathing/exercise tolerance, nasal congestion, sputum production), swallowing function (especially in infants), and exposure to others with respiratory illness. It is important to obtain information concerning the severity (hospitalizations, emergency department visits, missed school days) and pattern (acute, chronic, or intermittent) of symptoms. For infants, a feeding history should be obtained, including questions of coughing or choking with feeds. **Family history** should include questions about asthma and atopy, immune deficiencies, and CF. The **environmental history** queries exposure to smoke, pets, and pollutants. Travel history may also be relevant.

PHYSICAL EXAMINATION

Decision-Making Algorithms
Available @ StudentConsult.com

Stridor
Wheezing
Cyanosis

Clothing should be removed from the upper half of the child's body so that the thorax may be inspected, although maintaining modesty for adolescents should be respected. It is optimal to observe the respiratory pattern, rate, and work of breathing while the child is quiet, noting the shape and symmetry of the chest wall and the anteroposterior (AP) diameter.

Any factor that impairs respiratory mechanics is likely to increase the **respiratory rate**. However, nonrespiratory causes of tachypnea include fever, pain, and anxiety. Respiratory rates vary with age and activity (Table 133-2).

It is important to observe the respiratory **pattern** and **degree of effort** (work of breathing). **Hyperpnea** (increased depth of respiration) may be observed with fever, metabolic acidosis, pulmonary and cardiac disease, or extreme anxiety. Hyperpnea without signs of respiratory distress suggests an extrapulmonary etiology (metabolic acidosis, fever, pain). Increased work of breathing can be described as inspiratory **(intercostal, supraclavicular, or substernal retractions)** or

Table 133-2	Breathing Patterns
PATTERN	**FEATURES**
Normal rate (breaths/min)	Preterm: 40–60; term: 30–40; 5 yr: 25; 10 yr: 20; 15 yr: 16; adult: 12
Obstructive	
Mild	Reduced rate, increased tidal volume, slightly prolonged expiratory phase
Severe	Increased rate, increased use of accessory muscles, prolonged expiratory phase
Restrictive	Rapid rate, decreased tidal volume
Kussmaul respiration	Increased rate, increased tidal volume, regular deep respiration; consider metabolic acidosis or diabetic ketoacidosis
Cheyne-Stokes respiration	Cyclic pattern of waxing and waning of breathing interposed by central apneas/hypopneas; consider CNS injury, depressant drugs, heart failure, uremia (rare in children)
Biot respiration	Ataxic or periodic breathing with a respiratory effort followed by apnea; consider brainstem injury or posterior fossa mass
Gasping	Slow rate, variable tidal volume; consider hypoxia, shock, sepsis, or asphyxia

CNS, Central nervous system.

expiratory (use of abdominal muscles to actively exhale). In children, increased inspiratory effort is also manifested by **nasal flaring**. **Grunting** (forced expiration against a partially closed glottis) suggests respiratory distress, but it may also be a manifestation of pain.

Causes of increased work of breathing during inspiration include extrathoracic airway obstruction (laryngomalacia, croup, subglottic stenosis) and/or decreased pulmonary compliance (pneumonia, pulmonary edema). Increased expiratory work of breathing usually indicates intrathoracic airway obstruction (see Table 133-2).

Stridor is a harsh sound caused by a partially obstructed extrathoracic airway, more commonly heard on inspiration. **Wheezing** is produced by partial obstruction of the lower airways, more commonly heard during exhalation. Wheezes can be monophonic and low-pitched (usually from large, central airways) or high-pitched and musical (from small peripheral airways). Secretions in the intrathoracic airways may produce wheezing but more commonly result in irregular sounds called **rhonchi**. Fluid or secretions in small airways may produce sounds characteristic of crumpling cellophane (**crackles** or **rales**). Having the child take a deep breath and exhale forcefully will accentuate many abnormal lung sounds. Decreased breath sounds may be due to atelectasis, lobar consolidation (pneumonia), thoracic mass, or a pleural effusion. Observation of respiratory rate, work of breathing, tracheal and cardiac deviation, and chest wall motion, combined with percussion and auscultation, helps to identify intrathoracic disease (Table 133-3).

Digital clubbing is seen in CF and in other, less common chronic pulmonary diseases (such as interstitial lung disease). It is generally not seen in asthma, so its presence should heighten concern for other diagnoses. Clubbing may also be present in nonpulmonary chronic diseases (cardiac, gastrointestinal, or hematologic) or, rarely, as a familial trait.

Table 133-3	Physical Signs of Pulmonary Disease						
DISEASE PROCESS	**MEDIASTINAL DEVIATION**	**CHEST MOTION**	**VOCAL FREMITUS**	**PERCUSSION**	**BREATH SOUNDS**	**ADVENTITIOUS SOUNDS**	**VOICE SIGNS**
Consolidation	No	Reduced over area	Increased	Dull	Bronchial or reduced	None or crackles	Egophony* Pectoriloquy†
Bronchospasm	No	Hyperexpansion with limited motion	Normal or decreased	Hyperresonant	Normal to decreased	Wheezes, crackles	Normal to decreased
Atelectasis	Shift toward affected side	Reduced over area	Decreased	Dull	Reduced	None or crackles	None
Pneumothorax	With tension pneumothorax: shift to the opposite side	Reduced over PMI	None	Resonant	None	None	None
Pleural effusion	Deviation to opposite side	Reduced over area	None or reduced	Dull	None	Egophony Friction rub	Muffled
Interstitial process	No	Reduced	Normal to increased	Normal	Normal	Inspiratory crackles	None

Adapted from Andreoli TE, Bennett JC, Carpenter CJ, et al, editors: Cecil Essentials of Medicine, ed 4, Philadelphia, 1997, WB Saunders, p 115.
PMI, Point of maximum impulse.
*In egophony, e sounds like a (may be a sign of consolidation but also is associated with moderate-sized pleural effusions).
†In pectoriloquy, words/voice sounds clearer over the affected site (associated with consolidation and cavitary lesions).

Cough results from stimulation of irritant receptors in the airway mucosa. Acute cough generally is associated with respiratory infections or irritant exposure (smoke) and subsides as the infection resolves or the exposure is eliminated. The characteristics of the cough and the circumstances under which the cough occurs help in determining the cause. Sudden onset after a choking episode suggests foreign body aspiration. Morning cough may be due to the accumulation of excessive secretions during the night from sinusitis, allergic rhinitis, or bronchial infection. Nighttime coughing is a hallmark of asthma and can also be caused by gastroesophageal reflux disease. Cough exacerbated by lying flat may be due to postnasal drip, sinusitis, allergic rhinitis, or reflux. Recurrent coughing with exercise is suggestive of exercise-induced asthma/bronchospasm. Paroxysmal cough suggests pertussis or foreign body aspiration. A repetitive, staccato cough occurs in chlamydial infections in infants. A harsh, brassy, seal-like cough suggests croup, tracheomalacia, or psychogenic (habit) cough. The last, which is most common in teenagers, disappears during sleep. Younger children can develop a throat-clearing habit cough, which also disappears during sleep.

Chronic cough is defined as a daily cough lasting longer than 3 weeks. Common causes of chronic cough are asthma, postnasal drip (allergic rhinitis, sinusitis), and postinfectious tussive syndromes. It can also be caused by gastroesophageal reflux disease, swallowing dysfunction (infants), anatomic abnormalities (tracheoesophageal fistula, tracheomalacia), and chronic infection. Persistent cough may also be caused by exposure to irritants (tobacco and wood stove smoke) or foreign body aspiration, or it may be psychogenic in origin.

During the first several years of life, children experience frequent viral respiratory infections, especially if they have multiple older siblings or attend day care or preschool. Cough that resolves promptly and is clearly associated with a viral infection does not require further diagnostic workup. However, cough persisting longer than 3 weeks warrants further evaluation.

DIAGNOSTIC MEASURES
Imaging Techniques

Chest radiographs are useful in assessing respiratory disease in children. In addition to determining lung abnormalities, they provide information about the bony thorax (rib or vertebral abnormalities), the heart (cardiomegaly, pericardial effusion), and the great vessels (right aortic arch/vascular rings, rib notching). Chest radiographs should be obtained in both the posteroanterior (PA) and lateral projections and, if possible, following a full inspiration. Estimation of lung hyperinflation based on a single PA view is unreliable; flattened diaphragms and an increased AP diameter on lateral projection is a better indicator of hyperinflation. Crowding of the blood vessels with poor inspiration can be misinterpreted as increased markings or infiltrates. External skin folds, rotation, and motion may produce distorted or unclear images. Expiratory views and fluoroscopy may detect partial bronchial obstruction due to an aspirated foreign body that results in regional hyperinflation, because the affected lung or lobe does not deflate on exhalation. Fluoroscopy can also be used to evaluate diaphragm movement.

A **barium esophagram** may be valuable in diagnosing disorders of swallowing (dysphagia) and esophageal motility, vascular rings (esophageal compression), tracheoesophageal fistulas, and, to a lesser extent, gastroesophageal reflux. When evaluating for a tracheoesophageal fistula, contrast material must be instilled under pressure via a catheter with the distal tip situated in the esophagus (see Chapter 128).

A **computed tomography (CT) scan of the chest** is the imaging test of choice for evaluating pleural masses, bronchiectasis, and mediastinal lesions as well as delineating pleural from parenchymal lesions. CT scans with intravenous contrast provide excellent information about the pulmonary vasculature and great vessels and can detect pulmonary embolism. High-resolution CT scans are used to assess lung parenchyma (congenital pulmonary malformations, interstitial lung disease) and the airways (bronchiectasis). The speed of current

CT scanners makes it possible to scan most children without sedating them. However, sedation may be required in infants and toddlers to decrease motion artifact. **Magnetic resonance imaging (MRI)**, useful in visualizing cardiac and great vessel anatomy, is less useful for evaluation of pulmonary parenchymal lesions.

Ultrasonography can be used to delineate some intrathoracic masses and is the imaging procedure of choice for assessing parapneumonic effusion/empyema. It is useful for assessing diaphragmatic motion in small children.

Measures of Respiratory Gas Exchange
A properly performed **arterial blood gas** analysis provides information about the effectiveness of both oxygenation and ventilation. However, arterial samples are more difficult to obtain, so capillary and venous blood samples are more commonly used. The P_{CO_2} from a capillary sample is similar to that from arterial blood. The P_{CO_2} in venous samples is approximately 6 mm Hg higher than arterial P_{CO_2}. The ratio of the serum bicarbonate concentration to P_{CO_2} determines the pH. Capillary or venous samples should not be used to assess oxygenation.

There are both respiratory and metabolic causes of acidosis (see Chapter 37). In the presence of an alkalosis or acidosis, respiratory compensation (altering P_{CO_2} to maintain a normal pH) can occur within minutes, but renal compensation (altering the serum bicarbonate level) may not be complete for several days. Recall that both the respiratory and metabolic compensation are incomplete, so pH will remain on the side of the primary insult (whether acidosis or alkalosis).

Pulse oximetry measures the O_2 saturation of hemoglobin by measuring the blood absorption of two or more wavelengths of light. It is noninvasive, easy to use, and reliable. Because of the shape of the oxyhemoglobin dissociation curve, O_2 saturation does not decrease much until the P_{O_2} reaches approximately 60 mm Hg. Pulse oximetry may not accurately reflect true O_2 saturation when abnormal hemoglobin is present (carboxyhemoglobin, methemoglobin), when perfusion is poor, or if no light passes through to the photodetector (nail polish).

The measurement of P_{CO_2} is accomplished most reliably by blood gas analysis. However, there are noninvasive monitors that record exhaled P_{CO_2} (**end-tidal CO_2**), which is representative of alveolar P_{CO_2}. End-tidal P_{CO_2} measurements are most commonly used in intubated and mechanically ventilated patients, but some devices can measure P_{CO_2} at the nares. **Transcutaneous electrodes** can be used to monitor P_{CO_2} and P_{O_2} at the skin surface, but are less accurate. Noninvasive techniques of CO_2 measurement are best suited for detecting trends rather than for providing absolute values.

Pulmonary Function Testing
Measurement of lung volumes and airflow rates using **spirometry** are important in assessing pulmonary disease. The patient inhales to TLC and then forcibly exhales until no more air can be expelled. During the forced expiratory maneuver, forced vital capacity (**FVC**), forced expired volume in the first second (**FEV$_1$**), and **forced expiratory flow (FEF)** rates are measured. These are compared to predicted values based on patient age, gender, and race, but rely mostly on height. Most

children above 6 years of age can perform spirometry. Infant pulmonary function testing is possible, using sedation and sophisticated equipment.

Airway resistance, FRC, and RV cannot be measured with spirometry and require other techniques, such as **body plethysmography**. Helium dilution can also measure TLC and RV by determining the magnitude of dilution of inhaled helium in the air within the lung, but may underestimate air trapping.

Abnormal results on pulmonary function testing can be used to categorize **obstructive airway disease** (low flow rates and increased RV or FRC) or a **restrictive defect** (low FVC and TLC, with relative preservation of flow rates and FRC). When the FEV_1 and flow rates are decreased to a greater extent than the FVC, then airway obstruction is likely; however, a proportional decrease in FVC, FEV_1, and flow rates suggests a restrictive lung defect. The mean midexpiratory flow rate (**$FEF_{25-75\%}$**) is a more sensitive measure of small airways disease than the FEV_1, but is also more variable. Pulmonary function testing can detect reversible airway obstruction characteristic of asthma with a significant improvement in FEV_1 (>12%-15%) or in $FEF_{25-75\%}$ (>25%) following inhalation of a bronchodilator. Spirometry is also useful for longitudinal patient management. The **peak expiratory flow rate (PEFR)** can be obtained with a simple handheld device and may be useful for home monitoring of older children with asthma. However, it is highly dependent on patient effort, and values must be interpreted with caution. **Inhalation challenge tests** using methacholine, histamine, or cold, dry air are used to assess airway hyperreactivity, but require sophisticated equipment and special expertise and should be performed only in a pulmonary function laboratory with experienced technicians.

Endoscopic Evaluation of the Airways
Endoscopic evaluation of the upper airways (**nasopharyngoscopy**) is performed with a flexible fiberoptic nasopharyngoscope to assess adenoid size, patency of the nasal passages, and abnormalities of the glottis. It is especially useful in evaluating stridor and assessing vocal cord motion/function, and it does not require sedation. Endoscopic evaluation of the subglottic space and intrathoracic airways can be done with either a flexible or rigid bronchoscope under anesthesia. **Bronchoscopy** is useful in identifying airway abnormalities (stenosis, malacia, endobronchial lesions, excessive secretions) and in obtaining airway samples for culture (bronchoalveolar lavage), especially in immunocompromised patients. Rigid bronchoscopy is the method of choice for removing foreign bodies from the airways and performing other interventions, and flexible bronchoscopy is most useful as a diagnostic tool and for obtaining lower airway cultures. Transbronchial biopsies are rarely performed in children. There are few absolute contraindications to bronchoscopy. Relative contraindications include bleeding diatheses, thrombocytopenia (<50,000/cm^3), and clinical conditions when the patient is too unstable to tolerate the procedure.

Examination of Sputum
Sputum specimens may be useful in evaluating lower respiratory tract infections, but they are difficult to obtain in young children. In addition, an expectorated specimen may not

provide a representative sample of lower airway secretions. Specimens containing large numbers of squamous epithelial cells either are not from the lower airways or are heavily contaminated with upper airway secretions and may yield misleading results. Sputum in patients with lower respiratory tract bacterial infections often contains polymorphonucleated leukocytes and one predominant organism on culture. If sputum cannot be obtained, then bronchoalveolar lavage specimens may be used for microbiologic diagnosis in selected situations. In patients with CF who cannot produce sputum, specially processed throat cultures are often used as surrogates for lower airway cultures.

Lung Biopsy

When less invasive methods fail to provide diagnoses in patients with pulmonary disease, a lung biopsy may be required. Concern for childhood interstitial lung disease, atypical infection (especially in an immunocompromised host), and evaluation of a mass/malformation are the most common indications for biopsy. CT-guided needle biopsy performed by an interventional radiologist is an option if limited histology is needed and the lesion is amenable to percutaneous approach (e.g., fungal nodules). Either a **thoracoscopic procedure** or a **thoracotomy** is preferred if thorough histologic evaluation is desired. Thoracotomy allows the surgeon to inspect and palpate the lung, which aids in choosing the best site for biopsy, but it is more invasive than thoracoscopy. In most cases, infants and children tolerate lung biopsy well.

THERAPEUTIC MEASURES
Oxygen Administration

Any child in respiratory distress should be treated with **supplemental O_2** to maintain normal O_2 saturation levels. For long-term administration of O_2, a **nasal cannula** is the most widely used device, as it enables patients to eat and speak unhindered by the O_2 delivery system. Though nasal cannula is the easiest way to provide supplemental O_2, the actual fraction of inspired oxygen (**FIO_2**) delivered to the patient can be quite variable and affected by the child's size and respiratory pattern. Humidified **high flow nasal cannula** (HFNC) allows the provider to more comfortably deliver higher flow rates while controlling the FIO_2 and is now widely used in neonates as an alternative to noninvasive positive pressure. Supplemental O_2 may also be delivered by a variety of face-mask systems ranging from a simple face mask, which can provide 30% to 40% O_2, to a nonrebreather mask with reservoir that can provide nearly 100% O_2.

The concentration of administered O_2 should be high enough to relieve hypoxemia. The *acceptable* O_2 saturation depends on the patient and clinical situation. Generally, supplemental O_2 should be administered to achieve a goal saturation level above 90%. Normal oxygen saturation is greater than 95%. It is unnecessary to achieve 100% saturation, especially if this requires potentially toxic levels of inspired O_2 for extended periods of time.

Inspired O_2 concentrations less than 40% are usually safe for long-term use. Patients requiring supplemental O_2 should be monitored with pulse oximetry, either intermittently or continuously, or with arterial blood gas measurements of Po_2 to allow titration to the lowest possible O_2 concentration.

Aerosol Therapy

Delivering therapeutic agents to the lower respiratory tract can be accomplished by inhalation of aerosol forms of the agents via **dry powder inhaler** (DPI), **metered dose inhaler** (MDI), or **nebulizer**. All of these devices are designed to generate relatively small particles that can bypass the filtering action of the upper airway and deposit in the lower airways. Many factors influence drug deposition, including patient technique, device used, age of the child, and breathing pattern. Nebulizers should be used with a face mask (infants) or mouthpiece (children and teens) to minimize loss of drug to ambient air. Plastic holding chambers (**spacers**) are available for all ages and should always be used with MDIs. Dry powder inhalers require a single rapid deep inhalation for optimal drug delivery, which is difficult for children under 6 years of age. MDIs and nebulizers are equally effective in delivering medications only if the technique is correct, so it is important to review this frequently and carefully with families.

Chest Physiotherapy and Clearance Techniques

When disease processes impair clearance of pulmonary secretions, airway clearance techniques may help maintain airway patency. One method is **chest percussion**, which moves secretions toward the central airways, from which they can be expectorated. **Chest physiotherapy** can also be performed effectively with handheld devices that generate expiratory back-pressure and vibration (**TheraPEP**, **Flutter**, and **Acapella**) and **pneumatic vests**. Chest physiotherapy is most beneficial in children with chronic airway secretions, especially those with CF. Children who are too weak to generate an effective cough benefit from the use of a mechanical cough assist device, used in conjunction with chest physiotherapy. Chest physiotherapy is not generally beneficial for patients with asthma or pneumonia, and its effectiveness in patients with atelectasis has not been clearly established.

Intubation

If the upper airway is obstructed or mechanical ventilation is needed, it may be necessary to provide the patient with an **artificial airway**. This is best done by placing an endotracheal tube via the mouth or nose into the trachea (**intubation**). Intubation alters the physiology of the respiratory tract in many ways, not all of which are beneficial. It interferes with the humidification, warming, and filtration of inspired air and prevents phonation. Intubation also stimulates secretion production. However, in acute/impending respiratory failure, intubation with an endotracheal tube is lifesaving.

Endotracheal tubes can damage the larynx and the airways if the tubes are of improper size and are not carefully maintained. The cricoid ring is the narrowest segment of a child's airway and is completely surrounded by cartilage, which makes it vulnerable to damage, and may lead to subglottic stenosis. If the pressure created by the tube against the airway mucosa exceeds capillary filling pressure (roughly 35 cm H_2O), mucosal ischemia develops, leading to necrosis. Therefore, a small air leak should be maintained around the endotracheal tube to minimize the risk of mucosal damage.

Artificial airways must be kept clear of secretions as obstruction with mucous plugs can be fatal. Providing adequate humidification of inspired air and appropriate suctioning of the tube reduce the probability of occlusion by secretions. In addition to endotracheal tubes, the **laryngeal mask airway (LMA)** can be used to provide mechanical ventilation. This device consists of a tube with a soft mask at the distal end that is placed over the larynx, creating a seal without the trachea being instrumented. Although less invasive, the LMA is less secure, so it is generally limited to procedural anesthesia.

Tracheostomy

Tracheostomy is the surgical placement of an artificial airway into the trachea below the larynx. If prolonged intubation is anticipated, elective tracheostomy may be used to prevent laryngeal trauma, obviate the danger of accidental extubation, increase patient comfort, and facilitate nursing care. No clear guidelines are available as to how long patients can be intubated without sustaining airway damage or when a tracheostomy is indicated.

Children with severe chronic upper airway obstruction or those requiring long-term mechanical ventilation may benefit from tracheostomies. Because the tracheostomy tube hampers the ability to phonate and communicate, the child must be monitored carefully at all times. As with endotracheal tubes, tracheostomy tubes must be kept clear of secretions. Occlusion of the tube or accidental dislodgment of the tube can be fatal. Many children with tracheostomy tubes can be cared for at home provided the caregivers are well trained and adequately equipped.

Mechanical Ventilation

Patients who are unable to maintain adequate gas exchange may require mechanical ventilation. Most modes of mechanical ventilation involve inflation of the lungs with gas using positive pressure. The inspiratory phase is active (air is pushed in) and exhalation is passive.

Positive-pressure ventilation often requires an artificial airway, though it can be provided *noninvasively* via tight-fitting nasal or full face masks. **Noninvasive ventilation** is particularly useful in patients with obstructive sleep apnea and neuromuscular disease who require support only part of the day, but it can also be used to assist ventilation continuously for patients in acute respiratory failure from a variety of causes.

No method of mechanical ventilation truly simulates natural breathing. All methods have their drawbacks and complications. Positive pressure is transmitted to the entire thorax and may impede venous return to the heart during inspiration. The airways and lung parenchyma may be damaged by inflation pressures and high concentrations of inspired O_2. In general, inflation pressures should be limited to those necessary to provide sufficient lung expansion for adequate ventilation and the prevention of atelectasis. Pressure-cycled and volume-cycled ventilators (conventional ventilation) are the most widely used modalities in pediatrics; however, high-frequency jet ventilation and high-frequency oscillatory ventilation are used often in neonatology and may be used in patients with severe lung disease who are failing conventional mechanical ventilation.

CONTROL OF BREATHING

CONTROL OF VENTILATION

Ventilation is controlled primarily by **central chemoreceptors** located in the medulla that respond to intracellular pH and P_{CO_2} levels (Fig. 134-1). To a lesser extent, ventilation is modulated by **peripheral receptors** located in the carotid and aortic bodies, which respond predominantly to P_{O_2}. The central receptors are quite sensitive. Small acute changes in Pa_{CO_2} normally result in significant changes in **minute ventilation**. When the P_{CO_2} is chronically elevated, the intracellular pH returns to normal levels because of compensatory increases in the bicarbonate level, and ventilatory drive is not increased. The peripheral receptors do not stimulate ventilation until the Pa_{O_2} decreases to approximately 60 mm Hg. These receptors become important in patients with chronic Pa_{CO_2} elevation who may have a blunted ventilatory response to CO_2.

The output of the central respiratory center also is modulated by reflex mechanisms. Full lung inflation temporarily inhibits inspiratory effort in infants (**Hering-Breuer reflex**) through vagal afferent fibers. Other reflexes from the airways and intercostal muscles may influence the depth and frequency of respiratory efforts (see Fig. 134-1).

DISORDERS OF CONTROL OF BREATHING
Acute Life-Threatening Events
Etiology

An acute life-threatening event (ALTE) is defined as any unexpected and frightening change in condition characterized by

Figure 134-1 Schematic representation of the respiratory control system. The respiratory neurons in the brainstem receive information from the chemoreceptors, peripheral sensory receptors, and cerebral cortex. This information is integrated, and the resulting neural output is transmitted to the diaphragms and lungs. The sign denotes stimulation of the receptor. (*From Andreoli TE, Bennett JC, Carpenter CJ, et al, editors: Cecil Essentials of Medicine, ed 4, Philadelphia, 1997, WB Saunders, p 171.*)

apnea, color change (usually blue or pale), sudden limpness, choking, or gagging. The incidence of such events is 0.05% to 1%. Specific causes can be identified in more than 50% of the cases. Gastroesophageal reflux and laryngospasm are the most common causes of ALTE, and they are associated with emesis, choking, or gagging. Central nervous system (CNS) causes (e.g., seizures, breath-holding spells, intracranial bleeding from accidental or nonaccidental trauma) account for approximately 15% of cases, and cardiovascular events and metabolic derangements account for smaller percentages. Acute infection with respiratory viruses (respiratory syncytial virus [RSV] and others), pertussis, and serious bacterial infections (sepsis, meningitis) can also cause apnea in infants.

Diagnostic Studies

In most cases, a careful history can lead to a correct diagnosis. Questions should include history of premature birth, prior apnea, level of consciousness at the time of the event, presence or absence of respiratory effort, limpness or stiffness, jerking movements (seizure), feeding history, intercurrent illnesses, any trauma, and the social situation of the family. The physical examination should focus on bruising and injury, the general and neurologic condition of the infant, nutritional status, respiratory pattern, and cardiac status. The laboratory evaluation may include serum electrolytes, serum glucose, blood urea nitrogen, creatinine, hemoglobin, hematocrit, white blood cell count, a chest radiograph, and blood gas analysis. Testing for respiratory viruses and pertussis in patients with evidence of respiratory infection should occur. If gastroesophageal reflux is suspected, a barium swallow or pH probe study may be useful. Cardiorespiratory monitoring for 12 to 24 hours in the hospital can provide information on respiratory and cardiac patterns and feeding difficulties (choking, gagging, emesis); provide time to get more history and assess the home situation; and alleviate parental anxiety. Useful tests to determine CNS causes include a head computed tomography (CT) scan, magnetic resonance imaging of the brain, and an electroencephalogram (EEG) (for seizures).

Treatment and Prevention

There are no standard recommendations for when home monitoring should be prescribed. Polysomnography is not useful in predicting which children with ALTEs are likely to progress to sudden infant death syndrome (SIDS). The key to prevention of future events is to identify the underlying cause and treat it. Teaching parents infant cardiopulmonary resuscitation (CPR) and attempting to alleviate anxiety surrounding the event are recommended.

Sudden Infant Death Syndrome
Etiology and Epidemiology

SIDS is defined as the **unexpected death** of an infant younger than 1 year of age in which the cause remains unexplained after an autopsy, death scene investigation, and review of clinical history. The risk of SIDS is higher in premature and low birth weight infants, infants of young impoverished mothers who smoke cigarettes, African American and Native American infants, and in infants whose mothers have abused drugs. The risk of SIDS is increased three- to fivefold in siblings of

infants who have died of SIDS and is highest during the winter. SIDS is rare before 4 weeks or after 6 months of age and is most common between 2 and 4 months of age. The incidence of SIDS has decreased dramatically since the 1980s.

A variety of unproven mechanisms have been proposed to explain SIDS. SIDS is associated with prone position during sleep, especially on soft bedding. The widely advocated supine sleeping position explains, in part, the decreased incidence of SIDS during the past two decades. Current theories for a predisposition to SIDS include cellular brainstem abnormalities and maturational delay related to neural or cardiorespiratory control. A portion of SIDS deaths may be due to prolongation of the Q-T interval, abnormal CNS control of respiration, and CO_2 rebreathing from sleeping face down (especially in soft bedding).

Differential Diagnosis

See Table 134-1 for the differential diagnosis of SIDS.

Prevention

There has been a significant decline in SIDS with the **back-to-sleep program** and avoiding soft bedding. Thus, all parents should be instructed to place their infants in the supine position unless there are medical contraindications. All soft

Table 134-1	Differential Diagnosis of Sudden Infant Death Syndrome
INFECTIOUS DISEASE	
Fulminant infection[*,†]	
Infant botulism[*]	
NEUROLOGIC	
Seizure disorder[†]	
Brain tumor[*]	
Intracranial hemorrhage due to accidental or non-accidental trauma[*,‡]	
Drug intoxication[‡]	
METABOLIC	
Hypoglycemia[†]	
Medium-chain acyl-coenzyme A dehydrogenase deficiency[‡]	
Carnitine deficiency[*,‡]	
Urea cycle defect[‡]	
RESPIRATORY	
Laryngospasm	
Accidental suffocation[†]	
Hemosiderosis/pulmonary hemorrhage syndrome	
CARDIOVASCULAR	
Cardiac arrhythmia	
GASTROINTESTINAL	
Gastroesophageal reflux[*,‡]	
Midgut volvulus/shock[*]	

*Obvious or suspected at autopsy.
†Relatively common.
‡Diagnostic test required.

bedding should be avoided, and parents who share beds with their infants should be counseled on the risks. Decreasing maternal cigarette smoking, both during and after pregnancy, is recommended.

Apnea

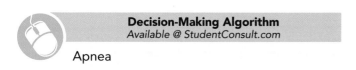

Decision-Making Algorithm
Available @ StudentConsult.com

Apnea

Etiology

Apnea is defined as the cessation of airflow due to either lack of respiratory effort (**central apnea**) or upper airway obstruction (**obstructive apnea**). Central apnea lasting less than 10 seconds is common in healthy infants and can be present in normal children during sleep, especially after a sigh breath. Central pauses lasting longer than 15 to 20 seconds are considered abnormal. Central apnea is more common in infants, and obstructive apnea, especially during sleep, is more common in older children.

Premature infants can have **apnea of prematurity**, which consists of recurrent apneic episodes that are often of central origin, though they can be mixed central/obstructive. Apnea of prematurity should resolve by 44 weeks postconceptional age. Older infants and children with apnea warrant thorough investigation (Table 134-2).

Central apnea outside of infancy is a rare occurrence and may be primary or secondary. Secondary causes of central hypoventilation, which are more common, include medications impairing central respiratory drive (narcotics), increased intracranial pressure, CNS tumors, myelomeningocele and/or Arnold-Chiari malformation, and mitochondrial/metabolic disorders. Genetic syndromes associated with abnormal central respiratory control and developmental delays include Rett, Joubert, and Prader-Willi syndromes and tuberous sclerosis.

Congenital central hypoventilation syndrome (**CCHS**) is a rare genetic disorder in which there is profound loss of respiratory control during sleep leading to central apnea, hypercarbia, and hypoxemia. Most patients with CCHS have a defect in the *PHOX2B* gene, which is necessary for autonomic nervous

system development. Most infants with CCHS have respiratory difficulties within the first several weeks of life, although it can also present later in childhood. CCHS is associated with an increased risk of Hirschsprung disease and neural crest tumors (neuroblastoma).

Obstructive sleep apnea syndrome (OSA), which affects 2% to 3% of young children with peak prevalence at 2 to 8 years, is caused by complete or partial upper airway obstruction during sleep. It presents as episodes of respiratory pauses, gasping, and restless sleep that can result in hypoxia and hypercarbia. Children may have difficulty awakening in the morning, daytime somnolence, behavioral changes, poor school performance, and poor somatic growth as a result of poor sleep quality. Nighttime hypoxia or hypercarbia can lead to morning headaches and, in severe cases, to pulmonary hypertension and cor pulmonale. Adenotonsillar hypertrophy is the most common cause of OSA in young children, but other risk factors for OSA include obesity, craniofacial malformations (Pierre Robin sequence, trisomy 21), glossoptosis, and neuromuscular diseases. Not all children who snore have OSA, and not all children who have OSA snore. Many young children with OSA do not have the classic findings of daytime somnolence and gasping respirations; restless sleep, behavioral problems, and inattention/hyperactivity are much more common. Thus, when the diagnosis is in question, it should be confirmed with a polysomnogram.

Polysomnogram (PSG) is the only definitive test for evaluation of obstructive and central sleep apnea. It involves continuous recording of EEG and electro-oculogram for sleep staging, oronasal airflow and pressure, audible snore, chest and abdominal wall excursion, leg and chin electromyogram, electrocardiogram, pulse oximetry, and capnography. The measured score from a PSG is the **apnea-hypopnea index** (AHI) or number of times in an hour of sleep that the child has cessation or reduction of airflow of a significant magnitude to negatively affect ventilation or sleep stage. An AHI less than 1 is the generally accepted norm for pediatric patients, although the decision to treat often hinges on the severity of daytime impairment. Measured AHI is typically worse in rapid eye movement (REM) sleep and when the child is supine, so an ideal study captures all sleep stages and positions.

Treatment of OSA starts with determining whether the child will benefit from an adenoidectomy, with or without a tonsillectomy. If surgical intervention is not indicated or fails

Table 134-2	Categories of Apnea			
DISEASE	**EXAMPLE(S)**	**MECHANISM**	**SIGNS**	**TREATMENT**
Apnea of prematurity	Premature (<36 wk)	Central control, upper airway obstruction	Apnea, bradycardia	Caffeine, HFNC, CPAP, intubation
Central apnea/ hypoventilation	CCHS, Arnold-Chiari malformation	Abnormal central control	Apnea	Mechanical ventilation
Obstructive sleep apnea	Obesity, adenotonsillar hypertrophy, Pierre Robin sequence, Down syndrome, cerebral palsy	Airway obstruction due to excess tissue, loss of pharyngeal tone or crowded anatomy	Snoring, restless sleep, enuresis, poor school performance, behavior problems, mouth breathing	Adenotonsillectomy, CPAP or BiPAP, uvuloveloplasty, tracheostomy
Breath-holding spells	<3 yr old who turns blue after crying, may have syncope	Prolonged expiratory apnea; reflex anoxic seizures	Cyanosis, syncope, brief tonic-clonic movements after cyanosis	Reassurance; condition is self-limiting. Must exclude seizure disorder

BiPAP, Bi-level positive airway pressure; *CCHS,* congenital central hypoventilation syndrome; *CPAP,* continuous positive airway pressure; *HFNC,* high flow nasal cannula.

to alleviate the problem, then the use of continuous positive airway pressure (**CPAP**) or bi-level positive airway pressure (**BiPAP**) via nasal interfaces can be used to distend the upper airway during sleep. This requires a tight-fitting nasal mask, which may not be well tolerated in young children. Supplemental oxygen can blunt hypoxemia in milder cases of OSA but does not alter obstruction and sleep fragmentation. In extreme cases, especially those associated with craniofacial abnormalities or hypotonia, tracheostomy may be indicated.

Chapter 135

UPPER AIRWAY OBSTRUCTION

ETIOLOGY

Upper airway obstruction (UAO), which is defined as blockage of any part of the airway located above the thoracic inlet, ranges from nasal obstruction due to the common cold to life-threatening obstruction of the larynx or upper trachea (subglottic space). In children, nasal obstruction is usually more of a nuisance than a danger because the mouth can serve as an airway, but it may be a serious problem for neonates, who breathe predominantly through their noses. The differential diagnosis of airway obstruction varies with patient age and can also be subdivided into **supraglottic**, **glottic**, and **subglottic** causes (Tables 135-1, 135-2, and 135-3).

CLINICAL MANIFESTATIONS

Decision-Making Algorithms
Available @ StudentConsult.com

Hoarseness
Stridor

UAO is more pronounced during inspiration because the negative pressure generated collapses the upper airway, increasing resistance to airflow and leading to inspiratory noise. The respiratory noise most commonly associated with UAO is **stridor**, a harsh sound caused by the vibration of the airway structures. Stridor often decreases during sleep, because of lower inspiratory flow rates, and increases during feeding, excitement, and agitation, because of higher flow rates. Occasionally stridor may also be present on exhalation. **Laryngomalacia** (floppy larynx) is the most common cause of inspiratory stridor in infants and may be aggravated by swallowing problems and gastroesophageal reflux. Hoarseness suggests **vocal cord** involvement. Children with UAO may have increased inspiratory work of breathing manifested by **suprasternal retractions**.

Table 135-1	Age-Related Differential Diagnosis of Upper Airway Obstruction

NEWBORN

Choanal atresia
Micrognathia (Pierre Robin syndrome, Treacher Collins syndrome, DiGeorge syndrome)
Macroglossia (Beckwith-Wiedemann syndrome, hypothyroidism, Pompe disease, trisomy 21, hemangioma)
Pharyngeal collapse
Laryngeal web, cleft, atresia
Vocal cord paralysis/paresis (weak cry; unilateral or bilateral, with or without increased intracranial pressure from Arnold-Chiari malformation or other central nervous system pathology)
Congenital subglottic stenosis
Nasal encephalocele

INFANCY

Laryngomalacia (most common non-infectious etiology)
Viral croup (most common infectious etiology)
Subglottic stenosis (congenital or acquired, e.g., after intubation)
Laryngeal web or cyst
Laryngeal papillomatosis
Vascular rings/slings
Airway hemangioma
Rhinitis

TODDLERS

Viral croup (most common etiology in children 6 mo to 4 yr of age)
Spasmodic/recurrent croup
Bacterial tracheitis (toxic, high fever)
Foreign body (airway or esophageal)
Laryngeal papillomatosis
Retropharyngeal abscess
Hypertrophied tonsils and adenoids

OLDER CHILDREN

Epiglottitis (infection, uncommon)
Inhalation injury (burns, toxic gas, hydrocarbons)
Foreign bodies
Angioedema (familial history, cutaneous angioedema)
Anaphylaxis (allergic history, wheezing, hypotension)
Trauma (tracheal or laryngeal fracture)
Peritonsillar abscess (adolescents)
Mononucleosis
Ludwig angina

DIAGNOSTIC STUDIES

Although **radiographic evaluation** of a child with stridor may not be helpful, lateral views of the neck and nasopharynx may provide information about adenoidal hypertrophy and airway swelling. On anteroposterior (AP) views of the neck taken with the head in extension, the subglottic space should be symmetrical and the lateral walls of the airway should fall away steeply. Asymmetry suggests subglottic stenosis or a mass lesion, whereas tapering suggests subglottic edema. However, these findings may be subtle. Computed tomography (CT) scans of the upper airway can help delineate the site of the obstruction but may require sedation in younger children. Flexible nasopharyngoscopy/laryngoscopy, which can be done without sedation, is extremely useful in assessing airway patency, the presence of adenoid tissue, vocal cord and other airway lesions, and laryngomalacia. Bronchoscopy can be useful in assessing the subglottic space and intrathoracic large airways, but this procedure requires sedation.

| Table 135-2 | Differential Diagnosis of Acute Upper Airway Obstruction |

CLINICAL/ HISTORICAL FEATURE	LARYNGOTRACHEOBRONCHITIS (CROUP)	LARYNGITIS	SPASMODIC CROUP	EPIGLOTTITIS	MEMBRANOUS CROUP (BACTERIAL TRACHEITIS)
Age	6 mo–3 yr	5 yr–teens	3 mo–3 yr	2–6 yr	Any age (3–10 yr)
Location Etiologic agent(s)	Subglottic Parainfluenza virus, influenza virus, RSV; rarely *Mycoplasma*, measles, adenovirus	Subglottic As per croup	Subglottic Noninfectious *Haemophilus influenzae* type b inflammation	Supraglottic Respiratory virus	Trachea with secondary bacterial infection (*Staphylococcus aureus, Moraxella catarrhalis*)
Prodrome/onset	Fever, URI	URI, sore throat at night	Sudden onset, short prodrome, prior episodes	Rapid onset High fever	High fever with rapid deterioration
Stridor	Yes	None	Yes	Rarely	Yes
Retractions	Yes	None	Yes	Yes	Yes
Voice	Hoarse	Hoarse	Hoarse	Muffled	Normal or hoarse
Body positioning	Normal	Normal	Normal	Tripod sitting; leaning forward	Normal
Appearance	Normal to anxious	Normal	Anxious	Agitated; toxic	Anxious; toxic
Swallowing	Normal	Normal	Normal	Drooling	Normal
Barking cough	Yes	Rare	Yes	No	Sometimes
Toxicity	Rare	No	No	Severe	Severe
Fever	Body temperature usually <38.5°C	Body temperature usually <38.5°C	None	Body temperature usually >39°C	Body temperature usually >39°C
Radiographic appearance	Subglottic narrowing; steeple sign	Normal	Subglottic narrowing of the epiglottis	Thumb sign of thickened epiglottis	Ragged irregular tracheal border; steeple sign
WBC count	Normal	Normal	Normal	Leukocytosis with elevated band count	Leukocytosis with elevated % bands
Therapy	Racemic epinephrine aerosol, systemic steroids, aerosolized steroids, cold mist	None	Same as for viral croup	Endotracheal intubation; antibiotics	Antibiotics; intubation if needed
Prevention	None	None	None	*H. influenzae* type b conjugated vaccine	None

CLINICAL/ HISTORICAL FEATURE	RETROPHARYNGEAL ABSCESS	FOREIGN BODY	ANGIOEDEMA	PERITONSILLAR ABSCESS	LARYNGEAL PAPILLOMATOSIS
Age	<6 yr	6 mo–5 yr	All ages	>10 yr	3 mo–3 yr
Location	Posterior pharynx	Supra- or subglottic, variable	Variable	Oropharynx	Larynx, vocal cords, trachea
Etiology	*Staphylococcus aureus Streptococcus pyogenes* respiratory anerobes	Small objects, vegetables, toys, coins	C1-esterase deficiency; anaphylaxis	Group A streptococci anaerobes	HPV
Prodrome/onset	Insidious or sudden	Sudden	Sudden	Biphasic with sudden worsening	Chronic
Stridor	None	Yes	Yes	No	Possible
Retractions	Yes	Yes—variable	Yes	No	No
Voice	Muffled	Complete obstruction—aphonic	Hoarse, may be normal	*Hot potato*, muffled	Hoarse
Body positioning	Arching of neck or normal	Normal	Normal; may have facial edema, anxiety	Normal	Normal

Continued

Table 135-2	Differential Diagnosis of Acute Upper Airway Obstruction—cont'd					
CLINICAL/ HISTORICAL FEATURE	**RETROPHARYNGEAL ABSCESS**	**FOREIGN BODY**	**ANGIOEDEMA**	**PERITONSILLAR ABSCESS**	**LARYNGEAL PAPILLOMATOSIS**
Appearance	Drooling	Variable, usually normal	Normal	Drooling, trismus	Normal
Cough	None	Variable; brassy if tracheal	Possible	None	Variable
Toxicity	Moderate to severe	None, but dyspneic	None, unless anaphylactic shock or severe anoxia is present	Dyspnea	None
Fever	Body temperature usually >38.5°C	None	None	Body temperature usually >38.5°C	None
Radiographic appearance	Thickened retropharyngeal space	Radiopaque object may be seen	Same as for viral croup	None needed	May be normal
WBC count	Leukocytosis with increased band count	Normal	Normal	Leukocytosis with increased % bands	Normal
Therapy	Antibiotics; surgical drainage of abscess	Endoscopic removal	Anaphylaxis: epinephrine, IV fluids, steroids; C1-esterase deficiency: danazol, C1-esterase infusion	Antibiotics; aspiration	Laser therapy, repeated excision, interferon
Prevention	None	Avoid small objects; supervision	Avoid allergens; FFP for congenital angioedema	Treat group A streptococcal infections promptly	Treat maternal genitourinary lesions; possible cesarean section?

Modified from Arnold JE: Airway obstruction in children. In Kliegman RM, Nieder ML, Super DM, editors: Practical Strategies in Pediatric Diagnosis and Therapy, Philadelphia, 1996, WB Saunders, p 126.
FFP, Fresh frozen plasma; HPV, human papillomavirus; RSV, respiratory syncytial virus; URI, upper respiratory tract infection (with coryza, sneezing); WBC, white blood cell.

Table 135-3	Differentiating Supraglottic from Subglottic Causes of Airway Obstruction	
FEATURE	**SUPRAGLOTTIC OBSTRUCTION**	**SUBGLOTTIC OBSTRUCTION**
Common clinical syndromes	Epiglottitis, peritonsillar and retropharyngeal abscess	Croup, angioedema, foreign body, tracheitis
Stridor	Quiet	Loud
Voice	Muffled	Hoarse
Dysphagia	Yes	No
Sitting-up or arching posture	Yes	No
Barking cough	No	Yes
Fever	High (temperature >39°C)	Low grade (temperature 38°–39°C)
Toxic	Yes	No, unless tracheitis is present
Trismus	Yes	No
Drooling	Yes	No
Facial edema	No	No, unless angioedema is present

Adapted from Davis H, Gartner JC, Galvis AG, et al: Acute upper airway obstruction: croup and epiglottitis, Pediatr Clin North Am 28:859–880, 1981.

DIFFERENTIAL DIAGNOSIS
Adenoidal and Tonsillar Hypertrophy
Etiology
The most common cause of chronic UAO in children is hypertrophy of the adenoids and tonsils. Adenoidal and tonsillar hyperplasia may be aggravated by recurrent infection, allergy, and inhaled irritants.

Clinical Manifestations
The signs of adenoidal and tonsillar hypertrophy are mouth breathing, snoring, and, in some patients, obstructive sleep apnea (see Chapter 134). The eustachian tubes enter the nasopharynx at the choanae and can be obstructed by enlarged adenoids, predisposing to recurrent or persistent otitis media.

Diagnostic Studies
Adenoidal hypertrophy is assessed by a lateral radiograph of the nasopharynx or by flexible nasopharyngoscopy.

Treatment
If the adenoids or tonsils are large and thought to be significantly contributing to UAO, then the most effective treatment is removal. Because the adenoids are not a discrete organ but rather consist of lymphoid tissue, regrowth is possible, especially in preschool children. If the tonsils are large and the obstruction is severe, then removing the tonsils in addition to the adenoids may be necessary.

Choanal Stenosis (Atresia)
Choanal stenosis/atresia is a congenital problem presenting in the neonatal period. It may be bilateral or unilateral and is relatively rare. Neonates are generally obligate nose breathers, so obstruction of nasal passages can cause significant respiratory distress, especially when feeding. Crying bypasses the obstruction because crying infants breathe though their mouths. Inability to easily pass a small catheter through the nostrils should raise the suspicion of choanal atresia. The diagnosis is confirmed by CT scan and by inspecting the area directly with a flexible nasopharyngoscope. An oral airway may be useful in the short term, but the definitive treatment is surgery.

Croup (Laryngotracheobronchitis)

Decision-Making Algorithm
Available @ StudentConsult.com
Stridor

SEE CHAPTER 107.

Epiglottitis

Decision-Making Algorithm
Available @ StudentConsult.com
Stridor

SEE CHAPTER 107.

Bacterial Tracheitis
SEE CHAPTER 107.

Laryngomalacia (Floppy Larynx)

Decision-Making Algorithm
Available @ StudentConsult.com
Stridor

Etiology
Laryngomalacia is due to exaggerated collapse of the glottic structures, especially the epiglottis and arytenoid cartilages, during inspiration. It may be due to decreased muscular tone of the larynx and surrounding structures or to immature cartilaginous structures. Inspiratory stridor beginning at or shortly after birth should raise the suspicion of laryngomalacia (see Table 135-1). This is the most common cause of stridor in infants. It usually does not result in significant respiratory distress, but occasionally it is severe enough to cause hypoventilation, with hypercarbia, hypoxemia, and difficulty with feeding.

Clinical Manifestations
The primary sign of laryngomalacia is **inspiratory stridor** with little or no expiratory component. The stridor is typically loudest when the infant is feeding or active and decreases when the infant is relaxed or placed prone, or when the neck is flexed. Any condition that increases upper airway inflammation will exacerbate laryngomalacia, including viral respiratory infections, dysphagia (swallowing dysfunction), and gastroesophageal reflux. Laryngomalacia normally peaks by 3 to 5 months of age and resolves between 6 and 12 months of age. However, occasionally it can persist in otherwise normal children up until 24 months of age and even longer in children with underlying conditions, especially those with neurologic diseases affecting control of upper airway muscles (such as cerebral palsy).

Diagnostic Studies
In many infants with presumed laryngomalacia, the diagnosis can be tentatively established by history and physical examination. If the patient follows the typical course for laryngomalacia, then no further workup is necessary. However, to firmly establish the diagnosis, which is important in more severe or atypical cases, the patient should undergo flexible nasopharyngoscopy to assess the patency and dynamic movement (collapse) of the larynx and surrounding structures. This procedure can also identify vocal cord abnormalities and airway lesions above the vocal cords.

Treatment
In most cases, no therapy is required for laryngomalacia. The infant should be observed closely during times of respiratory infection for evidence of respiratory compromise. Infants with severe laryngomalacia resulting in hypoventilation, hypoxia, or growth failure may benefit from a surgical procedure (aryepiglottoplasty) or, in extreme cases, a tracheostomy to bypass the upper airway.

Subglottic Stenosis

Decision-Making Algorithm
Available @ StudentConsult.com

Stridor

Etiology
Subglottic stenosis is the narrowing of the portion of the trachea immediately below the vocal cords. It may be congenital but more often is acquired. Endotracheal intubation, especially prolonged or repeated intubation required in some premature infants, can lead to inflammation and scarring of the subglottic space.

Clinical Manifestations
Subglottic stenosis can present as stridor that is frequently **biphasic** (on both inspiration and expiration). However, the stridor is usually more prominent on inspiration. With increasing respiratory effort, the stridor becomes louder. Very small infants may not be able to breathe with enough force to generate a sound. Subglottic stenosis may also be associated with a barky cough similar to that noted with croup. Respiratory infections can cause subglottic edema, exacerbating the clinical manifestations of subglottic stenosis.

Diagnostic Studies
Definitive diagnosis requires endoscopic evaluation, either by flexible or rigid bronchoscopy.

Treatment
Mild subglottic stenosis can be managed conservatively and may improve sufficiently with airway growth alone. More severe cases require surgical intervention. Depending on the nature of the lesion, endoscopic laser treatment may be effective. Other surgical options include tracheoplasty and cricoid split procedures. A tracheostomy tube may be required to bypass the subglottic space until the airway is patent enough to allow adequate airflow.

Mass Lesions
Upper airway mass lesions are relatively uncommon. The most common laryngeal tumor in childhood is the **hemangioma**, which usually presents before 6 months of age. (See Chapter 194.) Subglottic lesions produce asymmetrical narrowing of the subglottic space on AP radiographs of the larynx, but definitive diagnosis requires endoscopy. If the obstruction is severe, then a tracheostomy tube may be needed until the lesion spontaneously involutes or improves with therapy.

Laryngeal webs are the result of failed recanalization of the glottic airway in utero, whereas **laryngeal cysts** typically occur as a consequence of airway trauma (intubation). Both can produce biphasic stridor and are best identified by bronchoscopy. **Foreign body** should be considered in any infant or child capable of ingesting small objects who develops acute onset of stridor.

Juvenile laryngeal papillomatosis is a rare condition of benign tumors caused by human papillomavirus (HPV-6 and HPV-11) acquired at birth from maternal genital warts. Clinical manifestations usually start in infancy and include biphasic stridor and hoarse voice/cry. The lesions are most commonly located in the larynx, but they can spread distally into the trachea, large bronchi, and even to the lung parenchyma. Treatment options, which are limited and rarely curative, include laser therapy and interferon. Tracheostomy may be required to ensure an adequate airway, but should be avoided if possible as reports suggest a related seeding of the distal airways with tumor.

Vocal Cord Paralysis

Decision-Making Algorithm
Available @ StudentConsult.com

Stridor

Etiology
Vocal cord paralysis is an important cause of laryngeal dysfunction. Paralysis may be unilateral or bilateral and is more often caused by damage to the recurrent laryngeal nerve than by a central lesion. The left recurrent laryngeal nerve passes around the aortic arch and is more susceptible to damage than the right laryngeal nerve. Peripheral nerve injury may be caused by trauma (neck traction during delivery of infants or thoracic surgical procedures) and mediastinal lesions. Central causes include Arnold-Chiari malformation (meningomyelocele), hydrocephalus, and intracranial hemorrhage.

Clinical Manifestations
Vocal cord paralysis presents as biphasic stridor and alterations in voice and cry, including a weak cry (in infants), hoarseness, and aphonia. Children with vocal cord paralysis are at risk for aspiration, often manifested as coughing/choking with drinking and coarse airway sounds audibly and by auscultation.

Treatment and Prognosis
Patients with traumatic injury to the recurrent laryngeal nerve often have spontaneous improvement over time, usually within 3 to 6 months. If the paralyzed vocal cord has not recovered within 1 year of the injury, then it is likely to be permanently damaged. In some cases, Gelfoam injection of a paralyzed vocal cord can reposition the cord to improve phonation and airway protection. Patients with vocal cord paralysis resulting in severe airway obstruction and aspiration may require tracheostomy tube placement.

Chapter 136

LOWER AIRWAY, PARENCHYMAL, AND PULMONARY VASCULAR DISEASES

ETIOLOGY

There are many causes of lower airway diseases (Table 136-1). Lower airway diseases often result in airway obstruction. The most common lower airway disease in children is asthma, which results in diffuse bronchial obstruction from airway inflammation, constriction of bronchial smooth muscle, and excessive secretions. Virus-induced wheezing episodes are common, especially in children under 3 years of age. Wheezing that begins in the first weeks or months of life or that persists despite aggressive asthma therapy is likely not due to asthma, and further diagnostic evaluation may be warranted. Wheezing that is localized to one area of the chest suggests focal airway narrowing (foreign body aspiration or extrinsic compression by masses or lymph nodes).

CLINICAL MANIFESTATIONS

Decision-Making Algorithm
Available @ StudentConsult.com

Wheezing

In contrast to upper airway obstruction, obstruction below the thoracic inlet causes more wheezing on expiration than on inspiration. A wheeze is a continuous sound that is produced by vibration of airway walls and generally has a more musical quality than does stridor. Intrathoracic pressure is increased relative to atmospheric pressure during exhalation, which tends to collapse the intrathoracic airways and accentuates airway narrowing on expiration. This manifests as expiratory wheeze, prolonged expiratory phase, and increased expiratory work of breathing. In patients with chronic airway infection (e.g., cystic fibrosis), the bronchi become permanently damaged and dilated (bronchiectasis). Patients with bronchiectasis have episodes of cough, often productive of purulent sputum, and may have inspiratory crackles.

DIAGNOSTIC STUDIES

When asthma is suspected, empiric trials of therapy (bronchodilators, short courses of oral corticosteroids, long-term use of inhaled corticosteroids) are useful in arriving at a diagnosis. In children older than 6 years, pulmonary function tests (spirometry) can assess airflow obstruction and response to bronchodilators. **Radiographic evaluation** is not needed with each episode of wheezing, but those with significant respiratory distress, fever, history consistent with foreign body

Table 136-1	Causes of Wheezing in Childhood

ACUTE

Reactive airway disease
  Asthma
  Exercise-induced asthma
  Hypersensitivity reactions
Bronchial edema
  Infection (e.g., bronchiolitis)
  Inhalation of irritant gases or particulates
  Increased pulmonary venous pressure
Bronchial hypersecretion
  Infection
  Inhalation of irritant gases or particulates
  Cholinergic drugs
Aspiration
  Foreign body
  Aspiration of gastric contents

CHRONIC OR RECURRENT

Reactive airway disease (see under Acute)

Hypersensitivity reactions, allergic bronchopulmonary aspergillosis (seen only in children with either asthma or cystic fibrosis)

Dynamic airway collapse
  Bronchomalacia/tracheomalacia
  Vocal cord adduction (paradoxical vocal cord motion)
Airway compression by mass or blood vessel
  Vascular ring/sling
  Anomalous innominate artery
  Pulmonary artery dilatation (absent pulmonary valve)
  Bronchial or pulmonary cysts
  Lymph nodes (tuberculosis, lymphoma)
Aspiration
  Foreign body
  Gastroesophageal reflux
  Swallowing dysfunction (dysphagia)
  Tracheoesophageal fistula
Bronchial hypersecretion or failure to clear secretions
  Bronchitis, bronchiectasis
  Cystic fibrosis
  Primary ciliary dyskinesia
Intrinsic airway lesions
  Endobronchial tumors (carcinoid)
  Endobronchial granulation tissue
Endobronchial tuberculosis
  Bronchial or tracheal stenosis
  Bronchiolitis obliterans
Congestive heart failure

aspiration, or focal auscultatory findings should have postero-anterior (PA) and lateral chest radiographs obtained. Generalized **hyperinflation**, indicated by flattening of the diaphragms and an increased anteroposterior (AP) chest diameter, suggests diffuse obstruction of the small airways. Hyperinflation in association with patchy densities due to atelectasis is often seen in asthma and mistaken for pneumonia. Localized hyperinflation, especially on expiratory views, suggests localized bronchial obstruction (foreign body or an anatomic anomaly). Dysphagia leading to aspiration and airway inflammation can present with persistent wheezing. This is best assessed with a **videofluoroscopic swallowing study**. Gastroesophageal reflux may aggravate asthma and may lead to wheezing in very young children, especially if it is associated with aspiration.

DIFFERENTIAL DIAGNOSIS
Asthma

Decision-Making Algorithm
Available @ StudentConsult.com

Wheezing

SEE CHAPTER 78.

Tracheomalacia
Etiology
Tracheomalacia is a floppy trachea due to lack of structural integrity of the tracheal wall. The tracheal cartilaginous rings normally extend through an arc of approximately 320°, maintaining rigidity of the trachea during changes in intrathoracic pressure. With tracheomalacia, the cartilaginous rings may not extend as far around the circumference (leaving the membranous posterior trachea wider than usual), may be completely absent, or may be present but damaged. These abnormalities can result in excessive collapse of the trachea, most pronounced during expiration. Tracheomalacia may be congenital (tracheoesophageal fistula or bony dysplasia syndromes) or acquired (long-term mechanical ventilation). Tracheomalacia must be differentiated from extrinsic tracheal compression by masses or vascular structures. Localized tracheomalacia may persist after the trachea has been relieved of extrinsic compression. Viral infections may exacerbate tracheomalacia, leading to coarse expiratory wheezing and barky cough. The expiratory noises of tracheomalacia are often mistakenly ascribed to asthma or bronchiolitis, and the barky cough is often misdiagnosed as croup.

Clinical Manifestations
With tracheomalacia, the tracheal collapse may only be apparent during forced exhalation or with cough. It is commonly aggravated by respiratory infections. The airway collapse may cause recurrent coarse expiratory wheeze and a prolonged expiratory phase. Secretions may be retained behind the segment of malacia, predisposing to infection. Infants with severe tracheomalacia may completely collapse their tracheas during agitation, resulting in cyanotic episodes that resemble breath-holding spells. The voice is normal, as is inspiratory effort. In older children, the hallmark sign is a brassy, barky cough due to the vibration of the tracheal walls. This cough can be loud and persistent and is often misdiagnosed as croup.

Treatment
Infants with mild to moderate tracheomalacia usually require no intervention. Tracheomalacia improves with airway growth as the lumen increases in diameter and the tracheal wall becomes more firm. The treatment of older symptomatic children is geared toward treating any precipitating cause for cough and providing supportive care. Antibiotics may be necessary to treat concurrent infection. Children, especially infants, with severe tracheomalacia may require tracheostomy tubes to administer continuous positive airway pressure (CPAP), which serves to stent open the airway. Custom-length tracheostomy tubes have been used to stent open the airway when CPAP fails. Surgically placed airway stents are problematic in children because the stents cannot grow and thus serve as a source of fixed stenosis and obstruction.

Tracheoesophageal Fistula
SEE CHAPTER 128.

Extrinsic Tracheal Compression
Compression of the trachea by vascular structures or masses can cause significant respiratory compromise. Tracheal compression by aberrant great vessels (aorta, innominate artery) may cause wheezing, stridor, cough, and dyspnea. The most common cause of tracheal compression is anterior compression from an **anomalous innominate artery** that arises more distally than normal from the aortic arch. This usually results in mild respiratory symptoms, and surgical correction is rarely necessary. Complete vascular rings, which compress the esophagus posteriorly and the trachea anteriorly, include the double aortic arch and a right aortic arch with a persistent ligamentum arteriosum (most common). Both lesions have right-sided aortic arches, which may be visible on chest radiograph. In addition to respiratory symptoms, complete vascular rings may cause dysphagia as a result of esophageal compression. The diagnosis of vascular anomalies can often be made by a barium swallow, which identifies the esophageal compression. Bronchoscopy will identify a pulsatile compression of the airway, but the diagnostic procedure of choice is a computed tomography (CT) angiogram of the chest and great vessels. Complete vascular rings almost always require surgical repair. Other causes of extrinsic tracheal compression include enlarged mediastinal lymph nodes (tuberculosis), mediastinal masses (teratoma, lymphoma, thymoma, germ cell tumors), and, rarely, cystic hygromas.

Foreign Body Aspiration
Epidemiology
Aspiration of foreign bodies into the trachea and bronchi is relatively common. The majority of children who aspirate foreign bodies are under 4 years of age. Most deaths secondary to foreign body aspiration occur in this age group. Because the right mainstem bronchus takes off at a less acute angle than the left mainstem bronchus, foreign bodies tend to lodge in right-sided airways. Some foreign bodies, especially nuts, can

also lodge more proximally in the larynx or subglottic space, totally occluding the airway. Many foreign bodies are not radiopaque, which makes them difficult to detect radiographically. The most common foreign bodies aspirated by young children are food (especially nuts) and small toys. Coins more often lodge in the esophagus than in the airways. Older children have been known to aspirate rubber balloons, which can be life-threatening.

Clinical Manifestations

Decision-Making Algorithms
Available @ StudentConsult.com

Cough
Stridor
Hemoptysis

Many children who aspirate foreign bodies have clear histories of choking, witnessed aspiration, or physical or radiographic evidence of foreign body aspiration. However, a small percentage of patients have a negative history because the aspiration went unrecognized. Physical findings observed with acute foreign body aspiration may include cough, localized wheezing, unilateral absence of breath sounds, stridor, and, rarely, bloody sputum.

Most foreign bodies are small and quickly expelled, but some may remain in the lung for long periods of time and may come to medical attention because of persistent cough, sputum production, or recurrent unilateral pneumonia. Foreign body aspiration should be in the differential diagnosis of patients with persistent wheezing unresponsive to bronchodilator therapy, persistent atelectasis, recurrent or persistent pneumonia, or chronic cough without another explanation. Foreign bodies may also lodge in the esophagus and compress the trachea, thus producing respiratory symptoms. Therefore, esophageal foreign bodies should be included in the differential diagnosis of infants or young children with persistent stridor or wheezing, particularly if dysphagia is present.

Diagnostic Studies

Radiographic studies will reveal the presence of radiopaque objects and can also identify focal air trapping, especially on expiratory views. Thus, when foreign body aspiration is suspected, expiratory or lateral decubitus chest radiographs should be ordered. In addition, fluoroscopy may be helpful, especially in children who cannot perform expiratory views. If there is strong evidence (or history) of foreign body aspiration, the patient should undergo rigid bronchoscopy. Flexible bronchoscopy can be used to locate an aspirated foreign body and may be useful when the presentation is not straightforward, but foreign body removal is best performed via rigid bronchoscopy.

Prevention

The best approach to preventing foreign body aspiration is to educate parents and caregivers. Before molar teeth have erupted, infants and children should not be given nuts, uncooked carrots, or other foods that may be easily broken into small pieces and aspirated. Sound parental judgment is required to determine at what age and stage of development small objects should be accessible to children.

Bronchiolitis

Decision-Making Algorithm
Available @ StudentConsult.com

Wheezing

SEE CHAPTER 109.

Bronchopulmonary Dysplasia
SEE CHAPTER 61.

Endobronchial Mass Lesions
Endobronchial mass lesions are relatively uncommon in children. The most common lesion is **granulation tissue**, which usually results from local inflammation. Tuberculosis can cause endobronchial granulomas. Primary tumors of the lung are extremely rare in children. The most common airway malignancy is the nonsecreting carcinoid tumor. Endobronchial lesions that partially obstruct an airway present with wheezing or obstructive emphysema and occasionally with hemoptysis. If the lesion completely occludes the airway, then atelectasis may result. Radiographs and CT scans of the chest aid in making the diagnosis. Bronchoscopy is often used to confirm the diagnosis.

Congenital Lung Anomalies
Congenital lobar overdistention (formerly referred to as congenital lobar emphysema) consists of overinflation of one lobe of a lung. This overdistention may cause severe respiratory distress in the neonatal period due to compression of surrounding normal lung tissue, but it can also be asymptomatic and remain undiagnosed for years. Radiographically, it may be mistaken for a pneumothorax. Lobectomy may be required if respiratory distress is severe or progressive, but if the patient is asymptomatic, then surgical resection may not be indicated.

Pulmonary hypoplasia, or a relative decrease in amount of alveoli, may be the result of a number of congenital insults, such as **congenital diaphragmatic hernia** (see Chapter 61) or unilateral congenital absence of a pulmonary artery. Alveolar growth occurs after birth predominantly up to 3 years, but has been documented up to 8 years.

Emphysema
Emphysema is a condition due to disruption or destruction of alveolar septa. In pediatrics, the term *emphysema* often refers to hyperinflation or to leakage of air into the pulmonary interstitial spaces (interstitial emphysema, which may be seen in mechanically ventilated premature infants) or the subcutaneous tissue (subcutaneous emphysema). Although emphysema is common in adults, it is rare in children. However, generalized or localized **hyperinflation**, which can be

caused by airway obstruction from a variety of causes, is common. Emphysema is commonly observed in the disease **α₁-antitrypsin deficiency**, but it rarely appears before the second decade of life.

Primary Ciliary Dyskinesia
Etiology
Primary ciliary dyskinesia (PCD, immotile cilia syndrome) is an inherited disorder in which ultrastructural abnormalities in the cilia result in absent or disordered movement of the cilia. This disorder affects approximately 1 in 19,000 persons. There are many reported abnormalities in ciliary structure, but the most common are due to defects in the dynein arms, ultrastructural features that provide energy via adenosine triphosphatase (ATPase), which is necessary for ciliary motility.

Clinical Manifestations
The classic presentation is recurrent otitis media, chronic sinusitis, and bronchiectasis. Kartagener syndrome, the triad of **situs inversus**, **pansinusitis**, and **bronchiectasis**, accounts for approximately 50% of cases. Males are infertile as a result of immotile sperm. Because the cilia fail to beat normally, secretions accumulate in the airways, and endobronchial infection results. Chronic infection, if untreated, leads to bronchiectasis by early adulthood. Primary ciliary dyskinesia should be suspected in patients with early-onset chronic bronchitis or bronchiectasis associated with recurrent/persistent sinusitis and/or frequent otitis media.

Diagnostic Studies
PCD is confirmed by electron microscopy of respiratory cilia, obtained from scrapings/biopsy of nasal or airway epithelium. Results may be difficult to interpret as chronic infection and inflammation may lead to ultrastructural abnormalities in nasal cilia. The measurement of nasal nitric oxide has been used as a screening tool for PCD. Low nasal nitric oxide values (<200 parts per billion) are consistent with PCD, whereas values greater than 400 parts per billion make the diagnosis less likely. However, the validity of nasal nitric oxide assays as a diagnostic test for PCD has not been fully substantiated.

Treatment
Treatment is geared toward treating infections and improving clearance of respiratory secretions. High resolution chest CT scans are useful to confirm and monitor bronchiectasis. Surveillance cultures help identify organisms involved and guide antibiotic therapy. Sinus surgical procedures are often done to manage chronic sinusitis, but their benefit is questionable. Most children require placement of pressure equalization (PE) tubes for management of recurrent otitis media. Chest physiotherapy and prompt treatment of bacterial infections are helpful, but the course of the disease tends to be slowly progressive. Preventive antibiotics, such as thrice-weekly macrolides, may reduce the number of exacerbations per year.

Pneumonia

Decision-Making Algorithms
Available @ StudentConsult.com

Cough
Wheezing
Hemoptysis
Abdominal Pain
Acidemia

SEE CHAPTER 110.

Pulmonary Edema
Etiology
Pulmonary edema is the seepage of fluid into the alveolar and interstitial spaces. Capillary hydrostatic forces and interstitial osmotic pressures tend to push fluid into the airspaces, whereas plasma osmotic pressures and tissue mechanical forces tend to move fluid away from the airspaces. Under normal circumstances, the sum of these forces favors absorption, so the alveolar and interstitial spaces remain dry. Fluid entering the alveoli is normally removed by pulmonary lymphatics. Pulmonary edema forms when transcapillary fluid flux exceeds lymphatic drainage. Reduced left ventricular function leads to pulmonary venous hypertension and increased capillary hydrostatic pressure, and fluid moves into the interstitial space and alveoli. Fluid initially enters the interstitial space around the terminal bronchioles, alveoli, and arterioles (**interstitial edema**), causing increased lung stiffness and premature closure of bronchioles on expiration. If the process continues, fluid then enters the alveoli, further reducing compliance and resulting in **intrapulmonary shunting** (alveolar units that are perfused but not ventilated). Decreased ventilation (hypercarbia) is a late finding.

Pulmonary edema is most commonly due to heart failure from left ventricular or biventricular dysfunction. Pulmonary hypertension and associated cor pulmonale (right ventricular dysfunction) do not usually cause pulmonary edema as the increased vascular resistance is proximal to the capillary bed. Increased capillary permeability, seen in disease states such as sepsis and acute respiratory distress syndrome, can lead to pulmonary edema. Pulmonary edema may also occur with excessive swings in intrathoracic pressure, as seen after tracheal foreign body aspiration or severe obstruction from hypertrophied tonsils and adenoids (**postobstructive pulmonary edema**). Pulmonary edema may also be present in conditions with decreased serum oncotic pressure (hypoalbuminemia); after administration of large volumes of intravenous (IV) fluids, especially if there is capillary injury; with ascent to high altitude (**high altitude pulmonary edema**); and after central nervous system injury (**neurogenic pulmonary edema**).

Clinical Manifestations

Decision-Making Algorithm
Available @ StudentConsult.com

Cough

The clinical manifestations of pulmonary edema are **dyspnea**, tachypnea, and cough (often with frothy, pink-tinged sputum). As the edema worsens, there is increased work of breathing and hypoxemia; diffuse inspiratory crackles can be heard on auscultation.

Diagnostic Studies

Chest radiographs may reveal diffuse hazy infiltrates, classically in a perihilar pattern, but these findings may be obscured by underlying lung disease. Interstitial edema (**Kerley B lines**) may be seen, especially at the lung bases.

Treatment and Prognosis

Treatment and prognosis depend on the cause of the pulmonary edema and response to therapy. Patients should be positioned in an upright posture and given supplemental O_2. Diuretic therapy and rapidly acting IV inotropic agents may be helpful in cardiogenic pulmonary edema. Continuous positive airway pressure (CPAP) or intubation with positive pressure ventilation using high positive end-expiratory pressures (PEEP) may be required.

Acute Respiratory Distress Syndrome
SEE CHAPTER 39.

Pulmonary Arterial Hypertension and Cor Pulmonale
Etiology

Pulmonary hypertension (PH) is classified in five groups based on mechanism. Group 1 is pulmonary arterial hypertension (PAH) due to diseases within veins and small pulmonary muscular arteries such as persistent pulmonary hypertension of the newborn, congenital heart disease (including those with excessive pulmonary blood flow due to left-to-right cardiac shunting), exposure to various drugs (e.g., cocaine, amphetamines), and **idiopathic pulmonary arterial hypertension** (previously called primary pulmonary hypertension). Hereditary IPAH is also in this group and has been linked with the bone morphogenetic receptor-2 (BMPR2) gene. Group 2 is caused by dysfunction of the left heart such as valvular disease. Group 3 is secondary to lung disease or chronic hypoxia, including upper airway obstruction resulting in obstructive sleep apnea and hypoxemia. In Group 4, PH is secondary to chronic pulmonary thromboembolism. Group 5 includes PH of unclear but multifactorial diseases, including some autoimmune diseases and metabolic diseases. With prolonged PAH, irreversible changes may occur in the intima and media of the pulmonary arterioles.

Pulmonary arterial hypertension strains the right side of the heart, which leads to hypertrophy and dilation of the right ventricle. This may result in **cor pulmonale**, a condition in which right-sided heart failure leads to hepatic congestion, fluid retention, and tricuspid insufficiency. In severe cor pulmonale, the ventricular septum may be displaced toward the left ventricle, hindering left ventricular function. The most common causes of cor pulmonale in children are chronic lung diseases, especially severe bronchopulmonary dysplasia and scleroderma, and severe untreated obstructive sleep apnea (with chronic hypoxia).

Clinical Manifestations and Diagnostic Studies

Pulmonary arterial hypertension should be suspected whenever there is prolonged hypoxemia or hemodynamically significant left-to-right cardiac shunting. In addition to the other physical findings associated with pulmonary and cardiac diseases, an accentuated pulmonary component of the second heart sound may be heard. Definitive diagnosis is made by cardiac catheterization, but echocardiography may confirm the presence of right ventricular hypertrophy, ventricular dysfunction, interventricular septal flattening, and tricuspid insufficiency, which can be used to estimate the pulmonary artery pressures.

Treatment and Prognosis

For those with pulmonary hypertension in groups 2 through 5, treatment should focus on the underlying condition. In all conditions of PH and PAH, the relief of hypoxemia with supplemental O_2 therapy is essential. Heart failure may require treatment with diuretics and restrictions of salt and fluid intake. Vasodilator therapy (sildenafil) is helpful in some patients, and inhaled nitric oxide can be used short term. Continuous infusions of prostacyclin may be helpful both acutely and chronically and is available in inhaled, subcutaneous, and intravenous forms. Endothelium antagonists may be beneficial. Unfortunately, many patients with the idiopathic form of PAH have progressive courses, and lung or heart-lung transplantation may be the only treatment option.

Pulmonary Hemorrhage
Etiology

Pulmonary hemorrhage is a rare but potentially life-threatening condition in children. It can be due to bleeding from the airways (hemangiomas, bronchial vessel bleeds) or from diffuse capillary bleeding (alveolar hemorrhage). Alveolar hemorrhage is usually due to diffuse capillary disruption/inflammation caused by autoimmune disorders and after bone marrow transplantation. Airway bleeding can be due to airway hemangiomas, pulmonary arteriovenous malformations (as with hereditary hemorrhagic telangiectasia), and bronchial artery collaterals, which develop in some patients with chronic lung infections, especially cystic fibrosis. **Idiopathic pulmonary hemosiderosis** is a rare disorder characterized by recurrent alveolar bleeding, iron deficiency anemia, and hemosiderin-laden macrophages in the lung, which can be identified microscopically with the use of special iron-staining techniques in bronchoalveolar lavage or lung biopsy specimens. Although the term *hemosiderosis* is sometimes used interchangeably with pulmonary hemorrhage, it is a pathologic finding that results from bleeding anywhere in the lung, airway, pharynx, nasopharynx, or mouth leading to hemosiderin accumulation in the lung. **Pulmonary hemorrhage** is a preferable term for bleeding from an intrathoracic source.

Clinical Manifestations

Decision-Making Algorithm
Available @ StudentConsult.com

Hemoptysis

Most children with pulmonary hemorrhage present with **hemoptysis**. It is important to rule out extrapulmonary sources of bleeding, including hematemesis and bleeding from the nasopharynx or mouth, as these are more common than true pulmonary hemorrhage. In addition to hemoptysis, the presenting signs and symptoms of pulmonary hemorrhage include cough, wheeze, shortness of breath, pallor, fatigue, cyanosis, and fever. Episodic pulmonary hemorrhage frequently manifests as recurrent respiratory symptoms associated with pulmonary infiltrates on chest radiographs. Symptomatic **airway hemorrhage** may result in significant hemoptysis with few radiographic changes, whereas **alveolar bleeding** often causes profound respiratory symptoms, hypoxemia, diffuse infiltrates on radiographs, and minimal hemoptysis. Some patients experience a localized bubbling sensation in the chest, which may be helpful in differentiating local from diffuse sources of pulmonary bleeding. Physical examination findings may include locally or diffusely decreased breath sounds, cyanosis, and crackles on auscultation.

The **differential diagnosis** of pulmonary hemorrhage includes alveolar and airway bleeding. The causes of alveolar (capillary) bleeding include: idiopathic pulmonary hemosiderosis; diffuse alveolitis (capillaritis) secondary to autoimmune disease; clotting disorders; venoocclusive disease; diffuse alveolar injury; and cardiac conditions associated with elevated pulmonary venous and capillary pressures (Table 136-2). Rarely, a previously well infant will present with life-threatening acute alveolar hemorrhage. Often no cause is found, and, once the acute episode resolves, the infant returns to normal. Most of these infants never have a second bleeding episode. Hemoptysis can have cardiovascular, pulmonary, or immunologic causes (see Table 136-2).

Diagnostic Studies

It is important to perform a thorough upper airway examination to rule out epistaxis. Sometimes this requires nasopharyngoscopy. If extrapulmonary sources of bleeding have been excluded, then a chest radiograph, CT angiogram of the chest, bronchoscopy, echocardiogram, and evaluation for rheumatologic/autoimmune diseases, especially Goodpasture disease, granulomatosis with polyangiitis, Henoch-Schönlein purpura, and systemic lupus erythematosus, should be considered.

Treatment

The management of acute episodes of pulmonary bleeding includes the administration of supplemental O_2, blood transfusions, and, often with acute alveolar hemorrhages, mechanical ventilation with PEEP to tamponade the bleeding. Attempts should be made to identify the cause of the bleeding. Treatment is directed toward the underlying disorders and providing supportive care. In bronchial arterial bleeding, arteriography with vessel embolization has been shown to be successful.

Pulmonary Embolism
Etiology

Pulmonary embolism is rare in children. When it occurs, it is often associated with indwelling central venous catheters,

Table 136-2	Differential Diagnosis of Hemoptysis-Pulmonary Hemorrhage
CARDIOVASCULAR DISORDERS	
Heart failure	
Eisenmenger syndrome	
Mitral stenosis	
Venoocclusive disease	
Arteriovenous malformation (Osler-Weber-Rendu syndrome)	
Pulmonary embolism	
PULMONARY DISORDERS	
Respiratory distress syndrome	
Bronchogenic cyst	
Sequestration	
Pneumonia (bacterial, mycobacterial, fungal, or parasitic)	
Cystic fibrosis	
Tracheobronchitis	
Bronchiectasis	
Lung abscess	
Tumor (adenoma, carcinoid, hemangioma, metastasis)	
Foreign body retention	
Contusion—trauma	
IMMUNE DISORDERS	
Henoch-Schönlein purpura	
Idiopathic pulmonary hemosiderosis	
Goodpasture syndrome	
Wegener granulomatosis	
Systemic lupus erythematosus	
Polyarteritis nodosa	
OTHER CONDITIONS/FACTORS	
Hyperammonemia	
Kernicterus	
Intracranial hemorrhage (in preterm infant)	
Toxins	
Diffuse alveolar injury (smoke inhalation)	
Post–bone marrow transplantation	

oral contraceptives, or hypercoagulable states. In adolescents, trauma, obesity, abortion, and malignancy may lead to deep vein thromboses (DVTs) and pulmonary embolism.

Clinical Manifestations

Because the pulmonary vascular bed is distensible, small emboli, even if multiple, may be asymptomatic unless they are infected (septic emboli) and cause pulmonary infection. Large emboli may cause acute dyspnea, pleuritic chest pain, cough, and hemoptysis. **Hypoxia** is common, as are nonspecific ST-segment and T-wave changes on the electrocardiogram (ECG). The P_2 heart sound may be increased, and an S_4 sound may be present.

Diagnostic Studies

Although the chest x-ray is usually normal, atelectasis or cardiomegaly may be seen. The measurement of D-dimers can be used as a screening test, but it must be interpreted in light of the probability of a pulmonary embolism. If the D-dimer is normal and the probability for embolism is low, then no further workup may be necessary. However, if the D-dimer is elevated, or if it is normal but the probability of embolism is moderate or high, then the diagnostic test of choice is a **CT angiogram of the chest**. Ventilation-perfusion scans may revealing defects in perfusion without matching ventilation defects, but they are difficult to perform in young children. Doppler or compression ultrasonography can be useful in assessing patients for lower extremity DVTs. For definitive diagnosis of pulmonary embolism, the gold standard is still **pulmonary angiography**, though with the improvement in CT angiography, angiograms are now rarely necessary. Children with pulmonary embolism without an obvious cause should be evaluated for hypercoagulable states, the most common of which is factor V Leiden.

Treatment

Once a pulmonary embolism is suspected, the patient should be anticoagulated, usually with low-molecular-weight heparin. All patients should receive supplemental O_2, and it is important to treat the predisposing factors. Thrombolytic therapy and surgical resection of emboli are rarely indicated. Occasionally an inferior vena caval filter needs to be placed to prevent recurrent emboli.

Chapter 137

CYSTIC FIBROSIS

ETIOLOGY AND EPIDEMIOLOGY

Cystic fibrosis (CF) is an autosomal recessive disorder that is the most common life-limiting genetic disease in whites. In the United States, the incidence of CF is approximately 1 in 3200 whites, 1 in 15,000 African Americans, and 1 in 31,000 persons of Asian heritage. The gene for CF, located on the long arm of chromosome 7, encodes for a polypeptide, the **cystic fibrosis transmembrane regulator (CFTR)**, a chloride channel located on the apical surface of epithelial cells. CFTR is important for the proper movement of salt and water across cell membranes and maintaining the appropriate composition of various secretions, especially in the airways, liver, and pancreas. The most common mutation is a deletion of three base pairs resulting in the absence of phenylalanine at the 508 position (ΔF508). More than 1500 mutations of the *CFTR* gene have been identified.

The secretory and absorptive characteristics of epithelial cells are affected by abnormal CFTR, resulting in the clinical manifestations of CF. The altered chloride ion conductance in the sweat gland results in excessively high sweat sodium and chloride levels. This is the basis of the sweat chloride test, which is still the standard diagnostic test for this disorder. It is positive (elevated sweat chloride > 60 mEq/L) in 99% of patients with CF. Abnormal airway secretions make the airway more prone to colonization with bacteria. Defects in CFTR may also reduce the function of airway defenses and promote bacterial adhesion to the airway epithelium. This all leads to chronic airway infections and eventually to bronchial damage (bronchiectasis).

CLINICAL MANIFESTATIONS

Decision-Making Algorithms
Available @ StudentConsult.com

Neck Masses
Hoarseness
Hemoptysis
Chest Pain
Diarrhea
Constipation
Hepatomegaly
Eosinophilia
Polyuria
Failure to Thrive
Alkalemia
Hyponatremia

CF is a chronic progressive disease that can present with protein and fat malabsorption (failure to thrive, hypoalbuminemia, steatorrhea), liver disease (cholestatic jaundice), or chronic respiratory infection (Table 137-1). Many infants currently are diagnosed based on newborn screening, which has been available in all 50 states and the District of Columbia since 2010. Older children commonly present with pulmonary manifestations such as poorly controlled asthma and chronic respiratory infections. The respiratory epithelium of patients with CF exhibits marked impermeability to chloride and an excessive reabsorption of sodium. This leads to a relative dehydration of airway secretions, which results in airway obstruction and impaired mucociliary transport. This, in turn, leads to endobronchial colonization with bacteria, especially *Staphylococcus aureus* and *Pseudomonas aeruginosa*. Chronic bronchial infection results in persistent or recurrent cough that is often productive of sputum, especially in older children. Chronic airway infection leads to airway obstruction and bronchiectasis and, eventually, to pulmonary insufficiency and premature death. The median age of survival (years) is currently in the mid-30s. **Digital clubbing** is common in patients with CF, even in those without significant lung disease. Chronic sinusitis and **nasal polyposis** are common.

Pulmonary infections with virulent strains of *Burkholderia cepacia* are difficult to treat and may be associated with accelerated clinical deterioration. **Allergic bronchopulmonary aspergillosis (ABPA)** is a hypersensitivity reaction to *Aspergillus* in the CF airways. It causes airway inflammation/obstruction and aggravates CF lung disease. The treatment for ABPA is systemic corticosteroids (prednisone) and antifungal agents (itraconazole). Minor hemoptysis is usually due to airway infection, but major hemoptysis is often caused by bleeding from bronchial artery collateral vessels in damaged/chronically infected portions of the lung. Pneumothoraces can occur in patients with advanced lung disease.

| **Table 137-1** | Complications of Cystic Fibrosis |

RESPIRATORY COMPLICATIONS

Bronchiectasis, bronchitis, bronchiolitis, pneumonia

Atelectasis

Hemoptysis

Pneumothorax

Nasal polyps

Sinusitis

Airway reactivity

Cor pulmonale (associated with chronic hypoxemia)

Respiratory failure

Mucoid impaction of the bronchi

Allergic bronchopulmonary aspergillosis

GASTROINTESTINAL COMPLICATIONS

Meconium ileus (infants)

Meconium peritonitis (infants)

Volvulus (infants)

Intestinal atresia (infants)

Distal intestinal obstruction syndrome (non-neonatal obstruction)

Rectal prolapse

Intussusception

Fibrosing colonopathy (strictures)

Appendicitis

Pancreatitis

Hepatic cirrhosis (portal hypertension: esophageal varices, hypersplenism)

Neonatal obstructive jaundice

Hepatic steatosis

Gastroesophageal reflux

Cholelithiasis

Growth failure (malabsorption)

Fat soluble vitamin deficiency states (vitamins A, K, E, D)

Insulin deficiency, symptomatic hyperglycemia, diabetes

Malignancy (rare)

OTHER COMPLICATIONS

Infertility

Delayed puberty

Edema-hypoproteinemia (due to protein malabsorption)

Dehydration–heat exhaustion

Electrolyte disturbances (hyponatremia, hypokalemia, hypochloremia, and metabolic alkalosis)

Hypertrophic osteoarthropathy–arthritis

Digital clubbing

Ninety percent of patients with CF are born with **exocrine pancreatic insufficiency**. The inspissation of mucus and subsequent destruction of the pancreatic ducts result in the inability to excrete pancreatic enzymes into the intestine. This leads to malabsorption of proteins, sugars (to a lesser extent), and especially fat. Fat malabsorption manifests clinically as **steatorrhea** (large foul-smelling stools), deficiencies of fat-soluble vitamins (A, D, E, and K), and failure to thrive. Protein malabsorption can present early in infancy as hypoproteinemia and peripheral edema. Approximately 10% of patients with CF are born with intestinal obstruction caused by inspissated meconium (**meconium ileus**). In older patients, intestinal obstruction may result from thick inspissated mucus in the intestinal lumen (**distal intestinal obstruction syndrome**). In adolescent or adult patients, progressive pancreatic damage can lead to enough islet cell destruction to cause **insulin deficiency**. This initially presents as glucose intolerance, but true diabetes that requires insulin therapy (**CF-related diabetes**) may develop. The failure of the sweat ducts to conserve sodium and chloride may lead to hyponatremia and hypochloremic metabolic alkalosis, especially in infants. Inspissation of mucus in the reproductive tract leads to reproductive dysfunction in both males and females. In males, congenital absence of the vas deferens and azoospermia are nearly universal. In females, secondary amenorrhea is often present as a result of chronic illness and reduced body weight. Fertility is also diminished by abnormal secretions in the fallopian tubes and cervix, but women with CF can conceive.

All infants with a positive newborn screen and/or with meconium ileus should be evaluated for CF. The diagnosis of CF should be seriously considered in any infant presenting with failure to thrive, cholestatic jaundice, chronic respiratory symptoms, or electrolyte abnormalities (hyponatremia, hypochloremia, metabolic alkalosis). CF should be in the differential diagnosis of children with chronic respiratory or gastrointestinal symptoms, especially if there is digital clubbing. Any child with nasal polyps, especially those younger than 12 years, should be evaluated for CF. All siblings of patients with CF should also be evaluated.

DIAGNOSTIC STUDIES

Readily available commercial DNA tests detect many CF mutations, but because there are more than 1500 identified mutations (and others yet to be identified), DNA analysis will not detect all cases of CF. All U.S. states have newborn screening for CF, based either on elevated immunoreactive trypsinogen (IRT) levels or DNA tests, identifying the majority of infants with CF, but there are both false-positive and false-negative results. Therefore, the diagnostic test of choice is still the sweat test. Indications for performing a **sweat test** are listed in Table 137-2. The following criteria should be met to establish the diagnosis of CF:

The presence of one or more typical clinical features of CF (chronic pulmonary disease, characteristic gastrointestinal and nutritional abnormalities, salt loss syndromes, or obstructive azoospermia) AND

1. Two elevated sweat chloride tests performed at an accredited CF Foundation certified laboratory (positive if the value is >60 mEq/L, borderline if 40 to 60 mEq/L, and negative if <40mEq/L, with adequate sweat collection)

2. Two mutations known to cause CF identified by DNA analysis or

3. A characteristic abnormality in ion transport across nasal epithelium demonstrated in vivo (nasal potential difference testing)

For those identified by positive newborn screening or because a sibling has CF, positive sweat chloride testing or the

Table 137-2	Indications for Sweat Testing

RESPIRATORY

Chronic or recurrent cough

Chronic or recurrent pneumonia

Recurrent bronchiolitis
Recurrent wheezing/difficult to control asthma

Recurrent or persistent atelectasis

Hemoptysis

Pseudomonas aeruginosa in the respiratory tract (if not explained by other factors, e.g., tracheostomy or prolonged intubation)

GASTROINTESTINAL

Meconium ileus

Neonatal intestinal obstruction (meconium plug, atresia)

Steatorrhea, malabsorption

Hepatic cirrhosis in childhood (including any manifestations such as esophageal varices or portal hypertension)

Cholestatic jaundice in infancy

Pancreatitis

Rectal prolapse

Fat-soluble vitamin deficiency states (A, D, E, K)

Hypoproteinemia, hypoalbuminemia, peripheral edema unexplained by other causes

Prolonged, direct-reacting neonatal jaundice

MISCELLANEOUS

Digital clubbing

Failure to thrive

Family history of cystic fibrosis (e.g., in sibling or cousin)

Salty taste of skin (typically noted by parent on kissing affected child—from salt crystals formed after evaporation of sweat)

Hyponatremic hypochloremic alkalosis in infants

Nasal polyps

Recurrent sinusitis

Aspermia

Absent vas deferens

Table 137-3	Causes of False Positive and False Negative Results on Sweat Testing

FALSE POSITIVE

Adrenal insufficiency

Eczema

Ectodermal dysplasia

Nephrogenic diabetes insipidus

Hypothyroidism

Fucosidosis

Mucopolysaccharidosis

Dehydration

Malnutrition

Poor technique/inadequate sweat collection

Type I glycogen storage disease

Panhypopituitarism

Pseudohypoaldosteronism

Hypoparathyroidism

Prostaglandin E_1 administration

FALSE NEGATIVE

Edema

Poor technique/inadequate sweat collection

Atypical cystic fibrosis (unusual gene mutations—uncommon)

presence of known disease-causing DNA mutations are the only criteria required for diagnosis, as clinical symptoms may not be manifested early in life.

Although the sweat test is both specific and sensitive for CF, it is subject to technical problems, and there are false-positive and false-negative results (Table 137-3). Cutoff diagnostic measurements for infants less than 6 months may be lower. Other supportive tests include the measurement of bioelectrical potential differences across nasal epithelium (not widely available) and measurement of fecal elastase levels. Low fecal elastase levels indicate exocrine pancreatic insufficiency. CF genotyping done by commercial laboratories identifies approximately 95% of patients with CF, but there are mutations that are not identified by standard testing. Not all mutations in CFTR are considered disease-causing and have uncertain prognostic consequences. Some infants identified by newborn screening with borderline sweat tests and mutations of uncertain consequence are considered to have CFTR-related

metabolic syndrome (CRMS). Older children that present with atypical clinical features and borderline sweat tests may be considered non-classical CF or mild variant CF.

Identification of carriers (heterozygotes) and prenatal diagnosis of children with the ΔF508 and other common mutations is offered at most medical centers. Present testing techniques can identify more than 90% of carriers. Prenatal detection of a known CF genotype may be accomplished by amniocentesis or chorionic villus sampling.

TREATMENT

The treatment of CF is multifactorial, but it is primarily directed toward the gastrointestinal and pulmonary complications. Presently, there is no effective single cure for cystic fibrosis. Therapies targeted at correcting the underlying CFTR defect are under investigation. Recently, a landmark medication known as small-molecule potentiators targeted to improve function of defective CFTR has been approved for a small subset of CF patients who have an abnormal gating mechanism of their CFTR protein. Management of pulmonary complications is directed toward facilitating clearance of secretions from the airways and minimizing the effects of chronic bronchial infection. Airway secretion clearance techniques (**chest physiotherapy**) help remove mucus from the airways, and aerosolized DNAse and 7% hypertonic saline, both delivered by nebulizer, decrease the viscosity of mucus. **Antibiotic therapy** is important in controlling chronic infection. Monitoring pulmonary bacterial flora via airway cultures and providing aggressive therapy with appropriate antibiotics (oral, aerosolized, and IV) help to slow the progression of lung disease. Patients often require 2- to 3-week courses of high-dose intravenous antibiotics and aggressive chest physiotherapy to treat pulmonary exacerbations. Antibiotics are selected based on organisms identified by sputum culture. If patients are unable to provide sputum, then a throat culture for CF pathogens can be used to direct therapy. Common infecting organisms are *Pseudomonas aeruginosa* and *Staphylococcus aureus*.

Exocrine pancreatic insufficiency is treated with enteric-coated pancreatic enzyme capsules, which contain lipase and proteases. Patients with CF are encouraged to follow high-calorie diets, often with the addition of nutritional supplements. Even with optimal pancreatic enzyme replacement, stool losses of fat and protein may be high. Fat should not be withheld from the diet, even when significant steatorrhea exists. Rather, pancreatic enzyme doses should be titrated to optimize fat absorption, although there is a limit to the doses that should be used. Lipase dosages exceeding 2500 U/kg/meal are contraindicated because they have been associated with **fibrosing colonopathy**. Fat-soluble vitamins (A, D, E, and K) are recommended, preferably in a water-miscible form.

Newborns with **meconium ileus** may require surgical intervention, but some can be managed with contrast (Gastrografin) enemas. Intestinal obstruction in CF patients beyond the neonatal period is often due to distal intestinal obstruction syndrome (DIOS), which may need to be treated with courses of oral laxatives (polyethylene glycol) or, in more refractory cases, with balanced intestinal lavage solutions. Pancreatic enzyme dosage adjustment, adequate hydration, and dietary fiber may help prevent recurrent episodes. Patients with CF-related diabetes are treated with insulin, primarily to improve nutrition and prevent dehydration, as ketoacidosis is rare. Although transaminase elevation is common in patients with CF, only 1% to 3% of patients have progressive cirrhosis resulting in portal hypertension. Cholestasis is treated with the bile salt ursodeoxycholic acid. Portal hypertension and esophageal varices due to cirrhosis of the liver are managed, when necessary, with portal vein shunting procedures or liver transplantation. Patients with symptomatic sinus disease and nasal polyps may require sinus surgical procedures.

The management of CF is complex and is best coordinated by personnel at accredited CF centers. As with other severe chronic diseases, management of CF patients requires a multidisciplinary team working with patients and their families to maintain an optimistic, comprehensive, and aggressive approach to treatment.

Chapter 138

CHEST WALL AND PLEURA

SCOLIOSIS

Thoracic scoliosis, when it is severe (curve >60°), can be associated with chest wall deformity and limitation of chest wall movement. This, in turn, can lead to decreased lung volumes (restrictive lung disease), ventilation/perfusion mismatching, hypoventilation, and even respiratory failure (see Chapter 202). Surgical correction of scoliosis may prevent further loss of lung function, but it rarely improves pulmonary function above presurgical levels.

PECTUS EXCAVATUM AND CARINATUM
Pectus Excavatum

Sternal concavity (**pectus excavatum**), a common chest wall deformity in children, is usually not associated with significant pulmonary compromise. However, occasionally, if severe, it may result in restrictive lung disease, obstructive defects, and/or decreased cardiac function. Often it comes to medical attention because of concerns over the appearance of the chest. Adolescents with pectus excavatum may complain of exercise intolerance. Routine spirometry is often normal but may show decreased vital capacity consistent with restrictive lung disease. The main reason for surgical correction is generally to improve appearance (cosmetic reasons), although in some cases surgical repair is justified to improve cardiac function and exercise tolerance.

Pectus Carinatum

Pectus carinatum is an abnormality of chest wall shape in which the sternum bows out. It is not associated with abnormal pulmonary function. Underlying pulmonary disease may contribute to the deformity. It can be observed after cardiac surgery performed via midsternal approach. Surgical correction of this condition is rarely indicated, but occasionally is done for cosmetic purposes.

PNEUMOTHORAX
Etiology

Pneumothorax, which is the accumulation of air in the pleural space, may result from external trauma or from leakage of air from the lungs or airways. **Spontaneous primary pneumothorax** (no underlying cause) occurs in teenagers and young adults, more commonly in tall, thin males and smokers. Factors predisposing to **secondary pneumothorax** (underlying cause identified) include barotrauma from mechanical ventilation, asthma, cystic fibrosis, trauma to the chest, and severe necrotizing pneumonia.

Clinical Manifestations

Decision-Making Algorithm
Available @ StudentConsult.com

Chest Pain

The most common signs and symptoms of pneumothorax are chest and shoulder pain and dyspnea. If the pneumothorax is large and compresses functional lung (**tension pneumothorax**), severe respiratory distress and cyanosis may be present. Subcutaneous emphysema may result when the air leak communicates with the mediastinum. Physical findings associated with pneumothorax include decreased breath sounds on the affected side, a tympanitic percussion note, and evidence of mediastinal shift (deviation of the point of maximal impact [PMI] and trachea away from the side of the pneumothorax). If the pneumothorax is small, there may be few or no clinical findings. However, the patient's clinical condition can deteriorate rapidly if the pneumothorax expands, especially if the air in the pleural space is under pressure (**tension pneumothorax**). This is a life-threatening condition that can result in death if the pleural space is not decompressed by evacuation of the pleural air.

Diagnostic Studies
The presence of a pneumothorax can usually be confirmed by upright chest radiographs. Computed tomography (CT) scans of the chest are useful in quantifying the size of pneumothoraces and differentiating air within the lung parenchyma (cystic lung disease) from air in the pleural space and for identifying subpleural blebs that may be present in spontaneous recurrent pneumothoraces. In infants, transillumination of the chest wall may be of some use in making a rapid diagnosis of pneumothorax.

Treatment
The type of intervention depends on the size of the pneumothorax and the nature of the underlying disease. Small pneumothoraces (<20% of thorax occupied with pleural air) may not require intervention as they often resolve spontaneously. Inhaling high concentrations of supplemental O_2 may enhance reabsorption of pleural air by washing out nitrogen from the blood. Larger pneumothoraces and any tension pneumothorax require immediate drainage of the air, preferably via chest tube. In an emergency situation, a simple needle aspiration may suffice, although placement of a chest tube is often required for resolution. In patients with recurrent or persistent pneumothoraces, sclerosing the pleural surfaces to obliterate the pleural space (pleurodesis) may be necessary. This can be done either chemically, by instilling talc or sclerosis agents (doxycycline) through the chest tube, or mechanically, by surgical abradement. Surgical approaches, open thoracotomy and video-assisted thoracoscopic surgery (VATS), enable visualization of the pleural space and resection of pleural blebs, when indicated.

PNEUMOMEDIASTINUM
Pneumomediastinum results from the dissection of air from the pulmonary parenchyma into the mediastinum. It is usually a mild, self-limited process that does not require aggressive intervention. The most common causes in children are severe forceful coughing and acute asthma exacerbations. Common symptoms are chest pain and dyspnea. There are often no physical findings, although a crunching noise over the sternum can sometimes be appreciated on auscultation, and subcutaneous emphysema may be detected about the neck. The diagnosis is confirmed by chest radiograph, and treatment is directed toward the underlying lung disease.

PLEURAL EFFUSION
Etiology
Fluid accumulates in the pleural space when the local hydrostatic forces that are pushing fluid out of the vascular space

exceed the oncotic forces that are drawing fluid back into the vascular space. Pleural effusions can be transudates (intact membrane but abnormal hydrostatic or oncotic forces) or exudates (decreased integrity of the membrane due to inflammatory processes or impaired lymphatic drainage). There are relatively few causes of transudates, the primary ones being congestive heart failure and hypoproteinemia states, whereas the causes of exudates are legion. Almost any pulmonary inflammatory process can result in pleural fluid accumulation. Among the most common causes of exudates are infection (tuberculosis, bacterial pneumonia), collagen vascular diseases (systemic lupus erythematosus), and malignancy. Chylous pleural effusions (elevated triglyceride levels) are seen with thoracic duct injury and abnormalities of lymphatic drainage (lymphangiomyomatosis, lymphangiectasia). Bacterial pneumonia can lead to an accumulation of pleural fluid (**parapneumonic effusion**). When this fluid is purulent or infected, then it is called an **empyema**, although often the terms parapneumonic effusion and empyema are used interchangeably. Parapneumonic effusion/empyema is the most common effusion in children. Most parapneumonic effusions are due to pneumonia caused by *Streptococcus pneumoniae,* group A streptococci, or *Staphylococcus aureus.*

Clinical Manifestations

Decision-Making Algorithm
Available @ StudentConsult.com

Chest Pain

Small pleural effusions may be asymptomatic, but if they are large enough to compress lung tissue, then they can cause dyspnea, tachypnea, and occasionally chest pain. Effusions due to infection are usually associated with fever, malaise, poor appetite, pleuritic chest pain, and splinting. Physical findings include tachypnea, decreased breath sounds, dullness to percussion, and decreased tactile fremitus. Large effusions may occupy more than half the hemithorax and cause a mediastinal shift away from the affected side, compromising respiratory status, particularly in young children.

Diagnostic Studies
The presence of pleural fluid can often be confirmed by chest radiograph. In addition to anteroposterior and lateral projections, a decubitus view should be done to assess for layering of fluid. Chest ultrasonography is useful for confirming the presence of the effusion and quantifying its size. CT scans of the chest can help differentiate pleural fluid from parenchymal lesions and pleural masses. Both ultrasonography and CT scans can determine whether parapneumonic effusions contain loculations (fibrous strands that compartmentalize the effusion).

The analysis of pleural fluid is useful in differentiating a transudate from an exudate. Routine tests on pleural fluid such as cell count, pH, protein, lactose dehydrogenase, and glucose characterize the effusions. Triglyceride levels, cytology, hematocrit, gram and acid fast bacilli stain, culture, and adenosine deaminase levels can be useful in diagnosing

Table 138-1	Pleural Fluid Analysis

EXUDATIVE EFFUSION BY LIGHT'S TRADITIONAL CRITERIA

Pleural fluid protein/serum protein ratio greater than 0.5 **OR**

Pleural fluid LDH/serum LDH ratio greater than 0.6 **OR**

Pleural fluid LDH greater than two-thirds the upper limits of laboratory's normal serum LDH

CHYLOTHORAX

Triglycerides greater than 110 mg/dL

TUBERCULOUS

Positive acid fast bacilli stain, culture

Pleural fluid protein greater than 4 g/dL

Pleural fluid adenosine deaminase level greater than 35-50 U/L

Pleural fluid glucose 30-50 mg/dL

HEMOTHORAX

Pleural fluid hematocrit/serum hematocrit greater than 0.5

LDH, Lactate dehydrogenase.

chylous, malignant, and tuberculous effusions (Table 138-1). However, the yield of pleural fluid cultures is low. Transudative pleural effusions have a low specific gravity (<1.015) and protein content (<2.5 g/dL), low lactate dehydrogenase activity (<200 IU/L), and a low white blood cell (WBC) count with few polymorphonuclear cells. In contrast, exudates are characterized by high specific gravity and high protein (>3 g/dL) and lactate dehydrogenase (>250 IU/L) levels. They may also have a low pH (<7.2); low glucose level (<40 mg/dL); and a high WBC count with many lymphocytes or polymorphonuclear leukocytes.

Treatment

Therapy is directed at the underlying condition causing the effusion and at relief of the mechanical consequences of the fluid collection. For small effusions, especially if they are transudates, no pleural drainage is required. Large effusions that are causing respiratory compromise should be drained. Transudates and most exudates other than parapneumonic effusions can be drained with a **chest tube**. With parapneumonic effusions/empyema, a chest tube alone is often not sufficient because the fluid may be thick and loculated. In such cases, pleural drainage is best achieved with either the administration of fibrinolytic agents via chest tubes or **video-assisted thoracoscopic surgery (VATS)**. Both fibrinolytic therapy via chest tubes and VATS can reduce morbidity and length of hospital stay, but many patients with small to moderate-sized parapneumonic effusions can be managed conservatively with intravenous antibiotics alone.

Suggested Reading

Levitzky MG: *Pulmonary Physiology*, ed 7, New York, 2007, McGraw-Hill.

Kliegman RM, Stanton BF, St. Geme JW, et al: *Nelson Textbook of Pediatrics*, ed 19, Philadelphia, 2011, Saunders.

Taussig LN, Landau LI, et al: *Pediatric Respiratory Medicine*, ed 2, Philadelphia, 2008, Mosby.

Wilmott RW, Boat TF, Bush A, et al: *Kendig and Chernick's Disorders of the Respiratory Tract in Children*, ed 8, Philadelphia, 2012, Saunders.

The Cardiovascular System

Daniel S. Schneider

CARDIOVASCULAR SYSTEM ASSESSMENT

HISTORY

A **maternal history** of medication, drug, or alcohol use or excessive smoking may contribute to cardiac and other systemic findings. The **prenatal history** may reveal a maternal infection early in pregnancy (possibly teratogenic) or later in pregnancy (causing myocarditis or myocardial dysfunction in infants). Infants with heart failure exhibit poor **growth**, with weight being more significantly affected than height and head circumference.

Heart failure may present with **fatigue** or **diaphoresis** with feeds or fussiness. **Tachypnea** without significant dyspnea may be present. Older children with heart failure may have easy fatigability, **shortness of breath** on exertion, and sometimes orthopnea. Not keeping up with other children during play or exercise is a sign of **exercise intolerance**. Heart failure may be misdiagnosed as recurrent pneumonia, bronchitis, wheezing, or asthma.

A history of a **heart murmur** is important, but many well children have an innocent murmur at some time in their lives. Other cardiac symptoms include cyanosis, palpitations, chest pain, syncope, and near-syncope. A review of systems assesses for possible systemic diseases or congenital malformation syndromes that may cause cardiac abnormalities (Tables 139-1 and 139-2). Current and past medication use as well as history of drug use, is important. **Family history** should be reviewed for hereditary diseases, early atherosclerotic heart disease, congenital heart disease, sudden unexplained deaths, thrombophilia, rheumatic fever, hypertension, and hypercholesterolemia.

PHYSICAL EXAMINATION

A complete cardiovascular examination starts in the supine position and includes evaluation in sitting and standing positions when possible. **Inspection** is supplemented by **palpation** and **auscultation** to provide a complete examination.

The examination starts with vital signs. The normal **heart rate** varies with age and activity. Newborn resting heart rates are approximately 120 beats/minute, slightly higher in infants 3 to 6 months of age and then gradually declining through adolescence to near 80 beats/minute. The range of normal for any given age is approximately 30 beats/minute above or below the average. Tachycardia may be a manifestation of anemia, dehydration, shock, heart failure, or dysrhythmia. Bradycardia can be a normal finding in patients with high vagal tone (athletes), but may be a manifestation of atrioventricular block. The **respiratory rate** of infants is best assessed while the infant is quiet. Respiratory rate may be increased when there is a left-to-right shunt or pulmonary venous congestion.

Normal **blood pressure** also varies with age. A properly sized cuff should have a bladder width that is at least 90% and a length that is 80% to 100% of the arm circumference. Initially, blood pressure in the right arm is measured. If elevated, measurements in the left arm and legs are indicated to evaluate for possible coarctation of the aorta. The **pulse pressure** is determined by subtracting the diastolic pressure from the systolic pressure. It is normally below 50 mm Hg or half the systolic pressure, whichever is less. A wide pulse pressure

Table 139-1	Cardiac Manifestations of Systemic Diseases
SYSTEMIC DISEASE	**CARDIAC COMPLICATIONS**
Hunter-Hurler syndrome	Valvular insufficiency, heart failure, hypertension
Duchenne dystrophy	Cardiomyopathy, heart failure
Pompe disease	Short PR interval, cardiomegaly, heart failure, arrhythmias
Kawasaki disease	Coronary artery aneurysm, thrombosis, myocardial infarction, myocarditis
Marfan syndrome	Aortic and mitral insufficiency, dissecting aortic aneurysm
Juvenile rheumatoid arthritis	Pericarditis
Systemic lupus erythematosus	Pericarditis, Libman-Sacks endocarditis, congenital AV block
Lyme disease	Arrhythmias, myocarditis, heart failure
Graves disease (hyperthyroidism)	Tachycardia, arrhythmias, heart failure
Tuberous sclerosis	Cardiac rhabdomyoma
Neurofibromatosis	Pulmonic stenosis, coarctation of aorta

AV, atrioventricular.

Table 139-2	Congenital Malformation Syndromes Associated with Congenital Heart Disease
SYNDROME	**CARDIAC FEATURES**
Trisomy 21 (Down syndrome)	Endocardial cushion defect, VSD, ASD, PDA
Trisomy 18	VSD, ASD, PDA, PS
Trisomy 13	VSD, ASD, PDA, dextrocardia
XO (Turner syndrome)	Coarctation of aorta, aortic stenosis
CHARGE association (coloboma, heart, atresia choanae, retardation, genital and ear anomalies)	TOF, aortic arch and conotruncal anomalies*
22q11 (DiGeorge) syndrome	Aortic arch anomalies, conotruncal anomalies*
VACTERL association† (vertebral, anal, cardiac, tracheoesophageal, radial, renal, limb anomalies)	VSD
Marfan syndrome	Dilated and dissecting aorta, aortic valve regurgitation, mitral valve prolapse
William syndrome	Supravalvular aortic stenosis, peripheral pulmonary stenosis
Infant of diabetic mother	Hypertrophic cardiomyopathy, VSD, conotruncal anomalies
Asplenia syndrome	Complex cyanotic heart lesions, anomalous pulmonary venous return, dextrocardia, single ventricle, single AV valve
Polysplenia syndrome	Azygos continuation of inferior vena cava, pulmonary atresia, dextrocardia, single ventricle
Fetal alcohol syndrome	VSD, ASD
Fetal hydantoin syndrome	TGA, VSD, TOF

ASD, Atrial septal defect; *AV*, atrioventricular; *PDA*, patent ductus arteriosus; *PS*, pulmonic stenosis; *TGA*, transposition of great arteries; *TOF*, tetralogy of Fallot; *VSD*, ventricular septal defect.
*Conotruncal—tetralogy of Fallot, pulmonary atresia, truncus arteriosus, transposition of great arteries.
†VACTERL association is also known as VATER association, in which the limb anomalies are not included.

may be seen with aortopulmonary connections (patent ductus arteriosus [PDA], truncus arteriosus, arteriovenous malformations), aortic insufficiency, or relative intravascular volume depletion (anemia, vasodilation with fever or sepsis). A narrow pulse pressure is seen with pericardial tamponade, aortic stenosis, and heart failure.

Inspection includes general appearance, nutritional status, circulation, and respiratory effort. Many chromosomal abnormalities and syndromes associated with cardiac defects have dysmorphic features or failure to thrive (see Table 139-2). Skin color must be assessed for **cyanosis** and pallor. Central cyanosis (tongue, lips) is associated with arterial desaturation; isolated peripheral cyanosis (hands, feet) is associated with normal arterial saturation and increased peripheral extraction of oxygen. Perioral cyanosis is a common finding, especially in pale infants or when infants and toddlers become cold. Chronic arterial desaturation results in **clubbing** of the fingernails and toenails. Inspection of the chest may reveal asymmetry or a prominent left precordium suggesting chronic cardiac enlargement.

After inspection, **palpation** of pulses in all four extremities, the precordial activity, and the abdomen is performed. Pulses are assessed for rate, regularity, intensity, symmetry, and timing between upper and lower extremities. A good pedal pulse with normal right arm blood pressure effectively rules out coarctation of the aorta. The precordium should be assessed for apical impulse, **point of maximum impulse**, hyperactivity, and presence of a **thrill**. Abdominal palpation assesses liver and spleen size. The liver size provides an assessment of intravascular volume and is enlarged with systemic venous congestion. The spleen may be enlarged with infective endocarditis.

Auscultation is the most important part of the cardiovascular examination, but should supplement what already has been found by inspection and palpation. Systematic listening in a quiet room allows assessment of each portion of the cardiac cycle. In addition to heart rate and regularity, the heart sounds, clicks, and murmurs need to be timed and characterized.

Heart Sounds

S_1 is associated with closure of the mitral and tricuspid valves, is usually single, and is best heard at the lower left sternal border (LLSB) or apex (Fig. 139-1). Although it can normally be split, if a split S_1 is heard, the possibility of an ejection click or, much less commonly, an S_4 should be considered. S_2 is associated with closure of the aortic and pulmonary valves. It should normally split with inspiration and be single with exhalation. Abnormalities of splitting and intensity of the pulmonary component are associated with significant anatomic and physiologic abnormalities (Table 139-3). S_3 is heard in early diastole and is related to rapid ventricular filling. It is best heard at the LLSB or apex and may be a normal sound, but a loud S_3 is abnormal and heard in conditions with dilated ventricles. S_4 occurs late in diastole just before S_1, is best heard at the LLSB/apex, and is associated with decreased ventricular compliance. It is rare and is always abnormal.

Clicks

A click implies a valvular abnormality or dilated great artery. It may be ejection or midsystolic in timing and may or may not be associated with a murmur. A midsystolic click is associated with mitral valve prolapse. **Ejection clicks** occur early in systole. Pulmonary ejection clicks are best heard at the left upper sternal border and vary in intensity with respiration. Aortic clicks are often louder at the apex, left midsternal border, or right upper sternal border and do not vary with respiration.

Murmurs

Decision-Making Algorithm
Available @ StudentConsult.com

Heart Murmurs

Murmur evaluation should determine timing, duration, location, intensity, radiation, and frequency or pitch of the murmur. The timing determines a murmur's significance and can be used to develop a differential diagnosis (see Fig. 139-1).

Figure 139-1 Timing of heart murmurs. *AV,* Atrio-ventricular.

Table 139-3	Abnormal Second Heart Sound

SINGLE S₂

Pulmonary hypertension (severe)

One semilunar valve (aortic atresia, pulmonary atresia, truncus arteriosus)

Malposed great arteries (d-TGA, l-TGA)

Severe aortic stenosis

WIDELY SPLIT S₂

Increased flow across valve (ASD, PAPVR)

Prolonged flow across valve (pulmonary stenosis)

Electrical delay (right bundle branch block)

Early aortic closure (severe mitral regurgitation)

PARADOXICALLY SPLIT S₂

Severe aortic stenosis

ABNORMAL INTENSITY OF P2

Increased in pulmonary hypertension

Decreased in severe pulmonary stenosis, tetralogy of Fallot

ASD, Atrial septal defect; *d-TGA,* dextro-transposition of the great arteries; *l-TGA,* levo-transposition of the great arteries; *PAPVR,* partial anomalous pulmonary venous return.

Table 139-4	Heart Murmur Intensity	
GRADE	**DESCRIPTION**	
Grade I	Very soft, heard in quiet room with cooperative patient	
Grade II	Easily heard but not loud	
Grade III	Loud but no thrill	
Grade IV	Loud with palpable thrill	
Grade V	Loud with thrill, audible with stethoscope at 45° angle	
Grade VI	Loud with thrill, audible with stethoscope off chest 1 cm	

Murmurs should be classified as **systolic, diastolic**, or **continuous.** Most murmurs are systolic and can be divided further into systolic ejection murmurs or holosystolic (also called pansystolic or regurgitant) murmurs. **Ejection murmurs** are crescendo-decrescendo with a short time between S₁ and the onset of the murmur (isovolumic contraction). Systolic ejection murmurs require the ejection of blood from the ventricle and may occur with aortic stenosis, pulmonary stenosis, atrial septal defects (ASDs), and coarctation of the aorta. **Holosystolic murmurs** have their onset with S₁. The murmur has a plateau quality and may be heard with ventricular septal defects (VSDs) and mitral or tricuspid regurgitation. A *late regurgitant* murmur may be heard after a midsystolic click in mitral valve prolapse.

Murmurs are often heard along the path of blood flow. Ejection murmurs usually are best heard at the base of the heart, whereas holosystolic murmurs are louder at the LLSB and apex. Pulmonary ejection murmurs radiate to the back and axilla. Aortic ejection murmurs radiate to the neck. The **intensity** or loudness of a heart murmur is assessed as grade I through VI (Table 139-4). The **frequency** or pitch of a murmur provides information regarding the pressure gradient. The higher the pressure gradient across a narrowed area (valve, vessel, or defect), the faster the flow and higher the frequency of the murmur. Low-frequency murmurs imply low pressure gradients and mild obstruction or less restriction to flow.

Table 139-5	Normal or Innocent Heart Murmurs	
MURMUR	**TIMING/LOCATION/ QUALITY**	**USUAL AGE AT DIAGNOSIS**
Still's murmur/ vibratory murmur	Systolic ejection murmur LLSB or between LLSB and apex Grades I-III/VI Vibratory, musical quality Intensity decreases in upright position	3–6 yr
Venous hum	Continuous murmur Infraclavicular region (right > left) Grades I-III/VI Louder with patient in upright position Changes with compression of jugular vein or turning head	3–6 yr
Carotid bruit	Systolic ejection murmur Neck, over carotid artery Grade I-III/VI	Any age
Adolescent ejection murmur	Systolic ejection murmur LUSB Grade I-III/VI Usually softer in upright position Does not radiate to back	8–14 yr
Peripheral pulmonary stenosis	Systolic ejection murmur Axilla and back, LUSB/ RUSB Grade I-III/VI Harsh, short, high-frequency	Newborn to 6 mo

LLSB, Left lower scapular border; *LUSB*, left upper scapular border; *RUSB*, right upper scapular border.

Diastolic murmurs are much less common than systolic murmurs, and should be considered abnormal. Early diastolic murmurs occur when there is regurgitation through the aortic or pulmonary valve. Mid-diastolic murmurs are caused by increased flow (ASD, VSD) or anatomic stenosis across the mitral or tricuspid valves.

Continuous murmurs are heard when there is flow through the entire cardiac cycle and are abnormal with one common exception, the **venous hum.** A PDA is the most common abnormal continuous murmur. Continuous murmurs can also be heard with coarctation of the aorta when collateral vessels are present.

Normal physiologic or **innocent murmurs** are common, occurring in at least 80% of normal infants and children, heard most often during the first 6 months of life, from 3 to 6 years of age, and in early adolescence. They have also been called benign, functional, vibratory, and flow murmurs. Characteristic findings of innocent murmurs include the quality of the sound, lack of significant radiation, and significant alteration in the intensity of the murmur with positional changes (Table 139-5). Most important, the cardiovascular history and examination are otherwise normal. The presence of symptoms, including failure to thrive or dysmorphic features, should make one more cautious about diagnosing a *normal* murmur. Diastolic, holosystolic, late systolic, and continuous (except

for the venous hum) murmurs and the presence of a thrill are not normal.

LABORATORY AND IMAGING TESTS
Pulse Oximetry
Mild desaturation that is not clinically apparent may be the only early finding in complex congenital heart defects. Comparing pulse oximetry between the right arm and a lower extremity may allow diagnosis of a ductal dependent lesion in which desaturated blood flows right to left across a PDA to perfuse the lower body. This is now becoming a routine screening test in newborn infants to rule out congenital heart disease.

Electrocardiography
The 12-lead electrocardiogram (ECG) provides information about the **rate**, **rhythm**, **depolarization**, and **repolarization** of the cardiac cells and the size and wall thickness of the chambers. It should be assessed for rate, rhythm, axis (P wave, QRS, and T wave), intervals (PR, QRS, QTc) (Fig. 139-2), and voltages (left atrial, right atrial, left ventricular, right ventricular) adjusted for the child's age.

The **P wave** represents atrial depolarization. A criterion for right atrial enlargement is an increase of the amplitude of the P wave, reflected best in lead II. The diagnosis of left atrial enlargement is made by prolongation of the second portion of the P wave, exhibited best in the chest leads.

The **PR interval**, measured from the beginning of the P wave to the beginning of the QRS complex, increases with age. Conduction time is shortened when the conduction velocity is increased (glycogen storage disease) or when the atrioventricular node is bypassed (Wolff-Parkinson-White syndrome). A prolonged PR interval usually indicates slow conduction through the atrioventricular node. Diseases in the atrial myocardium, bundle of His, or Purkinje system may also contribute to prolonged PR intervals.

The **QRS complex** represents ventricular depolarization. A greater ventricular volume or mass causes a greater magnitude of the complex. The proximity of the right ventricle to the chest surface accentuates that ventricle's contribution to the complex. Changes in the normal ECG occur with age. Normative data for each age group must be known to make a diagnosis from the ECG.

The **QT interval** is measured from the beginning of the QRS complex to the end of the T wave. The corrected QT interval (corrected for rate) should be less than 0.45 second ($QTc = QT/\sqrt{precedingR\ to\ R\ interval}$). The interval may be prolonged in children with hypocalcemia or severe hypokalemia. It is also prolonged in a group of children at risk for severe ventricular arrhythmias and sudden death (**prolonged QT syndrome**). Drugs such as quinidine and erythromycin may prolong the QT interval.

Chest Radiography
A systematic approach to reading a chest radiograph includes assessment of extracardiac structures, the shape and size of the heart, and the size and position of the pulmonary artery and aorta (Fig. 139-3). Assessment of the location and size of the heart and **cardiac silhouette** may suggest a cardiac defect. On a good inspiratory film, the cardiothoracic ratio should be

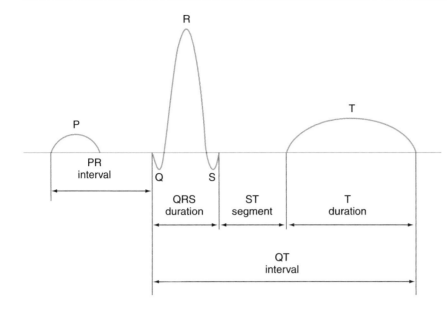

Figure 139-2 Nomenclature of electrocardiogram (ECG) waves and intervals.

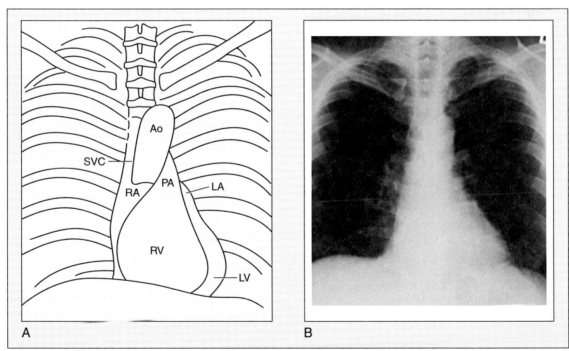

Figure 139-3 A, Parts of the heart whose outlines can be identified on a routine chest x-ray. B, Routine posteroanterior x-ray of the normal cardiac silhouette. *Ao,* Aorta; *LA,* left atrium; *LV,* left ventricle; *PA,* pulmonary artery; *RA,* right atrium; *RV,* right ventricle; *SVC,* superior vena cava. *(From Andreoli TE, Carpenter CCJ, Plum F, et al, editors: Cecil Essentials of Medicine, ed 2, Philadelphia, 1990, WB Saunders.)*

less than 55% in infants under 1 year of age and less than 50% in older children and adolescents. An enlarged heart may be due to an increased volume load (left-right shunt) or due to myocardial dysfunction (dilated cardiomyopathy). The shape of the heart may suggest specific congenital heart defects. The most common examples are the *boot-shaped* heart seen with tetralogy of Fallot, the *egg-on-a-string* seen with dextroposed transposition of the great arteries, and the "snowman" seen with supracardiac total anomalous pulmonary venous return. The chest x-ray can aid in the assessment of **pulmonary blood flow**. Defects associated with left-to-right shunting have increased pulmonary blood flow *(shunt vascularity)* on x-ray. Right-to-left shunts have decreased pulmonary blood flow.

Echocardiography

Echocardiography has become the most important noninvasive tool in the diagnosis and management of cardiac disease, providing a full anatomic evaluation in most congenital heart defects (Fig. 139-4). Physiologic data on the direction of blood flow can be obtained with the use of pulsed, continuous wave, and color flow Doppler. Imaging from multiple views provides an assessment of spatial relationships. Three-dimensional (3D) and four-dimensional (4D) imaging now allows reconstruction of the heart and manipulation of the images to provide more detail, especially with regard to valve structure and function. Prenatal or fetal echocardiography can diagnose congenital heart disease by 18 weeks of gestation and allows for

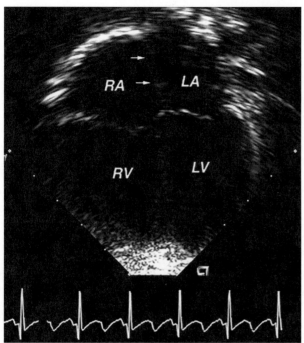

Figure 139-4 Four-chamber echocardiogram of an atrial septal defect. The defect margins are identified by the two *arrows*. *LA*, Left atrium; *LV*, left ventricle; *RA*, right atrium; *RV*, right ventricle.

Figure 139-5 The normal heart. *AO*, Aorta; *LA*, left atrium; *LV*, left ventricle; *PA*, pulmonary artery; *RA*, right atrium; *RV*, right ventricle. *Circled* values are oxygen saturations.

delivery of the infant at a tertiary care hospital, improving the timeliness of therapy. Many congenital heart defects now are surgically repaired based on the echocardiogram without need for cardiac catheterization.

Transesophageal echocardiography (TEE) provides better imaging when transthoracic imaging is inadequate. It is used intraoperatively to assess results and cardiac function after surgery. TEE and intracardiac echocardiography are used to guide interventional catheterization and radiofrequency ablation of dysrhythmias.

Cardiac Catheterization

Cardiac catheterization is performed in patients who need additional anatomic information or precise hemodynamic information before operating or establishing a management plan. Pressures, oxygen saturations, and oxygen content are measured in each chamber and blood vessel entered (Fig. 139-5). This information is used to calculate systemic and pulmonary blood flow and resistance. Angiography is performed by injecting contrast material into selected sites to define anatomy and supplement noninvasive information. An increasing percentage of cardiac catheterizations are done to perform an intervention, including balloon dilation of stenotic valves and vessels, ballooning and stenting of stenotic lesions, closure of collateral vessels by coil embolization, and device closure of PDAs, secundum ASDs, patent foramen ovales, and muscular VSDs. Catheterization with electrophysiologic studies allows for precise mapping of the electrical activity, can assess the risk of abnormal heart rhythms, and often is done in anticipation of radiofrequency ablation of the site of a dysrhythmia.

Chapter 140

SYNCOPE

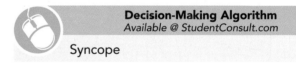

Decision-Making Algorithm
Available @ StudentConsult.com
Syncope

ETIOLOGY

Syncope is the transient loss of consciousness and muscle tone that, by history, does not suggest other altered states of consciousness. Presyncope or near-syncope has many or all of the prodromal symptoms without loss of consciousness. Syncope is relatively common (Table 140-1). The frequency of episodes, amount of stress, and functional impairment caused by syncope vary. Most syncopal events are relatively benign, but can represent a serious cardiac condition that may lead to death (Table 140-1). The differential diagnosis for typical syncope includes seizure, metabolic cause (hypoglycemia), hyperventilation, atypical migraine, and breath holding.

CLINICAL MANIFESTATIONS

Typical syncopal events usually occur in the upright position or are related to changing position. Syncope may be associated with anxiety, pain, blood drawing or the sight of blood, fasting, a hot environment, or crowded places. The patient often appears pale. A prodrome, consisting of *dizziness*, lightheadedness, nausea, diaphoresis, visual changes (blacking out), or possibly palpitations, warns the patient and often prevents

				HEART RATE/			
DIAGNOSIS	**HISTORY**	**SIGNS/ SYMPTOMS**	**DESCRIPTION**	**BLOOD PRESSURE**	**DURATION**	**POSTSYNCOPE**	**RECURRENCE**
Neurocardiogenic (vasodepressor)	At rest	Pallor, nausea, visual changes	Brief ± convulsion	↓/↓	<1 min	Residual pallor, sweaty, hot; recurs if child stands	Common
Other vagal							
Micturition	Postvoiding	Pallor, nausea	Brief; convulsions rare	↓/↓	< 1 min		(+)
Hair grooming	Standing getting hair done or ears touched	Pallor, nausea, visual changes, lightheaded	Brief		<1 min	Residual pallor, sweaty, hot, can recur if stands too soon	(+)
Cough (deglutition)	Paroxysmal cough	Cough	Abrupt onset	May not change	<5 min	Fatigue or baseline	(+)
Carotid sinus	Tight collar, turned head	Vague, visual changes	Sudden onset, pallor	Usually ↓/↓	<5 min	Fatigue or baseline	(+)
Cardiac syncope							
LVOT obstruction	Exercise	± Chest pain, SOB	Abrupt during or after exertion, pallor	↑/↓	Any duration	Fatigue, residual pallor, and sweating	(+)
Pulmonary hypertension	Any time, especially exercise	SOB	Cyanosis and pallor	↑/↓	Any duration	Fatigue, residual cyanosis	(+)
Myocarditis	Post–viral infection exercise	SOB, chest pain, palpitations	Pallor	↑/↓	Any duration	Fatigue	(+)
Tumor or mass	Recumbent, paroxysmal	SOB ± chest pain	Pallor	↑/↓	Any duration	Baseline	(+)
Coronary artery disease	Exercise	SOB ± chest pain	Pallor	↑/↓	Any duration	Fatigue, chest pain	(+)
Dysrhythmia	Any time	Palpitations ± chest pain	Pallor	↑ or ↑/↓	Usually <10 min	Fatigue or baseline	(+)

Table 140-1 Syncope and Dizziness: Etiology

From Lewis DA: Syncope and dizziness. In Kliegman RM, editor: Practical Strategies in Pediatric Diagnosis and Therapy, Philadelphia, 1996, WB Saunders.
LVOT, Left ventricular outflow tract; SOB, shortness of breath; ±, with or without; (+), yes but not consistent or predictable.

injury. Unconsciousness lasts for less than 1 minute. A return to normal consciousness occurs relatively quickly. Most of these syncopal episodes are vasovagal or neurocardiogenic in origin. The physical examination is normal.

DIAGNOSTIC STUDIES

Syncopal episodes may require no more than reassurance to the patient and family. If the episodes have a significant impact on daily activities, further evaluation may be indicated. An electrocardiogram (ECG) should be obtained with attention to the QTc and PR intervals (see Chapter 139). Although reassurance and increasing fluid and salt intake may be adequate to treat most cases of syncope, medical management is sometimes indicated.

Chapter **141**

CHEST PAIN

Decision-Making Algorithm
Available @ StudentConsult.com

Chest Pain

ETIOLOGY

Chest pain in the pediatric patient often generates a significant amount of patient and parental concern. Although chest pain is rarely cardiac in origin in children, common knowledge about atherosclerotic heart disease raises concerns about a child experiencing chest pain. Most diagnosable chest pain in childhood is musculoskeletal in origin. A significant amount

Table 141-1	Differential Diagnosis of Pediatric Chest Pain

COMMON

Musculoskeletal

Costochondritis

Trauma or muscle overuse/strain

Pulmonary

Asthma (often exercise-induced)

Severe cough

Pneumonia

Gastrointestinal

Reflux esophagitis

Psychogenic

Anxiety, hyperventilation

Miscellaneous

Precordial catch syndrome (Texidor's twinge)

Sickle cell vasoocclusive crisis

Idiopathic

UNCOMMON/RARE

Cardiac

Ischemia (coronary artery abnormalities, severe AS or PS, HOCM, cocaine)

Infection/inflammation (myocarditis, pericarditis, Kawasaki disease)

Dysrhythmia

Musculoskeletal

Abnormalities of rib cage/thoracic spine

Tietze syndrome

Slipping rib

Tumor

Pulmonary

Pleurisy

Pneumothorax, pneumomediastinum

Pleural effusion

Pulmonary embolism

Gastrointestinal

Esophageal foreign body

Esophageal spasm

Psychogenic

Conversion symptoms

Somatization disorders

Depression

AS, Aortic stenosis; *HOCM,* hypertrophic obstructive cardiomyopathy; *PS,* pulmonary stenosis.

remains idiopathic, however. Knowledge of the complete differential diagnosis is necessary to make an accurate assessment (Table 141-1).

CLINICAL MANIFESTATIONS

Assessment of a patient with chest pain includes a thorough history to determine activity at the onset; the location, radiation, quality, and duration of the pain; what makes the pain better and worse during the time that it is present; and any associated symptoms. A family history and assessment of how much anxiety the symptom is causing are important and often revealing. A careful general physical examination should focus on the chest wall, heart, lungs, and abdomen. A history of chest pain associated with exertion, syncope, or palpitations or acute onset associated with fever suggests a cardiac etiology. Cardiac causes of chest pain are generally ischemic, inflammatory, or arrhythmic in origin.

DIAGNOSTIC STUDIES

Tests rarely are indicated based on the history. A chest x-ray, electrocardiogram (ECG), 24-hour Holter monitoring, echocardiogram, and exercise stress testing may be obtained based on history and examination. Referral to a pediatric cardiologist is based on the history, physical examination findings, family history, and, frequently, the level of anxiety in the patient or family members regarding the pain.

Chapter **142**

DYSRHYTHMIAS

Decision-Making Algorithm
Available @ StudentConsult.com

Palpitations

ETIOLOGY AND DIFFERENTIAL DIAGNOSIS

Cardiac dysrhythmias or abnormal heart rhythms are uncommon in pediatrics but may be caused by infection and inflammation, structural lesions, metabolic abnormalities, and intrinsic conduction abnormalities (Table 142-1). Many pediatric dysrhythmias are normal variants that do not require treatment or even further evaluation.

Sinus rhythm originates in the sinus node and has a normal axis P wave (upright in leads I and AVF) preceding each QRS complex. Because normal rates vary with age, sinus bradycardia and sinus tachycardia are defined based on age. **Sinus arrhythmia** is a common finding in children and represents a normal variation in the heart rate associated with breathing. The heart rate increases with inspiration and decreases with expiration, producing a recurring pattern on the electrocardiogram (ECG) tracing. Sinus arrhythmia is normal and does not require further evaluation or treatment.

Table 142-1	Etiology of Dysrhythmias

DRUGS

Intoxication (cocaine, tricyclic antidepressants, and others)

Antiarrhythmic agents (proarrhythmic agents [quinidine])

Sympathomimetic agents (caffeine, theophylline, ephedrine, and others)

Digoxin

INFECTION AND POSTINFECTION

Myocarditis

Lyme disease

Endocarditis

Diphtheria

Guillain-Barré syndrome

Rheumatic fever

METABOLIC-ENDOCRINE

Electrolyte disturbances ($\downarrow\uparrow K^+$, $\downarrow\uparrow Ca^{2+}$, $\downarrow Mg^{2+}$)

Cardiomyopathy

Thyrotoxicosis

Uremia

Pheochromocytoma

Porphyria

Mitochondrial myopathies

STRUCTURAL LESIONS

Congenital heart defects

Ventricular tumor

Ventriculotomy

Arrhythmogenic right ventricle (dysplasia)

OTHER CAUSES

Adrenergic-induced

Prolonged QT interval

Maternal systemic lupus erythematosus

Idiopathic

Central venous catheter

Atrial Dysrhythmias

A **wandering atrial pacemaker** is a change in the morphology of the P waves with variable PR interval and normal QRS complex. This is a benign finding, requiring no further evaluation or treatment.

Premature atrial contractions are relatively common prenatally and in infants. A premature P wave, usually with an abnormal axis consistent with its ectopic origin, is present. The premature atrial activity may be blocked (no QRS following it), conducted normally (normal QRS present), or conducted aberrantly (a widened, altered QRS complex). Premature atrial contractions are usually benign and, if present around the time of delivery, usually disappear during the first few weeks of life.

Atrial flutter and **atrial fibrillation** are uncommon dysrhythmias in pediatrics and usually present after surgical repair of complex congenital heart disease. They may also be seen in patients with myocarditis or in association with drug toxicity.

Supraventricular tachycardia (SVT) is the most common symptomatic dysrhythmia in pediatric patients. The rhythm has a rapid, regular rate with a narrow QRS complex. SVT in infants is often 280 to 300 beats/minute with slower rates for older children and adolescents. The tachycardia has an abrupt onset and termination. In a child with a structurally normal heart, most episodes are relatively asymptomatic other than a pounding heartbeat. If there is structural heart disease or the episode is prolonged (>12 hours), there may be alteration in the cardiac output and development of symptoms of heart failure. Although most patients with SVT have structurally normal hearts and normal baseline ECGs, some children have Wolff-Parkinson-White syndrome or preexcitation as the cause of the dysrhythmia.

Ventricular Dysrhythmias

Premature ventricular contractions (PVCs) are less common than premature atrial contractions in infancy but more common in older children and adolescents (Table 142-2). The premature beat is not preceded by a P wave and the QRS complex is wide and bizarre. If the heart is structurally normal, and the PVCs are singleton, uniform in focus, and disappear with increased heart rate. The PVCs are usually benign and require no treatment. Any deviation from the presentation (history of syncope or a family history of sudden death) requires further investigation and possibly treatment with antiarrhythmic medications.

Ventricular tachycardia, defined as three or more consecutive PVCs, is also relatively rare in pediatric patients. Although there are multiple causes of ventricular tachycardia, it usually is a sign of serious cardiac dysfunction or disease. Rapid-rate ventricular tachycardia results in decreased cardiac output and cardiovascular instability. Treatment in symptomatic patients is synchronized cardioversion. Medical management with lidocaine or amiodarone may be appropriate in a conscious asymptomatic patient. Complete evaluation of the etiologic picture is necessary, including electrophysiologic study.

Heart Block

First-degree heart block is the presence of a prolonged PR interval. It is asymptomatic and, when present in otherwise normal children, requires no evaluation or treatment. **Second-degree heart block** is when some, but not all, of the P waves are followed by a QRS complex. Mobitz type I (also known as Wenckebach) is characterized by a progressive prolongation of the PR interval until a QRS complex is dropped. It is often seen during sleep, usually does not progress to other forms of heart block, and does not require further evaluation or treatment in otherwise normal children. Mobitz type II is present when the PR interval does not change, but a QRS is intermittently dropped. This form may progress to complete heart block and may require pacemaker placement. **Third-degree heart block**, whether congenital or acquired, is present when there is no relationship between atrial and ventricular activity. The ventricular rate is much slower than the atrial rate. **Congenital complete heart block** is associated with maternal collagen vascular disease (such as systemic lupus erythematosus or Sjögren syndrome) or congenital heart disease. The acquired form most often occurs after cardiac surgery but may be secondary to infection, inflammation, or drugs.

Table 142-2	Dysrhythmias in Children	
TYPE	**ECG CHARACTERISTICS**	**TREATMENT**
Supraventricular tachycardia	Rate usually >220 beats/min (range, 180–320 beats/min); abnormal atrial rate for age; P waves may be present and are related to QRS complex; normal, narrow QRS complexes unless aberrant conduction is present	Increase vagal tone (bag of ice water to face, Valsalva maneuver); adenosine; digoxin; sotalol; electrical cardioversion if acutely ill; catheter ablation
Atrial flutter	Atrial rate usually 300 beats/min, with varying degrees of block; sawtooth flutter waves	Digoxin, sotalol, cardioversion
Premature ventricular contraction	Premature, wide, unusually shaped QRS complex, with large inverted T wave	None if normal heart and if premature ventricular contractions disappear on exercise; lidocaine, procainamide
Ventricular tachycardia	>3 Premature ventricular beats; AV dissociation; fusion beats, blocked retrograde AV conduction; sustained if >30 sec; rate 120–240 beats/min	Lidocaine, amiodarone, procainamide, propranolol, cardioversion
Ventricular fibrillation	No distinct QRS complex or T waves; irregular undulations with varied amplitude and contour, no conducted pulse	Nonsynchronized cardioversion
Complete heart block	Atria and ventricles have independent pacemakers; AV dissociation; escape-pacemaker is at atrioventricular junction if congenital	Awake rate <55 beats/min in neonate or <40 beats/min in adolescent, or hemodynamic instability requires permanent pacemaker
First-degree heart block	Prolonged PR interval for age	Observe, obtain digoxin level if on therapy
Mobitz type I (Wenckebach) second-degree heart block	Progressive lengthening of PR interval until P wave is not followed by conducted QRS complex	Observe, correct underlying electrolyte or other abnormalities
Mobitz type II second-degree heart block	Sudden nonconduction of P wave with loss of QRS complex without progressive PR interval lengthening	Consider pacemaker
Sinus tachycardia	Rate <240 beats/min	Treat cause (fever), remove sympathomimetic drugs

AV, Atrioventricular; *ECG,* electrocardiogram.

Table 142-3	Classification of Drugs for Antiarrhythmia	
CLASS	**ACTION**	**EXAMPLE(S)**
I	Depression of phase of depolarization (velocity of upstroke of action potential); sodium channel blockade	
Ia	Prolongation of QRS complex and QT interval	Quinidine, procainamide, disopyramide
Ib	Significant effect on abnormal conduction	Lidocaine, mexiletine, phenytoin, tocainide
Ic	Prolongation of QRS complex and PR interval	Flecainide, propafenone, moricizine?
II	β blockade; slowing of sinus rate; prolongation of PR interval	Propranolol, atenolol, acebutolol
III	Prolongation of action potential; prolongation of PR, QT intervals, QRS complex; sodium and calcium channel blockade	Bretylium, amiodarone, sotalol
IV	Calcium channel blockade; reduction in sinus and AV node pacemaker activity and conduction; prolongation of PR interval	Verapamil and other calcium channel blocking agents

AV, Atrioventricular.

TREATMENT

Most atrial dysrhythmias require no intervention. Treatment of SVT depends on presentation and symptoms. Acute treatment of SVT in infants usually consists of **vagal maneuvers,** such as application of cold (ice bag) to the face. Intravenous (IV) **adenosine** usually converts the dysrhythmia because the atrioventricular node forms a part of the reentry circuit in most patients with SVT. In patients with cardiovascular compromise at the time of presentation, **synchronized cardioversion** is indicated using 1 to 2 J/kg. In patients with palpitations, it is important to document heart rate and rhythm during their symptoms before considering therapeutic options. The frequency, length, and associated symptoms during the episodes, as well as what is required to convert the rhythm, determine the need for treatment. Some patients require only education regarding the dysrhythmia and follow-up. Ongoing pharmacologic management with either digoxin or a β-blocker is usually the first choice. However, digoxin is contraindicated in patients with Wolff-Parkinson-White syndrome. Additional antiarrhythmic medications are rarely needed. In patients who are symptomatic or those not wanting to take daily medications, **radiofrequency ablation** may be performed.

A variety of antiarrhythmic agents are used to treat ventricular dysrhythmias that require intervention (Table 142-3). Management of third-degree heart block depends on the ventricular rate and presence of symptoms. Treatment, if needed, often requires placement of a pacemaker.

Chapter **143**

ACYANOTIC CONGENITAL HEART DISEASE

Decision-Making Algorithm
Available @ StudentConsult.com

Heart Murmurs

Table 143-1	Classification of Congenital Cardiac Defects			
	SHUNTING			
STENOTIC	**RIGHT → LEFT**	**LEFT → RIGHT**	**MIXING**	
Aortic stenosis	Tetralogy	Patent ductus arteriosus	Truncus	
Pulmonary stenosis	Transposition	Ventricular septal defect	TAPVR	
Coarctation of the aorta	Tricuspid atresia	Atrial septal defect	HLH	

HLH, Hypoplastic left heart syndrome; *TAPVR,* total anomalous pulmonary venous return.

ETIOLOGY AND EPIDEMIOLOGY

Congenital heart disease occurs in 8 per 1000 births. The spectrum of lesions ranges from asymptomatic to fatal. Although most cases of congenital heart disease are multifactorial, some lesions are associated with chromosomal disorders, single gene defects, teratogens, or maternal metabolic disease (see Table 139-2).

Congenital heart defects can be divided into three pathophysiologic groups (Table 143-1).
1. Left-to-right shunts
2. Right-to-left shunts
3. Obstructive, stenotic lesions

Acyanotic congenital heart disease includes left-to-right shunts resulting in an increase in pulmonary blood flow (patent ductus arteriosus [PDA], ventricular septal defect [VSD], atrial septal defect [ASD]) and obstructive lesions (aortic stenosis, pulmonary stenosis, coarctation of the aorta), which usually have normal pulmonary blood flow.

VENTRICULAR SEPTAL DEFECT
Etiology and Epidemiology

The ventricular septum is a complex structure that can be divided into four components. The largest component is the **muscular septum**. The inlet or posterior septum comprises **endocardial cushion tissue**. The subarterial or **supracristal septum** comprises conotruncal tissue. The **membranous septum** is below the aortic valve and is relatively small. VSDs occur when any of these components fails to develop normally (Fig. 143-1). VSD, the most common congenital heart defect, accounts for 25% of all congenital heart disease. **Perimembranous VSDs** are the most common of all VSDs (67%).

Although the location of the VSD is important prognostically and in approach to repair, the amount of flow crossing a VSD depends on the size of the defect and the pulmonary vascular resistance. Large VSDs are not symptomatic at birth because the pulmonary vascular resistance is normally elevated at this time. As the pulmonary vascular resistance decreases over the first 6 to 8 weeks of life, the amount of shunt increases, and symptoms may develop.

Clinical Manifestations

Small VSDs with little shunt are often asymptomatic but have a loud murmur. Moderate to large VSDs result in pulmonary

Figure 143-1 Ventricular septal defect. *AO,* Aorta; *LA,* left atrium; *LV,* left ventricle; *PA,* pulmonary artery; *RA,* right atrium; *RV,* right ventricle.

overcirculation and heart failure. The typical physical finding with a VSD is a **pansystolic murmur**, usually heard best at the lower left sternal border. There may be a thrill. Large shunts increase flow across the mitral valve causing a **mid-diastolic murmur** at the apex. The splitting of S_2 and intensity of P_2 depend on the pulmonary artery pressure.

Imaging Studies

Electrocardiogram (ECG) and chest x-ray findings depend on the size of the VSD. Small VSDs usually have normal studies. Larger VSDs cause volume overload to the left side of the heart, resulting in ECG findings of left atrial and ventricular enlargement and hypertrophy. A chest x-ray may reveal cardiomegaly, enlargement of the left ventricle, an increase in the pulmonary artery silhouette, and increased pulmonary blood flow. Pulmonary hypertension due to either increased flow or increased pulmonary vascular resistance may lead to right ventricular enlargement and hypertrophy.

Treatment

Approximately one third of all VSDs close spontaneously. Small VSDs usually close spontaneously and, if they do not

Figure 143-2 Atrial septal defect. *AO*, Aorta; *LA*, left atrium; *LV*, left ventricle; *PA*, pulmonary artery; *RA*, right atrium; *RV*, right ventricle.

Figure 143-3 Patent ductus arteriosus. *AO*, Aorta; *LA*, left atrium; *LV*, left ventricle; *PA*, pulmonary artery; *RA*, right atrium; *RV*, right ventricle.

close, surgical closure may not be required. Initial treatment for moderate to large VSDs includes **diuretics (± digoxin)** and **afterload reduction**. Continued poor growth or pulmonary hypertension despite therapy requires closure of the defect. Most VSDs are closed surgically, but some VSDs, especially muscular defects, can be closed with **devices** placed at cardiac catheterization.

ATRIAL SEPTAL DEFECT
Etiology and Epidemiology
During the embryologic development of the heart, a septum grows toward the endocardial cushions to divide the atria. Failure of septal growth or excessive reabsorption of tissue leads to ASDs (Fig. 143-2). ASDs represent approximately 10% of all congenital heart defects. A secundum defect, with the hole in the region of the foramen ovale, is the most common ASD. A **primum ASD**, located near the endocardial cushions, may be part of a complete atrioventricular canal defect or may be present with an intact ventricular septum. The least common ASD is the **sinus venosus defect**, which may be associated with anomalous pulmonary venous return.

Clinical Manifestations
The pathophysiology and amount of shunting depend on the size of the defect and the relative compliance of the both ventricles. Even with large ASDs and significant shunts, infants and children are rarely symptomatic. A prominent **right ventricular impulse** at the left lower sternal border (LLSB) often can be palpated. A soft (grade I or II) **systolic ejection murmur** in the region of the right ventricular outflow tract and a **fixed split S_2** (due to overload of the right ventricle with prolonged ejection into the pulmonary circuit) are often audible. A larger shunt may result in a mid-diastolic murmur at the LLSB as a result of the increased volume passing across the tricuspid valve.

Imaging Studies
ECG and chest x-ray findings reflect the **increased blood flow** through the right atrium, right ventricle, pulmonary arteries,

and lungs. The ECG may show **right axis deviation** and **right ventricular enlargement**. A chest radiograph may show cardiomegaly, right atrial enlargement, and a prominent pulmonary artery.

Treatment
Medical management is rarely indicated. If a significant shunt is still present at around 3 years of age, closure is usually recommended. Many secundum ASDs can be closed with an ASD **closure device** in the catheterization laboratory. Primum and sinus venosus defects require **surgical closure**.

PATENT DUCTUS ARTERIOSUS
Etiology and Epidemiology
The ductus arteriosus allows blood to flow from the pulmonary artery to the aorta during fetal life. Failure of the normal closure of this vessel results in a PDA (Fig. 143-3). With a falling pulmonary vascular resistance after birth, left-to-right shunting of blood and increased pulmonary blood flow occur. Excluding premature infants, PDAs represent approximately 5% to 10% of congenital heart disease.

Clinical Manifestations
Symptoms depend on the amount of pulmonary blood flow. The magnitude of the shunt depends on the size of the PDA (diameter, length, and tortuosity) and the pulmonary vascular resistance. Small PDAs are asymptomatic; moderate to large shunts can produce the symptoms of heart failure as the pulmonary vascular resistance decreases.

The physical examination findings depend on the size of the shunt. A **widened pulse pressure** is often present as a result of the runoff of blood into the pulmonary circulation during diastole. A **continuous, machine-like murmur** can be heard at the left infraclavicular area, radiating along the pulmonary arteries and often well heard over the left side of the back. Larger shunts with increased flow across the mitral valve may

Figure 143-4 Atrioventricular canal defects. *AO,* Aorta; *LA,* left atrium; *LV,* left ventricle; *PA,* pulmonary artery; *RA,* right atrium; *RV,* right ventricle.

result in a mid-diastolic murmur at the apex and a **hyperdynamic precordium**. Splitting of S$_2$ and intensity of P$_2$ depend on the pulmonary artery pressure. A thrill may be palpable.

Imaging Studies
ECG and chest x-ray findings are normal with small PDAs. Moderate to large shunts may result in a **full pulmonary artery silhouette** and **increased pulmonary vascularity**. ECG findings vary from normal to evidence of left ventricular hypertrophy. If pulmonary hypertension is present, there is also right ventricular hypertrophy.

Treatment
Spontaneous closure of a PDA after a few weeks of age is uncommon in full-term infants. Moderate and large PDAs may be managed initially with **diuretics**, but eventually require closure. Elective closure of small, hemodynamically insignificant PDAs is controversial. Most PDAs can be closed in the catheterization laboratory by either **coil embolization** or a PDA **closure device**.

ENDOCARDIAL CUSHION DEFECT
Etiology and Epidemiology
Endocardial cushion defects, also referred to as **atrioventricular canal defects**, may be complete or partial (Fig. 143-4). Failure of the septum to fuse with the endocardial cushion results in **abnormal atrioventricular valves** as well. The complete defect results in a primum ASD, a posterior or inlet VSD, and clefts in the anterior leaflet of the mitral and septal leaflet of the tricuspid valves. In addition to left-to-right shunting at both levels, there may be **atrioventricular valve insufficiency**.

Clinical Manifestations
The symptoms of heart failure usually develop as the pulmonary vascular resistance decreases over the first 6 to 8 weeks of life. Symptoms may be earlier and more severe with significant

atrioventricular valve insufficiency. Pulmonary hypertension resulting from increased pulmonary circulation often develops early. The presence of murmurs varies depending on the amount of shunting at both atrial and ventricular levels. If there is a large VSD component, S$_2$ will be single. Growth is usually poor. Complete endocardial cushion defects are most commonly seen in children with Down syndrome.

Imaging Tests
The diagnosis usually is made with echocardiography. A chest radiograph reveals cardiomegaly with enlargement of all chambers and the presence of **increased vascularity**. An ECG reveals **left axis deviation** and **combined ventricular hypertrophy** and may show combined atrial enlargement.

Treatment
Initial management includes diuretics (± digoxin) and afterload reduction for treatment of heart failure. **Surgical repair** of the defect ultimately is required.

PULMONARY STENOSIS
Etiology
Pulmonary stenosis accounts for approximately 10% of all congenital heart disease and can be **valvular**, **subvalvular**, or **supravalvular** in nature. Pulmonary stenosis results from the failure of the development, in early gestation, of the three leaflets of the valve, insufficient resorption of infundibular tissue, or insufficient canalization of the peripheral pulmonary arteries.

Clinical Manifestations
Symptoms depend on the degree of obstruction present. Mild pulmonary stenosis is asymptomatic. Moderate to severe stenosis results in **exertional dyspnea** and easy **fatigability**. Newborns with severe stenosis may be more symptomatic and even cyanotic because of right-to-left shunting at the atrial level.

Pulmonary stenosis causes a systolic ejection murmur at the second left intercostal space which radiates to the back. A thrill may be present. S$_2$ may be widely split with a quiet pulmonary component. With more severe pulmonary stenosis, an impulse at the lower left sternal border results from **right ventricular hypertrophy**. Valvular stenosis may result in a **click** that varies with respiration. Worsening stenosis causes an increase in the duration of the murmur and a higher frequency of the sound. The systolic ejection murmurs of **peripheral pulmonary stenosis** are heard distal to the site of obstruction in the pulmonary circulation, including radiation to the back.

Imaging Tests
ECG and chest x-ray findings are normal in mild stenosis. Moderate to severe stenosis results in **right axis deviation** and **right ventricular hypertrophy**. The heart size is usually normal on chest x-ray, although **dilation of the main pulmonary artery** may be seen. Echocardiography provides assessment of the site of stenosis, degree of hypertrophy, and valve morphology, as well as an estimate of the pressure gradient.

Treatment

Valvular pulmonary stenosis usually does not progress, especially if it is mild. **Balloon valvuloplasty** is usually successful in reducing the gradient to acceptable levels for more significant or symptomatic stenosis. **Surgical repair** is required if balloon valvuloplasty is unsuccessful or when subvalvular (muscular) stenosis is present.

AORTIC STENOSIS
Etiology and Epidemiology

Valvular, **subvalvular**, or **supravalvular** aortic stenosis represents approximately 5% of all congenital heart disease. Lesions result from failure of development of the three leaflets or failure of resorption of tissue around the valve.

Clinical Manifestations

Mild to moderate obstructions cause no symptoms. More severe stenosis results in easy fatigability, exertional chest pain, and syncope. Infants with critical aortic stenosis may present with symptoms of heart failure.

A **systolic ejection murmur** is heard at the right second intercostal space along the sternum and radiating into the neck. The murmur increases in length and becomes higher in frequency as the degree of stenosis increases. With valvular stenosis, a **systolic ejection click** often is heard, and a thrill may be present at the right upper sternal border or in the suprasternal notch. The aortic component of S_2 may be decreased in intensity.

Imaging Studies

ECG and chest x-ray findings are normal with mild degrees of stenosis. **Left ventricular hypertrophy** develops with moderate to severe stenosis and is detected on the ECG and chest x-ray. **Dilation** of the ascending aorta or aortic knob due to an intrinsic aortopathy may be seen on chest radiographs. Echocardiography shows the site of stenosis, valve morphology, and the presence of left ventricular hypertrophy, and it allows an estimate of the pressure gradient.

Treatment

The degree of aortic stenosis frequently progresses with growth and age. Aortic insufficiency often develops or progresses. Serial follow-up with echocardiography is indicated. **Balloon valvuloplasty** is usually the first interventional procedure for significant stenosis. It is not as successful as pulmonary balloon valvuloplasty and has a higher risk of significant valvular insufficiency. **Surgical management** is necessary when balloon valvuloplasty is unsuccessful or significant valve insufficiency develops.

COARCTATION OF THE AORTA
Etiology and Epidemiology

Coarctation of the aorta occurs in approximately 10% of all congenital heart defects. It is almost always **juxtaductal** in position. During development of the aortic arch, the area near the insertion of the ductus arteriosus fails to develop correctly, resulting in a narrowing of the aortic lumen.

Clinical Manifestations

Timing of presentation depends on the severity of obstruction and associated cardiac defects. Infants presenting with coarctation of the aorta frequently have hypoplastic aortic arches, abnormal aortic valves, and VSDs. They may be dependent on a patent ductus arteriosus to provide descending aortic flow. Symptoms develop when the aortic ampulla of the ductus closes. Less severe obstruction causes no symptoms.

Symptoms, including poor feeding, respiratory distress, and shock, may develop before 2 weeks of age. Classically the **femoral pulses** are weaker and delayed compared with the right radial pulse. The blood pressure in the lower extremities is lower than that in the upper extremities. If cardiac function is poor, however, these differences may not be as apparent until appropriate resuscitation is accomplished. In this situation, there may be no murmur, but an S_3 is often present.

Older children presenting with coarctation of the aorta are usually asymptomatic. There may be a history of **leg discomfort** with exercise, headache, or epistaxis. Decreased or absent lower extremity pulses, **hypertension** (upper extremity), or a murmur may be present. The murmur is typically best heard in the left interscapular area of the back. If significant collaterals have developed, continuous murmurs may be heard throughout the chest. An abnormal aortic valve is present approximately 50% of the time, causing a systolic ejection click and systolic ejection murmur of aortic stenosis.

Imaging Studies

The ECG and chest x-ray show evidence of right ventricular enlargement and hypertrophy in infantile coarctation with marked **cardiomegaly** and **pulmonary edema**. Echocardiography shows the site of coarctation and associated lesions. In older children, the ECG and chest x-ray usually show left ventricular hypertrophy and a mildly enlarged heart. **Rib notching** may also be seen in older children (>8 years of age) with large collaterals. Echocardiography shows the site and degree of coarctation, presence of left ventricular hypertrophy, and aortic valve morphology and function.

Treatment

Management of an infant presenting with cardiac decompensation includes intravenous infusion of **prostaglandin E_1** (chemically opens the ductus arteriosus), inotropic agents, diuretics, and other supportive care. **Balloon angioplasty** has been done, especially in critically ill infants, but **surgical repair** of the coarctation is most commonly performed. Ballooning and stenting of older patients with coarctation has become more accepted as primary therapy, but surgical repair remains a common form of management.

Chapter **144**

CYANOTIC CONGENITAL HEART DISEASE

Decision-Making Algorithms
Available @ StudentConsult.com

Cyanosis
Heart Murmurs

Cyanotic congenital heart disease occurs when some of the systemic venous return crosses from the right side of the heart to the left and returns to the body without going through the lungs (**right-to-left shunt**). **Cyanosis**, the visible sign of this shunt, occurs when approximately 5 g/100 mL of reduced hemoglobin is present in systemic blood. Thus, a polycythemic patient appears cyanotic with a lower percentage of reduced hemoglobin. A patient with anemia requires a higher percentage of reduced hemoglobin for the recognition of cyanosis.

The most common cyanotic congenital heart defects are the five *Ts*:

Tetralogy of Fallot
Transposition of the great arteries
Tricuspid atresia
Truncus arteriosus
Total anomalous pulmonary venous return

Other congenital heart defects that allow complete mixing of systemic and pulmonary venous return can present with cyanosis depending on the amount of pulmonary blood flow that is present. Many cyanotic heart lesions present in the neonatal period (Table 144-1).

TETRALOGY OF FALLOT
Etiology and Epidemiology

Tetralogy of Fallot is the most common cyanotic congenital heart defect, representing about 10% of all congenital heart defects (Fig. 144-1). There are four structural defects: **ventricular septal defect (VSD)**, **pulmonary stenosis**, **overriding aorta**, and **right ventricular hypertrophy**. Tetralogy of Fallot is due to abnormal septation of the truncus arteriosus into the aorta and pulmonary artery that occurs early in gestation (3 to 4 weeks). The VSD is large and the pulmonary stenosis is most commonly subvalvular or infundibular. It may also be valvular, supravalvular, or, frequently, a combination of levels of obstruction.

Clinical Manifestations

Infants initially may be acyanotic. A **pulmonary stenosis murmur** is the usual initial abnormal finding. The amount of right-to-left shunting at the VSD (and the degree of cyanosis) increases as the degree of pulmonary stenosis increases. With increasing severity of pulmonary stenosis, the murmur becomes shorter and softer. In addition to varying degrees of cyanosis and a murmur, a **single S$_2$** and **right ventricular impulse** at the left sternal border are typical findings.

When **hypoxic (Tet) spells** occur, they are usually progressive. During a spell, the child typically becomes restless and agitated and may cry inconsolably. An ambulatory toddler may

Table 144-1	Categories of Presenting Symptoms and Signs in the Neonate		
SYMPTOM/SIGN	**PHYSIOLOGIC CATEGORY**	**ANATOMIC CAUSE**	**LESION**
Cyanosis with respiratory distress	Increased pulmonary blood flow	Transposition	d-Transposition with or without associated lesions
Cyanosis without respiratory distress	Decreased pulmonary blood flow	Right heart obstruction	Tricuspid atresia Ebstein anomaly Pulmonary atresia Pulmonary stenosis Tetralogy of Fallot
Hypoperfusion	Poor cardiac output	Left heart obstruction	Total anomalous pulmonary venous return with obstruction Aortic stenosis Hypoplastic left heart syndrome
	Poor cardiac function	Normal anatomy	Cardiomyopathy Myocarditis
Respiratory distress with desaturation (not visible cyanosis)	Bidirectional shunting	Complete mixing	Truncus arteriosus AV canal Complex single ventricle (including heterotaxias) without pulmonary stenosis
Respiratory distress with normal saturation	Left-to-right shunting	Simple intracardiac shunt	ASD VSD PDA Aortopulmonary window AVM

ASD, Atrial septal defect; *AV,* atrioventricular; *AVM,* arteriovenous malformation; *PDA,* patent ductus arteriosus; *VSD,* ventricular septal defect.

Figure 144-1 Tetralogy of Fallot. *AO,* Aorta; *LA,* left atrium; *LV,* left ventricle; *PA,* pulmonary artery; *RA,* right atrium; *RV,* right ventricle.

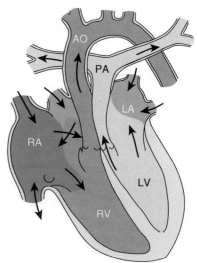

Figure 144-2 Transposition of the great vessels. *AO,* Aorta; *LA,* left atrium; *LV,* left ventricle; *PA,* pulmonary artery; *RA,* right atrium; *RV,* right ventricle.

squat. Hyperpnea occurs with gradually increasing cyanosis and loss of the murmur. In severe spells, prolonged unconsciousness and convulsions, hemiparesis, or death may occur. Independent of hypoxic spells, patients with unrepaired tetralogy of Fallot are at increased risk for cerebral thromboembolism and cerebral abscesses resulting, in part, from their right-to-left intracardiac shunt.

Imaging Studies

The electrocardiogram (ECG) usually has **right axis deviation** and **right ventricular hypertrophy**. The classic chest x-ray finding is a **boot-shaped heart** created by the small main pulmonary artery and upturned apex secondary to right ventricular hypertrophy. Echocardiography shows the anatomic features, including the anatomic level and quantification of pulmonary stenosis. Coronary anomalies, most commonly a left anterior descending coronary artery arising from the right coronary artery and crossing the anterior surface of the right ventricular outflow tract, are present in 5% of patients with tetralogy of Fallot.

Treatment

The natural history of tetralogy of Fallot is progression of pulmonary stenosis and cyanosis. Treatment of hypoxic spells consists of oxygen administration and placing the child in the knee-chest position (to increase venous return). Traditionally, morphine sulfate is given (to relax the pulmonary infundibulum and for sedation). If necessary, the systemic vascular resistance can be increased acutely through the administration of an α-adrenergic agonist (phenylephrine). The occurrence of a cyanotic spell is an indication to proceed with surgical repair.

Complete surgical repair with VSD closure and removal or patching of the pulmonary stenosis can be performed in infancy. Occasionally, **palliative shunt surgery** between the subclavian artery and pulmonary artery is performed for complex forms of tetralogy of Fallot and more complete repair is done at a later time. **Subacute bacterial endocarditis prophylaxis** is indicated until 6 months after complete repair unless there is a residual VSD. Prophylaxis is then continued as long as there is a residual VSD.

TRANSPOSITION OF THE GREAT ARTERIES
Etiology and Epidemiology

Although dextroposed transposition of the great arteries represents only about 5% of congenital heart defects, it is the most common cyanotic lesion to present in the newborn period (Fig. 144-2). Transposition of the great arteries is ventriculoarterial discordance secondary to abnormalities of septation of the truncus arteriosus. In dextroposed transposition, the aorta arises from the right ventricle, anterior and to the right of the pulmonary artery, which arises from the left ventricle. This results in desaturated blood returning to the right side of the heart and being pumped back out to the body, while well-oxygenated blood returning from the lungs enters the left side of the heart and is pumped back to the lungs. Without mixing of the two circulations, death occurs quickly. Mixing can occur at the atrial (patent foramen ovale/atrial septal defect [ASD]), ventricular [VSD], or great vessel (patent ductus arteriosus [PDA]) level.

Clinical Manifestations

A history of **cyanosis** is always present, although it depends on the amount of mixing. **Quiet tachypnea** and a **single S$_2$** are typically present. If the ventricular septum is intact, there may be no murmur.

Children with transposition and a large VSD have improved intracardiac mixing and less cyanosis. They may present with signs of heart failure. The heart is hyperdynamic, with palpable left and right ventricular impulses. A loud VSD murmur is heard. S$_2$ is single.

Imaging Studies

ECG findings typically include **right axis deviation** and **right ventricular hypertrophy**. The chest x-ray reveals **increased pulmonary vascularity**, and the cardiac shadow is classically an **egg on a string** created by the narrow superior mediastinum. Echocardiography shows the transposition of the great arteries, the sites and amount of mixing, and any associated lesions.

Figure 144-3 Tricuspid atresia with ventricular septal defect. *AO,* Aorta; *LA,* left atrium; *LV,* left ventricle; *PA,* pulmonary artery; *RA,* right atrium.

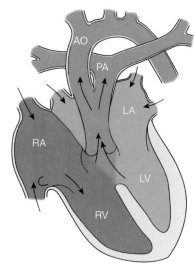

Figure 144-4 Truncus arteriosus. *AO,* Aorta; *LA,* left atrium; *LV,* left ventricle; *PA,* pulmonary artery; *RA,* right atrium; *RV,* right ventricle.

Treatment

Initial medical management includes **prostaglandin E₁** to maintain ductal patency. If significant hypoxia persists on prostaglandin therapy, a **balloon atrial septostomy** improves mixing between the two circulations. Complete surgical repair is most often an **arterial switch**. The arterial switch usually is performed within the first 2 weeks of life, when the left ventricle can still maintain systemic pressure.

TRICUSPID ATRESIA
Etiology and Epidemiology

Tricuspid atresia accounts for approximately 2% of all congenital heart defects (Fig. 144-3). The absence of the tricuspid valve results in a **hypoplastic right ventricle**. All systemic venous return must cross the atrial septum into the left atrium. A PDA or VSD is necessary for pulmonary blood flow and survival.

Clinical Manifestations

Infants with tricuspid atresia are usually **severely cyanotic** and have a **single S_2**. If a VSD is present, there may be a murmur. A diastolic murmur across the mitral valve may be audible. Frequently there is no significant murmur.

Imaging Studies

The ECG shows **left ventricular hypertrophy** and a **superior QRS axis** (between 0° and –90°). The chest x-ray reveals a normal or mildly enlarged cardiac silhouette with **decreased pulmonary blood flow**. Echocardiography shows the anatomy, associated lesions, and source of pulmonary blood flow.

Treatment

Management initially depends on the presence of a VSD and the amount of antegrade blood flow to the lungs. If there is no VSD, or it is small, prostaglandin E₁ maintains pulmonary

blood flow until surgery. Surgery is staged with an initial subclavian artery-to-pulmonary shunt (**Blalock-Taussig procedure**) typically followed by a two-stage procedure: **bidirectional cavopulmonary shunt (bidirectional Glenn)** and **Fontan procedure**. These surgeries direct systemic venous return directly to the pulmonary arteries.

TRUNCUS ARTERIOSUS
Etiology and Epidemiology

Truncus arteriosus occurs in less than 1% of all congenital heart disease (Fig. 144-4). It results from the failure of septation of the truncus during the first 3 to 4 weeks of gestation. A single arterial trunk arises from the heart with a large VSD immediately below the truncal valve. The pulmonary arteries arise from the single arterial trunk either as a single vessel that divides or individually from the arterial trunk to the lungs.

Clinical Manifestations

Varying degrees of cyanosis depend on the amount of pulmonary blood flow. If not diagnosed at birth, the infant may develop signs of heart failure as pulmonary vascular resistance decreases. The signs then include tachypnea and cough. Peripheral pulses are usually bounding as a result of the diastolic runoff into the pulmonary arteries. A single S_2 is due to the single valve. There may be a systolic ejection click, and there is often a **systolic murmur** at the left sternal border.

Imaging Studies

ECG findings include **combined ventricular hypertrophy** and **cardiomegaly**. A chest x-ray usually reveals **increased pulmonary blood** and may show displaced pulmonary arteries. Echocardiography defines the anatomy, including the VSD, truncal valve function, and origin of the pulmonary arteries.

Figure 144-5 Total anomalous pulmonary venous return. *AO,* Aorta; *IVC,* inferior vena cava; *LA,* left atrium; *LV,* left ventricle; *PA,* pulmonary artery; *PV,* pulmonary vein; *RA,* right atrium; *RV,* right ventricle; *SVC,* superior vena cava.

Figure 144-6 Hypoplastic left side of the heart. *AO,* Aorta; *LA,* left atrium; *LV,* left ventricle; *PA,* pulmonary artery; *PDA,* patent ductus arteriosus; *RA,* right atrium; *RV,* right ventricle.

Treatment

Medical management is usually needed and includes **anticongestive medications**. **Surgical repair** includes VSD closure and placement of a conduit between the right ventricle and pulmonary arteries.

TOTAL ANOMALOUS PULMONARY VENOUS RETURN
Etiology and Epidemiology

Total anomalous pulmonary venous return accounts for about 1% of congenital heart disease (Fig. 144-5). Disruption of the development of normal pulmonary venous drainage during the third week of gestation results in one of four abnormalities. All of the pulmonary veins fail to connect to the left atrium and return abnormally via the right side of the heart. They may have **supracardiac**, **infracardiac**, **cardiac**, or **mixed drainage**. An atrial-level communication is required for systemic cardiac output and survival.

Clinical Manifestations

The most important determinant of presentation is the presence or absence of **obstruction** to the pulmonary venous drainage. Infants without obstruction have minimal cyanosis and may be asymptomatic. There is a hyperactive **right ventricular impulse** with a **widely split S$_2$** (owing to increased right ventricular volume) and a **systolic ejection murmur** at the left upper sternal border. There is usually a mid-diastolic murmur at the lower left sternal border from the increased flow across the tricuspid valve. Growth is relatively poor. Infants with **obstruction** present with cyanosis, marked tachypnea and dyspnea, and signs of right-sided heart failure including hepatomegaly. The obstruction results in little, if any, increase in right ventricular volume, so there may be no murmur or changes in S$_2$.

Imaging Studies

For infants without obstruction, the ECG is consistent with right ventricular volume overload. Cardiomegaly with

increased pulmonary blood flow is seen on chest x-ray. Infants with obstructed veins have right axis deviation and right ventricular hypertrophy on ECG. On chest x-ray, the heart is normal or mildly enlarged with varying degrees of pulmonary edema that can appear similar to hyaline membrane disease or pneumonia. Echocardiography shows the volume-overloaded right side of the heart, right-to-left atrial level shunting, and common pulmonary vein site of drainage and degree of obstruction.

Treatment

At **surgery**, the common pulmonary vein is opened into the left atrium, and there is ligation of any vein or channel that had been draining the common vein.

HYPOPLASTIC LEFT HEART SYNDROME
Etiology and Epidemiology

Hypoplastic left heart syndrome accounts for 1% of all congenital heart defects (Fig. 144-6) but is the most common cause of death from cardiac defects in the first month of life. Hypoplastic left heart syndrome occurs when there is failure of development of the mitral or aortic valve or the aortic arch. A small left ventricle that is unable to support normal systemic circulation is a central finding, regardless of etiology. Associated degrees of hypoplasia of the ascending aorta and aortic arch are present. Left-to-right shunting occurs at the atrial level.

Clinical Manifestations

The newborn is dependent on right-to-left shunting at the ductus arteriosus for systemic blood flow. As the ductus arteriosus constricts, the infant becomes critically ill with signs and symptoms of heart failure from excessive pulmonary blood flow and obstruction of systemic blood flow. Pulses are diffusely weak or absent. S$_2$ is single and loud. There is usually no heart murmur. Cyanosis may be minimal, but **low cardiac output** gives a grayish color to the cool, mottled skin.

Table 144-2	Extracardiac Complications of Cyanotic Congenital Heart Disease	
PROBLEM	**ETIOLOGY**	**THERAPY**
Polycythemia	Persistent hypoxia	Phlebotomy
Relative anemia	Nutritional deficiency	Iron replacement
CNS abscess	Right-to-left shunting	Antibiotics, drainage
CNS thromboembolic stroke	Right-to-left shunting or polycythemia	Phlebotomy
Gingival disease	Polycythemia, gingivitis, bleeding	Dental hygiene
Gout	Polycythemia, diuretic agents	Allopurinol
Arthritis, clubbing	Hypoxic arthropathy	None
Pregnancy	Poor placental perfusion, poor ability to increase cardiac output	Bed rest
Infectious disease	Associated asplenia, DiGeorge syndrome	Antibiotics
	Fatal RSV pneumonia with pulmonary hypertension	Ribavirin, RSV immune globulin
Growth	Failure to thrive, increased oxygen consumption, decreased nutrient intake	Treat heart failure; correct defect early
Psychosocial adjustment	Limited activity, peer pressure; chronic disease, multiple hospitalizations, cardiac surgical techniques	Counseling

CNS, Central nervous system; *RSV,* respiratory syncytial virus.

Imaging Studies

ECG findings include **right ventricular hypertrophy** with **decreased left ventricular forces**. The chest x-ray reveals **cardiomegaly** (with right-sided enlargement) and pulmonary venous congestion or pulmonary edema. Echocardiography shows the small left side of the heart, the degree of stenosis of the aortic and mitral valves, the hypoplastic ascending aorta, and the adequacy of left-to-right atrial flow and right-to-left ductal flow.

Treatment

Medical management includes **prostaglandin E₁** to open the ductus arteriosus, correction of acidosis, and ventilatory and blood pressure support as needed. **Surgical repair** is staged with the first surgery (Norwood procedure) done in the newborn period. Subsequent procedures create a systemic source for the pulmonary circulation (bidirectional Glenn and Fontan procedures), leaving the right ventricle to supply systemic circulation. There have been many modifications to all three stages of the repair. Prognosis for survival has improved significantly over the past two decades.

COMPLICATIONS OF CONGENITAL HEART DISEASE

Extracardiac complications are summarized in Table 144-2.

Chapter 145

HEART FAILURE

ETIOLOGY AND EPIDEMIOLOGY

The force generated by the cardiac muscle fiber depends on its contractile status and basal length, which is equivalent to

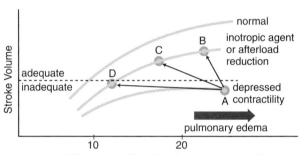

Figure 145-1 Ventricular function curve illustrating the effect of inotropic agents or arterial vasodilators. In contrast to diuretics, the effect of digitalis or arterial vasodilator therapy in a patient with heart failure is movement onto another ventricular function curve intermediate between the normal and the depressed curves. When the patient's ventricular function moves from *A* to *B* by the administration of one of these agents, the left ventricular end-diastolic pressure may also decrease because of improved cardiac function; further administration of diuretics or venodilators may shift the function further to the left along the same curve from *B* to *C* and eliminate the risk of pulmonary edema. A vasodilating agent that has arteriolar and venous dilating properties (e.g., nitroprusside) would shift this function directly from *A* to *C*. If this agent shifts the function from *A* to *D* because of excessive venodilation or administration of diuretics, the cardiac output may decrease too much, even though the left ventricular end-diastolic pressure would be normal (10 mm Hg) for a normal heart. Left ventricular end-diastolic pressures of 15 to 18 mm Hg are usually optimal in the failing heart to maximize cardiac output, but to avoid pulmonary edema. *(From Andreoli TE, Carpenter CCJ, Griggs RC, Loscalzo J, editors: Cecil essentials of medicine, ed 5, Philadelphia, Saunders, 2001.)*

the preload. As the preload (fiber length, left ventricular filling pressure, or volume) increases, myocardial performance (stroke volume and wall tension) increases up to a point (the normal Starling curve). The relationship is the **ventricular function curve** (Fig. 145-1). Alterations in the contractile state of the muscle lower the relative position of the curve, but retain the relationship of fiber length to muscle work. Heart rate is another important determinant of cardiac work because the cardiac output equals stroke volume times the heart rate. Additional factors also affect cardiac performance (Table 145-1).

Heart failure occurs when the heart is unable to pump blood at a rate commensurate with metabolic needs (oxygen delivery). It may be due to a change in **myocardial contractility** that results in low cardiac output or to **abnormal loading conditions** being placed on the myocardium. The abnormal loading conditions may be **afterload** (pressure overload, such as with aortic stenosis, pulmonary stenosis, or coarctation of the aorta) or **preload** (volume overload, such as in ventricular septal defect (VSD), patent ductus arteriosus (PDA), or valvular insufficiency. Volume overload is the most common cause of heart failure in children.

The age of presentation is helpful in creating the differential diagnosis (Table 145-2). In the first weeks of life, excessive afterload being placed on the myocardium is most common. Heart failure presenting around 2 months of age is usually due to increasing left-to-right shunts that become apparent as the pulmonary vascular resistance decreases. Acquired heart disease, such as myocarditis and cardiomyopathy, can present at any age.

Table 145-1	Factors Affecting Cardiac Performance
PRELOAD (LEFT VENTRICULAR DIASTOLIC VOLUME)	
Total blood volume	
Venous tone (sympathetic tone)	
Body position	
Intrathoracic and intrapericardial pressure	
Atrial contraction	
Pumping action of skeletal muscle	
AFTERLOAD (IMPEDANCE AGAINST WHICH THE LEFT VENTRICLE MUST EJECT BLOOD)	
Peripheral vascular resistance	
Left ventricular volume (preload, wall tension)	
Physical characteristics of the arterial tree (elasticity of vessels or presence of outflow obstruction)	
CONTRACTILITY (CARDIAC PERFORMANCE INDEPENDENT OF PRELOAD OR AFTERLOAD)	
Sympathetic nerve impulses*	
Circulating catecholamines*	
Digitalis, calcium, other inotropic agents*	
Increased heart rate or postextrasystolic augmentation*	
Anoxia, acidosis†	
Pharmacologic depression†	
Loss of myocardium†	
Intrinsic depression†	
HEART RATE	
Autonomic nervous system	
Temperature, metabolic rate	

From Andreoli TE, Carpenter CCJ, Griggs RC, Loscalzo J: Cecil Essentials of Medicine, ed 5, Philadelphia, 2001, Saunders.
*Increases contractility.
†Decreases contractility.

Table 145-2	Etiology of Heart Failure by Age Group
FETUS	
Severe anemia (hemolysis, fetal-maternal transfusion, hypoplastic anemia)	
Supraventricular tachycardia	
Ventricular tachycardia	
Complete heart block	
Atrioventricular valve insufficiency	
High-output cardiac failure (arteriovenous malformation, teratoma)	
PREMATURE NEONATE	
Fluid overload	
PDA	
VSD	
Cor pulmonale (BPD)	
FULL-TERM NEONATE	
Asphyxial cardiomyopathy	
Arteriovenous malformation (vein of Galen, hepatic)	
Left-sided obstructive lesions (coarctation of aorta, hypoplastic left heart, critical aortic stenosis)	
Transposition of great arteries	
Large mixing cardiac defects (single ventricle, truncus arteriosus)	
Viral myocarditis	
Anemia	
Supraventricular tachycardia	
Complete heart block	
INFANT/TODDLER	
Left-to-right cardiac shunts (VSD)	
Hemangioma (arteriovenous malformation)	
Anomalous left coronary artery	
Metabolic cardiomyopathy	
Acute hypertension (hemolytic uremic syndrome)	
Supraventricular tachycardia	
Kawasaki disease	
Postoperative repair of congenital heart disease	
CHILD/ADOLESCENT	
Rheumatic fever	
Acute hypertension (glomerulonephritis)	
Viral myocarditis	
Thyrotoxicosis	
Hemochromatosis/hemosiderosis	
Cancer therapy (radiation, doxorubicin)	
Sickle cell anemia	
Endocarditis	
Cor pulmonale (cystic fibrosis)	
Arrhythmias	
Chronic upper airway obstruction (cor pulmonale)	
Unrepaired or palliated congenital heart disease	
Cardiomyopathy	

BPD, Bronchopulmonary dysplasia; PDA, patent ductus arteriosus; VSD, ventricular septal defect.

CLINICAL MANIFESTATIONS

Decision-Making Algorithm
Available @ StudentConsult.com

Edema

Heart failure presents in infants as poor feeding, failure to thrive, tachypnea, and diaphoresis with feeding. Older children may present with shortness of breath, easy fatigability, and edema. The physical examination findings depend on whether pulmonary venous congestion, systemic venous congestion, or both are present. Tachycardia, a gallop rhythm, and thready pulses may be present with either cause. If left-sided

Table 145-3	Treatment of Heart Failure
THERAPY	**MECHANISM**
GENERAL CARE	
Rest	Reduces cardiac output
Oxygen	Improves oxygenation in presence of pulmonary edema
Sodium, fluid restrictions	Decreases vascular congestion; decreases preload
DIURETICS	
Furosemide	Salt excretion by way of ascending loop of Henle; reduces preload; afterload reduced with control of hypertension; may also cause venodilation
Combination of distal tubule and loop diuretics	Greater sodium excretion
INOTROPIC AGENTS	
Digitalis	Inhibits membrane Na+, K+-ATPase and increases intracellular Ca2+, improves cardiac contractility, increases myocardial oxygen consumption
Dopamine	Releases myocardial norepinephrine plus direct effect on β-receptor, may increase systemic blood pressure; at low infusion rates, dilates renal artery, facilitating diuresis
Dobutamine	β₁-Receptor agent; often combined with dopamine
Amrinone/ milrinone	Nonsympathomimetic, noncardiac glycosides with inotropic effects; may cause vasodilation
AFTERLOAD REDUCTION	
Hydralazine	Arteriolar vasodilator
Nitroprusside	Arterial and venous relaxation; venodilation reduces preload
Captopril/enalapril	Inhibition of angiotensin-converting enzyme; reduces angiotensin II production
OTHER MEASURES	
Mechanical counterpulsation	Improves coronary flow, afterload
Transplantation	Removes diseased heart
Extracorporeal membrane oxygenation	Bypasses heart
Carvedilol	β-Blocking agent

failure is predominant, tachypnea, orthopnea, wheezing, and pulmonary edema are seen. Hepatomegaly, edema, and distended neck veins are signs of right-sided failure.

IMAGING STUDIES

The absence of cardiomegaly on a chest x-ray usually rules out the diagnosis of heart failure. An echocardiogram assesses the heart chamber sizes, measures myocardial function, and diagnoses congenital heart defects when present.

TREATMENT

Initial treatment is directed at improving myocardial function and optimizing preload and afterload. Diuretics, inotropic support, and, often, **afterload reduction** are employed (Table 145-3). Long-term therapy usually consists of diuretics and afterload reduction is added. Long-term therapy with **β-blockers** also may be beneficial, although this remains somewhat controversial in pediatric patients. Spironolactone is usually added to the medical regimen because of its effect on cardiac remodeling.

Chapter **146**

RHEUMATIC FEVER

ETIOLOGY AND EPIDEMIOLOGY

Although uncommon in the United States, *acute* rheumatic fever remains an important preventable cause of cardiac disease. It is most common in children 6 to 15 years of age. It is due to an immunologic reaction that is a delayed sequela of group A beta-hemolytic streptococcal infections of the pharynx. A family history of rheumatic fever and lower socioeconomic status are additional factors.

CLINICAL MANIFESTATIONS

Decision-Making Algorithms
Available @ StudentConsult.com

Heart Murmurs
Arthritis
Involuntary Movements
Fever and Rash

Acute rheumatic fever is diagnosed using the clinical and laboratory findings of the **revised Jones criteria** (Table 146-1). The presence of either two **major criteria** or one major and two **minor criteria**, along with evidence of an antecedent **streptococcal infection**, confirm a diagnosis of acute rheumatic fever. The infection often precedes the presentation of rheumatic fever by 2 to 6 weeks. Streptococcal antibody tests, such as the antistreptolysin O titer, are the most reliable laboratory evidence of prior infection.

Table 146-1	Major Jones Criteria for Diagnosis of Acute Rheumatic Fever*,†
SIGN	**COMMENTS**
Polyarthritis	Common; swelling, limited motion, tender, erythema
	Migratory; involves large joints but rarely small or unusual joints, such as vertebrae
Carditis	Common; pancarditis, valves, pericardium, myocardium
	Tachycardia greater than explained by fever; new murmur of mitral or aortic insufficiency; Carey-Coombs mid-diastolic murmur; heart failure
Chorea (Sydenham disease)	Uncommon; manifests long after infection has resolved; more common in females; antineuronal antibody positive
Erythema marginatum	Uncommon; pink macules on trunk and proximal extremities, evolving to serpiginous border with central clearing; evanescent, elicited by application of local heat; nonpruritic
Subcutaneous nodules	Uncommon; associated with repeated episodes and severe carditis; located over extensor surface of elbows, knees, knuckles, and ankles or scalp and spine; firm, nontender

*Minor criteria include fever (temperatures of 101°–102°F [38.2°–38.9°C]), arthralgias, previous rheumatic fever, leukocytosis, elevated erythrocyte sedimentation rate/C-reactive protein, and prolonged PR interval.
†One major and two minor, or two major, criteria with evidence of recent group A streptococcal disease (e.g., scarlet fever, positive throat culture, or elevated antistreptolysin O or other antistreptococcal antibodies) strongly suggest the diagnosis of acute rheumatic fever.

Arthritis is the most common major manifestation. It usually involves the large joints and is migratory. Arthralgia cannot be used as a minor manifestation if arthritis is used as a major manifestation. **Carditis** occurs in about 50% of patients. Tachycardia, a new murmur (mitral or aortic regurgitation), pericarditis, cardiomegaly, and signs of heart failure are evidence of carditis. **Erythema marginatum**, a serpiginous, non-pruritic, and evanescent rash, is uncommon, occurs on the trunk, and is brought out by warmth. **Subcutaneous nodules** are seen predominantly with chronic or recurrent disease. They are firm, painless, nonpruritic, mobile nodules found on the extensor surfaces of the large and small joints, the scalp, and the spine. **Chorea** (Sydenham chorea or St. Vitus dance) consists of neurologic and psychiatric signs. It also is uncommon and often presents long after the infection.

TREATMENT AND PREVENTION

Management of acute rheumatic fever consists of **benzathine penicillin** to eradicate the beta-hemolytic streptococcus, anti-inflammatory therapy with **salicylates**, and **bed rest.** Additional supportive therapy for heart failure or chorea may be necessary. **Long-term penicillin prophylaxis**, preferably with intramuscular benzathine penicillin G, 1.2 million U every 28 days, is required. Oral regimens for prophylaxis generally are not as effective. The prognosis of acute rheumatic fever depends on the degree of permanent cardiac damage. Cardiac involvement may resolve completely, especially if it is

the first episode and the prophylactic regimen is followed. The severity of cardiac involvement worsens with each recurrence of rheumatic fever.

Chapter 147

CARDIOMYOPATHIES

ETIOLOGY

A cardiomyopathy is an intrinsic disease of the heart muscle and is not associated with other forms of heart disease (Table 147-1). There are three types of cardiomyopathy based on anatomic and functional features:
1. Dilated
2. Hypertrophic
3. Restrictive

Dilated cardiomyopathies are the most common. They are often idiopathic, but may be due to infection (echovirus or Coxsackie B virus) or be postinfectious, familial, or secondary to systemic disease or to cardiotoxic drugs. Hypertrophic cardiomyopathies are usually familial with autosomal dominant inheritance, but may occur sporadically. Restrictive cardiomyopathies are rare; they may be idiopathic or associated with systemic disease (Table 147-2).

CLINICAL MANIFESTATIONS

Decision-Making Algorithms
Available @ StudentConsult.com

Chest Pain
Palpitations
Edema

Dilated cardiomyopathies result in enlargement of the left ventricle only or of both ventricles. Myocardial contractility is variably decreased. Children with dilated cardiomyopathy present with signs and symptoms of inadequate cardiac output and **heart failure**. Tachypnea and tachycardia are present on examination. Peripheral pulses are often weak because of a **narrow pulse pressure**. Rales may be audible on auscultation. The heart sounds may be muffled, and an S_3 is often present. Concurrent infectious illness may result in circulatory collapse and shock in children with dilated cardiomyopathies.

Hypertrophic cardiomyopathy is initially difficult to diagnose. Infants, but not older children, frequently present with signs of heart failure. Sudden death may be the initial presentation in older children. Dyspnea, fatigue, chest pain, syncope or near-syncope, and palpitations may be present. A murmur is heard in more than 50% of children referred after identification of an affected family member. Restrictive cardiomyopathies are relatively rare in pediatrics. Presenting symptoms usually include dyspnea exacerbated by a respiratory illness, syncope, hepatomegaly, and an S_4 heart sound on examination.

Table 147-1	Etiology of Myocardial Disease

FAMILIAL/HEREDITARY	Mitochondrial myopathies and oxidative respiratory chain defects
Duchenne muscular dystrophy	Type II, X-linked 3-methylglutaconic aciduria
Other muscular dystrophies (Becker, limb-girdle)	**CONNECTIVE TISSUE/GRANULOMATOUS DISEASE**
Myotonic dystrophy	Systemic lupus erythematosus
Kearns-Sayre syndrome (progressive external ophthalmoplegia)	Scleroderma
Carnitine deficiency syndromes	Amyloidosis
Endocardial fibroelastosis	Rheumatic fever
Mitochondrial myopathy syndromes	Sarcoidosis
Familial dilated cardiomyopathy (dominant, recessive, X-linked)	Dermatomyositis
Familial hypertrophic cardiomyopathy	**DRUGS/TOXINS**
Familial restrictive cardiomyopathy	Doxorubicin (Adriamycin)
Pompe disease (glycogen storage)	Ipecac
INFECTIOUS (MYOCARDITIS)	Iron overload (hemosiderosis)
Viral (e.g., coxsackievirus infection, mumps, Epstein-Barr virus infection, influenza, parainfluenza infection, measles, varicella, HIV infection)	Irradiation
	Cocaine
Rickettsial (e.g., psittacosis, *Coxiella* infection, Rocky Mountain spotted fever)	Amphetamines
	CORONARY ARTERIES
Bacterial (e.g., diphtheria, *Mycoplasma* infection, meningococcal disease, leptospirosis, Lyme disease)	Anomalous left coronary artery
	Kawasaki disease
Parasitic (e.g., Chagas disease, toxoplasmosis)	**OTHER DISORDERS/CONDITIONS**
METABOLIC/NUTRITIONAL/ENDOCRINE	Idiopathic
Hypothyroidism	Sickle cell anemia
Hyperthyroidism	Endomyocardial fibrosis
Pheochromocytoma	Right ventricular dysplasia

HIV, Human immunodeficiency virus.

Table 147-2	Anatomic and Functional Features of Cardiomyopathies

FEATURE	DILATED	HYPERTROPHIC	RESTRICTIVE
Etiology	Infectious Metabolic Toxic Idiopathic	Sporadic Inherited (autosomal dominant)	Infiltrative (amyloidosis, sarcoidosis) Noninfiltrative (idiopathic, familial) Storage disease (hemochromatosis, Fabry disease) Endomyocardial disease
Hemodynamics	Decreased systolic function	Diastolic dysfunction (impaired ventricular filling)	Diastolic dysfunction (impaired ventricular filling)
Treatment	Positive inotropes Diuretics Afterload reduction β-Blockers Antiarrhythmics Anticoagulants Cardiac transplantation	β-Blockers Calcium channel blockers	Diuretics Anticoagulants Cardiac transplantation

IMAGING STUDIES

Decision-Making Algorithm
Available @ StudentConsult.com

Edema

Cardiomegaly usually is seen on chest radiographs for all three types of cardiomyopathies. The electrocardiogram (ECG) in dilated cardiomyopathy may have nonspecific ST-T wave changes and left ventricular hypertrophy. ECG evidence of right ventricular hypertrophy is present in 25% of children with cardiomyopathy. The ECG with hypertrophic cardiomyopathy is universally abnormal, but changes are nonspecific. Primary hypertrophic cardiomyopathy is associated with a prolonged QT interval. Children with restrictive cardiomyopathies may show atrial enlargement on the ECG. Echocardiography features vary by type of cardiomyopathy.

Dilated cardiomyopathies result in left atrial and ventricular dilation, a decreased shortening fraction, and globally depressed contractility. Asymmetrical septal hypertrophy and left ventricular outflow tract obstruction are seen in hypertrophic cardiomyopathies. Massive atrial dilation is seen in restrictive cardiomyopathies. Endomyocardial biopsy specimens, obtained while the patient is hemodynamically stable, identify histologic type and allow tests for mitochondrial or infiltrative diseases.

TREATMENT

Supportive therapy, including **diuretics**, **inotropic medications**, and **afterload reduction**, is provided for all three types of cardiomyopathy. If a specific etiology can be identified, treatment is directed at the etiology. Symptomatic therapy with close monitoring and follow-up is crucial. Because of the high mortality rate associated with all forms of cardiomyopathy, **cardiac transplantation** must be considered.

Chapter **148**

PERICARDITIS

ETIOLOGY AND EPIDEMIOLOGY

Pericarditis is inflammation of the parietal and visceral surfaces of the pericardium. It is most often viral in origin, with many viruses identified as causative agents. A bacterial etiology is rare but causes a much more serious and symptomatic pericarditis. *Staphylococcus aureus* and *Streptococcus pneumoniae* are the most likely bacterial causes. Pericarditis is associated with collagen vascular diseases, such as rheumatoid arthritis, and is seen with uremia (Table 148-1). **Postpericardiotomy syndrome** is a relatively common form of pericarditis that follows heart surgery.

Table 148-1	Etiology of Pericarditis and Pericardial Effusion
IDIOPATHIC (PRESUMED VIRAL) INFECTIOUS AGENTS	Sarcoidosis
Bacterial	Vasculitis
Group A streptococci	**TRAUMATIC**
Staphylococcus aureus	Cardiac contusion (blunt trauma)
Pneumococcus, meningococcus*	Penetrating trauma
*Haemophilus influenzae**	Postpericardiotomy syndrome
Mycobacterium tuberculosis	Radiation
Viral†	**CONTIGUOUS SPREAD**
Coxsackievirus (group A, B)	Pleural disease
Echovirus	Pneumonia
Mumps	Aortic aneurysm (dissecting)
Influenza	**METABOLIC**
Epstein-Barr	Hypothyroidism
Cytomegalovirus	Uremia
Fungal	Chylopericardium
Histoplasma capsulatum	**NEOPLASTIC**
Coccidioides immitis	Primary
Blastomyces dermatitidis	Contiguous (lymphoma)
Candida	Metastatic
COLLAGEN VASCULAR-INFLAMMATORY AND GRANULOMATOUS DISEASES	Infiltrative (leukemia)
Rheumatic fever	**OTHER ETIOLOGIC DISORDERS/FACTORS**
Systemic lupus erythematosus (idiopathic and drug-induced)	Drug reaction
Rheumatoid arthritis	Pancreatitis
Kawasaki disease	After myocardial infarction
Scleroderma	Thalassemia
Mixed connective tissue disease	Central venous catheter perforation
Inflammatory bowel disease	Heart failure
	Hemorrhage (coagulopathy)

From Sigman G: Chest pain. In Kliegman RM, Nieder ML, Super DM. editors: Practical Strategies in Pediatric Diagnosis and Therapy, Philadelphia, 1996, WB Saunders.
*Infectious or immune complex.
†Common (viral pericarditis or myopericarditis is probably the most common cause of acute pericarditis in a previously normal host).

Table 148-2	Manifestations of Pericarditis

SYMPTOMS

Chest pain (worsened if lying down or with inspiration)

Dyspnea

Malaise

Patient assumes sitting position

SIGNS

Nonconstrictive

Fever

Tachycardia

Friction rub (accentuated by inspiration, body position)

Enlarged heart by percussion and x-ray examination

Distant heart sounds

Tamponade

As above, plus:

Distended neck veins

Hepatomegaly

Pulsus paradoxus (>10 mm Hg with inspiration)

Narrow pulse pressure

Weak pulse, poor peripheral perfusion

Constrictive

Distended neck veins

Kussmaul sign (inspiratory increase in jugular venous pressure)

Distant heart sounds

Pericardial knock

Hepatomegaly

Ascites

Edema

Tachycardia

CLINICAL MANIFESTATIONS

Decision-Making Algorithm
Available @ StudentConsult.com

Chest Pain

The symptoms of pericarditis (Table 148-2) depend on the amount of fluid in the pericardial space and how fast it accumulates. A small effusion usually is well tolerated. A large effusion may be well tolerated if it accumulates slowly. The faster the fluid accumulates, the sooner the patient is hemodynamically compromised and develops symptoms.

IMAGING AND LABORATORY STUDIES

Echocardiography is the most specific and useful diagnostic test for detection of pericardial effusions. A chest x-ray may reveal cardiomegaly. A large effusion creates a rounded, globular cardiac silhouette. The electrocardiogram (ECG) may show tachycardia, elevated ST segments, reduced QRS voltage or electrical alternans (variable QRS amplitude). The causative organism may be identified through viral titers, antistreptolysin O (ASO) titers, or diagnostic testing of the pericardial fluid.

TREATMENT

Pericardiocentesis is indicated for treatment of hemodynamically significant effusions and to determine the etiology of the pericarditis. Additional treatment is directed at the specific etiology. There is no specific treatment for viral pericarditis other than **anti-inflammatory medications**.

Suggested Reading
Kliegman RM, Behrman RE, Jenson HB, et al: *Nelson Textbook of Pediatrics*, ed 19, Philadelphia, 2011, Saunders.

Lai WW, Mertens LL, Cohen MS, Geva T: *Echocardiography in Pediatric and Congenital Heart Disease: from Fetus to Adult*, Oxford, UK, 2009, Blackwell Publishing.

Moller JH, Hoffman JI, Benson DW, Van Hare GF, Wren C: *Pediatric Cardiovascular Medicine*, ed 2, West Sussex, UK, 2012, Wiley-Blackwell.

Shaddy RE: *Heart Failure in Congenital Heart Disease*, London, 2011, Springer.

Wren C: *Concise Guide to Pediatric Arrhythmias*, West Sussex, UK, 2012, Wiley-Blackwell.

Hematology

Julie A. Panepinto, Rowena C. Punzalan, and J. Paul Scott

Chapter 149

HEMATOLOGY ASSESSMENT

HISTORY

A detailed history of the onset, severity, progression, associated symptoms, presence of systemic complaints, and exacerbating factors is crucial to the diagnosis of a blood disorder. In many blood disorders, a **detailed pedigree** identifying a pattern of inheritance can point to the diagnosis.

PHYSICAL EXAMINATION AND COMMON MANIFESTATIONS

Decision-Making Algorithms
Available @ StudentConsult.com

Jaundice
Anemia
Bleeding
Petechiae/Purpura
Pancytopenia
Failure to Thrive

The physical examination of patients with blood disorders first focuses on hemodynamic stability. Acute episodes of anemia may be life-threatening, presenting with impairment of perfusion and cognitive status. The two most common findings of anemia include **pallor** and **jaundice**. The presence of **petechiae**, **purpura**, or deeper sites of **bleeding**, including generalized hemorrhage, indicates abnormalities of platelets, coagulation factors, or both. **Growth parameters** point to whether anemia is an acute or chronic process. Severe types of anemia, thrombocytopenia, and pancytopenia often are associated with congenital anomalies and a pattern of growth delay. Organ system involvement (especially **hepatosplenomegaly** and **lymphadenopathy**) or systemic illness point to a generalized illness as the cause for hematologic abnormalities (Table 149-1).

INITIAL DIAGNOSTIC EVALUATION

Diagnosis of pediatric blood disorders requires a detailed knowledge of normal hematologic values and varies according to age and, after puberty, according to sex (Table 149-2). Directed by the history, physical examination, and screening laboratory studies, specific diagnostic testing can confirm the diagnosis.

DEVELOPMENTAL HEMATOLOGY

Hematopoiesis begins by 3 weeks of gestation with **erythropoiesis** in the yolk sac. By 2 months' gestation, the primary site of hematopoiesis migrates to the liver. By 5 to 6 months' gestation, the process shifts from the liver to the bone marrow. An extremely premature infant may have significant **extramedullary hematopoiesis** due to limited bone marrow hematopoiesis. During infancy, virtually all marrow cavities are actively hematopoietic and the proportion of hematopoietic to stromal elements is quite high. As the child grows, hematopoiesis moves to the central bones of the body (vertebrae, sternum, ribs, and pelvis), and the marrow is gradually replaced with fat. Hemolysis or marrow damage may lead to marrow repopulation of cavities where hematopoiesis previously had ceased or may delay the shift of hematopoiesis. Hepatosplenomegaly in patients with chronic hemolysis may signify extramedullary hematopoiesis. When a patient with cytopenia is being evaluated, a **bone marrow examination** provides valuable information about processes that lead to underproduction of circulating cells. In addition, bone marrow infiltration by neoplastic elements or storage cells often occurs in concert with infiltration in the spleen, liver, and lymph nodes.

The hematopoietic cells consist of the following:

1. Small compartment of **pluripotential progenitor stem cells** that resemble small lymphocytes and are capable of forming all myeloid elements
2. Large compartment of committed, proliferating cells of myeloid, erythroid, and megakaryocytic lineage
3. Large compartment of postmitotic maturing cells (Fig. 149-1)

The bone marrow is the major storage organ for mature neutrophils and contains about seven times the intravascular pool of neutrophils. It contains 2.5 to 5 times as many cells of myeloid lineage as cells of erythroid lineage. Smaller numbers of megakaryocytes, plasma cells, histiocytes, lymphocytes, and stromal cells are also stored in the marrow.

Erythropoiesis (red blood cell [RBC] production) is controlled by erythropoietin, a glycoprotein that stimulates primitive pluripotential stem cells to differentiate along the

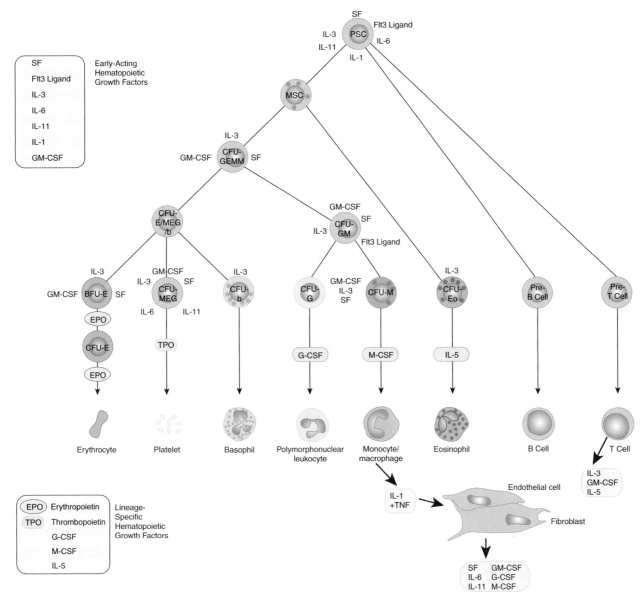

Figure 149-1 Major cytokine sources and actions to promote hematopoiesis. Cells of the bone marrow microenvironment, such as macrophages, endothelial cells, and reticular fibroblasts, produce macrophage colony-stimulating factor (M-CSF), granulocyte-macrophage colony-stimulating factor (GM-CSF), and granulocyte colony-stimulating factor (G-CSF) after stimulation. For all lineages, optimal development requires a combination of early and late acting factors. *BFU,* Burst-forming unit; *CFU,* colony-forming unit; *EPO,* erythropoietin; *IL,* interleukin; *MSC,* myeloid stem cell; *PSC,* pluripotent stem cell; *TNF,* tumor necrosis factor; *TPO,* thrombopoietin. *(From Sieff CA, Nathan DG, Clark SC: The anatomy and physiology of hematopoiesis. In Orkin SH, Nathan DG, editors:* Hematology of Infancy and Childhood, *ed 5, Philadelphia, 1998, WB Saunders, p 168.)*

Table 149-1	Presentation of Hematologic Disorders	
CONDITION	**SYMPTOMS AND SIGNS**	**COMMON EXAMPLES**
Anemia	Pallor, fatigue, heart failure, jaundice	Iron deficiency, hemolytic anemia
Polycythemia	Irritability, cyanosis, seizures, jaundice, stroke, headache	Cyanotic heart disease, infant of diabetic mother, cystic fibrosis
Neutropenia	Fever, pharyngitis, oral ulceration, cellulitis, lymphadenopathy, bacteremia, gingivitis	Congenital or drug-induced agranulocytosis, leukemia
Thrombocytopenia	Petechiae, ecchymosis, gastrointestinal hemorrhage, epistaxis	ITP, leukemia
Coagulopathy	Bruising, hemarthrosis, mucosal bleeding	von Willebrand disease, hemophilia, DIC
Thrombosis	Pulmonary embolism, deep vein thrombosis	Lupus anticoagulant; protein C, protein S, or antithrombin III deficiency; factor V Leiden, prothrombin 20210

DIC, Disseminated intravascular coagulation; *ITP,* idiopathic thrombocytopenic purpura.

Table 149-2 | Hematologic Values During Infancy and Childhood

AGE	HEMOGLOBIN (g/dL)		HEMATOCRIT (%)		RETICULOCYTES (%) MEAN	LEUKOCYTES (per mm³)		DIFFERENTIAL COUNTS					
								NEUTROPHILS (%)		LYMPHOCYTES (%) MEAN	EOSINOPHILS (%) MEAN	MONOCYTES (%) MEAN	NUCLEATED RED CELLS/100 WBCs
	MEAN	RANGE	MEAN	RANGE		MEAN	RANGE	MEAN	RANGE				
Cord blood	16.8	13.7–20.1	55	45–65	5	18,000	9000–30,000	61	40–80	31	2	6	7
2 wk	16.5	13–20	50	42–66	1	12,000	5000–21,000	40		48	3	9	3–10
3 mo	12.0	9.5–14.5	36	31–41	1	12,000	6000–18,000	30		63	2	5	0
6 mo–6 yr	12.0	10.5–14	37	33–42	1	10,000	6000–15,000	45		48	2	5	0
7–12 yr	13.0	11–16	38	34–40	1	8000	4500–13,500	55		38	2	5	0
Adult													
Female	14.0	12–16	42	37–47	1.6	7500	5000–10,000	55	35–70	35	3	7	0
Male	16.0	14–18	47	42–52									

From Behrman RE, editor: Nelson Textbook of Pediatrics, ed 14, Philadelphia, 1992, WB Saunders.
WBCs, White blood cells.

erythroid line and is made by the juxtaglomerular apparatus of the kidney in response to local tissue hypoxia. The normally high hemoglobin level of the fetus is a result of fetal erythropoietin production in the liver in response to low Po_2 in utero. Erythropoietin leads to production of the **erythroid colony-forming unit**. The earliest recognizable erythroid cell is the erythroblast, which forms eight or more daughter cells. The RBC nucleus becomes gradually pyknotic and eventually is extruded. The cell is then released from the marrow as a **reticulocyte** that maintains residual mitochondrial and protein synthetic capacity. These highly specialized RBC precursors are engaged primarily in the production of **globin chains, glycolytic enzymes**, and **heme**. Iron is taken up via transferrin receptors and incorporated into the heme ring, which combines with globin chains synthesized within the immature RBC. When the messenger RNA and mitochondria are gone from the RBC, heme or protein synthesis is no longer possible; however, the RBC continues to function for its normal life span of about 120 days.

Embryonic hemoglobins are produced during yolk sac erythropoiesis, then replaced by **fetal hemoglobin** (hemoglobin F, $\alpha_2\gamma_2$) during the hepatic phase. During the third trimester, gamma chain production gradually diminishes, replaced by beta chains, resulting in **hemoglobin A** ($a_2\beta_2$). Some fetal factors (e.g., infant of a diabetic mother) delay onset of beta chain production, but premature birth does not. Just after birth, with rapid increases in oxygen saturation, erythropoietin production stops and, thus, erythropoiesis ceases. Fetal RBCs have a shorter survival time (60 days).

During the first few months of postnatal life, rapid growth, shortened RBC survival, and cessation of erythropoiesis cause a gradual decline in hemoglobin levels, with a nadir at 8 to 10 weeks of life. This so-called **physiologic nadir** is accentuated in premature infants. Erythropoietin is produced in response to the decline in hemoglobin and decreased oxygen delivery. Erythropoiesis subsequently resumes with an increase in the reticulocyte count. The hemoglobin level gradually increases, accompanied by synthesis of increasing amounts of hemoglobin A. By 6 months of age in healthy infants, only trace gamma chain synthesis occurs.

Production of **neutrophil precursors** is controlled predominantly by two different colony-stimulating factors (see Fig. 149-1). The most immature neutrophil precursors are controlled by **granulocyte-macrophage colony-stimulating factor** (GM-CSF), produced by monocytes and lymphocytes. GM-CSF increases the entry of primitive precursor cells into the myeloid line of differentiation. **Granulocyte colony-stimulating factor** (G-CSF) augments the production of more mature granulocyte precursors. GM-CSF and G-CSF, working in concert, can augment production of neutrophils, shorten the usual 10- to 14-day production time from stem cell to mature neutrophil, and stimulate functional activity. The rapid increase in neutrophil count that occurs with infection is caused by release of stored neutrophils from the bone marrow, under the control of GM-CSF. During maturation, a mitotic pool of neutrophil precursors exists—myeloblasts, promyelocytes, and myelocytes possessing primary granules. The postmitotic pool consists of metamyelocytes, bands, and mature polymorphonuclear leukocytes containing secondary or specific granules that define the cell type. Only bands and mature neutrophils are fully functional with regard to phagocytosis, chemotaxis, and bacterial killing. Neutrophils migrate from the bone marrow, circulate for 6 to 7 hours, and enter the tissues, where they become end-stage cells that do not recirculate. Eosinophil production is under the control of a related glycoprotein hormone, interleukin 3. Eosinophils, which play a role in host defense against parasites, also are capable of living in tissues for prolonged periods.

Megakaryocytes are giant, multinucleated cells derived from the primitive stem cell and are polyploid (16 to 32 times the normal DNA content) because of nuclear but not cytoplasmic cell division. Platelets form by invagination of the megakaryocytic cell membrane and bud off from the periphery. **Thrombopoietin** is the primary regulator of platelet production. Platelets adhere to damaged endothelium and subendothelial surfaces via specific receptors for the adhesive proteins, von Willebrand factor (vWF), and fibrinogen. Platelets also have specific granules that readily release their contents after stimulation and trigger the process of platelet aggregation. Platelets circulate for 7 to 10 days and have no nucleus.

Lymphocytes are particularly abundant in the bone marrow of young children. These are primarily B lymphocytes arising in the spleen and lymph nodes, but T lymphocytes also are present.

Chapter **150**

ANEMIA

ETIOLOGY

The diagnosis of anemia is determined by comparison of the patient's hemoglobin level with age-specific and sex specific normal values (see Table 149-2). The production of androgens at the onset of puberty in boys causes males to maintain a normal hemoglobin value about 1.5 to 2 g/dL higher than girls. The easiest quantitative definition of anemia is any hemoglobin or hematocrit value that is 2 standard deviations (SDs) (95% confidence limits) below the mean for age and gender. However, in certain pathologic states, anemia may be present with a normal hemoglobin level (e.g., cyanotic cardiac or pulmonary disease or abnormally high hemoglobin affinity for oxygen). This is a physiologic definition of anemia. Anemia is often a manifestation of some other primary process and may accentuate other organ dysfunction.

Anemias are classified based on the size and hemoglobin content of the cells (Fig. 150-1). **Hypochromic, microcytic anemia** is caused by an inadequate production of hemoglobin. The most common causes of this type of anemia are iron deficiency and thalassemia. Most **normocytic anemias** are associated with a systemic illness that impairs

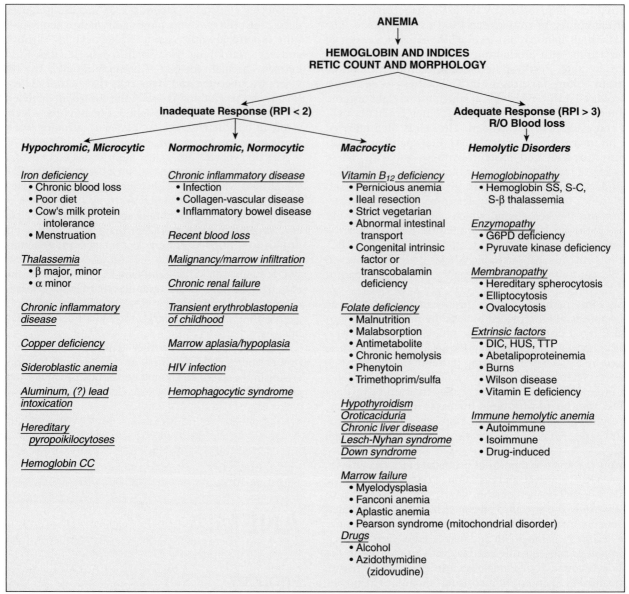

Figure 150-1 Use of the complete blood count, reticulocyte count, and blood smear in the diagnosis of anemia. *DIC,* Disseminated intravascular coagulation; *G6PD,* glucose-6-phosphate dehydrogenase; *HUS,* hemolytic uremic syndrome; *R/O,* rule out; *RPI,* reticulocyte production index; *TTP,* thrombotic thrombocytopenic purpura.

adequate marrow synthesis of red blood cells (RBCs). Vitamin B_{12} and folic acid deficiencies lead to **macrocytic anemia**. **Hemolytic diseases** are mediated either by disorders intrinsic or extrinsic to the RBC that increase cell destruction. The most common RBC membrane disorders are **hereditary spherocytosis** and **hereditary elliptocytosis**. In both of these disorders, abnormalities of proteins within the cytoskeleton lead to abnormal RBC shape and function. Numerous RBC enzyme deficiencies may lead to hemolysis, but only two are common: **glucose-6-phosphate dehydrogenase (G6PD) deficiency** and **pyruvate kinase deficiency**. Immune-mediated hemolysis may be extravascular when RBCs coated with antibodies or complement are phagocytosed by the reticuloendothelial system. The hemolysis may be intravascular when antibody binding leads to complement fixation and lysis of RBCs.

CLINICAL MANIFESTATIONS

Decision-Making Algorithms
Available @ StudentConsult.com

Heart Murmurs
Jaundice
Splenomegaly
Edema
Anemia

Acute onset of anemia can result in a poorly compensated state, manifested as an elevated heart rate, a flow murmur, poor exercise tolerance, headache, excessive sleeping (especially in infants) or fatigue, irritability, poor feeding, and syncope. In contrast, chronic anemia often is exceptionally well

Table 150-1	Historical Clues in Evaluation of Anemia
VARIABLE	**COMMENTS**
Age	Iron deficiency rare in the absence of blood loss before 6 mo or in term infants or before doubling of birth weight in preterm infants Neonatal anemia with reticulocytosis suggests hemolysis or blood loss; with reticulocytopenia, suggests bone marrow failure Sickle cell anemia and β-thalassemia appear as fetal hemoglobin disappears (4–8 mo of age)
Family history and genetic considerations	X-linked: G6PD deficiency Autosomal dominant: spherocytosis Autosomal recessive: sickle cell anemia, Fanconi anemia Family member with history of cholecystectomy (for bilirubin stones) or splenectomy at an early age Ethnicity (thalassemia in persons of Mediterranean origin; G6PD deficiency in blacks, Greeks, and people of Middle Eastern origin) Race (β-thalassemia in persons of Mediterranean, African, or Asian descent; α-thalassemia in those of African and Asian descent; SC and SS in African descent)
Nutrition	Cow's milk diet: iron deficiency Strict vegetarian: vitamin B$_{12}$ deficiency Goat's milk diet: folate deficiency Pica: plumbism, iron deficiency Cholestasis, malabsorption: vitamin E deficiency
Drugs	G6PD: oxidants (e.g., nitrofurantoin, antimalarials) Immune-mediated hemolysis (e.g., penicillin) Bone marrow suppression (e.g., chemotherapy) Phenytoin, increasing folate requirements
Diarrhea	Malabsorption of vitamin B$_{12}$ or E or iron Inflammatory bowel disease and anemia of inflammation (chronic disease) with or without blood loss Milk protein intolerance–induced blood loss Intestinal resection: vitamin B$_{12}$ deficiency
Infection	*Giardia lamblia* infection: iron malabsorption Intestinal bacterial overgrowth (blind loop): vitamin B$_{12}$ deficiency Fish tapeworm: vitamin B$_{12}$ deficiency Epstein-Barr virus, cytomegalovirus infection: bone marrow suppression, hemophagocytic syndromes *Mycoplasma* infection: hemolysis Parvovirus infection: bone marrow suppression HIV infection Chronic infection Endocarditis Malaria: hemolysis Hepatitis: aplastic anemia

G6PD, Glucose-6-phosphate dehydrogenase.

A history of jaundice, pallor, previously affected siblings, drug ingestion by the mother, or excessive blood loss at the time of birth provides important clues to the diagnosis in newborns. A careful **dietary history** is crucial. The key findings in patients with hemolytic anemias are **jaundice**, **pallor**, and **splenomegaly**. Because of increased bilirubin production, **gallstones** (bilirubinate), a result of chronic hemolysis, are a common complication. Systemic complaints suggest acute or chronic illnesses as probable causes of anemia. In later childhood and adolescence, the presence of constitutional symptoms, unusual diets, drug ingestion, or blood loss, especially from menstrual bleeding, often points to a diagnosis. **Congenital hemolytic disorders** (enzyme deficiencies and membrane problems) often present in the first 6 months of life and frequently are associated with neonatal jaundice, although these disorders often go undiagnosed. A careful **drug history** is essential for detecting problems that may be drug induced. Pure dietary iron deficiency is rare except in infancy, when cow's milk protein intolerance causes gastrointestinal blood loss and further complicates an already inadequate iron intake.

The physical examination may point to the potential causes (see Table 150-2). The **physiologic stability** of the patient may be abnormal with acute blood loss and acute hemolysis, manifesting as tachycardia, blood pressure changes, and, most ominously, an altered state of consciousness. The presence of **jaundice** suggests hemolysis. **Petechiae** and **purpura** indicate a coagulopathy. **Hepatosplenomegaly** and **adenopathy** suggest infiltrative disorders. **Growth failure** or poor weight gain suggests an anemia of chronic disease. An essential element of the physical examination is the investigation of the stool for the presence of **occult blood**.

LABORATORY STUDIES

A hemoglobin or hematocrit test indicates the severity of the anemia. Once anemia has been substantiated, the workup should include a complete blood count with differential, platelet count, indices, and reticulocyte count. Examination of the peripheral blood smear assesses the morphology of RBCs (Fig. 150-2), white blood cells (WBCs), and platelets. All cell lines should be scrutinized to determine whether anemia is the result of a process limited to the erythroid line or a process that affects other marrow elements. Using data obtained from the indices and reticulocyte count, the workup can be organized on the basis of whether RBC production is adequate or inadequate and whether the cells are microcytic, normocytic, or macrocytic (see Fig. 150-1).

An appropriate bone marrow response to anemia would be an elevated absolute reticulocyte number, suggesting increased production and implying either hemolysis or blood loss. Anemia with a normal reticulocyte number suggests decreased or ineffective production for the degree of anemia. Reticulocytopenia signifies an acute onset so that the marrow has not had adequate time to respond, that reticulocytes are being destroyed in the marrow (antibody-mediated), or that intrinsic bone marrow disease is present. The best indicators of the severity of hemolysis are the hemoglobin level and the elevation of the **reticulocyte count**. Biochemical evidence of hemolysis includes an increase in levels of bilirubin and lactate dehydrogenase and a decrease in haptoglobin.

tolerated in children because of their cardiovascular reserve. Usually, children with chronic anemia will have minimal tachycardia and a flow murmur on examination. The urgency of diagnostic and therapeutic intervention, especially the use of packed RBC transfusion, should be dictated by the extent of cardiovascular or functional impairment more than the absolute level of hemoglobin.

The causes of anemia often can be suspected from a careful history adjusted for the patient's age (Tables 150-1 and 150-2). Anemia at any age demands a search for **blood loss**.

Table 150-2	Physical Findings in the Evaluation of Anemia

SYSTEM/STRUCTURE	OBSERVATION	SIGNIFICANCE
Skin	Hyperpigmentation	Fanconi anemia, dyskeratosis congenita
	Cafe au lait spots	Fanconi anemia
	Vitiligo	Vitamin B_{12} deficiency
	Partial oculocutaneous albinism	Chediak-Higashi syndrome
	Jaundice	Hemolysis
	Petechiae, purpura	Bone marrow infiltration, autoimmune hemolysis with autoimmune thrombocytopenia, hemolytic uremic syndrome, hemophagocytic syndromes
	Erythematous rash	Parvovirus or Epstein-Barr virus infection
	Butterfly rash	SLE antibodies
	Bruising	Bleeding disorder, nonaccidental trauma, scurvy
Head	Frontal bossing	Thalassemia major, severe iron deficiency, chronic subdural hematoma
	Microcephaly	Fanconi anemia
Eyes	Microphthalmia	Fanconi anemia
	Retinopathy	Hemoglobin SS, SC disease (see Table 150-7)
	Optic atrophy	Osteopetrosis
	Blocked lacrimal gland	Dyskeratosis congenita
	Kayser-Fleischer ring	Wilson disease
	Blue sclera	Iron deficiency, osteopetrosis
Ears	Deafness	
Mouth	Glossitis	Vitamin B_{12} deficiency, iron deficiency
	Angular stomatitis	Iron deficiency
	Cleft lip	Diamond-Blackfan syndrome
	Pigmentation	Peutz-Jeghers syndrome (intestinal blood loss)
	Telangiectasia	Osler-Weber-Rendu syndrome (blood loss)
	Leukoplakia	Dyskeratosis congenita
Chest	Shield chest or widespread nipples	Diamond-Blackfan syndrome
	Murmur	Endocarditis: prosthetic valve hemolysis; severe anemia
Abdomen	Hepatomegaly	Hemolysis, infiltrative tumor, chronic disease, hemangioma, cholecystitis, extramedullary hematopoiesis
	Splenomegaly	Hemolysis, sickle cell disease, (early) thalassemia, malaria, leukemia/lymphoma, Epstein-Barr virus, portal hypertension
	Nephromegaly	Fanconi anemia
	Absent kidney	Fanconi anemia
Extremities	Absent thumbs	Fanconi anemia
	Triphalangeal thumb	Diamond-Blackfan syndrome
	Spoon nails	Iron deficiency
	Beau line (nails)	Heavy metal intoxication, severe illness
	Mees line (nails)	Heavy metals, severe illness, sickle cell anemia
	Dystrophic nails	Dyskeratosis congenita
Rectal	Hemorrhoids	Portal hypertension
	Heme-positive stool	Gastrointestinal bleeding
Nerves	Irritable, apathy	Iron deficiency
	Peripheral neuropathy	Deficiency of vitamins B_1, B_{12}, and E; lead poisoning
	Dementia	Deficiency of vitamins B_{12} and E
	Ataxia, posterior column signs	Vitamin B_{12} deficiency
	Stroke	Sickle cell anemia, paroxysmal nocturnal hemoglobinuria
General	Small stature	Fanconi anemia, HIV infection, malnutrition

HIV, Human immunodeficiency virus; *SLE*, systemic lupus erythematosus.

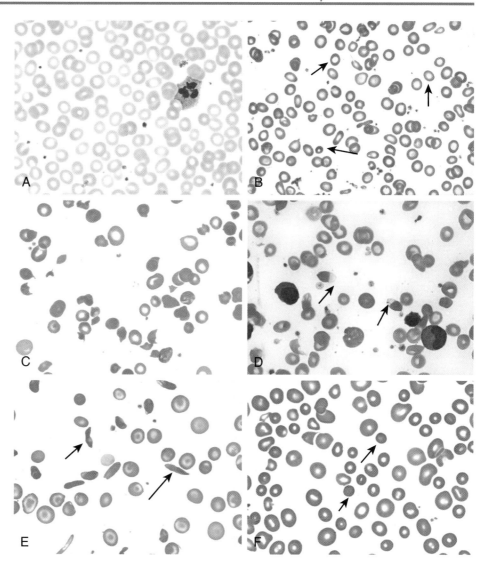

Figure 150-2 Morphologic abnormalities of the red blood cell. **A,** Normal. **B,** Hypochromic microcytes (iron deficiency). **C,** Schistocytes (hemolytic uremic syndrome. **D,** Blister cells (glucose-6-phosphate dehydrogenase deficiency). **E,** Sickle cells (hemoglobin SS disease). **F,** Spherocytes (autoimmune hemolytic anemia). (*Courtesy B. Trost and J. P. Scott.*)

DIFFERENTIAL DIAGNOSIS
Hypochromic, Microcytic Anemia
Iron Deficiency Anemia

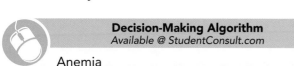

Decision-Making Algorithm
Available @ StudentConsult.com

Anemia

Etiology. Infants fed cow's milk when younger than 1 year of age, toddlers fed large volumes of cow's milk, and menstruating teenage girls who are not receiving supplemental iron are at high risk for iron deficiency. **Dietary** iron deficiency anemia is most common in bottle-fed toddlers who are receiving large volumes of cow's milk and eat minimal amounts of food high in iron content. (See Chapters 28 and 31.) Iron deficiency anemia also may be found in children with chronic inflammatory diseases, even without **chronic blood loss**.

Epidemiology. The prevalence of iron deficiency, the most common cause of anemia in the world, is about 9% in toddlers, 9% to 11% in adolescent girls, and less than 1% in teenage boys. Iron deficiency anemia occurs in about one third of children who are iron deficient (Table 150-3). Some underprivileged minority populations in the United States may be at increased risk for iron deficiency because of poor dietary intake (see Chapter 31). Breastfed infants are less likely to have iron deficiency than bottle-fed infants because, although there is less iron in breast milk, this iron is more efficiently absorbed.

Clinical Manifestations. In addition to cardiovascular manifestations of anemia, central nervous system (CNS) abnormalities (**apathy, irritability, poor concentration**) have been linked to iron deficiency, presumably resulting from alterations of iron-containing enzymes (monoamine oxidase) and cytochromes. Poor muscle endurance, gastrointestinal dysfunction, and impaired WBC and T-cell function have been associated with iron deficiency. Iron deficiency in infancy may be associated with later **cognitive deficits** and poor school performance.

Treatment. In an otherwise healthy child, a **therapeutic trial of iron** is the best diagnostic study for iron deficiency as long as the child is re-examined and a response is documented. The response to oral iron includes rapid subjective improvement, especially in neurologic function (within 24 to 48 hours) and reticulocytosis (48 to 72 hours); increase in hemoglobin levels (4 to 30 days); and repletion of iron stores (in 1 to 3 months). The usual therapeutic dose of 4 to 6 mg/day

Table 150-3	Stages in Development of Iron Deficiency Anemia				
HEMOGLOBIN (g/dL)	**PERIPHERAL SMEAR**	**SERUM IRON (µg/dL)**	**BONE MARROW IRON**		**SERUM FERRITIN (ng/mL)**
13+ (normal)	nc/nc	50–150	Fe^{2+}		*Male:* 40–340 *Female:* 40–150
10–12	nc/nc	↓	Fe^{2+} absent, erythroid hyperplasia		<12
8–10	hypo/nc	↓	Fe^{2+} absent, erythroid hyperplasia		<12
<8	hypo/micro*	↓	Fe^{2+} absent, erythroid hyperplasia		<12

From Andreoli TE, Bennett JC, Carpenter CC, et al: Cecil Essentials of Medicine, ed 4, Philadelphia, 1997, WB Saunders.
hypo/micro, Hypochromic, microcytic; hypo/nc, hypochromic, normocytic; nc/nc, normochromic, normocytic.
*Microcytosis, determined by a mean corpuscular volume (in fL) <2 SD below the mean, must be adjusted for age (e.g., –2 SD at 3–6 mo = 74; at 0.5–2 yr = 70; at 2–6 yr = 75; at 6–12 yr = 77; and at 12–18 yr = 78).

Table 150-4	Differentiating Features of Microcytic Anemias*			
TEST	**IRON DEFICIENCY ANEMIA**	**THALASSEMIA MINOR†**	**ANEMIA OF INFLAMMATION‡**
Serum iron	Low	Normal	Low
Serum iron-binding capacity	High	Normal	Low or normal
Serum ferritin	Low	Normal or high	Normal or high
Marrow iron stores	Low or absent	Normal or high	Normal or high
Marrow sideroblasts	Decreased or absent	Normal or increased	Normal or increased
Free erythrocyte protoporphyrin	High	Normal or slightly increased	High
Hemoglobin A_2 or F	Normal	High β-thalassemia; normal α-thalassemia	Normal
Red blood cell distribution width§	High	Normal	Normal/↑

*See Table 150-3 for definition of microcytosis.
†α-Thalassemia minor can be diagnosed by the presence of Bart hemoglobin on newborn screening.
‡Usually normochromic; 25% of cases are microcytic.
§Red blood cell distribution width quantitates the degree of anisocytosis (different sizes) of red blood cells.

of elemental iron induces an increase in hemoglobin of 0.25 to 0.4 g/dL/day (a 1%/day increase in hematocrit). If the hemoglobin level fails to increase within 2 weeks after institution of iron treatment, careful re-evaluation for ongoing blood loss, development of infection, poor compliance, or other causes of microcytic anemia is required (Table 150-4; see Fig. 150-1).

Prevention. Bottle-fed infants should receive an iron-containing formula until 12 months of age, and breastfed infants older than 6 months of age should receive an iron supplement. The introduction of iron-enriched solid foods at 6 months of age, followed by a transition to a limited amount of cow's milk and increased solid foods at 1 year, can help prevent iron deficiency anemia. Teenage girls who are menstruating should have a diet enriched with iron-containing foods. A vitamin with iron may also be used.

Thalassemia Minor

Etiology and Epidemiology. α-Thalassemia and β-thalassemia minor are common causes of microcytosis, either with or without a mild hypochromic, microcytic anemia. They are prevalent in certain ethnic groups (Mediterranean, Southeast Asian, African Americans). Individuals of Asian descent are at risk of having three or four α genes deleted, resulting in hemoglobin H disease (γ_4) or hydrops fetalis with only Bart (α_4) hemoglobin (Table 150-5 and Fig. 150-3).

Laboratory Testing. The thalassemia minor syndromes are characterized by a mild hypochromic, microcytic anemia

with a low absolute reticulocyte count (see Table 150-5). The RBC count is usually elevated. As a result, if the mean corpuscular volume (MCV) divided by the RBC count is less than 12.5 (Mentzer index), the diagnosis is suggestive of thalassemia trait. The blood smear reveals only microcytosis with α-thalassemia trait. Outside the neonatal period, when Bart hemoglobin is detectable, hemoglobin electrophoresis usually is normal in α-thalassemia minor (see Fig. 150-3). Blood smears of patients with β-thalassemia minor show microcytic RBCs. Target cells and basophilic stippled RBCs, caused by precipitation of alpha chain tetramers, also may be present. The diagnosis is based on an elevation of hemoglobin A_2 and F levels in **β-thalassemia**. **Molecular testing** is indicated for identification of more severe or unusual variants.

Treatment. No treatment is required for children with **thalassemia minor**. However, children with hemoglobin H disease (γ_4), especially the Constant Spring variant or hydrops fetalis with only Bart (α_4) hemoglobin, are likely to require chronic transfusion therapy.

Lead Poisoning

Lead poisoning may be associated with a hypochromic, microcytic anemia. Most patients have concomitant iron deficiency. The history of living in an older home (built before 1980) with chipped paint or lead dust should raise suspicion of lead poisoning, especially in a child with **pica**. **Basophilic stippling** on the blood smear is common. Lead intoxication

Table 150-5	Thalassemia Syndromes	
DISORDER	**GENOTYPIC ABNORMALITY**	**CLINICAL PHENOTYPE**
β-THALASSEMIA		
Thalassemia major (Cooley's anemia)	Homozygous β^0-thalassemia	Severe hemolysis, ineffective erythropoiesis, transfusion dependency, hepatosplenomegaly, iron overload
Thalassemia intermedia	Compound heterozygous β^0- and β^+-thalassemia	Moderate hemolysis, splenomegaly, moderately severe anemia, but not transfusion-dependent; main life-threatening complication is iron overload
Thalassemia minor	Heterozygous β^0- and β^+-thalassemia	Microcytosis, mild anemia
α-THALASSEMIA		
Silent carrier	α-/$\alpha\alpha$	Normal complete blood count
α-Thalassemia trait	$\alpha\alpha$/- - (α-thalassemia 1) or α -/α - (α-thalassemia 2)	Mild microcytic anemia
Hemoglobin H	α -/- -	Microcytic anemia and mild hemolysis; not transfusion-dependent*
Hydrops fetalis	- -/- -	Severe anemia, intrauterine anasarca from congestive heart failure; death in utero or at birth

From Andreoli T, Carpenter C, Griggs R, et al: Cecil Essentials of Medicine, ed 7, Philadelphia, 2007, Saunders.
*The Constant Spring variant may require chronic transfusion.

Figure 150-3 Genetic origins of the classic α-thalassemia syndromes due to gene deletions in the α-globin gene cluster. Hb Constant Spring (Hb CS) is an α-globin chain variant synthesized in such small amounts (1%–2% of normal) that it has the phenotypic impact of a severe non-deletion α-thalassemia allele; however, the α^{CS} allele is always linked to a functioning α-globin gene, so it has never been associated with hydrops fetalis. (From Hoffman R, Benz EJ, Shattil SS, et al, editors: Hematology: Basic Principles and Practice, ed 5, Philadelphia, 2008, Churchill Livingstone.)

rarely causes hemolytic anemia. Detection by routine screening, removal from exposure, chelation therapy, and correction of iron deficiency are crucial to the potential development of affected children.

Normocytic Anemia

Etiology and Treatment. Anemia is a common component of chronic inflammatory disease. Hepcidin, a protein made in the liver, plays a key role in iron homeostasis. Inflammation causes an increase in the production of hepcidin, interrupting the process of iron release by macrophages and the absorption of iron from the intestines leading to anemia. The **anemia of inflammation** may be normocytic or, less often, microcytic. This may pose a clinical challenge, when children with inflammatory disorders associated with blood loss (inflammatory bowel disease) exhibit a microcytic anemia. In these circumstances, only a bone marrow aspiration with staining of the sample for iron can differentiate the two entities clearly (see Table 150-4). Low ferritin levels indicate concurrent iron deficiency. A trial of iron therapy is not indicated without a specific diagnosis in children who appear to be systemically ill.

Bone marrow **infiltration by malignant cells** commonly leads to a normochromic, normocytic anemia. The mechanism

Table 150-6	Differentiation of Red Blood Cell Aplasias and Aplastic Anemias		
DISORDER	**AGE AT ONSET**	**CHARACTERISTICS**	**TREATMENT**
CONGENITAL			
Diamond-Blackfan syndrome (congenital hypoplastic anemia)	Newborn–1 mo; 90% of patients are <1 yr of age	Pure red blood cell aplasia, autosomal recessive trait, elevated fetal hemoglobin, fetal i antigen present, macrocytic, short stature, webbed neck, cleft lip, triphalangeal thumb; late-onset leukemia, mutation analysis	Prednisone, transfusion, hematopoietic stem cell transplant
ACQUIRED			
Transient erythroblastopenia	6 mo–5 yr of age; 85% of patients are >1 yr of age	Pure red blood cell defect; no anomalies, fetal hemoglobin, or i antigen; spontaneous recovery, normal MCV	Expectant transfusion for symptomatic anemia
Idiopathic aplastic anemia (status post hepatitis, drugs, unknown)	All ages	All cell lines involved; exposure to felbamate, chloramphenicol, radiation	Hematopoietic stem cell transplantation, antithymocyte globulin, cyclosporine, androgens
FAMILIAL			
Fanconi anemia	Usually before 10 yr of age; mean is 8 yr	All cell lines; microcephaly, absent thumbs, cafe au lait spots, cutaneous hyperpigmentation, short stature; chromosomal breaks, high MCV and hemoglobin F; horseshoe or absent kidney; leukemic transformation; autosomal recessive trait	Androgens, corticosteroids, hematopoietic stem cell transplantation
Paroxysmal nocturnal hemoglobinuria	After 5 yr	Initial hemolysis followed by aplastic anemia; increased complement-mediated hemolysis; thrombosis; iron deficiency; CD59 low	Iron, hematopoietic stem cell transplantation, androgens, steroids, eculizumab
Dyskeratosis congenita	Mean is 10 yr for skin; mean is 17 yr for anemia	Pancytopenia; hyperpigmentation, dystrophic nails, leukoplakia; X-linked recessive; lacrimal duct stenosis; high MCV and fetal hemoglobin	Androgens, splenectomy, hematopoietic stem cell transplantation
Familial hemophagocytic lymphohistiocytosis	Before 2 yr	Pancytopenia; fever, hepatosplenomegaly, hypertriglyceridemia, CSF pleocytosis	Transfusion; often lethal; VP-16, hematopoietic stem cell transplantation, IVIG, cyclosporine
INFECTIOUS			
Parvovirus	Any age	Any chronic hemolytic anemia, typically sickle cell; new-onset reticulocytopenia	Transfusion
Epstein-Barr virus (EBV)	Any age; usually <5 yr of age	X-linked immunodeficiency syndrome, pancytopenia	Transfusion, bone marrow transplantation
Virus-associated hemophagocytic syndrome (CMV, HHV-6, EBV)	Any age	Pancytopenia; hemophagocytosis in marrow, fever, hepatosplenomegaly	Transfusion, antiviral therapy, IVIG

CMV, Cytomegalovirus; *CSF,* cerebrospinal fluid; *HHV-6,* human herpesvirus 6; *IVIG,* intravenous immune globulin; *MCV,* mean corpuscular volume; *VP-16,* etoposide.

by which neoplastic cells interfere with RBC and other marrow cell synthesis is multifactorial. The reticulocyte count is often low. Immature myeloid elements may be released into the peripheral blood because of the presence of the offending tumor cells. An examination of the peripheral blood may reveal lymphoblasts; when solid tumors metastasize to the marrow, these cells are seldom seen in the peripheral blood. Teardrop cells may be seen in the peripheral blood. A bone marrow examination is frequently necessary in the face of normochromic, normocytic anemia.

Congenital pure RBC aplasia (Diamond-Blackfan syndrome), a lifelong disorder, usually presents in the first few months of life or at birth with severe anemia and mild macrocytosis or a normocytic anemia. It is due to a deficiency of bone marrow red blood cell precursors (Table 150-6). More than a third of patients have short stature. Many patients (50% to 66%) respond to corticosteroid treatment, but must receive therapy indefinitely. Patients who do not respond to

corticosteroid treatment are transfusion dependent and are at risk of the multiple complications of long-term transfusion therapy, especially iron overload. These patients have a higher rate of developing leukemia or other hematologic malignancies than the general population.

In contrast to the congenital hypoplastic anemias, **transient erythroblastopenia of childhood**, a normocytic anemia caused by suppression of RBC synthesis, usually appears after 6 months of age in an otherwise normal infant. Viral infections are thought to be the trigger, although the mechanism leading to RBC aplasia is poorly understood. The onset is gradual, but anemia may become severe. Recovery usually is spontaneous. Differentiation from Diamond-Blackfan syndrome, in which erythroid precursors also are absent or diminished in the bone marrow, may be challenging. Transfusion of packed RBCs may be necessary if the anemia becomes symptomatic before recovery.

Aplastic crises may complicate any chronic hemolytic anemia. These periods of severe reticulocytopenia, leading to an acute exacerbation of the anemia, may precipitate cardiovascular decompensation. Human parvovirus B19 (the cause of fifth disease) infects erythroid precursors and shuts down erythropoiesis. Transient erythroid aplasia is without consequence in individuals with normal RBC survival. Recovery from parvovirus infection in hemolytic disease is spontaneous, but patients may need transfusion if the anemia is severe.

Macrocytic Anemia
SEE FIGURE 150-1.

Marrow Failure/Pancytopenia

Decision-Making Algorithm
Available @ StudentConsult.com

Anemia

Etiology. Pancytopenia is a quantitative decrease in formed elements of the blood—erythrocytes, leukocytes, and platelets. Patients more often exhibit symptoms of infection or bleeding than anemia because of the relatively short life span of WBCs and platelets compared with the life span of RBCs. Causes of pancytopenia include failure of production (implying intrinsic bone marrow disease), sequestration (hypersplenism), and increased peripheral destruction.

Differential Diagnosis. Features that suggest **bone marrow failure** and mandate an examination of bone marrow include a low reticulocyte count, teardrop forms of RBCs (implying marrow replacement, not just failure), presence of abnormal forms of leukocytes or myeloid elements less mature than band forms, small platelets, and an elevated mean corpuscular volume in the face of a low reticulocyte count. Pancytopenia resulting from bone marrow failure is usually a gradual process, starting with one or two cell lines, but later involving all three cell lines. Features suggesting **increased destruction** include reticulocytosis, jaundice, immature erythroid or myeloid elements on the blood smear, large platelets, and increased serum bilirubin and lactic dehydrogenase.

Aplastic Anemia

Decision-Making Algorithm
Available @ StudentConsult.com

Anemia

Etiology and Epidemiology. In a child with aplastic anemia, pancytopenia evolves as the hematopoietic elements of the bone marrow disappear and the marrow is replaced by fat. In developed countries, aplastic anemia is most often idiopathic. The disorder may be induced by drugs such as chloramphenicol and felbamate or by toxins such as benzene. Aplastic anemia also may follow infections, particularly hepatitis and infectious mononucleosis (see Table 150-6). Immunosuppression of hematopoiesis is postulated to be an important mechanism in patients with postinfectious and idiopathic aplastic anemia.

Laboratory Studies. A **bone marrow biopsy** is crucial to determine cellularity or the extent of depletion of the hematopoietic elements.

Treatment. Survival rate is about 20% in severe aplastic anemia with supportive care alone, although the duration of survival may be years when vigorous blood product and antibiotic support is provided. For children with severe aplastic anemia—defined by an absolute reticulocyte count less than 50,000/µL, absolute neutrophil count less than 500/mm³, platelet count less than 20,000/mm³, and bone marrow cellularity on biopsy specimen less than 25% of normal—the treatment of choice is **hematopoietic stem cell transplantation (HSCT)** from a sibling with identical HLA and compatible mixed lymphocytes. When HSCT occurs before the recipient is sensitized to blood products, survival rate is greater than 80%. The treatment of aplastic anemia without an HLA-matched donor for HSCT is evolving, with two major options: potent immunosuppressive therapy or unrelated or partially matched HSCT. Results of trials using immunosuppressive therapy with antithymocyte globulin, cyclosporine, and corticosteroids in combination with hematopoietic growth factors have been encouraging. Such therapy is often toxic, and relapses often occur when therapy is stopped.

Fanconi Anemia

Decision-Making Algorithms
Available @ StudentConsult.com

Anemia
Petechiae/Purpura
Pancytopenia

Etiology and Epidemiology. Fanconi anemia is a constitutional form of aplastic anemia that usually presents in the latter half of the first decade of life and may evolve over years. A group of genetic defects in proteins involved in **DNA repair** have been identified in Fanconi anemia, which is inherited in an autosomal recessive manner. The diagnosis is based on demonstration of increased chromosomal breakage after exposure to agents that damage DNA. The repair mechanism for DNA damage is abnormal in all cells in Fanconi anemia, which may contribute to the increased risk of malignancies. Terminal acute leukemia develops in 10% of cases. Other malignancies include solid tumors of the head and neck, gastrointestinal tumors, and gynecologic tumors.

Clinical Manifestations. Patients with Fanconi anemia have numerous characteristic clinical findings (see Table 150-6).

Treatment. Hematopoietic stem cell transplantation can cure the pancytopenia caused by bone marrow aplasia. Many patients with Fanconi anemia and about 20% of children with aplastic anemia seem to respond for a time to **androgenic therapy**, which induces masculinization and may cause liver injury and liver tumors. Androgenic therapy increases RBC synthesis and may diminish transfusion requirements. The effect on granulocytes, and especially the platelet count, is less impressive.

Marrow Replacement. Marrow replacement may occur as a result of **leukemia**, **solid tumors** (especially neuroblastoma), **storage diseases**, **osteopetrosis** in infants, and **myelofibrosis**, which is rare in childhood. The mechanisms by which malignant cells impair marrow synthesis of normal hematopoietic elements are complex and incompletely understood. Bone marrow aspirate and biopsy are needed for precise diagnosis of the etiology of marrow synthetic failure.

Pancytopenia Resulting from Destruction of Cells. Pancytopenia resulting from destruction of cells may be caused by **intramedullary destruction** of hematopoietic elements (myeloproliferative disorders, deficiencies of folic acid and vitamin B_{12}) or by the **peripheral destruction** of mature cells. The usual site of peripheral destruction of blood cells is the spleen, although the liver and other parts of the reticuloendothelial system may participate. **Hypersplenism** may be the result of anatomic causes (portal hypertension or splenic hypertrophy from thalassemia); infections (including malaria); or storage diseases (Gaucher disease, lymphomas, or histiocytosis). Splenectomy is indicated only when the pancytopenia is of clinical significance.

Hemolytic Anemias
Major Hemoglobinopathies

Decision-Making Algorithms
Available @ StudentConsult.com

Jaundice
Splenomegaly
Red Urine and Hematuria
Anemia

Etiology. Because alpha chains are needed for fetal erythropoiesis and production of hemoglobin F ($\alpha_2\gamma_2$), **alpha chain hemoglobinopathies** are present in utero. Four alpha genes are present on the two number 16 chromosomes (see Fig. 150-3 and Table 150-5). Single gene deletions produce no disorder (silent carrier state), but can be detected by measuring the rates of α and β synthesis or by using molecular biologic techniques. Deletion of two genes produces **α-thalassemia minor** with mild or no anemia and microcytosis. In individuals of African origin, the gene deletions occur on different chromosomes (*trans*), and the disorder is benign. In the Asian population, deletions may occur on the same chromosome (*cis*), and infants may inherit two number 16 chromosomes lacking three or even four genes. Deletion of all four genes leads to hydrops fetalis, severe intrauterine anemia, and death, unless intrauterine transfusions are administered. Deletion of three genes produces moderate hemolytic anemia with γ_4 tetramers (**Bart hemoglobin**) in the fetus and β_4 tetramers (hemoglobin H) in older children and adults (see Table 150-5).

Beta chain hemoglobinopathies in the United States are more prevalent than alpha chain disorders, possibly because these abnormalities are not symptomatic in utero. The major beta hemoglobinopathies include those that alter hemoglobin function, including **hemoglobins S, C, E, and D,** and those that alter beta chain production, the β-thalassemias. Because each RBC has two copies of chromosome 11 and they express both β-globin genes, most disorders of beta chains are not clinically severe, unless both beta chains are abnormal. By convention, when describing β-thalassemia genes, β^0 indicates a thalassemic gene resulting in absent beta chain synthesis, whereas β^+ indicates a thalassemic gene that permits reduced but not absent synthesis of normal β chains. Disorders of the

beta chain usually manifest themselves clinically between 4 and 12 months of age, unless they have been detected prenatally or by cord blood screening.

β-Thalassemia Major (Cooley Anemia)

Etiology and Epidemiology. β-Thalassemia major is caused by mutations that impair **beta chain synthesis**. Because of unbalanced synthesis of alpha and beta chains, alpha chains precipitate within the cells, resulting in RBC destruction either in the bone marrow or in the spleen. β-Thalassemia major is seen most commonly in individuals of Mediterranean or Asian descent. The clinical severity of the illness varies on the basis of the molecular defect.

Clinical Manifestations. Signs and symptoms of β-thalassemia major result from the combination of chronic hemolytic disease, decreased or absent production of normal hemoglobin A, and ineffective erythropoiesis. The anemia is severe and leads to growth failure and high-output heart failure. **Ineffective erythropoiesis** causes increased expenditure of energy and expansion of the bone marrow cavities of all bones, leading to osteopenia, pathologic fractures, extramedullary erythropoiesis with resultant hepatosplenomegaly, and an increase in the rate of iron absorption.

Treatment. Treatment of β-thalassemia major is based on a **hypertransfusion program** that corrects the anemia and suppresses the patient's own ineffective erythropoiesis, limiting the stimulus for increased iron absorption. This suppression permits the bones to heal, decreases metabolic expenditures, increases growth, and limits dietary iron absorption. Splenectomy may reduce the transfusion volume, but it adds to the risk of serious infection. Chelation therapy with deferoxamine or deferasirox should start when laboratory evidence of iron overload (**hemochromatosis**) is present and before there are clinical signs of iron overload (nonimmune diabetes mellitus, cirrhosis, heart failure, bronzing of the skin, and multiple endocrine abnormalities). Hematopoietic stem cell transplantation in childhood, before organ dysfunction induced by iron overload, has had a high success rate in β-thalassemia major and is the treatment of choice.

Sickle Cell Disease

Decision-Making Algorithms
Available @ StudentConsult.com

Abdominal Pain
Jaundice
Hepatomegaly
Splenomegaly
Anemia
Pancytopenia
Fever without a Source
Irritable Infant

Etiology and Epidemiology. The common sickle cell syndromes are **hemoglobin SS disease, hemoglobin S-C disease, hemoglobin S-β thalassemia**, and rare variants (Table 150-7). The specific hemoglobin phenotype must be identified because the clinical complications differ in frequency, type, and severity. As a result of a single **amino acid substitution**

| Table 150-7 | Comparison of Sickle Cell Syndromes |

		PERCENT HEMOGLOBIN					
GENOTYPE	CLINICAL CONDITION	Hb A	Hb S	Hb A$_2$	Hb F	Hb C	OTHER FINDING(S)
SA	Sickle cell trait	55–60	40–45	2–3	–	–	Usually asymptomatic
SS	Sickle cell anemia	0	85–95	2–3	5–15	–	Clinically severe anemia; Hb F heterogeneous in distribution
S-β° thalassemia	Sickle cell–β° thalassemia	0	70–80	3–5	10–20	–	Moderately severe anemia; splenomegaly in 50%; smear: hypochromic, microcytic anemia
S-β+ thalassemia	Sickle cell-β+ thalassemia	10–20	60–75	3–5	10–20	–	Hb F distributed heterogeneously; mild microcytic anemia
SC	Hb SC disease	0	45–50	–	–	45–50	Moderately severe anemia; splenomegaly; retinopathy; target cells
S-HPFH	Sickle-hereditary persistence of Hb F	0	70–80	1–2	20–30	–	Often asymptomatic; Hb F is uniformly distributed

From Andreoli T, Carpenter C, Griggs R, et al: Cecil Essentials of Medicine, ed 7, Philadelphia, 2007, Saunders.

(valine for glutamic acid at the β6 position), sickle hemoglobin crystallizes and forms a gel in the deoxygenated state. When reoxygenated, the sickle hemoglobin is normally soluble. The so-called reversible sickle cell is capable of entering the microcirculation. As the oxygen is extracted and saturation declines, sickling may occur, occluding the microvasculature. The surrounding tissue undergoes infarction, inducing pain and dysfunction. This sickling phenomenon is exacerbated by hypoxia, acidosis, fever, hypothermia, and dehydration.

Clinical Manifestations and Treatment. A child with sickle cell anemia is vulnerable to **life-threatening infection** by 4 months of age. By that time, **splenic dysfunction** is caused by sickling of the RBCs within the spleen, resulting in an inability to filter microorganisms from the bloodstream in most patients. Splenic dysfunction is followed, eventually, by **splenic infarction**, usually by 2 to 4 years of age. The loss of normal splenic function makes the patient susceptible to overwhelming infection by encapsulated organisms, especially *Streptococcus pneumoniae* and other pathogens (Table 150-8). The hallmark of infection is fever. A febrile patient with a sickle cell syndrome (temperature >38.5°C) must be evaluated immediately (see Chapter 96). Current precautions to prevent infections include prophylactic daily oral penicillin begun at diagnosis and vaccinations against pneumococcus, *Haemophilus influenzae* type b, hepatitis B virus, and influenza virus.

The anemia of hemoglobin SS disease is usually a chronic, moderately severe, hemolytic anemia that is not routinely transfusion dependent. The severity depends in part on the patient's phenotype. Manifestations of chronic anemia include jaundice, pallor, variable splenomegaly in infancy, a cardiac flow murmur, and delayed growth and sexual maturation. Decisions about transfusion should be made on the basis of the patient's clinical condition, the hemoglobin level, and the reticulocyte count.

Sickle cell disease is complicated by sudden, occasionally severe and life-threatening events caused by the acute intravascular sickling of the RBCs, with resultant pain or organ dysfunction (so-called **crisis**). In two different clinical situations, an acute, potentially life-threatening decline in the hemoglobin level may be superimposed on the chronic compensated anemia. **Splenic sequestration crisis** is a life-threatening, hyperacute drop in the hemoglobin level (blood volume) secondary to splenic pooling of the patient's RBCs and sickling within the spleen. The spleen is moderately to markedly enlarged, and the reticulocyte count is elevated. In an **aplastic crisis**, parvovirus B19 infects RBC precursors in the bone marrow and induces transient RBC aplasia with reticulocytopenia and a rapid worsening of anemia because of the very short life span of sickle RBCs. Simple transfusion therapy is indicated for sequestration and aplastic crises when the anemia is symptomatic.

Vasoocclusive painful events may occur in any organ of the body and are manifested by pain and/or significant dysfunction (see Table 150-8). The **acute chest syndrome** is a vasoocclusive crisis within the lungs with evidence of a new infiltrate on chest radiograph. It is often associated with infection and infarction. The patient may first complain of chest pain but within a few hours develops cough, increasing respiratory and heart rates, hypoxia, and progressive respiratory distress. Physical examination reveals areas of decreased breath sounds and dullness on chest percussion. Treatment involves early recognition and prevention of arterial hypoxemia. Oxygen, fluids, judicious use of analgesic medications, antibiotics, bronchodilators, and RBC transfusion (rarely exchange transfusion) are indicated in therapy for acute chest syndrome. *Incentive spirometry* may help reduce the incidence of acute chest crisis in patients presenting with pain in the chest or abdomen.

Pain crisis is the most common type of vasoocclusive event. The pain usually localizes to the long bones of the arms or legs but may occur in smaller bones of the hands or feet in infancy (dactylitis) or in the abdomen. Painful crises usually last 2 to 7 days. Vasoocclusive crises within the femur may lead to avascular necrosis of the femoral head and chronic hip disease. Treatment of pain crises includes administration of fluids, analgesia (usually narcotics and nonsteroidal anti-inflammatory drugs), and oxygen if the patient is hypoxic. Although pain is often impossible to quantitate, the risk for drug dependency is highly overrated, and appropriate use of analgesics is necessary.

Priapism occurs in boys usually between 6 and 20 years old. The child experiences a sudden, painful onset of a

Table 150-8	Clinical Manifestations of Sickle Cell Anemia*

MANIFESTATION	COMMENTS
Anemia	Chronic, onset 3–4 mo of age; may require folate therapy for chronic hemolysis; hemoglobin usually 6-10 g/dL
Aplastic crisis	Parvovirus infection, reticulocytopenia; acute and reversible; may need transfusion
Sequestration crisis	Massive splenomegaly (may involve liver), shock; treat with transfusion
Hemolytic crisis	May be associated with G6PD deficiency
Dactylitis	Hand-foot swelling in early infancy
Painful crisis	Microvascular painful vasoocclusive infarcts of muscle, bone, bone marrow, lung, intestines
Cerebrovascular accidents	Large and small vessel occlusion → thrombosis/bleeding (stroke); requires chronic transfusion
Acute chest syndrome	Infection, asthma, atelectasis, infarction, fat emboli, severe hypoxemia, infiltrate, dyspnea, absent breath sounds
Chronic lung disease	Pulmonary fibrosis, restrictive lung disease, cor pulmonale, pulmonary hypertension
Priapism	Causes eventual impotence; treated with transfusion, oxygen, or corpora cavernosa-to-spongiosa shunt
Ocular	Retinopathy
Gallbladder disease	Bilirubin stones; cholecystitis
Renal	Hematuria, papillary necrosis, renal concentrating defect; nephropathy
Cardiomyopathy	Heart failure
Skeletal	Osteonecrosis (avascular) of femoral or humeral head
Leg ulceration	Seen in older patients
Infections	Functional asplenia, defects in properdin system; pneumococcal bacteremia, meningitis, and arthritis; deafness from meningitis; *Salmonella* and *Staphylococcus aureus* osteomyelitis; severe *Mycoplasma* pneumonia
Growth failure, delayed puberty	May respond to nutritional supplements
Psychological problems	Narcotic addiction (rare), dependence unusual; chronic illness, chronic pain syndrome

G6PD, Glucose-6-phosphate dehydrogenase.
*Clinical manifestations with sickle cell trait are unusual but include renal papillary necrosis (hematuria), sudden death on exertion, intraocular hyphema extension, and sickling in unpressurized airplanes.

tumescent penis that will not relax. Therapeutic steps for priapism include the administration of oxygen, fluids, analgesia, and transfusion when appropriate to achieve a hemoglobin S less than 30% (often by partial exchange transfusion). Fluid management requires recognition that renal medullary infarction results in loss of the ability to concentrate urine.

Overt **stroke** occurs in approximately 8% to 10% of patients with SS disease. These events may present as the sudden onset of an altered state of consciousness, seizures, or focal paralysis. **Silent stroke**, which is defined as evidence of cerebral

infarction on imaging studies but a normal neurologic examination, is more common and occurs in approximately 20% of patients with SS disease. A significant change in school performance or behavior has been associated with silent stroke. Children with Hg SS disease over 3 years of age should be screened for increased risk of stroke using transcranial Doppler (TCD).

Laboratory Diagnosis. The diagnosis of hemoglobinopathies is made by identifying the precise amount and type of hemoglobin using **hemoglobin electrophoresis**, **isoelectric focusing**, or **high-performance liquid chromatography**. Every member of an at-risk population should have a precise hemoglobin phenotype performed at birth (preferably) or during early infancy. Most states perform newborn screening for sickle cell disease.

Treatment. Direct therapy of sickle cell anemia is evolving. The mainstay of care is supportive measures. The use of chronic RBC transfusions to treat patients who have had a stroke has been very successful. Chronic RBC transfusions have also been used successfully for short time periods to prevent recurrent vasoocclusive painful events, including acute chest syndrome and priapism. **Hydroxyurea**, which increases hemoglobin F, decreases the number and severity of vasoocclusive events and frequency of acute chest syndrome in children as early as 1 year of age. **Hematopoietic stem cell transplantation**, using a haploidentical sibling match, has cured many children with sickle cell disease. HSCT using alternative donors for children, without a suitable sibling match, is being studied.

Enzymopathies

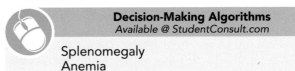

Decision-Making Algorithms
Available @ StudentConsult.com

Splenomegaly
Anemia

Etiology. Glucose-6-phosphate dehydrogenase (G6PD) deficiency is an abnormality in the **hexose monophosphate shunt pathway** of glycolysis that results in the depletion of reduced nicotinamide adenine dinucleotide phosphate (NADPH) and the inability to regenerate reduced glutathione. When a patient with G6PD is exposed to significant oxidant stress, hemoglobin is oxidized, forming precipitates of sulfhemoglobin (**Heinz bodies**), which are visible on specially stained preparations. The gene for G6PD deficiency is on the X chromosome.

The severity of hemolysis depends on the enzyme variant. In many G6PD variants, the enzymes become unstable with aging of the RBC and cannot be replaced because the cell is anucleated. Older cells are most susceptible to oxidant-induced hemolysis. In other variants, the enzyme is kinetically abnormal.

Epidemiology. The most common variants of G6PD deficiency have been found in areas where malaria is endemic. G6PD deficiency protects against parasitism of the erythrocyte. The most common variant with normal activity is termed **type B** and is defined by its electrophoretic mobility. The approximate gene frequencies in African Americans are 70% type B, 20% type A, and 10% type A–. Only the **A– variant**, termed the *African variant*, is unstable. Ten percent of black males are affected. A group of variants found in Sardinians, Sicilians, Greeks, Sephardic and Oriental Jews, and Arabs is termed the **Mediterranean variant** and is associated with chronic hemolysis and potentially life-threatening hemolytic disease. Because the gene for G6PD deficiency is carried on the X chromosome, clinical hemolysis is most common in males. Heterozygous females who have randomly inactivated a higher percentage of the normal gene may become symptomatic, as may homozygous females with the A– variant (0.5% to 1% of females of African descent).

Clinical Manifestations. G6PD deficiency has two common presentations. Individuals with the A– variant have normal hemoglobin values when well, but develop an **acute episode of hemolysis** triggered by serious (bacterial) infection or ingestion of an oxidant drug. The RBC morphology during episodes of acute hemolysis is striking, appearing to have "bites" taken out of them (cookie cells). These are areas of absent hemoglobin that are produced by phagocytosis of Heinz bodies by splenic macrophages; as a result, the RBCs appear blistered. Clinically evident jaundice, dark urine resulting from bilirubin pigments, hemoglobinuria when hemolysis is intravascular, and decreased haptoglobin levels are common during hemolytic episodes. Early on, the hemolysis usually exceeds the ability of the bone marrow to compensate, so the reticulocyte count may be low for 3 to 4 days.

Laboratory Studies. The diagnosis of G6PD deficiency is based on decreased NADPH formation. G6PD levels during an acute, severe hemolytic episode may be normal, however, because the most deficient cells have been destroyed and reticulocytes are enriched with G6PD. Repeating the test at a later time when the patient is in a steady-state condition, testing the mothers of boys with suspected G6PD deficiency, or performing electrophoresis to identify the precise variant present aids in diagnosis.

Treatment and Prevention. The treatment of G6PD deficiency is supportive. Transfusions are indicated when significant cardiovascular compromise is present. Maintaining hydration and urine alkalization protects the kidneys against damage from precipitated free hemoglobin. Hemolysis is prevented by avoidance of known oxidants, particularly long-acting sulfonamides, nitrofurantoin, primaquine, dimercaprol, and moth balls (naphthalene). Fava beans (favism) have triggered hemolysis, particularly in patients with the Mediterranean variant. Serious infection also is a potential precipitant of hemolysis in G6PD-deficient young children.

Pyruvate kinase deficiency is much less common than G6PD deficiency and represents a clinical spectrum of disorders caused by the functional deficiency of pyruvate kinase. Some individuals have a true deficiency state, and others have abnormal enzyme kinetics. The metabolic consequence of pyruvate kinase deficiency is adenosine triphosphate (ATP) depletion, impairing RBC survival. Pyruvate kinase deficiency is usually an autosomal disorder, and most children who are affected (and are not products of consanguinity) are double heterozygotes for two abnormal enzymes. Hemolysis is not aggravated by oxidant stress due to the profound reticulocytosis in this condition. Aplastic crises are potentially life-threatening. The spleen is the site for RBC removal in pyruvate kinase deficiency. Most patients have amelioration of the anemia and a reduction of transfusion requirements after splenectomy.

Membrane Disorders

Decision-Making Algorithms
Available @ StudentConsult.com

Anemia
Pancytopenia

Etiology. The biochemical basis of **hereditary spherocytosis** and **hereditary elliptocytosis** are similar. Both conditions appear to have a defect in the protein lattice (spectrin, ankyrin, protein 4.2, band 3) that underlies the RBC lipid bilayer and provides stability of the membrane shape. In hereditary spherocytosis, pieces of membrane bud off as microvesicles because of abnormal vertical interaction of the cytoskeletal proteins and uncoupling of the lipid bilayer from the cytoskeleton. When the RBC loses membrane, cell shape changes from a biconcave disk to a spherocyte. The RBC is less deformable when passing through narrow passages in the spleen. Hereditary elliptocytosis is a disorder of spectrin dimer interactions that occurs primarily in individuals of African descent. The transmission of the two variants is usually autosomal dominant, but spontaneous mutations causing hereditary spherocytosis are common. **Hereditary pyropoikilocytosis** (unusual instability of the erythrocytes when they are exposed to heat at 45°C) is the result of a structural abnormality of spectrin.

Clinical Manifestations. Hereditary spherocytosis varies greatly in clinical severity, ranging from an asymptomatic, well-compensated, mild hemolytic anemia that may be discovered incidentally to a severe hemolytic anemia with growth failure, splenomegaly, and chronic transfusion requirements in infancy necessitating early splenectomy. The most common variant of hereditary elliptocytosis is a clinically insignificant morphologic abnormality without shortened RBC survival. The less common variant is associated with spherocytes, ovalocytes, and elliptocytes with a moderate, usually compensated, hemolysis. Far more significant hemolysis occurs in hereditary pyropoikilocytosis. The peripheral blood smear in hereditary pyropoikilocytosis often includes elliptocytes, spherocytes, fragmented RBCs, and striking microcytosis. Such patients may have bizarre blood smears in the newborn period with small, fragmented RBCs.

Laboratory Diagnosis. The clinical diagnosis of hereditary spherocytosis should be suspected in patients with even a few spherocytes found on the blood smear because the spleen preferentially removes spherocytes. An incubated **osmotic fragility test** confirms the presence of spherocytes and increases the likelihood of the diagnosis. The osmotic fragility test result is abnormal in any hemolytic disease in which spherocytes are present—for example, in antibody-mediated hemolysis.

Treatment. Splenectomy corrects the anemia and normalizes the RBC survival in patients with hereditary spherocytosis, but the morphologic abnormalities persist. Splenectomy should be considered for any child with symptoms referable to anemia or growth failure, but should be deferred until age 5 years, if possible, to minimize the risk of overwhelming postsplenectomy sepsis and to maximize the antibody response to the polyvalent pneumococcal vaccine. In several reports, partial splenectomy seems to improve the hemolytic anemia and maintain splenic function in host defense.

A   B   C

Figure 150-4 Coombs or direct antiglobulin test (DAT). In the DAT, so-called Coombs serum that recognizes human immunoglobulin (Ig) or complement (C) is used to detect the presence of antibody or C on the surface of the red blood cells (RBCs) by agglutination. **A,** An IgM antibody can bind two RBCs simultaneously because of its multiple antigen-binding sites. The great size of the IgM allows it to bridge the surface repulsive forces (zeta potential) between RBCs and cause agglutination. **B,** An IgG antibody is too small to bridge the zeta potential and cause agglutination. **C,** On the addition of Coombs serum, the zeta potential is bridged successfully, and RBCs agglutinate. *(Modified from Ware RE, Rosse WF: Autoimmune hemolytic anemia. In Orkin SH, Nathan DG, Look AT, Ginsburg D, editors:* Hematology of Infancy and Childhood, *ed 6, Philadelphia, 2003, Saunders, p 530.)*

Hemolytic Anemia Caused by Disorders Extrinsic to the Red Blood Cell Etiology and Clinical Manifestations

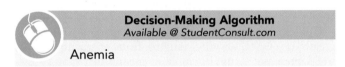

Decision-Making Algorithm
Available @ StudentConsult.com

Anemia

Isoimmune hemolysis is caused by active maternal immunization against fetal antigens that the mother's erythrocytes do not express (see Chapter 62). Examples are antibodies to the A, B, and Rh D antigens; other Rh antigens; and the Kell, Duffy, and other blood groups. Anti-A and anti-B hemolysis is caused by the placental transfer of naturally occurring maternal antibodies from mothers who lack A or B antigen (usually blood type O). Positive results of the direct antiglobulin (**Coombs**) test on the infant's RBCs (Fig. 150-4), the indirect antiglobulin test on the mother's serum, and the presence of spherocytes and immature erythroid precursors (erythroblastosis) on the infant's blood smear confirm this diagnosis. Isoimmune hemolytic disease varies in clinical severity. There may be no clinical manifestations, or the infant may exhibit jaundice, severe anemia, and hydrops fetalis.

Autoimmune hemolytic anemia is usually an acute, self-limited process that develops after an infection (*Mycoplasma,* Epstein-Barr, or other viral infections). Autoimmune hemolytic anemia may also be the presenting symptom of a chronic autoimmune disease (systemic lupus erythematosus, lymphoproliferative disorders, or immunodeficiency). Drugs may induce a Coombs-positive hemolytic anemia by forming a hapten on the RBC membrane (penicillin) or by forming immune complexes (quinidine) that attach to the RBC membrane. Antibodies then activate complement-induced intravascular hemolysis. The third type of drug-induced immune hemolysis occurs during treatment with α-methyldopa and a few other drugs. In this type, prolonged drug exposure alters the RBC membrane, inducing neoantigen formation. Antibodies are produced that bind to the neoantigen; this produces a positive antiglobulin test result far more commonly than it actually induces hemolysis. In each of these conditions, the erythrocyte is an *innocent bystander.*

A second form of acquired hemolytic disease is caused by mechanical damage to the RBC membrane during circulation. In **thrombotic microangiopathy**, the RBCs are trapped by fibrin strands in the circulation and physically broken by shear stress as they pass through these strands. Hemolytic uremic syndrome, disseminated intravascular coagulation (DIC), thrombotic thrombocytopenic purpura, malignant hypertension, toxemia, and hyperacute renal graft rejection can produce thrombotic microangiopathy. The platelets are usually large, indicating that they are young, but have a decreased survival even if the numbers are normal. Consumption of clotting factors is more prominent in DIC than in the other forms of thrombotic microangiopathy. The smear shows RBC fragments (schistocytes), microspherocytes, teardrop forms, and polychromasia. Other examples of mechanical injury to RBCs include damage by exposure to nonendothelialized surfaces (as in artificial heart valves) or as a result of high flow and shear rates in giant hemangiomas (**Kasabach-Merritt syndrome**).

Alterations in the plasma lipids, especially cholesterol, may lead to damage to the RBC membrane and shorten RBC survival. Lipids in the plasma are in equilibrium with lipids in the RBC membrane. High cholesterol levels increase the membrane cholesterol and the total membrane surface without affecting the volume of the cell. This condition produces **spur cells** that may be seen in abetalipoproteinemia and liver diseases. Hemolysis occurs in the spleen, where poor RBC deformability results in erythrocyte destruction. **Circulating toxins** (e.g., snake venoms and heavy metals) that bind sulfhydryl groups may damage the RBC membrane and induce hemolysis. Irregularly spiculated RBCs (burr cells) are seen in renal failure. **Vitamin E deficiency** can also cause an acquired hemolytic anemia as a result of abnormal sensitivity of membrane lipids to oxidant stress. Vitamin E deficiency may occur in premature infants who are not being supplemented with vitamin E or who have insufficient nutrition, in infants with severe malabsorption syndromes (including cystic fibrosis), and in infants with transfusional iron overload, which can lead to severe oxidant exposure.

Laboratory Diagnosis. The peripheral blood smear in autoimmune hemolytic anemia usually reveals spherocytes and occasionally nucleated RBCs. The reticulocyte count varies because some patients have relatively low reticulocyte counts as a result of autoantibodies that cross-react with RBC precursors.

Treatment and Prognosis. Transfusion for the treatment of autoimmune hemolysis is challenging because crossmatching is difficult, as the autoantibodies react with virtually all RBCs. In addition to **transfusion**, which may be lifesaving, management of autoimmune hemolytic anemia depends on antibody type. Management may involve administration of **corticosteroids** and, at times, **intravenous immunoglobulin**. Corticosteroids reduce the clearance of sensitized RBCs in the spleen. In drug-induced hemolysis, withdrawal of the drug usually leads to resolution of the hemolytic process. More than 80% of children with autoimmune hemolytic anemia recover spontaneously.

Chapter 151

HEMOSTATIC DISORDERS

NORMAL HEMOSTASIS
Hemostasis is the dynamic process of **coagulation** as it occurs in areas of vascular injury, involving the carefully modulated interaction of platelets, vascular wall, and procoagulant and anticoagulant proteins. After an injury to the vascular endothelium, subendothelial collagen induces a conformational change in von Willebrand factor (**vWF**), an adhesive protein to which platelets bind via their glycoprotein Ib receptor. After adhesion, platelets undergo activation and release numerous intracellular contents, including adenosine diphosphate (ADP). These **activated platelets** subsequently induce aggregation of additional platelets. Simultaneously, tissue factor, collagen, and other matrix proteins in tissue activate the coagulation cascade, leading to the formation of the enzyme **thrombin** (Fig. 151-1). Thrombin causes further aggregation of platelets, a positive feedback activation of factors 5 and 8, the conversion of fibrinogen to fibrin, and the activation of factor 11. A **platelet plug** forms, and bleeding ceases, usually within 3 to 7 minutes. The generation of thrombin leads to formation of a permanent clot by the activation of factor 13, which cross-links fibrin, forming a stable thrombus. Finally, contractile elements within the platelet mediate **clot retraction**. Thrombin also contributes to the eventual limitation of clot size by binding to the protein thrombomodulin on intact endothelial cells, converting protein C into activated protein C. Thrombin contributes to the eventual lysis of the thrombus by activating plasminogen to plasmin. All of the hemostatic processes are closely interwoven and occur on biologic surfaces that mediate coagulation by bringing the critical players—platelets, endothelial cells, and subendothelium—into close proximity with pro- and anticoagulant proteins.

Many think of coagulation as having **intrinsic and extrinsic pathways**, but the reality is that these pathways are closely interactive and do not react independently (Fig. 151-2). For ease of use, all coagulation factors are denoted using Arabic rather than Roman numerals to prevent misreading factor VII (7) as factor VIII (8). In vivo, factor 7 autocatalyzes to form small amounts of factor 7a. When tissue is injured, **tissue factor** is released and causes a burst of factor 7a generation. Tissue factor, in combination with calcium and factor 7a, activates factor 9 and factor 10. The activation of factor 9 by factor 7a results in eventual generation of thrombin, which feeds back on factor 11, generating factor 11a and accelerating thrombin formation. This process explains why deficiency of factor 8 or factor 9 leads to severe bleeding disorders, whereas deficiency of factor 11 is usually mild, and deficiency of factor 12 is asymptomatic.

A series of inhibitory factors serve to tightly regulate the activation of coagulation. **Antithrombin III** inactivates thrombin and factors 10a, 9a, and 11a. The **protein C and protein S** system inactivates activated factors 5 and 8, which are cofactors localized in the "tenase" and "prothrombinase" complexes. The **tissue factor pathway inhibitor**, an anticoagulant protein, limits activation of the coagulation cascade by factor 7a and factor 10a. **Fibrinolysis** is initiated by the action of tissue plasminogen activator on plasminogen, producing plasmin, the active enzyme that degrades fibrin into split products. Fibrinolysis eventually dissolves the clot and allows normal flow to resume. Deficiencies of anticoagulant proteins may predispose to thrombosis.

DEVELOPMENTAL HEMOSTASIS
In the fetus, fibrinogen, factor 5, factor 8, and platelets approach normal levels during the second trimester. Levels of other clotting factors and anticoagulant proteins increase gradually throughout gestation. The premature infant is simultaneously at increased risk of bleeding or clotting complications that are exacerbated by many of the medical interventions needed for care and monitoring, especially indwelling arterial or venous catheters. Most children attain normal levels of procoagulant and anticoagulant proteins by 1 year of age, although levels of protein C lag and normalize in adolescence.

HEMOSTATIC DISORDERS
Etiology and Epidemiology
A detailed **family history** is crucial for diagnosis of bleeding and thrombotic disorders. **Hemophilia** is X-linked, and almost all affected children are boys. **von Willebrand disease** usually is inherited in an autosomal dominant fashion. In the investigation of thrombotic disorders, a personal or family history of blood clots in the legs or lungs, early-onset stroke, or heart attack suggests a hereditary predisposition to thrombosis. The causes of bleeding may be hematologic in origin or due to vascular, nonhematologic causes (Fig. 151-3). Thrombotic disorders can be congenital or acquired (Table 151-1) and frequently present after an initial event (central catheter, trauma, malignancy, infection, pregnancy, treatment with estrogens) provides a nidus for clot formation or a procoagulant stimulus.

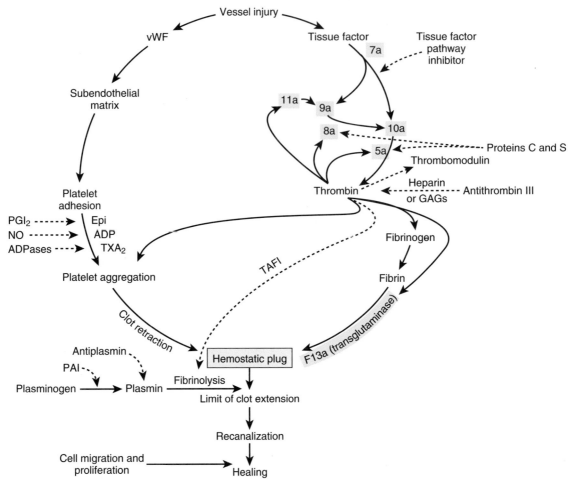

Figure 151-1 Diagram of the multiple interactions of the hemostatic mechanism. Solid lines indicate reactions that favor coagulation, and dashed lines indicate reactions that inhibit clotting. *Epi*, Epinephrine; *GAGs*, glycosaminoglycans; *NO*, nitric oxide; *PAI*, plasminogen activator inhibitor; *PGI₂*, prostaglandin I₂ (prostacyclin); *TAFI*, thrombin-activated fibrinolytic inhibitor; *TXA₂*, thromboxane A₂; *vWF*, von Willebrand factor. *(Modified from Scott JP, Montgomery RR: Hemorrhagic and thrombotic diseases. In Kliegman RM, Behrman RE, Jenson HB, Stanton BF, editors: Nelson Textbook of Pediatrics, ed 18, Philadelphia, 2007, Saunders, p 2062.)*

Clinical Manifestations

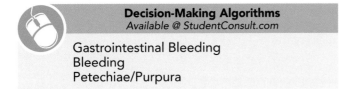

Decision-Making Algorithms
Available @ StudentConsult.com

Gastrointestinal Bleeding
Bleeding
Petechiae/Purpura

Patients with hemostatic disorders may have complaints of either bleeding or clotting. Age at onset of bleeding indicates whether the problem is congenital or acquired. The **sites of bleeding** (mucocutaneous or deep) and **degree of trauma** (spontaneous or significant) required to induce injury suggest the type and severity of the disorder. Certain medications (aspirin and valproic acid) are known to exacerbate preexisting bleeding disorders by interfering with platelet function.

The **physical examination** should characterize the presence of skin or mucous membrane bleeding and deeper sites of hemorrhage into the muscles and joints or internal bleeding sites. The term **petechia** refers to a non-blanching lesion less than 2 mm in size. **Purpura** is a group of adjoining petechiae, **ecchymoses** (bruises) are isolated lesions larger than petechiae, and **hematomas** are raised, palpable ecchymoses.

The physical examination should also search for manifestations of an underlying disease, lymphadenopathy, hepatosplenomegaly, vasculitic rash, or chronic hepatic or renal disease. **Deep venous thrombi** may cause warm, swollen (distended), tender, purplish discolored extremities or organs or no findings. **Arterial clots** cause acute, painful, pale, and poorly perfused extremities. Arterial thrombi of the internal organs present with signs and symptoms of infarction.

Laboratory Testing

Screening laboratory studies for bleeding patients include a **platelet count, prothrombin time, partial thromboplastin time, fibrinogen**, and **bleeding time** or other screening test of platelet function. Many laboratories have adopted the platelet function analyzer (PFA) to replace the bleeding time as a screening test for platelet function abnormalities and

Figure 151-2 Simplified pathways of blood coagulation. The area inside the solid black line is the intrinsic pathway measured by the activated partial thromboplastin time (APTT). The area inside the green line is the extrinsic pathway, measured by the prothrombin time (PT). The area encompassed by both lines is the common pathway. *AT-III,* Antithrombin III; *F,* factor; *HMWK,* high-molecular-weight kininogen; *P-C/S,* protein C/S; *PL,* phospholipid; *TFPI,* tissue factor pathway inhibitor. (*Modified from Scott JP, Montgomery RR: Hemorrhagic and thrombotic diseases. In Kliegman RM, Behrman RE, Jenson HB, Stanton BF, editors:* Nelson Textbook of Pediatrics, *ed 18, Philadelphia, 2007, Saunders, p 2061.*)

Figure 151-3 Common causes of bleeding. *TAR,* Thrombocytopenia with absence of radius (syndrome).

von Willebrand disease. The PFA has variable sensitivity and specificity for common bleeding disorders. No single laboratory test can screen for all bleeding disorders. The findings on screening tests for bleeding vary with the specific disorder (Table 151-2).

Table 151-1	Common Hypercoagulable States

CONGENITAL DISORDERS

Factor V Leiden (activated protein C resistance)

Prothrombin 20210

Protein C deficiency

Protein S deficiency

Antithrombin III deficiency

Plasminogen deficiency

Dysfibrinogenemia

Homocystinuria

ACQUIRED DISORDERS

Indwelling catheters

Lupus anticoagulant/antiphospholipid syndrome

Nephrotic syndrome

Malignancy

Pregnancy

Birth control pills

Autoimmune disease

Immobilization/surgery

Trauma

Infection

Inflammatory bowel disease

From Scott JP: Bleeding and thrombosis. In Kliegman RM, editor: Practical Strategies in Pediatric Diagnosis and Therapy, Philadelphia, 1996, WB Saunders.

Differential Diagnosis
Disorders of Platelets

Decision-Making Algorithms
Available @ StudentConsult.com

Bleeding
Petechiae/Purpura

Platelet counts less than 150,000/mm^3 constitute **thrombocytopenia.** Mucocutaneous bleeding is the hallmark of platelet disorders, including thrombocytopenia. The risk of bleeding correlates imperfectly with the platelet count. Children with platelet counts greater than 80,000/mm^3 are able to withstand all but the most extreme hemostatic challenges, such as surgery or major trauma. Children with platelet counts less than 20,000/mm^3 are at risk for spontaneous bleeding. These generalizations are modified by factors such as the age of the platelets (young, large platelets usually function better than old ones) and the presence of inhibitors of platelet function, such as antibodies, drugs (especially aspirin), fibrin degradation products, and toxins formed in the presence of hepatic or renal disease. The size of platelets is routinely measured as the mean platelet volume (MPV). The etiology of thrombocytopenia (Fig. 151-4) may be organized into three mechanisms:
1. Decreased platelet production
2. Increased destruction
3. Sequestration

Thrombocytopenia Resulting from Decreased Platelet Production

Primary disorders of megakaryopoiesis (platelet production) are rare in childhood, other than as part of an aplastic syndrome. **Thrombocytopenia with absent radii syndrome** is characterized by severe thrombocytopenia in association with orthopedic abnormalities, especially of the upper

Table 151-2	Screening Tests for Bleeding Disorders			
TEST	**MECHANISM TESTED**	**NORMAL VALUES**		**DISORDER**
Prothrombin time	Extrinsic and common pathway	<12 sec beyond neonate; 12–18 sec in term neonate		Defect in vitamin K–dependent factors; hemorrhagic disease of newborn, malabsorption, liver disease, DIC, oral anticoagulants, ingestion of rat poison
Activated partial thromboplastin time	Intrinsic and common pathway	25–40 sec beyond neonate; 70 sec in term neonate		Hemophilia; von Willebrand disease, heparin; DIC; deficient factors 12 and 11; lupus anticoagulant
Thrombin time	Fibrinogen to fibrin conversion	10–15 sec beyond neonate; 12–17 sec in term neonate		Fibrin split products, DIC, hypofibrinogenemia, heparin, uremia
Bleeding time	Hemostasis, capillary and platelet function	3–7 min beyond neonate		Platelet dysfunction, thrombocytopenia, von Willebrand disease, aspirin
Platelet count	Platelet number	150,000–450,000/mL		Thrombocytopenia differential diagnosis (see Fig. 151-4)
PFA	Closure time			
Blood smear	Platelet number and size; RBC morphology	–		Large platelets suggest peripheral destruction; fragmented, bizarre RBC morphology suggests microangiopathic process (e.g., hemolytic uremic syndrome, hemangioma, DIC)

DIC, Disseminated intravascular coagulation; PFA, platelet function analyzer-100; RBC, red blood cell.

extremity. The thrombocytopenia usually improves over time. **Amegakaryocytic thrombocytopenia** presents at birth or shortly thereafter with findings of severe thrombocytopenia, but no other congenital anomalies. The marrow is devoid of megakaryocytes and usually progresses to aplasia of all hematopoietic cell lines.

Acquired thrombocytopenia as a result of decreased production is rarely an isolated finding. It is seen more often in the context of **pancytopenia resulting from bone marrow failure** caused by infiltrative or aplastic processes. Certain chemotherapeutic agents may affect megakaryocytes selectively

more than other marrow elements. **Cyanotic congenital heart disease with polycythemia** often is associated with thrombocytopenia, but this is rarely severe or associated with significant clinical bleeding. Congenital (TORCH [toxoplasmosis, other agents, rubella, cytomegalovirus, herpes simplex]) and acquired **viral infections** (human immunodeficiency virus [HIV], Epstein-Barr virus, and measles) and some **drugs** (anticonvulsants, antibiotics, cytotoxic agents, heparin, and quinidine) may induce thrombocytopenia. Postnatal infections and drug reactions usually cause transient thrombocytopenia, whereas congenital infections may produce prolonged suppression of bone marrow function.

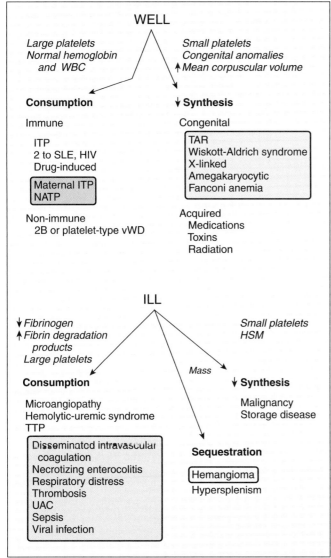

Figure 151-4 Differential diagnosis of childhood thrombocytopenic syndromes. The syndromes initially are separated by their clinical appearances. Clues leading to the diagnosis are presented in italics. The mechanisms and common disorders leading to these findings are shown in the lower part of the figure. Disorders that commonly affect neonates are listed in the shaded boxes. *HSM*, Hepatosplenomegaly; *ITP*, idiopathic immune thrombocytopenic purpura; *NATP*, neonatal alloimmune thrombocytopenic purpura; *SLE*, systemic lupus erythematosus; *TAR*, thrombocytopenia with absence of radius (syndrome); *TTP*, thrombotic thrombocytopenic purpura; *UAC*, umbilical artery catheter; *WBC*, white blood cell. *(From Scott JP: Bleeding and thrombosis. In Kliegman RM, Greenbaum LA, Lye PS, editors: Practical Strategies in Pediatric Diagnosis and Therapy, Philadelphia, 2004, Saunders, p 920.)*

Thrombocytopenia Resulting from Peripheral Destruction

Etiology. In a child who appears well, **immune-mediated mechanisms** are the most common cause of thrombocytopenia resulting from rapid peripheral destruction of antibody-coated platelets by reticuloendothelial cells. **Neonatal alloimmune thrombocytopenic purpura** (NATP) occurs as a result of sensitization of the mother to antigens present on fetal platelets. Antibodies cross the placenta and attack the fetal platelet (see Chapter 59). Many platelet alloantigens have been identified and sequenced, permitting prenatal diagnosis of the condition in an at-risk fetus. Mothers with idiopathic thrombocytopenic purpura (**maternal ITP**) or with a history of ITP may have passive transfer of antiplatelet antibodies, with resultant neonatal thrombocytopenia (see Chapter 59). The maternal platelet count is sometimes a useful indicator of the probability that the infant will be affected.

Clinical Manifestations. The infant with NATP is at risk for **intracranial hemorrhage** in utero and during the immediate delivery process. In ITP, the greatest risk seems to be present during passage through the birth canal, during which molding of the head may induce intracranial hemorrhage. Fetal scalp sampling or percutaneous umbilical blood sampling may be performed to measure the fetal platelet count.

Treatment. Administration of intravenous immunoglobulin (IVIG) before delivery increases fetal platelet counts and may alleviate thrombocytopenia in infants with NATP and ITP. Delivery by cesarean section is recommended to prevent central nervous system (CNS) bleeding (see Chapter 59). Neonates with severe thrombocytopenia (platelet counts <20,000/mm^3) may be treated with IVIG or corticosteroids or both until thrombocytopenia remits. If necessary, infants with NATP may receive washed maternal platelets.

Idiopathic Thrombocytopenic Purpura

Etiology. Autoimmune thrombocytopenic purpura of childhood (childhood ITP) is a common disorder that usually follows an acute viral infection. Childhood ITP is caused by an antibody (IgG or IgM) that binds to the platelet membrane. The condition results in Fc receptor–mediated splenic destruction of antibody-coated platelets. Rarely, ITP may be the presenting symptom of an autoimmune disease, such as systemic lupus erythematosus (SLE).

Clinical Manifestations. Young children typically exhibit ITP 1 to 4 weeks after viral illness, with abrupt onset of petechiae, purpura, and epistaxis. The thrombocytopenia usually is severe. Significant adenopathy or hepatosplenomegaly is unusual, and the red blood cell (RBC) and white blood cell (WBC) counts are normal.

Diagnosis. The diagnosis of ITP usually is based on clinical presentation and the platelet count and does not often require a bone marrow examination. If atypical findings are noted, however, marrow examination is indicated to rule out an infiltrative disorder (leukemia) or an aplastic process (aplastic anemia). In ITP, an examination of the bone marrow reveals increased megakaryocytes and normal erythroid and myeloid elements.

Treatment and Prognosis. Therapy is seldom indicated for platelet counts greater than 30,000/mm^3. Therapy does not affect the long-term outcome of ITP but is intended to increase the platelet count acutely. For moderate and severe clinical bleeding with severe thrombocytopenia (platelet count <10,000/mm^3), therapeutic options include **prednisone**, 2 to 4 mg/kg/24 hours for 2 weeks or IVIG, 1 g/kg/24 hours for 1 to 2 days. All of these approaches seem to decrease the rate of clearance of sensitized platelets, rather than decreasing production of antibody. The optimal choice for therapy (if any) is controversial. Splenectomy is indicated in acute ITP only for life-threatening bleeding. Approximately 80% of children have a spontaneous resolution of ITP within 6 months after diagnosis. Serious bleeding, especially intracranial bleeding, occurs in fewer than 1% of patients with ITP. There is no evidence that early treatment prevents intracranial bleeding.

ITP that persists for 6 to 12 months is classified as **chronic ITP**. Repeated treatments with IVIG, IV anti-D, or high-dose pulse steroids are effective in delaying the need for splenectomy. Secondary causes of chronic ITP, especially SLE and HIV infection, should be ruled out. Splenectomy induces a remission in 70% to 80% of childhood chronic ITP cases. The risks of splenectomy (surgery, sepsis from encapsulated bacteria, pulmonary hypertension) must be weighed against the risk of severe bleeding.

Other Disorders

Decision-Making Algorithms
Available @ StudentConsult.com

Petechiae/Purpura
Eosinophilia
Recurrent Infections

Wiskott-Aldrich syndrome is an X-linked disorder characterized by hypogammaglobinemia, eczema, and thrombocytopenia caused by a molecular defect in a cytoskeletal protein common to lymphocytes and platelets (see Chapter 74). Small platelets are seen on a peripheral blood smear. Nevertheless, thrombocytopenia often is improved by splenectomy. Hematopoietic stem cell transplantation cures the immunodeficiency and thrombocytopenia. Familial X-linked thrombocytopenia can be seen as a variant of Wiskott-Aldrich syndrome or a mutation in the *GATA1* gene. Autosomal macrothrombocytopenia is due to deletions in chromosomes 22q11 or mutations in 22q12.

Thrombotic microangiopathy causes thrombocytopenia, anemia secondary to intravascular RBC destruction, and, in some cases, depletion of clotting factors. Children with thrombotic microangiopathy usually are quite ill. In a child with disseminated intravascular coagulation (**DIC**), the deposition of

fibrin strands within the vasculature and activation of thrombin and plasmin result in a wide-ranging hemostatic disorder with activation and clearance of platelets. **Hemolytic uremic syndrome** occurs as a result of exposure to a toxin that induces endothelial injury, fibrin deposition, and platelet activation and clearance (see Chapter 164). In **thrombotic thrombocytopenic purpura**, platelet consumption, precipitated by a congenital or acquired deficiency of a metalloproteinase that cleaves von Willebrand factor, seems to be the primary process, with a modest deposition of fibrin and RBC destruction.

Disorders of Platelet Function

Etiology. Primary disorders of platelet function may involve receptors on platelet membranes for adhesive proteins. Deficiency of glycoprotein Ib complex (vWF receptor) causes **Bernard-Soulier syndrome**. A deficiency of glycoprotein IIb-IIIa (the fibrinogen receptor) causes **Glanzmann thrombasthenia**. Mild abnormalities of platelet aggregation and release, detectable by platelet aggregometry, are far more common. Secondary disorders caused by toxins and drugs (uremia, valproic acid, aspirin, nonsteroidal anti-inflammatory drugs, and infections) may cause a broad spectrum of platelet dysfunction.

Clinical Manifestations. Disorders of platelet function present with mucocutaneous bleeding and a prolonged bleeding time or long PFA closure time and may be primary or secondary. The bleeding time is an insensitive screen for mild and moderate platelet function disorders but is usually prolonged in severe platelet function disorders, such as Bernard-Soulier syndrome or Glanzmann thrombasthenia.

Disorders of Clotting Factors

Decision-Making Algorithm
Available @ StudentConsult.com

Bleeding

Etiology. Hereditary deficiencies of most procoagulant proteins lead to bleeding. The genes for factor 8 and factor 9 are on the X chromosome, whereas virtually all the other clotting factors are coded on autosomal chromosomes. **Factor 8 and factor 9 deficiencies** are the most common severe inherited bleeding disorders. **von Willebrand disease** is the most common congenital bleeding disorder. Of the procoagulant proteins, low levels of the so-called contact factors (prekallikrein, high-molecular-weight kininogen, and Hageman factor [factor 12]) cause a prolonged activated partial thromboplastin time but are not associated with a predisposition to bleeding.

Hemophilia

Etiology. Hemophilia A (factor 8 deficiency) occurs in 1 in 5000 males. **Hemophilia B** (factor 9 deficiency) occurs in approximately 1 in 25,000. Clinically the two disorders are indistinguishable other than by their therapy (Table 151-3). The lack of factor 8 or factor 9 delays the generation of thrombin, which is crucial to forming a normal, functional fibrin clot and solidifying the platelet plug that has formed in areas of vascular injury. The severity of the disorder is determined by the degree of clotting factor deficiency.

Table 151-3	Comparison of Hemophilia A, Hemophilia B, and von Willebrand Disease		
FEATURE	**HEMOPHILIA A**	**HEMOPHILIA B**	**VON WILLEBRAND DISEASE**
Inheritance	X-linked	X-linked	Autosomal dominant
Factor deficiency	Factor 8	Factor 9	vWF, factor 8
Bleeding site(s)	Muscle, joint, surgical	Muscle, joint, surgical	Mucous membranes, skin, surgical, menstrual
Prothrombin time	Normal	Normal	Normal
Activated partial thromboplastin time	Prolonged	Prolonged	Prolonged or normal
Bleeding time/PFA-100	Normal	Normal	Prolonged or normal
Factor 8 coagulant activity	Low	Normal	Low or normal
von Willebrand factor antigen	Normal	Normal	Low
von Willebrand factor activity	Normal	Normal	Low
Factor 9	Normal	Low	Normal
Ristocetin-induced platelet agglutination	Normal	Normal	Normal, low, or increased at low-dose ristocetin
Platelet aggregation	Normal	Normal	Normal
Treatment	DDAVP* or recombinant factor 8	Recombinant factor 9	DDAVP* or vWF concentrate

PFA, Platelet function analyzer-100; *vWF*, von Willebrand factor.
*Desmopressin (DDAVP) for mild to moderate hemophilia A or type 1 von Willebrand disease.

Clinical Manifestations. Patients with less than 1% (severe hemophilia) factor 8 or factor 9 may have **spontaneous bleeding** or bleeding with minor trauma. Patients with 1% to 5% (moderate hemophilia) factor 8 or factor 9 usually require moderate trauma to induce bleeding episodes. In mild hemophilia (>5% factor 8 or factor 9), significant trauma is necessary to induce bleeding; spontaneous bleeding does not occur. Mild hemophilia may go undiagnosed for many years, whereas severe hemophilia manifests in infancy when the child reaches the toddler stage. In severe hemophilia, spontaneous bleeding occurs, usually in the muscles or joints (**hemarthroses**).

Laboratory Studies. The diagnosis of hemophilia is based on a **prolonged activated partial thromboplastin time** (aPTT). In the aPTT, a surface-active agent activates the intrinsic system of coagulation, of which factors 8 and 9 are crucial components. In factor 8 or factor 9 deficiency, the aPTT is quite prolonged but should correct to normal when the patient's plasma is mixed 1:1 with normal plasma. When an abnormal aPTT is obtained, **specific factor assays** are needed to make a precise diagnosis (see Table 151-2) to determine the appropriate factor replacement therapy. Prenatal diagnosis and carrier diagnosis are possible using molecular techniques.

Treatment. Early, appropriate **replacement therapy** is the hallmark of excellent hemophilia care. Acute bleeding episodes are best treated in the home when the patient has attained the appropriate age and the parents have learned home treatment. Bleeding associated with surgery, trauma, or dental extraction often can be anticipated, and excessive bleeding can be prevented with appropriate replacement therapy. Prophylactic therapy starting in infancy has greatly diminished the likelihood of chronic arthropathy in children with hemophilia. For life-threatening bleeding, levels of 80% to 100% of normal factor 8 or factor 9 are necessary. For mild to moderate bleeding episodes (hemarthroses), a 40% level for factor 8 or a 30% to 40% level for factor 9 is appropriate. The dose can be calculated using the knowledge that 1 U/kg body weight of factor 8 increases the plasma level 2%, whereas 1.5 U/kg of recombinant factor 9 increases the plasma level 1%:

$$\text{Dose for factor } 8 = \text{desired level } (\%) \times \text{weight (kg)} \times 0.5$$

or

$$\text{Dose for recombinant factor } 9 = \text{desired level } (\%) \times \text{weight (kg)} \times 1.5$$

Desmopressin acetate is a synthetic vasopressin analog with minimal vasopressor effect. Desmopressin triples or quadruples the initial factor 8 level of a patient with mild or moderate (not severe) hemophilia A, but has no effect on factor 9 levels. When adequate hemostatic levels can be attained, desmopressin is the treatment of choice for individuals with mild and moderate hemophilia A. Aminocaproic acid is an inhibitor of fibrinolysis that may be useful for oral bleeding.

Patients treated with older factor 8 or 9 concentrates derived from large pools of plasma donors were at high risk for **hepatitis B, C, and D** and **HIV**. Recombinant factor 8 and factor 9 concentrates are safe from virally transmitted illnesses. Acquired immunodeficiency syndrome (AIDS) is the most common cause of death in older hemophilia patients (who received plasma-derived factors). Many older patients also have chronic hepatitis C.

Inhibitors are IgG antibodies directed against transfused factor 8 or factor 9 in congenitally deficient patients. Inhibitors arise in 15% of severe factor 8 hemophiliacs but are less common in factor 9 hemophiliacs. They may be high or low titer and show an anamnestic response to treatment. The treatment of bleeding patients with an inhibitor is difficult. For low titer inhibitors, options include continuous factor 8 infusions. For high titer inhibitors, it is usually necessary to administer a product that bypasses the inhibitor, preferably recombinant factor 7a. Activated prothrombin complex concentrates, used in the past to treat inhibitor patients, paradoxically increased the risks of thrombosis, resulting in fatal complications, such as myocardial infarction. For long-term treatment of inhibitor patients, induction of immune tolerance by repeated infusion of the deficient factor with or without immunosuppression may be beneficial.

Early institution of factor replacement and continuous prophylaxis beginning in early childhood should prevent the chronic joint disease associated with hemophilia.

von Willebrand Disease

Etiology. Von Willebrand disease is a common disorder (1% of the population) caused by a deficiency of **vWF**, an adhesive protein that serves two functions: acting as a bridge between sub-endothelial collagen and platelets and binding and protecting circulating factor 8 from rapid clearance from circulation. Von Willebrand disease usually is inherited as an autosomal dominant trait and rarely as an autosomal recessive trait. vWF may be either quantitatively deficient (partial = type 1 or absolute = type 3) or qualitatively abnormal (type 2 = dysproteinemia). Approximately 80% of patients with von Willebrand disease have classic (type 1) disease (i.e., a mild to moderate deficiency of vWF). Several other subtypes are clinically important, each requiring different therapy.

Clinical Manifestations. Mucocutaneous bleeding, epistaxis, gingival bleeding, cutaneous bruising, and menorrhagia occur in patients with von Willebrand disease. In severe disease, factor 8 deficiency may be profound, and the patient may also have manifestations similar to hemophilia A (hemarthrosis). Findings in classic von Willebrand disease differ from findings in hemophilia A and B (see Table 151-3).

Laboratory Testing. vWF testing involves measurement of the amount of protein, usually measured immunologically as the **vWF antigen** (vWF:Ag). vWF activity (vWF:Act) is measured functionally in the **ristocetin cofactor assay** (vWFR:Co), which uses the antibiotic ristocetin to induce vWF to bind to platelets.

Treatment. The treatment of von Willebrand disease depends on the severity of bleeding. **Desmopressin** is the treatment of choice for most bleeding episodes in patients with type 1 disease and some patients with type 2 disease. When high levels of vWF are needed but cannot be achieved satisfactorily with desmopressin, treatment with a virally attenuated, **vWF-containing concentrate** (Humate P) may be appropriate. The dosage can be calculated as for factor 8 in hemophilia. Cryoprecipitate should not be used because it is not virally attenuated. Hepatitis B vaccine should be given before the patient is exposed to plasma-derived products. As in all bleeding disorders, aspirin should be avoided.

Vitamin K Deficiency

For discussion of vitamin K deficiency, see Chapters 27 and 31.

Disseminated Intravascular Coagulation

Decision-Making Algorithms
Available @ StudentConsult.com

Bleeding
Petechiae/Purpura

Etiology. Disseminated intravascular coagulation (DIC) is a disorder in which widespread activation of the coagulation mechanism is usually associated with shock. Normal hemostasis is a balance between hemorrhage and thrombosis. In DIC,

Table 151-4	Causes of Disseminated Intravascular Coagulation

INFECTIOUS

Meningococcemia (purpura fulminans)
Other gram-negative bacteria (*Haemophilus, Salmonella, Escherichia coli*)
Rickettsiae (Rocky Mountain spotted fever)
Virus (cytomegalovirus, herpes, hemorrhagic fevers)
Malaria
Fungus

TISSUE INJURY

Central nervous system trauma (massive head injury)
Multiple fractures with fat emboli
Crush injury
Profound shock or asphyxia
Hypothermia or hyperthermia
Massive burns

MALIGNANCY

Acute promyelocytic leukemia
Acute monoblastic or myelocytic leukemia
Widespread malignancies (neuroblastoma)

VENOM OR TOXIN

Snake bites
Insect bites

MICROANGIOPATHIC DISORDERS

"Severe" thrombotic thrombocytopenic purpura
Hemolytic uremic syndrome
Giant hemangioma (Kasabach-Merritt syndrome)

GASTROINTESTINAL DISORDERS

Fulminant hepatitis
Severe inflammatory bowel disease
Reye syndrome

HEREDITARY THROMBOTIC DISORDERS

Antithrombin III deficiency
Homozygous protein C deficiency

NEONATAL PERIOD

Maternal toxemia
Group B streptococcal infections
Abruptio placentae
Severe respiratory distress syndrome
Necrotizing enterocolitis
Congenital viral disease (e.g., cytomegalovirus infection or herpes)
Erythroblastosis fetalis

MISCELLANEOUS CONDITIONS/DISORDERS

Severe acute graft rejection
Acute hemolytic transfusion reaction
Severe collagen vascular disease
Kawasaki disease
Heparin-induced thrombosis
Infusion of "activated" prothrombin complex concentrates
Hyperpyrexia/encephalopathy, hemorrhagic shock syndrome

From Scott JP: Bleeding and thrombosis. In Kliegman RM, editor: Practical Strategies in Pediatric Diagnosis and Therapy, Philadelphia, 1996, WB Saunders.

this balance is altered by the severe illness, so the patient has activation of coagulation (thrombosis) mediated by thrombin and fibrinolysis mediated by plasmin (bleeding). Coagulation factors—especially platelets, fibrinogen, and factors 2, 5, and 8—are consumed, as are the anticoagulant proteins, especially antithrombin, protein C, and plasminogen. Endothelial injury, tissue release of thromboplastic procoagulant factors, or, rarely, exogenous factors (snake venoms) directly activate the coagulation mechanism (Table 151-4).

Table 151-5	Differential Diagnosis of Coagulopathies That Can Be Confused with Disseminated Intravascular Coagulation					
	PROTHROMBIN TIME	PARTIAL THROMBOPLASTIN TIME	FIBRINOGEN	PLATELETS	D-DIMER	CLINICAL KEY(S)
DIC	↑	↑	↓	↓	↑	Shock
Liver failure	↑	↑	↓	Normal or ↓	↑	Jaundice
Vitamin K deficiency	↑	↑	Normal	Normal	Normal	Malabsorption, liver disease
Sepsis without shock	↑	↑	Normal	Normal	↑ or normal	Fever

From Scott JP: Bleeding and thrombosis. In Kliegman RM, editor: Practical Strategies in Pediatric Diagnosis and Therapy, Philadelphia, 1996, WB Saunders. DIC, Disseminated intravascular coagulation.

Clinical Manifestations. The diagnosis of DIC usually is suspected clinically and is confirmed by laboratory findings of a **decline in platelets and fibrinogen** associated with elevated prothrombin time, partial thromboplastin time, and elevated levels of D-dimer, formed when fibrinogen is clotted and then degraded by plasmin (Table 151-5). In some patients, DIC may evolve more slowly and there may be a degree of compensation. In a severely ill patient, the sudden occurrence of bleeding from a venipuncture or incision site, gastrointestinal or pulmonary hemorrhage, petechiae, or ecchymosis or evidence of peripheral gangrene or thrombosis suggests the diagnosis of DIC.

Treatment. The treatment of DIC is challenging. General guidelines include the following: treat the disorder inducing the DIC first; **support** the patient by correcting hypoxia, acidosis, and poor perfusion; and replace depleted blood-clotting factors, platelets, and anticoagulant proteins by transfusion.

Heparin may be used to treat significant arterial or venous thrombotic disease unless sites of life-threatening bleeding coexist.

Thrombosis

Etiology. A hereditary predisposition to **thrombosis** (see Table 151-1) may be caused by a deficiency of an anticoagulant protein (**protein C or S, antithrombin,** or **plasminogen**) (Fig. 151-5), by an abnormality of a procoagulant protein making it resistant to proteolysis by its respective inhibitor (**factor 5 Leiden**), by a mutation resulting in an increased level of a procoagulant protein (**prothrombin 20210**), or by damage to endothelial cells (**homocysteinemia**). Neonates with deficiency syndromes may be particularly vulnerable to thrombosis. Neonates with homozygous protein C deficiency present with purpura fulminans or thrombosis of the major arteries and veins or both. Many individuals with an inherited predisposition to thrombosis exhibit symptoms in adolescence or early adulthood. Protein C deficiency presenting in adulthood usually is inherited as an autosomal dominant trait, whereas the homozygous form usually is autosomal recessive. Protein S and antithrombin III deficiencies are inherited as autosomal dominant traits. Factor 5 Leiden is the most common hereditary cause of a predisposition to thrombosis, appearing in 3% to 5% of whites. **Acquired antiphospholipid antibodies** (anticardiolipin and lupus anticoagulant) also predispose to thrombosis.

Clinical Manifestations. Neonates and adolescents are the most likely pediatric patients to present with thromboembolic disease. Indwelling catheters, vasculitis, sepsis, immobilization, nephrotic syndrome, coagulopathy, trauma, infection, surgery, inflammatory bowel disease, oral contraceptive agents, pregnancy, and abortion all predispose to thrombosis.

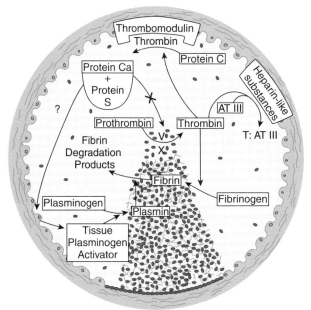

Figure 151-5 Formation of the hemostatic plug at the site of vascular injury. Three major physiologic anticoagulant mechanisms—antithrombin III (AT III), protein C, and the fibrinolytic system—are activated to limit clot formation to the site of damage and to prevent generalized thrombosis. T, Thrombin. (From Schafer A: The hypercoagulable state, Ann Intern Med 102:814–828, 1985.)

The manifestations of pulmonary emboli vary from no findings to chest pain, diminished breath sounds, a loud S_2, cyanosis, tachypnea, and hypoxemia.

Diagnostic and Imaging Studies. Venous thrombosis can be detected noninvasively by ultrasound Doppler flow compression studies. The gold standard for diagnosis is the venogram. An abnormal (high probability) ventilation-perfusion scan or detection of an intravascular thrombus on helical computed tomography (CT) is diagnostic of pulmonary emboli. There are no appropriate screening studies for thrombotic disorders. Diagnosis of a congenital or acquired predisposition to thrombosis requires a battery of specific assays.

Treatment. Therapy of thrombotic disorders depends on the underlying condition and usually involves standard or low-molecular-weight **heparin** and then longer term anticoagulation with **warfarin.** Major vessel thrombosis or life-threatening thrombosis may necessitate treatment with **fibrinolytic agents** (recombinant tissue plasminogen activator). In newborns, inherited deficiency syndromes may present as emergencies and necessitate **replacement** with plasma, antithrombin III concentrates, or protein C concentrates.

Chapter 152

BLOOD COMPONENT THERAPY

Transfusion of red blood cells (RBCs), platelets, plasma, cryoprecipitate, and granulocytes can be life-saving or life-maintaining (Table 152-1). **Whole blood** is rarely indicated and is most useful to provide both oxygen-carrying capacity and functional procoagulant and anticoagulant factors. Otherwise, **packed RBCs** are used to treat anemia to increase oxygen-carrying capacity. RBC transfusions should not be used to treat asymptomatic nutritional deficiencies that can be corrected by administering the appropriate deficient nutrient (iron or folic acid).

Blood component therapy requires proper anticoagulation of the component unit, screening for infectious agents and blood group compatibility testing before administration. Typical **transfusion reactions** are listed in Table 152-2. Transfusion may also result in circulatory overload, especially in the presence of cardiopulmonary deficiency. Filtering of blood products to remove white blood cells (WBCs) may prevent febrile reactions. Long-term complications of transfusions

Table 152-1	Commonly Used Transfusion Products			
COMPONENT	**CONTENT**	**INDICATION**	**DOSE**	**EXPECTED OUTCOME**
Packed RBCs	250–300 mL/unit	↓ Oxygen-carrying RBCs	10–15 mL/kg	↑ Hb by 2–3 g/dL
Platelet concentrate from whole blood donation	$5–7 \times 10^{10}$ platelets/unit	Severe thrombocytopenia ± bleeding	1 unit/10 kg	↑ Platelet count by 50,000/μL
Platelet concentrate	3×10^{11} platelets/unit	Severe thrombocytopenia ± bleeding	1 unit/70 kg	↑ Platelet count by 30,000-50,000/μL
Fresh frozen plasma	1 unit of each clotting factor /mL	Multiple clotting factor deficiency	10–20 mL/kg	Improvement in significantly prolonged prothrombin and partial thromboplastin times
Cryoprecipitate	Fibrinogen, factor 8, vWF, factor 13	Hypofibrinogenemia, factor 13 deficiency	1 unit/5-10 kg	↑ Fibrinogen by 50–100 mg/dL
Recombinant factor concentrates	Units as labeled	Hemophilic bleeding or prophylaxis	F8: 20–50 units/kg F9: 40–120 units/kg	F8: ↑ 2%/unit/kg F9: ↑ 0.7 unit/kg
Recombinant factor VIIa (NovoSeven)	Micrograms (μg)	Hemophilic bleeding in patient with inhibitor; also used for uncontrolled postoperative hemorrhage	30–90 μg/kg/dose	Cessation of bleeding

Hgb, Hemoglobin; *RBCs*, red blood cells; *vWF*, von Willebrand factor.

Table 152-2	Evaluation of Transfusion Reactions	
TYPE OF REACTION	**CLINICAL SIGNS**	**MANAGEMENT**
Acute hemolytic transfusion reaction (incidence of 1:250,000 to 1:1,000,000)	Acute shock, back pain, flushing, early fever, intravascular hemolysis, hemoglobinemia, hemoglobinuria (may be delayed 5–10 days and less severe if anamnestic response is present)	1. Stop transfusion; return blood to bank with fresh sample of patient's blood 2. Hydrate intravenously*; support blood pressure, maintain high urine flow, alkalinize urine 3. Check for and correct electrolyte abnormalities (hyperkalemia)
Delayed hemolytic transfusion reaction (incidence of 1:100,000)	Onset 7–14 days after transfusion: pain, fever, jaundice, hemoglobinuria; fall in hemoglobin; reticulocytopenia	Transfuse only antigen-negative RBCs if needed;
Febrile nonhemolytic transfusion reaction (incidence of 1:100)	Fever during or within 4 hours after end of transfusion, chills, usually from passively transfused cytokines or recipient reaction to leukocytes Bacterial contamination can occur in 1:100,000 platelet transfusions	Antipyretics for symptomatic treatment or pretreatment for future transfusions; leukocyte reduction has decreased incidence of febrile reactions Blood culture if high suspicion for bacterial infection
Allergic transfusion reaction (incidence of 1:100)	Urticaria, pruritus, maculopapular rash, edema, respiratory distress, hypotension during or within 4 hours of transfusion; often because recipient has preformed antibodies against donor antigens, occasionally from passive infusion of antibodies from atopic donor	Diphenhydramine ± hydrocortisone for acute management For future transfusions consider: 1. Pretreatment with diphenhydramine ± hydrocortisone 2. Volume reduction to reduce donor plasma 3. Washing cellular products to remove all donor plasma (for severe reactions)

Adapted from Andreoli TE, Bennett JC, Carpenter CC, Plum F, et al: Cecil Essentials of Medicine, ed 4, Philadelphia, 1997, WB Saunders.
HLA, Human leukocyte antigen; *RBCs*, red blood cells; *WBC*, white blood cell.
*Normal saline is the compatible intravenous fluid.

include graft-versus-host disease and **infectious diseases** such as **hepatitis B** (<1:250,000 units) **and C** (1:1,600,000 units), **human immunodeficiency virus** (<1:1,800,000 units), malaria, syphilis, babesiosis, brucellosis, and Chagas disease. Patients who are chronically transfused are more prone to iron overload and alloimmunization to RBCs and platelets.

Suggested Reading

Key NS, Negrier C, Klein HG, et al: Transfusion medicine 1, 2, 3, *Lancet* 370(9585):415–426, 2007, 427–438, 439–448.

Kliegman RM, Stanton BF, St. Geme JW, et al: *Nelson Textbook of Pediatrics*, ed 19, Philadelphia, 2011, Saunders, p 1648–1722.

Monagle P, Chan A, Goldenberg NA, et al: Antithrombotic therapy in neonates and children: antithrombotic therapy and prevention of thrombosis, 9th ed: American College of Chest Physicians evidence-based clinical practice guidelines, *Chest* 141(Suppl 2): 3737S–e801S, 2012.

Neunert C, Lim W, Crowther M, et al: American Society of Hematology: The American Society of Hematology 2011 evidence-based practice guideline for immune thrombocytopenia, *Blood* 117(16): 4190–4207, 2011.

Scheinberg P: Aplastic anemia: therapeutic updates in immunosuppression and transplantation, 2012, *Hematology Am Soc Hematol Educ Program* 292–300, 2012.

Tolar J, Mehta PA, Walters MC: Hematopoietic cell transplantation for nonmalignant disorders, *Biol Blood Marrow Transplant* 18(Suppl 1): S166–S171, 2012.

Oncology

Thomas W. McLean and Marcia M. Wofford

Chapter 153

ONCOLOGY ASSESSMENT

Childhood cancer is rare; only about 1% of new cancer cases in the United States occur among children younger than 19 years of age. Hematopoietic tumors (leukemia, lymphoma) are the most common childhood cancers, followed by brain/central nervous system (CNS) tumors and sarcomas of soft tissue and bone (Fig. 153-1). There is wide variability in the age-specific incidence of childhood cancers. Embryonal tumors, such as neuroblastoma and retinoblastoma, peak during the first 2 years of life; acute lymphoblastic leukemia peaks during early childhood (ages 2 to 5 years); osteosarcoma peaks during adolescence; and Hodgkin disease peaks during late adolescence (Fig. 153-2). The overall incidence of cancer among white children is higher than that among other ethnic groups and is twice that of African American children in the United States.

HISTORY

Many signs and symptoms of childhood cancer are nonspecific. Although most children with fever, fatigue, weight loss, or limp do not have cancer, each of these symptoms may be a manifestation of an underlying malignancy. Uncommonly a child with cancer will have no symptoms at all. An abdominal mass may be palpated on routine examination, or a complete blood count (CBC) may be unexpectedly abnormal. Some children have a genetic susceptibility to cancer and should be screened appropriately (Table 153-1).

It is important to explore quality, duration, location, severity, and precipitating events of the chief complaint. A prominent lymph node that does not resolve (with or without antibiotics) may warrant a biopsy. A limp that does not improve within weeks should prompt a CBC and a radiograph or a bone scan. Persistent headaches or morning vomiting should prompt a computed tomography (CT) or magnetic resonance imaging (MRI) scan of the head. Fever, night sweats, or weight loss should raise the concern for lymphoma. In addition it is important to obtain the birth history, medical and surgical history, growth history, developmental history, family history, and social history.

PHYSICAL EXAMINATION

Growth parameters and vital signs are important to obtain in all patients. Pulse oximetry should be obtained if respiratory symptoms are present. The overall appearance of the patient should be noted, particularly general appearance, pain, cachexia, pallor, and respiratory distress. Palpable masses should be measured. Lymphadenopathy and organomegaly should be quantified, if present. A thorough examination of the skin may reveal rashes, bruises, and petechiae. Careful neurologic and ophthalmologic examinations are crucial if headache or vomiting is present, because the vast majority of patients with CNS tumors have abnormal neurologic examinations.

COMMON MANIFESTATIONS

Decision-Making Algorithms
Available @ StudentConsult.com

Visual Impairment and Leukocoria
Vomiting Hepatomegaly
Splenomegaly
Headaches
Lymphadenopathy
Anemia
Petechiae/Purpura
Pancytopenia
Fever of Unknown Origin

The most common manifestations of childhood cancer are fatigue, anorexia, malaise, pain, fever, abnormal lump or mass, pallor, bruising, petechiae, bleeding, headache, vomiting, visual changes, weight loss, and night sweats (Table 153-2). Lymphadenopathy and organomegaly are common in leukemia, particularly with T-cell acute lymphoblastic leukemia (ALL) or non-Hodgkin lymphoma. Patients with solid tumors usually have a palpable or measurable mass. Other signs and symptoms may include limp, cough, dyspnea, cranial nerve palsies, and papilledema. In general malignant masses are firm, fixed, and nontender, whereas masses that are infectious or inflammatory in nature are relatively softer, mobile, and tender to palpation.

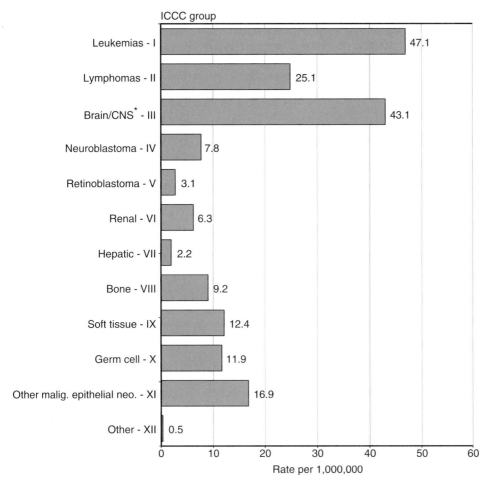

Figure **153-1** Childhood Cancer: SEER Incidence Rates 2005–2009 by ICCC Group (includes myelodysplastic syndromes and Group III benign brain). Under 20 years of age, both sexes, all races. Source: SEER 18 areas (San Francisco, Connecticut, Detroit, Hawaii, Iowa, New Mexico, Seattle, Utah, Atlanta, San Jose-Monterey, Los Angeles, Alaska Native Registry, Rural Georgia, California excluding SF/SJM/LA, Kentucky, Louisiana, New Jersey, and Georgia, excluding ATL/RG). Rates are age-adjusted to the 2000 U.S. Std Population (19 age groups - Census P25-1130). *International Classification of Childhood Cancer is based on ICD-O-3. (Steliarova-Foucher E, Stiller C, Lacour B, et al: International Classification of Childhood Cancer, ed 3. Cancer 103(7):1457–1467, 2005.) *Rate for Group III (Brain/CNS) includes benign brain tumors.*

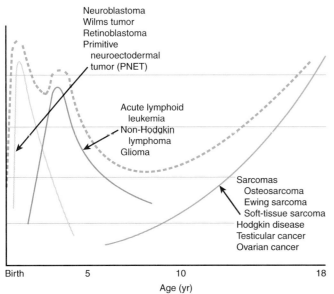

Figure **153-2** Incidence of the most common types of cancer in children by age. The cumulative incidence is shown as a dashed line. *(Courtesy of Archie Bleyer, MD).*

DIFFERENTIAL DIAGNOSIS

Distinguishing a malignant process from another disease can be difficult. Ultimately a tissue diagnosis (from bone marrow or solid tumor biopsy) with pathologic confirmation is required to confirm a diagnosis of cancer. Infection commonly masquerades as a potential malignancy. In particular Epstein-Barr virus, cytomegalovirus, and mycobacterial infections can mimic leukemia or lymphoma by causing fever, lymphadenopathy, organomegaly, weight loss, and abnormal blood counts. Trauma may produce swelling that can mimic solid tumors. Idiopathic thrombocytic purpura and iron deficiency can produce thrombocytopenia and anemia, respectively. Immune deficiencies or irregularities (autoimmune hemolytic anemia or neutropenia) can also produce cytopenias. Juvenile idiopathic arthritis and other collagen vascular disease can cause musculoskeletal pain and anemia, mimicking leukemia. Benign tumors are relatively common in children, including mature germ cell tumors/hamartomas, hemangiomas or other vascular tumors, mesoblastic nephromas, and bone cysts.

INITIAL DIAGNOSTIC EVALUATION
Screening Tests

A CBC with differential and review of the peripheral blood smear is the best screening test for many pediatric malignancies. Leukopenia (with or without neutropenia), anemia, or thrombocytopenia may be present in leukemia or any cancer that invades the bone marrow (e.g., neuroblastoma, rhabdomyosarcoma, and Ewing sarcoma). Leukemia may also produce leukocytosis, usually with blasts present on the peripheral blood smear. An isolated cytopenia (neutropenia, anemia, or thrombocytopenia) widens the differential diagnosis but still could be the only abnormal laboratory finding. Of note, a

| Table 153-1 | Known Risk Factors for Selected Childhood Cancers |

CANCER TYPE	RISK FACTOR	COMMENTS
Acute lymphoid leukemia	Ionizing radiation	Prenatal diagnostic x-ray exposure increases risk. Therapeutic irradiation for cancer treatment also increases risk.
	Genetic conditions	Down syndrome is associated with an estimated 10- to 20-fold increased risk. Neurofibromatosis 1, Bloom syndrome, and ataxia-telangiectasia, among others, are associated with an elevated risk.
Acute myeloid leukemias	Chemotherapeutic agents	Alkylating agents and epipodophyllotoxins increase risk.
	Genetic factors	Down syndrome and neurofibromatosis 1 are strongly associated. Familial monosomy 7 and several other genetic syndromes are also associated with increased risk. Patients treated with radiation therapy for other cancers.
Brain cancers	Therapeutic ionizing radiation to the head	
	Genetic factors	Neurofibromatosis 1 is strongly associated with optic gliomas and, to a lesser extent, with other central nervous system tumors. Tuberous sclerosis and several other genetic syndromes are associated with increased risk.
Hodgkin disease	Family history	Monozygotic twins and siblings are at increased risk.
	Infections	Epstein-Barr virus is associated with increased risk.
Non-Hodgkin lymphoma	Immunodeficiency	Acquired and congenital immunodeficiency disorders and immunosuppressive therapy increase risk.
	Infections	Epstein-Barr virus is associated with increased risk.
Osteosarcoma	Ionizing radiation	Cancer radiation therapy and high radium exposure increase risk.
	Genetic factors	Increased risk is apparent with Li-Fraumeni syndrome and hereditary retinoblastoma.
Ewing sarcoma	Race	Incidence is about nine times higher in white children than in black children in the United States.
Neuroblastoma	Genetic factors	Chromosome 6p22 variants and mutations in the ALK and PHOX genes are associated with increased risk.
Retinoblastoma	Genetic factors	Mutations in the Rb gene on chromosome 14
Wilms tumor	Congenital anomalies	Aniridia, Beckwith-Wiedemann syndrome, and other congenital and genetic conditions are associated with increased risk.
Renal medullary carcinoma	Sickle cell trait	Etiology is unknown.
Rhabdomyosarcoma	Congenital anomalies and genetic conditions	Li-Fraumeni syndrome and neurofibromatosis 1 are associated with increased risk.
Hepatoblastoma	Prematurity Genetic factors	Etiology unknown Beckwith-Wiedemann syndrome, hemihypertrophy, Gardner syndrome, and familial adenomatous polyposis are associated with increased risk.
Hepatocellular carcinoma	Infections	Hepatitis B virus infection increases risk.
Malignant germ cell tumors	Cryptorchidism	Cryptorchidism is a risk factor for testicular germ cell tumors.

Modified from Kliegman RM, Stanton BF, St. Geme JW III, editors: Nelson Textbook of Pediatrics, ed 19, Philadelphia, 2011, Saunders.

patient with leukemia may also have a normal CBC. Lactate dehydrogenase and uric acid are often elevated in fast-growing tumors (leukemia or lymphoma) and occasionally in sarcomas or neuroblastoma. In many cases, it is appropriate to assess electrolytes and renal and hepatic function in the screening process. Elevated blood pressure, if confirmed by repeat measurements, should prompt a urine analysis, as should the palpation of an abdominal mass.

Diagnostic Imaging

A chest x-ray (CXR) (posteroanterior and lateral) is the best screening radiographic study for a patient with suspicious cervical lymphadenopathy, fever, and weight loss. Mediastinal masses and pleural effusions can often be detected on CXR.

Abdominal signs or symptoms warrant an ultrasound or CT. Persistent headache, vomiting, or abnormal neurologic findings should lead to a head CT or MRI. For suspected bone tumors, plain radiographs are indicated and will usually reveal the lesion(s), if present. Radiographs may be normal when a bony pelvic lesion is suspected; a CT or MRI should be obtained. Other imaging studies to delineate a mass and to search for suspected metastases are often indicated, but these decisions are usually best left to the pediatric oncology team. Table 153-3 shows the general use of diagnostic imaging following confirmation of a diagnosis of cancer, assessing the primary tumor and for metastases. Positron emission tomography (PET) has proved useful for staging and assessing response for some pediatric cancers, especially lymphomas. Metaiodobenzylguanidine (mIBG) scans are useful for neuroblastoma.

Table 153-2 | Common Manifestations of Childhood Malignancies

SIGN/SYMPTOM	SIGNIFICANCE	EXAMPLE
Hematologic		
Pallor, anemia	Bone marrow infiltration	Leukemia, neuroblastoma
Petechiae, thrombocytopenia	Bone marrow infiltration	Leukemia, neuroblastoma
Fever, neutropenia	Bone marrow infiltration	Leukemia, neuroblastoma
Systemic		
Bone pain, limp, arthralgia	Primary bone tumor, metastasis to bone	Osteosarcoma, Ewing sarcoma, leukemia, neuroblastoma
Fever of unknown origin, weight loss, night sweats	Lymphoreticular malignancy	Hodgkin disease, non-Hodgkin lymphoma
Painless lymphadenopathy	Lymphoreticular malignancy, metastatic solid tumor	Leukemia, Hodgkin disease, non-Hodgkin lymphoma, Burkitt lymphoma, thyroid carcinoma
Cutaneous lesion	Primary or metastatic disease	Neuroblastoma, leukemia, Langerhans cell histiocytosis, melanoma
Abdominal mass	Abdominal/pelvic organ	Neuroblastoma, Wilms tumor, lymphoma, hepatoblastoma, germ cell tumor
Hypertension	Sympathetic nervous system tumor	Neuroblastoma, pheochromocytoma, Wilms tumor
Diarrhea	Vasoactive intestinal polypeptide	Neuroblastoma
Soft tissue mass	Local or metastatic tumor	Ewing sarcoma, osteosarcoma, neuroblastoma, thyroid carcinoma, rhabdomyosarcoma, germ cell tumor
Diabetes insipidus, galactorrhea, poor growth	Neuroendocrine involvement of hypothalamus or pituitary gland	Adenoma, craniopharyngioma, prolactinoma, Langerhans cell histiocytosis
Emesis, visual disturbances, ataxia, headache, papilledema, cranial nerve palsies	Increased intrathecal pressure	Primary brain tumor; metastasis
Ophthalmologic		
Leukocoria	White pupil	Retinoblastoma
Periorbital ecchymosis	Metastasis	Neuroblastoma
Miosis, ptosis, heterochromia	Horner syndrome: compression of cervical sympathetic nerves	Neuroblastoma
Opsomyoclonus, ataxia	Neurotransmitters (?) Autoimmunity (?)	Neuroblastoma
Exophthalmos, proptosis	Orbital tumor	Rhabdomyosarcoma, lymphoma
Thoracic		
Anterior mediastinal mass	Cough, stridor, pneumonia, tracheal-bronchial compression	Germ cell tumor, T-cell lymphoma, Hodgkin disease, primary mediastinal large B-cell lymphoma
Posterior mediastinal mass	Vertebral or nerve root compression; dysphagia	Neuroblastoma, ganglioneuroblastoma, ganglioneuroma

Table 153-3	Minimum Workup Required for Common Pediatric Malignancies to Assess Primary Tumor and Potential Metastases*							
MALIGNANCY	**BMA/bx**	**CXR**	**CT SCAN**	**MRI**	**BONE SCAN**	**CSF ANALYSIS**	**MARKER(S)**	**OTHER**
Leukemia	Yes	Yes				Yes		
Non-Hodgkin lymphoma	Yes	Yes	Yes		Yes	Yes		
Hodgkin lymphoma	Yes	Yes	Yes		Yes			PET or gallium scan
CNS tumors				Yes		Yes		
Neuroblastoma	Yes		Yes		Yes		VMA, HVA	mIBG scan
Wilms tumor		Yes	Yes					
Rhabdomyosarcoma	Yes	Yes	Yes		Yes	Yes, for parameningeal tumors only		
Osteosarcoma		Yes	Yes (chest)	Yes (primary)	Yes			
Ewing sarcoma	Yes	Yes	Yes (chest)	Yes (primary)	Yes			
Germ cell tumors		Yes	Yes				AFP, β-hCG	Consider brain MRI
Liver tumors		Yes	Yes				AFP	
Retinoblastoma	±		Yes, if MRI not available	Yes (brain)	±	Yes		Rb gene analysis

AFP, Alpha-fetoprotein; *BMA/bx*, bone marrow aspirate/biopsy; *CNS*, central nervous system; *CSF*, cerebrospinal fluid; *CT*, computed tomography; *CXR*, chest x-ray; *β-hCG*, beta-human chorionic gonadotropin; *HVA*, homovanillic acid; *mIBG*, metaiodobenzylguanidine; *MRI*, magnetic resonance imaging; *PET*, positron emission tomography; *Rb*, retinoblastoma; *VMA*, vanillylmandelic acid.
*Individual cases may require additional studies.

Chapter **154**

PRINCIPLES OF CANCER TREATMENT

The overall goal of pediatric oncology is to cure all patients with minimal toxicity. Treatment for children with cancer is often multimodal and may involve surgery, radiation therapy, and chemotherapy. Surgery and radiation are generally local treatment modalities (an exception is total body irradiation as part of a bone marrow or stem cell transplant), whereas chemotherapy has both local and systemic effects.

Primary prevention strategies for most pediatric malignancies are unknown. Two exceptions are the use of hepatitis B vaccine to lower the rates of hepatocellular carcinoma and the use of human papillomavirus vaccine to reduce the risk of cervical, vulvar, and vaginal cancers. Childhood malignancies are not associated with tobacco or alcohol use, dietary factors, or sun exposure. Treatment with certain chemotherapy agents and radiation therapy increases the rate of second malignancies. Secondary prevention may be accomplished by screening the at-risk child (e.g., a child with Beckwith-Wiedemann syndrome or twin of a leukemia patient), but these opportunities are rare.

ONCOLOGIC EMERGENCIES
Adverse effects of tumors and treatments may result in oncologic emergencies in children and adolescents (Table 154-1).

Mediastinal masses from lymphoma can cause life-threatening airway obstruction. Tumors with a large tumor burden (e.g., lymphoma, leukemia) may affect renal function adversely from tubular deposition of uric acid crystals. Allopurinol or rasburicase can be administered before chemotherapy to minimize this effect.

A common metabolic emergency is **tumor lysis syndrome,** often seen in treatment of leukemia and lymphoma. Large amounts of phosphate, potassium, and uric acid are released into the circulation from lysed cells. Overwhelming infection and spinal cord compression with neurologic compromise are other oncologic emergencies.

SURGERY
Appropriate imaging (usually with computed tomography [CT] or magnetic resonance imaging [MRI]) for solid tumors presenting as a palpable mass or mass-related symptoms (pain, respiratory distress, intestinal obstruction) should be obtained and followed by resection (when possible) or biopsy (if complete resection is not feasible). An exception to this is a suspected lymphoma, for which a biopsy may be needed. However, almost all pediatric lymphomas are chemosensitive and do not require surgical resection.

It is crucial to determine the amount of tissue required and the appropriate distribution of the tissue for testing so that all necessary studies are performed. A general oncologic surgery principle is to resect not just the tumor, but also, in most cases, a surrounding margin of normal tissue to ensure the entire tumor has been resected.

Table 154-1	Oncologic Emergencies			
CONDITION	**MANIFESTATIONS**	**ETIOLOGY**	**MALIGNANCY**	**TREATMENT**
Metabolic				
Hyperuricemia	Uric acid nephropathy; gout	Tumor lysis syndrome	Lymphoma, leukemia	Allopurinol, hydration, rasburicase
Hyperkalemia	Arrhythmias, cardiac arrest	Tumor lysis syndrome	Lymphoma, leukemia	Kayexalate; sodium bicarbonate, glucose, and insulin
Hyperphosphatemia	Hypocalcemic tetany; metastatic calcification, photophobia, pruritus	Tumor lysis syndrome	Lymphoma, leukemia	Hydration, diuresis; oral aluminum hydroxide to bind phosphate
Hypercalcemia	Anorexia, nausea, polyuria, pancreatitis, gastric ulcers; prolonged PR/shortened QT interval	Bone resorption; ectopic parathormone, vitamin D, or prostaglandins	Metastasis to bone, rhabdomyosarcoma	Hydration and furosemide diuresis; corticosteroids; mithramycin; calcitonin, diphosphonates
Hematologic				
Anemia	Pallor, weakness, heart failure	Bone marrow suppression or infiltration; blood loss	Any with chemotherapy	Packed red blood cell transfusion
Thrombocytopenia	Petechiae, hemorrhage	Bone marrow suppression or infiltration	Any with chemotherapy	Platelet transfusion
Disseminated intravascular coagulation	Shock, hemorrhage	Sepsis, hypotension, tumor factors	Promyelocytic leukemia, others	Fresh frozen plasma; platelets, treat infection
Neutropenia	Infection	Bone marrow suppression or infiltration	Any with chemotherapy	If patient is febrile, administer broad-spectrum antibiotics, with G-CSF if appropriate
Hyperleukocytosis (>50,000/mm^3)	Hemorrhage, thrombosis; pulmonary infiltrates, hypoxia; tumor lysis syndrome	Leukostasis; vascular occlusion	Leukemia	Leukapheresis; chemotherapy
Graft-versus-host disease	Dermatitis, diarrhea, hepatitis	Immunosuppression and nonirradiated blood products; bone marrow transplantation	Any with immunosuppression	Corticosteroids; cyclosporine; antithymocyte globulin
Space-occupying lesions				
Spinal cord compression	Back pain, motor and sensory deficits	Invasion of spinal canal by primary tumor or metastases	Neuroblastoma, medulloblastoma	MRI for diagnosis; corticosteroids; radiation therapy; laminectomy; chemotherapy
Increased intracranial pressure	Headache, confusion, coma, emesis, headache, hypertension, bradycardia, seizures, papilledema, hydrocephalus; cranial nerve III and VI palsies	Primary or metastatic brain tumor	Astrocytoma, medulloblastoma, others; neuroblastoma	CT or MRI for diagnosis; corticosteroids; ventriculoperitoneal shunt; radiation therapy; chemotherapy
Superior vena cava syndrome	Distended neck veins, plethora, edema of head and neck, cyanosis, proptosis; Horner syndrome	Superior mediastinal mass	Lymphoma	Chemotherapy; radiation therapy
Tracheal compression	Respiratory distress	Mediastinal mass compressing trachea	Lymphoma	Radiation therapy, corticosteroids

CNS, Central nervous system; *CT*, computed tomography; *G-CSF*, granulocyte colony-stimulating factor; *MRI*, magnetic resonance imaging.

CHEMOTHERAPY

Because most pediatric solid tumors have a high risk for micrometastatic disease at the time of diagnosis, chemotherapy is used in almost all cases (Table 154-2). Exceptions include low-stage neuroblastoma and Wilms tumor (particularly in infants) and low-grade central nervous system (CNS) tumors. For patients with localized solid tumors, chemotherapy administered after removal of the primary tumor is referred to as **adjuvant therapy.** Chemotherapy administered while the primary tumor is still present is referred to as **neoadjuvant chemotherapy.** Neoadjuvant chemotherapy has a number of potential benefits, including an early attack on

Table 154-2	Cancer Chemotherapy				
DRUG*	**ACTION**	**METABOLISM**	**EXCRETION**	**INDICATION**	**ACUTE TOXICITY**
Antimetabolites					
Methotrexate	Folic acid antagonist; inhibits dihydrofolate reductase	Hepatic	Renal, 50%–90% excreted unchanged; biliary	ALL, lymphoma, medulloblastoma, osteosarcoma	Myelosuppression (nadir 7–10 days), mucositis, dermatitis, hepatitis, renal and CNS effects with high-dose administration; prevent with hydration and leucovorin, monitor levels
6-Mercaptopurine	Purine analog	Hepatic	Renal	ALL	Myelosuppression; hepatitis; mucositis; allopurinol increases toxicity
Cytosine arabinoside (Ara-C)	Pyrimidine analog; inhibits DNA polymerase	Hepatic	Renal	ALL, AML, lymphoma	Myelosuppression, conjunctivitis, mucositis, neurotoxicity
Alkylating Agents					
Cyclophosphamide	Alkylates guanine; inhibits DNA synthesis	Hepatic	Renal	ALL, lymphoma, sarcoma, brain tumors	Myelosuppression; hemorrhagic cystitis
Ifosfamide	Similar to cyclophosphamide	Hepatic	Renal	Lymphoma, Wilms tumor, sarcoma, germ cell and testicular tumors	Similar to cyclophosphamide; neurotoxicity, cardiac toxicity
Antibiotics					
Doxorubicin and daunorubicin	Binds to DNA, intercalation	Hepatic	Biliary, renal	ALL, AML, osteosarcoma, Ewing sarcoma, lymphoma, neuroblastoma	Cardiomyopathy, red urine, tissue necrosis on extravasation, myelosuppression, conjunctivitis, radiation dermatitis, arrhythmia
Dactinomycin	Binds to DNA, inhibits transcription	—	Renal, stool, 30% excreted as unchanged drug	Wilms tumor, rhabdomyosarcoma, Ewing sarcoma	Tissue necrosis on extravasation, myelosuppression, hepatopathy with thrombocytopenia, stomatitis
Bleomycin	Binds to DNA, cuts DNA	Hepatic	Renal	Hodgkin disease, lymphoma, germ cell tumors	Pneumonitis, stomatitis, Raynaud phenomenon, pulmonary fibrosis, dermatitis
Vinca Alkaloids					
Vincristine	Inhibits microtubule formation	Hepatic	Biliary	ALL, lymphoma, Wilms tumor, Hodgkin disease, Ewing sarcoma, neuroblastoma, rhabdomyosarcoma, brain tumors	Local cellulitis, peripheral neuropathy, constipation, ileus, jaw pain, inappropriate ADH secretion, seizures, ptosis, minimal myelosuppression
Vinblastine	Inhibits microtubule formation	Hepatic	Biliary	Hodgkin disease, Langerhans cell histiocytosis	Local cellulitis, myelosuppression
Enzymes					
Asparaginase	Depletion of asparagine	—	Reticuloendothelial system	ALL, AML	Allergic reaction; pancreatitis, hyperglycemia, platelet dysfunction and coagulopathy, encephalopathy, stroke, thrombosis

Table 154-2	Cancer Chemotherapy—cont'd				
DRUG*	**ACTION**	**METABOLISM**	**EXCRETION**	**INDICATION**	**ACUTE TOXICITY**
			Antimetabolites		
			Hormones		
Prednisone	Direct lymphocyte cytotoxicity	Hepatic	Renal	ALL; Hodgkin disease, lymphoma	Cushing syndrome, cataracts, diabetes, hypertension, myopathy, osteoporosis, infection, peptic ulceration, irritability, psychosis, hunger, fluid retention
			Miscellaneous		
Carmustine BCNU, lomustine (CCNU)	Carbamylation of DNA; inhibits DNA synthesis	Hepatic	Renal	CNS tumors, lymphoma, Hodgkin disease	Delayed myelosuppression (4–6 wk); pulmonary fibrosis, carcinogenic, stomatitis
Cisplatin	Inhibits DNA synthesis	—	Renal	Osteosarcoma, neuroblastoma, CNS tumors, germ cell tumors	Nephrotoxic; myelosuppression, ototoxicity, neurotoxicity, hemolytic uremic syndrome
Carboplatin	Inhibits DNA synthesis	—	Renal	Same as for cisplatin	Myelosuppression
Etoposide (VP-16)	Topoisomerase-inhibitor	—	Renal	ALL, lymphoma, germ cell tumor, sarcoma	Myelosuppression, secondary leukemia, allergic reaction
Tretinoin (all-trans retinoic acid) and isotretinoin (cis-retinoic acid)	Promotes differentiation	Liver	Liver	M3 AML (ATRA); neuroblastoma (CRA)	Fever, respiratory distress, leukocytosis (ATRA); dry mouth, hair loss, pseudotumor cerebri (CRA)

ADH, Antidiuretic hormone; *ALL,* acute lymphoblastic leukemia; *AML,* acute myeloid leukemia; *CNS,* central nervous system.
*Many drugs produce nausea and vomiting during administration, and many cause alopecia with repeated doses.

presumed micrometastatic disease, shrinkage of the primary tumor to facilitate local control, and additional time to plan for definitive surgery.

Resistance to a particular chemotherapeutic agent can develop in a number of ways: decreased influx into or increased efflux of the chemotherapeutic agent from the malignant cell; mutation in the target tissue so that it cannot be inhibited by the drug; amplification of a drug target to overcome inhibition; and blockade of normal cellular processes leading to programmed cell death or apoptosis. Because mutation is an ongoing process in malignant tumors, it follows that certain subpopulations of tumor cells within a tumor may be more or less sensitive to any particular chemotherapy drug. Given this fact, combinations of chemotherapy drugs are used, as opposed to sequential single agents, to treat the various forms of childhood cancer.

The blood-brain barrier prevents the penetration of chemotherapeutic drugs into the CNS; instillation of the chemotherapeutic agent directly into the cerebrospinal fluid (by lumbar puncture) may be necessary. Radiation therapy also circumvents the blood-brain barrier.

RADIATION THERAPY

Radiation therapy is the process of delivering ionizing radiation to malignant cells in order to kill them directly or, more commonly, prevent them from dividing by interfering with DNA replication. Conventional radiation therapy uses photons, but atomic particles such as electrons, protons, and neutrons can also be used. Not all tumors are radiosensitive, and radiation therapy is not necessary in all tumors that are radiosensitive.

OTHER THERAPIES

Certain cancers have been treated with cytokines, biologic response modifiers, or monoclonal antibodies in addition to standard treatments. **Targeted therapies** specifically target the tumor cells, sparing normal host cells. Imatinib mesylate is a protein kinase inhibitor that targets the effects of the t(9;22) translocation of chronic myeloid leukemia and acute lymphoblastic leukemia. Rituximab is a monoclonal antibody directed against the cell surface antigen CD20 expressed in some lymphomas. Ch14.18 is an anti-GD2 monoclonal antibody used for neuroblastoma.

Supportive care also plays an important role in pediatric oncology, including the use of appropriate antimicrobial agents, blood products, nutritional support, intensive care, and integrative therapies.

ADVERSE EFFECTS

Because chemotherapy agents are cellular toxins, numerous adverse effects are associated with their use. Bone marrow suppression, immunosuppression, nausea, vomiting, and alopecia are general adverse effects of commonly used chemotherapy drugs. Each chemotherapy drug also has specific toxicities. Doxorubicin can cause cardiac damage; cisplatin can cause renal damage and ototoxicity; cyclophosphamide and ifosfamide can cause hemorrhagic cystitis; and vincristine can cause peripheral neuropathy. Radiation therapy produces many adverse effects such as mucositis, growth retardation, organ dysfunction, and the later development of secondary cancers. Significant therapy-related **late effects** may develop in pediatric cancer patients (Table 154-3).

Table 154-3	Long-Term Sequelae of Cancer Therapy
PROBLEM	**ETIOLOGIC AGENT(S)**
Infertility	Alkylating agents; radiation
Second cancers	Genetic predisposition; radiation; alkylating agents, etoposide, topoisomerase II inhibitors
Sepsis	Splenectomy
Hepatotoxicity	Methotrexate, 6-mercaptopurine; radiation
Hepatic venoocclusive disease	High-dose, intensive chemotherapy (busulfan, cyclophosphamide) ± bone marrow transplant
Scoliosis	Radiation
Pulmonary (fibrosis)	Radiation; bleomycin, busulfan
Cardiomyopathy	Doxorubicin, daunorubicin; radiation
Leukoencephalopathy	Cranial radiation ± methotrexate
Cognition/intelligence	Cranial radiation ± methotrexate
Pituitary dysfunction (growth hormone deficiency, panhypopituitarism)	Cranial radiation
Psychosocial	Stress, anxiety, death of peers; conditioned responses to chemotherapy
Thyroid dysfunction	Radiation
Osteonecrosis	Corticosteroids

Chapter 155

LEUKEMIA

ETIOLOGY

The etiology of childhood leukemia is unknown and is probably multifactorial. Genetics and environmental factors play important roles. There are many recurrent nonrandom chromosomal translocations in leukemia cells. A translocation may lead to the formation of a new gene, whose expression may lead to a novel protein with transforming capabilities. In **chronic myelogenous leukemia (CML)** and some cases of **acute lymphoblastic leukemia (ALL)**, a translocation between chromosomes 9 and 22 results in a fusion gene incorporating parts of two genes, *BCR* and *ABL*. The protein formed by this novel gene plays an important role in the development of the leukemias. In addition, certain constitutional genotypes can predispose a child to the development of acute leukemia. Patients with Down syndrome, Fanconi anemia, Bloom syndrome, ataxia-telangiectasia, Wiskott-Aldrich syndrome, and neurofibromatosis 1 all have an increased risk of acute leukemia. Siblings of children with leukemia are at increased risk of developing leukemia (approximately twofold to fourfold above the childhood population). This risk increases for twin siblings (up to 25% for monozygotic twins). In certain patients with leukemia, the unique antigen receptor gene rearrangement

or the specific chromosomal translocation characterizing the patient's leukemic clone can be demonstrated in cord blood cells and neonatal blood spots used for screening for metabolic diseases, suggesting a possible in utero etiology. There are reports of familial leukemia. Environmental factors that may increase the risk of leukemia include ionizing radiation and exposure to certain chemotherapy agents, particularly the topoisomerase II inhibitors.

EPIDEMIOLOGY

Each year 2500 to 3500 new cases of childhood leukemia occur in the United States. The disease affects about 40 per 1 million children under the age of 15 years. ALL accounts for approximately 75% of cases. **Acute myelogenous leukemia (AML)** accounts for 15% to 20%, and CML accounts for less than 5% of cases. Other chronic leukemias, including juvenile myelomonocytic leukemia, chronic myelomonocytic leukemia, and chronic lymphocytic leukemia, are rare in childhood.

ALL and AML are classified according to the World Health Organization system (Table 155-1), although many clinicians and pathologists still use the French-American-British system for AML. ALL is classified according to cell lineage as either B-lineage or T-lineage. The incidence of ALL peaks at 2 to 5 years of age and is higher in boys than in girls. T-cell ALL, in particular, is associated with male predominance as well as an older age of peak incidence. In the United States, ALL is more common in white than in African American children. The incidence of AML is relatively high in the neonatal period then drops and stabilizes until adolescence when there is a slight increase, which continues into adulthood, especially beyond 55 years of age. Males and females are equally affected by AML. Hispanic and African American children have slightly higher incidence rates than white children.

CLINICAL MANIFESTATIONS

Decision-Making Algorithms
Available @ StudentConsult.com

Arthritis
Extremity Pain
Lymphadenopathy
Anemia
Bleeding
Hypercalcemia

Signs and symptoms of acute leukemias are related to the infiltration of leukemic cells into normal tissues, resulting in either bone marrow failure (anemia, neutropenia, thrombocytopenia) or specific tissue infiltration (lymph nodes, liver, spleen, brain, bone, skin, gingiva, testes). Common presenting symptoms are fever, pallor, petechiae or ecchymoses, lethargy, malaise, anorexia, and bone or joint pain. **Physical examination** frequently reveals lymphadenopathy and hepatosplenomegaly. The testes and central nervous system (CNS) are common extramedullary sites for ALL; neurologic symptoms or a painless enlargement of one or both testes may be seen. Patients with **T-cell ALL** often have high white blood cell (WBC) counts, anterior mediastinal masses, bulky disease

Table 155-1	Classification of Acute Lymphoblastic and Acute Myeloid Leukemias

ACUTE LYMPHOBLASTIC LEUKEMIA (ALL)

ALL—L1/L2 morphology

    Precursor B-cell ALL

    Precursor T-cell ALL

ALL, B cell—L3 morphology (i.e., Burkitt leukemia)

ACUTE MYELOID LEUKEMIA (AML)

AMLs with recurrent cytogenetic translocations

    AML with t(8;21)(q22; q22), AML1(CBF-alpha)/ETO

    Acute promyelocytic leukemia—AML with t(15;17)(q22; q11–12) and variants, PML/RAR-alpha) (i.e., M3*)

    AML with abnormal bone marrow eosinophils—inv(16) (p13q22) or t(16;16)(p13; q11), CBFb/MYH11

    AML with 11q23/MLL abnormalities

AML with multilineage dysplasia

    With prior myelodysplastic syndrome

    Without prior myelodysplastic syndrome

AML and myelodysplastic syndromes, therapy-related

    Alkylating agent-related

    Epipodophyllotoxin-related (some may be lymphoid)

    Other types

AML not otherwise categorized

    AML minimally differentiated (M1)

    AML without maturation (M0)

    AML with maturation (M2)

    Acute myelomonocytic leukemia (M4)

    Acute monocytic leukemia (M5)

    Acute erythroid leukemia (M6)

    Acute megakaryocytic leukemia (M7)

    Acute basophilic leukemia

    Acute panmyelosis with myelofibrosis

Modified from World Health Organization Classification.
MLL, Mixed lineage leukemia.
*The designations M0 to M7 are those of the French-American- British classification system for AML, which predated the World Health Organization system and is still used by many clinicians and pathologists.

with cervical lymphadenopathy, hepatosplenomegaly, and CNS involvement. In patients with AML, extramedullary soft tissue tumors may be found in various sites.

LABORATORY AND IMAGING STUDIES

The diagnosis of acute leukemia is confirmed by findings of immature blast cells on either the peripheral blood smear, bone marrow aspirate, or both. Most patients have abnormal blood counts; anemia and thrombocytopenia are common. The WBC count may be low, normal, or high; 15% to 20% of patients have a WBC count greater than 50,000/mm³. Definitive diagnosis requires the evaluation of cell surface markers (**immunophenotype**) by flow cytometry and evaluation of cytochemical staining patterns. **Cytogenetic analysis** should

be undertaken in all cases of acute leukemia. Certain types of both lymphoid and myeloid leukemias have specific chromosomal abnormalities. In ALL, the t(12;21) translocation is most common (approximately 20% of all cases) and is associated with a favorable prognosis. The t(9;22) translocation occurs in less than 5% of cases and is associated with a poor prognosis. The t(4;11) translocation (and other translocations involving the *MLL* gene on chromosome 11) often occurs in infants and patients with secondary AML and is generally associated with a poor prognosis. Fluorescent in situ hybridization or polymerase chain reaction techniques are now used in most cases of leukemia because many chromosomal abnormalities may not be apparent on routine karyotypes. DNA microarray techniques are gaining relevance and will likely become standard in the future. A **lumbar puncture** should always be performed at the time of diagnosis to evaluate the possibility of CNS involvement. A chest x-ray should be obtained in all patients to exclude an anterior mediastinal mass, which is commonly seen in T-cell ALL. Electrolytes, calcium, phosphorus, uric acid, and renal and hepatic function should be monitored in all patients.

DIFFERENTIAL DIAGNOSIS

The differential diagnosis of acute leukemia includes nonmalignant and malignant diseases. Infection is probably the most common mimicker of acute leukemia, particularly the Epstein-Barr virus infection. Other infections (cytomegalovirus, pertussis, mycobacteria) also can produce signs and symptoms common to leukemia. Noninfectious diagnostic considerations include aplastic anemia, histiocytosis, juvenile rheumatoid arthritis, immune thrombocytopenic purpura, and congenital or acquired conditions that lead to neutropenia or anemia. Several malignant diagnoses also can mimic leukemia, including neuroblastoma, rhabdomyosarcoma, and Ewing sarcoma. Newborns with trisomy 21 may have a condition known as **transient myeloproliferative disorder,** which produces elevated WBC counts with peripheral blasts, anemia, and thrombocytopenia. It usually resolves with supportive care only, but these children have a significantly increased risk (30%) of developing true acute leukemia (ALL or AML) within the next few months and years of life.

TREATMENT

Patients with ALL generally receive three- or four-agent **induction chemotherapy** based on their initial risk group assignment. Low- and standard-risk patients receive vincristine, prednisone, and L-asparaginase for 4 weeks; high-risk patients also receive an anthracycline (daunorubicin or doxorubicin). During induction, intrathecal instillation of some combination of methotrexate, cytarabine, and hydrocortisone is given to treat existing CNS leukemia or prevent its development. Following induction of successful remission, which is achieved in nearly all patients with ALL, the remission is **consolidated** along with **CNS-directed therapy.** The intensity of therapy depends on risk factors with higher risk patients receiving more intensive chemotherapy. For patients with CNS disease detected at diagnosis and those with T-cell ALL, cranial radiation therapy is usually provided, although the omission of radiation therapy for all pediatric leukemia patients holds great promise. All patients receive **continuation** therapy for a total duration of therapy of 2 to 3 years. Continuation therapy generally consists of intermittent vincristine and short courses (5 to 7 days) of oral corticosteroid therapy, plus daily oral 6-mercaptopurine, and weekly methotrexate (orally or intramuscularly).

The **treatment of AML** is quite different from that of ALL because nonmyelosuppressive drugs (vincristine, prednisone, and asparaginase) are not effective. Several cycles of extremely intensive myelosuppressive chemotherapy are necessary to cure childhood AML; there is little evidence that low-dose continuation therapy is helpful in AML (with the exception of acute promyelocytic leukemia).

Induction therapy for AML usually consists of cytarabine, daunomycin, and etoposide (or 6-thioguanine). If a patient has an HLA-matched sibling donor, most experts recommend a stem cell transplantation in the first remission, except in patients with Down syndrome and those with relatively favorable cytogenetics such as inv(16), t(15;17), and t(8;21). Bortezomib, sorafenib and haploidentical natural killer cell transplantation are being studied as an adjuvant therapy for newly diagnosed childhood AML.

COMPLICATIONS

Major short-term complications associated with the treatment of leukemia result from bone marrow suppression caused by chemotherapy. Patients may have bleeding and significant anemia that necessitates transfusion of platelets or blood. Neutropenia with fewer than 500 neutrophils/mm^3, and especially fewer than 100 neutrophils/mm^3, greatly predispose the patient to significant bacterial and fungal infection. Cell-mediated immunosuppression increases the risk of *Pneumocystis jiroveci (carinii)* pneumonia. Prophylaxis with oral trimethoprim-sulfamethoxazole or aerosolized pentamidine is recommended. Prophylaxis with antibiotics and antifungal agents is under investigation. Long-term sequelae of therapy are less common than in previous treatment eras but are prevalent in long-term survivors treated in the 1980s and earlier. These sequelae include neurocognitive impairment, short stature, obesity, cardiac dysfunction, infertility, second malignant neoplasms, and psychosocial problems (see Table 154-3).

PROGNOSIS

Patients with ALL are classified into four prognostic risk groups (low, standard, high, and very high) based on age, initial WBC count, genetic characteristics, and response to induction therapy. Classification systems are complex and evolving (Table 155-2). In general low-risk patients are 1 to 9 years old with an initial WBC count less than 50,000/mm^3 and favorable cytogenetic findings such as t(12;21). High-risk patients are younger than 1 year of age or 10 years of age and older, have an initial WBC count greater than 50,000/mm^3, have CNS or testicular disease at diagnosis, or have unfavorable cytogenetics such as t(4;11). Very high-risk patients have a hypodiploid DNA index, a t(9;22) translocation, or fail to achieve remission after 4 weeks of therapy. All other patients are considered to have standard-risk ALL. Immunophenotype, minimal residual disease, and early response to therapy are other factors that influence risk stratification. Infants with ALL generally have a highly undifferentiated immunophenotype, often have a

Table 155-2	General Prognostic Factors in Acute Lymphoblastic Leukemia	
FACTOR	**FAVORABLE (LOWER RISK)**	**UNFAVORABLE (HIGHER RISK)**
Age	1–9.99 years	<1 or >10 years
Initial WBC count	<50,000/mm^3	>50,000/mm^3
CNS disease at diagnosis	Absent	Present
DNA index	>1.16	<1.16
Cytogenetics	t(12;21)	t(4;11), t(9;22)
Response to therapy	Rapid	Slow

CNS, Central nervous system; *WBC*, white blood cell.

translocation involving the mixed lineage leukemia gene (e.g., t(4;11)), and have a poor prognosis.

The overall **cure rate** for childhood **ALL** with current therapy approximates 80%. Relapse of ALL occurs most commonly in the bone marrow but also may occur in the CNS, testes, or other extramedullary sites. If relapse occurs while the patient is still receiving treatment, the prognosis is worse than if relapse occurs after discontinuation of therapy. Stem cell transplant from a matched sibling donor, matched unrelated donor, or cord blood currently is recommended for patients who have a relapse while receiving initial chemotherapy. The current overall **cure rate** for childhood **AML** is approximately 50%. It is slightly higher for patients who receive a matched sibling stem cell transplant in first remission than for patients treated with chemotherapy alone. The prognosis for relapsed AML is poor.

Chapter 156

LYMPHOMA

ETIOLOGY

Lymphomas, or malignancies of lymphoid tissues, are the third most common malignancy in childhood, behind leukemias and central nervous system (CNS) tumors. There are two major types of lymphoma: **Hodgkin disease** and **non-Hodgkin lymphoma (NHL).** The etiologies are unknown, but evidence in many cases suggests that the Epstein-Barr virus (EBV) plays a causal role in both conditions.

Almost all cases of NHL in childhood are diffuse, highly malignant, and show little differentiation. NHL has three histologic subtypes: small noncleaved cell (Burkitt lymphoma), lymphoblastic, and large cell. For simplicity, these may be regarded as B cell, T cell, and large cell (which may be of either B-cell or T-cell origin) (Table 156-1).

Chromosomal translocation may move an oncogene from its normal site to a new, unregulated site, leading to increased expression. In Burkitt lymphoma, translocation occurs

Table 156-1	Subtypes of Non-Hodgkin Lymphoma in Children		
HISTOLOGIC CATEGORY	**IMMUNOPHENOTYPE**	**USUAL PRIMARY SITE**	**MOST COMMON TRANSLOCATION(S)**
Small noncleaved (Burkitt lymphoma)	Mature B-cell (surface immunoglobulin present)	Abdomen (sporadic form) Head and neck (endemic form)	t(8;14)(q24;q32) t(2;8)(p11;q24) t(8;22)(q24;q11)
Lymphoblastic	T-cell (rarely pre-B-cell)	Neck and/or anterior mediastinum	Many
Large cell	T-cell, B-cell, or indeterminate	Lymph nodes, skin, soft tissue, bone	t(2;5)(p23;q35)

between chromosome 8 (*c-myc* oncogene) and the immuno-globulin gene locus on chromosome 2, 14, or 22, such that the *c-myc* oncogene comes to reside next to an immunoglobulin gene. The *c-myc* gene turns on the immunoglobulin gene, leading to a malignant B-cell lymphoma.

EPIDEMIOLOGY

The incidence of Hodgkin disease has a bimodal distribution with peaks in the adolescent/young adult years and again after age 50; it is rarely seen in children younger than 5 years of age. In children, boys are affected more commonly than girls; in adolescents, the gender ratio is approximately equal. The incidence of NHL increases with age. It is more common in whites than in African Americans and in males than in females. NHL has been described in association with congenital or acquired immunodeficiency states and after organ or stem cell transplantation. Burkitt lymphoma commonly is divided into two forms: a sporadic form commonly seen in North America and an endemic form commonly seen in Africa, which has a strong association to EBV.

CLINICAL MANIFESTATIONS

Decision-Making Algorithms
Available @ StudentConsult.com

Lymphadenopathy
Anemia
Bleeding
Neutropenia

The most common clinical presentation of Hodgkin disease is painless, firm lymphadenopathy often confined to one or two lymph node areas, usually the supraclavicular and cervical nodes. Mediastinal lymphadenopathy producing cough or shortness of breath is another frequent initial presentation. The presence of one of three **B symptoms** has prognostic value: fever (>38° C for 3 consecutive days), drenching night sweats, and unintentional weight loss of 10% or more within 6 months of diagnosis.

The **sporadic (North American) form** of Burkitt lymphoma more commonly has an abdominal presentation (typically with pain), whereas the **endemic (African) form** frequently presents with tumors of the jaw. The anterior mediastinum and cervical nodes are the usual primary sites for T-cell lymphomas. These lymphomas may cause airway or superior vena cava obstruction, pleural effusion, or both.

The **diagnosis** of lymphoma is established by tissue biopsy or examination of pleural or peritoneal fluid. Systemic symptoms, such as fever and weight loss, may be present and are particularly prominent in patients with anaplastic large cell lymphoma, which can be insidious in onset. If the bone marrow contains 25% or greater blasts, the disease is classified as acute leukemia (either B-cell acute lymphoblastic leukemia [ALL] or T-cell ALL). This distinction makes little prognostic or therapeutic difference because both require aggressive, systemic therapy in addition to CNS-directed therapy.

LABORATORY/IMAGING STUDIES

Patients suspected to have lymphoma should have a complete blood count, erythrocyte sedimentation rate, and measurement of serum electrolytes, calcium, phosphorus, lactate dehydrogenase, and uric acid. A chest x-ray assesses for a mediastinal mass (Fig. 156-1). The diagnosis ultimately requires a pathologic confirmation from tissue or fluid sampling. For staging purposes, a bone marrow aspirate, bone scan, and positron emission tomography or gallium scan also are indicated. The pathologic hallmark of Hodgkin disease is the identification of **Reed-Sternberg cells.** Histopathologic subtypes in childhood Hodgkin disease are similar to those in adults; 10% to 15% have lymphocyte predominant, 50% to 60% have nodular sclerosis, 30% have mixed cellularity, and less than 5% have lymphocyte depletion. All subtypes are responsive to treatment. Staging of Hodgkin disease is according to the Ann Arbor system. Staging laparotomy is no longer used in children because computed tomography scans often identify abdominal (lymph nodes, liver, spleen) involvement.

DIFFERENTIAL DIAGNOSIS

The differential diagnosis for lymphomas in children includes leukemia, rhabdomyosarcoma, nasopharyngeal carcinoma, germ cell tumors, and thymomas. Nonmalignant diagnoses include infectious mononucleosis (EBV infection), branchial cleft and thyroglossal duct cysts, cat scratch disease (*Bartonella henselae*), bacterial or viral lymphadenitis, mycobacterial infection, toxoplasmosis, and even tinea capitis, all of which can produce significant lymphadenopathy that can mimic lymphoma. Patients with acute abdominal pain from Burkitt lymphoma may be misdiagnosed as having appendicitis.

TREATMENT

The generally accepted treatment for childhood Hodgkin disease is a combination of chemotherapy and low-dose, involved-field radiation therapy. Chemotherapy usually consists of some

Figure 156-1 Chest x-ray of a 15-year-old boy demonstrating a large superior anterior mediastinal mass (*large arrows*) compressing the trachea and deviating it rightward (*arrowheads*). Biopsy revealed non-Hodgkin lymphoma.

combination of cyclophosphamide, vincristine, procarbazine, doxorubicin, bleomycin, vinblastine, prednisone, and etoposide. In general four to six courses of combination chemotherapy are given. Selected low-risk patients may be cured with chemotherapy alone, without radiation therapy.

Distant, noncontiguous metastases are common in childhood NHL. Systemic chemotherapy is mandatory and should be administered to all children with NHL, even those with clinically localized disease at diagnosis.

T-cell lymphoblastic lymphoma and anaplastic large cell lymphoma generally are treated with aggressive multidrug regimens similar to the regimens used in ALL. The main drugs used in the treatment of mature B-cell NHL are cyclophosphamide, moderate- to high-dose methotrexate, cytarabine, doxorubicin, ifosfamide, and etoposide. Surgery and radiation therapy rarely are used because the disease is rarely localized and is highly sensitive to chemotherapy.

COMPLICATIONS

The short-term complications from the treatment of lymphoma are similar to other pediatric malignancies and commonly include immunosuppression, related sequelae from myelosuppression, nausea, vomiting, and alopecia. **Late adverse effects** include second malignant neoplasms (acute myeloid leukemia or myelodysplasia, thyroid malignancies, and breast cancer), hypothyroidism, impaired soft tissue and bone growth, cardiac dysfunction, and pulmonary fibrosis.

PROGNOSIS

Children and adolescents with **Hodgkin disease** are classified as low, intermediate, or high risk according to stage and nodal bulk. The prognosis is generally excellent. There is an approximately 90% 5-year overall survival rate, approaching 100% for low-risk patients and 70% to 90% for high-risk patients. For **NHL** prognosis also is related to stage. The overall 3-year survival rates for B-cell, T-cell, and large cell NHL are 70% to 90%.

Chapter **157**

CENTRAL NERVOUS SYSTEM TUMORS

ETIOLOGY

Most central nervous system (CNS) tumors in children and adolescents are **primary tumors** that originate in the CNS and include low-grade astrocytomas or embryonic neoplasms (medulloblastoma, ependymoma, germ cell tumor). In contrast CNS tumors in adults are high-grade astrocytomas or **secondary tumors** that are metastatic from other carcinomas. CNS tumors also may arise in patients previously treated with radiation therapy. CNS tumors are likely multifactorial in etiology. The classification of CNS tumors is complex and evolving, with the World Health Organization classification being the most complete and accurate system.

EPIDEMIOLOGY

CNS tumors are the most common solid tumors in children and are second to leukemia in overall incidence during childhood. About 1700 new cases occur each year in the United States; the rate is approximately 33 cases per 1 million children under 15 years of age. The incidence peaks before age 10 years and then decreases until a second peak after age 70. For medulloblastoma and ependymoma, males are more affected than females; for other tumor types, no gender differences exist. In the first 2 to 3 years of life, whites are affected more than multiracial children; otherwise incidence rates are essentially equal for whites and multiracial children.

Children with certain inherited syndromes, including neurofibromatosis (types 1 and 2), Li-Fraumeni syndrome, tuberous sclerosis, Turcot syndrome, and von Hippel-Lindau syndrome, have an increased risk for developing a CNS tumor. Most CNS tumors arise in children with no known underlying disorder or risk factor.

CLINICAL MANIFESTATIONS

Decision-Making Algorithms
Available @ StudentConsult.com

Abnormal Head Size, Shape, and Fontanels
Visual Impairment and Leukocoria
Vomiting
Headaches

Brain tumors can cause symptoms by impingement on normal tissue (usually cranial nerves) or by an increase in intracranial pressure caused either by obstruction of cerebrospinal fluid (CSF) flow or by a direct mass effect. Tumors that obstruct the flow of CSF become quickly symptomatic. Symptoms of **increased intracranial pressure** are lethargy, headache, and vomiting (particularly in the morning on awakening). Irritability, anorexia, poor school performance, and loss of developmental milestones all may be signs of slow-growing CNS tumors. In young children with open cranial sutures, an increase in head circumference may occur. Optic pathway tumors may lead to loss of visual acuity or visual field defects. Inability to abduct the eye as the result of sixth cranial nerve palsy is a common sign of increased intracranial pressure. Cranial nerve deficits other than sixth nerve palsy suggest involvement of the brainstem. Seizures occur in 20% to 50% of patients with supratentorial tumors; focal weakness or sensory changes also may be seen. Pituitary involvement produces neuroendocrine effects (galactorrhea with prolactinoma, excessive growth with growth hormone secretory tumors, precocious puberty). Cerebellar tumors are associated with ataxia and diminished coordination. A history and physical examination are fundamental for evaluation, which should include a careful neurologic assessment, including visual fields and a funduscopic examination.

LABORATORY/IMAGING STUDIES

If an intracranial lesion is suspected, **magnetic resonance imaging (MRI)** is currently the examination of choice (Fig. 157-1). Examination of CSF by cytocentrifuge histologic testing is essential to determine the presence of metastatic disease in primitive neuroectodermal tumors, germ cell tumors, and pineal region tumors. A lumbar puncture should not be performed before imaging has been obtained to evaluate for evidence of increased intracranial pressure. If a tumor is

Figure 157-1 Magnetic resonance imaging scan of a 9-year-old boy showing a heterogeneously enhancing fourth ventricular mass (arrow). It was resected, and pathology revealed medulloblastoma.

suspected to have metastatic potential (medulloblastoma), MRI of the entire spine should be obtained before surgery to assess for neuraxial dissemination. A postoperative MRI study of the brain should be obtained within 24 to 48 hours of surgery to assess the extent of resection. During follow-up, magnetic resonance spectroscopy can help distinguish recurrent tumor from radiation necrosis.

DIFFERENTIAL DIAGNOSIS

The differential diagnosis of a CNS mass lesion includes malignant tumor, benign tumor, arteriovenous malformation, aneurysm, brain abscess, cysticercosis, granulomatous disease (tuberculosis, sarcoid), intracranial hemorrhage, pseudotumor cerebri, vasculitis, and, rarely, metastatic tumor.

TREATMENT

The therapy for children with CNS tumors is individualized and depends on the tumor type, location, size, and associated symptoms. High-dose **dexamethasone** often is administered immediately to reduce tumor-associated edema. Surgical objectives are complete excision, if possible, and maximal debulking if a complete excision is not possible. In children, radiation therapy often is combined with chemotherapy; in young children, radiation therapy may be delayed or avoided altogether. Primitive neuroectodermal tumors (including medulloblastoma) and germ cell tumors are sensitive to chemotherapy; gliomas are less sensitive to chemotherapy. Chemotherapy plays an especially important role, particularly in infants in whom the effects of high-dose CNS radiation may have devastating effects on growth and neurocognitive development.

COMPLICATIONS

Short-term adverse effects of therapy include nausea, vomiting, anorexia, fatigue, immunosuppression, and cushingoid features. Long-term adverse effects include neurocognitive deficits, endocrinologic sequelae, decreased bone growth, ototoxicity, renal insufficiency, cataracts, infertility, and second malignant neoplasms (including myelodysplasia). The neurocognitive deficits can be significant, particularly in infants and young children, and are the primary reason for the continued search for the lowest efficacious radiation therapy dose and the most conformal delivery methods for the radiation therapy boosts. **Cerebellar mutism syndrome** occurs in 25% of patients after resection of a posterior fossa tumor and is characterized by an acute decrease in speech (often mutism), behavioral changes (e.g., irritability, apathy, or both), diffuse cerebellar dysfunction, and other neurologic abnormalities. It may begin within hours to days of surgery and is usually self-resolving within weeks to months; cerebellar ataxia and dysmetria often persist. **Somnolence syndrome,** which is characterized by excessive fatigue and sleepiness, may occur in the months after completion of radiation therapy and is self-limited. **Posterior fossa syndrome** manifests as headache and aseptic meningitis days to weeks after surgery in this area.

PROGNOSIS

Improvements in neurodiagnosis, neurosurgical techniques, chemotherapy regimens, and radiation therapy techniques

Table 157-1	Location, Incidence, and Prognosis of CNS Tumors in Children	
LOCATION	**INCIDENCE (%)**	**5-YEAR SURVIVAL (%)**
Infratentorial (posterior fossa)	55–60	
Astrocytoma (cerebellum)	20	90
Medulloblastoma	20	50–80
Glioma (brainstem)	15	High grade: 0–5; low grade: 30
Ependymoma	5	50–60
Supratentorial (cerebral hemispheres)	40–55	
Astrocytoma	15	50–75
Glioblastoma multiforme	10	0–5
Ependymoma	2.5	50–75
Choroid plexus papilloma	1.5	95
Midline		
Craniopharyngioma	6	70–90
Pineal (germinoma)	1	65–75
Optic nerve glioma	3	90

have improved overall outcome. The 5-year overall survival rate associated with all childhood CNS tumors is approximately 50% to 60%, resulting in large measure from the high curability of cerebellar astrocytomas and the increasing cure rate for patients with medulloblastoma (Table 157-1). Intrinsic brainstem gliomas and glioblastoma multiforme have extremely poor prognoses.

Chapter 158

NEUROBLASTOMA

ETIOLOGY

Neuroblastoma is derived from **neural crest cells** that form the adrenal medulla and the sympathetic nervous system. The cause is unknown. Most cases occur in young children, thus it is likely that neuroblastoma results from prenatal and perinatal events. Neuroblastoma may rarely (1% to 2% of cases) be hereditary. Mutations in the ALK and PHOX2B genes are associated with most familial cases. In sporadic cases, several genetic mutations have been identified.

EPIDEMIOLOGY

Neuroblastoma is the most common extracranial solid tumor of childhood and the most common malignancy in infancy. The median age at diagnosis is 20 months. There are approximately 650 new cases of neuroblastoma in the United States

each year. The incidence is estimated to be 1 in 7000 live births. The tumor usually occurs sporadically, but, in 1% to 2% of cases, there is a family history of neuroblastoma.

CLINICAL MANIFESTATIONS

Decision-Making Algorithms
Available @ StudentConsult.com

Neck Masses
Abnormal Eye Movements
Involuntary Movements
Ataxia
Lymphadenopathy
Pancytopenia
Hypercalcemia

Neuroblastoma is remarkable for its broad spectrum of clinical prognosis ranging from spontaneous regression to rapid progression and metastasis resulting in death. Children with localized disease are often asymptomatic at diagnosis, whereas children with metastases often appear ill and have systemic complaints, such as fever, weight loss, and pain. The most common presentation is abdominal pain or mass. The mass is often palpated in the flank and is hard, smooth, and nontender. In the abdomen, 45% of tumors arise in the adrenal gland, and 25% arise in the retroperitoneal sympathetic ganglia. Other sites of origin are the paravertebral ganglia of the chest and neck. Paraspinal tumors may invade through the neural foramina and cause spinal cord compression. Horner syndrome sometimes is seen with neck or apical masses. Several **paraneoplastic syndromes,** including secretory diarrhea, profuse sweating, and **opsomyoclonus** *(dancing eyes and dancing feet),* are associated with neuroblastoma.

Neuroblastoma may metastasize to multiple organs, including the liver, bone, bone marrow, and lymph nodes. Periorbital ecchymoses is a sign of orbital bone involvement. A unique category of neuroblastoma, **stage 4S,** is defined in infants (<1 year old) with a small primary tumor and metastasis limited to skin, liver, or bone marrow. It is associated with a favorable outcome.

LABORATORY/IMAGING STUDIES

A complete blood count and plain films may help identify patients with neuroblastoma. Calcification within abdominal neuroblastoma tumors is often observed on plain films of the abdomen. About 90% of neuroblastomas produce **catecholamines (Vanillylmandelic acid; Homovanillic acid)** that can be detected in the urine. Definitive diagnosis of neuroblastoma requires tissue for light microscopic, electron microscopic, and immunohistologic examination. A computed tomography (CT) scan of the chest, abdomen, and pelvis; a bone scan and/or metaiodobenzylguanidine scan; bilateral bone marrow aspiration and biopsies; and urinary catecholamines complete the evaluation.

DIFFERENTIAL DIAGNOSIS

The abdominal presentation of neuroblastoma must be differentiated from Wilms tumor, which also presents as an abdominal flank mass. Ultrasound or CT examination usually differentiates the tumors. Periorbital ecchymoses from orbital metastases sometimes are mistaken for child abuse. Because children with bone marrow involvement may have anemia, thrombocytopenia, or neutropenia, leukemia is often considered in the differential.

TREATMENT

Treatment of neuroblastoma is based on surgical staging and biologic features (Table 158-1). Complete surgical excision is the initial treatment of choice for localized neuroblastoma. Children with favorable biology who undergo a gross total resection require no further therapy. In patients with advanced disease, combination chemotherapy usually is given after confirmation of the diagnosis. The most commonly used agents are vincristine, cyclophosphamide, doxorubicin, cisplatin, and etoposide. Delayed resection of the primary tumor is undertaken after numerous courses of chemotherapy. Radiation therapy often is administered to the primary tumor bed and areas of metastatic disease. **High-dose chemotherapy with autologous stem cell rescue** has improved the outcome for patients with high-risk neuroblastoma. Survival has also improved with the addition of **cis-retinoic acid** (isotretinoin) and anti-GD2 monoclonal antibody therapy after maximal reduction of tumor burden with chemotherapy, surgery, and radiation therapy.

COMPLICATIONS

Spinal cord compression from neuroblastoma may cause an irreversible neurologic deficit and is an oncologic emergency. Children with the opsomyoclonus syndrome may suffer from developmental delay or mental retardation. The aggressive chemotherapy and radiation therapies currently used to treat high-risk neuroblastoma may result in complications such as ototoxicity, nephrotoxicity, growth problems, and second malignancies.

PROGNOSIS

The prognosis for survival is affected by age at diagnosis, stage, primary site, presence or absence of metastasis, cytogenetics, DNA ploidy, *MYCN* status, and histopathology. Currently children with neuroblastoma can be divided into three groups: low, average, and high risk. Unfavorable biologic factors include lack of cell differentiation, amplification (>10 copies/cell) of the *MYCN* oncogene, lack of hyperdiploidy, and mutations of chromosome 1p, 11q, or 6p22. Patients with favorable biology tend to be younger and often have localized disease. Patients under 1 year of age generally have a better prognosis than older patients. Older patients with stage 4 disease most commonly have unfavorable biology, and more than 50% will relapse due to drug-resistant residual disease. Although neuroblastoma represents only 8% of cases of childhood cancer, it is responsible for 15% of cancer deaths in children.

Table 158-1	Proposed Children's Oncology Group Neuroblastoma Risk Stratification Schema, by Stage					
STAGE	AGE	MYCN	PLOIDY	HISTOLOGY	OTHER	RISK GROUP
1						Low
2A/2B		Not amplified			>50% resection	Low
		Not amplified			<50% resection	Intermediate
		Not amplified			Biopsy only	Intermediate
		Amplified				High
3	<547 days	Not amplified				Intermediate
	≥547 days	Not amplified		Favorable		Intermediate
		Amplified				High
	≥547 days	Not amplified		Unfavorable		High
4	<365 days	Amplified				High
	<365 days	Not amplified				Intermediate
	365–547 days	Amplified				High
	365–547 days		DI = 1			High
	365–547 days			Unfavorable		High
	365–547 days	Not amplified	DI > 1	Favorable		Intermediate
	≥547 days					High
4S	<365 days	Not amplified	DI > 1	Favorable	Asymptomatic	Low
	<365 days	Not amplified	DI = 1			Intermediate
	<365 days	Missing	Missing	Missing		Intermediate
	<365 days	Not amplified			Symptomatic	Intermediate
	<365 days	Not amplified		Unfavorable		Intermediate
	<365 days	Amplified				High

From Maris JM, Hogarty MD, Bagatell R, et al: Neuroblastoma, Lancet 369:2106–2120, 2007.
DI, DNA index.

Chapter 159

WILMS TUMOR

ETIOLOGY

Wilms tumor is thought to arise from primitive, metanephric blastema, the precursor of a normal kidney. Nephrogenic rests are foci of embryonal cells that may be rarely (<1%) found in normal infant kidneys and are commonly (25% to 40%) found in Wilms tumor-bearing kidneys. They may be perilobar, intralobar, or both, and are widely considered to be precursors to Wilms tumors. Although the cause of Wilms tumor is unknown, children with certain congenital anomalies or genetic conditions are at increased risk of developing the disease.

Multiple Wilms tumor or *WT* genes have been identified. The *WT1* gene at chromosomal band 11p13 is important in a minority of tumors, and other genes at 11p15, 16q, and 1p are also involved. The identification of several genes involved in the etiology or progression of Wilms tumor and the loss of heterozygosity (LOH) in normal tissues of some patients demonstrate that the genetic predisposition to Wilms tumor is heterogeneous.

EPIDEMIOLOGY

Wilms tumor is the most common malignant **renal tumor** of childhood, with approximately 500 new cases per year in the United States. The mean age at diagnosis is 3 to 3.5 years of age, and no gender predilection is apparent. A hereditary form of Wilms tumor may be associated with bilateral presentation and younger age at onset. Many congenital anomalies are associated with Wilms tumor, including sporadic aniridia, hemihypertrophy, and genitourinary abnormalities. Patients with the WAGR (Wilms tumor, aniridia, genitourinary malformation, mental retardation) syndrome have Wilms tumor as a manifestation of the syndrome itself, resulting from a germline deletion at chromosome 11p. Patients with Beckwith-Wiedemann syndrome and some other overgrowth syndromes are at increased risk for developing Wilms tumor and should be screened with periodic renal imaging.

CLINICAL MANIFESTATIONS

Decision-Making Algorithms
Available @ StudentConsult.com

Abdominal Pain
Abdominal Masses

Most children with Wilms tumor are brought to medical attention because they have an **abdominal mass** that is discovered by their parents. Although many children do not have complaints at the time that the mass is first noted, associated symptoms may include abdominal pain, fever, hypertension, and hematuria.

LABORATORY/IMAGING STUDIES

An abdominal ultrasound or computed tomography (CT) scan can usually distinguish an intrarenal mass from a mass in the adrenal gland or other surrounding structures. Evaluation of the inferior vena cava is crucial because the tumor may extend from the kidney into the vena cava. A complete blood count, urinalysis, liver and renal function studies, and a chest radiograph (to identify pulmonary metastases) should be obtained. In most cases, a CT scan of the chest, abdomen, and pelvis is obtained. The diagnosis is confirmed by histologic examination of the tumor. Although most cases of Wilms tumor are classified as *favorable histology,* the presence of anaplasia is predictive of a worse prognosis and is considered unfavorable.

DIFFERENTIAL DIAGNOSIS

The differential diagnosis of Wilms tumor includes hydronephrosis and polycystic disease of the kidney; benign renal tumors, such as mesoblastic nephroma and hamartoma; and other malignant tumors, such as renal cell carcinoma, neuroblastoma, lymphoma, and retroperitoneal rhabdomyosarcoma.

TREATMENT

The timing of nephrectomy for unilateral, resectable Wilms tumor remains controversial. The North American approach is for immediate nephrectomy followed by adjuvant chemotherapy, whereas the European approach is to make a diagnosis by imaging and sometimes a biopsy, give neoadjuvant chemotherapy followed by surgery and then adjuvant chemotherapy (plus radiation therapy, as indicated). The overall survival is comparable regardless of the approach. The Children's Oncology Group protocols for Wilms tumor with favorable histologic findings generally include vincristine and actinomycin, with or without doxorubicin. Radiation therapy is reserved for a minority of patients depending on stage, presence of metastases, response to therapy, and LOH status.

Bilateral Wilms tumor is present in about 5% of children on initial presentation, whereas recurrent disease affects the opposite kidney in 4% to 5% of patients. Treatment for patients with bilateral Wilms tumor should be individualized to retain as much normal kidney as possible.

COMPLICATIONS

Survivors of Wilms tumor are at risk for several late effects, including cardiomyopathy, scoliosis, hypertension and prehypertension, renal and bladder insufficiency, pulmonary dysfunction, hepatic dysfunction, infertility, and second malignancies. Patients with bilateral Wilms tumor are sometimes left with renal insufficiency or failure. Female survivors may have complicated pregnancies and deliveries.

PROGNOSIS

In general the prognosis for patients with Wilms tumor is very good. Prognostic factors include stage and histologic features. Anaplastic variants of Wilms tumor have a significantly worse outcome than classic Wilms tumor. In addition LOH at chromosomes 1p or 16q confers an increased risk of relapse and death compared to tumors without LOH at either site.

The 4-year relapse-free survival of patients with tumors of favorable histologic picture is directly related to stage. Cure rates for patients with localized Wilms tumor at diagnosis are greater than 85%, whereas patients with pulmonary metastases have event-free survival rates of approximately 70% to 80%.

Chapter 160

SARCOMAS

Sarcomas are divided into soft tissue sarcomas and bone cancers. Soft tissue sarcomas arise primarily from the connective tissues of the body, such as muscle tissue, fibrous tissue, and adipose tissue. **Rhabdomyosarcoma,** the most common soft tissue sarcoma in children, is derived from mesenchymal cells that are committed to skeletal muscle lineage. Less common soft tissue sarcomas include fibrosarcoma, synovial sarcoma, and extraosseous **Ewing sarcoma.** The most common malignant bone cancers in children are **osteosarcoma** and Ewing sarcoma. Osteosarcomas derive from primitive bone-forming mesenchymal stem cells. Ewing sarcomas are thought to be of neural crest cell origin.

ETIOLOGY

The cause is unknown for most children diagnosed with sarcoma, although a few observations have been made regarding risks. Individuals with **Li-Fraumeni syndrome** (associated with a germline *p53* mutation) and **neurofibromatosis** (associated with NF1 mutations) have an increased risk of soft tissue sarcomas. There is a 500-fold increased risk for osteosarcoma for individuals with hereditary retinoblastoma. Prior treatment for childhood cancer with **radiation therapy** or chemotherapy, specifically alkylating agents, or both, increases the risk for osteosarcoma as a second malignancy.

EPIDEMIOLOGY

In the United States, 850 to 900 children and adolescents under 20 years of age are diagnosed with soft tissue sarcomas each year; approximately 350 are rhabdomyosarcoma. The incidence of rhabdomyosarcoma peaks in children 2 to 6 years old and in adolescents. The early peak is associated with tumors in the genitourinary region, head, and neck; the later peak is associated with tumors in the extremities, trunk, and male genitourinary tract. Boys are affected 1.5 times more often than girls.

Of the 650 to 700 U.S. children and adolescents under 20 years of age diagnosed with bone tumors each year, approximately two thirds have osteosarcoma and one third have Ewing sarcoma. Osteosarcoma most commonly affects adolescents; the peak incidence occurs during the period of maximum growth velocity. The incidence of Ewing sarcoma peaks between ages 10 and 20 years but may occur at any age. Ewing sarcoma affects primarily whites; it rarely occurs in African American children or Asian children.

CLINICAL MANIFESTATIONS

Decision-Making Algorithms
Available @ StudentConsult.com

Neck Masses
Hoarseness
Scrotal Swelling (Painless)
Vaginal Discharge
Lymphadenopathy
Gynecomastia

The clinical presentation of **rhabdomyosarcoma** varies, depending on the site of origin, subsequent mass effect, and presence of metastatic disease. Periorbital swelling, proptosis, and limitation of extraocular motion may be seen with an orbital tumor. Nasal mass, chronic otitis media, ear discharge, dysphagia, neck mass, and cranial nerve involvement may be noted with tumors in other head and neck sites. Urethral or vaginal masses, paratesticular swelling, hematuria, and urinary frequency or retention may be noted with tumors in the genitourinary tract. Trunk or extremity lesions tend to present as rapidly growing masses that may or may not be painful. If there is metastatic disease to bone or bone marrow, limb pain and evidence of marrow failure may be present.

Osteosarcoma often is located at the epiphysis or metaphysis of anatomic sites that are associated with maximum growth velocity (distal femur, proximal tibia, proximal humerus), but any bone may be involved. It presents with pain and may be associated with a palpable mass. Because the pain and swelling often are initially thought to be related to trauma, radiographs of the affected region frequently are obtained, which usually reveal a lytic lesion, often associated with calcification in the soft tissue surrounding the lesion. While 75% to 80% of patients with osteosarcoma have apparently localized disease at diagnosis, the majority of patients are believed to have micrometastatic disease as well.

Although **Ewing sarcoma** can occur in almost any bone in the body, the femur and pelvis are the most common sites. In addition to local pain and swelling, clinical manifestations may include systemic symptoms, such as fever and weight loss.

LABORATORY/IMAGING STUDIES

Tissue biopsy is needed for a definitive diagnosis of sarcomas. Selection of the biopsy site is important and has implications for future surgical resection and radiation therapy. Under light microscopy, rhabdomyosarcoma and Ewing sarcoma appear as **small, round, blue cell tumors.** Osteosarcomas are distinguishable by the presence of **osteoid substance.**

Immunohistochemical staining for muscle-specific proteins, such as actin and myosin, helps confirm the diagnosis of rhabdomyosarcoma. Two major histologic variants exist for rhabdomyosarcoma: **embryonal** and **alveolar.** Embryonal histologic variant is most common in younger children with head, neck, and genitourinary primary tumors. Alveolar histologic variant occurs in older patients and is seen most commonly in trunk and extremity tumors. Alveolar rhabdomyosarcoma often is characterized by specific translocations: t(2;13) or t(1;13). Metastatic evaluation for patients with rhabdomyosarcoma should include a computed tomography (CT) scan of the chest, abdomen, and pelvis; a bone scan; and bone marrow aspiration and biopsy. A lumbar puncture is required in patients with a parameningeal primary site.

Definitive diagnosis of osteosarcoma often is established by carefully placed needle biopsy. The presence of osteoid and immunohistochemical analysis confirms the diagnosis of osteosarcoma. The extent of the primary tumor should be delineated carefully with magnetic resonance imaging (MRI) before starting chemotherapy. Osteosarcoma tends to metastasize to the lung, most commonly, and rarely to other bones. Metastatic evaluation includes a chest CT scan and a bone scan.

The diagnosis of Ewing sarcoma is established with immunohistochemical analysis and cytogenetic and molecular diagnostic studies of the biopsy material. Ewing sarcoma is characterized by a specific chromosomal translocation, **t(11;22),** which is seen in 95% of tumors. MRI of the primary lesion should be performed to delineate extent of the lesion and any associated soft tissue mass. Metastatic evaluation involves a bone scan, chest CT scan, and bone marrow aspiration and biopsy.

DIFFERENTIAL DIAGNOSIS

Patients with Ewing sarcoma may be misdiagnosed as having **osteomyelitis;** children with osteogenic sarcoma often are thought initially to have pain and swelling related to trauma. The differential diagnosis for rhabdomyosarcoma depends on the location of the tumor. Tumors of the trunk and extremities often present as a painless mass and may be initially thought to be benign tumors. Periorbital rhabdomyosarcoma may be misdiagnosed as orbital cellulitis, and other head and neck rhabdomyosarcoma may be confused with chronic infection of ears or sinuses. The differential diagnosis for intra-abdominal rhabdomyosarcoma includes other abdominal malignancies, such as Wilms tumor or neuroblastoma.

TREATMENT

Treatment of rhabdomyosarcoma is currently based on a staging system that incorporates both the primary site and histologic picture. The staging system also involves a local tumor group assessment based on the extent of disease and surgical result. In the intergroup rhabdomyosarcoma studies, the most common chemotherapy agents used are cyclophosphamide, vincristine, and actinomycin. Doxorubicin, etoposide, ifosfamide, topotecan, and irinotecan are also active against rhabdomyosarcoma. Radiation is administered to patients who have residual disease after initial surgery or who have only had a primary biopsy of the tumor.

The current treatment of osteosarcoma involves neoadjuvant chemotherapy followed by surgery and adjuvant chemotherapy. Agents effective against osteosarcoma are doxorubicin, cisplatin, high-dose methotrexate, ifosfamide, and etoposide. The treatment for Ewing sarcoma is similar to that for osteosarcoma; preoperative chemotherapy is given, followed by local control measures, and then further chemotherapy. In contrast to osteosarcoma, Ewing sarcoma is **radiation sensitive.** Chemotherapy includes vincristine, cyclophosphamide, ifosfamide, etoposide, and doxorubicin.

COMPLICATIONS

In addition to the risk of late effects from the chemotherapy, children with sarcomas have potential complications related to local control of the tumor. If the local disease is controlled with surgery, the long-term sequelae may include loss of limb or limitation of function. If local control is accomplished with radiation therapy, the late effects depend on the dose of radiation given, the extent of the site radiated, and the development of the child at the time of radiation therapy. Irradiating tissues interfere with growth and development, so significant adverse consequences may occur in young children.

PROGNOSIS

For all children with sarcoma, presence or absence of **metastatic disease** at presentation is the most important prognostic factor. The outlook remains poor for patients who have distant metastasis from Ewing sarcoma, rhabdomyosarcoma, or osteosarcoma at diagnosis. Patients with localized rhabdomyosarcomas in favorable sites have an excellent prognosis when treated with surgery followed by vincristine and actinomycin. In patients with osteosarcoma and Ewing sarcoma, another important prognostic factor is the **degree of tumor necrosis** after preoperative chemotherapy. In general, patients whose tumor specimens show a high degree (>90%) of necrosis following preoperative chemotherapy have an event-free survival rate greater than 80%. Patients who still have large amounts of viable tumor after presurgical chemotherapy have a much worse prognosis. The cure rate for patients with localized osteosarcoma and Ewing sarcoma is approximately 60% to 70%. Patients who have lung metastasis at diagnosis have a cure rate of approximately 30% to 35%. Patients with metastases to other bones have a poor prognosis.

Suggested Reading

Arndt CA, Rose PS, Folpe AL, et al: Common musculoskeletal tumors of childhood and adolescence, *Mayo Clin Proc* 87:475–487, 2012.

Davenport KP, Blanco FC, Sandler AD: Pediatric malignancies: neuroblastoma, Wilms tumor, hepatoblastoma, rhabdomyosarcoma and sacrococcygeal teratoma, *Surg Clin North Am* 92:745–767, 2012.

Kopp LM, Gupta P, Pelayo-Katsanis L, et al.: Late effects in adult survivors of pediatric cancer: a guide for the primary care physician, *Am J Med* 125:636–641, 2012.

Packer RJ, MacDonald T, Vezina G: Central nervous system tumors, *Pediatr Clin North Am* 55:121–145, 2008.

Pui CH, Mulligan CG, Evans WE, et al: Pediatric acute lymphoblastic leukemia: where are we going and how do we get there? *Blood* 120:1165–1174, 2012.

Nephrology and Urology

John D. Mahan and Hiren P. Patel

Chapter 161

NEPHROLOGY AND UROLOGY ASSESSMENT

The kidneys preserve homeostasis through multiple mechanisms: maintain fluid and electrolyte balance, excrete metabolic waste products through glomerular filtration and tubular secretion, generate energy (gluconeogenesis), and produce important endocrine hormones (renin, vitamin D metabolites, erythropoietin). Renal disorders, by disturbing homeostasis, can affect growth and development and result in a variety of clinical manifestations (Table 161-1). Renal disorders in children may represent intrinsic renal diseases or derive from systemic conditions (Table 161-2).

HISTORY

Fetal urine production contributes to amniotic fluid volume, lung maturation, and somatic development. Congenital renal disorders may be associated with reduced (oligohydramnios) or increased amniotic fluid volume (polyhydramnios). Pulmonary hypoplasia and fetal maldevelopment of the face and extremities may result from insufficient amniotic fluid (Potter syndrome) (see Chapters 58 and 60).

Risk factors for renal disease (e.g., perinatal hypoxia-ischemia, acute tubular necrosis, renal vein thrombosis) can be detected by a careful history. A detailed family history may identify hereditary renal conditions. Poor growth and/or feeding, abnormal fluid intake and/or output may indicate underlying renal dysfunction. Other common manifestations of renal and/or urinary tract disorders are listed in Table 161-1.

PHYSICAL EXAMINATION

Renal diseases in children may be initially asymptomatic and detected during routine visits. Abnormal growth, hypertension (HTN), dehydration, or edema may suggest occult renal disease (see Chapter 33). Abnormal facial features may suggest syndromes associated with renal disorders (fetal alcohol syndrome, Down syndrome). Preauricular tags, deformities of the external ear, or ophthalmologic abnormalities (keratoconus, aniridia, iridocyclitis, cataracts) can be associated with congenital renal defects. Abdominal examination may reveal renal masses. Bladder distention may suggest a urine-concentrating defect or urinary tract obstruction.

RENAL PHYSIOLOGY

Normal renal function depends on intact **glomerular filtration** and **tubular function** (**proximal tubule** [PT], **loop of Henle**, and **distal tubule** [DT]) that results in **urine formation** (Fig. 161-1). The net glomerular pressure favors movement of fluid out of the capillaries into Bowman's space. Intraglomerular pressure is regulated by afferent and, particularly, efferent arteriolar tone. **Renin** is generated by cells in the juxtaglomerular apparatus, located at the base of each glomerulus in proximity to the afferent/efferent arterioles and DT of that nephron and released in response to glomerular flow and perfusion.

The PT conducts isosmotic reabsorption (see Fig. 161-1) to reabsorb two thirds of the filtered volume, sodium, and chloride. Glucose, amino acids, potassium, and phosphate are almost completely reabsorbed. Approximately 75% of filtered bicarbonate is reabsorbed in the PT. When filtered bicarbonate exceeds the PT threshold, bicarbonate is spilled into the urine. The PT also secretes compounds such as organic acids, penicillins, and other drugs. The most potent vitamin D analog—1,25$(OH)_2$-cholecalciferol (**calcitriol**)—is produced by PT cells in response to parathyroid hormone and intracellular calcium/phosphorus concentrations.

The loop of Henle is the site of reabsorption of 25% of sodium chloride filtered in the glomerulus (see Fig. 161-1). Active chloride transport drives the countercurrent multiplier and composes the medullary interstitial hypertonic gradient required for urinary concentration.

The DT is composed of the **distal convoluted tubule** (DCT) and **collecting ducts (CD)**. The DCT is water impermeable and contributes to urine dilution by active sodium chloride absorption. The CD is the primary site of **antidiuretic hormone** (vasopressin) response, which leads to urine concentration. Sodium-potassium and sodium-hydrogen exchange in the CD is regulated by aldosterone. Active hydrogen ion secretion, which is responsible for the final acidification of the urine, also occurs in the CD.

Renal **ammonia** production and intraluminal generation of ammonium (NH_4^+) facilitate urine hydrogen ion excretion. Urinary NH_4^+ is not measured easily but can be inferred by calculation of the **urinary anion gap**. The *gap* between measured anions and cations largely consists of NH_4^+. Problems with renal acid excretion or ammonia production decrease the

Table 161-1	Common Manifestations of Renal Disease by Age

FINDING	SIGNIFICANCE
	NEONATE
Flank mass	Multicystic dysplasia, urinary tract obstruction (hydronephrosis), polycystic disease, tumor
Hematuria	Acute tubular/cortical necrosis, urinary tract malformation, trauma, renal vein thrombosis
Anuria and oliguria	Renal agenesis, obstruction, acute tubular necrosis, vascular thrombosis
	CHILD/ADOLESCENT
Cola red-colored urine	Hemoglobinuria (hemolysis); myoglobinuria (rhabdomyolysis); pigmenturia (porphyria, urate, beets, drugs); hematuria (infection, glomerulonephritis, Henoch-Schönlein purpura, hypercalciuria, stones)
Gross hematuria	Infection, glomerulonephritis, trauma, benign hematuria, nephrolithiasis, tumor
Edema	Nephrotic syndrome, glomerulonephritis, acute/chronic renal failure, cardiac/liver disease
Hypertension	Acute glomerulonephritis, acute/chronic renal failure, obstruction, cysts, dysplasia, coarctation of the aorta, renal artery stenosis
Polyuria	Diabetes mellitus, central and nephrogenic diabetes insipidus, obstruction, dysplasia, hypokalemia, hypercalcemia, psychogenic polydipsia, sickle disease/trait, polyuric renal failure, diuretic abuse
Oliguria	Dehydration, acute tubular necrosis, acute glomerulonephritis, interstitial nephritis, hemolytic uremic syndrome
Dysfunctional voiding/urgency	Neurogenic bladder, urinary tract infection, vaginitis, hypercalciuria, foreign body

Table 161-2	Primary and Systemic Causes of Renal Disease in Children

PRIMARY	SECONDARY (SYSTEMIC)
Minimal change nephrotic syndrome	Postinfectious glomerulonephritis
Focal segmental glomerulosclerosis	IgA nephropathy
Membranoproliferative glomerulonephritis	Henoch-Schönlein purpura-related nephritis Membranoproliferative glomerulonephritis
Membranous nephropathy	Hemolytic uremic syndrome Systemic lupus erythematosus Wegener granulomatosis and other vasculitides
Congenital nephrotic syndrome	Tubular toxins
Alport syndrome	Antibiotics
Intrinsic tubular disorders	Chemotherapeutic agents
Structural renal disorders	Hemoglobin/myoglobin
Congenital urinary tract abnormalities	Tubular disorders
Polycystic kidney disease	Cystinosis, oxalosis
Renal/urinary tract tumor	Galactosemia, hereditary fructose intolerance
	Stones
	Sickle disease/trait
	Trauma
	Extrarenal malignancy (leukemia, lymphoma)

urinary anion gap. A urinary gap of approximately 1 mEq/kg body weight is reasonable in normal children.

The maximum **urinary concentrating capacity** in a preterm newborn (~400 mOsm/L) is less than that in a full-term newborn (600 to 800 mOsm/L), which is less than that in older children and adults (~1200 mOsm/L). Neonates can dilute urine similar to adults (75 to 90 mOsm/L), but, because the **glomerular filtration rate** (GFR) is lower, the capacity to excrete a water load is less in infants. GFR reaches adult levels by 1 to 2 years of age. Tubular reabsorption of sodium, potassium, bicarbonate, and phosphate and excretion of hydrogen are all reduced in infants relative to adults. These functions mature independently and at different ages, so a neonate rapidly develops the ability to reabsorb sodium efficiently, but it takes 2 years for bicarbonate reabsorption to mature. **Erythropoietin** is secreted by interstitial cells in the renal medulla in response to low oxygen delivery and helps regulate bone marrow red blood cell production.

COMMON MANIFESTATIONS

Decision-Making Algorithms
Available @ StudentConsult.com

Dysuria
Enuresis
Red Urine and Hematuria

Renal disorders can be classified as **primary** or **secondary** (due to systemic illnesses) (see Table 161-2). Renal diseases may present with obvious signs, such as hematuria or edema, or with subtle signs detected on screening examinations (abdominal or flank mass, HTN, proteinuria). Fever,

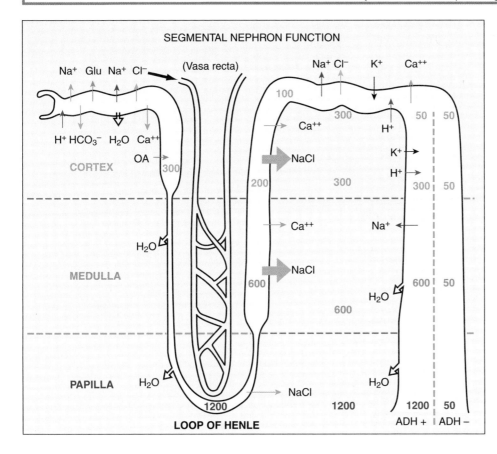

SEGMENTAL NEPHRON FUNCTION

Figure 161-1 Major transport functions of each nephron segment, including representative osmolalities in vasa recta, interstitium, and tubule at different levels within the kidney. *ADH*, Antidiuretic hormone; *Glu*, glucose; *OA*, organic acid. *(From Andreoli TE, Carpenter CCJ, Plum F, et al, editors:* Cecil Essentials of Medicine, *Philadelphia, 1986, WB Saunders.)*

irritability, and vomiting may be presenting symptoms in neonates and infants with **urinary tract infections** (UTIs), whereas frequency and dysuria suggest UTI in older children. Chronic kidney disease often is associated with poor growth and feeding but may be first detected on screening examinations (HTN, hematuria). An abnormal urine stream may indicate posterior urethral valves, other bladder disorders, or obstructive lesions.

DIAGNOSTIC STUDIES
Laboratory Studies

The GFR is measured most accurately by infusion of a substance that is *freely* filtered by the glomerulus but is not metabolized, reabsorbed, or secreted in or by the tubules. The GFR is calculated as follows:

$$GFR = [U] \, V/[P]$$

where $[U]$ is urine concentration, $[P]$ is serum concentration of a substance (mg/dL) used to measure clearance, and V is urine flow rate (mL/min).

By convention, GFR is corrected to a body surface area of 1.73 m² to allow comparison between different sized individuals. In a full-term newborn, an uncorrected GFR of 4 to 5 mL/min corrects to approximately 40 mL/min/1.73 m². GFR increases rapidly during the first 2 years of life when it achieves adult values (100 to 120 mL/min/1.73 m²). After that, GFR and body size increase proportionately, and GFR remains stable.

Plasma creatinine reflects muscle mass, increases with age, and is used to approximate GFR. Creatinine is also secreted by PT, resulting in a less accurate measurement of GFR with immature kidneys or with decreased renal function. **Blood urea nitrogen** is affected by renal function but is greatly altered by hydration, nutrition, catabolism, and tissue breakdown. The correlation between creatinine and GFR can be used to estimate GFR. The revised Schwartz formula is the following:

$$GFR = \frac{0.413 \times Ht}{Cr_{serum}}$$

Height is measured in centimeters. Serum creatinine is measured in milligram per deciliter. This formula is most useful when body habitus and muscle mass are reasonably normal and when renal function is relatively stable. This formula may be most accurate in the range of 15 to 75 mL/min per 1.73 m². Values greater than 75 should be reported as such rather than as a specific number. **Creatinine clearance** ($[U_{Cr}] V/[P_{Cr}]$) estimates GFR but overestimates GFR when renal function is decreased.

Urinalysis is a useful screen for renal abnormalities. In addition to urine color and turbidity, **macroscopic urinalysis** uses a **urine dipstick** for pH and the presence of protein, glucose, ketones, blood, and leukocytes. Dilute urine may result in a false-negative result for protein; false-positive results may occur with extremely alkaline or concentrated urine or if there is a delay in reading the test. Dipsticks are exquisitely sensitive to the presence of hemoglobin (or myoglobin); there are few false-negative test results but many false-positive results. **Glucose** is detected via a glucose oxidase-peroxidase reaction, and leukocytes are detected via a **leukocyte esterase** reaction. The **nitrite test** may detect bacteriuria if the bacteria reduce nitrate to nitrite and have long contact time with the urine. False-negative results occur with frequent voiding, low urine bacterial count, urinary tract obstruction, and infection with bacteria unable to generate nitrite. Gross hematuria or prolonged contact (uncircumcised boys) may result in a false-positive nitrite test. **Microscopic urinalysis** is used to confirm pyuria and hematuria and detect casts and crystals.

Proteinuria can be further defined by determination of a **spot urine protein/creatinine** ($U_{Pr}/_{Cr}$) in a single urine specimen. This unit-less value correlates very well with 24-hour urine protein excretion: spot $U_{Pr}/_{Cr}$ approximates 24-hour urine protein/m²/day (normal <0.20; nephrotic range >2.0 in children).

IMAGING STUDIES

Ultrasound reliably assesses kidney size, determines degree of dilation, and differentiates cortex and medulla. The bladder also can be visualized. **Pulsed Doppler studies** assess arterial and venous blood flow and can be used to calculate the kidneys' resistive index.

A **voiding cystourethrogram** involves repeated filling of the bladder to detect vesicoureteral reflux and to evaluate the urethra. **Computed tomography** and **magnetic resonance imaging** have mostly replaced the **intravenous pyelogram** to evaluate kidney structure and function. Radionuclide studies can define renal size, scars, and renal function/excretion.

Chapter 162

NEPHROTIC SYNDROME AND PROTEINURIA

ETIOLOGY AND EPIDEMIOLOGY

Small amounts of protein are found in the urine of healthy children (<4 mg/m²/hour or $U_{Pr}/_{Cr}$ <0.2). **Nephrotic proteinuria** in children is defined as protein greater than 40 mg/m²/hour or $U_{Pr/Cr}$ >2.0. Proteinuria between these levels is mildly to moderately elevated but not nephrotic.

Proteinuria may be **transient** or **persistent, asymptomatic** or **symptomatic,** and **orthostatic** (present in the upright position but not in the recumbent position) or **fixed** (present in all positions). Proteinuria may be **glomerular** (disruptions of the normal glomerular barrier to protein filtration) or **tubular** (increased filtration, impaired reabsorption, or secretion of proteins).

Nephrotic syndrome (NS) is characterized by persistent heavy **proteinuria** (mainly albuminuria) (>2 g/m²/24 h); **hypoproteinemia** (serum albumin <3.0 g/dL); **hypercholesterolemia** (>250 mg/dL); and **edema**. Age, race, and geography affect the incidence of NS. Certain HLA types (HLA-DR7, HLA-B8, and HLA-B12) are associated with an increased incidence of NS. Increased glomerular permeability is due to alterations in the normal glomerular cellular and basement membrane barrier that restrict filtration of serum proteins. The resultant massive proteinuria leads to decreased serum proteins, especially albumin. Plasma oncotic pressure is diminished, leading to fluid shifts from vascular to interstitial compartments and plasma volume contraction. Renal

Table 162-1	Primary and Secondary Forms of Nephrotic Syndrome
PRIMARY	**SECONDARY**
Minimal change nephrotic syndrome	Systemic lupus erythematosus
Primary focal glomerulosclerosis	Henoch-Schönlein purpura, Wegener and other vasculitides
Membranoproliferative glomerulonephritis	Chronic infections (hepatitis B, hepatitis C, malaria, human immunodeficiency virus)
Idiopathic membranous nephropathy	Allergic reactions
	Diabetes
	Amyloidosis
	Malignancies
	Congestive heart failure, constrictive pericarditis
	Renal vein thrombosis

blood flow and the glomerular filtration rate are not usually diminished. Edema results from reduction in effective circulating blood volume and increase in tubular sodium chloride reabsorption secondary to activation of the renin-angiotensin-aldosterone system. Hypoproteinemia stimulates hepatic lipoprotein synthesis and diminishes lipoprotein metabolism, leading to elevated serum lipids (cholesterol, triglycerides) and lipoproteins.

NS may be **primary** or **secondary** (Table 162-1). A child with apparent primary NS, prior to renal biopsy, is considered to have **idiopathic nephrotic syndrome. Minimal change nephrotic syndrome** (MCNS) is the most common histologic form of primary NS in children. More than 80% of children less than 7 years of age with NS have MCNS. Children 7 to 16 years old with NS have a 50% chance of having MCNS. Males are affected more frequently than females (2:1).

Focal segmental glomerulosclerosis (FSGS) accounts for approximately 10% to 20% of children with primary NS. It may present like MCNS or with less impressive proteinuria. FSGS may develop from MCNS or represent a separate entity. A circulating factor that increases glomerular permeability is found in some patients with FSGS. More than 35% of children with FSGS progress to renal failure.

Membranoproliferative glomerulonephritis (MPGN) is characterized by hypocomplementemia with signs of glomerular renal disease. MPGN represents 5% to 15% of children with primary NS, is typically persistent, and has a high likelihood of progression to renal failure over time.

Membranous nephropathy represents less than 5% of children with primary NS. It is seen most commonly in adolescents and children with systemic infections, such as hepatitis B, syphilis, malaria, and toxoplasmosis, or on specific medications (gold, penicillamine).

Congenital NS presents during the first 2 months of life. There are two common types. The Finnish type is an autosomal recessive disorder most common in persons of Scandinavian descent and is due to a mutation in the nephrin protein component in the glomerular filtration slit. The second type is a heterogeneous group of abnormalities, including diffuse mesangial sclerosis and conditions associated with drugs or infections. Prenatal onset is supported by elevated levels of maternal alpha-fetoprotein.

Secondary NS may result from many different causes in children and are listed in Table 162-1.

CLINICAL MANIFESTATIONS

Decision-Making Algorithms
Available @ StudentConsult.com

Abdominal Pain
Red Urine and Hematuria
Proteinuria
Edema

The sudden onset of dependent pitting edema or ascites is the most common presentation for children with NS. Anorexia, malaise, and abdominal pain are often present. Blood pressure may be elevated in up to 25% of children on presentation; acute tubular necrosis and significant hypotension may occur with sudden decline in serum albumin and significant volume depletion. Diarrhea (intestinal edema) and respiratory distress (pulmonary edema or pleural effusion) may be present. Typical MCNS is characterized by the *absence* of gross hematuria, renal insufficiency, hypertension (HTN), and hypocomplementemia.

DIAGNOSTIC STUDIES

Proteinuria of 1+ or higher on 2 to 3 random urine specimens suggests persistent proteinuria that should be further quantified. A $U_{Pr}/_{Cr} >0.2$ on a first morning specimen excludes orthostatic proteinuria. $U_{Pr}/_{Cr} >2.0$ indicates nephrotic range proteinuria.

In addition to a demonstration of proteinuria, hypercholesterolemia, and hypoalbuminemia, routine testing typically includes a serum C3 complement. A low serum C3 implies a lesion other than MCNS, and a renal biopsy is indicated before trial of steroid therapy. Microscopic hematuria may be present in up to 25% of cases of MCNS but does not predict response to steroids. Additional laboratory tests, including electrolytes, blood urea nitrogen, creatinine, total protein, and serum albumin level, are performed based on history and physical examination features. Renal ultrasound is often useful. Biopsy is performed when MCNS is not suspected.

DIFFERENTIAL DIAGNOSIS

Transient proteinuria can be seen after vigorous exercise, fever, dehydration, seizures, and adrenergic agonist therapy. Proteinuria usually is mild ($U_{Pr}/_{Cr}<1$), glomerular in origin, and always resolves within a few days. It does not indicate renal disease.

Postural (orthostatic) proteinuria is a benign condition defined by normal protein excretion while recumbent but significant proteinuria when upright. It is glomerular in nature, more common in adolescents and tall, thin individuals, and not associated with progressive renal disease. Many children with orthostatic proteinuria continue this process into adulthood.

Tubular proteinuria is characterized by preponderance of low-molecular-weight proteins in the urine and is suspected with acute tubular necrosis, pyelonephritis, structural renal disorders, polycystic kidney disease, and tubular toxins such as antibiotics or chemotherapeutic agents. The combination of tubular proteinuria with evidence of tubular electrolyte wasting and glycosuria is termed **Fanconi syndrome.**

Glomerular proteinuria is characterized by a combination of large- and small-molecular-weight proteins in the urine, variable levels of proteinuria, and often evidence of glomerular disease (hematuria, red blood cell casts, HTN, and renal insufficiency). Causes of glomerular proteinuria include glomerular capillary disruption (hemolytic uremic syndrome, crescentic glomerulonephritis); glomerular capillary immune complex deposition (poststreptococcal glomerulonephritis and lupus nephritis); and altered glomerular capillary permeability (MCNS, congenital NS).

TREATMENT

Because greater than 80% of children less than 13 years of age with primary NS have steroid-responsive forms (chiefly MCNS), steroid therapy may be initiated without a renal biopsy if a child has typical features of NS. Typical therapy for MCNS is prednisone, 2 mg/kg/day (60 mg/m²/24 h, maximum 60 mg/day), provided once a day or split into multiple doses. Over 90% of children who respond to steroids do so within 4 weeks. Responders should receive steroids for 12 weeks. A renal biopsy is indicated for nonresponders because steroid resistance decreases the chance that MCNS is the underlying disease. Frequent relapses or steroid resistance may necessitate additional immunosuppressive therapy.

No clearly effective therapy for FSGS has been identified. Approximately 35% respond to steroid therapy; others may respond to immunosuppressive therapy. MPGN and membranous glomerulonephritis may improve with chronic steroid or immunosuppressive therapy but do not reliably remit with standard NS steroid therapy. Aggressive medical therapy of familial congenital NS, with early nephrectomy, dialysis, and transplantation, is the only effective approach to this syndrome.

NS edema is treated by restricting salt intake. Severe edema may require the use of loop diuretics. When these therapies do not alleviate severe edema, cautious parenteral administration of 25% albumin (0.5 to 1.0 g/kg intravenously over 1 to 2 hours) with an intravenous loop diuretic usually results in diuresis. The administered albumin is excreted rapidly, and, thus, salt restriction and diuretics must be continued. Significant pleural effusions may require drainage. Acute HTN is treated with β-blockers or calcium channel blockers. Persistent HTN usually responds to angiotensin-converting enzyme inhibitors.

COMPLICATIONS

An increased incidence of serious infections, particularly **bacteremia** and **peritonitis** (particularly *Streptococcus pneumoniae, Escherichia coli,* or *Klebsiella),* is due to urinary loss of immunoglobulins and complement. Side effects of steroids are most common in steroid-dependent and frequently relapsing patients. Hypovolemia may result from diarrhea or diuretic use. The loss of coagulation factors, antithrombin, and plasminogen may lead to a hypercoagulable state with a risk of

thromboembolism (TE). Warfarin, Lovenox, low-dose aspirin, or dipyridamole may minimize the risk of clots in NS patients with a history of TE or high risk for TE. Hyperlipidemia promotes increased atherosclerotic vascular disease.

PROGNOSIS

Most children with NS eventually go into remission. Nearly 80% of children with MCNS experience NS relapse, defined as heavy proteinuria that persists for 3 or more consecutive days. Transient (up to 3 days) proteinuria may occur with intercurrent infection in children with MCNS and is not considered a relapse. Steroid therapy is typically effective for true relapse. Steroid-responsive patients have little risk of chronic renal failure. Patients with FSGS may initially respond to steroids but later develop resistance. Many children with FSGS progress to end-stage kidney failure (see Chapter 165). Recurrence of FSGS occurs in 30% of children who undergo renal transplantation.

Chapter **163**

GLOMERULONEPHRITIS AND HEMATURIA

ETIOLOGY AND EPIDEMIOLOGY

A child with **gross hematuria** may have a serious disease and requires prompt evaluation. **Microscopic hematuria,** defined as more than 3 to 5 red blood cells (RBCs) per high-power field on freshly voided and centrifuged urine, is often benign. Isolated asymptomatic microscopic hematuria is found in up to 4% of healthy children. In most cases this is a transient finding. Hematuria may originate from glomerular disease, tubulointerstitial processes, and lower urinary tract disorders (Table 163-1).

Immune-mediated inflammation is the mechanism of **glomerulonephritis** (GN). Poststreptococcal glomerulonephritis (PSGN) is the most common form of acute GN, and IgA nephropathy is the most common chronic GN, but many other types of GN can occur. The most common identifiable lower urinary tract causes of hematuria include urinary tract infection (UTI), kidney stones, and hypercalciuria.

CLINICAL MANIFESTATIONS

Decision-Making Algorithms
Available @ StudentConsult.com

Red Urine and Hematuria
Proteinuria
Edema
Hypertension

Table 163-1	Differential Diagnosis of Red Urine/ Hematuria

FACTITIOUS HEMATURIA

Nonpathologic (urate crystals in infants, ingested foods, medications, dyes)
Pathologic (hemoglobinuria from hemolytic anemia, myoglobinuria from rhabdomyolysis)

GLOMERULAR

Immunologic injury (GN—e.g., PSGN, IgA nephropathy, MPGN, systemic diseases)
Structural disorder (Alport syndrome, thin basement membrane disease)
Toxin-mediated injury (HUS)

TUBULOINTERSTITIAL/PARENCHYMAL

Inflammation (interstitial nephritis, pyelonephritis)
Vascular (sickle cell trait/disease, Nutcracker syndrome)
Structural (cyst rupture, Wilms tumor, urinary tract obstruction, renal trauma)

LOWER URINARY TRACT

Inflammation (cystitis, hemorrhagic cystitis, urethritis)
Injury (trauma, kidney stone)
Hypercalciuria

GN, Glomerulonephritis; HUS, hemolytic uremic syndrome; MPGN, membranoproliferative glomerulonephritis; PSGN, poststreptococcal glomerulonephritis.

Children with **acute GN** commonly present with hematuria (gross or microscopic) along with other cardinal features of glomerular injury (proteinuria, hypertension, edema, oliguria, renal insufficiency). **PSGN** occurs most frequently in children 2 to 12 years of age and is more common in boys. Manifestations of PSGN are typical of acute GN listed previously and develop 5 to 21 days (average 10 days) after streptococcal pharyngitis infections and 4 to 6 weeks after impetigo. **Acute postinfectious GN** presents in the same manner as PSGN and can occur following infections with other bacterial and viral pathogens. PSGN can develop regardless of whether the child was treated with antibiotics at the time of infection. Special attention must be paid to the blood pressure because hypertension may be severe enough to lead to complications such as heart failure, seizures, and encephalopathy.

The presentation of **IgA nephropathy** is more variable and may take the form of acute GN, asymptomatic microscopic hematuria, or recurrent gross hematuria concurrent with an upper respiratory infection as opposed to several days later, as with PSGN. Children with hematuria secondary to systemic disorders such as Henoch-Schönlein purpura nephritis, lupus nephritis, and vasculitis-associated GN will present with other systemic features typical of the respective disease.

A special form of GN is **rapidly progressive glomerulonephritis (RPGN)** that presents with typical features of acute GN, but the renal insufficiency progresses more quickly and severely. Renal biopsy shows glomerular epithelial cell proliferation with crescents. RPGN may be idiopathic or secondary to any of the known types of GN. Early recognition of RPGN is crucial to prevent the progression to end-stage renal disease (ESRD) that occurs without prompt treatment.

Alport syndrome is typically caused by X-chromosome mutations in type IV collagen leading to an abnormal glomerular basement membrane (GBM) and may present with either asymptomatic microscopic or gross hematuria. Males typically

Figure 163-1 Suggested algorithm for evaluation of red urine/hematuria. *GN*, Glomerulonephritis; *H&P*, history and physical; *Hgb*, hemoglobin; *RBCs*, red blood cells; *UTI*, urinary tract infection.

develop progressive renal failure and sensorineural hearing loss during adolescence and young adulthood. Females typically have a more benign course but usually have at least microscopic hematuria. **Thin basement membrane disease** (benign familial hematuria) is caused by more benign mutations leading to a thinning of the GBM. The mutation is often autosomal dominant, and therefore hematuria is often noted in first-degree relatives. As opposed to Alport syndrome, thin basement membrane disease is typically not progressive and usually has an excellent prognosis.

The presentation of nonglomerular causes of hematuria is more variable and related to the underlying etiology. Hematuria due to tubular disorders is usually only microscopic and may be associated with proteinuria, glycosuria, and polyuria. These children typically do not have hypertension and only develop renal insufficiency with more severe disease. Painless gross hematuria may be seen with sickle cell trait/disease, Wilms tumor, and strenuous exercise. Hematuria may or may not be associated with pain when due to cystic bleeding and Nutcracker syndrome. Gross hematuria following trauma may signify more severe renal or lower urinary tract injury. **UTI** is associated with typical symptoms such as dysuria and urinary frequency. **Urolithiasis** may be associated with asymptomatic hematuria or with flank or abdominal pain. **Hypercalciuria** can cause both gross and microscopic hematuria and may be associated with urinary tract symptoms such as dysuria and urinary frequency or may be asymptomatic.

DIAGNOSTIC STUDIES

All patients with hematuria should have a careful history and physical (including blood pressure) along with a

urinalysis, including microscopic examination to identify RBCs. Glomerular hematuria is suggested by a brownish (tea- or cola-colored) appearance of the urine and the presence of RBC casts and/or dysmorphic RBCs on urine microscopy. A urine color that is more bright red in appearance without RBC casts or dysmorphic RBCs is more suggestive of a lower urinary tract source. However there may be overlap of these findings.

A suggested algorithm for the evaluation of hematuria is given in Figure 163-1. Gross hematuria and microscopic hematuria with associated concerning findings should have additional laboratory evaluation. The presence of low C3 complement narrows the differential diagnosis to PSGN, membranoproliferative GN, and lupus nephritis. Children with isolated asymptomatic microscopic hematuria may be observed with repeat urinalyses. If the hematuria is persistent, additional evaluation may be appropriate.

THERAPY

Therapy for PSGN is supportive and involves dietary sodium restriction, diuretics, and antihypertensive agents as needed. Although treating the streptococcal infection does not prevent PSGN, antibiotic treatment is still warranted with active streptococcal infection. Therapies for children with other forms of GN depend on the underlying cause and severity. In some cases, anti-inflammatory therapy involving corticosteroids and/or other immunosuppressive agents may be used. Treatment with angiotensin-converting enzyme inhibitors may reduce proteinuria and glomerular hyperperfusion but should be used with caution in the setting of acute kidney injury.

PROGNOSIS AND PREVENTION

PSGN usually has a benign outcome. In typical cases, the gross hematuria, proteinuria, and edema decline quickly (in 5 to 10 days). Microscopic hematuria may persist for months or even years; over 95% of children recover completely with no long-term sequelae.

Children with IgA nephropathy and other forms of chronic GN have a greater risk of progression to ESRD. The prognosis for renal recovery in chronic GN and in RPGN is variable and related to the underlying disorder and disease severity. The presence of persistent, heavy proteinuria, hypertension, decreased kidney function, and severe glomerular lesions on biopsy is associated with poor outcomes.

Children with idiopathic isolated asymptomatic microscopic hematuria or suspected thin basement membrane disease typically have an excellent renal prognosis. Long-term follow-up, including yearly urinalysis (to rule out proteinuria) and blood pressure, is required to exclude progressive forms of renal disease.

Chapter **164**

HEMOLYTIC UREMIC SYNDROME

ETIOLOGY AND EPIDEMIOLOGY

Hemolytic uremic syndrome (HUS) is characterized by the triad of **microangiopathic hemolytic anemia, thrombocytopenia,** and **renal injury** and is an important cause of acute kidney injury in children. HUS typically occurs in children less than 5 years of age but can occur in older children. The most common type of HUS is associated with a prodromal diarrheal illness (**D+HUS**). Contamination of meat, fruit, vegetables, or water with verotoxin (VT)-producing *Escherichia coli* (most commonly *E. coli* **O157:H7**) is responsible for many outbreaks. VT may be produced by other *E. coli* strains as well as other bacteria such as *Shigella*. VT causes hemorrhagic enterocolitis of variable severity and results in HUS in 5% to 15% of affected children.

HUS presenting without a prodrome of diarrhea (**atypical HUS**) may occur at any age. The clinical course is usually more severe than that of D+HUS. Atypical HUS can be secondary to infection (*Streptococcus pneumonia*, human immunodeficiency virus), genetic and acquired defects in complement regulation, medications, malignancy, systemic lupus erythematosus, and pregnancy.

CLINICAL MANIFESTATIONS

Decision-Making Algorithms
Available @ StudentConsult.com

Diarrhea
Petechiae/Purpura

Classic D+HUS begins with enterocolitis, often with bloody stools, followed in 7 to 10 days by weakness, lethargy, and

Table 164-1	Common Laboratory Findings with Hemolytic Uremic Syndrome

EVIDENCE OF MICROANGIOPATHIC HEMOLYTIC ANEMIA

Anemia
Thrombocytopenia
Presence of schistocytes, helmet cells, and burr cells on peripheral blood smear
Increased LDH
Decreased haptoglobin
Increased indirect bilirubin
Increased AST
Elevated reticulocyte count

EVIDENCE OF RENAL INJURY

Elevated creatinine
Presence of hematuria, proteinuria, pyuria, casts on urinalysis

OTHER POTENTIAL FINDINGS

Leukocytosis
Positive stool culture for *E. coli* O157:H7
Positive stool test for shiga-toxin
Elevated amylase/lipase

AST, Aspartate aminotransferase; *LDH*, lactate dehydrogenase.

oliguria/anuria. Physical examination reveals irritability, pallor, and petechiae. Dehydration is often present; however some children have volume overload. Hypertension may be due to volume overload and/or renal injury. Central nervous system (CNS) involvement, including seizures, occurs in up to 25% of cases. Other potential organ involvement includes pancreatitis, cardiac dysfunction, and colonic perforation.

Children without evidence of a diarrheal prodrome may have a similar microangiopathic syndrome, identified as **thrombotic thrombocytopenic purpura** (TTP). Children with TTP typically have predominant CNS symptoms but may also have significant renal disease. Recurrent episodes are common. Because CNS involvement is also seen in HUS, TTP can be difficult to distinguish from HUS in some cases. Deficiencies of ADAMTS13, a von Willebrand factor-cleaving protease, have been identified in children affected with TTP.

DIAGNOSTIC STUDIES

Common laboratory findings in HUS are listed in Table 164-1. Peripheral blood smear reveals evidence of microangiopathic hemolysis. Coombs test is negative. The diarrhea and presence of toxin-producing *E. coli* may have resolved by the time HUS is diagnosed.

TREATMENT AND PROGNOSIS

Therapy for HUS is supportive and includes volume repletion, control of hypertension, and managing complications of renal insufficiency, including dialysis when indicated. Red blood cell transfusions are provided as needed. Platelet transfusions should be avoided because they may add to the thrombotic microangiopathy and are indicated only by active hemorrhage or in anticipation of a procedure. Antibiotics and antidiarrheal agents may increase the risk of developing HUS. Early hydration during the diarrheal phase may lessen the severity of renal insufficiency. Most children (>95%) with D+HUS survive the acute phase and recover normal renal function, although some may have evidence of long-term morbidity.

ACUTE AND CHRONIC RENAL FAILURE

ACUTE KIDNEY INJURY
Etiology

Acute kidney injury (AKI), formerly termed *acute renal failure,* refers to an abrupt decrease in glomerular filtration rate (GFR) and tubular function. This may lead to decreased excretion of waste products (e.g., urea) and a disturbance in fluid and electrolyte homeostasis. Early recognition and management of AKI are crucial.

AKI may be **oliguric** (<1 mL/kg/h in neonates and infants, <0.5 mL/kg/h in children) or **nonoliguric**, which is more difficult to recognize. Although urine output in nonoliguric AKI is normal or polyuric, electrolyte disturbances and uremia may become significant. The major causes of AKI may be divided into **prerenal** (renal hypoperfusion), **intrinsic renal** (tubular, glomerular, or vascular injury), and **postrenal** (urinary tract obstruction) categories (Table 165-1). In many cases the cause of AKI is multifactorial.

Prerenal azotemia is most commonly due to **dehydration** but may be secondary to other mechanisms of glomerular hypoperfusion. Tubular injury encompasses the most common causes of intrinsic AKI in children. Tubular injury may occur from hypoxia-ischemia (**acute tubular necrosis**), infection (**sepsis**), **nephrotoxic agents** (medications, contrast, myoglobin) and inflammation (**interstitial nephritis**). Postrenal AKI may be due to either structural or functional **urinary tract obstruction**.

Clinical Manifestations

Decision-Making Algorithm
Available @ StudentConsult.com

Hypertension

History, physical examination, and basic studies usually allow proper classification of the child with AKI (Table 165-2). Prerenal azotemia is characterized by precipitating factors and oliguria. Intrinsic tubular injury is associated with precipitating factors but urine output may be low, normal, or high, depending on the severity of the injury. Glomerular and vascular disorders may present with hematuria, edema, hypertension, and oliguria. The urine output with postrenal AKI may be low or normal and may be associated with flank masses or a distended bladder on examination. Depending on the underlying cause and severity of illness, AKI can be associated with signs of dehydration or volume overload.

Diagnostic Studies

A **urinalysis** (UA) should be obtained in all children with AKI. In prerenal azotemia, the UA is unremarkable with a high specific gravity reflecting appropriate renal retention of water in the setting of renal hypoperfusion. However neonates are not able

Table 165-1	Causes of Acute Kidney Injury
PRERENAL	
Dehydration	
Hemorrhage	
Septic shock	
Burns	
Heart failure	
Cirrhosis	
POSTRENAL (OBSTRUCTION)	
Urethral obstruction (stricture, posterior urethral valves)	
Ureteral obstruction	
Ureterocele	
Extrinsic tumor compressing bladder outlet	
Neurogenic bladder (myelomeningocele, spinal cord injury)	
INTRINSIC	
Acute tubular necrosis	
Nephrotoxins (medications, contrast, myoglobin)	
Infection (sepsis)	
Interstitial nephritis	
Glomerular injury (primary glomerulonephritis, vasculitis, hemolytic uremic syndrome)	
Vascular (renal vein thrombosis, arterial emboli, malignant hypertension)	

to concentrate urine as well. With intrinsic tubular injury and postrenal AKI, the UA may show mild hematuria and/or proteinuria with a specific gravity of 1.015 or less. With glomerular and vascular injury, the amount of hematuria and proteinuria is usually moderate to severe. In oliguric states, differentiation between prerenal azotemia and acute tubular necrosis may be aided by determining the urine osmolality and fractional excretion of sodium (see Table 165-2). **Renal ultrasound** is often helpful in determining the AKI category (see Table 165-2). Renal biopsy is indicated in select cases only.

Common electrolyte abnormalities seen with AKI include hyperkalemia, metabolic acidosis, hypocalcemia, and hyperphosphatemia. These labs may need to be monitored frequently, depending on the initial results and clinical course. A complete blood count should be obtained as anemia is frequently observed. Other studies may be obtained as clinically indicated.

Treatment

In some cases the underlying disorder can be treated. Examples include volume repletion in dehydration, stopping an offending nephrotoxic medication, and relieving urinary tract obstruction. In all cases efforts should be made to limit additional renal injury (e.g., ensuring adequate renal perfusion and avoiding nephrotoxic medications). Medication dosages should be adjusted for decreased renal function as appropriate.

Fluid therapy depends on the volume status and urine output. If hypovolemia is present, intravascular volume should be expanded by intravenous administration of saline. If hypervolemia is present, 1 to 2 mg/kg of furosemide and fluid restriction may be attempted. If the patient is relatively euvolemic, then the total fluid input should be adjusted to meet the total

Table 165-2	Laboratory and Clinical Evaluation of Acute Kidney Injury					
	PRERENAL			**RENAL**		**POSTRENAL**
LABORATORY/ CLINICAL FEATURE	**CHILD**	**NEONATE**	**CHILD**	**NEONATE**		
Urine output	Low		Low, normal, or high			Low or normal
Urinalysis	Normal		RBCs, WBCs, protein, casts			Variable
Urine Na⁺ (mEq/L)	<15	<20–30	>40	>50		Variable, may be >40
FE_{Na}* (%)	<1	<2.5	>2	>2.5		Variable, may be >2
Urine osmolality (mOsm/L)	>500	>350	~300	~300		Variable, may be <300
Renal ultrasound	Normal		Increased echogenicity, decreased corticomedullary differentiation			Hydronephrosis

FE_{Na}, Fractional excretion of sodium; RBCs, red blood cells; WBCs, white blood cells.
*FE_{Na} (%) = [(urine sodium/plasma sodium) ÷ (urine creatinine/plasma creatinine)] × 100.

Table 165-3	Indications for Renal Replacement Therapy
ACUTE AND/OR CHRONIC DIALYSIS	
Volume overload Metabolic acidosis Electrolyte abnormalities Uremia	
ACUTE DIALYSIS	
Certain ingestions Hyperammonemia	
CHRONIC DIALYSIS	
Poor growth Stage 5 chronic kidney disease (end-stage renal disease)	

output, which may be higher or lower than normal, depending on the urine output. Assessment of intake and output should be augmented with serial measurements of body weight.

A large part of AKI treatment involves management of its complications. Electrolyte disorders are treated as appropriate. Potassium intake and medications that increase potassium should be restricted. Intravenous calcium will lower risk of arrhythmia while measures are initiated to shift potassium into cells (bicarbonate, beta-agonists, insulin/dextrose) and hasten removal (diuretics, sodium-potassium exchange resins, dialysis). Preferred treatment of hypocalcemia involves oral supplementation and calcitriol, and IV supplementation is reserved for severe cases. Hypertension may be treated with diuretics, calcium channel blockers, and vasodilators. Angiotensin-converting enzyme (ACE) inhibitors are usually avoided in the setting of AKI.

Major indications for **acute dialysis** are listed in Table 165-3. Medical therapy may be attempted before initiating renal replacement therapy. There is no set blood urea nitrogen or creatinine level at which dialysis is started for uremia. Renal replacement options in children include peritoneal dialysis, hemodialysis, and continuous renal replacement therapy. The mode used is chosen on an individual basis.

Prognosis
Recovery from AKI depends on the etiology, severity, availability of specific treatments, and other aspects of the patient's course. Nonoliguric AKI usually recovers well, whereas the outcome with oliguric AKI is more variable. Even with a seemingly good recovery, history of AKI may place the child at increased risk for future renal complications, including chronic kidney disease (CKD).

CHRONIC KIDNEY DISEASE
Etiology and Epidemiology
Congenital anomalies of the kidney and urinary tract (CAKUT) are the most common causes of CKD that present between birth and 10 years of age. After age 10 acquired diseases, such as focal segmental glomerulosclerosis and glomerulonephritis (GN), are more common causes of incident CKD. The risk of progression to end-stage renal disease (ESRD) is related to the underlying cause and severity of CKD. During puberty, renal function may deteriorate if the damaged kidneys are not able to grow and adapt to increased demands. CKD is staged to facilitate appropriate evaluation and monitoring (Table 165-4). The GFR can be estimated in children using the Schwartz formula (see Chapter 161). Most complications of CKD do not manifest until at least stage 3 CKD. In stage 4 CKD, the complications become more numerous and severe. Children with stage 5 CKD (ESRD) are typically treated with either dialysis or renal transplantation.

Clinical Manifestations
The clinical presentation of a child with CKD may be related to both the underlying diagnosis and complications of CKD. A child with CAKUT may have polyuria, polydipsia, and recurrent urinary tract infections. A child with glomerular disease may have hematuria, proteinuria, edema, and hypertension. Common complications of CKD in children are listed in Table 165-5. Most of these complications are multifactorial in etiology. For example, factors associated with **growth failure** include poor nutrition, **renal osteodystrophy (ROD)**, metabolic acidosis, hormonal abnormalities, and resistance to growth hormone. **Anemia** results primarily from a failure to produce adequate **erythropoietin** and iron deficiency. ROD is usually due to **secondary hyperparathyroidism** as a result of diminished 1,25-dihydroxyvitamin D production in the kidney, hypocalcemia, and hyperphosphatemia (from decreased renal excretion). If prolonged and/or severe, ROD may eventually lead to rickets and bone deformities. **Hypertension** and

Table 165-4	Classification of the Stages of Chronic Kidney Disease	
STAGE	**GFR (ml/min/ 1.73 m²)***	**DESCRIPTION**
1	>90	Minimal kidney damage
2	60–89	Kidney damage with mild reduction of GFR
3	30–59	Moderate reduction of GFR
4	15–29	Severe reduction of GFR
5	<15 (or dialysis)	End-stage renal disease

From National Kidney Foundation Kidney Disease Outcomes Quality Initiative.
GFR, Glomerular filtration rate.
*GFR ranges apply for children 2 years of age and older.

Table 165-5	Common Complications and Treatments of CKD
COMPLICATION	**TREATMENT**
1. Poor growth	Increased caloric intake, treat acidosis, treat renal osteodystrophy, recombinant GH
2. Anemia	Erythropoietin, iron supplementation
3. Renal osteodystrophy/ secondary hyperparathyroidism	1,25-Dihydroxyvitamin D supplementation, calcium supplementation, dietary phosphorous restriction, phosphate binders
4. Cardiovascular 4a. Hypertension 4b. Left ventricular hypertrophy	Antihypertensive medications Volume control
5. Electrolyte abnormalities 5a. Hyperkalemia 5b. Hyponatremia 5c. Metabolic acidosis	Low K diet, furosemide, sodium polystyrene sulfonate Sodium supplementation Alkali replacement

CKD, Chronic kidney disease; GH, growth hormone; K, potassium.

left ventricular hypertrophy are commonly seen cardiovascular complications. Delayed puberty results from altered gonadotropin secretion and feedback patterns. Learning and school performance may also be impaired in CKD.

Treatment

The management of children with advanced CKD requires a multidisciplinary team of pediatric practitioners. Adequate nutrition should be provided even if this requires dietary supplements and tube feedings. In infants a low-solute formula may be indicated. Unless a child is oliguric, fluid restriction is not necessary. Many children with CAKUT require supplemental salt due to urine sodium wasting. Conversely children with GN tend to retain sodium and may become hypertensive or edematous if given excess salt. Common treatment considerations for other CKD complications are given in Table 165-5.

Measures can be taken to preserve kidney function or slow down the progression of CKD. Hypertension and proteinuria can be treated with ACE inhibitors or angiotensin receptor blockers. Potentially nephrotoxic medications should be avoided when feasible, and medication adjustment for reduced kidney function should be made as appropriate. Protein intake is typically not restricted in pediatric CKD.

The optimal treatment of ESRD is **renal transplantation.** Both deceased and living donors can be used for renal transplantation, but living donors are preferred when available. **Maintenance dialysis** is effective for a child awaiting renal transplantation or for whom renal transplantation is not possible. Indications for chronic dialysis are given in Table 165-3. **Peritoneal dialysis** is done at home by the family. **Hemodialysis** is typically done three times a week at a dialysis facility.

Prognosis

Children with mild CKD (stages 1 and 2) may do well but need to be monitored for progressive loss of kidney function. Children with stages 3 and 4 CKD have a high likelihood of progressing to ESRD at some point, although the timing can vary. Children with kidney transplants generally do well but have to take immunosuppressive medications associated with a variety of side effects, including infections, nephrotoxicity, cardiovascular complications, and increased risk for certain malignancies. Unfortunately most transplanted kidneys fail over time but can last for several years. Children on maintenance dialysis have the highest morbidity and mortality, especially with longer time spent on dialysis. Thus, their primary goal is to receive a kidney transplant.

Chapter **166**

HYPERTENSION

DEFINITION

In children, hypertension (HTN) is defined as blood pressure (BP) greater than the 95th percentile for age, gender, and height on at least three different occasions. The context of the BP measurement (e.g., cuff size, pain, anxiety) is important. The staging of HTN is given in Table 166-1. Hypertensive emergency is defined as severe elevation in BP associated with target organ damage (encephalopathy, heart failure).

ETIOLOGY

Pediatric HTN has many causes (Table 166-2) that are either **primary** (essential) *or* **secondary. Essential HTN** is the most common cause of HTN in adolescents. Obese children are more likely to develop essential HTN. Secondary HTN should be suspected with younger age and more severely elevated BP. **Renal disease** is the most common cause of secondary HTN in children.

CLINICAL MANIFESTATIONS

Decision-Making Algorithms
Available @ StudentConsult.com

Red Urine and Hematuria
Hypertension
Headaches
Obesity
Alkalemia

Table 166-1	Classification of Blood Pressure
BLOOD PRESSURE CATEGORY	**BLOOD PRESSURE PERCENTILE (%)**
Normal	<90th
Prehypertension	*90th to 95th
Stage 1 hypertension	95th to (99th + 5 mm Hg)
Stage 2 hypertension	>99th + 5 mm Hg

*If 90th % is >120/80, use 120/80 as the lower limit.

Table 166-2	Causes of Hypertension
PRIMARY HYPERTENSION	
Essential hypertension	
Metabolic syndrome	
RENAL CAUSES	
Congenital anomalies (renal dysplasia, obstructive uropathy)	
Structural disorders (Wilms tumor, polycystic kidney disease)	
Glomerulonephritis	
Acquired injury (renal scarring, acute tubular necrosis)	
ENDOCRINE CAUSES	
Catecholamine-secreting tumors (pheochromocytoma, neuroblastoma)	
Hypercortisolism (Cushing syndrome)	
Hyperaldosteronism	
Hyperthyroidism	
NEUROLOGIC CAUSES	
Increased sympathetic activity (stress, anxiety, pain)	
Dysautonomia	
Increased intracranial pressure	
VASCULAR CAUSES	
Coarctation of the aorta	
Renal artery embolism (from umbilical artery catheter)	
Renal vein thrombosis	
Renal artery stenosis	
Vasculitis	
OTHER CAUSES	
Obstructive sleep apnea	
Medications, illicit drugs	

Most children with HTN have no symptoms. Signs and symptoms associated with severe HTN include encephalopathy (headache, vomiting, seizures), heart failure, stroke, and retinopathy (blurred vision, flame hemorrhage, and cotton wool spots on retinal exam). Neonatal history (low birth weight or use of umbilical artery catheter); family history of HTN, stroke, or heart disease; and dietary history (excessive salt or caffeine, drugs) are important. Additional findings that may suggest specific causes include abdominal bruit; diminished leg pressure and weak femoral pulse (coarctation of aorta); cafe-au-lait spots (neurofibromatosis associated renal artery stenosis); flank mass (hydronephrosis, Wilms tumor); tachycardia with flushing and diaphoresis (pheochromocytoma); and truncal obesity, acne, striae, and buffalo hump (Cushing syndrome). Signs of underlying kidney disease may be present.

DIAGNOSTIC STUDIES

In addition to history and physical examination, the evaluation of children with confirmed HTN includes the following:
1. Baseline etiologic assessment (urinalysis, electrolytes, blood urea nitrogen, creatinine, and renal ultrasound)
2. Focused studies based on clinical suspicion (e.g., plasma metanephrines, thyroid studies, vascular imaging)
3. Assessment for target organ damage (echocardiogram for left ventricular hypertrophy)
4. Assessment of other cardiovascular risk factors (lipids, fasting glucose, uric acid)

TREATMENT

Therapeutic lifestyle changes (diet, exercise) should be initiated for asymptomatic stage 1 HTN without target organ damage or systemic disease. Medication should be started for stage 2 or symptomatic HTN and stage 1 HTN, which fails to respond to lifestyle changes. Calcium channel blockers or angiotensin-converting enzyme inhibitors are the most frequently chosen first-line options in children. Angiotensin receptor blockers, β-blockers, or diuretics are also recommended as first-line antihypertensive agents. More than one agent may be needed. Hypertensive emergency requires prompt hospitalization and may require parenteral antihypertensive treatment with nicardipine, labetalol, esmolol, or sodium nitroprusside.

PROGNOSIS

Prognosis depends on the underlying etiology and BP control. Essential HTN, when present in adolescents, is usually not associated with morbidity at presentation. Left untreated, however, even asymptomatic stage 1 HTN may increase risk for cardiovascular, central nervous system, and renal morbidity in adults.

Chapter **167**

VESICOURETERAL REFLUX

ETIOLOGY AND EPIDEMIOLOGY

Vesicoureteral reflux (VUR) is the retrograde flow of urine from the bladder up to the ureter or even up to the kidney. Most VUR results from congenital incompetence of the ureterovesical (UV) junction, a structure that matures through early childhood. In a significant minority of children, structural UV abnormalities exist that never resolve. VUR may be familial; 30% to 40% of siblings of a child with VUR also have VUR. VUR may also be secondary to distal bladder obstruction or other urinary tract anomalies.

VUR exposes the kidney to increased hydrodynamic pressure during voiding and increases the likelihood of renal infection due to incomplete emptying of the ureter and bladder (see Chapter 114). **Reflux nephropathy** refers to development and progression of renal scarring. This is a particular risk if VUR is associated with a urinary tract infection (UTI) or obstruction. Although a single UTI may result in renal scarring, the incidence is higher in children with recurrent UTIs. Renal dysplasia is associated with congenital VUR. Because of increasing use of maternal-fetal ultrasonography, a number of newborns are now identified with VUR before UTI has occurred, creating opportunities for early intervention and prevention strategies. **Duplication of the ureters,** with or without an associated ureterocele, may obstruct the upper collecting system. Often the ureter draining the lower pole of a duplicated renal unit has VUR. **Neurogenic bladder** is accompanied by VUR in up to 50% of affected children. VUR may also be due to increased intravesicular pressure when the bladder outlet is obstructed from inflammation of the bladder (cystitis) or by acquired bladder obstruction.

CLINICAL MANIFESTATIONS

VUR is most often identified during radiologic evaluation following a UTI (see Chapter 114). The younger the patient with UTI, the more likely VUR is present. No clinical signs reliably differentiate children with UTI with and without VUR.

DIAGNOSTIC STUDIES

An imaging study can be performed after initiation of UTI treatment with no need to wait days or weeks before performing the test. **Renal ultrasound** (RUS) is the best study to evaluate the urinary tract in children. A **voiding cystourethrogram** (VCUG) or **radionuclide cystogram** (NCG) is performed to detect urethral/bladder abnormalities and/or VUR. Recent American Academy of Pediatrics guidelines for infants with a first UTI between 2 and 24 months of age recommend a VCUG if an RUS reveals hydronephrosis, scarring, or other findings suggestive of either high grade VUR or obstructive uropathy and in other atypical or complex clinical circumstances. VCUG should also be performed if there is a recurrence of a febrile UTI. Although the VCUG provides additional anatomic detail, the NCG may detect more children with mild VUR and involves less radiation. An international grading system has been used to describe reflux (Fig. 167-1). The incidence of renal scarring in patients with low-grade VUR is low (15%) and increases with grade IV or V reflux (65%). Grade I or II VUR is likely to resolve without surgical intervention, but VUR resolves in less than 50% grade IV or V. **Nuclear renal scanning** best identifies renal scars.

TREATMENT

Controversy remains about whether long-term prophylactic antibiotic therapy (trimethoprim-sulfamethoxazole or nitrofurantoin) is indicated in mild to moderate VUR. It is optional in this population and may be particularly useful in children with high-grade VUR and/or recurrent symptomatic

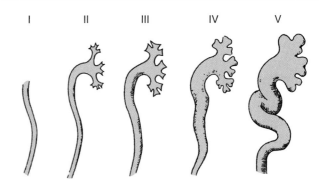

Figure 167-1 International classification of vesicoureteral reflux. Grade I: into a nondilated ureter; grade II: into the pelvis and calyces without dilation; grade III: mild to moderate dilation of the ureter, renal pelvis, and calyces with minimal blunting of the fornices; grade IV: moderate ureteral tortuosity and dilation of the pelvis and calyces; grade V: gross dilation of the ureter, pelvis, and calyces; loss of papillary impressions; and ureteral tortuosity. *(From Wein A, Kavoussi L, Novick A, et al: Campbell-Walsh Urology, ed 9, Philadelphia, 2007, Saunders.)*

UTI. Pivotal studies are under way. **Complications** of reflux nephropathy are hypertension and chronic kidney disease (CKD). CKD is typically heralded by mild proteinuria and involves the development of focal and segmental glomerulosclerosis as well as interstitial scarring. Indications for surgical repair of VUR are controversial and have been made more complex by the development of dextranomer/hyaluronic acid copolymer (Deflux procedure), which appears to be a very successful minimally invasive correction of mild to moderate VUR.

Chapter **168**

CONGENITAL AND DEVELOPMENTAL ABNORMALITIES OF THE URINARY TRACT

ETIOLOGY AND EPIDEMIOLOGY

Anomalies of the urinary tract (UT) occur in up to 4% of infants. **Bilateral renal agenesis** occurs in 1 in 4000 births. Renal agenesis is a component of **Potter syndrome** (flat facies, clubfoot, and pulmonary hypoplasia). Any intrauterine UT disorder that results in little fetal urine and, therefore, little amniotic fluid can lead to Potter syndrome. **Unilateral renal agenesis** occurs in 1 in 3000 births and is more common in infants of diabetic mothers and African Americans. It is accompanied by normal or minimally reduced renal function. This condition can also be found with vesicoureteral reflux (VUR) and other anomalies of the genital tract, ear, skeletal system, and cardiovascular system. Unilateral renal agenesis can be a component of the Turner syndrome, Poland syndrome, or VACTERL association (vertebral abnormalities, anal atresia, cardiac abnormalities, tracheoesophageal fistula, renal agenesis and dysplasia, and limb defects).

Renal hypoplasia/dysplasia refers to kidneys that are congenitally small, malformed, or both. Over time many affected children progress to chronic kidney disease (CKD) because of reduced nephron number. The kidneys are often unable to fully reabsorb sodium and water, and these children require salt and water supplementation to optimize growth.

Multicystic renal dysplasia (MCD) is due to abnormal nephron development that occurs in 1 in 4000 births. There is minimal or no functioning renal tissue in the affected kidney; bilateral disease is lethal. There is an association with VUR in the contralateral kidney. MCD often spontaneously involutes over the first few years of life and is rarely associated with hypertension (HTN) or recurrent urinary tract infection (UTI).

Polycystic kidney diseases (PKDs) are a group of genetic diseases affecting the kidneys and other tissues. PKD may be primary (autosomal recessive or autosomal dominant) or associated with other syndromes. Autosomal recessive PKD occurs in 1 in 10,000 to 40,000 children and is due to genetic defects in fibrocystin. Autosomal dominant PKD, due to defects in polycystin 1 or 2, occurs in 1 in 1000 individuals, making it the most common inherited kidney disease. Although there is some overlap clinically, the two conditions differ morphologically. Both may appear in infancy or in older children. Renal cysts also are observed in other inherited disorders, such as von Hippel–Lindau syndrome, tuberous sclerosis, and Bardet-Biedl syndrome.

Urinary tract obstruction can occur at any anatomic level of the genitourinary system (Table 168-1). Early in gestation, severe obstruction results in renal dysplasia. Ureteral obstruction later in fetal life or after birth results in dilation of the ureter and collecting system, often with subsequent renal parenchymal alterations. An obstructed UT is susceptible to infections, which may worsen renal injury. **Posterior urethral valves** are the most common cause of **bladder outlet obstruction** in males, present in 1 in 50,000 boys. Parents may note a poor urine stream in affected children. The valves are sail-shaped membranes that arise from the verumontanum and attach to the urethral wall. The prostatic urethra becomes dilated, VUR may be present, and hypertrophied detrusor muscle develops. Renal dilation varies in severity. Some degree of renal dysplasia is often present. Severe obstruction may be associated with oligohydramnios, resulting in lethal pulmonary hypoplasia. Intrauterine rupture of the renal pelvis produces **urinary ascites,** which is the most common cause of ascites in the newborn period.

CLINICAL MANIFESTATIONS

Decision-Making Algorithms
Available @ StudentConsult.com

Red Urine and Hematuria
Hyponatremia

Bilateral renal agenesis results in insufficient lung development and Potter syndrome. Respiratory distress is severe, pneumothoraces can occur, and severe pulmonary hypoplasia is fatal. Unilateral renal agenesis may be asymptomatic because the nonaffected kidney undergoes compensatory growth and provides normal renal function.

Autosomal recessive PKD is characterized by marked bilateral renal enlargement. Interstitial fibrosis and tubular atrophy progress over time. Kidney failure usually occurs in early childhood. **Hepatic fibrosis** is present and may lead to portal HTN. Bile duct ectasia and biliary dysgenesis occur. Many affected infants display flank masses, hepatomegaly, pneumothorax, proteinuria, and/or hematuria.

Autosomal dominant PKD typically presents in middle adulthood but may present in infancy or childhood. Infants may have a clinical picture similar to autosomal recessive PKD, but older children show a pattern similar to that of adults, with large isolated cysts developing over time. The defect may occur anywhere along the nephron unit. Hepatic cysts are often present, and pancreatic, splenic, and ovarian cysts can also develop. **Cerebral aneurysms** may develop, and the risk of hemorrhage depends on size, blood pressure, and family history of intracranial hemorrhage.

UT obstruction may be silent but usually is discovered during prenatal ultrasound or with UTI or flank mass in early childhood. In a newborn, the most common type of abdominal mass is renal (most commonly **ureteropelvic junction obstruction**).

DIAGNOSTIC IMAGING

Renal ultrasound (RUS) and **radionuclide renography** (usually with a diuretic administered) are the standard tests for diagnosis of UT obstruction. RUS allows identification of renal agenesis, hypoplasia, dysplasia, cysts, and UT dilation. Obstruction may be suggested but a dilated UT may also result from VUR, ureteral hypoplasia, or neurogenic bladder. A voiding cystourethrogram (VCUG) is also a part of the evaluation. Many boys with posterior urethral valves are identified by prenatal ultrasound. Postnatally the

Table 168-1	Site and Etiology of Urinary Tract Obstruction
SITE	**ETIOLOGIC CONDITION/DISORDER**
Infundibula/pelvis	Congenital, calculi, infection, trauma/hemorrhage, tumor
Ureteropelvic junction	Congenital stenosis,* calculi, trauma/hemorrhage
Ureter	Obstructive megaureter,* ectopic ureter, ureterocele, calculi,* inflammatory bowel disease
	Retroperitoneal tumor (lymphoma), retroperitoneal fibrosis, chronic granulomatous disease
Bladder	Neurogenic dysfunction,* tumor (rhabdomyosarcoma), diverticula, ectopic ureter
Urethra	Posterior valves,* diverticula, strictures, atresia, ectopic ureter, foreign body, phimosis,* priapism

*Relatively common.

diagnosis and extent of renal damage are established by RUS and VCUG.

TREATMENT

Infants and children with bilateral dysplasia often require additional sodium and water due to renal wasting. With MCD surgical removal of the kidney is rarely indicated unless severe HTN or recurrent UTI occurs.

Treatment of HTN can prolong maintenance of renal function. General therapy of CKD (see Chapter 165) can improve growth and development.

UT obstruction often requires drainage or surgical correction. Treatment of posterior urethral valve consists of either primary valve ablation or diversion (usually via vesicostomy) if ablation is not possible. Ectopic ureters are frequently obstructed; when this happens, surgical intervention is required.

Children with neurogenic bladder are prone to UTI and renal impairment from poor urine emptying. Clean intermittent catheterization or a urinary diversion is used to help minimize these complications.

Chapter 169

OTHER URINARY TRACT AND GENITAL DISORDERS

URINARY TRACT STONES
Etiology

Urinary tract calculi are called **nephrolithiasis** or **urolithiasis.** Primary bladder stones can be seen with recurrent urinary tract infections (UTIs), neurogenic bladder or bladder surgery (sutures serve as a nidus), and intestinal bladder augmentation. Renal stones can result from obstructive abnormalities or an underlying metabolic predisposition. In industrialized societies, most stones (>90%) in children arise in the urinary tract (UT) and become symptomatic with passage or if lodged (commonly at the ureteropelvic junction or the ureterovesical junction). Metabolic causes include idiopathic familial hypercalciuria (IHC), hyperoxaluria, uric acid disorders, distal renal tubular acidosis, cystinuria, hypercalcemic hypercalciuria, and primary hyperparathyroidism. Some children with UT abnormalities and stones have a concomitant metabolic predisposition.

Clinical Manifestations

Decision-Making Algorithm
Available @ StudentConsult.com

Red Urine and Hematuria

Acute obstruction of urine flow is the cause of renal colic, a severe sharp intermittent pain in the flank or lower abdomen often radiating to the groin. Vomiting, distress, and inability to relieve pain with position changes are characteristic. In younger children, classic symptoms may not be apparent; fussiness and vomiting may be the only symptoms. Hematuria may be gross or microscopic and typically clears rapidly with passage of gravel or stone material.

Diagnostic Studies

Renal ultrasound may identify kidney stones in the kidney but can easily miss UT stones. Computed tomography (CT), particularly a helical CT, can identify stones throughout the UT, but stones can be obscured by oral or intravenous contrast material. Etiologic diagnosis is facilitated when stone material can be obtained and sent for analysis. Spot or 24-hour urine studies for mineral and electrolyte determinations, obtained on a typical diet for the child, are important to characterize any underlying metabolic predisposition and are valuable even when a stone is available for analysis.

Treatment

Acute treatment of urinary calculi consists of hydration and analgesia. Chronic treatment for all types of metabolic stones involves vigorous fluid intake, usually twice maintenance rates. Infection-related stones require treatment of infection and often removal of the stone as well as correction of any predisposing anatomic abnormality. Specific metabolic conditions require specific treatments; for IHC, normal calcium intake with low sodium and low oxalate intake is prescribed. For some children with IHC, potassium citrate or thiazides are required to minimize stone recurrence. Lithotripsy or surgery by a pediatric urologist may be required for children with large, infected, or obstructing stones.

VOIDING DYSFUNCTION
Etiology

Voiding difficulties are frequent in preschool age children due to delay in maturation of bladder and micturition pathways. Normal micturition and continence rely on structural UT integrity, neurologic maturation, and coordination between somatic and autonomic nervous system units, including the central nervous system, spinal cord pathways, nerves innervating the bladder/urinary sphincter, and the autonomic system. Daytime continence is usually achieved before nighttime continence. Most children are dry, day and night, by 4 to 5 years of age. Nocturnal enuresis is the involuntary loss of urine during sleep. Children with primary enuresis have never had a prolonged (usually >3 months) span of nighttime continence. Up to 10% of 5-year-old children have primary enuresis with 15% spontaneous resolution per year. Boys are affected more than girls with increased incidence in families (40% at 6 years of age if one affected parent, 70% if two affected parents). Secondary enuresis involves loss of nighttime control after an extended period of dryness and generally requires evaluation to uncover the cause.

Clinical Manifestations

Dysfunctional voiding (DV) may manifest as incontinence, frequency, urgency, hesitancy, dysuria, lower abdominal pain, or recurrent UTI. Symptoms may vary over time and be associated with obvious neurologic problems (spinal cord injury, encephalitis), constipation, and/or behavioral problems. DV symptoms may vary, depending on recent UTI or changes in family or school life/stressors. The majority of children with DV are anatomically, neurologically, and psychologically normal.

Diagnostic Studies

Evaluation for DV may be performed at any age, but isolated urinary incontinence in an otherwise normal child is not usually evaluated until 5 years of age. A urinalysis and urine culture should be done to exclude occult infection and renal disease. Children with daytime incontinence should undergo renal/bladder ultrasound to exclude structural abnormalities. Urodynamic evaluation is typically reserved for children with a suspicion of neurogenic bladder or known neurologic etiology.

Treatment

For children with recurrent UTI, prophylactic antibiotics may be useful. Timed voiding and anticholinergic medications are used to treat bladder hyperactivity and sensory defects. More complicated treatment regimens include biofeedback, α-blockers, and intermittent catheterization. For children with simple primary enuresis, the bed wetting alarm provides safe and effective resolution of the problem for greater than 70% of affected children; medical therapy with anticholinergics, imipramine, or DDAVP may also be used in selected children.

ANOMALIES OF THE PENIS
Etiology

Hypospadias occurs in approximately 1 in 500 newborn infants. In this condition the urethral folds fail to fuse completely over the urethral groove leaving the urethral meatus located ventrally and proximally to its normal position. The ventral foreskin is also lacking, and the dorsal portion gives the appearance of a hood. Severe hypospadias with undescended testes is a form of ambiguous genitalia. Etiologies include congenital adrenal hyperplasia with masculinization of females or androgen insensitivity. UT anomalies are uncommon in association with hypospadias. Hypospadias may occur alone, but in severe cases can be associated with a **chordee** (a fixed ventral curvature of the penile shaft). Rarely when the urethra opens onto the perineum, the chordee is extreme, and the scrotum is bifid and sometimes extends to the dorsal base of the penis.

In 90% of uncircumcised males, the foreskin should be retractable by adolescence. Before this age, the prepuce may normally be tight and not need treatment. After this age, the inability to retract the prepuce is termed **phimosis.** The condition may be congenital or the result of inflammation. **Paraphimosis** occurs when the prepuce has been retracted behind the coronal sulcus, cannot resume its normal position, and causes swelling of the glans or pain.

Clinical Manifestations and Treatment

The meatal opening in **hypospadias** may be located anteriorly (on the glans, coronal, or distal third of the shaft); on the middle third of the shaft; or posteriorly (near the scrotum). Testes are undescended in 10% of boys with hypospadias. Inguinal hernias are common. Males with hypospadias should not be circumcised, particularly if the meatus is proximal to the glans, because the foreskin may be necessary for later repair. Most pediatric urologists repair hypospadias before the patient is 18 months old.

Phimosis is rarely symptomatic. Parents should be reassured that loosening of the prepuce usually occurs during puberty. Treatment, if needed, is topical steroids. If the narrowing is severe, gentle stretching may be useful. Circumcision is reserved for the most severe cases. **Paraphimosis** with venous stasis and edema leads to severe pain. When paraphimosis is discovered early, reduction of the foreskin may be possible with lubrication. In some cases, emergent circumcision is needed.

DISORDERS AND ABNORMALITIES OF THE SCROTUM AND ITS CONTENTS
Etiology

Undescended testes (cryptorchidism) are found in about 1% of boys after 1 year of age. It is more common in full-term newborns (3.4%) than in older children. In neonates, cryptorchidism is more common with shorter gestation (20% in 2000- to 2500-g infants and 100% in <900-g infants). Cryptorchidism is bilateral in 30% of cases. Spontaneous testicular descent does not tend to occur after 1 year of age, but failure to find one or both testes in the scrotum does not indicate undescended testicles. **Retractile testes,** absent testes, and ectopic testes may resemble cryptorchidism in presentation.

Clinical Manifestations

Decision-Making Algorithms
Available @ StudentConsult.com

Scrotal Pain
Scrotal Swelling (Painless)

A history of maternal drug use (steroids) and family history are important in the evaluation of a child for apparent cryptorchidism. Whether the testis was ever noted in the scrotum should be asked. The true undescended testis is found along the normal embryologic path of descent, usually in the presence of a patent processus vaginalis. An undescended testis is often associated with an inguinal hernia; it is also subject to **torsion.** There is a high incidence of infertility in adulthood. When bilateral and untreated, infertility is uniform. There is an increased malignancy risk (five times the normal rate) with undescended testis, usually presenting between the ages of 20 and 30. The risk is greater in untreated males or those with surgical correction during or after puberty.

Retractile testes are normal testes that retract into the inguinal canal from an exaggerated cremasteric reflex. The diagnosis of retractile testes is likely if testes are palpable in the newborn period but not at later examination. Frequently parents describe seeing their son's testes in his scrotum when he is in the bath and seeing one or both "disappear" when he gets cold.

Complications

Decision-Making Algorithm
Available @ StudentConsult.com

Scrotal Pain

Torsion of the testis is an emergency requiring prompt diagnosis and treatment to save the affected testis. Torsion accounts for 40% of cases of acute scrotal pain and swelling and is the major cause of the acute scrotum in boys less than 6 years of age. It is thought to arise from abnormal fixation of the testis to the scrotum. On examination the testicle is swollen and tender, and the cremasteric reflex is absent. The absence of blood flow on nuclear scan or Doppler ultrasound is consistent with torsion.

The differential diagnosis of testicular pain includes trauma, an incarcerated hernia, and torsion of the testicular epididymal appendix. Torsion of the appendix testis is associated with point tenderness over the lesion and minimal swelling. In adolescents, the differential diagnosis of testicular torsion also must include **epididymitis,** the most common cause of acute scrotal pain and swelling in older adolescents. Diagnosis is aided by an antecedent history of sexual activity or UTI. Testicular torsion must be considered as the principal diagnosis when severe acute testicular pain is present.

Treatment

The undescended testis is usually histologically normal at birth. Atrophy and dysplasia are found after the first year of life. Some boys have congenital dysplasia in the contralateral descended testis. Surgical correction at an early age results in greater chance of adult fertility. Administration of human chorionic gonadotropin causes testosterone release from functioning testes and may result in descent of retractile testes.

Orchidopexy is usually done in the second year of life. Most extra-abdominal testes can be brought into the scrotum with correction of the associated hernia. If the testis is not palpable, ultrasound or magnetic resonance imaging may determine its location. The closer the testis is to the internal inguinal ring, the better the chance of successful orchidopexy.

Surgical correction of testicular torsion is called *detorsion and fixation of the testis.* If performed within 6 hours of torsion, there is greater than a 90% chance of testicular salvage. The contralateral testis usually is fixed to the scrotum to prevent possible torsion. If torsion of the appendix is found, the necrotic tissue is removed.

ACKNOWLEDGMENT
We gratefully acknowledge the invaluable contributions of Rama Jayanthi, MD, Pediatric Urology, Nationwide Children's Hospital, Columbus, Ohio.

Suggested Reading
Brady TM: Hypertension, *Pediatr Rev* 33:541–552, 2012.
Gipson DS, Massengil SF, Yao L, et al: Management of childhood onset nephrotic syndrome, *Pediatrics* 124:747–757, 2009.
Massengill SF: Hematuria, *Pediatr Rev* 29:342–348, 2008.
McKay CP: Renal stone disease, *Pediatr Rev* 31:179–188, 2010.
Schwartz GJ, Munoz A, Schneider MF, et al: New equation to estimate GFR in children with CKD, *J Am Soc Nephrol* 20:629–637, 2009.
Urinary tract infection: clinical practice guideline for the diagnosis and management of the initial UTI in febrile infants and children 2 to 24 months. Subcommittee on Urinary Tract Infection, Steering Committee on Quality Improvement and Management, *Pediatrics* 128:595–610, 2011.
Whyte DA, Fine RN: Acute renal failure in children, *Pediatr Rev* 29:299–307, 2008.
Whyte DA, Fine RN: Chronic kidney disease in children, *Pediatr Rev* 29:335–341, 2008.

Endocrinology

Paola A. Palma Sisto and MaryKathleen Heneghan

Chapter 170

ENDOCRINOLOGY ASSESSMENT

The endocrine system regulates vital body functions by means of hormonal messengers. **Hormones** are defined as circulating messengers, with action at a distance from the organ **(gland)** of origin of the hormone. Hormones can be regulated by nerve cells; endocrine agents can serve as neural messengers. There is also a relationship between the endocrine system and the immune system; autoantibodies may cause an organ to produce an excess or deficiency of a hormone. Manifestations of an endocrine disorder are related to the response of the peripheral tissue to a hormone excess or deficiency.

Hormone action also may be **paracrine** (acting on adjacent neighboring cells to the cell of origin of the hormone) or **autocrine** (acting on the cell of origin of the hormone itself); agents acting in these ways are called *factors* rather than hormones (Fig. 170-1). Hormones generally are regulated in a feedback loop so that the production of a hormone is linked to its effect or its circulating concentration. Endocrine disorders generally manifest from one of four ways:

1. By **excess hormone:** In Cushing syndrome, there is an excess of glucocorticoid present; if the excess is secondary to autonomous glucocorticoid secretion by the adrenal gland, the trophic hormone adrenocorticotropic hormone (ACTH) is suppressed.
2. By **deficient hormone:** In glucocorticoid deficiency, the level of cortisol is inadequate; if the deficiency is at the adrenal gland, the trophic hormone is elevated (ACTH).
3. By an abnormal **response of end organ** to hormone: In pseudohypoparathyroidism, defects in the gene (GNAS1) encoding the alpha subunit of the stimulatory G protein (Gsa) is manifested by elevated PTH levels in the face of deficient PTH function (PTH resistance).
4. By **gland enlargement** that may have effects as a result of size rather than function: With a large nonfunctioning pituitary adenoma, abnormal visual fields and other neurologic signs and symptoms result even though no hormone is produced by the tumor.

Peptide hormones act through specific cell membrane receptors; when the hormone is attached to the receptor, the complex triggers various intracellular second messengers that cause the biologic effects. Peptide hormone receptor number and avidity may be regulated by hormones. **Steroid hormones** exert their effects by attachment to intranuclear receptors, and the hormone-receptor complex translocates to the nucleus, where it binds with DNA, and leads to further gene activation.

The interpretation of serum hormone levels must be related to their controlling factors. For example, a given value of parathyroid hormone may be normal in a eucalcemic patient but inadequate in a hypocalcemic patient with partial hypoparathyroidism or excessive in a hypercalcemic patient with hyperparathyroidism.

HYPOTHALAMIC-PITUITARY AXIS

The **hypothalamus** controls many endocrine systems either directly or through the pituitary gland. Higher central nervous system (CNS) centers control the hypothalamus. Hypothalamic releasing or inhibiting factors travel through capillaries of the pituitary portal system to control the anterior pituitary gland, regulating the hormones specific for the factor (Fig. 170-2). The pituitary hormones enter the peripheral circulation and exert their effects on target glands, which produce other hormones that feed back to suppress their controlling hypothalamic and pituitary hormones. Insulin-like growth factor-1 (IGF-1), growth hormone (GH), cortisol, sex steroids, and thyroxine (T_4) all feed back on the hypothalamic-pituitary system. Prolactin is the only pituitary hormone that is suppressed by a hypothalamic factor, dopamine. The hypothalamus is also the location of vasopressin-secreting axons that either terminate in the posterior pituitary gland and exert their effect via vasopressin secretion

Figure 170-1 Schematic representation of mechanisms of action of hormones and growth factors. Although traditional hormones are formed in endocrine glands and transported to distant sites of action through the bloodstream (endocrine mechanism), peptide growth factors may be produced locally by the target cells themselves (autocrine modality of action) or by neighboring cells (paracrine action). *(From Wilson JD, Foster DW, editors:* Williams Textbook of Endocrinology, *ed 8, Philadelphia, 1992, WB Saunders, p 1007.)*

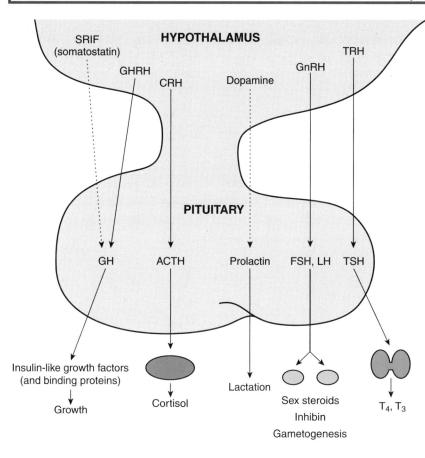

Figure 170-2 Hormonal influences of the hypothalamus and pituitary gland. *Solid line* represents stimulatory influence; *dotted line* represents inhibitory influence. *ACTH,* Adrenocorticotropic hormone; *CRH,* corticotropin-releasing hormone or CRF; *FSH,* follicle-stimulating hormone; *GH,* growth hormone; *GHRH,* GH-releasing hormone or GRF; *GnRH,* gonadotropin-releasing hormone or luteinizing hormone releasing factor, LRF or LHRH; *LH,* luteinizing hormone; *SRIF,* somatotropin release-inhibiting factor, somatostatin or SS; *TRH,* thyrotropin-releasing hormone or TRF; *TSH,* thyroid-stimulating hormone; T_3, triiodothyronine; T_4, thyroxine.

Table 170-1	Diagnostic Evaluation for Hypopituitarism	
MANIFESTATION	**CAUSE**	**TESTS***
Growth failure, hypothyroidism, or both	GH deficiency, TRH/TSH deficiency, or both	Provocative GH tests, free T_4, bone age, IGF-1, IGFBP3
Hypoglycemia	GH deficiency, ACTH insufficiency, or both	Provocative GH tests, test of ACTH secretion, IGF-1, IGFBP3
Micropenis, pubertal delay, or arrest	Hypogonadotropic hypogonadism with or without GH deficiency	Sex steroids (E_2, testosterone), basal LH and FSH (analyzed by ultrasensitive assays) or after GnRH administration, provocative GH tests, IGF-1, IGFBP3
Polyuria, polydipsia	ADH deficiency	Urine analysis (specific gravity), serum electrolytes, urine and serum osmolality, water deprivation test

ADH, Antidiuretic hormone; *CNS,* central nervous system; E_2, estradiol; *FSH,* follicle-stimulating hormone; *GH,* growth hormone; *GnRH,* gonadotropin-releasing hormone; *IGF-1,* insulin-like growth factor; *IGFBP3,* insulin-like growth factor-binding protein 3; *LH,* luteinizing hormone; *MRI,* magnetic resonance imaging; *TRH,* thyrotropin-releasing hormone; *TSH,* thyroid-stimulating hormone; T_4, thyroxine.
*Each patient with hypopituitarism should have CNS MRI as part of evaluation to determine the etiology of the condition.

from this area or terminate in the mediobasal hypothalamus, from which they can exert effects on water balance, even in the absence of the posterior pituitary gland.

The **assessment** of pituitary function may be determined by measuring some of the specific pituitary hormone in the basal state; other assessments require the measurement after stimulation. Indirect assessment of pituitary function can be obtained by measuring serum concentrations of the target gland hormones (Table 170-1). Several tests of pituitary function are listed in Table 170-2.

DISORDERS OF THE HYPOTHALAMIC-PITUITARY AXIS

Decision-Making Algorithms
Available @ StudentConsult.com

Visual Impairment and Leukocoria
Amenorrhea
Pubertal Delay
Polyuria

Table 170-2	Anterior Pituitary Hormone Function Testing	
RANDOM HORMONE MEASUREMENTS	**PROVOCATIVE OR OTHER TESTS**	**TARGET HORMONE MEASUREMENT**
GH (not useful as a random determination except in newborns, and in GH resistance or in pituitary gigantism)	Arginine (a weak stimulus) L-Dopa (useful clinically) Insulin-induced hypoglycemia (a dangerous but accurate test)	IGF-1, IGFBP3 (affected by malnutrition as well as GH excess)
	Clonidine (useful clinically) GHRH	
	12- to 24-h integrated GH levels (of questionable utility)	
ACTH (early AM sample useful only if in high-normal range)	Cortisol after insulin-induced hypoglycemia (a dangerous test but accurate)	8 AM cortisol
		24-h urinary free cortisol
	ACTH stimulation test (may differentiate ACTH deficiency from primary adrenal insufficiency)	
TSH* LH, FSH*	TRH GnRH (difficult to interpret in prepubertal subjects)	FT$_4$ Testosterone/estradiol
Prolactin (elevated in hypothalamic disease and decreased in pituitary disease)	TRH	None

ACTH, Adrenocorticotropic hormone; *CRH*, corticotropin-releasing hormone; *FSH*, follicle-stimulating hormone; *FT$_4$*, free thyroxine; *GH*, growth hormone; *GnRH*, gonadotropin-releasing hormone; *GRH*, growth hormone-releasing hormone; *IGF-1*, insulin-like growth factor-1; *IGF-BP3*, insulin-like growth factor-binding protein 3; *L-dopa*, L-dihydroxyphenylalanine; *LH*, luteinizing hormone; *TRH*, thyrotropin-releasing hormone; *TSH*, thyroid-stimulating hormone.
*New supersensitive assays allow determination of abnormally low values found in hypopituitarism.

Hypothalamic deficiency leads to a decrease in most pituitary hormone secretions but may lead to an increase in prolactin secretion. Destructive lesions of the pituitary gland or hypothalamus are more common in childhood than increased pituitary secretion of various hormones. A **craniopharyngioma**, a tumor of the Rathke pouch, may descend into the sella turcica, causing erosion of the bone and destruction of pituitary and hypothalamic tissue. **Acquired hypopituitarism** also may result from pituitary infections; from infiltration (Langerhans cell histiocytosis [histiocytosis X], lymphoma, and sarcoidosis); after radiation therapy or trauma to the CNS; and as a consequence of autoimmunity against the pituitary gland.

Congenital hypopituitarism can be caused by the absence of hypothalamic releasing factors. Without hypothalamic stimulation, the pituitary gland does not release its hormones. Congenital defects associated with hypopituitarism range from **holoprosencephaly** (cyclopia, cebocephaly, orbital hypotelorism), to cleft palate (6% of cases of cleft palate are associated with GH deficiency). **Septo-optic dysplasia** (optic nerve hypoplasia, absent septum pellucidum, or variations of both) may result in significant visual impairment with pendular ("roving") nystagmus (inability to focus on a target) in addition to varying degrees of hypopituitarism. The magnetic resonance imaging (MRI) findings of congenital hypopituitarism may include an ectopic posterior pituitary gland *bright spot,* the appearance of a *pituitary stalk transection,* and/or small pituitary gland.

Chapter 171

DIABETES MELLITUS

Diabetes mellitus (DM) is characterized by hyperglycemia and glycosuria and is an end point of a few disease processes (Table 171-1). The most common type occurring in childhood is type 1 DM (DM1), which is caused by autoimmune destruction of the insulin-producing beta cells (islets) of the pancreas leading to permanent insulin deficiency. Type 2 DM (DM2) results from insulin resistance and relative insulin deficiency, usually in the context of exogenous obesity. The incidence of DM1 and DM2 in the United States is increasing. Less common types of diabetes result from genetic defects of the insulin receptor or inherited abnormalities in sensing of ambient glucose concentration by pancreatic beta cells (see Table 171-1).

DEFINITION

A **diagnosis** of DM is made based on four glucose abnormalities that may need to be confirmed by repeat testing: (1) Fasting serum glucose concentration ≥126 mg/dL, (2) a random venous plasma glucose ≥200 mg/dL with symptoms of hyperglycemia, (3) an abnormal oral glucose tolerance test (OGTT) with a 2-hour postprandial serum glucose concentration ≥200 mg/dL, and (4) a HgbA1c ≥6.5%.

A patient is considered to have **impaired fasting glucose** if fasting serum glucose concentration is 100 to 125 mg/dL or **impaired glucose tolerance** if 2-hour plasma glucose following an OGTT is 140 to 199 mg/dL. Sporadic hyperglycemia can occur in children, usually in the setting of an intercurrent illness. When the hyperglycemic episode is clearly related to

Table 171-1	Classification of Diabetes Mellitus in Children and Adolescents
TYPE	**COMMENT**
TYPE 1 (INSULIN-DEPENDENT)	
Transient neonatal	Manifests immediately after birth; lasts 1–3 months
Permanent neonatal	Other pancreatic defects possible
Classic type 1	Glycosuria, ketonuria, hyperglycemia, islet cell positive; genetic component
TYPE 2 (NON-INSULIN-DEPENDENT)	
Secondary	Cystic fibrosis, hemochromatosis, drugs (L-asparaginase, tacrolimus)
Adult type (classic)	Associated with obesity, insulin resistance; genetic component
OTHER	
Gestational diabetes	Abnormal glucose tolerance during pregnancy only, which reverts to normal postpartum; increased risk for later onset of diabetes
Maturity-onset diabetes of youth	Autosomal dominant, onset before age of 25 years; not associated with obesity or autoimmunity
Mitochondrial diabetes	Single-gene mutations include hepatocyte nuclear factors 1β,1α, 4α; glucokinase; insulin promoter factor 1 Associated with deafness and other neurologic defects, maternal transmission—mtDNA point mutations

an illness or other physiologic stress, the probability of incipient diabetes is small (<5%).

INSULIN-DEPENDENT (TYPE 1) DIABETES MELLITUS
Etiology

DM1 results from the autoimmune destruction of insulin-producing beta cells (islets) of the pancreas. In addition to the presence of diabetes susceptibility genes, an unknown environmental insult presumably triggers the autoimmune process. A variety of studies has produced conflicting data regarding a host of environmental factors. These include cow's milk feeding at an early age, viral infectious agents (Coxsackie virus, cytomegalovirus, mumps, rubella), vitamin D deficiency, and perinatal factors. DM1 is thought to be primarily a T cell–mediated disease.

Antibodies to islet cell antigens may be seen months to years before the onset of beta cell dysfunction (Fig. 171-1). These include islet cell antibodies, insulin autoantibodies, antibodies to tyrosine phosphatase IA-2, antibodies to glutamic acid decarboxylase, and others. The risk for diabetes increases with the number of antibodies detected in the serum. In individuals with one detectable antibody only, the risk is only 10% to 15%; in individuals with three or more antibodies, the risk is 55% to 90%. When 80% to 90% of the beta cell mass have been destroyed, the remaining beta cell mass is insufficient to maintain euglycemia and clinical manifestations of diabetes result (see Fig. 171-1).

Epidemiology

The annual incidence of DM1 is increasing steadily but with significant geographic differences. In the United States, the annual incidence is approximately 20 in 100,000. The annual incidence in children ranges from a high of 40 in 100,000 among Scandinavian populations to less than 1 in 100,000 in China. The prevalence of DM1 in the United States is highest in non-Hispanic whites followed by African Americans, Hispanic, and American Indians.

Genetic determinants play a role in the susceptibility to DM1, although the mode of inheritance is complex and multigenic. Siblings or offspring of patients with diabetes have a risk of 2% to 8% for the development of diabetes; an identical twin has a 30% to 50% risk. The human leukocyte antigen (HLA) region on chromosome 6 provides the strongest determinant of susceptibility, accounting for approximately 40% of familial inheritance of DM1. Specific class II DR and DQ HLA alleles (HLA DR3 and HLA DR4) increase the risk of developing DM1, whereas other specific HLA alleles exert a protective effect. More than 90% of children with DM1 possess HLA DR3 alleles, HLA DR4 alleles, or both. The insulin gene region variable number tandem repeat on chromosome 11 is also linked to DM1 susceptibility. There is evidence for association, beyond HLA, of more than 100 other loci with DM1. Genetic factors do not fully account for susceptibility to DM1; environmental factors also play a role.

Clinical Manifestations

Decision-Making Algorithms
Available @ StudentConsult.com

Polyuria
Failure to Thrive

Hyperglycemia results when insulin secretory capacity becomes inadequate to enhance peripheral glucose uptake and to suppress hepatic and renal glucose production. Insulin deficiency usually first causes postprandial hyperglycemia and then fasting hyperglycemia. Ketogenesis is a sign of more complete insulin deficiency. Lack of suppression of gluconeogenesis and glycogenolysis further exacerbates hyperglycemia while fatty acid oxidation generates the ketone bodies: β-hydroxybutyrate, acetoacetate, and acetone. Protein stores in muscle and fat stores in adipose tissue are metabolized to provide substrates for gluconeogenesis and fatty acid oxidation.

Glycosuria occurs when the serum glucose concentration exceeds the renal threshold for glucose reabsorption (from 160 to 190 mg/dL). Glycosuria causes an osmotic diuresis (including obligate loss of sodium, potassium, and other electrolytes), leading to dehydration. Polydipsia occurs as the patient attempts to compensate for the excess fluid losses. Weight loss results from the persistent catabolic state and the loss of calories through glycosuria and ketonuria. The classic presentation of DM1 includes polyuria, polydipsia, polyphagia, and weight loss.

DIABETIC KETOACIDOSIS

If the clinical features of new-onset DM1 are not detected, **diabetic ketoacidosis (DKA)** will occur. DKA may also occur in patients with known DM1 if insulin injections are omitted

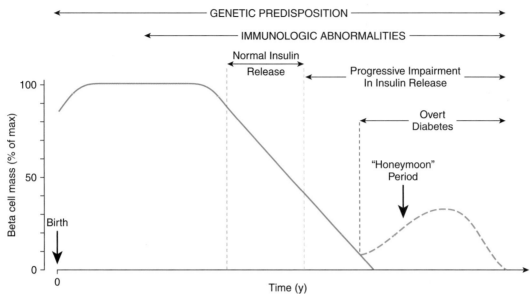

Figure 171-1 Schematic representation of the autoimmune evolution of diabetes in genetically predisposed individuals.

or during an intercurrent illness when greater insulin requirements are unmet in the presence of elevated concentrations of the counter-regulatory and stress hormones (glucagon, growth hormone [GH], cortisol, and catecholamines). DKA can be considered to be present if (1) the arterial pH is below 7.3, (2) the serum bicarbonate level is below 15 mEq/L, and (3) ketones are elevated in serum or urine.

Pathophysiology

In the absence of adequate insulin secretion, persistent partial hepatic oxidation of fatty acids to ketone bodies occurs. Two of these three ketone bodies are organic acids and lead to metabolic acidosis with an elevated anion gap. Lactic acid may contribute to the acidosis when severe dehydration results in decreased tissue perfusion. Hyperglycemia causes an osmotic diuresis that is initially compensated for by increased fluid intake. As the hyperglycemia and diuresis worsen, most patients are unable to maintain the large fluid intake, and dehydration occurs. Vomiting, as a result of increasing acidosis, and increased insensible water losses caused by tachypnea can worsen the dehydration. Electrolyte abnormalities occur through a loss of electrolytes in the urine and transmembrane alterations resulting from acidosis. As hydrogen ions accumulate as a result of ketoacidosis, intracellular potassium is exchanged for hydrogen ions. Serum concentrations of potassium increase initially with acidosis then decrease as serum potassium is cleared by the kidney. Depending on the duration of ketoacidosis, serum potassium concentrations at diagnosis may be increased, normal, or decreased, but intracellular potassium concentrations are depleted. A decreased serum potassium concentration is an ominous sign of total body potassium depletion. Phosphate depletion also can occur as a result of the increased renal phosphate excretion required for elimination of excess hydrogen ions. Sodium depletion is also common ketoacidosis, resulting from renal losses of sodium caused by osmotic diuresis and from gastrointestinal losses from vomiting (Fig. 171-2).

Clinical Presentation

Decision-Making Algorithms
Available @ StudentConsult.com

Abdominal Pain
Polyuria
Acidemia
Hypernatremia

Patients with DKA present initially with polyuria, polydipsia, nausea, and vomiting. Abdominal pain occurs frequently and can mimic an acute abdomen. The abdomen may be tender from vomiting or distended secondary to a paralytic ileus. The presence of polyuria, despite a state of clinical dehydration, indicates osmotic diuresis and differentiates patients with DKA from patients with gastroenteritis or other gastrointestinal disorders. Respiratory compensation for acidosis results in tachypnea with deep (**Küssmaul**) respirations. The *fruity* odor of acetone frequently can be detected on the patient's breath. An altered mental status can occur, ranging from disorientation to coma.

Laboratory studies reveal hyperglycemia (serum glucose concentrations ranging from 200 mg/dL to >1000 mg/dL). Arterial pH is below 7.30, and the serum bicarbonate concentration is less than 15 mEq/L. Serum sodium concentrations may be elevated, normal, or low, depending on the balance of sodium and free water losses. The measured serum sodium concentration is artificially low, however, because of hyperglycemia. Hyperlipidemia also contributes to the decrease in measured serum sodium. The level of blood urea nitrogen (BUN) can be elevated with prerenal azotemia secondary to dehydration. The white blood cell count is usually elevated and can be left-shifted without implying the presence of infection. Fever is unusual and should prompt a search for infectious sources that may have triggered the episode of DKA.

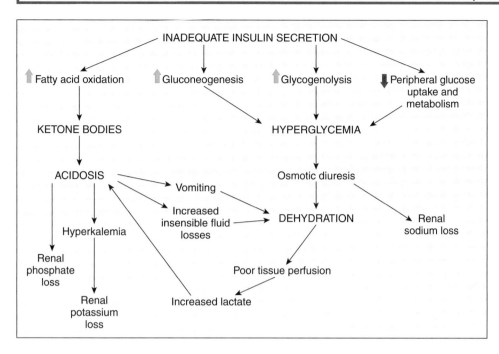

Figure 171-2 Pathophysiology of diabetic ketoacidosis.

Treatment

Decision-Making Algorithms
Available @ StudentConsult.com

Altered Mental Status
Acidemia
Hypokalemia

Therapy for patients with DKA involves careful replacement of fluid deficits, correction of acidosis and hyperglycemia via insulin administration, correction of electrolyte imbalances, and monitoring for complications of treatment. The optimal approach to management of DKA must strike a balance between adequate correction of fluid losses and avoidance of rapid shifts in osmolality and fluid balance. The most serious complication of DKA and its treatment is **cerebral edema** and cerebral herniation.

A patient with severe DKA is assumed to be approximately 10% dehydrated. If a recent weight measurement is available, the precise extent of dehydration can be calculated. An initial intravenous (IV) fluid bolus of a glucose-free isotonic solution (normal saline, lactated Ringer solution) at 10 to 20 mL/kg should be given to restore intravascular volume and renal perfusion. The remaining fluid deficit after the initial bolus should be added to maintenance fluid requirements, and the total should be replaced slowly over 36 to 48 hours. Ongoing losses resulting from osmotic diuresis usually do not need to be replaced unless urine output is large or signs of poor perfusion are present. Osmotic diuresis is usually minimal when the serum glucose concentration decreases to less than 300 mg/dL. To avoid rapid shifts in serum osmolality, 0.9% sodium chloride can be used as the replacement fluid for the initial 4 to 6 hours, followed by 0.45% sodium chloride.

Hyperglycemia. Fast-acting soluble insulin should be administered as a continuous IV infusion (0.1 U/kg/hour). Serum glucose concentrations should decrease at a rate no faster than 100 mg/dL/hour. When serum glucose concentrations decrease to less than 250 to 300 mg/dL, glucose should be added to the IV fluids. If serum glucose concentrations decrease to less than 200 mg/dL before correction of acidosis, the glucose concentration of the IV fluids should be increased, but the insulin infusion should not be decreased by more than half, and it should never be discontinued before resolution of acidosis.

Acidosis. Insulin therapy decreases the production of free fatty acids and protein catabolism and enhances glucose usage in target tissues. These processes correct acidosis. Bicarbonate therapy should be avoided. Potential adverse effects of bicarbonate administration include paradoxical increases in central nervous system (CNS) acidosis caused by increased diffusion of carbon dioxide across the blood-brain barrier, potential tissue hypoxia caused by shifts in the oxyhemoglobin dissociation curve, abrupt osmotic changes, and increased risk of the development of cerebral edema.

As acidosis is corrected, urine ketone concentrations may appear to rise. β-Hydroxybutyrate, which is not detected in urine ketone assays, is converted with treatment to what the assay most detects, acetoacetate. Hence minute-to-minute urine ketone concentrations are not a required index of the adequacy of therapy.

Electrolyte imbalances. Regardless of the serum potassium concentration at presentation, total body potassium depletion is likely. Serum potassium concentrations can decrease rapidly as insulin and then glucose therapy improves acidosis, and potassium is exchanged for intracellular hydrogen ions. When adequate urine output is shown, potassium should be added to the IV fluids. Potassium replacement should be given as 50% potassium chloride and 50% potassium phosphate at a concentration of 20 to 40 mEq/L. This combination provides phosphate for replacement of deficits but avoids excess phosphate administration, which may precipitate hypocalcemia. If the serum potassium level is greater than 6 mEq/L, potassium should not be added to IV fluids until the potassium level decreases.

Monitoring. Initial laboratory measurements should include serum glucose, sodium, potassium, chloride, bicarbonate, BUN, creatinine, calcium, phosphate and magnesium concentrations; arterial or venous pH; and a urinalysis. Serum glucose measurement should be repeated every hour during therapy; electrolyte concentrations should be repeated every 2 to 3 hours. Calcium, phosphate, and magnesium concentrations should be measured every 4 to 6 hours during therapy. Neurologic and mental status should be assessed at frequent intervals. Any complaints of headache or deterioration of mental status should prompt rapid evaluation for possible **cerebral edema.** Indicative symptoms include a decreased sensorium, sudden severe headache, vomiting, change in vital signs (bradycardia, hypertension, apnea), a dilated pupil, ophthalmoplegia, or seizure.

Complications

Clinically apparent **cerebral edema** occurs in 1% to 5% of cases of DKA. Cerebral edema is the most serious complication of DKA, with a mortality rate of 20% to 80%. The pathogenesis of cerebral edema likely involves osmolar shift resulting in fluid accumulation in the intracellular compartment and cell swelling. Subclinical cerebral edema is common in patients with DKA, but the factors that exacerbate this process leading to symptomatic brain swelling and possible cerebral herniation are not clearly defined. Cerebral edema typically occurs 6 to 12 hours after therapy for DKA is begun, often following a period of apparent clinical improvement. Factors that correlate with increased risk for cerebral edema include higher initial BUN concentration, lower initial Pco_2, failure of the serum sodium concentration to increase as glucose concentration decreases during treatment, and treatment with bicarbonate.

Signs of advanced cerebral edema include obtundation, papilledema, pupillary dilation or inequality, hypertension, bradycardia, and apnea. **Treatment** involves the rapid use of IV mannitol, endotracheal intubation, and ventilation and may require the use of a subdural bolt. Other complications of DKA are intracranial thrombosis or infarction, acute tubular necrosis with acute renal failure caused by severe dehydration, pancreatitis, arrhythmias caused by electrolyte abnormalities, pulmonary edema, and bowel ischemia. Peripheral edema occurs commonly 24 to 48 hours after therapy is initiated and may be related to residual elevations in antidiuretic hormone and aldosterone.

Transition to Outpatient Management

When the acidosis has been corrected and the patient tolerates oral feedings, the IV insulin infusion can be discontinued, and a regimen of subcutaneous (SC) insulin injections can be initiated. The first SC insulin dose should be given 30 to 45 minutes before discontinuation of the IV insulin infusion. Further adjustment of the insulin dose should be made over the following 2 to 3 days. A patient already diagnosed with DM1 may be restarted on the prior doses if they were adequate. For a patient with new-onset DM1, typical starting total daily doses are approximately 0.5 to 0.7 U/kg/24 hours for prepubertal patients and approximately 0.7 to 1 U/kg/24 hours for adolescents, using any number of the available insulin combinations. The best and most common choice for making the transition to SC insulin is to begin by giving injections of fast-acting

(bolus) insulin (lispro, aspart, or glulisine insulin) with each meal and long-acting (basal) insulin (glargine or detemir) at bedtime. This regimen of multiple daily injections provides the most flexibility but requires the patient to administer many injections per day and to count carbohydrates in food. An alternative is a fixed mixed split dosing regimen (neutral protamine Hagedorn [NPH] and fasting-acting insulin) with two daily injections.

Externally worn pumps that provide a continuous SC infusion of fast-acting insulin are available, although not usually used at the very onset of DM1. Insulin pumps provide fast-acting insulin in small basal amounts continuously every hour and will provide bolus insulin when instructed. Insulin pumps may be used by all age groups who are highly motivated to achieve tight control. The absence of SC depot insulin (glargine or detemir) can increase the risk of DKA.

Serum glucose concentrations should be assessed before each meal, at bedtime, and periodically at 2 to 3 AM to provide information for adjustment of the regimen. Patients and their families should begin learning the principles of diabetes care as soon as possible. Demonstration of the ability to administer insulin injections and test glucose concentrations using a glucose meter is necessary before discharge, as is knowledge of hypoglycemia management. Meal planning is crucial to control glucose in DM1. Nutrition services must be part of the care delivered to the families from diagnosis.

Honeymoon Period

In some patients with new onset of DM1, the beta cell mass has not been completely destroyed. The remaining functional beta cells seem to recover function with insulin treatment. When this occurs, exogenous insulin requirements decrease. This is a period of stable blood glucose control, often with nearly normal glucose concentrations. This phase of the disease, known as the honeymoon period, usually starts in the first weeks of therapy, often continues for 3 to 6 months, and can last 2 years.

Outpatient Type 1 Diabetes Mellitus Management

Management of DM1 in children requires a comprehensive approach with attention to medical, nutritional, and psychosocial issues. Therapeutic strategies should be flexible with the individual needs of each patient and the family taken into account. Optimal care involves a team of diabetes professionals, including a physician, a diabetes nurse educator, a dietitian, and a social worker or psychologist.

Goals

The Diabetes Control and Complications Trial established that intensive insulin therapy, with the goal of maintaining blood glucose concentrations as close to normal as possible, can delay the onset and slow the progression of complications of diabetes (retinopathy, nephropathy, neuropathy). Attaining this goal using intensive insulin therapy can increase the risk of hypoglycemia. The adverse effects of hypoglycemia in young children may be significant because the immature CNS may be more susceptible to glycopenia. Although the risk for diabetic complications increases with duration of diabetes, there is controversy as to whether the increase of risk is slower in the prepubertal years than in adolescence and adulthood.

The goals of therapy differ, depending on the age of the patient. For children younger than 5 years old, an appropriate goal is maintenance of blood glucose concentrations between 80 and 180 mg/dL. For school-age children, 80 to 150 mg/dL is a reasonable target range. For adolescents, the goal is 70 to 130 mg/dL. Goals of therapy also should take into account other individual characteristics, such as a past history of severe hypoglycemia and the abilities of the patient and family.

Insulin Regimens

Many types of insulin differ in duration of action and time to peak effect (Table 171-2). These insulins can be used in various combinations, depending on the needs and goals of the individual patient. The most commonly used regimen is that of multiple injections of fast-acting insulin given with meals in combination with long-acting basal insulin given at bedtime. This regimen provides flexibility but requires administration of many injections per day and will require assistance for young children. After the total daily dose of insulin is determined, 30% to 50% are given as long-acting insulin, and the remainder is given as fast-acting insulin, divided according to the need for corrections of high glucose levels and for meals. To correct for hyperglycemia, one can determine the insulin sensitivity using the 1800 rule; dividing 1800 by the total daily dose of insulin to determine how many milligrams per deciliter of glucose will decrease with one unit of insulin. The insulin:carbohydrate ratio is used to calculate insulin for the carbohydrate content of food; 450 divided by the total daily dose determines the number of grams of carbohydrate that requires one unit of insulin.

Pumps that provide a continuous SC infusion of short-acting insulin also are available and are being used by children and adolescents who are highly motivated to achieve tight control.

Lispro, aspart, and glulisine insulin are synthetic human insulin analogs in which amino acid alterations result in fast absorption and onset of action (see Table 171-2). Because of the short duration of action, these are used in combination with long-acting insulin. Glargine and detemir are insulin analogs with increased solubility at acidic pH and decreased solubility at physiologic pH. They have a duration of greater than 24 hours and act as a basal insulin.

Newly diagnosed patients in the honeymoon period may require 0.4 to 0.6 U/kg/24 hours. Prepubertal patients with diabetes longer than 1 to 2 years typically require 0.5 to 1 U/kg/24 hours. During middle adolescence when elevated GH concentrations produce relative insulin resistance, insulin requirements increase by 40% to 50%, and doses of 1 to 2 U/kg/24 hours are typical.

Nutrition

Balancing the daily meal plan with the dosages of insulin is crucial for maintaining serum glucose concentrations within the target range and avoiding hypoglycemia or hyperglycemia. The content and schedule of meals vary according to the type of insulin regimen used. It is recommended that carbohydrates contribute 50% to 65% of the total calories, protein 12% to 20%, and fat <30%. Saturated fat should contribute <10% of the total caloric intake, and cholesterol intake should be less than 300 mg/24 hours. High fiber content is recommended.

Patients using multiple daily injections or the insulin pump can maintain a more flexible meal schedule with regard to the timing of meals and the carbohydrate content. These patients give an injection of insulin before or immediately after each meal with the total dose calculated according to the carbohydrate content of the meal. Further adjustments in the dose can be made based on the measured serum glucose concentration and plans for activity during the day. Children using a twice-a-day combination of intermediate-acting and fast-acting insulins need to maintain a relatively consistent meal schedule so that carbohydrate absorption and insulin action peaks correspond. A typical meal schedule for a patient using this type of regimen involves three meals and three snacks daily. The total carbohydrate content of the meals and snacks should be kept constant.

Blood Glucose Testing

Blood glucose should be routinely monitored before each meal and at bedtime. Hypoglycemia during the night or excessive variability in the morning glucose concentrations should prompt additional testing at 2 or 3 AM to ensure that there is no consistent hypoglycemia or hyperglycemia. During periods of illness or when blood glucose concentrations are higher than 300 mg/dL, urine ketones also should be tested. Continuous glucose monitors, which provide minute-to-minute blood glucose concentration information, can be useful in following

Table 171-2	Representative Profiles of Insulin		
INSULIN	**ONSET**	**PEAK ACTION**	**DURATION**
Very Short Acting Lispro, aspart, glulisine	5–15 minutes	30–90 minutes	3–5 hours
Short Acting Regular	30–60 minutes	2–3 hours	5–8 hours
Intermediate Acting Neutral protamine Hagedorn (NPH) (isophane)	2–4 hours	4–10 hours	10–16 hours
Long Acting Glargine Detemir	2–4 hours 2–4 hours	None 6–14 hours	20–24 hours 16–20 hours

Data from Wolfsdorf JI, editor: Intensive Diabetes Management, ed 4, Alexandria, VA, 2009, American Diabetes Associations.

trends of blood glucose concentrations but should not be used in calculations of mealtime insulin doses.

Long-Term Glycemic Control

Measurements of glycohemoglobin or hemoglobin A_{1c} (HgbA1c) reflect the average blood glucose concentration over the preceding 3 months and provide a means for assessing long-term glycemic control. HgbA1c should be measured four times a year, and the results should be used for counseling of patients. The American Diabetes Association has set HgbA1c targets based on age with children less than 6 years having an HgbA1c target of 7.5% to 8.5%, ages 6 to 13 years HgbA1c target of less than 8%, and ages 13 to 18 years HgbA1c target of less than 7.5%. Measurements of HgbA1c are inaccurate in patients with hemoglobinopathies. Glycosylated albumin or fructosamine can be used in these cases.

Complications

Patients with DM1 for more than 3 to 5 years should receive an annual ophthalmologic examination for retinopathy. Urine should be collected annually for assessment of microalbuminuria, which suggests early renal dysfunction and indicates a high risk of progression to nephropathy. Treatment with angiotensin-converting enzyme inhibitors may halt the progression of microalbuminuria. In children with DM1, annual cholesterol measurements and periodic assessment of blood pressure are recommended. Early detection of hypertension and hypercholesterolemia with appropriate intervention can help limit future risk of coronary disease.

Other Disorders

Chronic autoimmune lymphocytic thyroiditis is particularly common and can result in hypothyroidism. Because symptoms can be subtle, thyroid function tests should be performed annually. Other disorders that occur with increased frequency in children with DM1 include celiac disease, IgA deficiency, Addison disease, and peptic ulcer disease.

Special Problems: Hypoglycemia

Hypoglycemia occurs commonly in patients with DM1. For patients in adequate or better control, it is expected to occur on average once or twice a week. Severe episodes of hypoglycemia, resulting in seizures or coma or requiring assistance from another person, occur in 10% to 25% of these patients per year.

Hypoglycemia in patients with DM1 results from a relative excess of insulin in relation to the serum glucose concentration. This excess can be caused by alterations in the dose, timing, or absorption of insulin; alterations of carbohydrate intake; or changes in insulin sensitivity resulting from activity. Defective counterregulatory responses also contribute to hypoglycemia. Abnormal glucagon responses to falling serum glucose concentrations develop within the first few years of the disease, and abnormalities in epinephrine release occur after a longer duration.

Lack of awareness of hypoglycemia occurs in approximately 25% of patients with diabetes. Recent episodes of hypoglycemia may play a role in the pathophysiology of *hypoglycemia unawareness*; after an episode of hypoglycemia, autonomic responses to subsequent episodes are reduced. A return of symptoms of hypoglycemia can be exhibited in these patients after 2 to 3 weeks of strict avoidance of hypoglycemic episodes.

Symptoms of hypoglycemia include symptoms resulting from neuroglycopenia (headache, visual changes, confusion, irritability, or seizures) and symptoms resulting from the catecholamine response (tremors, tachycardia, diaphoresis, or anxiety). Mild episodes can be treated with administration of rapidly absorbed oral glucose (glucose gel or tablets or fruit juices). More severe episodes that result in seizures or loss of consciousness at home should be treated with glucagon injections. IV glucose should be given in hospital settings.

Prognosis

Long-term complications of DM1 include retinopathy, nephropathy, neuropathy, and macrovascular disease. Evidence of organ damage caused by hyperglycemia is rare in patients with diabetes of less than 5 to 10 years' duration; clinically apparent disease rarely occurs before 10 to 15 years' duration. Diabetic retinopathy is the leading cause of blindness in the United States. Nephropathy eventually occurs in 30% to 40% and accounts for approximately 30% of all new adult cases of end-stage renal disease. Neuropathy occurs in 30% to 40% of postpubertal patients with DM1 and leads to sensory, motor, or autonomic deficits. Macrovascular disease results in an increased risk of myocardial infarction and stroke among individuals with diabetes.

Intensive control of diabetes, using frequent blood glucose testing and multiple daily injections of insulin or an insulin pump, can reduce the development or progression of diabetic complications, including a 76% reduction of risk for retinopathy, a 39% reduction in microalbuminuria, and a 60% reduction in clinical neuropathy. For pubertal and adult patients, the benefits of intensive therapy likely outweigh the increased risk for hypoglycemia. For younger patients, in whom the risks for hypoglycemia are greater and the benefits of tight glucose control may be lower, a less intensive regimen may be appropriate.

NON-INSULIN–DEPENDENT (TYPE 2) DIABETES MELLITUS
Pathophysiology

DM2 can occur as the result of various pathophysiologic processes; however the most common form results from peripheral insulin resistance and compensatory hyperinsulinemia, followed by failure of the pancreas to maintain adequate insulin secretion (see Table 171-1).

Epidemiology

The prevalence of DM2 in children is increasing in parallel with childhood obesity and is highest in children of ethnic groups with a high prevalence of DM2 in adults, including Native Americans, Hispanic Americans, and African Americans. Obesity, the metabolic syndrome, ethnicity, and a family history of DM2 are risk factors. Auto-antibodies to the pancreas are present among some clinically assumed to have DM2, compounding the difficulty in differentiating DM1 from DM2 at the time of diagnosis.

Clinical Manifestations and Differential Diagnosis

Fasting and postprandial glucose levels for diagnosis of DM2 are the same as those for DM1. The diagnosis of DM2 may be suspected on the basis of polyuria and polydipsia in a background of the metabolic syndrome. Differentiating DM2 from DM1 in children on only clinical grounds can be challenging. The possibility of DM2 should be considered in patients who are obese, have a strong family history of DM2, have other characteristics of the metabolic syndrome, or have absence of antibodies to beta cell antigens at the time of diagnosis of diabetes. **Acanthosis nigricans,** a dermatologic manifestation of hyperinsulinism and insulin resistance, presents as hyperkeratotic pigmentation in the nape of the neck and in flexural areas and is noted as a sign in the metabolic syndrome. Although ketoacidosis occurs far more commonly in DM1, it also can occur in patients with DM2 under conditions of physiologic stress and cannot be used as an absolute differentiating factor. DM2 can be confirmed by the evaluation of insulin or C-peptide responses to stimulation with oral carbohydrate and in the absence of islet cell autoreactivity.

Therapy

DM2 is the result of a combination of insulin resistance, relative insulin deficiency, and a secretory beta cell defect. Asymptomatic patients with mildly elevated glucose values (slightly >126 mg/dL for fasting or slightly >200 mg/dL for random glucose) may be managed initially with lifestyle modifications, including nutrition therapy (dietary adjustments) and increased exercise. Exercise has been shown to decrease insulin resistance. In most children with new-onset, uncomplicated DM2, oral agents are usually the first line of therapy. Only metformin, an insulin secretagogue, is approved by the U.S. Food and Drug Administration for use in children. A rare side effect of metformin is lactic acidosis, occurring mainly in patients with compromised renal function. The most common side effect is gastrointestinal upset. If ketonuria or ketoacidosis occurs, insulin treatment is necessary to first achieve adequate glycemic control but may be discontinued within weeks with continuation of oral medications. Insulin therapy may be required if adequate glycemic control is not achieved with lifestyle modifications and metformin.

Because DM2 may have a long preclinical course, early diagnosis is possible in subjects at risk who have the **metabolic syndrome.** Significant lifestyle modifications, such as improved eating habits and increased exercise, have a role in preventing or decreasing the morbidity of DM2. Finally it is critical to monitor and manage the other components of metabolic syndrome, such as advanced pubertal development, hypertension, hyperlipidemia, and polycystic ovary syndrome in females.

MATURITY-ONSET DIABETES OF YOUTH (MODY)

MODY comprises a group of dominantly inherited forms of relatively mild diabetes. Insulin resistance does not occur in these patients; instead the primary abnormality is an insufficient insulin secretory response to glycemic stimulation. Treatment depends on the type and can include the use of sulfonylureas.

Chapter 172

HYPOGLYCEMIA

Hypoglycemia in infancy and childhood can result from a large variety of hormonal and metabolic defects (Table 172-1). Hypoglycemia occurs most frequently in the early neonatal period, often as a result of transient neonatal hyperinsulinemia in infants of diabetic mothers or as a result of inadequate energy stores to meet the disproportionately large metabolic needs of premature or small for gestational age newborns. Hypoglycemia during the first few days of life in an otherwise normal newborn is less frequent and warrants concern (see Chapter 6). After the initial 2 to 3 days of life, hypoglycemia is far less common and is more frequently the result of endocrine or metabolic disorders (although sepsis must always be ruled out).

DEFINITION

The **diagnosis** of hypoglycemia should be made on the basis of a low serum glucose concentration, symptoms compatible with hypoglycemia, and resolution of the symptoms after administration of glucose.

Serum glucose concentrations less than 45 mg/dL are considered to be abnormal and necessitate treatment. Serum glucose concentrations greater than 55 mg/dL occasionally can occur in normal individuals, especially with prolonged fasting, but should be considered suspect, particularly if there are concurrent symptoms of hypoglycemia (Table 172-2).

CLINICAL MANIFESTATIONS

Decision-Making Algorithms
Available @ StudentConsult.com

Hypotonia and Weakness
Altered Mental Status
Irritable Infant

The symptoms and signs of hypoglycemia result from direct depression of the central nervous system owing to lack of energy substrate and the counterregulatory adrenergic response to low glucose via catecholamine secretion designed to correct hypoglycemia (see Table 172-2). Compared with older children, infants do not usually show adrenergic symptoms. The signs and symptoms of hypoglycemia in infants are relatively nonspecific and include jitteriness, feeding difficulties, pallor, hypotonia, hypothermia, episodes of apnea and bradycardia, depressed levels of consciousness, and seizures. In older children, signs and symptoms include confusion, irritability, headaches, visual changes, tremors, pallor, sweating, tachycardia, weakness, seizures, and coma.

Failure to recognize and treat severe, prolonged hypoglycemia can result in serious long-term morbidity, including mental retardation and nonhypoglycemic seizures. Younger infants and patients with more severe or prolonged hypoglycemia are at greatest risk for adverse outcomes.

PATHOPHYSIOLOGY
Hormonal Signal

Normal regulation of serum glucose concentrations requires appropriate interaction of a number of hormonal signals and metabolic pathways (Figure 172-1). In a normal individual, a decrease in serum glucose concentrations leads to a suppression of insulin secretion and increased secretion of the counterregulatory hormones (growth hormone [GH], cortisol, glucagon, and epinephrine) (see Fig. 172-1). This hormonal signal promotes the release of amino acids (particularly alanine) from muscle to fuel gluconeogenesis and the release of triglyceride from adipose tissue stores to provide free fatty acids (FFAs) for hepatic ketogenesis. FFAs and ketones serve as alternate fuels for muscle. This hormonal signal also stimulates the breakdown of hepatic glycogen and promotes gluconeogenesis. Failure of any of the components of this hormonal signal can lead to hypoglycemia.

Hyperinsulinemia

	Decision-Making Algorithm
	Available @ StudentConsult.com
Obesity	

A lack of suppression of insulin secretion in response to low serum glucose concentrations can occur in infants but is uncommon beyond the neonatal period. This situation arises most frequently in infants of diabetic mothers who were exposed to high concentrations of maternally derived glucose in utero, resulting in fetal islet cell hyperplasia. The hyperinsulinemic state is transient, usually lasting hours to days.

Hyperinsulinism that persists beyond a few days of age can result from distinct genetic disorders affecting glucose-regulated insulin release. These were previously referred to

Table 172-1	Classification of Hypoglycemia in Infants and Children

ABNORMALITIES IN THE HORMONAL SIGNAL INDICATING HYPOGLYCEMIA	FATTY ACID OXIDATION
COUNTERREGULATORY HORMONE DEFICIENCY	Long-, medium-, or short-chain fatty acid acyl-CoA dehydrogenase deficiency
Panhypopituitarism	Carnitine deficiency (primary or secondary)
Isolated growth hormone deficiency	Carnitine palmitoyltransferase deficiency
ACTH deficiency	**Other**
Addison disease	Enzymatic defects
Glucagon deficiency	Galactosemia
Epinephrine deficiency	Hereditary fructose intolerance
HYPERINSULINISM	Propionic acidemia
Infant of a diabetic mother	Methylmalonic acidemia
Infant with erythroblastosis fetalis	Tyrosinosis
Persistent hyperinsulinemic hypoglycemia of infancy	Glutaric aciduria
Beta cell adenoma (insulinoma)	Global hepatic dysfunction
Beckwith-Wiedemann syndrome	Reye syndrome
Anti-insulin receptor antibodies	Hepatitis
INADEQUATE SUBSTRATE	Heart failure
Prematurity/small for gestational age infant	Sepsis, shock
Ketotic hypoglycemia	Carcinoma/sarcoma (IGF-2 secretion)
Maple syrup urine disease	Malnutrition/starvation
DISORDERS OF METABOLIC RESPONSE PATHWAYS	Hyperviscosity syndrome
Glycogenolysis	**DRUGS/INTOXICATIONS**
Glucose-6-phosphatase deficiency	Oral hypoglycemic agents or insulin
Amylo-1,6-glucosidase deficiency	Alcohol
Liver phosphorylase deficiency	Salicylates
Glycogen synthase deficiency	Propranolol
Gluconeogenesis	Valproic acid
Fructose-1,6-diphosphatase deficiency	Pentamidine
Pyruvate carboxylase deficiency	Ackee fruit (unripe)
Phosphoenolpyruvate carboxykinase deficiency	Quinine
	Trimethoprim-sulfamethoxazole (with renal failure)

ACTH, Adrenocorticotropic hormone; *acyl-CoA,* acyl coenzyme A; *IGF-2,* insulin-like growth factor-2.

as *nesidioblastosis,* or **persistent hyperinsulinemic hypoglycemia of the newborn.** In these infants, hyperplasia of the pancreatic islet cells develops in the absence of excess stimulation by maternal diabetes. Some of these patients have genetic abnormalities of the islet cell sulfonylurea receptor or other genetic defects that alter the function of the adenosine triphosphate–sensitive potassium channel that regulates insulin secretion. Hyperinsulinism also can occur in **Beckwith-Wiedemann syndrome,** a condition characterized by neonatal somatic gigantism: macrosomia, macroglossia, omphalocele, visceromegaly, and earlobe creases.

Regardless of the cause, neonates with hyperinsulinism are characteristically large for gestational age (see Chapter 60). Hypoglycemia is severe and frequently occurs within 1 to 3 hours of a feeding. Glucose requirements are increased, often two to three times the normal basal glucose requirement of 6 to 8 mg/kg/min. The *diagnosis* of hyperinsulinism is confirmed by the detection of serum insulin concentrations greater than 5 μU/mL during an episode of hypoglycemia. The absence of serum and urine ketones at the time of hypoglycemia is an important diagnostic feature, distinguishing hyperinsulinism from defects in counterregulatory hormone secretion.

Treatment initially involves the infusion of intravenous (IV) glucose at high rates and of diazoxide to suppress insulin secretion. If diazoxide therapy is unsuccessful, long-acting somatostatin analogs can be tried. Often medical therapy for persistent hyperinsulinemic hypoglycemia of the newborn is unsuccessful, and subtotal (90%) pancreatectomy is required to prevent long-term neurologic sequelae of hypoglycemia.

In children hyperinsulinemia is a rare condition characterized by a voracious appetite, obesity, and accelerated linear growth and usually results from an **islet cell adenoma.** Computed tomography, magnetic resonance imaging, or radioisotope imaging of the pancreas should be attempted, but visualization of an adenoma is usually difficult. Surgical removal of the adenoma is curative.

Factitious Hyperinsulinemia
In rare cases insulin or a hypoglycemic medication is administered by a parent or caregiver to a child as a form of child abuse, which is a condition referred to as **Munchausen syndrome by proxy.** This *diagnosis* should be suspected if extremely high insulin concentrations are detected (>100 μU/mL). C-peptide concentrations are low or undetectable, which confirms that the insulin is from an exogenous source.

Defects in Counterregulatory Hormones
Abnormalities in the secretion of counterregulatory hormones that produce hypoglycemia usually involve GH, cortisol, or both. Deficiencies in glucagon and epinephrine secretion are rare. GH and cortisol deficiency occur as a result of hypopituitarism. Hypopituitarism results from congenital hypoplasia or aplasia of the pituitary or, more commonly, from deficiency of hypothalamic releasing factors (see Chapter 173). Clues to this diagnosis in infants include the presence of hypoglycemia in association with midline facial or neurologic defects (e.g., cleft lip and palate or absence of the corpus callosum), pendular (roving) nystagmus (indicating visual impairment from possible abnormalities in the development of the optic nerves,

Table 172-2	Symptoms and Signs of Hypoglycemia
FEATURES ASSOCIATED WITH EPINEPHRINE RELEASE*	**FEATURES ASSOCIATED WITH CEREBRAL GLYCOPENIA**
Perspiration	Headache
Palpitation (tachycardia)	Mental confusion
Pallor	Somnolence
Paresthesia	Dysarthria
Trembling	Personality changes
Anxiety	Inability to concentrate
Weakness	Staring
Nausea	Hunger
Vomiting	Convulsions
	Ataxia
	Coma
	Diplopia
	Stroke

*These features and perceptions of the features may be blunted if the patient is receiving β blocking agents.

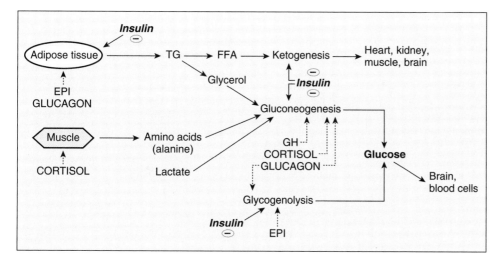

Figure 172-1 Regulation of serum glucose. ⊖ represents inhibitions. *EPI,* Epinephrine; *FFA,* free fatty acid; *GH,* growth hormone; *TG,* triglyceride.

which can occur in septo-optic dysplasia), and the presence of microphallus and cryptorchidism in boys (indicating abnormalities in gonadotropin secretion). Jaundice and hepatomegaly also can occur, simulating neonatal hepatitis. Despite the presence of GH deficiency, these infants are usually of normal size at birth.

Deficient cortisol secretion also can occur in primary adrenal insufficiency, resulting from a variety of causes. In infants it often results from congenital adrenal hyperplasia, most frequently as a result of 21-hydroxylase deficiency (see Chapters 177 and 178). In older children, primary adrenal insufficiency is seen most frequently in **Addison disease** and other disorders (see Chapter 178).

Confirmation of GH or cortisol deficiency as the cause of hypoglycemia requires the detection of low serum GH and cortisol concentrations during an episode of hypoglycemia or after other stimulatory testing. In contrast to hyperinsulinism, serum and urine ketones are positive at the time of hypoglycemia and FFAs are elevated. Treatment involves supplementation of the deficient hormones in physiologic doses.

ENERGY STORES

Sufficient energy stores in the form of glycogen, adipose tissue, and muscle are necessary to respond appropriately to hypoglycemia. Deficiencies in these stores are a common cause of hypoglycemia in neonates who are small for gestational age or premature (see Chapter 60). Beyond the early neonatal period, energy stores are usually sufficient to meet the metabolic requirements except in malnourished children.

IDIOPATHIC KETOTIC HYPOGLYCEMIA

A common cause of new-onset hypoglycemia is idiopathic ketotic hypoglycemia, usually seen in children between 18 months and 5 years of age. Patients have symptoms of hypoglycemia after a period of prolonged fasting, often in the setting of an intercurrent illness with decreased feeding. Children with this disorder are often thin and small and may have a history of being small for gestational age. Defective mobilization of alanine from muscle to fuel gluconeogenesis is thought to be the cause, although the condition may derive mostly from having lower fuel reserves. Because there are no specific diagnostic tests for this disorder, ketotic hypoglycemia is a *diagnosis of exclusion*.

Treatment involves avoidance of fasting and frequent feedings of a high-protein, high-carbohydrate diet. Patients may require hospitalization for IV glucose infusion if they cannot maintain adequate oral intake during a period of illness. The disorder usually resolves spontaneously by 7 to 8 years of age.

DISRUPTED METABOLIC RESPONSE PATHWAYS

Maintenance of normal serum glucose concentrations in the fasting state requires glucose production via glycogenolysis and gluconeogenesis and the production of alternative energy sources (FFAs and ketones) via lipolysis and fatty acid oxidation.

Glycogenolysis

Glycogen storage diseases occur in a variety of subtypes that differ in severity (see Chapter 52). Among the subtypes that result in hypoglycemia, the most severe form is

glucose-6-phosphatase deficiency, which is characterized by severe hypoglycemia, massive hepatomegaly, growth retardation, and lactic acidosis. In contrast, deficiencies in the glycogen phosphorylase enzymes may cause isolated hepatomegaly with or without hypoglycemia.

The *diagnosis* of glycogen storage disease is suggested by a finding of hepatomegaly without splenomegaly. Confirmation of the diagnosis requires specific biochemical studies of leukocytes or liver biopsy specimens. *Treatment* involves frequent high-carbohydrate feedings during the day and continuous feedings at night via nasogastric tube. Feedings of uncooked cornstarch overnight are sufficient to maintain serum glucose concentrations in some patients.

Gluconeogenesis

Defects in gluconeogenesis are uncommon and include fructose-1,6-diphosphatase deficiency and phosphoenolpyruvate carboxykinase deficiency. Affected patients exhibit fasting hypoglycemia, hepatomegaly, lactic acidosis, and hyperuricemia. Ketosis occurs, and FFA and alanine concentrations are high. *Treatment* involves frequent high-carbohydrate, low-protein feedings (see Chapter 52).

Fatty Acid Oxidation

Fatty acid oxidation disorders of ketogenesis include the fatty acid acyl-coenzyme A (CoA) dehydrogenase deficiencies; long-chain, medium-chain, and short-chain acyl-CoA dehydrogenase deficiencies; and hereditary carnitine deficiency (see Chapter 55). Of these disorders, medium-chain acyl-CoA dehydrogenase deficiency is the most common; it occurs in 1 in 9000 to 15,000 live births. Patients often are well in infancy and have the first episode of hypoglycemia at 2 years of age or older. Episodes of hypoglycemia usually occur with prolonged fasting or during episodes of intercurrent illness.

Mild hepatomegaly may be present along with mild hyperammonemia, hyperuricemia, and mild elevations in hepatic transaminases. Ketone concentrations are low or undetected. The *diagnosis* is confirmed by the finding of elevated concentrations of dicarboxylic acids in the urine. *Treatment* involves avoidance of fasting.

OTHER METABOLIC DISORDERS

Many metabolic disorders can lead to hypoglycemia, including galactosemia, hereditary fructose intolerance, and disorders of organic acid metabolism (see Table 172-1). Hypoglycemia in these disorders is usually a reflection of global hepatic dysfunction secondary to the buildup of hepatotoxic intermediates. Many of these disorders present with low concentrations of ketone bodies because ketogenesis also is affected. The finding of non–glucose-reducing substances in the urine suggests a diagnosis of galactosemia or hereditary fructose intolerance. Occurrence of symptoms after ingestion of fructose or sucrose suggests **hereditary fructose intolerance.** *Treatment* requires dietary restriction of the specific offending substances.

MEDICATIONS AND INTOXICATION

Hypoglycemia can occur as an adverse effect of numerous medications (see Table 172-1). Valproate toxicity can cause a disorder similar to that seen in the fatty acid oxidation defects. Ethanol ingestion also can cause hypoglycemia, especially in younger children, because the metabolism of ethanol results in the depletion of cofactors necessary for gluconeogenesis.

DIAGNOSIS

Although the list of causes of hypoglycemia is long and complex, establishing the *etiology* in a particular patient is important. Frequently it is difficult to make an accurate diagnosis until one can obtain a *critical sample* of blood and urine at the time of the hypoglycemic episode. In a child with unexplained hypoglycemia, a serum sample should be obtained before treatment for the measurement of glucose and insulin, GH, cortisol, FFAs, and β-hydroxybutyrate and acetoacetate. Measurement of serum lactate levels also should be considered. A urine specimen should be obtained for measuring ketones and reducing substances. *Hypoglycemia without ketonuria suggests hyperinsulinism or a defect in fatty acid oxidation.* The results of this initial testing can establish whether endocrine causes are responsible and, if not, provide initial information regarding which types of metabolic disorders are most likely. Whenever possible, additional samples of blood and urine should be frozen for further analysis, if necessary.

EMERGENCY MANAGEMENT

Acute care of a patient with hypoglycemia consists of rapid administration of IV glucose (2 mL/kg of 10% dextrose in water). After the initial bolus, an infusion of IV glucose should provide approximately 1.5 times the normal hepatic glucose production rate (8 to 12 mg/kg/min in infants, 6 to 8 mg/kg/min in children). This infusion allows for suppression of the catabolic state and prevents further decompensation in patients with certain metabolic disorders. If adrenal insufficiency is suspected, stress doses of glucocorticoids should be administered.

Chapter 173

SHORT STATURE

GROWTH

Normal growth is the final common pathway of many factors, including endocrine, environmental, nutritional, and genetic influences (see Chapter 5). A normal linear growth pattern is good evidence of overall health and can be considered a *bioassay* for the well-being of the whole child. The effects of certain hormones on growth and ultimate height are listed in Table 173-1. Just as various factors influence stature, stature itself influences psychological, social, and potentially economic well-being. Parental concern about the psychosocial consequences of abnormal stature often causes a family to seek medical attention.

Growth Hormone Physiology

Growth hormone (GH) secretion is pulsatile, stimulated by hypothalamic GH-releasing factor (GRF) and inhibited by GH release inhibitory factor (somatostatin, somatotropin release-inhibiting factor [SRIF]), which interact with their individual receptors on the somatotrope in a noncompetitive manner. GH is also stimulated by ghrelin, produced in the stomach. GH circulates bound to a GH-binding protein (GHBP); GHBP abundance reflects the abundance of GH receptors. GH has direct effects on tissue and also causes production and secretion of insulin-like growth factor-1 (IGF-1) in many tissues. GH stimulates IGF-1 production in liver along with production of the acid-labile subunit and the IGF-binding protein (IGF-BP3); this forms the complex that delivers IGF-1 to tissue.

IGF-1 acts primarily as a paracrine and autocrine agent and is most closely associated with postnatal growth. When IGF-1 attaches to its membrane-bound receptor, second messengers are stimulated to change the physiology of the cell and produce growth effects. IGF-1 production is influenced by disease states such as malnutrition, chronic renal and liver disease, hypothyroidism, or obesity.

IGF-BP3 is measurable in clinical assays and is less influenced by nutrition and age than is IGF-1; measuring IGF-1 and IGF-BP3 is useful in evaluating GH adequacy, particularly in infancy and early childhood.

Measurement of Growth

The correct measurement of an infant's length requires one adult to hold the infant's head still and another adult to extend the feet with the soles perpendicular to the lower legs. A caliper-like device, such as an infantometer, or the movable plates on an infant scale are used so that the exact distance between the two calipers or plates can be determined. Marking the position of the head and feet of an infant lying on a sheet of paper on the examining table leads to inaccuracies and may miss true disorders of growth or create false concerns about a disorder of growth in a normal child. Accurate measurements of height (standing), or length (lying down), and weight should be plotted on the Centers for Disease Control and Prevention growth charts for the timely diagnosis of growth disorders (http://www.cdc.gov/growthcharts/).

After 2 years of age, the height of a child should be measured in the standing position. Children measured in the standing position should be barefoot against a hard surface. A Harpenden stadiometer or equivalent device is optimal for the measurement of stature. A decrease of roughly 1.25 cm in height measurement may occur when the child is measured in the standing position rather than in the lying position, leading to the inappropriate referral of many children who appear to be *not growing* to a subspecialist.

Measurement of the **arm span** is essential when the diagnoses of Marfan or Klinefelter syndrome, short-limbed dwarfism, or other dysmorphic conditions are considered. Arm span is measured as the distance between the tips of the fingers when the patient holds both arms outstretched horizontally while standing against a solid surface. The **upper-to-lower segment ratio** is the ratio of the upper segment (determined by subtraction of the measurement from the symphysis pubis to the floor [known as the lower segment] from the total height) to the lower segment. This ratio changes with age. A normal term

Table 173-1	Hormonal Effects on Growth		
HORMONE	**BONE AGE**	**GROWTH RATE**	**ADULT HEIGHT***
Androgen excess	Advanced	Increased	Diminished
Androgen deficiency	Normal or delayed	Normal or decreased	Increased slightly or normal
Thyroxine excess	Advanced	Increased	Normal or diminished
Thyroxine deficiency	Retarded	Decreased	Diminished
Growth hormone excess	Normal or advanced	Increased	Excessive
Growth hormone deficiency	Retarded	Decreased	Diminished
Cortisol excess	Retarded	Decreased	Diminished
Cortisol deficiency	Normal	Normal	Normal

Adapted from Underwood LE, Van Wyk JJ: Normal and aberrant growth. In Wilson JD, Foster DW, editors: Textbook of Endocrinology, ed 8, Philadelphia, 1992, WB Saunders.
*Effect in most patients with treatment.

infant has an upper-to-lower ratio of 1.7:1, a 1-year-old has a ratio of 1.4:1, and a 10-year-old has a ratio of 1:1. Conditions of hypogonadism, not commonly discerned or suspected until after the normal age for onset of puberty, lead to greatly decreased upper-to-lower ratio in an adult, whereas long-lasting and untreated hypothyroidism leads to a high upper-to-lower ratio in the child.

Endocrine Evaluation of Growth Hormone Secretion

Decision-Making Algorithm
Available @ StudentConsult.com

Short Stature

GH is a 191–amino acid protein secreted by the pituitary gland under the control of GRF and SRIF (see Fig. 170-2). GH secretion is enhanced by α-adrenergic stimulation, hypoglycemia, starvation, exercise, early stages of sleep, and stress and inhibited by β-adrenergic stimulation and hyperglycemia. Because concentrations of GH are low throughout the day, except for brief secretory peaks in the middle of the night or early morning, the daytime ascertainment of GH deficiency or sufficiency on the basis of a single determination of a random GH concentration is impossible. Adequacy of GH secretion may be determined by a stimulation test to measure peak GH secretion. A normal response is a vigorous secretory peak after stimulation; the lack of such a peak is consistent with GH deficiency. However there is a high false-positive rate (on any day, about 10% or more of normal children may not reach the normal GH peak after even two stimulatory tests). Indirect measurements of GH secretion, such as serum concentrations of IGF-1 and IGF-BP3, are considered better screens for GH deficiency.

The factors responsible for postnatal growth are not the same as the factors that mediate fetal growth. **Thyroid hormone** is essential for normal postnatal growth, although a thyroid hormone–deficient fetus achieves a normal birth length; similarly a GH-deficient fetus has a normal birth length, although in IGF-1 deficiency resulting from GH resistance **(Laron dwarfism),** fetuses are shorter than control subjects. Adequate thyroid hormone is necessary to allow the secretion

of GH. Hypothyroid patients may appear falsely to be GH deficient; with thyroid hormone repletion, GH secretion normalizes. Gonadal steroids are important in the pubertal growth spurt. The effects of other hormones on growth are noted in Table 173-1.

ABNORMALITIES OF GROWTH
Short Stature of Nonendocrine Causes

Decision-Making Algorithm
Available @ StudentConsult.com

Short Stature

Short stature is defined as subnormal height relative to other children of the same gender and age, taking family heights into consideration. It can be caused by numerous conditions (Table 173-2). The Centers for Disease Control and Prevention growth charts use the 3rd percentile of the growth curve as the demarcation of the lower limit. **Growth failure** denotes a slow growth rate regardless of stature. Ultimately a slow growth rate leads to short stature, but a disease process is detected sooner if the decreased growth rate is noted before the stature becomes short. Plotted on a growth chart, growth failure appears as a curve that crosses percentiles downward and is associated with a height velocity below the 5th percentile of height velocity for age (Fig. 173-1). A corrected midparental, or genetic target, height helps determine whether the child is growing well for the family (see Chapter 6). To determine a range of normal height for the family under consideration, the corrected midparental height is bracketed by 2 standard deviations (SDs), which, for the United States, is approximately 10 cm (4 in.). The presence of a height 3.5 SDs below the mean, a height velocity below the 5th percentile for age, or a height below the target height corrected for midparental height requires a diagnostic evaluation.

Nutrition is the most important factor affecting growth on a worldwide basis (see Chapter 28). Failure to thrive may develop in the infant as a result of **maternal deprivation** (nutritional deficiency or aberrant psychosocial interaction) or as a result of organic illness (anorexia, nutrient losses through a form of malabsorption, or hypermetabolism caused

Table 173-2	Causes of Short Stature

VARIATIONS OF NORMAL	SYNDROMES OF SHORT STATURE
Constitutional (delayed bone age)	Turner syndrome (syndrome of gonadal dysgenesis)
Genetic (short familial height)	Noonan syndrome (pseudo-Turner syndrome)
ENDOCRINE DISORDERS	Autosomal trisomy 13, 18, 21
GH deficiency	Laurence-Moon-Bardet-Biedl syndrome
Congenital	Prader-Willi syndrome
Isolated GH deficiency	Autosomal abnormalities
With other pituitary hormone deficiencies	Dysmorphic syndromes (e.g., Russell-Silver or Cornelia de Lange syndrome)
With midline defects	Pseudohypoparathyroidism
Pituitary agenesis	**CHRONIC DISEASE**
With gene deficiency	Cardiac disorders
Acquired	Left-to-right shunt
Hypothalamic/pituitary tumors	Heart failure
Langerhans cell histiocytosis (X cell histiocytosis)	Pulmonary disorders
CNS infections and granulomas	Cystic fibrosis
Head trauma (birth and later)	Asthma (severe steroid dependent)
Hypothalamic/pituitary irradiation	Gastrointestinal disorders
CNS vascular accidents	Malabsorption (e.g., celiac disease)
Hydrocephalus	Disorders of swallowing
Autoimmune	Inflammatory bowel disease
Psychosocial dwarfism (functional GH deficiency)	Hepatic disorders
Amphetamine treatment for hyperactivity*	Hematologic disorders
Laron dwarfism (increased GH and decreased IGF-1)	Sickle cell anemia
Pygmies (normal GH and IGF-2 but decreased IGF-1)	Thalassemia
Hypothyroidism	Renal disorders
Glucocorticoid excess	Renal tubular acidosis
Endogenous	Chronic uremia
Exogenous	Immunologic disorders
Diabetes mellitus under poor control	Connective tissue disease
Diabetes insipidus (untreated)	Juvenile idiopathic arthritis
Hypophosphatemic vitamin D-resistant rickets	Chronic infection
Virilizing congenital adrenal hyperplasia (tall child, short adult) P-450$_{c21}$, P-450$_{c11}$ deficiencies	AIDS
SKELETAL DYSPLASIAS	Hereditary fructose intolerance
Osteogenesis imperfecta	Malnutrition
Osteochondrodysplasias	Kwashiorkor, marasmus
LYSOSOMAL STORAGE DISEASES	Iron deficiency
Mucopolysaccharidoses	Zinc deficiency
Mucolipidoses	Anorexia caused by chemotherapy for neoplasms
	Cerebral palsy

Modified from Styne DM: Growth disorder. In Fitzgerald PA, editor: Handbook of Clinical Endocrinology, Norwalk, CT, 1986, Appleton & Lange.
AIDS, Acquired immunodeficiency syndrome; *CNS,* central nervous system; *GH,* growth hormone; *IGF,* insulin-like growth factor.
*Only if caloric intake is severely diminished.

by hyperthyroidism or other causes) (see Chapter 21). Psychological difficulties also can affect growth, as in **psychosocial** or **deprivation dwarfism,** in which the child develops functional temporary GH deficiency and poor growth as a result of psychological abuse; when placed in a different, healthier psychosocial environment, GH physiology normalizes, and growth occurs.

The common condition known as **constitutional delay** in growth or puberty or both is considered a variation of normal growth, caused by a reduced tempo, or cadence, of physiologic

Figure 173-1 Patterns of linear growth. Normal growth percentiles (5th, 50th, and 95th) are shown along with typical growth curves for **A,** Constitutional delay of growth and adolescence (short stature with normal growth rate for bone age, delayed pubertal growth spurt, and eventual achievement of normal adult stature). **B,** Familial short stature (short stature in childhood and as an adult). **C,** Acquired pathologic growth failure (e.g., acquired untreated primary hypothyroidism) (see Chapter 5).

development (see Fig. 173-1). Usually a family member had delayed growth or puberty but achieved a normal final height. The bone age is delayed, but the growth rate remains mostly within the lower limits of normal. Constitutional delay usually leads to a delay in secondary sexual development. **Genetic or familial short stature** (Table 173-3) refers to the stature of a child of short parents, who is expected to reach a lower than average height and yet normal for these parents. If the parents were malnourished as children, grew up in a zone of war, or suffered famine, the heights of the parents are less predictive. Although there are differences in height associated with ethnicity, the most significant difference in stature between ethnic groups is the result of nutrition.

Phenotypic features suggesting an underlying chromosomal disorder can occur in many syndromes. These syndromes can be suspected by attending to arm spans and upper-to-lower segment ratios. Genetic syndromes often combine obesity and decreased height, whereas otherwise normal obese children are usually taller than average and have advanced skeletal development and physical maturation (see Table 173-2). The **Prader-Willi syndrome** includes fetal and infantile hypotonia, small hands and feet (acromicria), postnatal acquired obesity with an insatiable appetite, developmental delay, hypogonadism, almond-shaped eyes, and abnormalities of the snRNP (small nuclear ribonucleic particle) portion of the 15th chromosome at 15q11-q13. Most cases have deletion of the paternal sequence, but about 20% to 25% have uniparental disomy, in which both chromosomes 15 derive from the mother. **Laurence-Moon-Bardet-Biedl syndrome** is characterized by retinitis pigmentosa, hypogonadism, and developmental delay with an autosomal dominant

inheritance pattern. Laurence-Moon syndrome is associated with spastic paraplegia; Bardet-Biedl syndrome is associated with obesity and polydactyly. **Pseudohypoparathyroidism** leads to short stature and developmental delay with short fourth and fifth digits (Albright hereditary osteodystrophy phenotype), resistance to parathyroid hormone and resultant hypocalcemia, and elevated levels of serum phosphorus. **Turner syndrome** is characterized by a karyotype of 45XO or by a mosaic karyotype and clinically presents with short stature, shield chest, wide-spaced nipples, wide-carrying angle of the upper extremities, high-arched palate, gonadal failure, kidney dysplasias with normal function, and aortic arch abnormalities. Affected girls are often susceptible to autoimmune disorders.

Decision-Making Algorithms
Available @ StudentConsult.com

Hypotonia and Weakness
Short Stature
Pubertal Delay
Obesity
Hypocalcemia

Short Stature Caused by Growth Hormone Deficiency
Etiology and Epidemiology

Decision-Making Algorithm
Available @ StudentConsult.com

Short Stature

Classic congenital or **idiopathic GH deficiency** occurs in about 1 in 4000 to 1 in 10,000 children. Idiopathic GH deficiency, of unidentified specific etiology, is the most common cause of both congenital and acquired GH deficiency. Less often GH deficiency is caused by anatomic defects of the pituitary gland, such as pituitary aplasia or other midline defects, with variable degrees of deficiency of other pituitary functions. Hereditary forms of GH deficiency that affect pituitary differentiation are the result of heterogeneous defects of the gene for GH, GRF, or GH receptor. *Classic GH deficiency* refers to very reduced to absent secretion of GH; numerous short children may have intermediate forms of decreased GH secretion. Acquired GH deficiency causing late-onset growth failure suggests the possibility of a **tumor** of the hypothalamus or pituitary causing compression of the area (see Tables 173-2 and 173-3).

Clinical Manifestations
Infants with congenital GH deficiency achieve a normal or near-normal birth length and weight at term, but the growth rate slows after birth, most noticeably after age 2 to 3 years. These children become progressively shorter for age and tend to have an elevated weight-to-height ratio, appearing chubby and short. Careful measurements in the first year of life may suggest the diagnosis, but most patients elude diagnosis until several years of age. A patient with classic GH deficiency has the appearance of a **cherub (a chubby, immature appearance)**, with a high-pitched voice resulting from an immature

Table 173-3 | Differential Diagnosis and Therapy of Short Stature

DIAGNOSTIC FEATURE	HYPOPITUITARISM GH DEFICIENCY*	CONSTITUTIONAL DELAY	FAMILIAL SHORT STATURE	DEPRIVATIONAL DWARFISM	TURNER SYNDROME	HYPOTHYROIDISM	CHRONIC DISEASE
Family history positive	Rare	Frequent	Always	No	No	Variable	Variable
Gender	Both	Males more often affected than females	Both	Both	Female	Both	Both
Facies	Immature or with midline defect (e.g., cleft palate or optic hypoplasias)	Immature	Normal	Normal	Turner facies or normal	Coarse (cretin if congenital)	Normal
Sexual development	Delayed	Delayed	Normal	May be delayed	Female prepubertal	Usually delayed, may be precocious if hypothyroidism is severe	Delayed
Bone age	Delayed	Delayed	Normal	Usually delayed; growth arrest lines present	Delayed	Delayed	Delayed
Dentition	Delayed	Normal; delay usual	Normal	Variable	Normal	Delayed	Normal or delayed
Hypoglycemia	Variable	No	No	No	No	No	No
Karyotype	Normal	Normal	Normal	Normal	45,X or partial deletion of X chromosome or mosaic	Normal	Normal
Free T_4	Low (with TRH deficiency) or normal	Normal	Normal	Normal or low	Normal: hypothyroidism may be acquired	Low	Normal
Stimulated GH	Low	Normal for bone age	Normal	Possibly low, or high if patient malnourished	Usually normal	Low	Usually normal
Insulin-like growth factor-1	Low	Normal or low for chronologic age	Normal	Low	Normal	Low	Low or normal (depending on nutritional status)
Therapy	Replace deficiencies	Reassurance; sex steroids to initiate secondary sexual development in selected patients	None	Change or improve environment	Sex hormone replacement, GH; oxandrolone may be useful	T_4	Treat malnutrition, organ failure (e.g., dialysis, transplant, cardiotonic drugs, insulin)

ACTH, Adrenocorticotropic hormone; *CRH,* corticotropin-releasing hormone; *GH,* growth hormone; *GnRH,* gonadotropin-releasing hormone; *TRH,* thyrotropin-releasing hormone; *T_4,* thyroxine.
*Possibly with GnRH, CRH, or TRH deficiency.

Table 173-4	Growth Failure: Screening Tests
TEST	**RATIONALE**
CBC	*Anemia:* nutritional, chronic disease, malignancy
	Leukopenia: bone marrow failure syndromes
	Thrombocytopenia: malignancy, infection
ESR, CRP	Inflammation of infection, inflammatory diseases, malignancy
Metabolic panel (electrolytes, liver enzymes, BUN)	Signs of acute or chronic hepatic, renal, adrenal dysfunction; hydration and acid-base status
Carotene, folate, and prothrombin time; celiac antibody panel	Assess malabsorption; detect celiac disease
Urinalysis with pH	Signs of renal dysfunction, hydration, water and salt homeostasis; renal tubular acidosis
Karyotype	Determines Turner (XO) or other syndromes
Cranial imaging (MRI)	Assesses hypothalamic-pituitary tumors (craniopharyngioma, glioma, germinoma) or congenital midline defects
Bone age	Compare with height age and evaluate height potential
IGF-1, IGF-BP3	Reflects growth hormone status or nutrition
Free thyroxine	Detects panhypopituitarism or isolated hypothyroidism
Prolactin	Elevated in hypothalamic dysfunction or destruction, suppressed in pituitary disease

BUN, Blood urea nitrogen; *CBC,* complete blood count; *CRP,* C-reactive protein; *ESR,* erythrocyte sedimentation rate; *IGF-1,* insulin-like growth factor-1; *IGF-BP3,* insulin-like growth factor-binding protein 3; *MRI,* magnetic resonance imaging.

larynx. Unless severe hypoglycemia occurs or dysraphism (midline defects) of the head includes a central nervous system (CNS) defect that affects mentation, the patient has normal intellectual growth and age-appropriate speech. Male neonates with isolated GH deficiency with or without gonadotropin deficiency may have a microphallus (a stretched penile length of <2 cm [normal is 3 to 5 cm]) and fasting hypoglycemia. Patients who lack the adrenocorticotropic hormone (ACTH, stimulates cortisol) in addition to GH may have more profound hypoglycemia because cortisol also stimulates gluconeogenesis.

A very rare cause of growth failure is GH resistance or GH insensitivity, caused by abnormal number or function of GH receptors or by a postreceptor defect. Patients with the autosomal recessive **Laron syndrome,** involving mutations of the GH receptor, have a prominent forehead, hypoplastic nasal bridge, delayed dentition, sparse hair, blue sclerae, delayed bone maturation and osteoporosis, progressive adiposity, hypercholesterolemia, and low blood glucose. They have elevated serum GH concentrations, although serum IGF-1 and

IGF-BP3 concentrations are low. Malnutrition, medications (corticosteroids), or severe liver disease may cause **acquired GH resistance** because serum GH is elevated and IGF-1 is decreased.

Diagnosis

If family or other medical history does not provide a likely diagnosis, screening tests should include a metabolic panel to evaluate kidney and liver function, a complete blood count (CBC) to rule out anemia, a celiac panel to rule out celiac disease, and carotene and folate levels to reflect nutrition and rule out malabsorption. A urinalysis aids in the evaluation of renal function. Urinary pH and serum bicarbonate can assess for renal tubular acidosis. In a girl without another explanation for short stature, a karyotype may rule out **Turner syndrome.** A bone age will establish skeletal maturation.

If chronic disease or familial short stature are ruled out and routine laboratory testing is normal (Table 173-4), two GH stimulatory tests are commonly performed (see Table 170-2). GH testing should be offered to a patient who is short (<5th percentile and usually >3.5 SDs below the mean), growing poorly (<5th percentile growth rate for age), or whose height projection, based on bone age, is considerably below the target height when corrected for family height.

Classic GH-deficient patients do not show an increase in serum GH levels after stimulation. Some patients release GH in response to secretagogue testing but cannot release GH spontaneously during the day or night. Measuring serum IGF-1 and IGF-BP3 is suggested but not consistently helpful in establishing a diagnosis of GH deficiency. Tests for GH secretion are insensitive, not very specific, and fairly variable. In equivocal cases, an operational definition of GH deficiency might be that patients grow significantly faster when administered a normal dose of GH than before treatment.

Treatment

GH deficiency is treated with biosynthetic recombinant DNA–derived GH. Dosage is titrated to the growth rate. Treatment with GH carries the risk of an increased incidence of slipped capital femoral epiphysis, especially in rapidly growing adolescents, and of pseudotumor cerebri.

Administration of GH to patients with normal GH responsiveness to secretagogues is controversial, but, as noted earlier, diagnostic tests are imperfect; if the patient is growing extremely slowly without alternative explanation, GH therapy is sometimes used. GH is effective in increasing the growth rate and final height in Turner syndrome and in chronic renal failure; GH also is used for treatment of short stature and muscle weakness of Prader-Willi syndrome. Other indications include children born small for gestational age who have not exhibited catch-up growth by 2 years of age and the long-term treatment of idiopathic short stature with height 2.25 SDs or less below the mean. Psychological support of children with severe short stature is important. Although there is controversy, marital status, satisfaction with life, and vocational achievement may be decreased in children of short stature who are not given supportive measures.

Chapter 174

DISORDERS OF PUBERTY

PHYSIOLOGY

The staging of pubertal changes and the sequence of events are discussed in Chapter 67. The onset of puberty is marked by pubarche and gonadarche. **Pubarche** results from adrenal maturation or adrenarche and is marked with the appearance of pubic hair; other features include oiliness of hair and skin, acne, axillary hair, and body odor. **Gonadarche** is characterized by increasing secretion of gonadal sex steroids as a result of the maturation of the hypothalamic-pituitary-gonadal axis. These sex steroids differ by gender, consisting of testosterone from the testes and estradiol and progesterone from the ovaries. In males physical signs are pubic hair, axillary hair, facial hair, increased muscularity, deeper voice, increased penile size, and increased testicular volume. In females the physical signs are breast development, development of the female body habitus, increased size of the uterus, and menarche with regular menstrual cycles. The third component is the growth spurt of puberty.

Hypothalamic gonadotropin-releasing hormone (GnRH), produced by cells in the arcuate nucleus, is secreted from the median eminence of the hypothalamus into the pituitary portal system and reaches the membrane receptors on the pituitary gonadotropes to cause the production and release of luteinizing hormone (LH) and follicle-stimulating hormone (FSH) into the circulation. The hypothalamic-pituitary-gonadal axis is active in the fetus and newborn but is suppressed in the childhood years until activity increases again at the onset of puberty.

In females FSH stimulates the ovarian production of estrogen and, later in puberty, causes the formation and support of corpus luteum. In males LH stimulates the production of testosterone from the Leydig cells; later in puberty, FSH stimulates the development and support of the seminiferous tubules. The gonads also produce the protein inhibin. Both sex steroids and inhibin suppress the secretion of gonadotropins. The interplay of the products of the gonads and GnRH modulates the serum concentrations of gonadotropins. GnRH is released in episodic pulses that vary during development and during the menstrual period. These pulses ensure that gonadotropins are released in a pulsatile manner. With the onset of puberty, the amplitude of the pulses of gonadotropins and, in turn, the sex steroids increases, first at night and then throughout the day. Adrenarche generally occurs several years earlier than gonadarche and is heralded by increasing circulating dehydroepiandrosterone (DHEA) or androstenedione. Serum DHEA increases years before the appearance of its effects.

The normal developmental sequence in girls is **thelarche** (due to gonadarche) followed closely by **pubarche** (due to adrenarche) and finally **menarche,** 2 to 3 years later. In boys the first normal event is scrotal thinning followed by the enlargement of testes and by the appearance of pubic hair

(long diameter of the testis greater than 2.5 cm, volume greater than 4 mL). Most of the enlargement of testes during puberty is the result of seminiferous tubule maturation.

DELAYED PUBERTY

Decision-Making Algorithm
Available @ StudentConsult.com

Pubertal Delay

Puberty is delayed when there is no sign of pubertal development by age 13 years in girls and 14 years in boys living in the United States (Tables 174-1 and 174-2).

Constitutional Delay in Growth and Adolescence

Patients with constitutional delay have delayed onset of pubertal development and significant bone age delay (2 standard deviations below the mean, which is equal to a 1.5- to 2-year delay as a teenager). The height of the patient should remain close to the genetic potential, based on the parental heights, when reinterpreted for bone age (see Chapter 173). Usually height gain is below, although fairly parallel to, the normal percentiles on the growth curve. The prepubertal nadir, or deceleration before their pubertal growth spurt, is prolonged or protracted. A family history of delayed puberty in a parent or sibling is reassuring. Spontaneous puberty usually begins in these patients by the time the bone age reaches 12 years in boys and 11 years in girls. Other causes of delayed puberty must be eliminated before a diagnosis of constitutional delay in puberty is made. Observation and reassurance are appropriate. Adult height normal for the genetic potential is generally attained. In some cases, boys may be treated with low-dose testosterone for a few months if the bone age is at least 11 to 12 years. Treatment is not required for longer than 4 to 8 months because endogenous hormone production usually ensues. Boys who do not initiate endogenous hormone production should be evaluated for other causes of hypogonadism. Estrogen treatment has been used in girls with constitutional delay, but there are no clear studies showing the added benefits. Young women with delayed puberty may need to be evaluated for primary amenorrhea.

Hypogonadotropic Hypogonadism

As a cause of delayed or absent puberty, hypogonadotropic hypogonadism may be difficult to distinguish from constitutional delay (see Tables 174-1 and 174-2). Hypogonadotropic hypogonadism precludes spontaneous entry into gonadarche; adrenarche usually occurs to some degree. Throughout childhood and in early puberty, patients with hypogonadotropic hypogonadism have normal proportions and growth. When these patients reach adulthood, *eunuchoid* proportions may ensue because their long bones grow for longer than normal, producing an upper-to-lower ratio below the lower limit of normal of 0.9 and an arm span greater than their height. If a patient has concurrent growth hormone (GH) deficiency, however, stature is exceptionally short, and the condition may have been diagnosed in infancy with a microphallus.

Table 174-1	Classification of Delayed Puberty and Sexual Infantilism

Constitutional delay in growth and puberty

Hypogonadotropic hypogonadism

CNS disorders

   Tumors (craniopharyngioma, germinoma, glioma, prolactinoma)

   Congenital malformations

   Radiation therapy

   Other causes

Isolated gonadotropin deficiency

   Kallmann syndrome (anosmia-hyposmia)

   Other disorders

Idiopathic and genetic forms of multiple pituitary hormone deficiencies

Miscellaneous disorders

   Prader-Willi syndrome

   Laurence-Moon-Bardet-Biedl syndrome

   Functional gonadotropin deficiency

      Chronic systemic disease and malnutrition

      Hypothyroidism

      Cushing disease

      Diabetes mellitus

      Hyperprolactinemia

      Anorexia nervosa

      Psychogenic amenorrhea

Impaired puberty and delayed menarche in female athletes and ballet dancers (exercise amenorrhea)

Hypergonadotropic hypogonadism

Klinefelter syndrome (syndrome of seminiferous tubular dysgenesis) and its variants

Other forms of primary testicular failure

Anorchia and cryptorchidism

Syndrome of gonadal dysgenesis and its variants (Turner syndrome)

Other forms of primary ovarian failure

XX and XY gonadal dysgenesis

   Familial and sporadic XX gonadal dysgenesis and its variants

   Familial and sporadic XY gonadal dysgenesis and its variants

Noonan syndrome

Galactosemia

Modified from Grumbach MM, Styne DM: Puberty. In Wilson JD, Foster DW, editors: Williams Textbook of Endocrinology, ed 9, Philadelphia, 1998, WB Saunders.
CNS, Central nervous system.

Isolated Gonadotropin Deficiency

Decision-Making Algorithms
Available @ StudentConsult.com

Pubertal Delay
Obesity

Disorders that can cause hypogonadism include congenital hypopituitarism, such as midline defects, tumors, infiltrative disease (hemochromatosis), and many syndromes, including Laurence-Moon-Bardet-Biedl, Prader-Willi, and Kallmann syndromes. If there is an inability to release gonadotropins but no other pituitary abnormality, the patient has isolated gonadotropin deficiency (almost universally a result of absent GnRH). Patients grow normally until the time of the pubertal growth spurt, when they fail to experience the accelerated growth characteristic of the normal growth spurt.

Kallmann syndrome combines isolated gonadotropin deficiency with disorders of olfaction. There is genetic heterogeneity; some patients have a decreased sense of smell, others have abnormal reproduction, and some have both. Most cases are sporadic but a number of patients may have mutations in the *KAL1* gene at Xp 22.3 (X chromosome) or *KAL2* gene. The mutation causes the GnRH neurons to remain ineffectually located in the primitive nasal area, rather than migrating to the correct location at the medial basal hypothalamus. Olfactory bulbs and olfactory sulci are often absent on magnetic resonance imaging (MRI). Other symptoms include disorders of the hand, with one hand copying the movements of the other hand, shortened fourth metacarpal bone, and an absent kidney.

Abnormalities of the Central Nervous System

Decision-Making Algorithms
Available @ StudentConsult.com

Amenorrhea
Pubertal Delay

Central nervous system (CNS) tumors, including pituitary adenoma, glioma, prolactinoma, or craniopharyngioma, are important causes of gonadotropin deficiency. Craniopharyngiomas have a peak incidence in the teenage years and may cause any type of anterior or posterior hormone deficiency. Craniopharyngiomas usually calcify, eroding the sella turcica when they expand. They may impinge on the optic chiasm, leading to bitemporal hemianopsia and optic atrophy. Other tumors that may affect pubertal development include astrocytomas and gliomas.

Idiopathic hypopituitarism is the congenital absence of various combinations of pituitary hormones. Although this disorder may occur in family constellations, in X-linked or autosomal recessive patterns, sporadic types of congenital idiopathic hypopituitarism are more common. Congenital hypopituitarism may manifest in a male with GH deficiency and associated gonadotropin deficiency with a microphallus or with hypoglycemia with seizures, especially if adrenocorticotropic hormone and GH deficiency occurs as well.

Syndromes of Hypogonadotropic Hypogonadism

Decision-Making Algorithms
Available @ StudentConsult.com

Amenorrhea
Pubertal Delay

| Table 174-2 | Differential Diagnostic Features of Delayed Puberty and Sexual Infantilism |

CAUSATIVE CONDITION/ DISORDER	STATURE	PLASMA GONADOTROPINS	GnRH TEST: LH RESPONSE	PLASMA GONADAL STEROIDS	PLASMA DHEAS	KARYOTYPE	OLFACTION
Constitutional delay in growth and adolescence	Short for chronologic age, usually appropriate for bone age	Prepubertal, later pubertal	Prepubertal, later pubertal	Prepubertal, later normal	Low for chronologic age, appropriate for bone age	Normal	Normal
HYPOGONADOTROPIC HYPOGONADISM							
Isolated gonadotropin deficiency	Normal, absent pubertal growth spurt	Low	Prepubertal or no response	Low	Appropriate for chronologic age	Normal	Normal
Kallmann syndrome	Normal, absent pubertal growth spurt	Low	Prepubertal or no response	Low	Appropriate for chronologic age	Normal	Anosmia or hyposmia
Idiopathic multiple pituitary hormone deficiencies	Short stature and poor growth since early childhood	Low	Prepubertal or no response	Low	Usually low	Normal	Normal
Hypothalamic-pituitary tumors	Decrease in growth velocity of late onset	Low	Prepubertal or no response	Low	Normal or low for chronologic age	Normal	Normal
PRIMARY GONADAL FAILURE							
Syndrome of gonadal dysgenesis and variants	Short stature since early childhood	High	Hyperresponsive for age	Low	Normal for chronologic age	XO or variant	Normal
Klinefelter syndrome and variants	Normal to tall	High	Hyperresponsive at puberty	Low or normal	Normal for chronologic age	XXY or variant	Normal
Familial XX or XY gonadal dysgenesis	Normal	High	Hyperresponsive for age	Low	Normal for chronologic age	XX or XY	Normal

From Grumbach MM, Styne DM: Puberty. In Wilson JD, Foster DW, editors: Williams Textbook of Endocrinology, ed 9, Philadelphia, 1997, WB Saunders.
DHEAS, Dehydroepiandrosterone sulfate; GnRH, gonadotropin-releasing hormone; LH, luteinizing hormone.

Decreased gonadotropin function occurs when voluntary dieting, malnutrition, or chronic disease results in weight loss to less than 80% of ideal weight. **Anorexia nervosa** is characterized by striking weight loss and psychiatric disorders (see Chapter 70). Primary or secondary amenorrhea frequently is found in affected girls, and pubertal development is absent or minimal, depending on the level of weight loss and the age at onset. Regaining weight to the ideal level may not immediately reverse the condition. Increased physical activity, even without weight loss, can lead to decreased menstrual frequency and gonadotropin deficiency in **athletic amenorrhea;** when physical activity is interrupted, menstrual function may return. Chronic or systemic illness (e.g., cystic fibrosis, diabetes mellitus, inflammatory bowel disease, or hematologic diseases) can lead to pubertal delay or to amenorrhea from hypothalamic dysfunction. **Hypothyroidism** inhibits the onset of puberty and delays menstrual periods. Conversely severe primary hypothyroidism may lead to precocious puberty.

Hypergonadotropic Hypogonadism

Decision-Making Algorithms
Available @ StudentConsult.com

Pubertal Delay
Gynecomastia

Hypergonadotropic hypogonadism is characterized by elevated gonadotropins and low sex steroid levels resulting from primary gonadal failure. This permanent condition is almost always diagnosed following the lack of entry into gonadarche and is not suspected throughout childhood. Gonadotropins do not increase to greater than normal until shortly before or around the normal time of puberty.

Ovarian failure is diagnosed by elevated gonadotropins. Turner syndrome, the syndrome of gonadal dysgenesis, is a common cause of ovarian failure and short stature. The karyotype is classically 45,XO, but other abnormalities of the

X chromosome or mosaicism are possible. The incidence of Turner syndrome is 1 in 2000 to 1 in 3000 births. The features of a girl with Turner syndrome need not be evident on physical examination or by history. The diagnosis must be considered in any girl who is short without a contributory history. Patients with other types of gonadal dysgenesis and galactosemia as well as patients treated undergoing radiation therapy or chemotherapy for malignancy may develop ovarian failure.

Klinefelter syndrome (seminiferous tubular dysgenesis) is the most common cause of **testicular failure**. The karyotype is 47,XXY, but variants with more X chromosomes are possible. The incidence is approximately 1 in 500 to 1 in 1000 in males. Testosterone levels may be close to normal, at least until mid-puberty, because Leydig cell function may be spared; however seminiferous tubular function characteristically is lost, causing infertility. Commonly LH levels may be normal to elevated, whereas FSH levels are usually more unequivocally elevated. The age of onset of puberty is usually normal, but secondary sexual changes may not progress because of inadequate Leydig cell function.

Primary Amenorrhea

Decision-Making Algorithms
Available @ StudentConsult.com

Amenorrhea
Pubertal Delay

In addition to other diagnoses mentioned, other conditions need to be considered when evaluating girls with lack of menses. The Mayer-Rokitansky-Kuster-Hauser syndrome of congenital absence of the uterus occurs in 1 in 4000 to 5000 female births. Anatomic obstruction by imperforate hymen or vaginal septum also presents with normal secondary sexual development without menstruation. The complete syndrome of **androgen insensitivity** includes normal feminization, absence of pubic or axillary hair, and primary amenorrhea. In this syndrome, all müllerian structures, including ovaries, uterus, fallopian tubes, and upper third of the vagina, are lacking; the karyotype is 46,XY, and subjects have intra-abdominal testes.

Evaluation

When no secondary sexual development is present after the upper age limits of normal pubertal development, serum gonadotropin levels should be obtained to determine whether the patient has a hypogonadotropic or hypergonadotropic hypogonadism (see Table 174-2). Based on gonadotropin measurements only, the differentiation between constitutional delay in growth and hypogonadotropic hypogonadism is difficult; the gonadotropin levels are low in both conditions. Sometimes observation for months or years is necessary before the diagnosis is confirmed. Ultrasound of the pelvic structures in females would be helpful in the workup of delayed puberty.

Treatment

If a permanent condition is apparent, replacement with sex steroids is indicated. Females are given transdermal estradiol, low-dose ethinyl estradiol (5 to 10 μg) or conjugated estrogens

(starting at 0.3 mg daily, increasing to 0.625 mg or 0.9 mg by 6 to 12 months later) in low daily doses until breakthrough bleeding occurs, at which time cycling is started with a dose for 25 days; on days 20 to 25, a progestational agent, such as medroxyprogesterone acetate (5 mg), is added to mimic the normal increases in gonadal hormones and to induce a normal menstrual period. Alternatively combined estrogen and progesterone agents (oral contraceptives) may be used after breakthrough bleeding occurs. In males testosterone enanthate or cypionate (50 to 100 mg monthly with a progressive increase to 100 to 200 mg) is given intramuscularly once every 4 weeks. This starting regimen is appropriate for patients with hypogonadotropic or hypergonadotropic hypogonadism, and doses are increased gradually to adult levels. Oral agents are not used for fear of hepatotoxicity. Patients with apparent constitutional delay in puberty who have, by definition, passed the upper limits of normal onset of puberty may be given a 3- to 6-month course of low-dose, sex-appropriate gonadal steroids to see whether spontaneous puberty occurs. This course of therapy might be repeated once without undue advancement of bone age. All patients with any form of delayed puberty are at risk for decreased bone density; adequate calcium intake is essential. Patients with hypogonadotropic hypogonadism may be able to achieve fertility by the administration of gonadotropin therapy or pulsatile hypothalamic-releasing hormone therapy administered by a programmable pump on an appropriate schedule. Subjects with hypergonadotropic hypogonadism have, by definition, a primary gonadal problem and are unlikely to achieve spontaneous fertility.

In subjects with **Turner syndrome**, the goals of therapy include promoting growth with exogenous human GH supplementation and induction of the secondary sexual characteristics and of menses with low-dose cyclic estrogen/progesterone replacement therapy. Patients with Turner syndrome have had successful pregnancies after in vitro fertilization with a donor ovum and endocrine support.

SEXUAL PRECOCITY

Decision-Making Algorithms
Available @ StudentConsult.com

Precocious Puberty in the Male
Precocious Puberty in the Female

Classification

Sexual precocity (**precocious puberty**) is classically defined as secondary sexual development occurring before the age of 9 years in boys or 8 years in girls (Tables 174-3 and 174-4). During the past 15 to 20 years, studies from the United States and Europe reported earlier breast development in girls, as compared to historical data. Studies clearly suggest an earlier age at puberty onset in American girls in the 1980s to 1990s compared to the 1930s and 1940s. However age at menarche occurred at the same time or slightly earlier. Thus the time span from breast development to menarche seemed to have increased. The findings could reflect that exogenous or lifestyle factors may influence the typical sequence of pubertal events.

Central precocious puberty, resulting in gonadarche, emanates from premature activation of the hypothalamic-pituitary-gonadal axis (GnRH-dependent). **Peripheral precocious**

Table 174-3 | Classification of Sexual Precocity

TRUE PRECOCIOUS PUBERTY OR COMPLETE ISOSEXUAL PRECOCITY

Idiopathic true precocious puberty

    CNS tumors

    Hamartomas (ectopic GnRH pulse generator)

    Other tumors

Other CNS disorders

True precocious puberty after late treatment of congenital virilizing adrenal hyperplasia

INCOMPLETE ISOSEXUAL PRECOCITY (GNRH-INDEPENDENT SEXUAL PRECOCITY)

Males

Chorionic gonadotropin-secreting tumors (hCG-dependent sexual precocity)

CNS tumors (e.g., germinoma, chorioepithelioma, teratoma)

Tumors in locations outside of the CNS (hepatoblastoma)

LH-secreting pituitary adenoma

Increased androgen secretion by adrenal or testis

Congenital adrenal hyperplasia (21-hydroxylase deficiency, 11-hydroxylase deficiency)

Virilizing adrenal neoplasm

Leydig cell adenoma

Familial testotoxicosis (familial premature gonadotropin-independent Leydig cell and germ cell maturation)

Females

Estrogen-secreting ovarian or adrenal neoplasms

Ovarian cysts

Males and females

McCune-Albright syndrome

Primary hypothyroidism

Peutz-Jeghers syndrome

Iatrogenic sexual precocity

VARIATIONS OF PUBERTAL DEVELOPMENT

Premature thelarche

Premature menarche

Premature adrenarche

Adolescent gynecomastia

CONTRASEXUAL PRECOCITY

Males (feminization)

Adrenal neoplasm

Increased extraglandular conversion of circulating steroids to estrogen

Females (virilization)

(Congenital adrenal hyperplasia, P-450$_{c21}$ deficiency, P-450$_{c11}$ deficiency, 3β-Hydroxysteroid dehydrogenase deficiency)

Virilizing adrenal neoplasms

Virilizing ovarian neoplasms (e.g., arrhenoblastomas)

From Grumbach MM, Styne DM: Puberty. In Wilson JD, Foster DW, editors: Williams Textbook of Endocrinology, ed 9, Philadelphia, 1998, WB Saunders. CNS, Central nervous system; GnRH, gonadotropin-releasing hormone; hCG, human chorionic gonadotropin; LH, luteinizing hormone.

puberty, gonadarche or adrenarche, does not involve the hypothalamic-pituitary-gonadal axis (GnRH-independent).

Central Precocious Puberty (GnRH-Dependent Precocious Puberty)

In central precocious puberty, every endocrine and physical aspect of pubertal development is normal but too early; this includes tall stature, advanced bone age consistent with somatic age, increased sex steroid and pulsatile gonadotropin secretion, and increased response of LH to GnRH. The clinical course of central precocious puberty may wax and wane. Benign precocious puberty is the presumptive diagnosis in individuals who begin puberty early on a **constitutional** or **familial** basis. If no cause can be determined, the diagnosis is idiopathic precocious puberty, which occurs much more often in girls than in boys. Obese girls have earlier adrenarche, and sometimes menarche as well, than appropriate-weight girls. Compared with girls, boys with precocious puberty have a higher incidence of CNS disorders, such as tumors and hamartomas, precipitating the precocious puberty.

Almost any condition that affects the CNS, including hydrocephalus, meningitis, encephalitis, suprasellar cysts, head trauma, epilepsy, mental retardation, and irradiation, can precipitate central precocious puberty and must be considered before central precocious puberty is diagnosed. **Hamartomas** are nonmalignant tumors of the tuber cinereum with a characteristic appearance on computed tomography (CT) or MRI; biopsy is rarely required. The mass of GnRH neurons secrete GnRH and cause precocious puberty. Although hamartomas are not true neoplasms, they may require neurosurgical attention. The resulting precocious puberty is responsive to medical therapy with GnRH agonists, and surgery is rarely indicated.

Other masses that cause precocious puberty are not benign. **Germinomas** are noncalcifying hypothalamic or pineal tumors that frequently produce human chorionic gonadotropin (hCG), which may cause sexual precocity in prepubertal boys (hCG cross-reacts with the LH receptor because of the similarity of structure between LH and hCG). **Optic** or **hypothalamic gliomas** (with or without neurofibromatosis), astrocytomas, and ependymomas may cause precocious puberty by disrupting the negative restraint of the areas of the CNS that normally inhibit pubertal development throughout childhood. These tumors may require radiotherapy, which contributes to a significant risk for hypopituitarism.

GnRH-Independent Precocious Puberty

Decision-Making Algorithm
Available @ StudentConsult.com

Precocious Puberty in the Female

The most common cause of GnRH-independent precocious puberty, **McCune-Albright syndrome,** is more frequent in girls than boys and includes precocious gonadarche, a bone disorder with polyostotic fibrous dysplasia, and hyperpigmented cutaneous macules (café au lait spots). The precocious gonadarche results from ovarian hyperfunction and sometimes cyst formation, leading to episodic estrogen secretion. This disorder results from a post-conception somatic

Table 174-4	Differential Diagnosis of Sexual Precocity				
CAUSATIVE DISORDER	**SERUM GONADOTROPIN CONCENTRATION***	**LH RESPONSE TO GNRH**	**SERUM SEX STEROID CONCENTRATIONS**	**GONADAL SIZE**	**MISCELLANEOUS**
True precocious puberty	Pubertal values	Pubertal	Pubertal values of testosterone or estradiol	Normal pubertal testicular enlargement or ovarian and uterine enlargement (by sonography)	MRI scan of brain to rule out CNS tumor or other abnormality; bone scan for McCune-Albright syndrome
Incomplete sexual precocity (pituitary gonadotropin-independent)					
Males					
Chorionic gonadotropin-secreting tumor in males	High hCG (low LH)	Prepubertal (suppressed)	Pubertal values of testosterone	Slight to moderate uniform enlargement of testes	Hepatomegaly suggests hepatoblastoma; MRI scan of brain if chorionic gonadotropin-secreting CNS tumor suspected
Leydig cell tumor in males	Suppressed	Suppressed	Very high testosterone	Irregular asymmetric enlargement of testes	
Familial testotoxicosis	Suppressed	Suppressed	Pubertal values of testosterone	Testes symmetric and >2.5 cm but smaller than expected for pubertal development; spermatogenesis may occur	Familial; probably sex-linked, autosomal dominant trait
Premature adrenarche	Prepubertal	Prepubertal	Prepubertal testosterone; DHEAS values appropriate for pubic hair stage 2	Testes prepubertal	Onset usually after 6 yr of age; more frequent in brain-injured children
Females					
Granulosa cell tumor (presentation may be similar to that with follicular cysts)	Suppressed	Suppressed	Very high estradiol	Ovarian enlargement on physical examination, MRI, CT, or sonography	Tumor often palpable on abdominal examination
Follicular cyst	Suppressed	Suppressed	Prepubertal to very high estradiol values	Ovarian enlargement on physical examination, MRI, CT, or sonography	Single or repetitive episodes; exclude McCune-Albright syndrome (e.g., perform skeletal survey and inspect skin)
Feminizing adrenal tumor	Suppressed	Suppressed	High estradiol and DHEAS values	Ovaries prepubertal	Unilateral adrenal mass
Premature thelarche	Prepubertal	Prepubertal	Prepubertal or early pubertal estradiol	Ovaries prepubertal	Onset usually before 3 yr of age
Premature adrenarche	Prepubertal	Prepubertal	Prepubertal estradiol; DHEAS values appropriate for pubic hair Tanner stage 2	Ovaries prepubertal	Onset usually after 6 yr of age; more frequent in brain-injured children

Modified from Grumbach MM, Styne DM: Puberty. In Wilson JD, Foster DW, editors: Williams Textbook of Endocrinology, ed 9, Philadelphia, 1997, WB Saunders.
CNS, Central nervous system; CT, computed tomography; DHEAS, dehydroepiandrosterone sulfate; GnRH, gonadotropin-releasing hormone; hCG, human chorionic gonadotropin; LH, luteinizing hormone; MRI, magnetic resonance imaging.
*In supersensitive assays.

mutation in the G protein intracellular signaling system (specifically G_{sa}, which leads to unregulated constitutive activation of adenylate cyclase, and of cAMP in the absence of trophic hormone stimulation), in the affected cells in ovary, bone, and skin; other endocrine organs may also autonomously hyperfunction for the same reason. Hyperthyroidism, hyperadrenalism, or acromegaly may occur. **Adrenal carcinomas** usually secrete adrenal androgens, such as DHEA; **adrenal adenomas** may virilize a child as a result of the production of androgen or may feminize a child as a result of the production of estrogen.

Boys may have precocious gonadarche on the basis of a rare entity called **familial GnRH-independent sexual precocity with premature Leydig cell maturation.** This condition, with germ cell maturation caused by an X-limited dominant defect, produces constitutive activation of the LH receptor that leads to continuous production and secretion of testosterone without requiring LH or hCG.

The **hCG-secreting tumors** stimulate LH receptors and increase testosterone secretion. These tumors may be found in various places, including the pineal gland (dysgerminomas) or the liver (hepatoblastoma).

Ovarian cysts may occur once or may be recurrent. High serum estrogen values may mimic ovarian tumors. **Congenital adrenal hyperplasia (CAH)** is a cause of virilization in girls (see Chapter 178).

Evaluation of Sexual Precocity

The first step in evaluating sexual precocity is to determine which characteristics of normal puberty are apparent (see Chapter 67) and whether estrogen effects, androgen effects, or both are present (see Table 174-4). In girls the estrogen effect manifests as breast development, uterine increase, and, eventually, menarche. Both boys and girls manifest the androgen effect as adult body odor, pubic and axillary hair, and facial skin oiliness and acne. In boys it is also important to note whether the testes are enlarged more than 2.5 cm in length (4 mL volume), which implies gonadarche. If the testes are not enlarged but virilization is progressing, the source of the androgens may be the adrenal glands or exogenous sources.

Laboratory evaluation includes determination of sex steroid levels (testosterone, estradiol, DHEAS [dehydroepiandrosterone sulfate], or androstenedione) and baseline gonadotropin concentrations. The inherent nature of gonadotropin secretion is characterized by low secretory rates throughout childhood and pulsatile secretion in adolescents and adults. If baseline gonadotropin values are elevated into the normal pubertal range, central precocious puberty is likely. If baseline gonadotropins are low, however, no immediate conclusion may be drawn as to GnRH-dependent versus GnRH-independent precocious puberty. This distinction often requires the assessment of gonadotropin responsiveness to GnRH stimulation. A prepubertal GnRH response is FSH predominant, whereas a pubertal response is more LH predominant. Thyroid hormone determination also is useful because severe primary hypothyroidism can cause incomplete precocious puberty. If there is a suggestion of a CNS anomaly or a tumor (CNS, hepatic, adrenal, ovarian, or testicular), MRI of the appropriate location is indicated. The diagnosis of central precocious puberty mandates that an MRI of the CNS be performed.

Treatment

Long-acting, superactive analogs of GnRH (leuprolide depot, histrelin depot) are the treatment of choice for central precocious puberty. They suppress gonadotropin secretion by downregulating GnRH receptors in the pituitary gonadotropes (Table 174-5), causing gonadal secretion to revert to the prepubertal state. Boys with GnRH-independent premature Leydig cell and germ cell maturation do not respond to GnRH analogs but require treatment with an inhibitor of testosterone synthesis (e.g., ketoconazole), an antiandrogen (e.g., spironolactone), or an aromatase inhibitor (e.g., testolactone or letrozole). Patients with precocious puberty from a hormone-secreting tumor require surgical removal, if possible. The precocious puberty of the McCune-Albright syndrome is GnRH independent and unresponsive to therapy with GnRH

Table 174-5	Pharmacologic Therapy of Sexual Precocity	
DISORDER	**TREATMENT**	**ACTION AND RATIONALE**
GnRH-dependent true or central precocious puberty	GnRH agonists	Desensitization of gonadotropes; blocks action of endogenous GnRH
GnRH-independent incomplete sexual precocity *Girls*		
Autonomous ovarian cysts	Medroxyprogesterone acetate	Inhibition of ovarian steroidogenesis; regression of cyst (inhibition of FSH release)
McCune-Albright syndrome	Medroxyprogesterone acetate*	Inhibition of ovarian steroidogenesis; regression of cyst (inhibition of FSH release)
Boys	Testolactone*	Inhibition of P-450 aromatase; blocks estrogen synthesis
Familial GnRH-independent sexual precocity with premature Leydig cell maturation	Ketoconazole* Spironolactone* or flutamide *and* testolactone or fadrozole Medroxyprogesterone acetate*	Inhibition of P-450$_{c17}$ (mainly 17,20-lyase activity) Antiandrogen inhibition of aromatase; blocks estrogen synthesis Inhibition of testicular steroidogenesis

Modified from Grumbach MM, Kaplan SL: Recent advances in the diagnosis and management of sexual precocity, Acta Paediatr Jpn *30(Suppl):155, 1988.*
FSH, Follicle-stimulating hormone; GnRH, gonadotropin-releasing hormone.
*If true precocious puberty develops, a GnRH agonist can be added.

analog. Therapy is provided with testolactone and antiandrogens or antiestrogen, such as tamoxifen.

VARIATIONS IN PUBERTAL DEVELOPMENT
Isolated Premature Thelarche (Premature Breast Development)

Decision-Making Algorithm
Available @ StudentConsult.com

Precocious Puberty in the Female

Benign **premature thelarche** is the isolated appearance of unilateral or bilateral breast tissue in girls, usually at ages 6 months to 3 years. There are no other signs of puberty and no evidence of excessive estrogen effect (vaginal bleeding, thickening of the vaginal secretions, increased height velocity, or bone age acceleration). Ingestion or dermal application of estrogen-containing compounds must be excluded. Laboratory investigations are not usually necessary, but a pelvic ultrasound study rarely may be indicated to exclude ovarian disease. Girls with this condition should be re-evaluated at intervals of 6 to 12 months to ensure that apparent premature thelarche is not the beginning of progression into precocious puberty. The prognosis is excellent; if no progression occurs, no treatment other than reassurance is necessary.

Gynecomastia

Decision-Making Algorithm
Available @ StudentConsult.com

Gynecomastia

In males breast tissue is termed *gynecomastia,* and it may occur to some degree in 45% to 75% of normal pubertal boys (see Chapter 67). Androgens normally are converted to estrogen by aromatization; in early puberty, only modest amounts of androgens are produced, and the estrogen effect can overwhelm the androgen effects at this stage. Later in pubertal development, the androgen production is so great that there is little effect from the estrogen produced by aromatization. Gynecomastia also can suggest the possibility of Klinefelter syndrome as puberty progresses. Prepubertal gynecomastia suggests an unusual source of estrogen either from exogenous sources (oral or dermal estrogen administration is possible from contamination of food or ointments) or from endogenous sources (from abnormal function of adrenal gland or ovary or from increased peripheral aromatization).

Isolated Premature Adrenarche (Pubarche)

Decision-Making Algorithms
Available @ StudentConsult.com

Amenorrhea
Precocious Puberty in the Male
Precocious Puberty in the Female

The isolated appearance of pubic hair before age 6 to 7 years in girls or before age 9 years in boys is termed **premature pubarche,** usually resulting from adrenarche. It is relatively common. If the pubic hair is associated with any other feature of virilization (clitoral or penile enlargement or advanced bone age) or other signs (acne, rapid growth, or voice change), a detailed investigation for a pathologic cause of virilization is indicated. Measurements of serum testosterone, 17-hydroxyprogesterone, and DHEAS are indicated to investigate the possibility of CAH. Ultrasound studies may reveal a hyperplastic adrenal gland or a virilizing adrenal or ovarian tumor. Most patients with isolated pubic hair do not have progressive virilization and simply have premature adrenarche (*pubarche*) resulting from premature activation of DHEA secretion from the adrenal gland. The skeletal maturation, as assessed by bone age, may be slightly advanced and the height slightly increased, but testosterone concentrations are normal. DHEA levels usually are high for prepubertal age but are consistent with Tanner (sexuality maturity rating) stages II and III.

Chapter 175

THYROID DISEASE

THYROID PHYSIOLOGY AND DEVELOPMENT

Thyrotropin-releasing hormone (TRH), a tripeptide synthesized in the hypothalamus, stimulates the release of pituitary thyroid-stimulating hormone (TSH). Pituitary TSH is a glycoprotein that stimulates the synthesis and release of thyroid hormones by the thyroid gland. Thyroid function develops in three stages. At the end of the first trimester, the gland descends from the floor of the primitive oral cavity to its definitive position in the anterior lower neck. The hypothalamic-pituitary-thyroid axis becomes functional in the second trimester. Peripheral metabolism of thyroid hormones matures in the third trimester.

Thyroxine (T_4), triiodothyronine (T_3), and TSH do not cross the placenta in significant amounts. Concentrations in fetal serum reflect primarily fetal secretion and metabolism. Maternal thyroid antibodies, iodides (including radioactive iodides), and medications given to mothers to treat hyperthyroidism (methimazole and propylthiouracil) cross the placenta and affect fetal thyroid function. An infant born prematurely or with intrauterine growth restriction may have an interruption of the normal maturational process and appear to have hypothyroidism by standard tests.

The thyroid gland concentrates iodine and binds it to tyrosine molecules to produce either monoiodotyrosine or diiodotyrosine, with subsequent coupling of two tyrosines, T_4 or T_3. The major fraction of circulating T_3 (approximately two thirds) is derived from peripheral deiodination of T_4 to T_3, but some is produced by the thyroid gland itself. The conversion of T_4 to T_3 requires the removal of one iodine from the outer ring

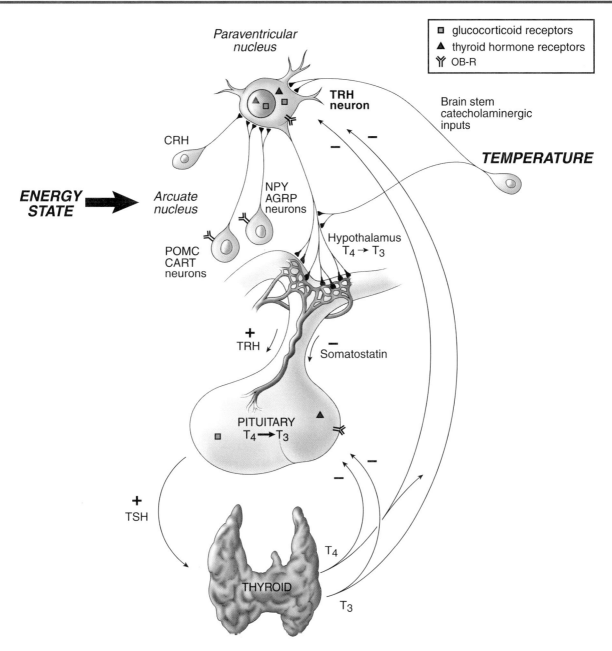

Figure 175-1 Interrelationships of the hypothalamic-pituitary-thyroid axis. Thyroid-stimulating hormone (TSH) from the pituitary gland stimulates the secretion of thyroxine (T_4) and triiodothyronine (T_3) from the thyroid gland. These act at the pituitary gland level to control secretion of TSH by a negative feedback mechanism. In addition, T_4 is metabolized to the potent T_3 within the pituitary gland by a deiodinase. Secretion of TSH is stimulated by thyrotropin-releasing hormone (TRH) from the hypothalamus and inhibited by somatostatin. Thyroid hormone acts at the hypothalamus to stimulate secretion of somatostatin (somatostatin acts as a negative signal to the pituitary secretion of TSH). *CRH*, Corticotropin-releasing hormone; *OB-R*, leptin receptor. *(From Melmed S, Polonsky K, Kronenberg H, Larsen R, editors: Williams Textbook of Endocrinology, ed 10, Philadelphia, 2003, Saunders, p 101.)*

of tyrosine; removing an iodine from the inner ring results in reverse T_3, which has little biologic effect. Preferential conversion of T_4 to reverse T_3 rather than T_3 occurs in utero and in all forms of severe illness, including respiratory distress syndrome, fevers, anorexia, cachexia, and starvation. Conversion from T_4 to T_3 increases immediately after birth and throughout life. T_4 and T_3 are noncovalently bound to a specific serum carrier protein, **thyroxine-binding globulin,** and, to a lesser extent, albumin. Only small (<0.02%) fractions of T_4 and T_3 are not bound; free T_4 (as it is converted to free T_3) and free T_3 are biologically active. Free T_3 exerts metabolic effects and negative feedback on TSH release (Fig. 175-1).

Serum TSH increases just after birth but soon decreases to lower values considered normal for later life. T_4 secretion increases after birth as a result of the peak in TSH and because of maturation of thyroid metabolism. It is important to refer to age-adjusted normative data to interpret thyroid function tests properly, whether relative to making diagnoses of hyperthyroidism or hypothyroidism or when adjusting therapy. Free T_4 is the test of choice because it eliminates the effects of variation in protein binding, which can be substantial.

Table 175-1 summarizes laboratory test results in various types of thyroid abnormalities. In usual circumstances, plasma concentrations of TSH above the normal range indicate

Table 175-1	Laboratory Test Results in Various Types of Thyroid Function Abnormalities in Children*			
	SERUM			
ABNORMALITY	**TOTAL T$_4$**	**FREE T$_4$**	**SERUM TSH**	**SERUM TBG**
Primary hypothyroidism	↓	↓	↑	N
Hypothalamic (TRH) tertiary hypothyroidism	↓	↓	↓	N
Pituitary (TSH) secondary hypothyroidism	↓	↓	↓	N
TBG deficiency	↓	N	N	↓
TBG excess	↑	N	N	↑

↓, decreased; *↑*, increased; *N*, Normal; *T$_4$*, thyroxine; *TBG*, thyroxine-binding globulin; *TRH*, thyrotropin-releasing hormone; *TSH*, thyroid-stimulating hormone.
*TSH may be slightly elevated.

primary hypothyroidism, and concentrations below the normal range most often indicate the presence of hyperthyroidism. Thyroid scans with 99m-pertechnetate or 123-I-iodine are occasionally indicated in the evaluation of pediatric thyroid disease. They can be useful in identifying thyroid agenesis or ectopic thyroid tissue.

THYROID DISORDERS
Hypothyroidism

Decision-Making Algorithms
Available @ StudentConsult.com

Short Stature
Pubertal Delay
Precocious Puberty in the Male
Precocious Puberty in the Female

Hypothyroidism is diagnosed by a decreased serum free T$_4$ and may be the result of diseases of the thyroid gland (primary hypothyroidism), abnormalities of the pituitary gland (secondary), or abnormalities of the hypothalamus (tertiary). Hypothyroidism is congenital or acquired and may be associated with a goiter (Table 175-2).

Congenital Hypothyroidism
Congenital hypothyroidism occurs in approximately 1 in 2000 to 4000 live births and is caused by dysgenesis (agenesis, aplasia, ectopia) or, less often, dyshormonogenesis (e.g., enzyme defects). Thyroid tissue usually is not palpable in these sporadic nongoitrous conditions. Dyshormonogenesis, disorders of intrathyroid metabolism, or goitrous congenital hypothyroidism occurs in about 1 in 30,000 live births. A goiter reflects an inborn error of metabolism in the pathway of iodide incorporation or thyroid hormone biosynthesis or reflects the transplacental passage of antithyroid drugs given to the mother. The free T$_4$ concentration is low, and the TSH level is elevated. Routine neonatal screening programs to measure cord blood or, more often, heel-stick TSH values occur in every state in the United States. An immediate confirmatory serum sample should be obtained from any infant having a positive result on a **screening test**. A low free T$_4$ and high TSH confirm the finding.

Table 175-2	Causes of Hypothyroidism in Infancy and Childhood	
AGE GROUP	**MANIFESTATION**	**CAUSE**
Newborn	No goiter	Thyroid gland dysgenesis or ectopic location Exposure to iodides TSH deficiency TRH deficiency
	+/– Goiter	Inborn defect in hormone synthesis* or effect Maternal goitrogen ingestion, including propylthiouracil, methimazole, iodides Severe iodide deficiency (endemic)
Child	No goiter	Thyroid gland dysgenesis Cystinosis Hypothalamic-pituitary insufficiency Surgical after thyrotoxicosis or other thyroid surgery
	Goiter	Hashimoto thyroiditis: chronic lymphocytic thyroiditis Inborn defect in hormone synthesis or effect Goitrogenic drugs infiltrative (sarcoid, lymphoma)

TRH, Thyrotropin-releasing hormone; *TSH*, thyroid-stimulating hormone.
*Impaired iodide transport, defective thyroglobulin iodination, defective iodotyrosine dehalogenase, or defective thyroglobulin or its coupling to iodotyrosine.

Isolated secondary or tertiary hypothyroidism occurs in 1 in 100,000 live births; the free T$_4$ is normal to low. When tertiary or secondary hypothyroidism is detected, assessment of other pituitary hormones and investigation of pituitary-hypothalamic anatomy via magnetic resonance imaging are indicated. Although not a hypothyroid condition, **congenital thyroxine-binding globulin deficiency** occurs in about 1 in 10,000 live births and is associated with low serum total T$_4$ concentration, normal TSH, and normal serum free T$_4$. This is a euthyroid condition and does not require treatment with thyroid hormone because it is merely a binding protein abnormality. It is commonly X-linked dominant.

Clinical manifestations of congenital hypothyroidism in the immediate newborn period usually are subtle but become more evident weeks or months after birth. By then it is too late to ensure that there is not a detriment to the infant's cognitive development. Newborn screening is crucial to make an early diagnosis and initiate thyroid replacement therapy by younger than 1 month of age. Findings at various stages after birth include hypothermia, acrocyanosis, respiratory distress, large fontanels, abdominal distention, lethargy and poor feeding, prolonged jaundice, edema, umbilical hernia, mottled skin, constipation, large tongue, dry skin, and hoarse cry. Thyroid hormones are crucial for maturation and differentiation of tissues, such as bone and brain (most thyroid-dependent brain maturation occurs 2 to 3 years after birth) (Table 175-3).

When **treatment** (with levothyroxine) is initiated within 1 month or less after birth, the prognosis for normal intellectual development is excellent; screening programs usually offer therapy within 1 to 2 weeks of birth. If therapy is instituted after 6 months, when the signs of severe hypothyroidism are present, the likelihood of normal intellectual function is markedly decreased. Growth improves after thyroid replacement even in late diagnosed cases. The dose of levothyroxine changes with age; 10 to 15 µg/kg of levothyroxine is used for a newborn, but about 3 µg/kg is used later in childhood. In neonatal hypothyroidism, the goal is to bring the serum free T_4 rapidly into the upper half of the range of normal. Suppression of TSH is not seen and not necessary in all cases because such suppression may lead to excessive doses of levothyroxine.

Acquired Hypothyroidism

The **etiology** of acquired hypothyroidism is presented in Table 175-2. The clinical manifestations may be subtle. Hypothyroidism should be suspected in any child who has a decline in growth velocity, especially if **not** associated with weight loss (see Table 175-3). The most common cause of acquired hypothyroidism in older children in the United States is lymphocytic autoimmune thyroiditis (**Hashimoto thyroiditis**). In many areas of the world, iodine deficiency is the etiology of endemic goiter (**endemic cretinism**). The failure of the thyroid gland may be heralded by an increase of TSH before T_4 levels decrease. In contrast to untreated congenital hypothyroidism, acquired hypothyroidism is not a cause of permanent developmental delay.

Hashimoto thyroiditis. Also known as autoimmune or *lymphocytic thyroiditis,* Hashimoto thyroiditis is a common cause of goiter and acquired thyroid disease in older children and adolescents. A family history of thyroid disease is present in 25% to 35% of patients. The *etiology* is an autoimmune process targeted against the thyroid gland with lymphocytic infiltration and lymphoid follicle and germinal center formation preceding fibrosis and atrophy.

Clinical manifestations include a firm, nontender euthyroid, hypothyroid, or, rarely, hyperthyroid (hashitoxicosis) diffuse goiter with a pebble-like surface. See Table 175-3 for signs and symptoms, which can be diverse. Onset typically occurs after 6 years of age with a peak incidence in adolescence with a female predominance. Associated autoimmune diseases include diabetes mellitus type 1 (DM1), adrenal insufficiency, and hypoparathyroidism. **Autoimmune polyglandular syndrome type I** consists of hypoparathyroidism, Addison disease, mucocutaneous candidiasis and, often, hypothyroidism. **Autoimmune polyglandular syndrome type II** consists of Addison disease, DM1, and frequently autoimmune

Table 175-3	Symptoms and Signs of Hypothyroidism

ECTODERMAL

Poor growth

Dull facies: thick lips, large tongue, depressed nasal bridge, periorbital edema

Dry scaly skin

Sparse brittle hair

Diminished sweating

Carotenemia

Vitiligo

CIRCULATORY

Sinus bradycardia/heart block

Cold extremities

Cold intolerance

Pallor

ECG changes: low-voltage QRS complex

NEUROMUSCULAR

Muscle weakness

Hypotonia: constipation, potbelly

Umbilical hernia

Myxedema coma (carbon dioxide narcosis, hypothermia)

Pseudohypertrophy of muscles

Myalgia

Physical and mental lethargy

Developmental delay

Delayed relaxation of reflexes

Paresthesias (nerve entrapment: carpal tunnel syndrome)

Cerebellar ataxia

SKELETAL

Delayed bone age

Epiphyseal dysgenesis, increased upper-to-lower segment ratio

METABOLIC

Myxedema

Serous effusions (pleural, pericardial, ascites)

Hoarse voice (cry)

Weight gain

Menstrual irregularity

Arthralgia

Elevated CK

Macrocytosis (anemia)

Hypercholesterolemia

Hyperprolactinemia

Precocious puberty in severe cases

CK, Creatine kinase; ECG, electrocardiographic.

hypothyroidism. Trisomy 21 and Turner syndrome are predisposed to the development of autoimmune thyroiditis.

The **diagnosis** may be confirmed by serum antithyroid peroxidase (previously antimicrosomal) and antithyroglobulin antibodies. Neither biopsy nor thyroid scan is indicated in

Hashimoto thyroiditis, although the thyroid scan with reduced uptake may differentiate hashitoxicosis from Graves disease.

Treatment with thyroid hormone sufficient to normalize TSH and free T_4 is indicated for hypothyroidism in Hashimoto thyroiditis. Patients without manifestation of hypothyroidism require thyroid function testing (serum TSH and free T_4) every 6 to 12 months to detect the later development of hypothyroidism. Goiter with a normal TSH usually is not an indication for treatment.

Hyperthyroidism

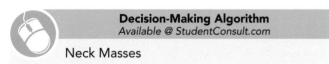

Decision-Making Algorithm
Available @ StudentConsult.com

Neck Masses

Graves Disease

Most children with hyperthyroidism have Graves disease, the autonomous functioning of the thyroid caused by autoantibodies [thyroid stimulating immunoglobulins (TSIs)] stimulating the thyroid. The resulting excessive synthesis, release, and peripheral metabolism of thyroid hormones produce the clinical features. Hashimoto thyroiditis and thyrotoxicosis are on a continuum of autoimmune diseases; there is overlap in their immunologic findings. Antithyroid peroxidase and antithyroglobulin antibodies may be present in thyrotoxicosis, although the values are usually lower than in Hashimoto thyroiditis. Exceptionally high titers of antibodies may indicate the thyrotoxic phase of Hashimoto thyroiditis with the subsequent evolution toward permanent hypothyroidism. In Graves disease, serum free T_4 or T_3 or both levels are elevated, whereas TSH is suppressed. Rare causes of hyperthyroidism include McCune-Albright syndrome, thyroid nodule (often an adenoma), TSH hypersecretion, subacute thyroiditis, and iodine or thyroid hormone ingestion.

Clinical manifestations. Graves disease presents as hyperthyroidism (Table 175-4) and is about five times more common in girls than in boys, with a peak incidence in adolescence. Personality changes, mood instability, and poor school performance are common initial problems. Tremor, anxiety, inability to concentrate, and weight loss may be insidious and confused with a psychological disorder until thyroid function tests reveal the elevated serum free T_4 level. In rare cases, serum free T_4 may be near-normal whereas serum T_3 is selectively elevated (T_3 toxicosis). A firm homogeneous goiter is usually present. Many patients complain of neck fullness. Thyroid gland enlargement is best visualized with the neck only slightly extended and with the examiner lateral to the patient. Palpation of the thyroid gland is best performed with the examiner's hands around the neck from the back. The patient swallows so that the examiner can feel and examine the size, consistency, nodularity and motion of the gland. The examiner should watch the patient swallow to note any discernible enlargement or asymmetry of the thyroid lobes. Auscultation may reveal a bruit over the gland that needs to be differentiated from a carotid bruit.

Treatment. Three treatment choices are available: pharmacologic, radioactive iodine, and surgical.

Drugs. Medical therapy to block thyroid hormone synthesis consists of methimazole (0.4 to 0.6 mg/kg/day once or

Table 175-4	Clinical Manifestations of Hyperthyroidism
ASSOCIATED CHANGE	**SIGN/SYMPTOM**
Increased catecholamine effects	Nervousness
	Palpitations
	Tachycardia
	Atrial arrhythmias
	Systolic hypertension
	Tremor
	Brisk reflexes
Hypermetabolism	Increased sweating
	Shiny, smooth skin
	Heat intolerance
	Fatigue
	Weight loss—increased appetite
	Increased bowel movement (hyperdefecation)
	Hyperkinesis
Myopathy	Weakness
	Periodic paralysis
	Cardiac failure—dyspnea
Miscellaneous	Proptosis, stare, exophthalmos, lid lag, ophthalmopathy
	Hair loss
	Inability to concentrate
	Personality change (emotional lability)
	Goiter
	Thyroid bruit
	Onycholysis
	Painful gland*
	Acute thyroid storm (hyperpyrexia, tachycardia, coma, high-output heart failure, shock)

*Unusual except in subacute thyroiditis with hyperthyroid phase.

twice daily) or propylthiouracil (5 to 7 mg/kg/day divided every 8 hours). Both medications are equally effective, however, propylthiouracil is no longer a first-line therapy secondary to concerns of severe liver injury and acute liver failure. A beta blocker, such as propranolol or atenolol, is started if symptoms are severe to control cardiac manifestations and is tapered as the methimazole takes effect. Antithyroid medication is usually continued for 1 to 2 years because the remission rate is approximately 25% per year. In patients complying with the treatment regimen, the 2-year course of treatment can be repeated. Medication should suppress thyroid function to normal, without the need to add thyroid hormone replacement to normalize serum free T_4. Complications of methimazole are muscle pain, rash, granulocytopenia, and jaundice. The granulocytopenia is an idiosyncratic complication of rapid onset, which is observed only in the early months after institution of antithyroid medication and requires monitoring the complete blood count. If a suppressed white blood cell count is observed, antithyroid therapy must be discontinued. This potentially lethal rare complication affects 3 in 10,000 users a year. After resolution, the other of the two antithyroid medications can be started because there is usually less than a 50% chance of a similar reaction from the other medication. Iodine administration, which may suppress thyroid function but becomes ineffective in a few weeks, is sometimes used as a preparation for surgery but never for long-term therapy.

Radioiodine. Radioiodine (^{131}I) is slower in exerting therapeutic effects, may require repeated dosing, and is likely to cause permanent hypothyroidism. Hypothyroidism is the desired outcome because it is easier and safer to treat than continued hyperthyroidism. Although studies reveal no long-term consequences, concern remains about possible sequelae in children. This method of treatment is entering the mainstream for children and adolescents. Radioiodine given to a pregnant teenager renders the fetus hypothyroid and is contraindicated.

Surgery. Surgical treatment consists of partial or complete thyroidectomy. Risks associated with thyroidectomy include the use of anesthesia and the possibility that the thyroid removal will be excessive causing hypothyroidism or that it will be inadequate resulting in persistent hyperthyroidism. In addition, keloid formation, recurrent laryngeal nerve palsy, and hypoparathyroidism (transient postoperative or permanent) may occur. Thyroid storm caused by the release of large amounts of preformed hormone is a serious but rare complication. Even with optimal immediate postoperative results, patients may become hypothyroid within 10 years.

Thyroid Storm

Thyroid storm (see Table 175-4) is a rare medical emergency consisting of tachycardia, disorientation, elevated blood pressure, and hyperthermia. Treatment includes reducing the hyperthermia with a cooling blanket and administering a beta blocker to control the tachycardia, hypertension, and autonomic hyperfunction symptoms. Iodine may be given to block thyroid hormone release after an antithyroid medication is started. Hydrocortisone may be indicated for relative adrenal insufficiency, and therapy for heart failure includes diuretics and digoxin.

Congenital Hyperthyroidism

This disorder results from transplacental passage of maternal TSIs and may be masked for several days until the short-lived effects of transplacental maternal antithyroid medication wear off (assuming the mother was receiving such medication), at which time the effects of TSIs are observed. Irritability, tachycardia (often with signs of cardiac failure simulating *cardiomyopathy*), polycythemia, craniosynostosis, bone age advancement, poor feeding, and failure to thrive are the clinical hallmarks. This condition may be anticipated if the mother is known to be thyrotoxic in pregnancy. Cure of hyperthyroidism before pregnancy (surgery or radioiodine treatment) limits or curtails T_4 production but not the underlying immune disturbance producing TSIs; thus the infant still may be affected, at least transiently.

Treatment for a severely affected neonate includes methimazole and, as needed, a beta blocker to help decrease symptoms. Because the half-life of the immunoglobulin is several weeks, spontaneous resolution of neonatal thyrotoxicosis resulting from transplacental passage of TSIs usually occurs by 2 to 3 months of age. Observation without treatment is indicated in patients who are minimally affected.

NODULES/TUMORS OF THE THYROID

About 2% of children develop solitary thyroid nodules, most of which are benign. Evaluation of a nodule includes thyroid function tests, neck ultrasound, and, if needed, fine-needle aspiration (FNA). Ultrasound guidance may be needed for aspiration of small nodules or those not palpable. Nodules found to be benign on FNA may be monitored through clinical exam and ultrasound.

Carcinoma of the thyroid is rare in children (1% of all pediatric cancers in the 5- to 9-year-old age group and up to 7% of cancers in the 15- to 19-year-old age group). Papillary and follicular carcinomas represent 90% of childhood thyroid cancers. A history of therapeutic head or neck irradiation or radiation exposure from nuclear accidents predisposes a child to thyroid cancer. Carcinoma usually presents as a firm to hard, painless nonfunctional solitary nodule and may spread to adjacent lymph nodes. Rapid growth, hoarseness (recurrent laryngeal nerve involvement), and lung metastasis may be present. If the nodule is solid on ultrasound, is *cold* on radioiodine scanning, and feels hard, the likelihood of a carcinoma is high. Excisional biopsy usually is performed, but FNA biopsy also may be diagnostic.

Treatment includes total thyroidectomy, selective regional node dissection, and radioablation with ^{131}I for residual or recurrent disease. The **prognosis** is usually good if the disease is diagnosed early.

Medullary carcinoma of the thyroid may be asymptomatic except for a mass. Diagnosis is based on the presence of elevated calcitonin levels, either in the basal state or after pentagastrin stimulation (difficult to obtain) and histologic examination. This tumor most often occurs with multiple endocrine neoplasia 2a or 2b (MEN), possibly in a familial pattern. In some families, the presence of mutations of the *RET* proto-oncogene is predictive of the development of medullary carcinoma of the thyroid. The location of the mutation can help determine when removal of the thyroid is warranted. Genetic screening of other members of the family is indicated after a proband is recognized. Prophylactic thyroidectomy is indicated for the family members with the same allele.

Chapter 176

DISORDERS OF PARATHYROID BONE AND MINERAL ENDOCRINOLOGY

PARATHYROID HORMONE AND VITAMIN D

Calcium and phosphate are regulated mainly by diet and three hormones: parathyroid hormone (PTH), vitamin D, and calcitonin. PTH is secreted in response to a decrease in serum ionized calcium level. PTH attaches to its membrane receptor then acts via adenylate cyclase to mobilize calcium from bone into the serum and to enhance fractional reabsorption of calcium by the kidney while inducing phosphate excretion; all increase the serum calcium concentration and decrease serum phosphate. Lack of PTH effect is heralded by low serum calcium in the presence of elevated phosphate for age. PTH stimulates vitamin D secretion by increasing renal 1α-hydroxylase activity and acts indirectly to elevate serum calcium concentration by stimulating the production of 1,25-dihydroxyvitamin D from 25-hydroxyvitamin D. Calcitonin increases the deposition of calcium into bone; in normal states the effect is subtle, but calcitonin may be used temporarily to suppress extremely elevated serum calcium values.

1,25-dihydroxyvitamin D enhances calcium absorption from the gastrointestinal tract, increasing serum calcium levels and bone mineralization. Vitamin D is derived from exposure of the skin to ultraviolet rays (usually via the sun) or from oral ingestion. It is modified first to 25-hydroxyvitamin D in the liver and then 1α-hydroxylated to the metabolically active form (1,25-dihydroxyvitamin D) in the kidney. The serum concentration of 25-hydroxyvitamin D is a better reflection of vitamin D sufficiency than the measurement of 1,25-hydroxyvitamin D (see Chapter 31).

HYPOCALCEMIA

Decision-Making Algorithm
Available @ StudentConsult.com

Hypocalcemia

The **clinical manifestations** of hypocalcemia result from increased neuromuscular irritability and include muscle cramps, carpopedal spasm (tetany), weakness, paresthesia, laryngospasm, and seizure-like activity. Tetany can be detected by the *Chvostek sign* (facial spasms produced by lightly tapping over the facial nerve just in front of the ear) or by the *Trousseau sign* (carpal spasms exhibited when arterial blood flow to the hand is occluded for 3 to 5 minutes with a blood pressure cuff inflated to 15 mm Hg above systolic

blood pressure). Total serum calcium concentration is usually measured, although a determination of serum ionized calcium, the biologically active form, is preferable. Albumin is the major reservoir of protein-bound calcium. Disorders that alter plasma pH or serum albumin concentration must be considered when circulating calcium concentrations are being evaluated. The fraction of ionized calcium is inversely related to plasma pH; **alkalosis** can precipitate hypocalcemia by lowering ionized calcium without changing total serum calcium. Alkalosis may result from hyperpnea caused by anxiety or from hyperventilation related to physical exertion. Hypoproteinemia may lead to a false suggestion of hypocalcemia because the serum total calcium level is low even though the ionized Ca^{2+} remains normal. It is best to measure serum ionized calcium if hypocalcemia or hypercalcemia is suspected.

Primary hypoparathyroidism causes hypocalcemia but does not cause rickets. The etiology of primary hypoparathyroidism includes the following:

1. Congenital malformation (e.g., DiGeorge syndrome or other complex syndromes) resulting from developmental abnormalities of the third and fourth branchial arches (see Chapters 143 and 144)
2. Surgical procedures, such as thyroidectomy or parathyroidectomy, in which parathyroid tissue is removed either deliberately or as a complication of surgery for another goal
3. Autoimmunity, which may destroy the parathyroid gland

Pseudohypoparathyroidism (all with hypocalcemia and hyperphosphatemia) may occur in one of four forms as follows:

1. *Type Ia:* an abnormality of the G_{sa} protein linking the PTH receptor to adenylate cyclase; biologically active PTH is secreted in great quantities but does not stimulate its receptor
2. *Type Ib:* normal phenotype, normal G_{sa} with abnormalities in the production of adenylate cyclase
3. *Type Ic:* abnormal phenotype, normal production of adenylate cyclase, but a distal defect eliminates the effects of PTH
4. *Type II:* normal phenotype, normal production of adenylate cyclase, with a postreceptor defect, close to type Ib

Pseudohypoparathyroidism is an autosomal dominant condition that may present at birth or later. Pseudohypoparathyroidism is associated with **Albright hereditary osteodystrophy** whose clinical manifestations include short stature, stocky body habitus, round facies, short fourth and fifth metacarpals, calcification of the basal ganglia, subcutaneous calcification, and developmental delay. Albright hereditary osteodystrophy may be inherited separately so that a patient may have a normal appearance with hypocalcemia or may have the Albright hereditary osteodystrophy phenotype with normal serum calcium, phosphate, PTH, and response to PTH.

Transient neonatal hypocalcemia. During the first 3 days after birth, serum calcium concentrations normally decline in response to withdrawal of the maternal calcium supply via the placenta. Sluggish PTH response in a neonate may result in a transient hypocalcemia. Hypocalcemia caused by attenuated PTH release is found in infants of mothers with hyperparathyroidism and hypercalcemia; the latter suppresses fetal PTH release, causing **transient hypoparathyroidism** in the neonatal period.

Table 176-1	Important Physiologic Changes in Bone and Mineral Diseases			
CONDITION	**CALCIUM**	**PHOSPHATE**	**PARATHYROID HORMONE**	**25(OH)D**
Primary hypoparathyroidism	↓	↑	↓	Nl
Pseudohypoparathyroidism	↓	↑	↑	Nl
Vitamin D deficiency	Nl(↓)	↓	↑	↓
Familial hypophosphatemic rickets	Nl	↓	Nl (sl↑)	Nl
Hyperparathyroidism	↑	↓	↑	Nl
Immobilization	↑	↑	↓	Nl

25(OH)D, 25-Hydroxyvitamin D; *Nl*, normal; *sl*, slight; *↑*, high; *↓*, low.

Normal serum magnesium concentrations are required for normal parathyroid gland function and action. **Hypomagnesemia** may cause a secondary hypoparathyroidism, which responds poorly to therapies other than magnesium replacement.

The **etiology** of hypocalcemia usually can be discerned by combining features of the clinical presentation with determinations of serum ionized calcium, phosphate, alkaline phosphatase, PTH (preferably at a time when the calcium is low), magnesium, and albumin. If the PTH concentration is not appropriately elevated in relation to the low serum calcium, hypoparathyroidism (transient, primary, or caused by hypomagnesemia) is present. Vitamin D stores can be estimated by measuring serum 25-hydroxyvitamin D. Renal function is assessed by a serum creatinine measurement or determination of creatinine clearance (Table 176-1).

Treatment of severe tetany or seizures resulting from hypocalcemia consists of intravenous calcium gluconate (1 to 2 mL/kg of a 10% solution) given slowly over 10 minutes while cardiac status is monitored by electrocardiogram for bradycardia, which can be fatal. Long-term treatment of hypoparathyroidism involves administering vitamin D, preferably as 1,25-dihydroxyvitamin D and calcium. Therapy is adjusted to keep the serum calcium in the lower half of the normal range to avoid episodes of hypercalcemia that might produce nephrocalcinosis and to avoid pancreatitis.

RICKETS

Decision-Making Algorithm
Available @ StudentConsult.com

Hypocalcemia

Rickets is defined as decreased or defective bone mineralization in growing children; **osteomalacia** is the same condition in adults. The proportion of osteoid (the organic portion of bone) is excessive. As a result, the bone becomes soft and the metaphyses of the long bones widen. In older infants, poor linear growth, bowing of the legs on weight bearing (which can be painful), thickening at the wrists and knees, and prominence of the costochondral junctions (rachitic rosary) of the rib cage occur. At this stage, x-ray findings are diagnostic.

In **nutritional vitamin D deficiency,** calcium is not absorbed adequately from the intestine (see Chapter 31). Poor vitamin D intake or avoidance of sunlight in infants exclusively breastfed may contribute to the development of rickets. Fat malabsorption resulting from hepatobiliary disease (biliary atresia, neonatal hepatitis) or other causes (cystic fibrosis) also may produce vitamin D deficiency because vitamin D is a fat-soluble vitamin. Defects in vitamin D metabolism by the kidney (renal failure, autosomal recessive deficiency of 1α-hydroxylation, **vitamin D–dependent rickets**) or liver (defect in 25-hydroxylation) also can cause rickets.

In **familial hypophosphatemic rickets,** the major defect in mineral metabolism is failure of the kidney to adequately reabsorb filtered phosphate so that serum phosphate decreases and urinary phosphate is high. The *diagnosis* of this X-linked disease usually is made within the first few years of life and is typically more severe in males.

The **etiology** of rickets usually can be determined by an assessment of the mineral and vitamin D status (25-hydroxyvitamin D <8 ng/mL suggests nutritional vitamin D deficiency) (see Table 176-1). Further testing of mineral balance or measurement of other vitamin D metabolites may be required.

Several chemical forms of vitamin D can be used for **treatment** of the different rachitic conditions, but their potencies vary widely. Required dosages depend on the condition being treated (see Chapter 31). Rickets may also be treated with 1,25-hydroxyvitamin D and supplemental calcium. In hypophosphatemic rickets, phosphate supplementation (not calcium) must accompany vitamin D therapy, which is given to suppress secondary hyperparathyroidism. Adequate therapy restores normal skeletal growth and produces resolution of the radiographic signs of rickets. Nutritional rickets is treated with vitamin D given as one large dose, in weekly larger doses, or multiple smaller replacement doses. Surgery may be required to straighten legs in untreated patients with long-standing disease.

Chapter 177

DISORDERS OF SEXUAL DEVELOPMENT

NORMAL SEXUAL DEVELOPMENT

The successive sequence of chromosomal sex, gonadal sex, and phenotypic sex leads to gender identity of the individual. Genes usually determine the morphology of internal organs and of gonads (gonadal sex); this directs the appearance of the external genitalia that form the secondary sex characteristics (phenotypic sex); self-perception of the individual (gender identity) and the perception of the individual by others (gender role) follow last. In most children, these features blend and conform, but, in some patients, one or more features may not follow this sequence, leading to the disorder of sexual development (DSD) (see Chapter 23).

The internal and external genitalia are formed between 6 and 13 weeks of gestation. Fetal gonad and external genitalia are bipotential and have the capacity to support development of a normal male or female phenotype (Fig. 177-1). In the presence of a gene called *SRY* for sex-determining region on the Y chromosome, the primitive fetal gonad differentiates into a testis (Fig. 177-2). The Leydig cells of the testis secrete testosterone, which has direct effects (stimulating development of the wolffian ducts) but also is locally converted to dihydrotestosterone (DHT) by the 5α-reductase enzyme. DHT causes enlargement, rugation, and fusion of the labioscrotal folds into a scrotum; fusion of the ventral surface of the penis to enclose a penile urethra; and enlargement of the

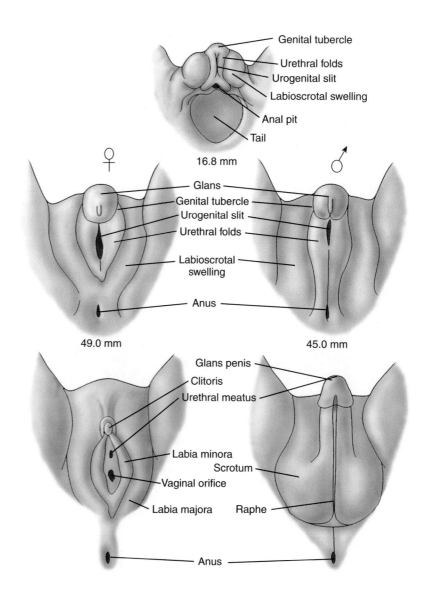

Figure 177-1 Differentiation of male and female external genitalia as proceeding from a common embryonic anlage. Testosterone acts at 9 to 13 weeks of gestation to virilize the bipotential anlage. In the absence of testosterone action, the female phenotype develops. *(From Grumbach MM, Conte FA: Disorders of sexual differentiation. In Wilson JD, Foster DW, editors: Textbook of Endocrinology, ed 8, Philadelphia, 1990, WB Saunders, p 873; adapted from Spaulding MH, Contrib Embryol Instit 13:69–88, 1921.)*

phallus with ultimate development of male external genitalia. Testicular production and secretion of müllerian-inhibitory substance by Sertoli cells cause the regression and disappearance of the müllerian ducts and their derivatives, such as the fallopian tubes and uterus. In the presence of testosterone, the wolffian ducts develop into the vas deferens, seminiferous tubules, and prostate.

The female phenotype develops unless specific *male* influences alter development. In the absence of *SRY*, an ovary spontaneously develops from the bipotential, primitive gonad. In the absence of fetal testicular secretion of müllerian-inhibitory substance, a normal uterus, fallopian tubes, and posterior third of the vagina develop out of the müllerian ducts, and the wolffian ducts degenerate. In the total absence of androgens, the external genitalia appear female.

Classification

The terms *intersex, hermaphroditism,* and *pseudohermaphroditism* are not useful. DSDs are categorized under three main subgroups according to karyotype (XX, XY, and sex chromosome for mosaic karyotypes).

Figure 177-2 A diagrammatic scheme of male sex determination and differentiation. *SRY* is the master gene controlling male sex differentiation, but there are many other genes and their products that control male and female sexual differentiation. *DHT,* Dihydrotestosterone; *SRY,* the gene for the testis-determining factor. *(From Wilson JD, Foster DW, editors: Williams Textbook of Endocrinology, ed 8, Philadelphia, 1992, WB Saunders, p 918.)*

ABNORMAL SEXUAL DEVELOPMENT
46,XX Disorders of Sexual Development

Decision-Making Algorithms
Available @ StudentConsult.com

Hypertension
Amenorrhea
Precocious Puberty in the Male
Precocious Puberty in the Female
Ambiguous Genitalia
Alkalemia

Masculinization of the external genitalia of genotypic females (except for isolated enlargement of the clitoris, which can occur from later androgen exposure) is always caused by the presence of excessive androgens during the critical period of development (8 to 13 weeks of gestation) (Table 177-1). The degree of virilization can range from mild clitoral enlargement to the appearance of a *male* phallus with a penile urethra and fused scrotum with raphe. Congenital virilizing adrenal hyperplasia is the most common cause of female ambiguous genitalia; it is most commonly the result of an enzyme deficiency that impairs synthesis of glucocorticoids but does not affect androgen production. The impaired cortisol secretion leads to adrenocorticotropic hormone (ACTH) hypersecretion, which stimulates hyperplasia of the adrenal cortex and excessive adrenal production of androgens (see Chapter 178).

46,XY Disorders of Sexual Development

Decision-Making Algorithms
Available @ StudentConsult.com

Amenorrhea
Pubertal Delay
Ambiguous Genitalia
Gynecomastia

Underdevelopment of the male external genitalia occurs because of a relative deficiency of testosterone production or action (Table 177-2). The penis is small, with various degrees

Table 177-1	Causes of Virilization in the Female
CONDITION	**ADDITIONAL FEATURE(S)**
P-450$_{c21}$ deficiency (21 hydroxylase)	Salt loss in some
3β-Hydroxysteroid dehydrogenase deficiency	Salt loss
P-450$_{c11}$ deficiency (11 hydroxylase)	Salt retention/hypertension
Androgenic drug exposure (e.g., progestins)	Exposure between 9 and 12 weeks of gestation
Mixed gonadal dysgenesis or mosaic Turner syndrome	Karyotype = 46,XY/45,X
Ovotesticular DSD	Testicular and ovarian tissue present
Maternal virilizing adrenal or ovarian tumor	Rare, positive history

of hypospadias (penile or perineal) and associated chordee or ventral binding of the phallus; unilateral, but more often bilateral, cryptorchidism may be present. The testes should be sought carefully in the inguinal canal or labioscrotal folds by palpation or ultrasound. Rarely a palpable gonad in the inguinal canal or labioscrotal fold represents a herniated ovary or an ovotestis. The latter patients have ovarian and testicular tissue and usually ambiguous external genitalia. Production of testosterone by a gonad implies that testicular tissue is present and that at least some cells carry the *SRY* gene.

Testosterone production can be reduced by specific deficiencies of the enzymes needed for androgen biosynthesis or by dysplasia of the gonads. In the latter, if müllerian-inhibiting substance production also is reduced, a rudimentary uterus and fallopian tubes are present.

The complete form of **androgen resistance** or **androgen insensitivity syndrome** is the most dramatic example of resistance to hormone action by defects in the androgen receptor. Affected patients have a **46,XY** karyotype, normally formed testes (usually located in the inguinal canal or labia majora), and female external genitalia with a short vagina and no internal müllerian structures. At the time of puberty, testosterone concentrations increase to normal or above normal male range. Because a portion of the testosterone is normally converted to estradiol in peripheral tissues and the estrogen cannot be opposed by the androgen, breast development ensues at the normal age of puberty without growth of pubic, facial, or axillary hair or the occurrence of menstruation.

5α-Reductase deficiency presents at birth with predominantly female phenotype or with ambiguous genitalia, including perineoscrotal hypospadias. The defect is in 5α reduction of testosterone to its metabolite DHT. At puberty spontaneous secondary male sexual development occurs. Gender identity and gender role are significant psychological issues with these patients if diagnosed at puberty.

Table 177-2	Causes of Inadequate Masculinization in the Male
CONDITION	**ADDITIONAL FEATURE(S)**
P-450scc (StAR) deficiency	Salt loss
3β-Hydroxysteroid dehydrogenase deficiency	Salt loss
P-450$_{c17}$ deficiency	Salt retention/hypokalemia/hypertension
Isolated P-450$_{c17}$ deficiency with 17,20-desmolase deficiency	Adrenal function normal
17β-Hydroxysteroid oxidoreductase deficiency	Adrenal function normal
Dysgenetic testes	Possible abnormal karyotype; possible mutations in DAX1, SOX9, GATA4, WT1
Leydig cell hypoplasia	Rare
Complete androgen insensitivity	Female external genitalia, absence of müllerian structures
Partial androgen insensitivity	As previous with ambiguous external genitalia
5α-Reductase deficiency	Autosomal recessive, virilization at puberty

StAR, Steroid acute regulatory protein.

Sex Chromosome and Ovotesticular Disorders of Sexual Development

Decision-Making Algorithms
Available @ StudentConsult.com

Short Stature
Pubertal Delay
Gynecomastia

Turner syndrome and **Klinefelter syndrome** and their mosaic variants are classified as sex chromosome DSD. Mixed gonadal dysgenesis (45,X; 46,XY) often may present with genital ambiguity, asymmetric external genitalia, and inguinal hernias. There may be virilization on one side and none on the other. Similar findings may be seen with **ovotesticular DSD,** another classification of DSD.

APPROACH TO THE INFANT WITH GENITAL AMBIGUITY

Decision-Making Algorithms
Available @ StudentConsult.com

Pubertal Delay
Ambiguous Genitalia

Ambiguous genitalia in a newborn must be attended to with as little delay as possible and with informed sensitivity to the psychosocial context as required. The laboratory evaluations required might take days or weeks to complete, delaying a sex assignment and naming of the infant, such that choice often precedes diagnosis. Beyond infancy and childhood, and to offset any gender uncertainty in the patient and confusion in the parents, health care providers must help families come to an appropriate closure and gender choice.

On physical examination, it is essential to note where the urethral opening lies and whether there is fusion of the anterior portion of the labioscrotal folds. Endogenous excessive production of androgen (as in congenital adrenal hyperplasia [CAH]) in a female fetus between 9 and 13 weeks of gestation leads to ambiguous genitalia. If the vaginal opening is normal, and there is no fusion, but the clitoris is enlarged without ventral fusion of the ventral urethra, the patient had later exposure to androgens. A patient with a fully formed scrotum, even if small, and a normally formed but small penis, termed a *microphallus,* must have had normal exposure to and action of androgen during 9 to 13 weeks of gestation.

The major goal is a rapid identification of any life-threatening disorders (salt loss and shock caused by the salt-losing form of CAH). Although the classic approach to sex assignment has been based on the feasibility of genital reconstruction and potential fertility rather than on karyotype or gonadal histology, the effects of prenatal androgen must be considered. Yet it may be inappropriate to raise a female infant who is severely virilized from virilizing CAH as a male; nonetheless in most reported cases, sex assignment and adult gender role remain female, and fertility can be retained because the internal organs are female. A 46,XY male with ambiguous genitalia and an extremely small phallus that does not increase in size with androgen therapy (partial androgen resistance) traditionally has been raised as a female because surgical construction of a fully functional phallus is difficult. Some of these patients frequently revert spontaneously to a male gender identity. Present management of ambiguous genitalia involves extensive open discussion with parents involving the biology of the infant and the likely prognosis. Treatment should be individualized and managed by a team, including an experienced pediatric endocrinologist, urologist or gynecologist, psychologist, geneticist, and the primary care physician.

Diagnosis

The first step toward diagnosis is to determine whether the disorder represents virilization of a genetic female (androgen excess) or underdevelopment of a genetic male (androgen deficiency) (see Fig. 177-2). Inguinal gonads that are evident on palpation usually are testes and indicate that incomplete development of a male phenotype has occurred; this pattern is not consistent, and ovaries and ovotestes may feel similar. Similarly absence of female internal genitalia (detected by ultrasound) implies that müllerian-inhibiting substance was present and secreted by fetal testes. Karyotype determination is only one of many factors in deciding the sexual identity for purposes of rearing; the *SRY* gene may be found on chromosomes other than the Y chromosome, and, conversely, a Y chromosome may lack an *SRY* gene (it may have been translocated to an X chromosome, leading to the development of a 46,XX male- XX sex reversal, testicular DSD).

Statistically most virilized females have CAH; 90% of these females have 21-hydroxylase deficiency. The diagnosis is established by measuring the plasma concentration of 17-hydroxyprogesterone and androstenedione (see Chapter 178), which typically is hundreds of times above the normal range. Other enzymatic defects also may be diagnosed by quantifying circulating levels of the adrenal steroid precursor proximal to the defective enzyme block.

Establishing an accurate diagnosis is more difficult in underdeveloped males. When certain types of adrenal hyperplasia coexist with defects in androgen production of the testes, excessive ACTH secretion elevates substantially levels of specific adrenal steroid precursors, allowing a diagnosis. If the defect is restricted to testosterone biosynthesis, the measurement of testosterone and its precursors in the basal state and after stimulation by hCG may be required. Patients with normal levels of testosterone either have persistent androgen resistance or have had an interruption of normal morphogenesis of the genitalia. Abnormalities of the sex chromosomes may be associated with dysgenetic gonads, which may be associated with persistence of müllerian structures.

Treatment

Treatment consists of replacing deficient hormones (cortisol in adrenal hyperplasia or testosterone in a child with androgen biosynthetic defects who will be raised as male), surgical restoration to make the individual look more appropriate for the gender of rearing, and psychological support of the whole family. Gonads and internal organs discordant for the gender of rearing are often removed. Dysgenetic gonads with Y-genetic material always should be removed because

gonadoblastomas or dysgerminomas may develop in the organ. Reconstructive surgery is usually performed by 2 years of age so that genital structure reflects gender of rearing. This recommendation for reconstructive surgery is controversial; some advocate that surgery not be performed in infancy or early childhood so that the child or young adolescent can be involved in the decision. A decision for gender of rearing is recommended from birth; however the knowledge that the person with a DSD may change gender later on is shared with parents from the outset.

Chapter **178**

ADRENAL GLAND DYSFUNCTION

PHYSIOLOGY

The adrenal gland consists of an outer cortex, which is responsible for the synthesis of steroids, and an inner medulla derived from neuroectodermal tissue, which synthesizes catecholamines. The *adrenal cortex* consists of three zones: an outer glomerulosa (end product is the mineralocorticoid aldosterone, which regulates sodium and potassium balance), a middle fasciculata (end product is cortisol), and an inner reticularis (synthesizes sex steroids). The general scheme of these synthetic steps is shown in Figure 178-1.

Hypothalamic corticotropin-releasing hormone (CRH) stimulates the release of pituitary adrenocorticotropic hormone (ACTH, corticotropin), derived by selective processing from pro-opiomelanocortin. ACTH governs the synthesis and release of cortisol and adrenal androgens. Primary adrenal insufficiency or cortisol deficiency from any defect in the adrenal gland results in an oversecretion of ACTH; cortisol deficiency also may occur from ACTH (secondary) or CRH (tertiary) deficiency, causing low serum ACTH concentrations and low cortisol. Endogenous (or exogenous) glucocorticoids feed back to inhibit ACTH and CRH secretion. The renin-angiotensin system and potassium regulate aldosterone secretion; ACTH has little effect on aldosterone production except in excess, when it may increase aldosterone secretion.

Steroids that circulate in the free form (not bound to cortisol-binding protein [transcortin]) may cross the placenta from mother to fetus, but ACTH does not. The placenta plays an important role in steroid biosynthesis in utero, acting as a metabolic mediator between mother and child. Because the fetal CRH-ACTH-adrenal axis is operational in utero, deficiencies in cortisol synthesis lead to excessive ACTH secretion. If a virilizing adrenal enzyme defect is present, such as 21-hydroxylase deficiency, the fetal adrenal gland secretes excess androgens, virilizing the fetus. Normal variation of serum cortisol and ACTH levels leads to values that are high early in the morning and lower at night. This normal diurnal variation may take months to years to fully develop.

Figure 178-1 Diagram of the steroid biosynthetic pathways and the biosynthetic defects that result in congenital hyperplasia. The defect in patients with lipoid adrenal hyperplasia is not (except for one reported case) in the CYP11A1 (cholesterol side-chain cleavage) enzyme, but in StAR, the steroidogenic acute regulatory protein. This protein is involved in the transport of cholesterol from the outer mitochondrial membrane to the inner membrane, where the CYP11A1 enzyme is located. CYP11B1 (11β-hydroxylase) catalyzes 11β-hydroxylation of deoxycorticosterone and 11β-deoxycortisol primarily. CYP17 (17α-hydroxylase/17,20-lyase) catalyzes 17α-hydroxylation and splitting of the 17,20 bond, but for the latter it has preferential D5-17,20-lyase activity. CYP19 (aromatase) catalyzes the conversion of corticosterone to aldosterone. 3β-HSD I and 3β-HSD II, 3β-hydroxysteroid dehydrogenase/$\Delta^{4,5}$-isomerase types I and II; CYP21 (P450c21), 21-hydroxylase; 17β-HSD 3, 17β-hydroxysteroid dehydrogenase type 3. In the human, deletion of a homozygous null mutation of CYP11A (P450$_{ccc}$) is probably lethal in utero, but a heterogeneous mutation caused congenital lipoid adrenal hyperplasia. *(From Melmed S, Polonsky K, Kronenberg H, et al, editors:* Williams Textbook of Endocrinology, *ed 10, Philadelphia, 2003, Saunders, p 917.)*

ADRENAL INSUFFICIENCY

Decision-Making Algorithms
Available @ StudentConsult.com

Ambiguous Genitalia
Hyponatremia
Hyperkalemia

The **clinical manifestations** of inadequate adrenal function result from inadequate secretion or action of glucocorticoids, mineralocorticoids, or both (Table 178-1). In the case of enzyme defects that affect the gonad and the adrenal gland, overproduction or underproduction of potent androgens can occur, depending on the site of enzyme blockade (see Fig. 178-1). Progressive prenatal virilization of the external genitalia may occur in females; incomplete virilization may occur in males. Ambiguity of the external genitalia is a common manifestation of disordered fetal adrenal enzyme function. Precise *diagnosis* is essential for the prescription of appropriate therapy, long-term outlook, and genetic counseling. In patients with enzyme defects, an elevation in the precursor steroid is present proximal to the enzyme block and is metabolized through remaining normal alternate enzyme pathways, whereas a deficiency of steroids is present subsequent to the block.

The dominant clinical features of congenital adrenal mineralocorticoid deficiency are hyponatremia and hyperkalemia, usually developing by 5 to 7 days after birth but not immediately after birth. Vomiting, dehydration, and acidosis soon follow, as does hypotensive shock from glucocorticoid deficiency. Death may occur if the disorder remains undiagnosed and untreated. In females the ambiguity of the external genitalia is an obvious clue that salt-losing congenital adrenal hyperplasia (CAH) or simple virilizing CAH must be ruled out. Because these forms cannot be distinguished clinically, all presentations of ambiguous genitalia should involve evaluation for mineralocorticoid deficiency. In males the most common form of CAH, 21-hydroxylase deficiency, does not cause abnormal genitalia. There may be hyperpigmentation of the scrotal skin, but this is a subtle sign. In all infants, the diagnosis of adrenal insufficiency may be overlooked or confused with pyloric stenosis. In pyloric stenosis, in contrast to salt-losing CAH, vomiting of stomach contents results in hypochloremia, serum potassium is normal or low, and alkalosis is present. This distinction may be lifesaving in preventing unnecessary investigations or inappropriate therapy.

Not all forms of adrenal hyperplasia present at birth; the spectrum of disorder ranges from severe (classic) to mild (late-onset) or nonclassic. Milder forms may manifest in childhood, adolescence, or even young adulthood (not as

Table 178-1	Clinical Manifestations of Adrenal Insufficiency

Cortisol deficiency

    Hypoglycemia

    Inability to withstand stress

    Vasomotor collapse

    Hyperpigmentation (in primary adrenal insufficiency with excess of adrenocorticotropic hormone)

    Apneic spells

    Muscle weakness, fatigue

Aldosterone deficiency

    Hyponatremia

    Hyperkalemia

    Vomiting

    Urinary sodium wasting

    Salt craving

    Acidosis

    Failure to thrive

    Volume depletion

    Hypotension

    Dehydration

    Shock

    Diarrhea

    Muscle weakness

Androgen excess or deficiency (caused by adrenal enzyme defect)

Ambiguous genitalia in certain conditions

glucocorticoid or mineralocorticoid deficiencies, but as androgen excess).

In patients with **congenital adrenal hypoplasia** or **adrenal hemorrhage**, the secretion of all adrenal steroids is low. In contrast CAH leads to a diagnostic steroid pattern in blood and urine (see Fig. 178-1). Deficiency of 21-hydroxylase is the most common form (95%) and serves as a paradigm for these disorders.

21-HYDROXYLASE DEFICIENCY

Decision-Making Algorithms
Available @ StudentConsult.com

Hypertension
Precocious Puberty in the Male
Precocious Puberty in the Female
Ambiguous Genitalia
Hirsutism

The incidence of classic 21-hydroxylase deficiency is about 1 in 15,000 among various white populations. Nonclassic CAH may occur with an incidence of 1 in 50 in certain populations. The gene for 21-hydroxylase lies on the short arm of chromosome 6; the genotype may be determined in a proband, permitting prenatal diagnosis in a subsequent pregnancy.

Deficient 21-hydroxylase activity (P-450$_{c21}$ deficiency) impairs the conversion of 17-hydroxyprogesterone (17-OHP) to 11-deoxycortisol and in the salt-losing form, of progesterone to deoxycorticosterone, a mineralocorticoid proximal in the pathway to the production of aldosterone. The decreased production of cortisol causes hypersecretion of ACTH, which stimulates the synthesis of steroids immediately proximal to the block and shunting of these to overproduction of androgens. The primary clinical manifestation is the virilization of the external genitalia of the affected female fetus; the development of the uterus, ovaries, and fallopian tubes remains unaffected by the androgens. The degree of virilization varies, ranging from mild clitoromegaly to complete fusion of labioscrotal folds, with severe clitoromegaly simulating a phallus (see Chapter 177). A male infant with this defect appears normal at birth, although penile enlargement may be apparent thereafter. The deficiency in aldosterone, found in about 75% of patients, causes salt wasting with shock and dehydration until the diagnosis is established and appropriate treatment is given.

The treatment of 21-hydroxylase deficiency requires hydrocortisone and fludrocortisone in the case of the salt-losing form. Therapy must be adjusted throughout childhood at regular intervals. Overtreatment will cause growth stunting and weight gain (cushingoid features), whereas undertreatment will cause excessive height gain, skeletal advance, and early appearance puberty, ultimately jeopardizing adult height potential.

Late-onset CAH is typically noted years after birth. Affected subjects have milder manifestations without ambiguous genitalia, but they may have acne, hirsutism, and in girls irregular menstrual cycles or amenorrhea. Late-onset CAH in girls may be confused with **polycystic ovarian syndrome**.

Biochemical diagnostic studies show elevated levels of serum 17-OHP, the substrate for the defective 21-hydroxylase enzyme activity. In newborns with CAH, the values are elevated a hundredfold to a thousandfold. In late-onset CAH, an ACTH stimulation test is necessary to show an abnormally high response of 17-OHP. Serum cortisol and aldosterone levels (in salt losers) are low, renin levels are high, whereas the testosterone level is elevated because it is derived from 17-OHP.

The goals of **treatment** are to achieve normal linear growth and bone age advancement. Long-term therapy consists of providing glucocorticoids at a dose of approximately 10 to 15 mg/m^2/24 hours in three divided doses of oral hydrocortisone or its equivalent. Mineralocorticoid therapy for salt losers consists of fludrocortisone at a dose of 0.1 to 0.2 mg/24 hours, often with sodium chloride supplementation in infancy and early childhood. Surgical correction of ambiguous external genitalia may be considered. The adequacy of glucocorticoid replacement therapy is monitored by determining serum concentrations of adrenal precursors, including androstenedione and 17-OHP for 21-hydroxylase deficiency. In addition, the assessment of linear growth and skeletal age, by bone age determination, is required as a reflection of appropriate therapy. To avoid adrenal insufficiency, threefold higher doses of glucocorticoids are given during **stressful states** such as febrile illnesses and surgery. Intramuscular hydrocortisone is used in severe emergencies or with illnesses involving emesis. Mineralocorticoid therapy is monitored with serum sodium, potassium, and plasma renin activity levels. Prenatal treatment with dexamethasone to suppress fetal ACTH-induced

Table 178-2 Clinical and Biochemical Features in Newborn Adrenal Insufficiency

FEATURE	ELECTROLYTE DISTURBANCE*	AMBIGUOUS GENITALIA		SERUM CORTISOL	URINE 11-DEOXYCORTISOL	17-OHP	DHEA	ALDOSTERONE	17-OHCS	17-KS	PRE-GNANETRIOL
		VIRILIZED FEMALE	UNDER-VIRILIZED MALE								
Hypoplasia	Severe	No	No	D	D	D	D	D	D	D	D
Hemorrhage	Moderate to severe	No	No	D	D	D	D	D	D	D	D
StAR deficiency	Severe	No	Yes	D	D	D	D	D	D	D	D
3β-HSD	Severe	Yes	Yes	D	D	D	I	D	D	I	D
P-450$_{c21}$ deficiency	Absent to severe	Yes	No	D	D	I	I	D	D	I	I
Aldosterone synthesis block	Severe	No	No	NI	NI	NI	NI	D	NI	NI	NI
Pseudohypo-aldosteronism	Severe	No	No	NI	NI	NI	NI	I	NI	NI	NI
P-450$_{c11}$ deficiency	None	Yes	No	D	I	NI or I	NI	D	I	I	NI-sl I
P-450$_{c17}$ deficiency	†	No	Yes	D	NI-D	D	D	NI-D	D	D	D
Unresponsiveness to ACTH	†	No	No	D	NI-D	NI-D	NI-D	NI-D	D	D	NI-D

17-KS, 17-Ketosteroid; 17-OHCS, 17-hydroxycorticosteroid; ACTH, adrenocorticotropic hormone; D, decrease; HSD, hydroxysteroid dehydrogenase; I, increase; NI, normal; StAR, steroid acute regulatory protein.
*Usually manifested after 5 days of age.
†High normal Na$^+$ and low normal to low K$^+$.

androgen production can reduce or eliminate the ambiguity of the external genitalia in affected female fetuses, if begun at approximately 7 weeks of gestation; this remains controversial.

OTHER ENZYME DEFECTS

Other enzyme defects are rare in contrast to 21-hydroxylase deficiency. In **11-hydroxylase deficiency,** the next most common cause of CAH, virilization occurs with salt retention and hypokalemia, as a result of the buildup of deoxycorticosterone (see Fig. 178-1), a potent mineralocorticoid. Hypertension develops as a result of excessive mineralocorticoid production. Table 178-2 summarizes the clinical and biochemical features of adrenal insufficiency in infancy.

ADDISON DISEASE

Decision-Making Algorithms
Available @ StudentConsult.com

Hyponatremia
Hyperkalemia

Addison disease is a rare acquired disorder of childhood, usually associated with autoimmune destruction of the adrenal cortex. It is a form of primary adrenal insufficiency with absence of glucocorticoid and mineralocorticoid.

Clinical manifestations are hyperpigmentation, salt craving, postural hypotension, fasting hypoglycemia, anorexia, weakness, and episodes of shock during severe illness. Baseline and ACTH-stimulated cortisol values are subnormal, confirming the diagnosis; hyponatremia, hyperkalemia, and elevated plasma renin activity indicate mineralocorticoid deficiency. Addison disease may occur within the context of autoimmune polyglandular syndromes (APS I and APS II). Other rare causes of adrenal insufficiency include adrenal leukodystrophy and conditions that affect the hypothalamus-pituitary whether acquired, such as in craniopharyngioma, or iatrogenic, such as in irradiation for treatment of malignancy.

Replacement **treatment** with 10 to 15 mg/m^2/24 hours of hydrocortisone is indicated, with supplementation during stress at three times the maintenance dosage or the use of intramuscular hydrocortisone. The dose is titrated to allow a normal growth rate. Mineralocorticoid replacement with fludrocortisone is monitored by plasma renin activity and serum sodium and potassium determinations.

CUSHING SYNDROME

Decision-Making Algorithms
Available @ StudentConsult.com

Short Stature
Hirsutism
Obesity
Alkalemia
Hyponatremia
Hypokalemia

Classic **clinical manifestations** of Cushing syndrome in children include progressive central or generalized obesity, marked failure of longitudinal growth, hirsutism, weakness, a nuchal fat pad, acne, striae, hypertension, and often hyperpigmentation when ACTH is elevated. The most frequent cause is exogenous administration in the context of numerous conditions requiring long-term pharmacologic doses of glucocorticoids. Endogenous causes include adrenal adenoma, carcinoma, nodular adrenal hyperplasia, an ACTH-secreting pituitary microadenoma resulting in bilateral adrenal hyperplasia (**Cushing disease**), or an extremely rare ACTH-secreting tumor. **Diagnostic tests** include 24-hour urinary cortisol excretion, low-dose dexamethasone suppression test, high-dose dexamethasone suppression test (helps distinguish Cushing syndrome from Cushing disease), and late evening salivary cortisol sampling.

Treatment of Cushing syndrome is directed to the etiology and may include excision of autonomous adrenal, pituitary, or ectopic ACTH-secreting tumors. Rarely adrenalectomy is needed to control the symptoms. Parenteral glucocorticoid therapy is necessary during and immediately after surgical treatment to avoid acute adrenal insufficiency.

Suggested Reading

Backeljauw PF, Chernausek SD: The insulin-like growth factors and growth disorders of childhood, *Endocrinol Metab Clin North Am* 41(2):265–282, 2012.

Kliegman RM, Stanton B, St Geme III J, et al: *Nelson Textbook of Pediatrics*, ed 19, Philadelphia, 2011, Elsevier.

Nimkarn S, Lin Su K, New MI: Steroid 21 hydroxylase deficiency congenital adrenal hyperplasia, *Pediatr Clin North Am* 58(5):1281–1300, 2011.

Palmert MR, Dunkel L: Clinical practice: delayed puberty, *N Engl J Med 2* 366(5):443–453, 2012.

Péter F, Muzsnai A: Congenital disorders of the thyroid: hypo/hyper, *Pediatr Clin North Am* 58(5):1099–1115, 2011.

Romero CJ, Nesi-França S, Radovick S: The molecular basis of hypopituitarism, *Trends Endocrinol Metab* 20(10):506–516, 2009.

Schatz DA, Haller MJ, Atkinson MA: Type 1 diabetes. Preface, *Endocrinol Metab Clin North Am* 39(3), 2010 481–667.

Williams RM, Ward CE, Hughes IA: Premature adrenarche, *Arch Dis Child* 97(3):250–254, 2012.

Neurology

Jocelyn Huang Schiller and Renée A. Shellhaas

Chapter 179

NEUROLOGY ASSESSMENT

A neurologic evaluation, including history, physical examination, and judicious use of ancillary studies, allows the localization and diagnosis of nervous system pathology. The process and interpretation of the neurologic examination varies with age; the newborn is unique with many transient and primitive reflex patterns, whereas the examination of adolescents and adults is similar. Careful evaluation of social, cognitive, language, fine motor and gross motor skills, and their age appropriateness is key.

HISTORY

Gathering neurologic history follows the traditional medical model with two additions: the **pace** of the process and the **localization** of the problem. The symptom evolution provides clues to the underlying process as symptoms may evolve in a **progressive**, **static**, or **episodic** fashion. Progressive symptoms may evolve suddenly (seizures, stroke); acutely over minutes or hours (epidural hemorrhage); subacutely over days or weeks (brain tumor); or slowly over years (hereditary neuropathies). Static neurologic abnormalities are observed early in life and do not change in character over time (cerebral palsy). Static lesions are often caused by congenital brain abnormalities or prenatal/perinatal brain injury. Intermittent attacks of recurrent, stereotyped episodes suggest epilepsy or migraine syndromes, among others. Episodic disorders are characterized by periods of symptoms, followed by partial or complete recovery (demyelinating, autoimmune, vascular diseases).

PHYSICAL EXAMINATION

Observation of the child's appearance, movement, and behavior begins at the start of the encounter. For example, the child may display an unusual posture, abnormal gait, or lack of awareness of the environment.

Because the brain and skin have the same embryonic origin (ectoderm), abnormalities of hair, skin, teeth, and nails are associated with congenital brain disorders (neurocutaneous disorders) such as neurofibromatosis (NF type 1) in which **café au lait macules** (flat, light brown macules) are characteristic.

Adenoma sebaceum, fibrovascular lesions that look like acne on the nose and malar regions, nail fibromas, ash-leaf spots (hypopigmented macules), and Shagreen patches (flesh-colored soft plaques with prominent follicular openings) are commonly seen in older children and adults with tuberous sclerosis.

The **head circumference** is measured in its largest occipitofrontal circumference and plotted against standard growth curves (Chapter 5). **Microcephaly** and **macrocephaly** represent an occipitofrontal circumference 2 standard deviations (SDs) below or above the mean, respectively. Measurements plotted over time may show an accelerating pattern (hydrocephalus) or decelerating pattern (brain injury, degenerative neurologic disorder). The anterior fontanelle is slightly depressed and pulsatile when a calm infant is placed upright. A tense or bulging fontanelle may indicate increased intracranial pressure (ICP) but may also be seen in a crying or febrile infant. Premature closure of one or more sutures (**craniosynostosis**) results in an unusual shape of the head. Abnormal shape, location, and condition of the face, eyes, nares, philtrum, lips, or ears are found in many genetic syndromes.

A careful **ocular examination** is essential and should include a search for epicanthal folds, coloboma, conjunctival telangiectasias, and cataracts. Direct ophthalmoscopy assesses the optic disks and macula for abnormalities such as papilledema or a cherry-red spot. A complete examination of the retina involves dilating the pupil and use of indirect ophthalmoscopy, typically requiring ophthalmologic consultation.

Examination of the hands and feet may reveal abnormal creases or digits (Chapters 50, 201). The neck and spine should be examined for obvious (myelomeningocele) or subtle (cutaneous dimples, sinus tracts, hair tufts, subcutaneous lipomas) midline defects. Nervous system abnormalities may result in kyphosis or scoliosis (Chapter 202).

NEUROLOGIC EXAMINATION OF A NEONATE

Because of the developmental immaturity of infants, the neonatal neurologic examination primarily assesses the function of the basal ganglia, brainstem, and more caudal structures. The plasticity of the developing nervous system means that examination results should be used cautiously in predicting developmental outcomes.

Mental Status

A healthy newborn infant should have periods of quiet, sustained wakefulness interspersed with active and quiet sleep.

Table 179-1	Central Nervous System (CNS) Reflexes of Infancy		
REFLEX	**DESCRIPTION**	**AGE AT APPEARANCE**	**AGE AT DISAPPEARANCE**
Moro	Light drop of head produces sudden extension followed by flexion of the arms and legs	Birth	6 mo
Grasp	Placing finger in infant's palm results in flexing of infant's fingers	Birth	6 mo
Rooting	Tactile stimulus about infant's mouth results in the mouth pursuing the stimulus	Birth	4–6 mo
Trunk incurvation (Gallant)	Stroking the skin along the edge of vertebrae produces curvature of the spine with concavity on the side of the stroke	Birth	4 mo
Placing	When dorsum of foot is brought into contact with the edge of a surface, infant places foot on the surface	Birth	4–6 mo
Asymmetrical tonic neck	With infant supine, turning of the head results in ipsilateral extension of the arm and leg with flexion of opposite extremities in a "fencing" posture	Birth	3 mo
Parachute	Infant is suspended face down by the chest. When infant is moved toward a table, the arms extend as if to protect self	8–10 mo	Never
Babinski	Stroking lateral aspect of sole from heel up results in dorsiflexion of the great toe and fanning of the remaining toes	Birth	12–18 mo

Irritability, lethargy, or more severely depressed consciousness are nonspecific signs of abnormal brain function.

Reflexes

Examination of the **primitive reflexes** provides assessment of the functional integrity of the brainstem and basal ganglia (Table 179-1). Many of these stereotyped motor responses are present at birth. They are symmetrical and disappear at 4 to 6 months of age, indicating the normal maturation of descending inhibitory cerebral influences. The **grasp** and **rooting** reflexes are inhibited by maturation of frontal lobes but may reappear later in life with acquired frontal lobe lesions. Asymmetry or persistence of the primitive reflexes may indicate focal brain or peripheral nerve lesions.

Posture

Posture is the position that a calm infant naturally assumes when placed supine. An infant at 28 weeks of gestation shows an extended posture. By 32 weeks, there is a slight trend toward increase in tone and flexion of the lower extremities. At 34 weeks, the lower extremities are flexed; the upper extremities are extended. The term infant flexes lower and upper extremities. **Recoil**, the readiness with which an arm or leg springs back to its original position after passive stretching and release, is essentially absent in very premature infants but is brisk at term. Because of the asymmetric tonic neck reflex, it is essential to maintain the infant's head in a neutral position (not turned to the side) during assessment of posture and tone.

Movement and Tone

Spontaneous movements of premature infants are slow and writhing; those of term infants are more rapid.

NEUROLOGIC EXAMINATION OF A CHILD

The purpose of the neurologic examination is to *localize* or identify the region within the neuraxis from which the

symptoms arise. The **mental status examination** assesses the cerebral cortex. The **cranial nerve examination** evaluates the integrity of the brainstem. The **motor examination** evaluates upper and lower motor neuron function. The **sensory examination** assesses the peripheral sensory receptors and their central reflections. **Deep tendon reflexes** assess upper and lower motor connections. **Gait** assessment evaluates the motor system in a dynamic state for better functional assessment.

Mental Status Evaluation

Alertness is assessed in infants by observing spontaneous activities, feeding behavior, and visual ability to fix and follow objects. Response to tactile, visual, and auditory stimuli is noted. If consciousness is altered, the response to painful stimuli is noted. Observation of toddlers at play allows a nonthreatening assessment of developmentally appropriate skills. In addition to language function, older children can be tested for reading, writing, numerical skills, fund of knowledge, abstract reasoning, judgment, humor, and memory.

The simplest way to assess intellectual abilities is through language skills. **Language function** is receptive (understanding speech or gestures) and expressive (speech and use of gestures). Abnormalities of language resulting from cerebral hemisphere disorders are referred to as **aphasias**. Anterior, expressive, or *Broca aphasia* is characterized by sparse, nonfluent language. Posterior, receptive, or *Wernicke aphasia* is characterized by an inability to understand language, with speech that is fluent but nonsensical. Global aphasia refers to impaired expressive and receptive language.

CRANIAL NERVE EVALUATION

The cranial nerve evaluation assesses brainstem integrity but depends on the stage of brain maturation and the ability to cooperate. A colorful toy may capture a young child's attention and permit observation of coordination, movement, and cranial nerve function.

Cranial Nerve I

Smell can be assessed in verbal, cooperative children older than 2 years of age. Aromatic substances (perfumes, vanilla) should be used instead of volatile substances (ammonia), which irritate the nasal mucosa and stimulate the trigeminal nerve.

Cranial Nerve II

Full-term newborns in a quiet awake state follow human faces, lights in a dark room, or large, opticokinetic strips. Visual acuity has been estimated to be 20/200 in newborns and 20/20 in 6-month-old infants. Standard visual charts displaying pictures instead of letters can be used to assess visual acuity in toddlers. Peripheral vision is tested by surreptitiously bringing objects into the visual field from behind. A reduced pupillary reaction to light suggests anterior visual pathway lesions, including the retina, optic nerves, and chiasm. Unilateral optic nerve lesions are identified by the *swinging flashlight test*. With an optic nerve abnormality, both pupils constrict when light is directed into the normal eye. When light is swung over to the abnormal eye, both pupils dilate inappropriately; this is called an *afferent pupillary defect* or **Marcus Gunn pupil**. Interruption of the sympathetic innervation to the pupil produces **Horner's syndrome** (ptosis, miosis, and unilateral facial anhidrosis). In this instance, anisocoria (unequal pupils) is more pronounced in a dark room, because the affected pupil is unable to dilate appropriately. Lesions of the posterior visual pathway, including the lateral geniculate, optic radiations, and occipital cortex, have normal pupillary light reactions but are expressed by loss of visual fields.

Cranial Nerves III, IV, and VI

These three cranial nerves control eye movement and are most easily examined with the use of a colorful toy to capture the child's attention. For infants too young to fix and follow, rotating the infant's head assesses oculocephalic vestibular reflexes (**doll's eye maneuver**). If the brainstem is intact, rotating a newborn or comatose patient's head to the right causes the eyes to move to the left, and vice versa. In awake, older patients, voluntary eye movements mask the reflex.

Abnormalities of these cranial nerves may cause diplopia (double vision). With unilateral third cranial nerve (oculomotor nerve) palsy, the involved eye deviates down and out (infraducted, abducted), with associated ptosis and a dilated, mydriatic pupil. Injury to cranial nerve IV (trochlear nerve) causes weakness of downward eye movement with consequent vertical diplopia. Cranial nerve VI (abducens nerve) palsy results in the inability to move the eye outward. Because cranial nerve VI has a long intracranial route within the subarachnoid space, failure of abduction of one or both eyes is a frequent, but nonspecific, sign of increased ICP.

Cranial Nerve V

The muscles of mastication can be observed as an infant sucks and swallows. The **corneal reflex** can test cranial nerves V ophthalmic division and VII at any age. Facial sensation of light touch and pain can be determined with cotton gauze and pinprick. Facial sensation can be functionally assessed in an infant by gently brushing the cheek, which will produce the **rooting reflex** (turns head and neck with mouthing movement, as if seeking to nurse).

Cranial Nerve VII

Facial muscles are assessed by observing the face during rest, crying, and blinking. At older, cooperative ages, children can be asked to smile, blow out their cheeks, blink forcibly, and furrow their foreheads. Weakness of all unilateral muscles of the face, including the forehead, eye, and mouth, indicates a lesion of the ipsilateral peripheral facial nerve (**Bell palsy**). Because the upper third of the face receives bilateral cortical innervation, if the weakness affects only the lower face and mouth, a contralateral lesion of upper motor neuron in the brain (tumor, stroke, abscess) must be considered.

Cranial Nerve VIII

Lesions of cranial nerve VIII cause deafness, tinnitus, and vertigo. Normally, alert neonates blink in response to a bell or other abrupt, loud sound. Four-month-old infants turn their head and eyes to localize a sound. Hearing can be tested in a verbal child by whispering a word in one ear while covering the opposite ear. If there are any concerns about hearing, formal audiologic assessment is indicated.

Lesions of the vestibular component of cranial nerve VIII produce symptoms of vertigo, nausea, vomiting, diaphoresis, and nystagmus. Nystagmus is an involuntary beating eye movement with a rapid phase in one direction and a slow phase in the opposite direction. By convention, the direction of the nystagmus is defined by the fast phase and may be horizontal, vertical, or rotatory.

Cranial Nerves IX and X

The gag reflex is brisk at all ages except the very immature neonate. An absent gag reflex suggests a lower motor neuron lesion of the brainstem, cranial nerves IX or X, neuromuscular junction, or pharyngeal muscles. Weak, breathy, or nasal speech; weak sucking; drooling and inability to handle secretions; gagging and nasal regurgitation of food are additional symptoms of cranial nerve X dysfunction.

Cranial Nerve XI

Observing the infant's posture and spontaneous activity assesses the functions of the trapezius and sternocleidomastoid muscles. Head tilt and drooping of the shoulder suggest lesions involving cranial nerve XI. In later childhood, strength in these muscles can be tested directly and individually.

Cranial Nerve XII

Atrophy and fasciculation of the tongue, usually indicating a lesion of the anterior horn cells (spinal muscular atrophy [SMA]), can be observed at any age and are assessed most reliably when the infant is asleep. The tongue deviates toward the weak side in unilateral lesions.

MOTOR EXAMINATION
Power

In infants, power is assessed by observation of spontaneous movements and movements against gravity. Arm and leg movements should be symmetrical, seen best when the infant is held supine with one hand supporting the buttocks and one supporting the shoulders. The limbs should easily lift up. Power is graded as follows:

5 Normal
4 Weak but able to provide resistance
3 Able to move against gravity but not against resistance
2 Unable to move against gravity
1 Minimal movement
0 Complete paralysis

Strength in toddlers is assessed by observing functional abilities, such as walking, stooping to pick up an object, and standing up from the floor. An older child should be able to easily reach high above his or her head, wheelbarrow walk, run, hop, go up and down stairs, and arise from the ground. **Gower sign** (child arises from lying on the floor by using his arms to *climb up* his legs and body) is a sign of significant proximal weakness. Subtle asymmetry can be detected when the child extends arms out in front with the palms upward and eyes closed. The hand on the weaker side cups and begins to pronate slowly (**pronator drift**). Cooperative children can undergo individual muscle strength testing. **Muscle fasciculations** indicate denervation from disease of the anterior horn cell or peripheral nerve.

Tone

Tone represents the dynamic resistance of muscles to passive stretch. Lower motor and cerebellar lesions produce decreased tone (**hypotonia**). Upper motor lesions produce increased tone (**spasticity**). In extrapyramidal disease, an increase in resistance is present throughout passive movement of a joint (**rigidity**).

Bulk

Muscle bulk represents the volume of muscle tissue. In many lower motor neuron conditions (neuropathies, SMA), muscle bulk is diminished or atrophic. Excessive muscle bulk is seen in rare conditions, such as myotonia congenita; boys with Duchenne muscular dystrophy have *pseudohypertrophy* of their calves.

Coordination

Ataxia is the lack of coordination of movement, which is typically due to a dysfunction of the cerebellar pathways. Observation and functional analysis help assess coordination in infants and toddlers. Watching the child sit or walk assesses truncal stability. Exchanging toys or objects with the child permits assessment of intention tremor and **dysmetria** (errors in judging distance), signs of cerebellar dysfunction. Cooperative children can do repetitive finger or foot tapping to test rapid alternating movements. Cerebellar and corticospinal tract dysfunction produce slowing and irregularity during tests of rapid alternating movements.

Gait

Watching a child creep, crawl, cruise, or walk is the best global assessment for the motor and coordination systems (Chapter 197). Subtle deficits and asymmetries in power, tone, or balance may be observed. The toddler gait is normally wide-based and unsteady. The base of the gait narrows with age. By 6 years, a child is able to walk on toes, walk on heels, and tandem walk (heel to toe). Cerebellar dysfunction results in a broad-based, unsteady gait accompanied by difficulty in executing turns. Corticospinal tract dysfunction produces a stiff, scissoring gait and toe walking. Arm swing is decreased, and the affected arm is flexed across the body. Extrapyramidal dysfunction produces a slow, stiff, shuffling gait with dystonic postures. A waddling gait occurs with hip weakness due to lower motor neuron or neuromuscular disorders. A steppage gait results from weakness of ankle dorsiflexors (common peroneal palsy).

Reflexes

Deep tendon reflexes can be elicited at any age and are reported on a 5-point scale:

0 Absent
1 Trace
2 Normal
3 Exaggerated reflex, with spread to contiguous areas (tapping a patellar reflex and observing a bilaterally brisk quadriceps response)
4 Clonus (self-limited or sustained)

These reflexes are decreased in lower motor neuron diseases and increased in upper motor neuron disease. **Babinski response**, or extensor plantar reflex, is an upward movement of the great toe and flaring of the toes on stimulation of the lateral foot and is a sign of corticospinal tract dysfunction. This reflex is unreliable in neonates except when asymmetrical because the "normal" response at this age varies. By 12 to 18 months of age, the plantar response should consistently be flexor (toes flexing down).

SENSORY EXAMINATION

The sensory examination of newborns and infants is limited to observing the behavioral response to light touch or gentle sterile pinprick. Stimulation of the limb should produce a facial grimace. A spinal reflex alone may produce withdrawal movement of the limb. In a cooperative child, the senses of pain, touch, temperature, vibration, and joint position can be tested individually. The cortical areas of sensation must be intact to identify an object placed in the hand (**stereognosis**) or a number written in the hand (**graphesthesia**) or to distinguish between two sharp objects applied simultaneously and closely on the skin (**two-point discrimination**).

SPECIAL DIAGNOSTIC PROCEDURES
Cerebrospinal Fluid Analysis

Analysis of cerebrospinal fluid (CSF) is essential when central nervous system (CNS) infection is suspected and provides important clues to other diagnoses (Table 179-2). Differentiating hemorrhagic CSF caused by a traumatic lumbar puncture (LP) from a true subarachnoid hemorrhage may be difficult. In most cases of traumatic LP, the fluid clears significantly as the sequence of tubes is collected. If there is clinical evidence of increased ICP (papilledema, depression of consciousness, focal neurologic deficits), caution must be exercised before performing an LP to limit risk of cerebral herniation. A computed tomography (CT) scan should be performed and confirmed to be normal before the LP if increased ICP is suspected. If increased ICP is present, it must be treated before an LP is performed.

Table 179-2 | Analysis of Cerebrospinal Fluid (CSF)

CSF FINDING	NORMAL CSF VALUES	
	Newborn	**>1 Month Old**
Cell count*	10–25/mm³	5/mm³
Protein	65–150 mg/dL	<40 mg/dL
Glucose	>2/3 blood glucose	>2/3 blood glucose
	or >40 mg/dL	or >60 mg/dL

CSF change	Significance
Increased polymorphonuclear and decreased CSF glucose	Bacterial infection Partially treated bacterial meningitis Brain or parameningeal abscess Parasitic infection Leak of dermoid contents
Increased lymphocytes and decreased CSF glucose	Mycobacterial infection (tuberculosis) Fungal infection Carcinomatous meningitis Sarcoidosis
Increased lymphocytes and normal CSF glucose	Viral meningitis Post–infectious disease (ADEM) Vasculitis
Increased CSF protein	Infection Guillain-Barré syndrome Inflammatory disease (ADEM, multiple sclerosis) Leukodystrophy Venous thrombosis Hypertension Spinal block (Froin syndrome) Carcinomatous meningitis
Decreased glucose (without pleocytosis)	GLUT-1 transporter deficiency (epilepsy and ataxia)
Mild CSF pleocytosis	Tumor Infarction Multiple sclerosis Subacute bacterial endocarditis
Bloody CSF	Subarachnoid hemorrhage Subdural hemorrhage Intraparenchymal hemorrhage Hemorrhagic meningoencephalitis (group B streptococci, HSV) CNS trauma Vascular malformation Coagulopathy Traumatic lumbar puncture

ADEM, Acute disseminated encephalomyelitis; CNS, central nervous system; HSV, herpes simplex virus.
*In normal children, cells present should be lymphocytes.

Electroencephalography

The electroencephalogram (EEG) records electrical activity generated by the cerebral cortex. EEG rhythms mature throughout childhood. There are three key features present: background patterns, behavioral state modulation, and presence or absence of epileptiform patterns. The background varies with age, but there should be general symmetry and synchrony between the background of the two hemispheres without any localized area of higher amplitude or slower frequencies (focal slowing). Fixed slow wave foci (1 to 3 Hz) delta rhythms suggest an underlying structural abnormality (brain tumor, abscess, stroke). Bilateral disturbances of brain activity (increased ICP, metabolic encephalopathy) must be suspected when there is diffuse slow wave activity (delta frequency). Spikes, polyspikes, and spike-and-wave abnormalities, either in a localized region (focal) or distributed bihemispherically (generalized), indicate an underlying seizure tendency.

Electromyography and Nerve Conduction Studies

Electromyography and nerve conduction velocities (NCVs) assess for abnormalities of the neuromuscular apparatus, including anterior horn cells, peripheral nerves, neuromuscular junctions, and muscles. Normal muscle is electrically silent at rest. Spontaneous discharge of motor fibers (**fibrillations**) or groups of muscle fibers (**fasciculation**) indicates denervation, revealing dysfunction of anterior horn cells or peripheral nerves. Abnormal muscle responses to repetitive nerve stimulation are seen with neuromuscular junction disorders, such as myasthenia gravis and botulism. The amplitude and duration of the muscle compound action potentials are decreased in primary diseases of muscle. NCVs assess the action potential transmission along peripheral nerves. NCVs are slowed in demyelinating neuropathies (Guillain-Barré syndrome). The amplitude of the signal is diminished in axonal neuropathies.

Neuroimaging

Imaging the brain and spinal cord is accomplished using CT or magnetic resonance imaging (MRI). CT is quick and accessible for emergency purposes. MRI provides fine detail and, with different sequences, permits detection of posterior fossa lesions, subtle cerebral abnormalities, vascular anomalies, low-grade tumors, and ischemic changes. For a child with a head injury or sudden headache, cranial CT is the study of choice because it can rapidly reveal intracranial hemorrhage or other large lesions. For a child with new-onset complex partial seizures, MRI is the study of choice, because an area of focal cortical dysplasia or other subtle lesions might not be apparent on CT. MRI also provides excellent views of the spinal cord. Cranial ultrasonography is a noninvasive bedside procedure used to visualize the brain and ventricles of infants and young children with open fontanelles.

Chapter **180**

HEADACHE AND MIGRAINE

ETIOLOGY AND EPIDEMIOLOGY

Headache is a common symptom among children and adolescents. Headaches can be a primary problem (migraines, tension-type headaches) or secondary to another condition. Secondary headaches are most often associated with minor illnesses such as viral upper respiratory infections or sinusitis, but may be the first symptom of serious conditions (meningitis, brain tumors), so a systematic approach is necessary.

CLINICAL MANIFESTATIONS

Decision-Making Algorithm
Available @ StudentConsult.com

Headaches

The temporal pattern of the headache must be clarified. Each pattern (acute, recurrent-episodic, chronic-progressive, chronic-nonprogressive) has its own differential diagnosis (Table 180-1).

Tension-type headaches are the most common recurrent pattern of primary headaches in children and adolescents. They are generally mild and lack associated symptoms, so are not typically disruptive to patients' lifestyle or activities. The pain is global and squeezing or pressing in character, but can last for hours or days. There is no associated nausea, vomiting, phonophobia, or photophobia. Headaches can be related to environmental stresses or symptomatic of underlying psychiatric illnesses, such as anxiety or depression.

Migraine headaches are another common type of recurrent headaches and frequently begin in childhood. Headaches are stereotyped attacks of frontal, bitemporal, or unilateral, moderate to severe, pounding or throbbing pain that are aggravated by activity and last 1 to 72 hours. Associated symptoms include nausea, vomiting, pallor, photophobia, phonophobia, and an intense desire to seek a quiet dark room for rest. Toddlers may be unable to verbalize the source of their discomfort and exhibit episodes of irritability, sleepiness, pallor, and vomiting. Migraines can be associated with auras that may be typical (visual, sensory, dysphagic) or atypical. Aura can precede or coincide with the headache and typically persists for 15 to 30 minutes. Visual auras consist of spots, flashes, or lines of light that flicker in one or both visual fields. Atypical auras may also consist of brief episodes of unilateral or perioral numbness, unilateral weakness, or vertigo that persist for hours, then resolve completely. Complex, atypical symptoms (e.g., hemiparesis, monocular blindness, ophthalmoplegia, or confusion), accompanied by a headache, warrant careful diagnostic investigation, including a combination of neuroimaging, electroencephalogram, and appropriate metabolic studies.

Common causes of **secondary headaches** include head trauma, intercurrent viral illness, and sinusitis. Medication overuse headaches may complicate primary and secondary headaches. Serious causes of secondary headache include increased intracranial pressure (ICP) caused by a mass (tumor, vascular malformation) or intrinsic increase in pressure (pseudotumor cerebri). Increased ICP should be suspected if the headache and associated vomiting are worse when lying down or on first awakening; awaken the child from sleep; remit on arising; or are exacerbated by coughing, Valsalva maneuver, or bending over. Papilledema (Figure 180-1) or focal neurological deficits such as cranial nerve VI palsy may be seen on examination.

DIAGNOSTIC STUDIES

For most children, a thorough history and physical examination provide an accurate diagnosis and obviate the need for further testing. Neuroimaging is usually not necessary. Imaging is warranted, however, when the neurologic examination is abnormal, there are unusual neurologic features during the headache, or the child has signs or symptoms of increased ICP. Focal neurological deficits, alteration of consciousness, or a chronic progressive headache pattern may warrant imaging. In these cases, brain magnetic resonance imaging, with and without gadolinium contrast, is the study of choice, providing the highest sensitivity for detecting posterior fossa lesions and other, more subtle abnormalities. When the headache has a sudden, severe onset, emergent computed tomography (CT) can quickly evaluate for intracranial bleeding. If the CT

Table 180-1	Four Temporal Patterns of Childhood Headache

Acute: Single episode of pain without a history of such episodes. The "first and worst" headache, which raises concerns for aneurysmal subarachnoid hemorrhage in adults, is commonly due to *febrile illness* related to upper respiratory tract infection in children. Regardless, more ominous causes of acute headache (hemorrhage, meningitis, tumor) must be considered.

Acute recurrent: Pattern of attacks of pain separated by symptom-free intervals. Primary headache syndromes, such as *migraine or tension-type* headache, usually cause this pattern. Infrequently recurrent headaches can sometimes also be attributed to certain epilepsy syndromes (benign occipital epilepsy), substance abuse, or recurrent trauma.

Chronic progressive: Most ominous of the temporal patterns—implies a gradually increasing frequency and severity of headache. The pathologic correlate is *increasing ICP.* Causes of this pattern include pseudotumor cerebri, brain tumor, hydrocephalus, chronic meningitis, brain abscess, and subdural collections.

Chronic nonprogressive or chronic daily: Pattern of frequent or constant headache. Chronic daily headache generally is defined as >4-month history of >15 headaches/month, with headaches lasting >4 hours. Affected patients have normal neurologic examinations; psychological factors and anxiety about possible underlying organic causes are common.

Figure 180-1 Papilledema with dilation of the vessels, obliteration of the optic cup, loss of disc margin, and hemorrhages around disc. *(From Kliegman RE, Behrman, RM, Jenson HB, editors:* Nelson Textbook of Pediatrics, *ed 18, Philadelphia, 2007, Saunders, p 2107.)*

is negative, a lumbar puncture should be performed, with measurement of opening pressure and evaluation for red and white blood cells, protein, glucose, or xanthochromia.

TREATMENT

Treating migraines requires an individually tailored regimen to address the frequency, severity, and disability produced by the headache. Intermittent *symptomatic,* or abortive, analgesics are the mainstay for treatment of infrequent, intense episodes of migraine. Symptomatic therapy requires early administration of an analgesic, rest, and sleep in a quiet, dark room. Acetaminophen or a nonsteroidal anti-inflammatory drug such as ibuprofen or naproxen sodium is often effective. Hydration and antiemetics are also useful adjunctive therapies. If these first-line medications are insufficient, *triptan* agents may be considered. Triptans, available in injectable, nasal spray, oral disintegrating, and tablet form, are serotonin receptor agonists that may alleviate migraine symptoms promptly. Triptans are contraindicated for patients with focal neurological deficits associated with their migraines or signs consistent with basilar migraine (syncope) because of the risk of stroke.

Many children suffer with severe and frequent migraines that disrupt their daily lives. Children with more than one disabling headache per week may require daily preventive agents to reduce both attack frequency and severity. Preventative medications include tricyclic antidepressants (amitriptyline, nortriptyline), anticonvulsants (topiramate, valproic acid), antihistamines (cyproheptadine), beta-blockers (propranolol), and calcium channel blockers (flunarizine, verapamil).

Before initiating daily medications, lifestyle modifications must be put into place to regulate sleep, daily routines, and exercise and identify any precipitating or aggravating influences, eliminating as many as possible (caffeine, certain foods, stress, missed meals, dehydration). Other adjunctive treatment options include psychological support, counseling, stress management, and biofeedback.

Chapter 181

SEIZURES (PAROXYSMAL DISORDERS)

A seizure is a transient occurrence of signs or symptoms resulting from abnormal excessive or synchronous neuronal activity in the brain.

ETIOLOGY AND EPIDEMIOLOGY

Decision-Making Algorithm
Available @ StudentConsult.com

Seizures and Other Paroxysmal Disorders

Table 181-1	Paroxysmal Disorders of Childhood

Seizures/epilepsy

Migraine and variants
    Paroxysmal torticollis of infancy
    Paroxysmal vertigo (benign)

Syncope
    Vasovagal syncope
    Breath-holding spells
    Cardiac syncope (arrhythmias, long QT syndrome)
    Apnea

Transient ischemic attack

Metabolic disorders
    Hypoglycemia
    Inborn errors of metabolism

Sleep disorders
    Narcolepsy, cataplexy
    Night terrors

Paroxysmal dyskinesias and other movement disorders
    Tics

Shudder attacks

Sandifer syndrome (gastroesophageal reflux causing paroxysmal stiffening and posturing)

Conversion disorder

Malingering

Normal behavior
    Neonatal jitteriness
    Benign sleep myoclonus

Self-stimulatory behavior

The differential diagnosis of paroxysmal disorders includes **seizures** and **nonepileptic events** (Table 181-1). Nonseizure paroxysmal events are often normal or benign phenomena, although some are clinically significant and consequential. A thorough medical history from the patient and primary witnesses is the most reliable tool for establishing the correct diagnosis.

Acute symptomatic seizures are secondary to an acute problem affecting brain excitability, such as electrolyte imbalance or infection (Table 181-2). **Epilepsy** is defined as recurrent, *unprovoked* seizures. Epileptic seizures are generally classified as *focal* (or partial), arising from one region of the cortex, or *generalized* seizures, which arise from both hemispheres, simultaneously (Table 181-3). Approximately 4% to 10% of children experience at least one seizure. The incidence of childhood epilepsy is 1% to 2%.

FOCAL SEIZURES

Simple focal (or **partial**) **seizures** arise from a specific anatomic focus and may or may not spread to surrounding brain regions. Clinical symptoms include motor (tonic, clonic, myoclonic), sensory, psychic, or autonomic abnormalities, but consciousness is preserved. The location and direction of spread of the seizure focus determine the clinical symptoms.

Complex partial seizures can have similar sensorimotor signs but also have associated alteration of consciousness. Although the child may not be completely unresponsive, subtle slowing or alteration of mental status (*dyscognitive* features) may occur. Along with altered responsiveness, patients may have staring

Table 181-2	Causes of Seizures

PERINATAL CONDITIONS

Malformation of cortical development

Intrauterine infection

Hypoxic-ischemic encephalopathy*

Trauma

Hemorrhage*

INFECTIONS

Encephalitis*

Meningitis*

Brain abscess

METABOLIC CONDITIONS

Hypoglycemia*

Hypocalcemia

Hypomagnesemia

Hyponatremia

Hypernatremia

Storage diseases

Reye syndrome

Degenerative disorders

Porphyria

Pyridoxine dependency and deficiency

POISONING

Lead

Drug toxicity

Drug withdrawal

NEUROCUTANEOUS SYNDROMES

Tuberous sclerosis

Neurofibromatosis

Sturge-Weber syndrome

Incontinentia pigmenti

SYSTEMIC DISORDERS

Vasculitis

Systemic lupus erythematosus

Hypertensive encephalopathy

Hepatic encephalopathy

OTHER CAUSATIVE DISORDERS/CONDITIONS

Accidental trauma*

Child abuse*

Increased intracranial pressure

Tumor

Remote brain injury

Febrile illnesses*

Cryptogenic* (no underlying disorder found)

Familial*

*Common.

Table 181-3	Classification of Seizures and Epilepsy Syndromes

FOCAL/PARTIAL SEIZURES

Simple partial (consciousness not impaired)
  Motor signs (can be tonic, clonic, myoclonic)
  Special sensory (visual, auditory, olfactory, gustatory, vertiginous, somatosensory)
  Autonomic

Complex partial/focal dyscognitive (consciousness impaired)
  Psychic (déjà vu, fear)
  Impaired consciousness at onset
  Development of impaired consciousness

Focal seizures with secondarily generalized convulsions
  Jacksonian seizures

GENERALIZED SEIZURES

Absence (staring, unresponsiveness)

Tonic (sustained contraction)

Clonic (rhythmic contractions)

Tonic-clonic (tonic phase followed by clonic phase)

Atonic (loss of tone)

Myoclonic (rapid, shock-like contraction)

Spasms (flexion or extension of trunk and extremities for <2 seconds)

EPILEPSY SYNDROMES

Symptomatic
  Underlying cause is identified
  Example: Focal epilepsy associated with a remote stroke
Idiopathic
  Presumed to have a *genetic* etiology
  Example: Benign childhood epilepsy with centrotemporal spikes, childhood absence epilepsy, juvenile myoclonic epilepsy
Cryptogenic
  Epilepsy of uncertain etiology
  Example: Infantile spasms with no identifiable cause

and automatisms during complex partial seizures. Automatisms are automatic semipurposeful movements of the mouth (lip smacking, chewing) or extremities (rubbing of fingers, shuffling of feet). Focal seizures that manifest only with psychic or autonomic symptoms, such as a feeling of déjà vu during a temporal lobe seizure, can be difficult to recognize. When focal seizures spread to involve the whole brain and produce a generalized seizure, they are said to have *secondarily generalized*. Such spread is classically described as progression from face to arm to leg (*Jacksonian* march). It is often difficult to distinguish primary generalized tonic and clonic seizures from secondarily generalized focal seizures on purely clinical grounds. This distinction is important, however, because evaluation and treatment for focal or generalized epilepsy syndromes are quite different.

GENERALIZED SEIZURES

Tonic, **clonic**, and biphasic **tonic-clonic** seizures may occur alone or in association with other seizure types. Typically the seizure begins abruptly but occasionally is preceded by a series of myoclonic jerks. During a tonic-clonic seizure, consciousness and control of posture are lost, followed by tonic stiffening and upward deviation of the eyes. Pooling of secretions,

Table 181-4	Differentiating Absence Seizure and Complex Partial Seizure	
FEATURE	**ABSENCE SEIZURE**	**COMPLEX PARTIAL SEIZURE**
Duration	Seconds	Minutes
Provoking maneuver	Hyperventilation Photic stimulation	Variable, but often none
Postictal phase	None (return immediately to baseline)	Confusion, sleepiness
Number of seizures	Many per day	Infrequent (rarely more than one per day)
EEG features	Interictal: normal Ictal: 3-Hz generalized spike-wave	Interictal: focal slowing or sharp waves Ictal: Focal discharges (with or without secondary generalization)
Neurological examination	Normal	Normal, or focal deficits
Neuroimaging	Normal*	Normal, or focal abnormalities (mesial temporal sclerosis, focal cortical dysplasia, neoplasm, encephalomalacia)
First-line treatment	Ethosuximide or valproic acid†	Oxcarbazepine

*In the proper clinical context, and with an appropriate EEG, a diagnosis of absence epilepsy should be made without neuroimaging.
†Oxcarbazepine and carbamazepine are relatively contraindicated for children with typical absence epilepsy, as their seizures can be exacerbated by these medications.

pupillary dilation, diaphoresis, and hypertension are common. Clonic jerks follow the tonic phase. In the post-ictal phase, the child might be hypotonic. Irritability and headache are common as the child awakens.

Absence Seizures

Seizures in which the primary clinical feature is staring can be either absence (generalized) or complex partial seizures. The clinical hallmark of absence seizures is a brief (less than 15 seconds) loss of environmental awareness accompanied by eye fluttering or simple automatisms, such as fumbling with the fingers and lip smacking. Absence seizures usually begin between 4 and 6 years of age. Neurologic examination and brain imaging are normal. The characteristic electroencephalographic (EEG) patterns consist of generalized **3-Hz spike-and-wave activity**. A clinical seizure can be provoked by **hyperventilation** or strobe light stimulation. Differentiating absence from complex partial seizures can be difficult, but is essential for appropriate evaluation and treatment (Table 181-4).

Atypical Absence, Myoclonic, and Atonic Seizures

Atypical absence seizures manifest as episodes of impaired consciousness with automatisms, autonomic phenomena, and motor manifestations, such as eye opening, eye deviation, and body stiffening. They are associated with slower EEG discharges (2 Hz) and other seizure types. **Myoclonus** is

a sudden jerk of all or part of the body; not all myoclonus is epileptic in nature. Nonepileptic myoclonus may be benign, as in sleep myoclonus, or indicate serious disease. Myoclonic epilepsy usually is associated with multiple seizure types. The underlying disorder producing myoclonic epilepsy may be static (juvenile myoclonic epilepsy) or progressive and associated with neurologic deterioration (neuronal ceroid lipofuscinosis). Myoclonic absence refers to the body jerks that commonly accompany absence seizures and atypical absence seizures. Although **atonic seizures** are typically brief (lasting 1 to 2 seconds), they are quite disabling because of a sudden loss of postural tone, resulting in falls and injuries.

Febrile Seizures

Seizures in the setting of fever may be caused by infections of the nervous system (meningitis, encephalitis, brain abscess), unrecognized epilepsy triggered by fever, or **febrile seizures**. The latter represents the most common cause of seizures among children between 6 months and 6 years of age, occurring in about 4% of all children. By definition, a febrile seizure occurs in the presence of fever. **Simple febrile seizures** are generalized at onset, last less than 15 minutes, and occur only once in a 24-hour period in a neurologically and developmentally normal child. If there are focal features, the seizure lasts longer than 15 minutes or recurs within 24 hours, or if the child has preexisting neurologic challenges, the seizure is referred to as a **complex** or **atypical febrile seizure**.

The prognosis of children with simple febrile convulsions is excellent. Intellectual achievements are normal. Febrile seizures recur in 30% to 50% of children. The risk of subsequent epilepsy is not substantially greater than that for the general population (approximately 2%). Factors that increase the risk for the development of epilepsy include abnormal neurologic examination or development, family history of epilepsy, and complex febrile seizures. Because febrile seizures are brief and the outcome is benign, most children require no treatment. Rectal diazepam can be administered during a seizure to abort a prolonged event and is a reasonable option for children with a history of prolonged febrile seizures. Because of the potential for side effects, daily administration of anticonvulsant medication is not recommended. Administration of antipyretics during febrile illnesses does not prevent febrile seizures.

Psychogenic Nonepileptic Seizures (PNES)

PNES (previously termed pseudoseizures) may be the manifestation of conversion disorders or malingering. Additionally, children with genuine epilepsy may, consciously or subconsciously, exhibit concurrent nonepileptic spells. Although the clinical differentiation can be difficult, PNES often differ from epileptic seizures in that the patient's eyes are often closed (typically eyes are open during epileptic seizures) and the movement is tremulousness or thrashing rather than true tonic-clonic activity. Verbalization and pelvic thrusting are seen more commonly in PNES, urinary and fecal continence is usually preserved, and injury does not occur. If the tongue is bitten, more often the tip of the tongue is injured (as opposed to the sides of the tongue in epileptic seizures). PNES can often be initiated or terminated by suggestion. An EEG performed during PNES does not show epileptiform patterns. The diagnosis is critical, because appropriate mental health care, and not anticonvulsant medications, is the crux of treatment.

EPILEPSY SYNDROMES

The epilepsy syndromes represent clinical entities in which age, pattern of clinical events, EEG features, natural history, and prognosis are distinctive (see Table 181-3).

Benign childhood epilepsy with centrotemporal spikes, also known as **benign Rolandic epilepsy**, is among the most common epilepsy syndromes and usually begins between ages 5 and 10 years. The seizures typically occur only during sleep or on awakening in more than half of patients. Affected children usually have focal motor seizures involving the face and arm (abnormal movement or sensation around the face and mouth, drooling, rhythmic guttural sound). Speech and swallowing may be impaired. Seizures sometimes secondarily generalize. The interictal EEG demonstrates independent bilateral centrotemporal sharp waves but is otherwise normal. With a classic history and EEG, and a normal neurological examination, the diagnosis can be made with confidence and neuroimaging is not required. Seizures usually respond promptly to anticonvulsant therapy. Intellectual outcome is normal, and the epilepsy resolves after puberty. Comorbid learning difficulties and attention deficit/hyperactivity disorder (ADHD) are common.

Childhood absence epilepsy is another common syndrome. Absence seizures typically begin in the early school years and usually resolve by late childhood or adolescence. If absence does not remit, 44% will go on to develop juvenile myoclonic epilepsy (see later discussion). Ethosuximide is the first-choice therapy. A subset of patients also has generalized tonic-clonic seizures. For these children, valproic acid is the first choice as it can prevent both absence and convulsive seizures. Comorbid learning disabilities and ADHD are common. There is no contraindication to treating these children's ADHD with stimulant medication.

Juvenile myoclonic epilepsy (of Janz) is the most common generalized epilepsy among adolescents and young adults. Onset is typically in early adolescence with myoclonic jerks (exacerbated in the morning, often causing the patient to drop objects), generalized tonic-clonic seizures, and absence seizures. Seizures usually resolve promptly with anticonvulsant medication (classically valproic acid, but several medications have been shown to be efficacious), but therapy must be maintained for life.

Infantile spasms are brief contractions of the neck, trunk, and arm muscles, followed by a phase of sustained muscle contraction lasting less than 2 seconds. Spasms occur most frequently when the child is awakening from or going to sleep. Each jerk is followed by a brief period of relaxation with repeated spasms in clusters of variable duration. Many clusters occur each day. **West syndrome** is the triad of infantile spasms, developmental regression, and a dramatically abnormal EEG pattern (hypsarrhythmia). **Hypsarrhythmia** consists of chaotic high-voltage slow waves, spikes, and polyspikes. The peak age at onset is 3 to 8 months. When flexion of the thighs and crying are prominent, the syndrome may be mistaken for colic or gastroesophageal reflux. The underlying etiology of the spasms dictates the prognosis. More than 200 different etiologies have been identified, including tuberous sclerosis, malformations of cortical

development (lissencephaly), genetic syndromes (trisomy 21), acquired brain injury (stroke, perinatal hypoxic-ischemic encephalopathy), and metabolic disorders (phenylketonuria). Infants for whom an etiology is determined are classified as having *symptomatic* infantile spasms and are at very high risk for long-term neurodevelopmental difficulties. The etiology is not determined for a small subset of children. These patients with *cryptogenic* spasms have a somewhat better long-term prognosis but remain at high risk for adverse outcomes. First-line treatment options for infantile spasms include adrenocorticotropic hormone, high-dose oral corticosteroids, and vigabatrin. For infants with underlying tuberous sclerosis, vigabatrin is considered the treatment of choice. For other patients, treatment determinations are made on a case-by-case basis.

Lennox-Gastaut syndrome is a severe epilepsy syndrome with variable age of onset. Most children present before age 5 years. Frequent, multiple seizure types, including atonic, focal, atypical absence, and generalized tonic, clonic, or tonic-clonic varieties, characterize the disorder. Many children have underlying brain injury or malformations. The seizures usually respond poorly to treatment, and most patients have significant intellectual disability.

Benign neonatal convulsions are an autosomal dominant genetic disorder linked to abnormal neuronal potassium channels. Otherwise well newborns present with focal seizures toward the end of the first week of life, leading to the colloquial term *fifth-day fits*. Response to treatment is generally excellent, and the long-term outcome is typically favorable.

Acquired epileptic aphasia (Landau-Kleffner syndrome) is characterized by the abrupt loss of previously acquired language in young children. The language disability is an acquired cortical auditory deficit (auditory agnosia). The EEG is highly epileptiform in sleep, the peak area of abnormality often being in the dominant perisylvian region (language areas). This diagnosis should be considered for young patients with clear autistic regression, as it is a potentially treatable entity.

STATUS EPILEPTICUS

Status epilepticus is a neurologic emergency and is defined as ongoing seizure activity or repetitive seizures without return of consciousness for greater than 30 minutes. Status epilepticus carries an approximately 14% risk of new neurologic deficits, most secondary to the underlying pathology. Similarly, the mortality rate of status epilepticus (4% to 5%) is related to the underlying etiology. Etiologies include new-onset epilepsy of any type, drug intoxication, drug withdrawal (especially missed anticonvulsant doses among children with preexisting epilepsy), hypoglycemia, electrolyte imbalance, acute head trauma, infection, ischemic stroke, intracranial hemorrhage, metabolic disorders, and hypoxia.

The first priority of treatment is to ensure an adequate airway, breathing, and circulation (Chapter 38). Vital signs should be obtained and oxygen administered if needed. If respirations are inadequate, positive-pressure ventilation may be required. Intravenous (IV) access should be obtained. In patients with no history of seizures, laboratory evaluation should be undertaken (see below). Several pharmacologic options exist for management of status epilepticus (Table 181-5). Initial management is usually with a benzodiazepine. Lorazepam, diazepam, and midazolam all are effective agents. Diazepam distributes rapidly to the brain but has a short duration of action. If IV access is not available, liquid preparations may be administered per rectum. If the seizure does not resolve after two doses of benzodiazepine, a second-line agent must be administered. Either IV phenytoin or fosphenytoin is effective, but cardiac monitoring is required to evaluate for arrhythmia. If the seizures persist, a loading dose of phenobarbital or valproic acid is appropriate (see Table 181-5). Alternatively, continuous infusions, such as midazolam or pentobarbital, can be employed as third-line agents (with appropriate airway protection, blood pressure support, and strong consideration of continuous video-EEG monitoring to evaluate for ongoing subclinical seizures). If this approach is ineffective, preparations for general anesthesia are undertaken. When status epilepticus stops, maintenance therapy is initiated with the appropriate anticonvulsant.

LABORATORY AND DIAGNOSTIC EVALUATION

For an otherwise healthy child with an unprovoked seizure and a normal physical and neurological examination, no laboratory evaluation is required. Children with *simple febrile seizures* who have recovered completely require little or no laboratory evaluation other than studies necessary to evaluate the source of the fever. If the clinical presentation does not meet these criteria and acute symptomatic seizures are suspected, potentially life-threatening causes such as meningitis, sepsis, head trauma, and toxins should be pursued. A complete laboratory evaluation for new onset of seizures includes a complete blood count and measurement of glucose, calcium, sodium, potassium, chloride, bicarbonate, urea nitrogen, creatinine, magnesium, and phosphorus, as well as blood or urine toxicology

Table 181-5	Management of Status Epilepticus

STABILIZATION

ABCs (airway, breathing, circulation)

Cardiac monitoring

Oxygen and pulse oximetry

Intravenous access

Immediate laboratory tests
  Glucose
  Basic metabolic panel—sodium, calcium, magnesium
  Anticonvulsant drug levels
  Toxicology studies as appropriate
  Complete blood counts, platelets, and differential

PHARMACOLOGIC MANAGEMENT

Benzodiazepine (max rate of administration = 1 mg/min)
  Lorazepam 0.05–0.1 mg/kg (maximum 2–4mg per dose)
  Diazepam 0.2–0.5 mg/kg
  Midazolam 0.1–0.2 mg/kg

Standard anticonvulsant medications
  Fosphenytoin 10–20 mg/kg (phenytoin equivalents)
  Phenobarbital 10–20 mg/kg
  Valproic acid 20 mg/kg

Continuous infusions
  Pentobarbital
  Midazolam
  General anesthesia

screening. Children with clinical signs and symptoms of meningitis (neck stiffness, Kernig sign, Brudzinski sign), or history or physical examination suggestive of intracranial infection, should undergo a lumbar puncture. Cerebrospinal fluid (CSF) should be analyzed for cell counts, culture, protein, and glucose levels. In children less than 18 months old, particularly young infants, the clinical symptoms of meningitis may be subtle. Neonates also may require testing for inborn errors of metabolism; blood ammonia; CSF glycine and lactate, as well as herpes simplex polymerase chain reaction; urine and stool culture (cytomegalovirus and enterovirus); and a clinical trial of pyridoxine.

The **EEG** is the most useful neurodiagnostic test for distinguishing seizures from nonepileptic paroxysmal disorders and for classifying seizures as having focal or generalized onset. The EEG must be interpreted in the context of the clinical history, because some normal children have focal or epileptiform EEG patterns. Children with seizures may have normal interictal EEGs. When the diagnosis is unclear, more sophisticated EEGs with prolonged recordings and simultaneous video monitoring of the patient in an attempt to capture a typical event may be necessary.

Magnetic resonance imaging (MRI) is superior to computed tomography (CT) in showing most brain pathology, but in the emergency department setting, CT can be performed rapidly and often shows acute intracranial hemorrhage more clearly than MRI. MRI is unnecessary in patients with the primary generalized epilepsies, such as typical absence and juvenile myoclonic epilepsy. Lesions (tumors, arteriovenous malformations, cysts, strokes, gliosis, focal atrophy) may be identified in 25% of patients, even when the clinical examination and EEG do not suggest focal features. Identification of some lesions, such as focal cortical dysplasia, hamartoma, and mesial temporal sclerosis, can assist in consideration of surgical treatment of pharmacoresistant epilepsy.

LONG-TERM THERAPY

The decision to institute daily seizure medications for a first unprovoked seizure is based on the likelihood of recurrence balanced against the risk of long-term drug therapy. Determination of the recurrence risk is based on the clinical history and neurodiagnostic testing (Table 181-6). If the recurrence risk is 75% or greater, it is usually suggested that daily medication be prescribed. Absence seizures, infantile spasms, atypical absence seizures, and atonic seizures are universally recurrent at the time of diagnosis, indicating the need for therapy.

Table 181-6	Recurrence Risk after a First Unprovoked Seizure*		
SEIZURE TYPE	EEG NORMAL, EXAM NORMAL	EEG EPILEPTIFORM OR EXAM ABNORMAL	BOTH EEG AND EXAM ABNORMAL
Generalized	25%	50%	75%
Focal	50%	75%	>90%

*Most recurrences occur within 2 years

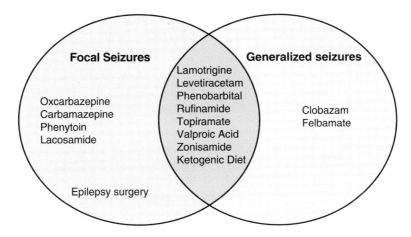

Special circumstances:
1. For absence epilepsy, ethosuximide is the first line treatment.
2. Adrenocorticotropic hormone, oral corticosteroids, or vigabatrin are used to treat infantile spasms.

Figure 181-1 Treatment for epilepsy.

The goal of treatment is to maintain an optimal functional state. Medication toxicity should be weighed against the risk of seizure itself. Initial drug selection is based on the mechanism of the seizure (Fig. 181-1). A single agent limits toxicity, contains cost, and improves compliance. Approximately 60% of children obtain satisfactory seizure control and minimal side effects with the initial drug. If seizure control is not achieved, despite good compliance, addition of a second drug is considered. When available, measuring anticonvulsant blood levels can be helpful in adjusting dosing and monitoring compliance. Levels should be interpreted in light of the patient's clinical state; a patient with a "low" drug level who is seizure free does not necessarily need a higher dose. Anticonvulsant drug levels should be drawn at trough, usually before the morning doses. When hepatic or renal disease is present, drug binding is likely to be altered. In this instance, free and bound anticonvulsant levels can be helpful.

The duration of anticonvulsant treatment varies according to seizure type and epilepsy syndrome. For most children, anticonvulsant medications can be weaned off after 2 years without seizures. There are some exceptions. For example, children with juvenile myoclonic epilepsy, progressive myoclonic epilepsy, atypical absence seizures, and Lennox-Gastaut syndrome usually require treatment for life. Children who have other neurological comorbidities, seizures that were initially difficult to control, or persistently epileptiform EEGs are at highest risk for recurrence when therapy is discontinued.

Although cognitively normal children with epilepsy have the same rates of injury as normal healthy children, there are important safety considerations for people with epilepsy. The risk of drowning is high, so swimming and bathing must only occur under direct adult supervision. Children should use appropriate helmets for sports such as bicycling or ice skating. There is no contraindication to participation in contact sports, but scuba diving, hang gliding, and free climbing are not safe for people with epilepsy. Each country and individual states have specific laws regarding driving for people with epilepsy. Most require a period of seizure freedom before issuing a driving permit.

Chapter 182

WEAKNESS AND HYPOTONIA

Weakness is a decreased ability to voluntarily and actively move muscles. This may be generalized or localized to one aspect of the body. Hypotonia is a state of low muscle resistance to movement. Hypotonia can be associated with weakness, but in some cases is present with normal motor strength. The differential diagnosis for weakness is extensive (Table 182-1).

ETIOLOGY

Weakness and hypotonia may be due to disorders of **upper motor neurons** or **lower motor neurons**. *Upper motor neurons* originate in the cerebral motor cortex; their axons form the corticospinal tract ending in the spinal cord and control voluntary motor activity. The anterior horn cells, their motor roots, peripheral motor nerves, neuromuscular junctions, and muscles represent the *lower motor neurons* and muscle units. Maintenance of normal strength, tone, and coordination requires integrated communication throughout this complex system, including the cerebral cortex, cerebellum, brainstem, thalamus, basal ganglia, and spinal cord.

CLINICAL MANIFESTATIONS

Decision-Making Algorithm
Available @ StudentConsult.com

Hypotonia and Weakness

Weakness caused by upper motor neuron disease differs from weakness produced by lower motor units (Table 182-2). Dysfunction of the upper motor neuron causes loss of voluntary

Table 182-1	Disorders Causing Weakness in Infants and Children
ANATOMIC REGION	**CORRESPONDING DISORDERS**
Central nervous system—brain	Brain tumor Trauma (accidental, nonaccidental) Infection (meningitis, encephalitis, abscess) Ischemia (arterial or venous) Hemorrhage Metabolic disease (leukodystrophy; inborn error of metabolism; mitochondrial encephalomyopathy, lactic acidosis, and stroke-like episodes) Degenerative disease
Central nervous system—spinal cord	Transverse myelitis Tumor Abscess Trauma Infarction
Anterior horn cell	Spinal muscular atrophy Poliomyelitis
Peripheral nerve	Guillain-Barré syndrome Hereditary motor sensory neuropathy Tick paralysis Bell palsy
Neuromuscular junction	Myasthenia gravis (juvenile, transient neonatal, congenital) Botulism
Muscle	Muscular dystrophies (Duchenne, Becker, limb-girdle) Myotonic dystrophies Congenital myopathies Metabolic myopathies Dermatomyositis Polymyositis

Table 182-2	Clinical Distinction between Upper Motor Neuron and Lower Motor Neuron Lesions	
CLINICAL SIGN	**UPPER MOTOR NEURON (CORTICOSPINAL TRACT)**	**LOWER MOTOR NEURON (NEUROMUSCULAR)**
Tone	Increased (spastic)	Decreased
Reflexes	Increased	Decreased
Babinski reflex	Present	Absent
Atrophy	Possible	Possible
Fasciculations	Absent	Possible

neuron, the final common pathway producing muscle activity, leads to total absence of movement with hypotonia. Function is best tested by measuring the strength of individual muscle groups or, in a young child, by observing the ability to perform tasks requiring particular muscle groups (e.g., walk up or down stairs, arise from the ground, walk on toes or heels, raise the hands above the head, squeeze a ball).

DISEASE OF THE UPPER MOTOR NEURON
Etiology and Epidemiology
Tumors, trauma, infections, demyelinating syndromes, infarction, metabolic diseases, and degenerative diseases may injure the corticospinal tract, producing an upper motor neuron pattern of weakness coupled with increased deep tendon reflexes, spasticity, and extensor plantar responses (Babinski sign).

Clinical Manifestations
The distribution of weakness depends on the location of the lesion. A tumor in the left parietal region may produce a right hemiparesis. A brainstem glioma may produce a slowly progressive quadriparesis. A diffuse disorder of myelin synthesis, such as a leukodystrophy, would produce a progressive symmetrical quadriparesis.

DISEASES OF THE SPINAL CORD

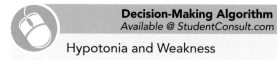

Decision-Making Algorithm
Available @ StudentConsult.com

Hypotonia and Weakness

Acute spinal cord lesions, such as infarction or compression, may produce a **flaccid, areflexic paralysis** that mimics lower motor neuron disease. A child who exhibits an acute or subacute flaccid paraparesis is most likely to have either an acute cord syndrome or Guillain-Barré syndrome. The hallmarks of spinal cord disease are a sensory level, a motor level, disturbance of bowel and bladder function, and local spinal pain or tenderness. The acute cord syndrome may be the result of transverse myelitis, cord tumor, infarction, demyelination, or trauma. **Transverse myelitis**, an acute postinfectious demyelinating disorder of the spinal cord, is treated with high-dose steroids. Trauma and tumors (neuroblastoma, lymphoma, sarcoma) compressing the spinal cord necessitate immediate neurosurgical management to preserve vital function.

DISEASES OF THE LOWER MOTOR NEURON
Neuromuscular disease affects any component of the lower motor neuron unit. The distribution of muscle weakness can point toward specific diseases (Table 182-3).

Spinal Muscular Atrophy
Etiology
Progressive degeneration of anterior horn cells is the key manifestation of spinal muscular atrophy (SMA), a genetic disease that may begin in intrauterine life or any time thereafter. About

control, but not total loss of movement because motor nuclei of the basal ganglia, thalamus, and brainstem have tracts that produce simple or complex stereotyped patterns of movement. The corticospinal tract permits fine motor activity and is best tested by rapid alternating movements of the distal extremities. Mild dysfunction produces slowed, stiff motions. More severe dysfunction produces stiff, abnormal involuntary postures (spasticity) consisting of forearm flexion at the elbow and wrist and adduction close to the chest, with leg extension and adduction.

Damage to the spinal cord leaves residual simple, stereotyped reflex movements coordinated by local spinal reflexes below the level of the lesion. Destruction of the lower motor

Table 182-3	Topography of Neuromuscular Diseases
LOCATION	**CLINICAL SYNDROMES/DISORDERS**
Proximal muscle weakness	Muscular dystrophy
	Duchenne / Becker
	Limb-girdle
	Dermatomyositis; polymyositis
	Kugelberg-Welander disease (spinal muscular atrophy type 2)
Distal limb weakness	Polyneuropathy (Guillain-Barré syndrome)
	Hereditary motor sensory neuropathy I
	Hereditary motor sensory neuropathy II
	Myotonic dystrophy
	Distal myopathy
Ophthalmoplegia and limb weakness	Myasthenia gravis
	Botulism
	Myotonic dystrophy
	Congenital myotubular myopathy
	Miller Fisher variant of Guillain-Barré syndrome
Facial and bulbar weakness	Myasthenia gravis
	Botulism
	Polio
	Miller Fisher variant of Guillain-Barré syndrome
	Myotonic dystrophy
	Congenital myopathy
	Facioscapulohumeral dystrophy

25% of patients have a severe infantile form (SMA type 1/**Werdnig-Hoffmann disease**), 50% have a late infantile and more slowly progressive form (SMA type 2/**Kugelberg-Welander syndrome**), and 25% have a more chronic, juvenile form (SMA type 3). SMA is one of the most frequent autosomal recessive diseases, with a carrier frequency of 1 in 50.

Clinical Manifestations

Decision-Making Algorithm
Available @ StudentConsult.com

Hypotonia and Weakness

The earlier in life the process starts, the more severe the progression. Infants with SMA type 1 present in early infancy with severe hypotonia, generalized weakness, and facial involvement. Infants have normal cognitive, social, and language skills and sensation. **Fasciculations** (quivering of the lateral aspect of the tongue) are best identified by inspecting the mouth when the child is asleep. Deep tendon reflexes are absent. With progression, breathing becomes rapid, shallow, and predominantly abdominal. In an extremely weak child, respiratory compromise leads to atelectasis, pulmonary infection, and death. Most infants with SMA type 1 die within the first 2 years. Children with SMA type 2 may survive to adulthood. Children with SMA type 3 can appear normal, with slower progression of weakness and a normal life expectancy.

Laboratory and Diagnostic Studies

The diagnosis is made by genetic testing. Creatine phosphokinase (CK) may be normal or mildly elevated. The electromyelogram (EMG) shows fasciculations, fibrillations, and other signs of denervation. Muscle biopsy specimens show grouped atrophy.

Treatment

No specific treatment delays progression of SMA, although a number of promising agents are being studied. Symptomatic therapy is directed toward minimizing contractures, preventing scoliosis, maximizing nutrition, and avoiding infections. Respiratory infections are managed early and aggressively with pulmonary hygiene, oxygen, and antibiotics. The use or nonuse of artificial ventilation and tube feedings must be individualized for each patient in each stage of the illness.

Peripheral Neuropathy

There are many peripheral nerve diseases in childhood, but the most classic presentations are: Guillain-Barré syndrome, chronic inflammatory demyelinating polyneuropathy (CIDP), hereditary motor sensory neuropathy (HMSN), and tick paralysis. Peripheral neuropathies produced by diabetes mellitus, alcoholism, chronic renal failure, exposure to toxins, vasculitis, and the effects of neoplasm are common in adults but are rare in children.

Guillain-Barré Syndrome

Guillain-Barré syndrome (acute inflammatory demyelinating polyradiculoneuropathy) is a postinfectious autoimmune peripheral neuropathy that can occur about 10 days after a respiratory or gastrointestinal infection (classically *Mycoplasma pneumonia* or *Campylobacter jejuni*). It occurs in people of all ages and is the most common cause of acute flaccid paralysis in children.

The characteristic symptoms are *areflexia*, *flaccidity*, and *symmetrical ascending weakness*. Progression can occur rapidly, in hours, or more indolently over weeks. Typically symptoms start with numbness or paresthesia in the hands and feet, then a heavy, weak feeling in the legs. Weakness ascends to involve the arms, trunk, and bulbar muscles (tongue, pharynx, larynx). Deep tendon reflexes are absent even when strength is relatively preserved. Objective signs of sensory loss are usually minor compared with the dramatic weakness. Bulbar and respiratory insufficiency may progress rapidly. Dysfunction of autonomic nerves can lead to blood pressure changes, tachycardia and other arrhythmias, urinary retention or incontinence, or stool retention. This polyneuropathy can be difficult to distinguish from an acute spinal cord syndrome. Preservation of bowel and bladder function, loss of arm reflexes, absence of a sensory level, and lack of spinal tenderness point toward Guillain-Barré syndrome. A cranial nerve variant of Guillain-Barré syndrome called the **Miller Fisher variant** manifests with ataxia, partial ophthalmoplegia, and areflexia.

The cerebrospinal fluid in Guillain-Barré syndrome is sometimes normal early in the illness but classically shows elevated protein levels without significant pleocytosis. Magnetic resonance imaging (MRI) with gadolinium may reveal enhancement of the spinal nerve roots. Electrophysiology studies (EMG, nerve conduction velocity [NCV]) are not always required but can provide corroborative diagnostic evidence and prognostic indicators.

Children in early stages of the disease should be admitted to the hospital. Those with moderate, severe, or rapidly progressive weakness should be cared for in an intensive care unit. Pulmonary and cardiac functions are monitored continuously. Endotracheal intubation should be performed in patients with impending respiratory failure or an inability to clear secretions. Most patients are treated initially with intravenous immunoglobulin (IVIG). Plasma exchange and immunosuppressive drugs are alternatives when IVIG treatment is unsuccessful or in rapidly progressive disease. Physical, occupational, and speech therapies are mainstays of treatment.

The illness usually resolves spontaneously, albeit slowly; 80% of patients recover normal function within 1 to 12 months. Twenty percent of patients are left with mild to moderate residual weakness. Some children will suffer acute relapse or chronic symptoms.

Chronic Inflammatory Demyelinating Polyneuropathy

CIDP is an immune-mediated peripheral neuropathy and can affect patients of all ages. Patients present with both proximal and distal weakness (usually in an episodic, relapsing-remitting pattern) affecting the extremities. Patients may also experience sensation changes such as numbness, tingling, or pain. The diagnosis is clinical, although EMG or nerve biopsy may confirm the diagnosis. The mainstays of treatment for CIDP are IVIG, glucocorticoids, and plasmapheresis. Prognosis varies, with some patients undergoing complete remission, whereas others experience partial remission or severe disability.

Hereditary Motor Sensory Neuropathy

HMSN (also called Charcot-Marie-Tooth Disease [CMT]) is a group of progressive peripheral nerve diseases. Motor components generally dominate the clinical picture, with sensation and autonomic functions affected later. The most common HMSN is CMT type 1A. Other forms may have milder symptoms. Some subtypes present with severe symptoms starting in infancy.

The peroneal and tibial nerves are the earliest and most severely affected. Most often, complaints begin in the preschool to early adolescent years, with weakness of the ankles and frequent tripping. Examination shows **pes cavus deformity of the feet** (high-arched feet), bilateral weakness of foot dorsiflexors, and normal sensation despite occasional complaints of paresthesia. Peripheral nerves can become markedly enlarged and may be palpable on exam. Progression of HMSN is slow, extending over years and decades. Eventually, patients develop weakness and atrophy of the entire lower legs and hands and mild to moderate sensory loss in the hands and feet. Some patients never have more than a mild foot deformity, loss of ankle reflexes, and electrophysiologic abnormalities. Others

in the same family may be confined to a wheelchair and have difficulties performing everyday tasks with their hands.

HMSN can be either demyelinating (CMT1, with severely decreased NCV and hypertrophic changes on sural nerve biopsy) or axonal (CMT2, with normal NCV but decreased action potential amplitudes and axonal degeneration on biopsy). Specific genetic testing is available for many subtypes of HMSN. Specific treatment for HMSN is not available, but braces that maintain the feet in dorsiflexion can improve function.

Tick Paralysis

Decision-Making Algorithm
Available @ StudentConsult.com

Hypotonia and Weakness

Tick paralysis produces an acute lower motor neuron pattern of weakness, clinically similar to Guillain-Barré syndrome. An attached female tick releases a toxin, similar to botulism, blocking neuromuscular transmission. Affected patients present with a severe generalized flaccid weakness, including ocular, papillary, and bulbar paralysis. A methodical search for an affixed tick, particularly in hairy areas, must be made in any child with acute weakness. Removal of the tick results in a prompt return of motor function.

Myasthenia Gravis

Decision-Making Algorithm
Available @ StudentConsult.com

Hypotonia and Weakness

Myasthenia gravis is an autoimmune condition. Most commonly, antibodies block the acetylcholine receptors (AChR) at the neuromuscular junction, decreasing the number of effective receptors, which results in rapid fatigability of striated muscle, though other types of auto-antibodies exist. The three childhood varieties are **juvenile myasthenia gravis** in late infancy and childhood, **transient neonatal myasthenia**, and **congenital myasthenia**.

Juvenile Myasthenia

Variable ptosis, diplopia, ophthalmoplegia, and facial weakness are the presenting symptoms. Dysphagia, poor head control, and extremity weakness may occur. Rapid fatigue of muscles distinguishes myasthenia from other neuromuscular disorders, with progressive worsening over the day or with repetitive activity. In some children, the disease never advances beyond ophthalmoplegia and ptosis (ocular myasthenia). Others have a progressive and potentially life-threatening illness that involves all musculature, including that of respiration and swallowing. Treatment includes pyridostigmine, an inhibitor of acetylcholinesterase, and, depending on severity, various forms of immunosuppression.

Transient Neonatal Myasthenia Gravis

A transient myasthenic syndrome develops in 10% to 20% of neonates born to mothers with myasthenia gravis, presenting in the first hours to days after birth. Almost all infants born to mothers with myasthenia have maternal anti-AChR antibodies. Signs include ptosis, ophthalmoplegia, weak facial movements, poor feeding, hypotonia, respiratory difficulty, and variable extremity weakness. Neonates with transient myasthenia gravis require cholinesterase inhibitors and supportive care for a few days to weeks until the weakness remits.

Congenital Myasthenia Gravis

A variety of rare disorders of the neuromuscular junction have been reported that are not autoimmune mediated. The congenital myasthenic syndromes (CMS) are due to gene mutations in the components of the neuromuscular junction. They typically present in infancy with hypotonia, ophthalmoparesis, facial diplegia, and extremity weakness, although they can present throughout childhood. Respiratory function and feeding may be compromised. Children with CMS usually have lifelong disability. Some children will respond to pyridostigmine or other drugs that improve neuromuscular junction function.

Diagnostic Studies

Autoimmune myasthenia is most commonly diagnosed through the combination of clinical symptoms and antibody testing. The majority of individuals have antibodies to the AChR, although some have antibodies to other components of the neuromuscular junction. Neurophysiology may exhibit the classic feature of electrodecrement with 3-Hz repetitive stimulation during nerve conduction studies. Administration of a cholinesterase inhibitor (edrophonium chloride) can result in transient improvement in strength, particularly of ptosis, and thus can additionally be used for diagnostic verification.

Infant Botulism

Decision-Making Algorithm
Available @ StudentConsult.com

Hypotonia and Weakness

Infant botulism results from intestinal infection by *Clostridium botulinum*, which produces a neurotoxin that blocks presynaptic cholinergic transmission. Young age and the absence of competitive bowel flora predispose infants to this disease. Infants may ingest dust, soil, or food (honey or poorly canned foods) contaminated with spores. The progressive neuromuscular blockade ranges from mild to severe. Infants often present with constipation and poor feeding. Hypotonia and weakness develop, along with cranial nerve dysfunction manifested by decreased gag reflex, diminished eye movements, decreased pupillary contraction, and ptosis. Heart rate and blood pressure may fluctuate. Affected infants may develop respiratory failure. The diagnosis is made by the presence of *C. botulinum* spores and toxin in stool samples. Therapy with botulism IVIG should be administered as soon as the diagnosis is suspected.

With prompt treatment and respiratory and supportive care, the prognosis is good.

Duchenne Muscular Dystrophy

Muscular dystrophies are a group of genetic muscle diseases characterized by progressive myofiber degeneration and the gradual replacement of muscle by fibrotic tissue. Duchenne muscular dystrophy is the most common muscular dystrophy and one of the most common genetic disorders of childhood.

Etiology

Duchenne muscular dystrophy is an X-linked disorder (Xp21) affecting approximately 1 in 3500 boys and resulting from a gene mutation of dystrophin. **Becker muscular dystrophy** is an allelic disorder associated with more mild symptoms; its mutations at least partially preserve the function of the resulting gene product.

Clinical Manifestations

Decision-Making Algorithm
Available @ StudentConsult.com

Hypotonia and Weakness

Infant boys are only rarely symptomatic in early infancy. At about 2 to 3 years of age, boys develop an awkward gait and an inability to run properly. Some have an antecedent history of mild slowness in attaining motor milestones or poor head control during infancy. Examination shows firm calf hypertrophy and mild to moderate proximal leg weakness with a hyperlordotic, waddling gait. The child typically arises from a lying position on the floor by using his arms to *climb up* his legs and body (**Gower sign**). Arm weakness is evident by age 6 years, and most boys are wheelchair dependent by age 12 years. Other manifestations include cardiomyopathy, scoliosis, respiratory decline, and, in some boys, cognitive and behavioral dysfunction. Many boys with Duchenne live into adulthood. Most die in their 20s or early 30s, usually as a result of progressive respiratory decline or cardiac dysfunction.

Laboratory and Diagnostic Studies

Serum CK levels are always markedly elevated. Diagnosis is established by genetic testing for the dystrophin gene mutation. Prenatal diagnosis is possible. Approximately one third of cases represent new mutations. Occasionally, the diagnosis is not made until a muscle biopsy shows muscle fiber degeneration and regeneration accompanied by increased intrafascicular connective tissue.

Treatment

Steroid therapy is now instituted to slow the pace of the disease and delay motor disability. Supportive care includes physical therapy, bracing, proper wheelchairs, and treatment of cardiac dysfunction or pulmonary infections. A multidisciplinary approach is recommended. Through improvements in management, patients are now living significantly longer than in the pre-steroid era.

Myotonic Dystrophy
Etiology and Epidemiology

Myotonic dystrophy (DM) is the second most common muscular dystrophy and the most common form to present in adulthood. An autosomal dominant genetic disease, DM is caused by progressive expansion of a triplet repeat, CTG, in the myotonic dystrophy protein kinase gene. Presentation is roughly correlated with the number of CTG repeats, and the disease is characterized by genetic anticipation, where each generation presents with earlier and more severe symptoms.

Clinical Manifestations

Although DM most typically presents in adulthood, it can present at any age. Clinical features of childhood-onset "classic" DM include slowly progressive facial and *distal* extremity weakness as well as **myotonia**. Myotonia is a disorder of muscle relaxation after contraction. Patients grasp onto an object and have difficulty releasing their grasp, peeling their fingers away slowly. The facial appearance is characteristic, with hollowing of muscles around temples, jaw, and neck; ptosis; facial weakness; and drooping of the lower lip. The voice is nasal and mildly dysarthric. Not only is the striated muscle affected, but smooth muscle of the alimentary tract, uterus, and cardiac tissue are involved. Patients have variable arrhythmias, endocrinopathies, immunologic deficiencies, cataracts, and intellectual impairment.

A severe congenital form of DM can appear in infants of mothers with myotonic dystrophy because of rapid expansion of the CTG repeat length. Infants are immobile and hypotonic, with ptosis, absence of sucking and Moro reflexes, poor feeding, and respiratory difficulties. Often, weakness and atony of uterine smooth muscle during labor lead to associated hypoxic ischemic encephalopathy and its sequelae, which make the clinical diagnosis more difficult. The presence of congenital contractures, clubfoot, or a history of poor fetal movements indicates intrauterine neuromuscular disease. Those requiring prolonged ventilation have an infant mortality of 25%. Individuals with congenital DM often make significant gains in terms of motor skills, and nearly all children eventually ambulate independently. However, approximately 50% of DM patients have mental retardation. In addition, children with congenital DM experience a second progressive phase of the disease in the teen years, including potentially fatal cardiac arrhythmias.

Diagnosis

Diagnosis is established by genetic testing.

Other Forms of Childhood Muscle Disease

Congenital muscular dystrophies (CMDs) refer to a group of genetically determined conditions that present in infancy or early childhood. The most common subtypes include merosin-deficient congenital muscular dystrophy, Ullrich congenital muscular dystrophy, and the dystroglycanopathies. The characteristic clinical features include hypotonia, extremity weakness, delayed motor development, and congenital contractures. Diagnosis is established through the combination of elevated serum CK and dystrophic changes detected on muscle biopsy. In most individuals, the disease course is slow or nonprogressive, although many children with CMD are wheelchair dependent and require some type of respiratory support. Contractures and scoliosis are often progressive and severely worsen; respiratory status diminishes with age.

Emery-Dreifuss muscular dystrophy (EDMD), also known as humeroperoneal muscular dystrophy, can be inherited as an X-linked recessive, autosomal dominant, or autosomal recessive disorder. Symptoms typically begin in childhood, although adult onset has been noted. Patients may experience early contractures, slowly progressive humeroperoneal muscle weakness or wasting, and cardiac disease with conduction defects and arrhythmias. EDMD is associated with mild elevations of serum CK levels, abnormal electrocardiograms (ECG), characteristic changes on muscle imaging, and abnormal but nonspecific muscle biopsies. There are no disease-specific modifying therapies for EDMD, although early placement of defibrillators in patients with abnormal ECGs reduces the incidence of sudden death.

Several forms of **limb-girdle muscular dystrophy** (LGMD) have been described, which are usually inherited in an autosomal recessive pattern. Depending on the subtype of LGMD, presentation can be throughout childhood. A subset of children will have a Duchenne-like presentation. LGMD primarily affects muscles of the hip and shoulder girdles. Distal muscles may later become weak and atrophic. Many children with LGMD will lose the ability to ambulate. Some may also have progressive cardiac and respiratory failure.

Facioscapulohumeral dystrophy is an autosomal dominant myopathy. Weakness first appears in the facial and shoulder girdle muscles. Shoulder weakness results in the characteristic observation of scapular winging, which can often be asymmetric. Patients have mild ptosis, a decrease in facial expression, inability to pucker the lips or close eyes during sleep, neck weakness, difficulty in fully elevating the arms, and thinness of upper arm musculature. Progression is slow, although children often have a more severe presentation and can have significant disability related to upper extremity weakness and dysfunction.

Congenital myopathies (CM) are a relatively common group (prevalence approximately 1:20,000) of nondystrophic muscle disorders that, like congenital muscular dystrophies, most typically present in infancy with hypotonia and weakness. Additional signs and symptoms include congenital contractures, hip subluxation/dislocation, small/atrophic muscles, thin body habitus, and characteristic facial appearance (the "myopathic facies"). Symptoms are often nonprogressive or only slowly progressive, although children often have severe lifelong disabilities including wheelchair dependence, severe scoliosis, and respiratory failure. Clinical finding may distinguish CMDs and other dystrophies (e.g., involvement of the facial musculature in congenital myopathies). Diagnosis is ultimately established based on laboratory studies, biopsy findings, and genetic test results. Histopathologic subtypes are distinguished by characteristic features on muscle biopsy, the most common being nemaline myopathy, centronuclear myopathy, and core myopathy. More than 15 different genetic causes have been established for CMs. However, nearly 50% of cases are genetically unresolved. Although no specific therapies currently exist for any CM subtype, several promising therapies have shown efficacy in preclinical models of disease.

Metabolic Myopathies

Glycogen storage disease type II (Pompe disease) and muscle carnitine deficiency are discussed in Chapters 52 and 55. **Several mitochondrial myopathies** may present with hypotonia, ophthalmoplegia, and progressive weakness, but the phenotype of these disorders is broad (Chapter 57). **Endocrine myopathies**, including hyperthyroidism, hypothyroidism, hyperparathyroidism, and Cushing syndrome, are associated with proximal muscle weakness. **Periodic paralysis** due to familial forms of hypokalemia or hyperkalemia produces episodic weakness.

Laboratory and Diagnostic Studies

The diagnostic evaluation should be guided by the clinical history and physical examination (Chapter 179).

Malignant Hyperthermia

Malignant hyperthermia is a life-threatening syndrome manifested by a rapid increase of body temperature, muscle rigidity, metabolic and respiratory acidosis, hypotension, arrhythmias, and convulsions. Acute episodes are precipitated by exposure to anesthetic agents in patients with a genetic predisposition. Patients with Duchenne muscular dystrophy, central core myopathy, and other myopathies are susceptible, although malignant hyperpyrexia can also occur in children without muscle disease as an autosomal dominant genetic disorder. A family history of unexplained death during anesthesia is often noted. Serum CK levels rise and myoglobinuria can result in tubular necrosis and acute renal failure. Diagnosis of idiopathic malignant hyperthermia is possible with genetic testing or an in vitro muscle contraction test that reveals excessive tonic contracture on exposure to halothane and caffeine. Treatment consists of IV dantrolene, sodium bicarbonate, and cooling.

Neonatal and Infantile Hypotonia

The clinical distinction between upper and lower motor neuron disorders in infants is blurred because incomplete myelinization of the developing nervous system limits expression of many of the cardinal signs, such as spasticity. The two critical clinical points are whether the child is weak and the presence or absence of deep tendon reflexes. Hypotonia and weakness coupled with depressed or absent deep tendon reflexes suggest a neuromuscular disorder. A stronger child with brisk reflexes suggests an upper motor neuron source for the hypotonia. Causes of neonatal weakness are outlined earlier. A diagnostic algorithm for infants with hypotonia or weakness is presented in Figure 182-1.

Hypotonia without Significant Weakness (Central Hypotonia)

Decision-Making Algorithm
Available @ StudentConsult.com

Hypotonia and Weakness

Some infants who appear to move well when supine in their cribs are *floppy* when handled or moved. When lifted, their

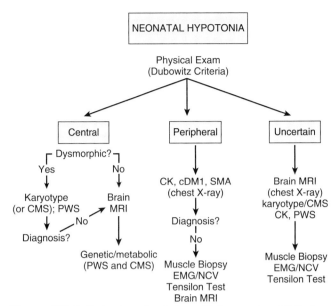

Figure 182-1 Evaluation of an infant with hypotonia. *cDM1*, Congenital myotonic dystrophy; *CK*, creatine kinase; *CMS*, chromosomal microarray analysis; *EMG*, electromyogram; *MRI*, magnetic resonance imaging; *NCV*, nerve conduction velocity; *PWS*, Prader-Willi syndrome; *SMA*, spinal muscular atrophy. (*Courtesy James Dowling, MD.*)

heads flop, they *slip through* at the shoulders, do not support weight on their legs, and form an *inverted* U in prone suspension (**Landau posture**). When placed prone as neonates, they may lie flat instead of keeping their arms and legs flexed. Passive tone is decreased, but reflexes are normal. Hypotonia may be associated with significant cerebral disease or may be a benign phenomenon that is outgrown (Table 182-4). The most common cause of hypotonia is hypoxic-ischemic encephalopathy.

Prader-Willi syndrome (PWS) presents with severe neonatal hypotonia; severe feeding problems leading to failure to thrive; small hands and feet; and, in boys, a small penis, small testicles, and cryptorchidism. Severe hyperphagia and obesity develop in early childhood. Approximately 60% to 70% of affected individuals have an interstitial deletion of *paternal* chromosome 15q11q13. PWS and trisomy 21 are the most common genetic causes of neonatal hypotonia.

Infants who have a connective tissue disorder, such as **Ehlers-Danlos syndrome**, **Marfan syndrome**, or familial laxity of the ligaments, may exhibit marked passive hypotonia, *ligamentous laxity*, and increased skin elasticity. They have normal strength and cognition and achieve motor and mental milestones normally. They may have peculiar postures of their feet or unusual gaits.

Infants with **benign congenital hypotonia** typically exhibit the condition at 6 to 12 months old with delayed gross motor skills. They are unable to sit, creep, or crawl, but have good verbal, social, and manipulative skills. Strength appears normal, and the infants can kick arms and legs briskly and bring their toes to their mouths. The children often display head lag, slip-through in ventral suspension, and floppiness of passive tone. The infant seems floppy from birth. The differential diagnosis includes upper and motor neuron disorders and connective tissue diseases. Extensive laboratory investigation is often unrevealing. Most of these children catch up to peers and

Table 182-4	Approach to Differential Diagnosis in the Floppy Infant

HYPOTONIA WITH WEAKNESS

Awareness Intact

Neuromuscular disease

    Spinal muscular atrophy*

    Myasthenic syndromes

    Congenital neuropathy or myopathy

Spinal cord disease (cervical cord trauma or compression)

    Tumor

    Spinal cord infarct

    Malformation

    Spina bifida

    Syringomyelia

Consciousness Depressed

Severe brain illness*

Structural (hydrocephalus)

Infectious

Metabolic (e.g., anoxia or hypoglycemia)

Intoxication through mother

    Magnesium sulfate

    Barbiturates

    Narcotics

    Benzodiazepines

    General anesthesia

Metabolic abnormality

    Hypoglycemia

    Kernicterus

HYPOTONIA WITHOUT WEAKNESS

Acute systemic illness*

Specific syndromes

    Down syndrome*

    Cerebrohepatorenal (Zellweger peroxisomal disorder)

    Oculocerebrorenal (Lowe syndrome)

    Kinky hair disease (Menkes syndrome—copper metabolism disorder)

    Neonatal adrenal leukodystrophy

    Prader-Willi syndrome

Connective tissue disorder

    Ehlers-Danlos syndrome

    Marfan syndrome

    Congenital laxity of ligaments

Nutritional-metabolic disease

    Rickets

    Renal tubular acidosis

    Celiac disease

    Biliary atresia

Congenital heart disease

Benign congenital hypotonia*

*Common.

Table 182-5	Causes of Stroke in Childhood

ARTERIAL ISCHEMIC STROKE

Arteriopathic

    Idiopathic arterial stenosis

    Vasculitis (autoimmune or infectious)

    Arterial dissection (traumatic or spontaneous)

    Moyamoya disease

Cardiac

    Cyanotic congenital heart disease

    Valvular disease

    Patent foramen ovale

    Arrhythmias

    Cardiomyopathy

    Infective endocarditis

Hematologic

    Sickle cell anemia

    Iron deficiency anemia

    Hypercoagulable state

    Hereditary prothrombotic states (factor V Leiden)

    Acquired prothrombotic states (antiphospholipid antibodies)

    Prothrombotic medications (oral contraception)

CEREBRAL SINOVENOUS THROMBOSIS

Hematologic

    Hypercoagulable state (see above)

    Iron deficiency anemia

    Severe dehydration

Infections

    Meningitis

    Otitis media

    Mastoiditis

Systemic disease

    Leukemia

    Inflammatory bowel disease

    Nephrotic syndrome

Trauma

HEMORRHAGIC STROKE

Head trauma (accidental or abusive)

Vascular malformations

    Arteriovenous malformations

    Cerebral aneurysms

Brain tumor

Vasculitis

Moyamoya disease

appear normal by 3 years of age. Often, other family members have exhibited a similar developmental pattern.

STROKE IN CHILDHOOD
Etiology

The incidence of pediatric stroke is 2.5 to 10 per 100,000 children and is higher among neonates, approaching that of elderly patients. A wide spectrum of conditions can produce stroke in childhood (Table 182-5). Pediatric strokes may be due to ischemia (arterial ischemic stroke, cerebral sinovenous thrombosis) or hemorrhage. **Arterial ischemic stroke** (AIS) is focal brain infarction that results from occlusion of the arteries in the brain. The most common causes are vasculitis resulting in abnormal cerebral arteries (either autoimmune or infectious, such as vasculitis associated with meningitis) and cardioembolic infarcts due to congenital heart disease, sickle cell anemia, or coagulation disorders. Coagulation disorders also increase the risk of **cerebral sinovenous thrombosis** (CSVT), the occlusion of venous structures in the brain, which can result in ischemia as the cerebral venous pressure rises.

CSVT can also be caused by infections or dehydration. **Hemorrhagic strokes** (HS) may be intraparenchymal (primary, or secondary bleeding after AIS) or associated with intraventricular, subarachnoid, subdural, or epidural bleeds. The most common causes of HS are vascular malformations, head trauma, and vasculitis.

Clinical Manifestations

The acute onset of focal neurologic deficits in a child is stroke until proven otherwise. Symptoms may be subtle and nonspecific, which can lead to a delay in diagnosis. AIS typically presents with acute, focal neurologic deficits. Hemiparesis is most common, but visual, speech, sensory, or balance deficits may be present. Unlike AIS in adults, focal seizures are quite common in childhood presentation of AIS. Similarly, neonatal AIS most often presents with acute symptomatic focal seizures (typically in the first day of life) or with encephalopathy.

Symptoms of CSVT may progress more gradually and be more variable and nonspecific than AIS. In CSVT, acute focal deficits may be present, or the child may have progressive signs of elevated intracranial pressure, including headache, papilledema, diplopia (most often from cranial nerve VI palsy), seizures, lethargy, or confusion.

HS tends to present acutely, with a sudden "thunderclap" headache. HS may also present with loss of consciousness, nuchal rigidity, focal deficits, or seizures and can be rapidly fatal.

Congenital hemiplegia becomes apparent as infants develop, with decreased use of one side of the body, early handedness, or ignoring one side. Neuroimaging reveals an area of encephalomalacia in the contralateral cerebral hemisphere. The details of the child's intrauterine, labor, delivery, and postnatal history often are unremarkable. The area of encephalomalacia may predispose the child to epilepsy.

Differential Diagnosis

There are many conditions that mimic pediatric stroke, most of which are more common than AIS, HS, or CSVT. Some of these mimics are benign (migraine, psychogenic weakness, musculoskeletal abnormalities), but others require specific, prompt diagnosis and/or treatment (e.g., transient postictal weakness, intracranial infection, inflammatory disease of the central nervous system, tumor, or posterior reversible leukoencephalopathy syndrome).

Diagnostic Tests and Imaging

On initial presentation, acute neuroimaging is necessary. A noncontrast head computed tomography (CT) scan is highly sensitive to acute HS and can reveal larger, mature AIS; acute, nonhemorrhagic stroke may not be seen on routine CT. Therefore, MRI with diffusion-weighted imaging is required for most presentations. Angiography by magnetic resonance angiography (MRA) or CT angiography is used to confirm arterial occlusion in AIS and can identify underlying arteriopathy, vascular malformations, and aneurysms. Diagnosis of CSVT requires a high clinical suspicion and purposeful imaging of the cerebral venous system with venography by MRI or CT. If clinical assessment does not reveal the cause of the stroke, a complete laboratory investigation should be undertaken promptly based on suspected etiologies (see Table 182-5). Many children with AIS have more than one predisposing factor, so identifying one risk factor does not obviate the need for a complete evaluation.

Treatment

Treatment must focus on limiting secondary neuronal injury and prevention of future strokes. Neuroprotection by maintaining control of temperature, blood pressure, glucose, and seizures is essential. Emergency thrombolysis with medications or catheterization is not yet established for children, but this is an area of active clinical research. Anticoagulants (IV heparin, subcutaneous low-molecular-weight heparin, oral warfarin) and platelet antiaggregants (aspirin) are used for secondary stroke prevention in some instances. For those with progressive CSVT, anticoagulation is the mainstay of therapy. Long-term rehabilitation programs are required for most survivors.

Chapter **183**

ATAXIA AND MOVEMENT DISORDERS

ATAXIA

Ataxia is the inability to make accurate, smooth and coordinated movements, usually due to a dysfunction of the cerebellar pathways. If either the afferent (joint position senses) or efferent cerebellar connections (cerebellum through thalamus to cerebral cortex) are disturbed, the patient has ataxia. **Truncal ataxia** reflects disturbances of the midline cerebellar vermis (e.g., medulloblastoma, acute postinfectious cerebellar ataxia, or ethanol intoxication). **Appendicular ataxia** reflects disturbances of the ipsilateral cerebellar hemisphere (e.g., cystic cerebellar astrocytoma). The most common causes of acute ataxia in childhood are postinfectious acute cerebellar ataxia and drug intoxications. Discrete lesions within the posterior fossa, tumors (e.g., medulloblastoma, ependymoma, cerebellar astrocytoma), multiple sclerosis, strokes, and hemorrhages may cause ataxia. Other causes include benign paroxysmal vertigo, head trauma, seizures, postictal states, migraine, paraneoplastic opsoclonus-myoclonus syndrome associated with neuroblastoma, and inborn errors of metabolism. Congenital disorders also may produce chronic, nonprogressive ataxia. There are a number of inherited ataxia syndromes (Table 183-1).

Clinical Manifestations

Decision-Making Algorithm
Available @ StudentConsult.com

Ataxia

Table 183-1	Causes of Ataxia

Brain tumors	Inhalants
Medulloblastoma*	Drugs of abuse
Ependymoma	Vascular disorders
Cerebellar astrocytoma*	Cerebellar hemorrhage or infarction
Brainstem glioma	Vertebral artery dissection
Paraneoplastic disease	Demyelinative disorders
Neuroblastoma (opsoclonus-myoclonus-ataxia)	Multiple sclerosis
Infectious disorders	Acute disseminated encephalomyelitis
Encephalitis*	Structural or congenital disorders
Brainstem encephalitis	Cerebellar hypoplasia
Meningitis	Vermal aplasia
Labrynthitis*	Dandy-Walker malformation
Cerebellar abscess	Arnold-Chiari malformation
Postinfectious disorders	Hydrocephalus
Acute cerebellar ataxia (acute postinfectious cerebellitis)*	Hereditary ataxic disorders
Guillain-Barré syndrome	Episodic ataxia
Migrainous disorders	Friedreich ataxia
Basilar migraine*	Ramsay Hunt syndrome
Benign paroxysmal vertigo	Spinocerebellar ataxia 1 and 2
Trauma	Ataxia-telangiectasia
Cerebellar hemorrhage	Marinesco-Sjögren syndrome
Cerebellar contusion	Genetic and metabolic disorders
Concussion	Metachromatic leukodystrophy
Postconcussive syndrome*	Adrenoleukodystrophy
Vertebrobasilar occlusion	Maple syrup urine disease
Toxic ingestions*	Hartnup disease
Ethanol	GM_2 gangliosidosis (juvenile)
Anticonvulsants	Refsum disease
Antihistamines	Vitamin E deficiency
Benzodiazepines	Leigh disease
Carbon monoxide	Wilson disease
	Abetalipoproteinemia

*Common.

The usual symptoms of ataxia are a broad-based, unsteady gait (truncal ataxia) and intention tremor or **dysmetria** (over- or undershooting of the target due to abnormal distance perception). An intention tremor worsens as the arm/hand approaches the target. Classically, these symptoms stem from disorders of the cerebellar pathways, but peripheral nerve lesions causing loss of proprioceptive inputs to the cerebellum (Guillain-Barré syndrome) may present with similar symptoms. In addition, weakness may intensify or mimic ataxia, so strength must be assessed, along with coordination.

Etiologies

Decision-Making Algorithm
Available @ StudentConsult.com

Ataxia

Drug intoxication is the most common cause of acute ataxia among children. Overdosage with any sedative-hypnotic agent can produce acute ataxia and lethargy, but ataxia without lethargy usually results from intoxication with ethanol or anticonvulsant drugs. It is important to ask about any medications or drugs of abuse the patient may have access to. Treatment is supportive.

Postinfectious acute cerebellar ataxia may occur 1 to 3 weeks following varicella, infectious mononucleosis, mild respiratory or gastrointestinal viral illnesses, or other infections. The pathogenesis is uncertain and may represent either a direct viral infection of the cerebellum or, more likely, an autoimmune response precipitated by the viral infection and directed at the cerebellar white matter. Symptoms begin abruptly, causing truncal ataxia, staggering, and frequent falling. Dysmetria of the arms, dysarthria, nystagmus, vomiting, irritability, and lethargy may be present. Symptoms, which may be severe enough to prevent standing or sitting, usually peak within 2 days, then stabilize and resolve over several weeks. Cerebrospinal fluid (CSF) examination sometimes shows a mild lymphocytic pleocytosis or mild elevation of protein content. Brain magnetic resonance imaging may reveal cerebellar enhancement. No specific therapy is available except to prevent injury during the ataxic phase.

Brain tumors are the second most common neoplasm in children. About 50% arise from within the posterior fossa. Tumors that arise in the posterior fossa or brainstem produce progressive ataxia with headache that may be acute or gradual in onset. There is a progressive worsening over days, weeks, or months, typically with associated signs and symptoms of elevated intracranial pressure. The ataxia and dysmetria may result from primary cerebellar invasion or from obstruction of the CSF pathways (aqueduct of Sylvius or fourth ventricle) with resultant hydrocephalus. The most common tumors in this region include medulloblastoma, ependymoma, cerebellar astrocytoma, and brainstem glioma.

Rarely, a **neuroblastoma** located in the adrenal medulla or anywhere along the paraspinal sympathetic chain in the thorax or abdomen is associated with degeneration of Purkinje cells and the development of severe ataxia, dysmetria, irritability, **myoclonus**, and **opsoclonus**. An immunologic reaction directed toward the tumor may be misdirected to attack Purkinje cells and other neuronal elements. The myoclonic movements are irregular, lightning-like movements of a limb or the head. Opsoclonus is a rapid, multidirectional, conjugate movement of the eyes, which suddenly dart in random directions. The presence of **opsoclonus-myoclonus** in a child should prompt a vigorous search for an occult neuroblastoma.

Several rare **inborn errors of metabolism** can present with intermittent episodes of ataxia and somnolence. These include Hartnup disorder, maple syrup urine disease, mitochondrial disorders, abetalipoproteinemia, and vitamin E deficiency.

Difficulty walking with a severe staggering gait is one manifestation of **acute labrynthitis**, but the diagnosis usually is clarified by the associated symptoms of a severe sense of spinning dizziness (vertigo), nausea and vomiting, and associated signs of pallor, sweating, and nystagmus.

Ataxia-telangiectasia, an autosomal recessive genetic disorder, is the most common of the degenerative ataxias. Affected patients present with ataxia around age 2 years, progressing to loss of ambulation by adolescence. In mid-childhood, telangiectasia is evident over the sclerae, nose, ears, and extremities. Abnormalities in immune function and greatly increased risk of lymphoreticular tumors result in early death.

Friedreich ataxia is a relentlessly progressive, autosomal recessive disorder. Children present in the late elementary years with ataxia, dysmetria, dysarthria, diminished proprioception and vibration, absent deep tendon reflexes, and nystagmus, and many develop hypertrophic cardiomyopathy and skeletal abnormalities (high-arched feet, hammer toes, kyphoscoliosis).

MOVEMENT DISORDERS

Decision-Making Algorithm
Available @ StudentConsult.com

Involuntary Movements

Movement disorders or **dyskinesias** are a diverse group of entities associated with abnormal excessive, exaggerated, chaotic, or explosive movements of voluntary muscles. They are generally the result of abnormalities of the extrapyramidal system or the basal ganglia. Movement disorders in children are typically **hyperkinetic** (increased movement) patterns. The abnormal movements are activated by stress and fatigue and often disappear in sleep. They are typically diffuse and migratory (chorea) but may be isolated to specific muscle groups (segmental myoclonus, palatal myoclonus) and may not disappear in sleep.

Chorea is a hyperkinetic, rapid, unsustained, irregular, purposeless movement that seems to flow from one body part to another. Affected patients demonstrate difficulty keeping the tongue protruded or maintaining grip (*milkmaid grip*). Patients often attempt to incorporate the involuntary movements into more purposeful movements, making them appear fidgety. Choreiform movement abnormalities may be autoimmune/parainfectious, infectious, genetic, structural, metabolic or toxic in origin (Table 183-2). The movements may occur

Table 183-2	Causes of Movement Disorders

CHOREA

Autoimmune/parainfectious (acute rheumatic fever,* systemic lupus erythematosus)
Infectious (human immunodeficiency virus, neurosyphilis, scarlet fever, encephalitis)
Genetic (Huntington disease, ataxia-telangiectasia)
Structural (stroke, neoplasm)
Metabolic/toxic (hepatic/renal failure, hyperthyroidism)
Drug induced

ATHETOSIS

Cerebral palsy*
Kernicterus
Hypoxic-ischemic encephalopathy
Drug induced
Pantothenate kinase-associated neurodegeneration
Pelizaeus-Merzbacher disease

DYSTONIA

Inherited primary dystonias
Acute dystonic reaction*
Tardive dyskinesia
Cerebral palsy*
Metabolic disorders (Wilson disease)

TREMOR

Physiologic*
Essential tremor*
Hereditary, degenerative (Huntington disease, Wilson disease)
Stroke
Metabolic (hyperthyroidism, hepatic encephalopathy, electrolyte disturbances)
Drugs/toxins* (caffeine, bronchodilators, amphetamines, tricyclic antidepressants)
Psychogenic tremor

MYOCLONUS

Epilepsy
Benign*
Infection
Toxin
Metabolic encephalopathies

TICS*

Transient
Chronic motor tic disorder
Tourette syndrome

*Common

alone or as part of a more extensive neurologic disorder (e.g., Sydenham chorea, Huntington chorea, systemic lupus erythematosus, or encephalitis).

Athetosis is a hyperkinetic, slow, coarse, writhing movement that is more pronounced in distal muscles. Athetosis is seen frequently in combination with chorea (choreoathetosis) and usually is present in conjunction with other neurologic signs. It may be seen in virtually all the disorders mentioned for chorea. Many children with mixed forms of cerebral palsy have spasticity and choreoathetosis.

Dystonia is characterized by abnormally sustained muscle contraction, causing twisting motion (torsion spasm) and repetitive movements or abnormal postures. Cerebral palsy is the most common cause of dystonia among children, usually associated with basal ganglia or thalamic lesions. Many genetic mutations have been implicated in primary dystonias. Antipsychotics and antiemetics can produce **acute dystonic reactions**, typically involving the face and neck with torticollis, retrocollis, tongue protrusions, and oculogyric crises (eye rotation). **Tardive dyskinesia** usually is associated with chronic antipsychotic drug use and presents with characteristic face involvement (tongue thrusting, chewing).

Tremor is a hyperkinetic, rhythmic, oscillatory movement caused by simultaneous contractions of antagonistic muscles. The amplitude and frequency are regular. In children, tremor is usually due to a physiologic tremor, or essential tremor. Essential tremor is the most common movement disorder in adults, and half report onset in childhood. Other causes of tremor include thyrotoxicosis, hypoglycemia, or drugs (caffeine, bronchodilators, amphetamines, tricyclic antidepressants).

Myoclonus is a hyperkinetic, brief flexion contraction of a muscle group, resulting in a sudden jerk. Myoclonus may be epileptic or nonepileptic. Nonepileptic myoclonus is distinguished from tremor in that it is a simple contraction of an agonist muscle, whereas tremor is a simultaneous contraction of agonist and antagonist muscles. Myoclonus is seen as a manifestation of various epilepsies and of infectious, toxic, and metabolic encephalopathies. Benign myoclonus is commonly observed during sleep and may be particularly pronounced in neonates.

Tics are rapid, purposeless, involuntary, stereotyped movements and typically involve the face, eyes, shoulder, and arm. Examples of simple motor tics include blinking, nose twitching, and extremity jerking. Complex motor tics are more orchestrated movements, including head shaking, gesturing, or jumping. Phonic tics may be simple (grunting, throat clearing) or complex (uttering words, phrases). Approximately 25% of children have transient tics. Most tic disorders in children are transient and not intrusive into the child's life, but may be a source of parental anxiety. Occasionally, tics may be unmasked by stimulant agents. Persistent motor tics (>12 months) in association with vocal tics are characteristic of **Tourette syndrome**, a chronic tic disorder that usually begins before age 7 years. The pathophysiology underlying tics is unknown, but a family history of tics is elicited in more than 50% of cases. Comorbid features, such as obsessive-compulsive disorder and attention-deficit/hyperactivity disorder, may be present in half of children with Tourette disorder (Chapters 13, 19). Tic disorders are clinical diagnoses, and neurodiagnostic studies have limited value. Many children with tic disorders or Tourette syndrome are unperturbed by their tics and require

no therapy. Others may benefit from psychological support, including habit reversal training, and pharmacologic therapy with α-adrenergic receptor agonists (clonidine) or neuroleptics (pimozide, haloperidol, risperidone). Chronic tic disorders wax and wane regardless of intervention and most often improve substantially or resolve entirely by late adolescence.

Chapter **184**

ALTERED MENTAL STATUS

DISORDERS OF CONSCIOUSNESS

Consciousness represents awareness of self and environment (place and time). **Arousal** represents the system that initiates and maintains consciousness. Consciousness is mediated by the cerebral cortex; arousal is mediated by the reticular activating system extending from the mid pons through the midbrain and hypothalamus to the thalamus.

Lethargic patients have difficulty maintaining an aroused state. Patients who are **obtunded** have decreased arousal but are responsive to stimuli. **Stupor** is a state of responsiveness to pain but not to other stimuli. **Coma** is a state of unresponsive unconsciousness and is caused by dysfunction of the cerebral hemispheres (bilaterally), the brainstem, or both simultaneously.

Acute Disorders of Consciousness

Decision-Making Algorithm
Available @ StudentConsult.com

Altered Mental Status

Acute changes in consciousness vary in degree from mild lethargy and confusion to deep coma. In childhood, the most common causes of coma are toxins, infections, head trauma, hypoxia-ischemia (cardiac arrest, near-drowning), and seizure (postictal state, subclinical status epilepticus) (Table 184-1).

Assessment

The most common cause of long-term morbidity in a patient with depressed consciousness is **hypoxia**; therefore, airway, breathing and circulation are addressed first. Vital signs, including pulse oximetry, must be assessed. A glucose level should also be checked immediately because hypoglycemia is a rapidly treatable cause of altered mental status. Physical examination searches for clues as to the cause of altered consciousness, such as unusual odors, needle tracts, trauma, or signs of dehydration or organ system failure.

Breathing patterns may provide important clues to the depth, neurologic localization, and etiology of the depressed consciousness. In **Cheyne-Stokes respiration**, a period of

Table 184-1 | Causes of Coma and Diagnostic Approach

CAUSES

Infection

Meningitis
Encephalitis
Brain abscess
Herpes simplex virus meningoencephalitis
Human immunodeficiency virus
Tubercular meningitis
Toxic shock syndrome
Postinfectious (acute disseminated encephalomyelitis)

Trauma

Shaken baby syndrome
Epidural hemorrhage
Subdural hemorrhage
Subarachnoid hemorrhage
Concussion

Toxins (intoxication or withdrawal)

Ethanol
Narcotics
Barbiturates
Antihistamines
Anticonvulsants
Iron
Acetaminophen
Aspirin (Reye syndrome)
Illicit drugs
Lead poisoning
Thiamine deficiency (Wernicke encephalopathy)

Hypoxia-ischemia

Near-drowning
Post–cardiopulmonary arrest
  Cardiac arrhythmia
  Obstructive cardiomyopathy
Carbon monoxide intoxication
Perinatal asphyxia
Strangulation

Epilepsy

Subclinical (or nonconvulsive) status epilepticus
Postictal states

Stroke

Arterial ischemic stroke
Cerebral sinovenous thrombosis
Hemorrhage

Increased intracranial pressure

Brain tumor
Cerebral edema
Hydrocephalus

Migraine

Systemic disorders

Gastrointestinal (intussusception)
Vasculitis (systemic lupus erythematosus)
Hepatic failure
Hypertensive encephalopathy
Reye syndrome
Endocrine disorders (adrenal insufficiency, thyroid disorders)
Renal disorders (uremia)

Metabolic derangements

Hypoglycemia
Hyponatremia or its correction
Hypernatremia or its correction
Hyperosmolality or its correction
Hypercapnia
Hyperammonemia
Inborn errors of metabolism
Diabetes mellitus—ketoacidosis or hypoglycemia

DIAGNOSTIC APPROACH

Routine laboratory testing
  Glucose
  Sodium, potassium, chloride, bicarbonate, BUN, creatinine, AST, ALT, blood gases, ammonia
  Blood and urine analyses for toxic substances

CSF analysis including opening pressure, white and red blood cell counts, protein, glucose, and culture (± viral PCR testing)
Neuroimaging
  Head CT
  Brain MRI, MRA, MRV
Electrodiagnostic studies
  Routine-length EEG
  Video-EEG monitoring
Secondary laboratory testing (if cause remains unknown)
  Lead level, pyruvate, lactate, serum amino acids, urine organic acids, acylcarnitine profile

ALT, Alanine aminotransferase; *AST,* aspartate aminotransferase; *BUN,* blood urea nitrogen; *CSF,* cerebrospinal fluid; *CT,* computed tomography; *EEG,* electroencephalogram; *MRI/MRA/MRV,* magnetic resonance imaging/angiography/venography; *PCR,* polymerase chain reaction; *PT,* prothrombin time; *PTT,* partial thromboplastin time.

hyperventilation with a crescendo-decrescendo pattern alternates with a shorter period of apnea and is due to the loss of cerebral, thalamic, or hypothalamic modulation of respiration. This pattern also can be seen in patients with metabolic disorders, heart failure, or primary respiratory disease. A mid-brain lesion yields **central neurogenic hyperventilation**, which consists of sustained rapid deep breathing. **Gasping** respirations are irregularly irregular and indicate dysfunction of the lower brainstem (medulla). Gasping is ominous and usually is followed by terminal apnea.

The **Glasgow Coma Scale** (see Table 42-2) can be used to assess unresponsive patients regarding their best verbal and motor responses and eye opening to stimulation with a score of 3 to 15 points.

The detailed neurologic examination of a comatose patient focuses on the integrity of the brainstem which is the location of the reticular activating system, mediating arousal. Pupillary responses assess the midbrain function. Eye movements are observed or elicited with the **doll's eye maneuver** (oculocephalic response) (Chapter 179) or cold caloric stimulation (**oculovestibular response**). If the oculocephalic responses are not elicited or unclear, cold water is flushed into the external ear canal. In a conscious person, this maneuver elicits nystagmus to the opposite side and extreme vertigo with vomiting. In a comatose patient, cold water irrigation into the ear canal elicits a tonic eye deviation toward the ear irrigated if the brainstem is functioning and the patient is not brain dead. With complete loss of oculomotor function, the eyes remain in the center of the orbit regardless of any stimulation, indicating brainstem failure.

Body posture at rest and after noxious stimulation can indicate the anatomic level responsible for the alteration of consciousness. Mildly altered mental status may be manifested by a comfortable *sleeping* posture. Frequent spontaneous readjustments of position, yawns, and sighs are observed. Patients who lie in a flat, extended, unvarying position with eyes half-open exhibit a deeper coma. An asymmetrical posture suggests motor dysfunction of one side. This asymmetry may be subtle, such as mild external rotation of the affected leg.

Posturing in response to noxious stimulation indicates more serious neurologic conditions. **Decorticate posturing** consists of rigid extension of the legs and feet, flexion and supination of the arms, and fisting of the hands. It indicates bilateral cortical or subcortical abnormalities or herniation, with preserved brainstem function. **Decerebrate posturing** (rigid extension and internal rotation of legs and arms) indicates a midbrain abnormality and is classically associated with herniation or toxic-metabolic abnormalities. These postures may be exhibited unilaterally or bilaterally. A structural cause is likely when posturing is asymmetric, whereas symmetric posturing may be more likely with underlying toxic-metabolic etiologies.

Etiology

The evolution of change in consciousness is an important clue to the etiology. A detailed history and physical examination usually provide sufficient clues to differentiate among the three major diagnostic categories producing coma: **metabolic/toxic**, **infectious**, and **structural**. In most clinical situations, the cause of coma is readily identified.

Metabolic derangements are common causes of altered mental status. Disturbances of blood chemistries (glucose, sodium, calcium, bicarbonate, blood urea nitrogen, ammonia) may produce depressed mental status. Metabolic causes of acute coma are suggested by spontaneous fluctuations in the level of consciousness, tremors, myoclonus, asterixis, visual and tactile hallucinations, and deep coma with preservation of pupillary light reflexes. Acute metabolic or toxic disorders usually produce a hypotonic, limp state, but hypertonia, rigidity, and decorticate and decerebrate posturing are sometimes observed in coma caused by hypoglycemia, hepatic encephalopathy, and short-acting barbiturates. A subacute course of somnolence progressing to difficulty arousing from a deep *sleep* (stupor) over hours suggests drug intoxication or organ system failure (kidney, liver) producing a metabolic encephalopathy. Care must be taken to investigate background medical conditions that may produce a decline in consciousness (e.g., diabetes mellitus, leukemia, kidney failure, liver disease). Intoxication and ingestion are common causes of acute alteration of consciousness, and a thorough history must be taken to search for the offending agent (Chapter 45). A history of social and emotional difficulties, drug abuse, or depression raises concern for self-inflicted injury or toxic ingestion.

Central nervous system infection, such as meningitis or encephalitis, usually causes abrupt alteration of mental status, although viral meningoencephalitis (particularly herpes simplex virus) can present with subacute alterations in mental status. The presence of fever, petechiae, chills, and sweats suggests infection. Prodromal photophobia and pain on movement of the head or eyes are symptoms of meningeal irritation. Premonitory symptoms, such as abdominal pain, diarrhea, sore throat, conjunctivitis, cough, or rash, point toward viral encephalitis or a postinfectious syndrome as the cause of the altered consciousness.

Structural processes, such as hemorrhage, infarction, or acute hydrocephalus, can cause sudden depressed consciousness in children. An evolution of headache and morning vomiting suggests increased intracranial pressure (ICP). A gradual fading of alertness or declining school performance over preceding weeks suggests an expanding intracranial mass, subdural hematoma, or chronic infection (e.g., tuberculous meningitis, human immunodeficiency virus). Deprivation of oxygen to the brain, caused by either deficient oxygen in the blood (hypoxemia) or deficient delivery of blood to the brain (ischemia), impairs consciousness.

Clinical Manifestations

Papilledema or paralysis of cranial nerves III or VI in a patient with depressed consciousness is strong evidence of elevated ICP, a medical and neurosurgical emergency. **Herniations** occur under the falx, through the tentorial notch, or into the foramen magnum (Table 184-2). Recognition of the signs associated with the major herniation syndromes can be lifesaving, if emergent neuroimaging and treatment are initiated. **Uncal herniation** implies displacement of the mesial temporal lobe over the tentorial edge, producing a unilateral third

Table 184-2	Herniation Syndromes		
LOCATION	**ETIOLOGY**	**DESCRIPTION**	**CLINICAL FINDING(S)**
Transtentorial Unilateral (uncal) or bilateral	Supratentorial mass lesions, diffuse brain swelling, focal edema, or acute hydrocephalus	Downward displacement of supratentorial brain tissue into infratentorial compartment (below tentorium), compressing the cerebral peduncles, midbrain, third cranial nerve, and posterior circulation	Headache Altered consciousness Dilated ipsilateral pupil Cranial nerve III palsy Hemiparesis Decerebrate posturing Cushing triad Respiratory arrest
Subfalcian	Increased pressure in one hemisphere (mass, focal edema)	Brain tissue displaced under the falx cerebri, compressing the anterior cerebral artery	Weakness, bladder incontinence, coma
Foremen magnum	Cerebellar mass or edema	Downward displacement of cerebellar tonsils, compressing the medulla oblongata and upper spinal cord	Bradycardia, bradypnea, hypertension, death

nerve palsy ("blown pupil") and hemiparesis (which can be ipsilateral, because of compression of the contralateral cerebral peduncle, or contralateral if the uncus compresses the ipsilateral peduncle). **Transtentorial (or central) herniation** occurs with gradual downward pressure from the diencephalon through the tentorium, resulting in compression of the brainstem (first midbrain, then progressing to pons and medulla). A progressive loss of consciousness accompanied by a characteristic progression of motor, oculomotor, pupillary, and respiratory signs indicates incipient transtentorial herniation.

Laboratory and Diagnostic Imaging

Evaluation is guided by the history and physical examination (see Table 184-1). Computed tomography (CT) remains the preferred imaging technique in emergency situations because it can be performed rapidly and accurately identifies acute hemorrhages, large space-occupying lesions, edema, and shifts of the midline. The initial head CT scan is done without contrast to identify blood and calcifications. Contrast can be administered to identify inflammatory and neoplastic lesions, but is not usually required for identification of major lesions. Several metabolic derangements (hepatic encephalopathy, Reye syndrome, hyponatremia, lead encephalopathy, diabetic ketoacidosis, and hypoxic-ischemic injury) may give rise to severe elevations of ICP without producing obvious CT abnormalities. Lumbar puncture (LP) in a patient with elevated ICP can result in transtentorial herniation, so imaging should be performed before LP if elevated ICP is suspected, especially if there are any focal neurological deficits on exam. If trauma or immersion injuries are suspected, neck manipulation should be avoided until cervical spine imaging excludes vertebral fracture or subluxation.

Examination of the cerebrospinal fluid (CSF) may establish the cause of the alteration of consciousness. Appropriate neuroimaging should be performed to ensure that no added injury is likely to be inflicted with LP. The presence of red blood cells in the CSF may suggest primary subarachnoid hemorrhage, parenchymal hemorrhage, or hemorrhagic infection (herpes simplex virus), or it may be due to a traumatic procedure. White blood cells in the CSF usually denote infectious meningitis or meningoencephalitis but may also be associated with vasculitis or parainfectious syndrome. Elevated CSF protein is seen in patients with meningeal inflammation or tumors, and abnormal CSF glucose levels are also markers of infection and inflammation.

Treatment

The etiology of altered mental status determines the treatment. Ingestions may necessitate gastric lavage, charcoal administration, forced diuresis, dialysis, or specific antidotes (Chapter 45). Infections are treated with appropriate antibiotics or antiviral agents (Chapter 95). If mental status changes are due to increased ICP, acute medical interventions (osmotic agents, steroids, hyperventilation) must be instituted, emergent neuroimaging performed, and urgent neurosurgical consultation obtained. Structural brain lesions may necessitate medical treatment of increased ICP or surgical excision.

Prognosis

The outcome of altered mental status relates to many variables, including etiology. Intoxication typically carries a good prognosis, whereas hypoxia carries a poor prognosis. Other prognostic factors include the duration of coma and the age of the patient; children have better outcomes than adults. Complete recovery from traumatic coma of several days' duration is possible in children; however, many survivors of prolonged coma are left in a persistent vegetative state or with severe neuropsychiatric disability.

Transient, Recurrent Depression of Consciousness

Episodic alteration or depression of consciousness with full recovery is usually due to seizure, migraine, syncope, or metabolic abnormality (hypoglycemia). Consciousness can be impaired during seizures or in the postictal state. Nonconvulsive (subclinical) status epilepticus (generalized or focal) can directly impair consciousness and is a common complicating factor for patients with acute neurological disorders (head trauma, meningitis, following convulsive status epilepticus). Some patients may have a prolonged postictal state after an unrecognized seizure.

Basilar artery or **confusional migraines** can last hours and be accompanied by agitation, ataxia, cortical blindness, vertigo, or cranial nerve palsies. Headache may precede or follow the neurologic signs.

Syncope is one of the most common causes of abrupt, episodic loss of consciousness. Neurocardiogenic syncope, cardiac arrhythmia, or an obstructive cardiomyopathy can cause recurrent episodes of loss of consciousness. Two thirds of children with syncope have irregular, myoclonic movements as they lose consciousness (anoxic seizures), which much be distinguished from epilepsy (unprovoked seizures). Children with unexplained syncope require a complete cardiac examination (Chapter 140).

Metabolic derangements, particularly **hypoglycemia**, give rise to episodes of lethargy, confusion, seizures, or coma. Several other metabolic disorders cause recurrent bouts of **hyperammonemia** (Chapter 53). Symptoms include nausea, vomiting, lethargy, confusion, ataxia, hyperventilation, and coma.

TRAUMATIC BRAIN INJURY

Following head injury, children may have immediate depression of consciousness and neurologic deficits or may be completely alert without any immediate signs of neurologic injury. Most serious trauma results from motor vehicle crashes, sports, recreation-related injuries, and violence. Head trauma may result in concussion, posttraumatic intracranial hemorrhage, skull fractures, or cranial nerve or cervical spine injuries. Head injury, or other injuries, with associated retinal hemorrhages in infants and young children should raise the suspicion of abusive head trauma.

Concussion

Concussion is the process in which traumatic forces on the brain result in the rapid onset of short-lived neurologic impairment that typically resolves spontaneously. Patients may have signs or symptoms in one or more domain: somatic (headache), cognitive (slowed reaction times, feeling like they are in a fog, poor attention), emotional (lability, irritability), sleep

Table 184-3	Protocol for Return to Sport after Concussion

Return to play protocol follows a stepwise progress with each step taking 24 hours. The athlete should continue to the next level if asymptomatic at the current level.

1. No activity, complete physical and mental rest.
2. Light aerobic exercise such as walking or stationary cycling; no resistance training.
3. Sport-specific exercise (skating in hockey, running in soccer).
4. Noncontact, more progressive training drills; resistance training.
5. Full-contact practice after medical clearance.
6. Game play.

Modified from McCrory P, Meeuwisse W, Johnston K, et al: Consensus statement on concussion in sport: the 3rd International Conference on Concussion in Sport, held in Zurich, November 2008. Br J Sports Med 2009;43:i76-i84.

disturbance (drowsiness), or physical signs (loss of consciousness, amnesia). Acute symptoms usually reflect a functional disturbance rather than structural injury, and no abnormalities are seen on standard imaging. The majority of concussions resolve within 10 days, although the recovery may be slower in children, and in a small percentage of cases, the symptoms are prolonged.

Repeated concussions, especially within a short time frame (days or weeks) carry a significant risk of permanent brain injury (**second impact syndrome**). Children must not be permitted to resume physical activities until well after the symptoms resolve (Table 184-3).

Traumatic Intracranial Hemorrhage

Head trauma can result in epidural, subdural, parenchymal, and subarachnoid intracranial hemorrhages, as well as brain contusions (Table 184-4). Symptoms include headache, vomiting lethargy, decreased consciousness and seizures. The classic presentation of epidural hemorrhages involves a lucid interval, where, following primary brain injury, a child has a decreased level of consciousness, then returns to normal for several hours before developing rapidly progressive neurologic symptoms. Subdural hemorrhages may result from direct trauma or rotational forces from vigorous shaking (shaken baby syndrome). In neonates and infants with open fontanelles, signs and symptoms may be absent or nonspecific. Occasionally, epidural, subdural, or intracranial hemorrhage or a rapid, life-threatening increase in ICP develops unexpectedly in children due to cerebral edema.

Skull Fractures

Skull fractures may be linear, diastatic (spreading the suture), depressed (an edge displaced inferiorly), or compound (bone fragments breaking the skin surface). Linear and diastatic fractures necessitate no treatment, but indicate trauma capable of producing an underlying hematoma. Small, depressed fractures have the same significance as linear fractures, but if the depression is more than 0.5 to 1 cm, surgical elevation of bone fragments and repair of associated dural tears are generally recommended. Compound fractures or penetrating injuries necessitate emergent surgical debridement and tetanus

Table 184-4	Syndromes of Posttraumatic Intracranial Hemorrhage

SYNDROME	CLINICAL AND RADIOLOGIC CHARACTERISTICS	TREATMENT
Epidural	Onset over minutes to hours; Lucid interval followed by progressive neurologic deficits; Lens-shaped extracerebral hemorrhage compressing brain	Surgical evacuation or observation; Prognosis good with prompt treatment, otherwise poor
Acute subdural	Onset over hours; Focal neurologic deficits; Crescentic extracranial hemorrhage compressing brain	Surgical evacuation; Prognosis guarded
Chronic subdural	Onset over weeks to months; Anemia, macrocephaly; Seizures, vomiting; Crescentic, low-density mass on CT	Subdural taps or subdural shunt as necessary; Prognosis can be good
Intraparenchymal	Depressed consciousness; Focal neurologic deficits; ± Additional multiple contusions	Supportive care; Prognosis guarded
Subarachnoid	Stiff neck; Worst headache of life; Late hydrocephalus	Supportive care; Prognosis variable
Contusion	Focal neurologic deficits; Brain swelling with transtentorial herniation; CT findings: multifocal low-density areas with punctate hemorrhages	Medical treatment of elevated intracranial pressure*; Prognosis guarded

CT, Computed tomography.
*Mannitol, elevation of head of bed, diuresis, hyperventilation, steroids.

prophylaxis. The risk of associated brain contusion and early seizures is high in compound fractures.

Skull fractures may present with localized swelling and pain; subcutaneous bleeding over the mastoid process (**Battle sign**) or around the orbit (**raccoon eyes**); blood behind the tympanic membrane (**hemotympanum**); or CSF leak from the nose (rhinorrhea) or ear (otorrhea). Rarely, a few weeks to months after linear skull fractures, a soft, pulsatile scalp mass is palpable; radiographically, the fracture edges are separated by a soft tissue mass that consists of fibrotic tissue and accumulated brain and meningeal tissue and, possibly a **leptomeningeal cyst**. The recommended treatment of leptomeningeal cysts involves surgical excision of abnormal tissue and dural repair.

CSF leak occurs when a skull fracture tears adjacent dura, creating communications between the subarachnoid space and the nose, paranasal sinuses, mastoid air cells, or ear. Clear fluid that leaks from the nose or ear after head trauma is presumed to be CSF until proved otherwise. The presence of air within the subdural, subarachnoid, or ventricular space also indicates a dural tear and open communication between the nose or paranasal sinuses and brain. In most cases, the dura heals spontaneously when the patient's head is kept elevated. Patients with CSF leaks are at risk for the development of meningitis or extradural abscesses. If the leak persists or recurs or if meningitis develops, the dura is surgically repaired. **Cranial nerve palsies**, secondary to a laceration or contusion of the cranial nerves, may result from a skull fracture and may be transitory or permanent. Longitudinal fracture of the petrous bone produces a conductive hearing loss and facial palsy, which begin hours after the injury and usually resolve spontaneously. Transverse petrous fractures produce sensorineural hearing loss and immediate facial palsy with a poor prognosis for spontaneous recovery. Disruption of the ossicular chain can cause hearing loss and may necessitate surgery. Vestibular disturbances, producing prolonged posttraumatic vertigo, are extremely common. Permanent loss of olfaction after a head injury is the result of a rupture of the thin olfactory nerves within the cribriform plate. Disruption of cranial nerves III, IV, and VI produces ophthalmoplegia, diplopia, and head tilt. Even seemingly minor head injuries can produce sixth nerve palsy with medial deviation (or incomplete abduction) of one or both eye(s).

Other Complications of Head Trauma

Cervical spine injuries must be suspected in any unconscious child, especially if bruises are present on the head, neck, or back. In conscious children, findings of neck or back pain, burning or stabbing pains radiating to the arms, paraplegia, quadriplegia, or asymmetrical motor or sensory responses of arms or legs suggest spinal cord injury. Cervical spine injury (displaced or fractured vertebra) may result in complete transection of the cord with spinal shock, loss of sensation, and flaccid paralysis. A contused cord (without vertebral abnormality) may present in a similar manner. Any patient with a clinical or radiologic abnormality of the spine requires immediate spine and cardiopulmonary stabilization and neurosurgical consultation.

Posttraumatic seizures are divided into one of three patterns: impact seizures, early posttraumatic seizures, and late posttraumatic seizures. Impact seizures occur within seconds of the injury and are presumed to reflect a direct mechanical stimulation to the cortex. The prognosis is excellent, and likelihood of later epilepsy is negligible. Early posttraumatic seizures occurring within the first week of the head injury are likely the result of a localized area of cerebral contusion or edema. The long-term prognosis for these seizures is quite favorable. Late posttraumatic seizures arise more than a week after the trauma and most likely indicate an area of cortical gliosis or scarring that will be a source for long-term epilepsy. These patients often require long-term antiepileptic drug therapy.

Transient neurologic disturbances may develop a few minutes after head trauma and last for minutes to hours before clearing. The most common symptoms are cortical blindness and confusional states, but hemiparesis, ataxia, or any other neurologic deficit may appear. These symptoms may represent a trauma-triggered migraine in susceptible children, but care must be exercised to exclude intracranial pathology.

Drowsiness, **headache**, and **vomiting** are common after head trauma. They are not, by themselves, of concern if consciousness is preserved, the clinical trend is one of improvement, and results of the neurologic examination are normal. Children are especially susceptible to somnolence after head trauma but should be easily arousable. If symptoms worsen or persist for more than 1 to 2 days, neuroimaging may be indicated to look for subdural hematoma or cerebral edema.

Evaluation and Treatment

Children who have been unconscious or have amnesia following a head injury should be evaluated in an emergency department. High-risk patients include those with persistent depressed or decreasing level of consciousness, focal neurologic signs, penetrating skull injury, depressed skull fractures, or worsening symptoms. Because patients with intracranial hemorrhage may progressively deteriorate and require immediate neurosurgical care, these patients warrant care in a skilled trauma center.

The **Glasgow Coma Scale** is a valuable tool for monitoring the course of patients after trauma for signs of deterioration (Chapter 42). Management includes ensuring an appropriate airway, breathing, and circulation. Neuroimaging with CT or magnetic resonance imaging (MRI), and skull and cervical spine radiographs are obtained emergently. Neuroimaging is not necessary for uncomplicated concussions but should be employed whenever suspicion of structural intracranial lesion exists.

The observation period varies with the severity of the injury and may include hospitalization even for children without neurologic deficits who have sustained a concussion. Any patient demonstrating any features of a concussion should be medically evaluated, and disposition (return to play) must be determined by a health care provider (see Table 184-3). The child should be monitored for deterioration over the initial few hours after injury and not left alone. If the child appears well after several hours and is discharged home, parents should be instructed to call their physician for any change in alertness, orientation, or neurologic functioning. An increase in somnolence, headache, or vomiting is cause for concern and neuroimaging.

Patients with intracranial hemorrhage may require emergent surgical intervention for decompression and drainage of the blood collection. Increased ICP may require monitoring, placement of a ventricular drain, and aggressive medical management, including intubation and ventilation, osmotic therapy, and sedation (see later discussion).

Prognosis

Children with concussion without subsequent neurologic deficits have a favorable long-term prognosis, and late sequelae are rare. Children with moderate contusions usually make good recoveries even when neurologic signs persist for weeks. Long-term sequelae may include poor memory, slowing of motor skills, generalized decrease in cognitive skills, behavioral alterations, or attention deficits. Language function, especially in a young child, frequently makes a good recovery. Rehabilitation programs with physical therapy, behavioral management, and appropriate education may be necessary. Poor prognostic signs include a Glasgow Coma Scale score of less than 4 on admission without improvement in 24 hours, absent pupillary light reflexes, and persistent extensor plantar reflexes.

Children with cerebral contusion who survive acute cerebral swelling may improve gradually or may remain vegetative. Extracranial trauma also contributes to the morbidity of these patients (aspiration pneumonia, acute respiratory distress syndrome, sepsis, emboli). Maximal recovery may take weeks or months. Coma lasting for weeks after head trauma may be compatible with a good outcome, although the risk of late sequelae is significant. Patients who remain in a vegetative state for months after head injury are unlikely to improve.

INCREASED INTRACRANIAL PRESSURE
Etiology

When the cranial sutures are fused, the skull becomes a rigid container enclosing a fixed volume, including the brain (80% to 85%), CSF (10% to 15%), and blood (5% to 10%). The exponential relationship between the volume within a closed container and pressure results in a massive increase in ICP as intracranial volume increases. The brain accommodates increased ICP initially by expelling CSF and blood from the intracranial compartment into the spinal subarachnoid space. When the limits of this accommodation are reached, the brain itself begins to shift in response to the continuing elevation of ICP. Brain shifts may cause herniations across the dural extensions or skull barriers (see Table 184-2).

The causes of increased ICP include mass lesion, hydrocephalus, cerebral edema due to trauma or infection and idiopathic intracranial hypertension (Tables 184-5, 184-6).

Mass lesions (brain tumor, abscess, hemorrhage) may produce increased ICP not only by virtue of large size, but by blockage of CSF pathways, blockage of venous outflow, or production of vasogenic cerebral edema. Brain abscesses usually present as mass lesions, producing focal neurologic signs and increased ICP. Symptoms of infection, including fever, malaise, anorexia, and stiff neck, may be subtle or absent. Brain edema around an abscess is usually severe and extends into the surrounding white matter. Children with chronic cardiac or pulmonary disease may embolize infected material to their brains, predisposing them to brain abscesses. Brain tumors in children are most often located in the posterior fossa and can result in elevated ICP due to obstruction of CSF flow through the cerebral aqueduct and fourth ventricle.

Hydrocephalus from congenital abnormalities or due to an intracranial mass is typically characterized by a slowly evolving syndrome of increased ICP extending over weeks or months. CSF is continuously produced by the choroid plexus within the lateral, third, and fourth ventricles. CSF flows from the lateral ventricles through the intraventricular foramen of Monro to the third ventricle, then passes through the cerebral aqueduct to the fourth ventricle. CSF exits the fourth ventricle from the foramen of Magendie and foramina of Luschka. Subarachnoid flow occurs superiorly to the cisterns of the brain and inferiorly to the spinal subarachnoid space. Absorption of CSF is accomplished predominantly by the arachnoid villi into the large dural sinuses. Hydrocephalus is due to the obstruction of CSF flow anywhere along its course (see Table 184-6). **Obstructive hydrocephalus** is caused by a block before the CSF flows to the subarachnoid space, usually within the fourth ventricle or at the level of the aqueduct. Impairment of CSF flow within the subarachnoid space or impairment of

Table 184-5	Causes of Increased Intracranial Pressure

MASS EFFECT

Hydrocephalus
Infarction with edema
Hemorrhage
Tumor
Abscess
Cyst
Inflammatory mass
Arterial ischemic stroke
Intracranial venous sinus thrombosis

DIFFUSE EDEMA

Hypoxic-ischemic injury
Trauma
Infection
   Meningitis
   Encephalitis
Hypertension
Metabolic derangement or toxin
   Hyponatremia
   Diabetic ketoacidosis
   Dialysis dysequilibrium syndrome
   Reye syndrome
   Fulminant hepatic encephalopathy
   Pulmonary insufficiency with hypercarbia
   Lead intoxication
Idiopathic intracranial hypertension (pseudotumor cerebri)
   Drugs
   Withdrawal of long-term steroid administration
   Endocrinologic disturbance
   Obesity

Table 184-6	Causes of Hydrocephalus	
PATHOGENIC MECHANISM	**ETIOLOGIC DISORDER/ CONDITION**	
Obstruction of CSF pathways	Intraventricular foramina (Monro) obstruction	
	Parasellar mass (craniopharyngioma, germinoma, pituitary tumor)	
	Intraventricular tumor (ependymoma)	
	Tuberous sclerosis with subependymal giant cell astrocytoma	
	Aqueduct of Sylvius (cerebral aqueduct) obstruction	
	Aqueductal stenosis	
	Midbrain or pineal region tumor	
	Postinfectious or postinflammatory	
	Posthemorrhagic	
	Impaired flow from the fourth ventricle foramina of Luschka and Magendie	
	Basilar impression	
	Platybasia	
	Dandy-Walker malformation	
	Arnold-Chiari malformation	
	Bone lesions of the cranial base (achondroplasia, rickets)	
Overproduction of CSF	Choroid plexus papilloma	
Defective reabsorption of CSF (extraventricular obstruction or communicating hydrocephalus)	Hypoplasia of the arachnoid villi Postinfectious or posthemorrhagic destruction of arachnoid villi or subarachnoid fibrosis Extensive cerebral sinovenous thrombosis	

CSF, Cerebrospinal fluid.

absorption is known by the misnomer *communicating hydrocephalus*, where there is actually extraventricular obstruction of CSF flow (*external hydrocephalus*). Hydrocephalus caused by overproduction of CSF without true obstruction is seen in choroid plexus papillomas, which account for 2% to 4% of childhood intracranial tumors.

Bacterial meningitis may produce increased ICP by blockage of CSF pathways, toxic cerebral edema, increase in cerebral blood flow, or multifocal cerebral infarctions (Chapter 100). Most children with bacterial meningitis can undergo LP safely because the brain swelling is diffuse and distributed evenly throughout the brain and spinal CSF compartments. A few patients with meningitis, however, develop transtentorial herniation within a few hours of LP. Focal neurologic signs, poorly reactive pupils, and a tense fontanelle are contraindications to LP in a patient with suspected bacterial meningitis.

Idiopathic intracranial hypertension (pseudotumor cerebri) is a cause of increased ICP with normal brain imaging. Patients exhibit a daily debilitating headache associated with diplopia, abducens palsy, transient visual obscurations, and papilledema. If untreated, permanent visual field loss may develop. The syndrome has been associated with ingestion of medications (tetracycline, vitamin A, oral contraceptive agents) and endocrine disturbances (thyroid disease, Addison disease). Most commonly, this condition is idiopathic and affects children who are otherwise well except for being overweight, with rapid weight gain being a predisposing factor. **Treatment** including acetazolamide or other diuretic, topiramate, or corticosteroids, is generally effective. Weight loss and cessation of triggering medications are also mainstays of treatment. Infrequently, chronic papilledema from persistent idiopathic intracranial hypertension produces visual impairment, and more aggressive management is required (optic nerve fenestration) to preserve visual function.

Clinical Manifestations

Decision-Making Algorithms
Available @ StudentConsult.com

Strabismus
Vomiting
Headaches
Altered Mental Status

The symptoms and signs of increased ICP include headache, vomiting, lethargy, irritability, altered consciousness, sixth nerve palsy, strabismus, diplopia, and papilledema. Headaches suggestive of increased ICP are those associated with nocturnal wakening; worse in the morning; with cough, micturition, defecation, or Valsalva maneuver; or progressively worsening. Infants who have an open fontanelle usually do not develop papilledema or abducens palsy. Specific signs of increased ICP in infants consist of a bulging fontanelle, suture diastasis, distended scalp veins, a persistent downward deviation of the eyes (*sunsetting*), and rapid growth of head circumference. Specific signs of increased ICP in the infratentorial compartment (posterior fossa) include stiff neck and head tilt. Focal neurologic deficits reflect the site of the lesion that is producing the increased ICP and may include hemiparesis from supratentorial lesions, or ataxia and cranial nerve palsies from infratentorial lesions. Critically increased ICP may result in herniation syndromes, as

discussed earlier. In addition, the **Cushing triad** of elevated blood pressure, bradycardia, and irregular respirations is a late sign of critically elevated ICP.

The clinical manifestations of hydrocephalus are caused by ventricular distention and increased ICP. Dilation of the lateral ventricles stretches the corticopontocerebellar and corticospinal pathways, resulting in ataxia and spasticity that initially are most marked in the lower extremities because the leg fibers are closest to the ventricles. Distention of the third ventricle may compress the hypothalamic regions and result in endocrine dysfunction. The optic nerves, chiasm, and tracts also are in proximity to the anterior third ventricle, and visual dysfunction results when these structures are compressed. Dilation of the cerebral aqueduct compresses the surrounding periaqueductal vertical gaze center, causing downward deviation of the eyes. Manifestations of increased ICP may evolve slowly when obstruction is not complete and there is time for transependymal absorption of CSF into the veins, or rapidly when obstruction is abrupt and complete (subarachnoid hemorrhage) and compensation cannot occur.

Laboratory and Diagnostic Studies

The cause of increased ICP is determined by brain imaging with either head CT or brain MRI. CT is rapid, readily available, and provides clear visualization of an acute hemorrhage or dilated ventricles. Mass lesions, hydrocephalus, and trauma are easily recognized. Diffuse brain swelling produced by hypoxic-ischemic injury, meningitis, encephalitis, metabolic abnormalities, or toxins may be better delineated by MRI. MRI is also superior to CT for visualizing the posterior fossa and cortical contusions. LP is the diagnostic test for infection and for documentation of elevated ICP (essential for patients with idiopathic intracranial hypertension). However, LP is contraindicated in the setting of an intracranial mass lesion or clear hydrocephalus, because withdrawal of CSF can change pressures between the intracranial compartments and promote brainstem shifts and herniation. Idiopathic intracranial hypertension is diagnosed when direct measurement of ICP with a manometer during LP reveals elevated ICP in the absence of other CSF or imaging abnormalities.

Treatment of Elevated ICP

The treatment of acute increased ICP should be carried out in an intensive care setting with continuous monitoring and vigilant attention to vital signs. The patient's response to specific interventions must be carefully assessed. The head is placed at midline and the head of the bed elevated 30°. Immediate endotracheal intubation and hyperventilation (to a Paco$_2$ not lower than 35 mm Hg) produces rapid, but transient, reduction in ICP by cerebral vasoconstriction, leading to decreased cerebral blood volume. Mannitol or 3% saline may be used acutely to produce an osmotic shift of fluid from the brain to the plasma. A ventricular catheter may be used to remove CSF and to monitor the ICP continuously. Pentobarbital-induced coma reduces pressure by severely suppressing cerebral metabolism and cerebral blood flow. Acetazolamide and furosemide may transiently decrease CSF production. Because acute interventions such as hyperventilation, osmotic therapies, and barbiturates can have negative impacts on systemic and cerebral perfusion and have only transient effects on ICP, they must be used judiciously.

The **treatment of hydrocephalus** may be medical or surgical, depending on the etiology. After subarachnoid hemorrhage or meningitis, the flow or absorption of CSF may be transiently impaired. In this circumstance, the use of medication that decreases CSF production, such as acetazolamide, may be beneficial. Surgical management consists of removing the obstructive lesion, placing a shunt, or both. A shunt consists of polyethylene tubing extending usually from a lateral ventricle to the peritoneal cavity (**ventriculoperitoneal shunt**). Shunts carry the hazards of infection or sudden occlusion with signs and symptoms of acute hydrocephalus.

Vasopressor drugs may be necessary to maintain adequate arterial pressure and cerebral perfusion pressure. Serum electrolytes and osmolarity should be monitored because of risk of the syndrome of inappropriate antidiuretic hormone or cerebral salt wasting. Maintaining normoglycemia may have a positive impact on outcomes. Other supportive measures include controlling agitation, fever, and seizures.

All treatments for increased ICP are temporary measures intended to prevent herniation until the underlying disease process either is treated or resolves spontaneously. Timely intervention can reverse cerebral herniation. Complete neurologic recovery is possible, but rare, after signs of transtentorial or foramen magnum herniation have begun. When these signs are complete, however, with bilaterally dilated, unreactive pupils, absent eye movements, and flaccid quadriplegia, recovery is no longer possible.

Chapter 185

NEURODEGENERATIVE DISORDERS

Children typically acquire developmental milestones in a variable but predictable sequence (Chapter 7). Rarely, children present with stagnation of development or frank loss of previously acquired skills. These **neurodegenerative disorders** encompass a large heterogenous group of diseases that result from specific genetic and biochemical defects and varied unknown causes. Neurodegenerative disorders can present at any age. Clinical phenotypes also vary, but neurologic deterioration may be demonstrated as loss of speech, vision, hearing, and intellectual or motor abilities—sometimes in concert with seizures, feeding difficulties, and mental retardation. Progression may be slow over many years, or may lead to death in early childhood.

HEREDITARY AND METABOLIC DEGENERATIVE DISEASES

Degenerative diseases may affect gray matter (**neuronal degenerative disorders**), white matter (**leukodystrophies**), both gray and white matter, or specific, focal regions of the brain. Early seizures and intellectual impairment mark grey matter disorders, whereas upper motor neuron signs and progressive spasticity are the hallmarks of white matter disorders. Many neurodegenerative illnesses result from enzymatic disorders within subcellular organelles, including lysosomes, mitochondria, and peroxisomes (Table 185-1). Therefore, any

Table 185-1	Selected Clinical Features of Neurodegenerative Disorders and Relevant Diagnostic Tests

SPHINGOLIPIDOSES

Niemann-Pick Disease

Cognitive regression, hepatosplenomegaly, jaundice, seizures

    Test: acid sphingomyelinase (ASM) enzyme activity

Gaucher Disease

Hepatosplenomegaly, cytopenia, spasticity, hyperextension, extraocular palsies, trismus, difficulty swallowing

    Test: glucosylceramidase enzyme activity

GM1 Gangliosidoses

Infantile form—early feeding difficulties, global retardation, seizures, coarse facial features, hepatosplenomegaly, cherry red spot

Juvenile form—incoordination, weakness, language regression; later, seizures, spasticity, blindness

Adult form

    Test: GM1 ganglioside enzyme activity; *GLB1* gene testing

GM2 Gangliosidoses

Tay-Sachs—progressive weakness, marked startle reaction, blindness, convulsions, spasticity, and cherry red spots

    Test: β-hexosaminidase A (HEX A) enzymatic activity

Sandhoff disease—phenotype similar to Tay-Sachs

    Test: hexosaminidase A and B enzyme activity (both deficient)

Krabbe Disease/Globoid Cell Leukodystrophy

Irritability, hyperpyrexia, vomiting, seizures, hypertonia, blindness

    Test: galactocerebrosidase (GALC) enzyme activity

Metachromic Leukodystrophy

Late infantile form—stiffening and ataxia of gait, spasticity, optic atrophy, intellectual deterioration, absent reflexes

Juvenile and adult forms

    Test: 1. arylsulfatase A (ARSA) enzyme activity

    2. If ARSA activity is <10% of controls, exclude ARSA pseudodeficiency with genetic testing of *ARSA* and/or abnormal urinary sulfatide excretion

NEURONAL CEROID LIPOFUSCINOSES

Visual loss, progressive dementia, seizures, motor deterioration

    Test: Diagnostic algorithm depends on age of symptom onset, and replies on stepwise testing for palmitoyl-protein thioesterase 1 (PPT1) and tripeptidyl-peptidase 1 (TPP-1) enzyme activity

X-LINKED ADRENOLEUKODYSTROPHY

Classic Adrenoleukodystrophy

Academic difficulties, behavioral disturbances, hypoadrenalism, seizures, spasticity, ataxia, and swallowing difficulties.

Adrenomyeloneuropathy

Spastic paraparesis, urinary incontinence, adrenal insufficiency

    Test: very long chain fatty acids

MUCOPOLYSACCHARIDOSES (MPS)

Short stature, kyphoscoliosis, coarse facies, hepatosplenomegaly, cardiovascular abnormalities, and corneal clouding

Hurler (MPS type I-H)

Continued

Table 185-1	Selected Clinical Features of Neurodegenerative Disorders and Relevant Diagnostic Tests—cont'd

Hunter (MPS type II)

Sanfilippo Disease (MPS type III)

Sly Syndrome (MPS type VII)

Test: 1. lysosomal enzymes

2. urinary glycosaminoglycan excretion

MITOCHONDRIAL DISORDERS

MELAS

Mitochondrial myopathy, encephalopathy, lactic acidosis, and stroke-like episodes

MERRF

Myoclonus, epilepsy, and ragged red fibers, dementia, hearing loss, optic nerve atrophy, ataxia, and loss of deep sensation

NARP

Neuropathy, ataxia, and retinitis pigmentosa

Tests: testing for mitochondrial disorders is complex and must be tailored to the individual clinical scenario; screening for blood and serum lactate and pyruvate is reasonable

SUBACUTE NECROTIZING ENCEPHALOMYELOPATHY (LEIGH DISEASE)

Hypotonia, feeding difficulties, respiratory irregularity, weakness of extraocular movements, and ataxia

Test: depends on clinical phenotype

RETT SYNDROME

Loss of purposeful hand movements and communication skills, social withdrawal, gait apraxia, seizures, spasticity, and kyphoscoliosis

Test: *MECP2* gene testing

WILSON DISEASE

Inborn error of copper metabolism resulting in signs of cerebellar and basal ganglia dysfunction

Test: serum ceruloplasmin levels, urinary copper excretion

patient with a degenerative neurologic condition of unknown cause should have leukocytes or skin fibroblasts harvested for measurement of a standard battery of lysosomal, peroxisomal, and mitochondrial enzymes (Chapters 56, 57). Neuroimaging, usually with brain magnetic resonance imaging (MRI), is also typically warranted. The diagnosis of leukodystrophy usually can be made confidently on the basis of extensive cerebral white matter changes on MRI. Histologic and biochemical studies may be normal in gray matter encephalopathy, making the diagnosis much less secure. Acquired lesions (infectious, inflammatory, vascular, toxic) are difficult to exclude completely. Brain biopsy is not likely to be helpful.

Sphingolipidoses

The sphingolipidoses are characterized by intracellular storage of lipid substrates resulting from defective catabolism of the sphingolipids comprising cellular membranes. They are inherited in an autosomal recessive pattern. In most cases, there are several forms of these diseases, typically corresponding to the amount of residual activity in the relevant enzyme.

The infantile forms are generally the most severe, usually presenting in the first or second year of life with rapid disease progression; affected individuals have virtually no normal enzyme activity. Juvenile and chronic forms are manifest somewhat later in childhood or even adulthood and have a less fulminant disease course because of some residual enzyme activity.

Classic **Niemann-Pick disease** is caused by a deficiency of sphingomyelinase and should be suspected in infants who exhibit the combination of hepatosplenomegaly, developmental delay, interstitial lung disease, and **retinal cherry-red spots**. The ganglion cells of the retina and macula are distended and appear as a large area of white surrounding a small red fovea that is not covered by ganglion cells. Cognitive regression, myoclonic seizures, hypotonia, and jaundice are also noted within the first year of life. Genetic testing for *SMPD1* mutations is clinically available.

Although the most common form of **Gaucher disease** is an indolent illness of adults, there is a rapidly fatal infantile form featuring severe neurologic involvement caused by deficiency of the enzyme glucocerebrosidase. Glucoceramide accumulates in the liver, spleen, and bone marrow. The characteristic neurologic signs are opisthotonos (arching of the trunk), trismus (difficulty opening mouth), eye movement abnormalities, and bulbar signs including difficulty swallowing.

Decision-Making Algorithm
Available @ StudentConsult.com

Splenomegaly

Tay-Sachs disease (GM_2 gangliosidosis) is caused by deficiency of hexosaminidase A and results in the accumulation of GM_2 ganglioside in cerebral gray matter and cerebellum. Infants are typically normal except for a marked startle response until 6 months of age, when they develop listlessness, irritability, hyperacusis, intellectual retardation, and retinal cherry-red spots. Within months, blindness, convulsions, spasticity, and opisthotonos develop.

Metachromatic leukodystrophy (MLD) is a lipidosis caused by deficiency of arylsulfatase that results in demyelination of the central nervous system (CNS) and peripheral nervous system. Children with the late-infantile form present between 1 and 2 years of age. After a period of normal development, progressive stiffening and ataxia of gait, spasticity, optic atrophy, intellectual deterioration, and absent reflexes occur. Diagnostic testing reveals increased cerebral spinal fluid protein (a sign of CNS demyelination) and slowing of motor nerve conduction velocity (a sign of peripheral demyelination). Older school-age children with the juvenile form of MLD may present with gradual onset of behavior difficulties and declining academic abilities, succeeded by gait difficulties, clumsiness, slurred speech, and sometimes seizures. Relentless progression is the rule. Bone marrow transplant is a treatment option, particularly if a sibling is diagnosed with MLD before symptom onset.

Krabbe disease (globoid cell leukodystrophy) is caused by a deficiency of galactocerebrosidase. Individuals with the infantile form (85% to 90% of cases) appear to be normal during the first months of life. Symptoms begin by 6 months of age and include extreme irritability, hyperpyrexia, vomiting, seizures, hypertonia, and blindness. Demyelination of the CNS and peripheral nervous system results in upper and lower motor neuron signs.

Neuronal Ceroid Lipofuscinoses

The neuronal ceroid lipofuscinoses are a group of inherited, neurodegenerative lysosomal storage disorders characterized by progressive vision loss, seizures, declining cognitive abilities, motor deterioration, and early death. Ten different types have been characterized, including infantile, late-infantile, and juvenile types.

Adrenoleukodystrophy

The adrenoleukodystrophies (ALD) are a group of X-linked neurodegenerative disorders that are often associated with adrenocortical insufficiency. ALD is caused by accumulation of very long chain fatty acids in neuronal and adrenal tissue (Chapter 178) and is diagnosed by abnormal very long chain fatty acid testing. The most common leukodystrophy is **classic X-linked adrenoleukodystrophy**, caused by a mutation in the *ABCD1* gene. Boys present between ages 5 and 15 years with academic difficulties, behavioral disturbances, and gait abnormalities, progressing to seizures, spasticity, ataxia, and swallowing difficulties. Brain MRI demonstrates a classic pattern of symmetric abnormal white matter signal in the parietal-occipital regions, with contrast enhancement at the anterior margin. Symptomatic *adrenocortical insufficiency* with fatigue, vomiting, and hypotension develops in 20% to 40% of patients with X-linked ALD. ALD should be considered in any male with primary adrenocortical insufficiency, even in the absence of clear-cut neurological abnormalities. **Adrenomyeloneuropathy**, a chronic disorder of spinal cord and peripheral nerves, presents in the third decade of life. Female carriers of the *ABCD1* mutation may also have symptoms similar to adrenomyeloneuropathy, beginning later in life (>35 years of age).

Mucopolysaccharidoses

Mucopolysaccharidoses are caused by defective lysosomal hydrolases resulting in the accumulation of mucopolysaccharides within lysosomes (see Chapter 56). The clinical manifestations include coarse facies, short stature, kyphoscoliosis, hepatosplenomegaly, cardiovascular abnormalities, and corneal clouding. Neurologic involvement is seen in mucopolysaccharidosis types I (**Hurler syndrome**), II (**Hunter syndrome**), III (**Sanfilippo syndrome**), and VII (**Sly syndrome**). Children with Hurler syndrome, the most severe of these illnesses, appear normal during the first 6 months of life, then develop the characteristic skeletal and neurologic features. Intellectual disability, spasticity, deafness, and optic atrophy are progressive. Hydrocephalus frequently occurs because of obstruction to cerebrospinal fluid (CSF) flow by thickened leptomeninges.

Mitochondrial Disorders

Mitochondrial diseases represent a clinically heterogeneous group of disorders that fundamentally share a disturbance in oxidative phosphorylation (adenosine triphosphate synthesis) (Chapter 57). Abrupt symptoms are often manifest concurrent with periods of physiologic stress such as febrile illness or fasting. Specific genetic diagnoses are often difficult to identify because clinical features are pleotropic within individual defects and overlap between different defects, and because analysis of mitochondrial protein function is technically demanding. Specific syndromes include **MELAS** (mitochondrial myopathy, encephalopathy, lactic acidosis, and stroke-like episodes); **MERRF** (myoclonus, epilepsy, and ragged red fibers) which can also manifest as combinations of dementia, sensorineural hearing loss, optic nerve atrophy, peripheral neuropathy, and occasionally cardiomyopathy with Wolff-Parkinson-White syndrome; and **NARP** (neuropathy, ataxia, and retinitis pigmentosa).

Rett Syndrome

Rett syndrome is a neurodevelopmental disorder that classically affects girls. Typically, development appears normal during the first 6 to 18 months of life, followed by *regression*, loss of purposeful hand movements, loss of verbal communication skills, gait apraxia, and stereotypic repetitive hand movements that resemble washing, wringing, or clapping of the hands. Girls also develop acquired microcephaly. Episodic apnea and/or hyperpnea, peripheral vasomotor disturbances, growth retardation, abnormal muscle tone, and prolonged QTc interval often occur. The regression plateaus and stabilizes, but seizures, spasticity, and kyphoscoliosis develop. The etiology is a mutation on an X chromosome gene coding for methyl-CpG-binding protein 2 transcription factor. Boys with *MECP2* mutations usually do not survive to delivery, but can present with severe neonatal encephalopathy, seizures, microcephaly, abnormal tone, and respiratory insufficiency.

Degenerative Diseases with Focal Manifestations

Some neurodegenerative disorders have predilections to target specific regions or systems within the neuraxis, producing symptoms referable to the affected region.

Wilson disease is a treatable degenerative condition that exhibits signs of cerebellar and basal ganglia dysfunction. It is an autosomal recessive inborn error of copper metabolism. Serum ceruloplasmin levels are low. Abnormal copper deposition is found in the liver, producing cirrhosis; in the peripheral cornea, producing a characteristic green-brown (Kayser-Fleischer) ring; and in the CNS, producing neuronal degeneration and protoplasmic astrocytosis. Neurologic symptoms characteristically begin in the early teenage years with dysarthria, dysphasia, drooling, fixed smile, tremor, dystonia, and emotional lability. MRI shows abnormalities of the basal ganglia. Treatment is with a copper-chelating agent, such as oral penicillamine.

Decision-Making Algorithms
Available @ StudentConsult.com

Jaundice
Hepatomegaly
Involuntary Movements
Hypocalcemia

Subacute necrotizing encephalomyelopathy, or Leigh disease, is a neuropathologically defined, degenerative inherited CNS disease primarily involving the periaqueductal region of the brainstem, caudate, and putamen. Symptoms usually begin before 2 years of age and consist of hypotonia, feeding difficulties, respiratory irregularity, weakness of extraocular movements, and ataxia. Blood and CSF lactate and pyruvate levels are elevated. Several alterations of mitochondrial function produce this clinical syndrome.

ACQUIRED ILLNESSES MIMICKING DEGENERATIVE DISEASES

Children with poorly controlled epilepsy may be continuously in either an ictal or a postictal state and may appear stuporous because of their *epileptic encephalopathy*. Antiepileptic drugs that are sedating or affect mood, memory, motivation, or attention may contribute to the lack or loss of developmental abilities and school failure. Use of high doses or multiple anticonvulsants may compound this problem.

Chronic drug use or overuse (sedatives, tranquilizers, anticholinergics) can bring about progressive confusion, lethargy, and ataxia. Intoxications with heavy metals, such as lead, may cause chronic learning difficulties or may present acutely with irritability, listlessness, anorexia, and pallor, progressing to fulminant encephalopathy. Vitamin deficiency of thiamine, niacin, vitamin B_{12}, and vitamin E can produce encephalopathy, peripheral neuropathy, and ataxia.

Congenital and acquired hypothyroidism impairs cognition and retards developmental progress. Unrecognized congenital hypothyroidism produces irreversible damage if it is not treated immediately after birth (Chapter 175).

Structural brain diseases, such as hydrocephalus and slowly growing tumors, may mimic dementia. Certain indolent brain infections, such as rubeola (measles, causing subacute sclerosing panencephalitis), rubella (German measles), syphilis, and some fungal infections, cause neurologic deterioration over months and years. Congenital human immunodeficiency virus infection causes failure of normal development and regression of acquired skills.

Psychiatric disorders, such as depression and severe psychosocial deprivation in infancy, can give rise to apathy and failure to attain developmental milestones (Chapter 21). Children with autism spectrum disorder may go through a phase of developmental stagnation or disintegration at about 12 to 18 months of age after a period of early normal milestones. Depression in older children can lead to blunting of affect, social withdrawal, and poor school performance, which raise the question of encephalopathy or dementia.

Chapter 186

NEUROCUTANEOUS DISORDERS

The skin, teeth, hair, nails, and brain are derived embryologically from ectoderm. Abnormalities of these surface structures may indicate abnormal brain development. Not all of the so-called neurocutaneous disorders have characteristic cutaneous lesions, however, and not all are of ectodermal origin. Neurofibromatosis (types 1 and 2), tuberous sclerosis, Sturge-Weber syndrome, von Hippel–Lindau disease, and ataxia-telangiectasia are the most common of the more than 40 neurocutaneous disorders.

NEUROFIBROMATOSIS TYPE 1
Etiology

Neurofibromatosis type 1 (NF1), also known as von Recklinghausen disease, is an autosomal-dominant disorder with an incidence of approximately 1 in 3000. It is caused by mutations of the *NF1* gene, which codes for a tumor suppressor gene, neurofibromin. Neurofibromin is a major negative regulator of a key signal transduction pathway, the Ras pathway. Mutations results in increased downstream mitogenic signaling. Somatic mosaicism, in which an abnormality in one copy of the *NF1* gene is present in some cells but not others, indicates a postzygotic mutation and is called **segmental neurofibromatosis**.

Clinical Manifestations

Decision-Making Algorithms
Available @ StudentConsult.com

Hearing Loss
Gynecomastia

The cardinal features of neurofibromatosis are café au lait spots, axillary or inguinal freckling, cutaneous neurofibromas, and iris hamartomas (Lisch nodules). **Café au lait spots** are present in more than 90% of patients who have NF1 (Fig. 186-1). They typically appear in the first few years of life and increase in number and size over time. The presence of six or

FIGURE 186-1 Cafe au lait macules. *(From Kliegman RE, Behrman RE, Jenson HB, editors: Nelson Textbook of Pediatrics, ed 19, Philadelphia, 2007, Saunders, p 2680.)*

more café-au-lait spots larger than 5 mm in a prepubescent child suggests the diagnosis. **Lisch nodules** also increase in frequency with age and are present in more than 90% of adults who have NF1.

Neurofibromas are composed of various combinations of Schwann cells, fibroblasts, mast cells, and vascular elements. Dermal neurofibromas are nearly universal and consist of discrete, small, soft lesions that lie within the dermis and epidermis and move passively with the skin. They rarely cause any symptoms, but can cause significant cosmetic concerns. Neurofibromas may also be situated within viscera or along blood vessels and peripheral nerves. Plexiform neurofibromas are large, occasionally nodular, subcutaneous lesions that lie along the major peripheral nerve trunks. They often cause symptoms including pain, weakness, and invasion of adjacent viscera, bone, or spinal cord. Sarcomatous degeneration may occur. Surgical treatment may be attempted, but results are often unsatisfactory.

Common complications are learning disability, scoliosis, seizures, and cerebral vasculature abnormalities. Other tumors that occur in NF1 are optic nerve gliomas, astrocytomas of brain and spinal cord, and malignant peripheral nerve tumors. T2-weighted magnetic resonance images (MRI) reveal hyperintense lesions (hamartomas) in the optic tracts, internal capsule, thalamus, cerebellum, and brainstem that are common and distinctive for the disease. They are benign and disappear in adulthood.

The average life expectancy of patients with NF1 may be reduced by 10 to 15 years. Malignancy is the most common cause of death. Genetic and psychological counseling are important components of care for this chronic disorder. Although it is an autosomal dominant disorder, spontaneous mutations account for 30% to 50% of cases.

Neurofibromatosis Type 2

Neurofibromatosis type 2 (NF2) is an autosomal-dominant disorder with an incidence of 1 in 25,000. Half the cases have no family history. The *NF2* gene is a tumor suppressor gene, and disease results in neurologic, eye, and skin lesions. NF2 predisposes patients to multiple intracranial and spinal tumors, including bilateral acoustic schwannomas, schwannomas of other cranial and spinal nerves, meningiomas, and gliomas. Posterior capsular or cortical cataracts are common, and skin lesions include plaque-like lesions, subcutaneous nodules, and cutaneous schwannomas. Lisch nodules, cafe au lait spots, and axillary freckling are *not* features of NF2.

TUBEROUS SCLEROSIS COMPLEX
Etiology

Tuberous sclerosis complex (TSC), an autosomal dominant disorder, is characterized by hamartomas in many organs, especially the brain, eyes, skin, kidneys, and heart. The incidence is 1 in 10,000 births. Two thirds of cases are sporadic and thought to represent new mutations. Germline mosaicism is uncommon, but explains how parents who apparently do not have the disease can have multiple children with tuberous sclerosis. Mutations affecting either of the presumed tumor suppressor genes, *TSC1* or *TSC2*, cause tuberous sclerosis. The *TSC1* and *TSC2* genes encode distinct proteins, hamartin and tuberin, which are widely expressed in the brain and result in

constitutive activation of the protein kinase mTOR (mammalian target of rapamycin), leading to the formation of numerous benign tumors (hamartomas).

Clinical Manifestations

TSC is an extremely heterogeneous disease with variable expression and a wide clinical spectrum varying from normal intelligence without seizures to severe mental retardation with refractory seizures, often within the same family. Tuberous sclerosis is one of the most common causes of infantile spasms. These children often develop intractable epilepsy, mental retardation, autism, and hyperactivity. Patients may have retinal lesions (retinal hamartomas, white depigmented patches) and brain lesions (cortical tubers, subependymal nodules, hydrocephalus). **Tubers** in the cerebral cortex are areas of dysplasia that, in combination with other microscopic areas of abnormal development, are responsible for the symptoms of mental retardation and epilepsy. **Subependymal nodules** are hamartomas that may mutate into a growth phase and become **subependymal giant cell astrocytomas** causing obstruction of cerebrospinal fluid outflow and resultant hydrocephalus.

Extracerebral manifestations include typical skin findings of hypomelanotic macules (**ash leaf spots**) which are easiest to visualize under a Wood ultraviolet lamp and are apparent in infancy. Facial angiofibromas (**adenoma sebaceum**) appear as small red nodules over the nose and cheeks that are sometimes confused with acne. **Shagreen patches** are elevated, rough plaques of skin with a predilection for the lumbar and gluteal regions that develop in late childhood or early adolescence. Cardiac rhabdomyomas are largest during prenatal life and infancy and are rarely symptomatic. Occasionally, they may cause arrhythmias or cardiac outflow obstruction. Renal angiomyolipomas may undergo malignant transformation and are the most common cause of death in adults with TSC. Interstitial pulmonary disease also affects adults with TSC (pulmonary lymphangioleiomyomatosis).

STURGE-WEBER SYNDROME

Sturge-Weber syndrome is sporadic (not inherited) and characterized by abnormal blood vessels (**angiomas**) of the leptomeninges overlying the cerebral cortex in association with an ipsilateral facial **port-wine stain** involving the ophthalmic division of the trigeminal nerve (forehead and upper eyelid) and, often, glaucoma. The port-wine stain, also known as nevus flammeus, is due to an ectasia of superficial venules and may have a much more extensive and even bilateral distribution. Not all children with a facial port-wine stain have Sturge-Weber syndrome.

MRI with contrast demonstrates leptomeningeal angioma and white matter abnormalities thought to be due to chronic hypoxia and atrophy. Angiomas produce venous engorgement and, presumably, stasis within the involved areas, which are thought to result in hypoxia. Patients present with seizures, hemiparesis, stroke-like episodes, headaches, mental retardation, and learning disabilities. Seizures are the most common associated neurologic abnormality, occurring in 75% of patients, and develop because of ischemic injury to the brain. Many children with Sturge-Weber syndrome are intellectually normal, and seizures are well controlled with standard anticonvulsants. However, progressive ischemia of the underlying brain develops in some children with Sturge-Weber syndrome, resulting in hemiparesis, hemianopia, intractable focal seizures, and cognitive impairment. Hemispherectomy has been proposed for individuals with unilateral disease whose seizures are difficult to control. Intellectual and motor outcome seems improved, compared with ongoing anticonvulsant drug treatment, but the surgical risks and sequelae of the procedure are considerable. Pulse dye laser surgery is the most promising therapeutic option for cosmetic management of the facial nevus flammeus. Expert ophthalmologic management of glaucoma is required. Endocrinology evaluations are also necessary, as these patients often have growth hormone deficiency and/or hypothyroidism.

Chapter 187

CONGENITAL MALFORMATIONS OF THE CENTRAL NERVOUS SYSTEM

Central nervous system malformations include disorders of spinal cord and neural tube formation, structure specification (neuronal migration, gray matter), brain growth and size, and skull growth and shape.

The precursor of the nervous system is the neural plate of the embryonic ectoderm, which develops at 18 days of gestation. The neural plate gives rise to the neural tube, which forms the brain and spinal cord, and neural crest cells, which form the peripheral nervous system, meninges, melanocytes, and adrenal medulla. The neural tube begins to form on day 22 of gestation. The rostral end forms the brain, and the caudal region forms the spinal cord. The lumen of the neural tube forms the ventricles of the brain and the central canal of the spinal cord. Most brain malformations are produced by a variety of injuries occurring during a vulnerable period of gestation. Precipitating factors include chromosomal, genetic, and metabolic abnormalities; infections (toxoplasmosis, rubella, cytomegalovirus, herpes); and exposure to irradiation, certain drugs, and maternal illness during pregnancy.

CONGENITAL ANOMALIES OF THE SPINAL CORD
Etiology and Clinical Manifestations
Defective closure of the caudal neural tube at the end of week 4 of gestation results in anomalies of the lumbar and sacral vertebrae or spinal cord called **spina bifida**. These anomalies range in severity from clinically insignificant defects of the L5 or S1 vertebral arches to major malformations, leaving the spinal cord uncovered by skin or bone on the infant's back. The latter severe defect, called a **myelomeningocele**, results

in flaccid paralysis and loss of sensation in the legs and incontinence of bowel and bladder, with the extent and degree of neurologic deficit dependent on the location of the myelomeningocele. In addition, affected children usually have an associated **Chiari type II malformation** (downward displacement of the cerebellar tonsils and medulla), resulting in hydrocephalus and weakness of face and swallowing. In a **meningocele**, the spinal canal and cystic meninges are exposed on the back, but the underlying spinal cord is anatomically and functionally intact. In **spina bifida occulta**, the skin of the back is apparently intact, but defects of the underlying bone or spinal canal are present. Meningoceles and spina bifida occulta may be associated with a lipoma, dermoid cyst, or tethering of the cord to a thick filum terminale. A dimple or tuft of hair may be present over the affected area. Patients may also have an associated dermoid sinus, an epithelial tract extending from the skin surface to the meninges; this increases the risk of meningitis. Patients with spina bifida occulta or meningocele may have weakness and numbness in the feet that can result in recurrent ulcerations, or difficulties controlling bowel or bladder function that may result in recurrent urinary tract infections, reflux nephropathy, and renal insufficiency. In **diastematomyelia**, a bone spicule or fibrous band divides the spinal cord into two longitudinal sections. An associated lipoma that infiltrates the cord and tethers it to the vertebrae may be present. Symptoms include weakness and numbness of the feet and urinary incontinence.

Diagnostic Studies
Myelomeningocele in the fetus is suggested by an elevated **alpha-fetoprotein** in the mother's blood and confirmed by ultrasound and high concentrations of alpha-fetoprotein and acetylcholinesterase in the amniotic fluid. After birth, screening ultrasound may be used with magnetic resonance imaging to confirm less dramatic underlying spinal abnormalities.

Treatment and Prevention
Neonates with myelomeningocele must undergo operative closure of the open spinal defects (fetal or postnatal surgery) and often require treatment of hydrocephalus by placement of a ventriculoperitoneal shunt. Toddlers and children with lower spinal cord dysfunction require physical therapy, bracing of the lower extremities, and intermittent bladder catheterization. In the absence of associated brain anomalies, most survivors have normal intelligence, but learning problems and epilepsy are more common than in the general population.

Spina bifida can be prevented in many cases by **folate** administration to the pregnant mother. Because the defect occurs so early in gestation, all women of childbearing age are advised to take oral folic acid daily.

CONGENITAL MALFORMATIONS OF THE BRAIN
Defective closure of the rostral neural tube produces anencephaly or encephaloceles. Neonates with **anencephaly** have a rudimentary brainstem or midbrain, but no cortex or cranium. This is rapidly fatal after delivery. Patients with **encephalocele** usually have a skull defect and exposure of meninges alone or meninges and brain. The recurrence risk in subsequent

pregnancies for either cranial or spinal neural tube defects is 3% to 4%. Within a family, an anencephalic birth may be followed by the birth of a child affected with a lumbosacral myelomeningocele. The inheritance of neural tube defects is polygenic.

Agenesis of the corpus callosum may be partial or complete and may occur in an isolated fashion or in association with other anomalies of cellular migration. **Dandy-Walker malformation** is diagnosed on the basis of the classic triad: complete or partial agenesis of the cerebellar vermis, cystic dilation of the fourth ventricle, and enlarged posterior fossa. There may be associated hydrocephalus, absence of the corpus callosum, and neuronal migration abnormalities. Intelligence may be normal or impaired, depending on the degree of associated cerebral dysgenesis.

Holoprosencephaly represents varying degrees of failure of the forebrain (prosencephalon) to divide into two distinct cerebral hemispheres. Holoprosencephaly is often associated with midline facial defects (hypotelorism, cleft lip, cleft palate). This anomaly may be isolated or associated with a chromosomal or genetic disorder. The prognosis for infants with severe (*alobar*) holoprosencephaly is uniformly poor, but those with milder forms (*semilobar*, or *lobar*) may have less severe neurological outcomes. Children with trisomy 13 and trisomy 18 characteristically have varying degrees of holoprosencephaly.

Hydranencephaly is a condition in which the brain presumably develops normally, but then is destroyed by an intrauterine, probably vascular, insult. The result is virtual absence of the cerebrum with an intact skull. The thalamus, brainstem, and some occipital cortex are typically present. Children may have a normal external appearance at the time of birth, but do not achieve developmental milestones.

Macrocephaly and Microcephaly

Macrocephaly represents a head circumference above the 97th percentile and may be the result of **macrocrania** (increased skull thickness), **hydrocephalus** (enlargement of the ventricles; see Chapter 184), or **megalencephaly** (enlargement of the brain). Diseases of bone metabolism or hypertrophy of the bone marrow cause macrocrania. Megalencephaly may be the result of a significant disorder of brain development or an accumulation of abnormal metabolic substances (Table 187-1). Most often, however, macrocephaly is a familial trait of no clinical significance. If the child is developmentally normal but has macrocephaly, plotting the parents' head circumference on a growth chart can provide reassurance and help to avoid unnecessary neurodiagnostic testing.

Microcephaly represents a head circumference below the 3rd percentile. Myriad syndromes and metabolic disorders are associated with microcephaly, some of which are hereditary (Table 187-2). In most instances, a small head circumference is a reflection of a small brain. Brain growth is rapid during the perinatal period, and any insult (infectious, metabolic, toxic, vascular) sustained during this period or during early infancy is likely to impair brain growth and result in microcephaly. Rarely, a small head is the result of premature closure of one or more skull sutures, called **craniosynostosis**. This diagnosis is readily made by the abnormal shape of the skull. As a rule, macrocephaly and microcephaly raise a concern about cognitive ability, but head circumference alone should never be used to establish a prognosis for intellectual development.

Table 187-1	Causes of Macrocephaly

Macrocrania (increased skull thickness)
  Achondroplasia
  Hypochondroplasia
  Fragile X syndrome
  Osteopetrosis
  Chronic, severe anemia
Hydrocephalus (enlargement of the ventricles; see Chapter 184)
Masses
  Cysts
  Arteriovenous malformations
  Subdural fluid collections/hematoma
  Neoplasm
Megalencephaly (enlargement of the brain)
  Embryologic disorder causing abnormal proliferation of brain tissue
    Neurofibromatosis
    Tuberous sclerosis
    Sturge-Weber syndrome
    Sotos syndrome
    Riley-Smith syndrome
    Hemi-megalencephaly
  Accumulation of abnormal metabolic substances
    Alexander disease
    Canavan disease
    Gangliosidoses
    Mucopolysaccharidoses
Benign causes
  Benign extracerebral collections of infancy
  Familial macrocephaly

Disorders of Neuronal Migration

Many malformations result from the failure of normal migration of neurons from the periventricular germinal matrix zone to the cortical surface at 1 to 5 months of gestation. Multiple malformations may exist in the same patient. Neurologic development with these anomalies varies and depends on the type and extent of the malformation.

Schizencephaly is characterized by clefts within the cerebral hemispheres that extend from the cortical surface to the ventricular cavity. Unilateral clefts can cause isolated congenital hemiparesis, whereas bilateral schizencephaly causes spastic quadriparesis and associated intellectual disability. Affected individuals are at high risk for focal epilepsy.

A severe defect in cortical migration, **lissencephaly** results in a smooth brain without sulcation (agyria). The normal six-layered cortex does not develop. Affected children have difficult-to-control seizures and profound developmental retardation. This anomaly most commonly is part of a genetic disorder, which may be x-linked (*DCX* mutations) or caused by de novo autosomal dominant gene mutations (*Lis-1* mutations). In **pachygyria**, the gyri are few in number and too

Table 187-2	Causes of Microcephaly	
PRIMARY MICROCEPHALY	**SECONDARY (ACQUIRED) MICROCEPHALY**
Microcephaly vera	Infections (congenital)
Chromosomal disorders	Rubella
Trisomy 21	Cytomegalovirus
Trisomy 13	Toxoplasmosis
Trisomy 18	Syphilis
5p microdeletion	Human immunodeficiency virus (HIV)
Angelman syndrome	Infections (noncongenital)
Prader-Willi syndrome	Meningitis
Central nervous system (CNS) malformation	Encephalitis
Holoprosencephaly	Stroke
Encephalocele	Toxic
Hydranencephaly	Radiation exposure—fetal
CNS migrational disorder	Fetal alcohol syndrome
Lissencephaly	Maternal phenylketonuria
Schizencephaly	Hypoxic-ischemic or other severe brain injury
Pachygyria	Periventricular leukomalacia
Micropolygyria	Systemic disease
Agenesis of the corpus callosum	Chronic cardiac or pulmonary disease
Sex-linked microcephaly syndromes	Chronic renal disease
Smith-Lemli-Opitz syndrome	Malnutrition
Cornelia de Lange syndrome	Craniosynostosis totalis
Seckel dwarfism syndrome	
Cockayne syndrome	
Rubinstein-Taybi syndrome	
Hallermann-Streiff syndrome	

broad. In **polymicrogyria**, the gyri are too many and too small. Sometimes pachygyria and polymicrogyria affect an entire hemisphere, producing enlargement of that hemisphere and a clinical syndrome of severe, medically intractable seizures that begin in early infancy. **Gray matter heterotopias** are abnormal islands within the central white matter of neurons that have never completed the migratory process.

ACKNOWLEDGMENT

The authors thank Dr. James Dowling for his generous help in preparing Chapter 182 on weakness and hypotonia.

Suggested Reading

Fenichel GM: *Clinical Pediatric Neurology: a Signs and Symptoms Approach,* ed 6, Philadelphia, 2009, Saunders.

Jacobs H, Gladstein J: Pediatric headache: a clinical review, *Headache* 52:333–339, 2012.

Kliegman RM, Behrman RE, Jenson HB, et al: *Nelson Textbook of Pediatrics,* ed 19, Philadelphia, 2011, Saunders.

Mink JW, Zinner SH: Movement disorders II: chorea, dystonia, myoclonus and tremor, *Pediatr Rev* 31:287–295, 2010.

Peredo DE, Hannibal MC: The floppy infant: evaluation of hypotonia, *Pediatr Rev* 30:e66–e76, 2009.

Schunk JE, Schutzman SA: Pediatric head injury, *Pediatr Rev* 33:398–411, 2012.

Zinner SH, Mink JW: Movement disorders I: tics and stereotypies, *Pediatr Rev* 31:223–233, 2010.

Dermatology

Yvonne E. Chiu

Chapter 188

ASSESSMENT

Approximately one in three Americans of any age has at least one recognizable skin disorder at any time. The most common cutaneous diseases encountered in community settings are dermatophytosis, acne vulgaris, seborrheic dermatitis, atopic dermatitis (eczema), verrucae (warts), tumors, psoriasis, vitiligo, and infections such as herpes simplex and impetigo. In children attending pediatric dermatology clinics, atopic dermatitis, impetigo, tinea capitis, acne vulgaris, verrucae vulgaris, and seborrheic dermatitis are the most common diagnoses.

HISTORY

The age of the patient, onset, duration, progression, associated cutaneous symptoms (pain, pruritus), and associated systemic signs or symptoms (fever, malaise, weight loss) are important clues. Obtaining an accurate description of the original lesion improves diagnostic accuracy. Over-the-counter remedies may alter the appearance of a rash dramatically. Patients often do not consider a topical antibiotic or anti-itch medication as treatment. Thus it is important to probe deeply with related questions in the history. Other important information includes a history of allergies, environmental exposure, travel history, previous treatment, affected contacts, and family history.

PHYSICAL EXAMINATION

A careful examination of the skin requires a visual and a tactile assessment. Examination of the skin over the entire body must be performed systematically. Mucous membranes, hair, nails, and teeth, all of ectodermal origin, also may be involved in cutaneous disorders and should be assessed.

COMMON MANIFESTATIONS

Decision-Making Algorithms
Available @ StudentConsult.com

Alopecia
Vesicles and Bullae
Fever and Rash

A descriptive nomenclature of skin lesions helps with generating a differential diagnosis and also with communication between health care providers. Determination of the primary lesion and secondary change is the cornerstone of dermatologic diagnosis. A **primary lesion** is defined as the basic lesion that arises de novo and is most characteristic of the disease process (Table 188-1 and Fig. 188-1). Primary lesions are rarely seen on a patient at the time of presentation, as most lesions are altered by time or external factors such as

Table 188-1	Primary Skin Lesions
LESION	**DESCRIPTION**
Macule	Flat, nonpalpable lesion <1 cm in diameter
Patch	Similar to macule, but >1 cm in diameter
Papule	Elevated, solid lesion <1 cm in diameter
Plaque	Similar to papule, but >1 cm in diameter; has a flat and broad surface in contrast to a nodule
Nodule	Similar to papule, but >1 cm in diameter; has a rounded surface in contrast to a plaque
Tumor	Similar to nodule, but implies a neoplastic growth rather than an inflammatory process
Vesicle	Fluid-filled (usually clear or straw-colored) epidermal lesion <1 cm in diameter
Bulla	Similar to vesicle, but >1 cm in diameter
Pustule	Pus-filled epidermal lesion, which may have an initial papular phase and often is surrounded by erythema
Purpura	Macule or papule resulting from extravasated blood into the skin; does not blanch with pressure
Petechia	Similar to purpura, but less than a few millimeters in diameter
Ecchymosis	Larger, hemorrhagic patch or plaque resulting from extravasated blood
Wheal (hive)	Pink, edematous papules and plaques that vary greatly in size and configuration; characterized by transient nature with individual lesions resolving within 24 hours
Telangiectasia	Collection of small superficial red blood vessels
Milia	Superficial, white, small epidermal keratin cysts
Comedo	Plug of keratin and sebum within the orifice of a hair follicle, which can be open (whitehead) or closed (blackhead); characteristic lesion of acne vulgaris
Cyst	Papule or nodule with an epidermal lining composed of fluid or solid material

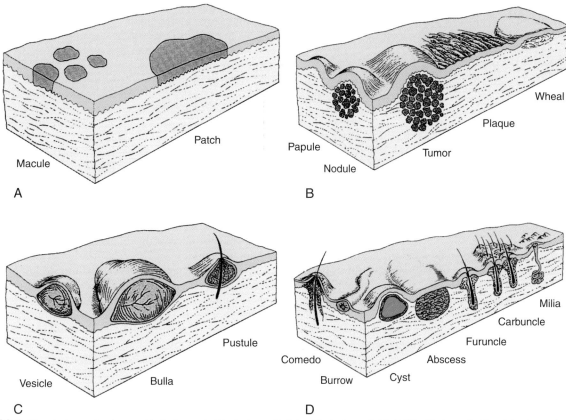

A, Macule, Patch

B, Papule, Nodule, Tumor, Plaque, Wheal

C, Vesicle, Bulla, Pustule

D, Comedo, Burrow, Cyst, Abscess, Furuncle, Carbuncle, Milia

Figure 188-1 Morphology of primary skin lesions. **A**, Flat lesions. **B**, Palpable lesions. **C**, Fluid-filled lesions. **D**, Special primary lesions. *(From Swartz MH:* Textbook of Physical Diagnosis: History and Examination, *Philadelphia, 1989, WB Saunders.)*

medication applied, secondary infection, or physical manipulation (e.g., scratching). A search for the primary lesion often proves worthwhile and focuses the differential diagnosis to a category of lesion that is specific for the underlying diagnosis. On occasion, two different types of primary lesions may be present. In most cases, **secondary lesions** are the residue, or result, of the effects of the primary lesion. They may be created by scratching or secondary infection and may be seen in the absence of a primary lesion (Table 188-2).

The color, texture, configuration, location, and distribution of the lesion should be recorded. A localized or grouped eruption may suggest a cutaneous infection, whereas widespread, symmetrical involvement of extensor surfaces may suggest a primary skin disorder, such as psoriasis. Herpesvirus lesions are usually grouped lesions. Annular lesions may suggest Lyme disease, syphilis, and fungal infections. Lesions on mucous membranes are usually short-lived, and lesions in thick-skinned areas, such as the palms and soles, may be particularly difficult to characterize.

INITIAL DIAGNOSTIC EVALUATION AND TESTS

A thorough history and physical examination are usually sufficient for diagnosis because of the visibility of the skin. Adjunctive tests at the time of examination include potassium hydroxide (KOH) examination for fungi and dermatophytes, skin scrapings for scabies, cytologic examination (Tzanck test) for herpesvirus and varicella-zoster virus infection, and Wood light examination for the yellowish gold fluorescence

Table 188-2	Secondary Skin Lesions
LESION	**DESCRIPTION**
Scale	Results from abnormal keratinization; may be fine or sheetlike
Crust	Dried collection of serum and cellular debris
Erosion	Shallow depression with loss of the superficial epidermis
Ulcer	Deeper depression with loss of the entire epidermis into dermis; heals with scarring
Atrophy	Thinning of epidermis (surface appears shiny and translucent) or dermis (skin is depressed)
Scar	Thickened, firm, and discolored collection of connective tissue that results from dermal damage; initially pink, but lightens with time
Sclerosis	Circumscribed or diffuse hardening of skin
Lichenification	Accentuated skin lines/markings that result from thickening of the epidermis
Excoriation	Superficial linear erosion that is caused by scratching
Fissure	Linear break within the skin surface that usually is painful

of tinea versicolor. A skin biopsy may be performed to help with the diagnosis. The biopsy specimen can be accomplished by either shave or punch biopsy, and both are simple, in-office procedures. Occasionally, laboratory or imaging studies are necessary.

Chapter 189

ACNE

ETIOLOGY

Acne vulgaris (or acne) is a chronic inflammatory disorder that affects areas with the greatest concentration of sebaceous glands, such as the face, chest, and back. The pathogenesis of acne is multifactorial. Gender, age, genetic factors, and environment are all major contributing factors. Stress may trigger acne, possibly by affecting hormone levels. There is no evidence linking chocolate, candy, or fried foods to acne.

Acne is caused by chronic inflammation of the pilosebaceous unit (hair follicle with an associated sebaceous gland). The primary event in all acne lesions is the development of the **micro-comedo**, which results from the obstruction of the hair follicle with keratin, increased sebum production from sebaceous glands, and overgrowth of normal skin flora, leading to pilosebaceous occlusion and enlargement. Androgens are a potent stimulus of the sebaceous gland. The subsequent inflammatory component and pustule formation results from proliferation of *Propionibacterium acnes*, a commensal organism of the skin. The pathogenesis of acne thus involves three components: increased sebum production, hyperkeratosis, and bacterial proliferation. Effective treatment focuses on minimizing these factors.

EPIDEMIOLOGY

Acne is the most common skin disorder in adolescents, occurring in 85% of teenagers. The incidence is similar in both sexes, although boys often are more severely affected. Acne may begin as early as 8 years of age and may continue into adulthood.

CLINICAL MANIFESTATIONS

Acne primarily affects areas with increased sebaceous gland density, such as the face, upper chest, and back. Superficial plugging of the pilosebaceous unit results in noninflammatory small (1- to 2-mm) **open (blackhead)** and **closed (whitehead) comedones**. An open comedo is less likely to become inflammatory than a closed comedo. Rupture of a comedo into adjacent dermis and proliferation of *P. acnes* induce an inflammatory response and development of inflammatory **papules** and **pustules**. Larger, skin-colored or red cysts and nodules represent deeper plugging and **cystic acne**. Increased and persistent inflammation, especially with rupture of a deep cyst, increases the risk of scarring.

The diagnosis of acne is usually not difficult because of the characteristic and chronic lesions. Laboratory studies and imaging studies are usually not necessary to diagnose acne. Screening tests may be necessary if there are signs of hyperandrogenism due to polycystic ovarian syndrome (irregular menses, hirsutism, insulin resistance) or an underlying androgen-secreting tumor (irregular menses, hirsutism, deepening voice, clitoromegaly).

TREATMENT

The mainstays of treatment of acne are topical keratolytic agents and topical antibiotics. Creams, lotions, gels, foams, and solutions are available. Gels and solutions are commonly used because acne skin is generally greasier and these agents tend to be drying, but they have the tendency to be irritating and may not be as well tolerated. Creams and lotions are better tolerated but may not be as effective.

The keratolytic agents (salicylic acid, azelaic acid, tretinoin, adapalene, tazarotene) produce superficial desquamation and, subsequently, relieve follicular obstruction. They are a mainstay of first-line therapy. The topical retinoids (tretinoin, adapalene, tazarotene) are based on the vitamin A molecule. They decrease keratin and sebum production and have some anti-inflammatory and antibacterial activity; thus they can be the most effective when used as monotherapy.

Topical antimicrobials (benzoyl peroxide, dapsone, sulfur-sulfacetamide) and topical antibiotics (erythromycin, clindamycin) are anti-inflammatory and inhibit *P. acnes* proliferation. Erythromycin efficacy has decreased as *P. acnes* has become increasingly resistant to this antibiotic; topical antibiotics should be combined with an antimicrobial such as benzoyl peroxide to prevent the development of resistance. Combination therapy of a topical keratolytic agent and a topical antimicrobial is more effective than either agent alone for inflammatory acne.

Oral antibiotics (tetracycline, doxycycline, minocycline) are typically used for deeper cystic lesions but should always be used in combination with a topical regimen. Tetracyclines are the most effective antibiotics because of their significant anti-inflammatory activity. As with topical erythromycin, oral erythromycin is rarely used because of bacterial resistance.

For recalcitrant or severe nodulocystic acne, oral isotretinoin may be instituted. Isotretinoin, an oral analog of vitamin A, normalizes follicular keratinization, reduces sebum production, and decreases 5α-dihydrotestosterone formation and androgen receptor–binding capacity. A course of isotretinoin (0.5 to 1 mg/kg/day to reach a cumulative dose of 120 mg/kg) is the only medication that can permanently alter the course of acne and induce a durable remission. Because of the high incidence of adverse effects, it should be used only by physicians familiar with this medication. Isotretinoin therapy requires careful patient selection, pretreatment counseling, and monthly laboratory monitoring. It is teratogenic and must not be used immediately before or during pregnancy.

COMPLICATIONS

Acne has significant and frequently devastating effects on an adolescent's body image and self-esteem. There may be little correlation between severity and psychosocial impact. Scarring may result in permanent morbidity.

PROGNOSIS

Classically, acne lasts 3 to 5 years, although some individuals may have disease for 15 to 20 years. Only early treatment with isotretinoin may alter the natural course of acne. Acne lesions often heal with temporary postinflammatory erythema and hyperpigmentation. Depending on the severity, chronicity, and depth of involvement, pitted, atrophic, or hypertrophic scars may develop. **Cystic acne** has the highest incidence of scarring because rupture of a deep cyst induces the greatest inflammation, though scarring may be caused by milder pustular or even comedonal acne.

PREVENTION

Greasy hair and cosmetic preparations should be avoided because they exacerbate preexisting acne. There are no effective means for preventing acne, and there is little evidence that diet is associated with acne. Repetitive cleansing with soap and water or use of astringents or abrasives removes only surface lipids. Their use makes the skin appear less oily but does not prevent formation of microcomedones and may paradoxically worsen acne.

Chapter **190**

ATOPIC DERMATITIS

ETIOLOGY

Atopic dermatitis is a chronic inflammatory disease with no known cure. It is associated with significant psychosocial morbidity and decreased health-related quality of life. For many affected individuals, atopic dermatitis is the skin manifestation of atopy accompanied by asthma and allergic rhinitis.

Atopic dermatitis manifests with a defective skin barrier, reduced innate immune responses, and exaggerated immune responses to allergens and microbes. Both genetic predisposition and environmental factors play a role in the development of atopic dermatitis. Genes associated with skin barrier dysfunction and inflammation have been linked with atopic dermatitis. Inflammatory mediators involved include predominantly T helper cells, with the T_H2 pathway implicated early in acute lesions and a T_H1 predominance found in chronic lesions. Langerhans cells, IgE, and eosinophils play a prominent role, as well as many other inflammatory mediators. Environmental and contact allergens, infections, irritants, extremes of temperature, sweat, and lack of humidity can exacerbate the condition, as can scratching or rubbing. Triggers are somewhat variable from individual to individual.

EPIDEMIOLOGY

Atopic dermatitis is the most common skin disease in children, with an estimated prevalence of up to 20% of children. Only 1% to 2% of adults manifest disease. In addition to genetic factors, an environmental influence contributes. Atopic dermatitis occurs more frequently in urban areas and in higher socioeconomic classes. Prevalence is lower in areas where industrial pollution is less and where eosinophil-mediated infections such as helminthic infections are endemic.

Patients generally have a family history of atopy. Children with atopic dermatitis are predisposed to the development of allergy and allergic rhinitis, referred to as the *atopic march*. Asthma develops in up to half of children with atopic dermatitis, and allergic rhinitis even more frequently. Food allergies are commonly associated with atopic dermatitis.

CLINICAL MANIFESTATIONS

Atopic dermatitis is a chronic, relapsing skin disease characterized by xerosis, pruritus, and characteristic skin findings. The condition generally improves with age and remits in adulthood, although some childhood cases will continue into adulthood.

Characteristic lesions of atopic dermatitis are erythematous papules or plaques with ill-defined borders and overlying scale or hyperkeratosis. Lesions can be secondarily excoriated or have an overlying crust that is yellow or hemorrhagic. Weeping may be present in acute stages. Lichenification is found in older lesions. Formation of fissures is common in both acute and chronic lesions. Temporary hypo- and hyperpigmentation can be seen after lesions resolve, but atopic dermatitis is not usually scarring unless secondary features become severe (e.g., infection or physical manipulation [scratching]).

Characteristic locations vary with the age of the patient. Infantile atopic dermatitis typically affects the face and extensor surfaces of the extremities and is often generalized. Childhood lesions predominate in flexural surfaces (antecubital and popliteal fossae), wrists, ankles, hands, and feet (Fig. 190-1). The adult phase occurs after puberty and manifests in the flexural areas including the neck, as well as predominant involvement on the face, dorsa of the hands, fingers and toes, and the upper arms and back.

Secondary bacterial infection, most commonly with *Staphylococcus aureus* or less commonly with *Streptococcus pyogenes*, is frequently present. Patients are at increased risk for infections with cutaneous viruses and can develop disseminated skin infections with viruses such as herpes simplex virus (eczema herpeticum), varicella-zoster virus, smallpox virus (eczema vaccinatum), and molluscum contagiosum. Atopic skin is more susceptible to fungal infections as well.

Figure 190-1 Atopic dermatitis (arm).

Signs of concomitant infection include acute worsening of disease in an otherwise well-controlled patient, resistance to standard therapy, fever, and presence of pustules, fissures, or exudative or crusted lesions (Fig. 190-2). Eczema herpeticum and eczema vaccinatum can be life threatening if not treated.

LABORATORY AND IMAGING STUDIES

Diagnosis of atopic dermatitis is based on clinical signs and symptoms. Skin biopsy findings are generally characteristic but not exclusively diagnostic and can overlap with other skin conditions. Peripheral blood eosinophilia and elevated IgE levels can be found but are not specific. Skin prick testing or measurement of specific IgE antibody levels can detect sensitization to food and environmental allergens, although false-positive findings occur.

DIFFERENTIAL DIAGNOSIS

The differential diagnosis of atopic dermatitis is extensive, but the history of a relapsing pruritic condition in the setting of atopy and skin lesions in a characteristic distribution is typical.

The lesions of **seborrheic dermatitis** have circumscribed and well-defined borders. The scale or hyperkeratosis is thicker, greasy, and yellowish. The distribution of seborrheic dermatitis is different from that of atopic dermatitis, typically involving the scalp, eyebrows, perinasal region, upper chest, and back. Occasionally the two conditions coexist.

Psoriasis tends to localize on the elbows, knees, lower back, and scalp. The lesions of psoriasis on exposed surfaces are salmon color at the base with an overlying hyperkeratosis that is much thicker with silver coloration. They are generally very well demarcated, oval or round, thick plaques.

Allergic contact dermatitis has a distribution limited to one area of the body corresponding to contact with the allergen. The lesions generally make bizarre, linear, square, or angulated shapes corresponding to the source. **Nickel dermatitis** is common and results from contact sensitization to nickel in metals. It occurs in characteristic locations, such as the periumbilical area (where metal from pant buttons rub against skin); on the ear lobule or neck (where earrings contact skin); circumferentially around the neck (necklaces); and under rings or

Figure 190-2 Atopic dermatitis with *Staphylococcus* superinfection.

wristbands. Patients with atopic dermatitis can have concomitant contact dermatitis as well.

TREATMENT

Ideal therapy for atopic dermatitis includes three main components: frequent liberal use of bland emollients to restore the skin barrier, avoidance of triggers of inflammation, and use of topical anti-inflammatory medication to affected areas of skin when needed. Control of pruritus and infection should be considered on an individual basis. If topical therapy and these measures are inadequate, systemic therapy with immunosuppressive agents or ultraviolet light therapy may be indicated.

A daily short bath with warm but not hot water is generally recommended, although this is controversial and there are some who advocate less frequent bathing. A moisturizing cream or ointment should be applied to the entire body immediately afterward to trap moisture. Application of topical medications is also most effective immediately after bathing. Additional information for patients and families can be found at the website of the National Eczema Association for Science and Education (http://www.nationaleczema.org).

Common triggers of inflammation in atopic dermatitis include rubbing or scratching, contact with saliva or foods that are acidic, soaps and detergents, fabric softeners, wool or other harsh materials, fragranced personal care products, sweat, highly chlorinated pools, low humidity, tobacco smoke, dust mites, animal dander, environmental pollens, and molds. Exposure to these triggers should be limited whenever possible. Infections that are unrelated to skin disease, such as an upper respiratory infection, can also exacerbate atopic dermatitis. Food allergy is commonly seen in patients with atopic dermatitis but typically presents with urticaria or anaphylaxis rather than exacerbation of the atopic dermatitis.

Topical corticosteroids are the mainstay of anti-inflammatory therapy for atopic dermatitis. Hundreds of topical corticosteroids are available and are classified according to strength from I to VII. Class I is the highest potency and class VII is the lowest potency. Potency varies according to the steroid molecule (active ingredient), and, for a given ingredient, strength can vary according to relative concentration and vehicle base. Enhanced penetration occurs in areas of natural occlusion (flexures such as axillae and groin), with external occlusion (diapers or bandages), in areas of open skin (excoriations), and with heat or hydration. Use of wet wraps with topical corticosteroid application takes advantage of this principle of heat and hydration for enhanced penetration for recalcitrant lesions. Class I and II steroids are typically avoided in young children or in areas of thinner skin or enhanced penetration.

Corticosteroids are available in different vehicles. In general, ointments are preferred because of their increased efficacy, occlusive nature, and tolerability. Creams may be slightly less effective for a given steroid ingredient but may be more cosmetically acceptable for older patients or in warmer climates. Lotions may have more preservatives that can cause irritation and are generally less potent. Sprays, foams, solutions, and gels can be especially useful for hair-bearing areas. Creams, lotions, sprays, solutions, and gels can be particularly irritating when applied to atopic skin and should generally be avoided on areas of open skin.

Topical corticosteroids should be used in conjunction with adequate skin care, such as avoiding triggers of inflammation and frequent application of emollients. Twice-daily application of corticosteroids is recommended. The goal is to limit the need for anti-inflammatory medications and thereby avoid potential for adverse effects. Local side effects such as skin atrophy, striae, acne, and hypopigmentation are related to corticosteroid potency, site of application, and duration of application. Systemic side effects of adrenal suppression or Cushing syndrome can result with application of a potent topical corticosteroid to large surface areas or occluded areas at risk of enhanced penetration.

Topical **calcineurin inhibitors** (also referred to as topical immune modulators) such as topical tacrolimus and pimecrolimus may be part of the treatment regimen for atopic dermatitis. These agents selectively inhibit T-cell proliferation by inhibiting calcineurin and subsequent interleukin 2 production. There is no potential for skin atrophy; thus these agents are particularly useful for face or genital lesions. They are currently approved for intermittent therapy as second-line treatments for mild to moderate atopic dermatitis. Long-term studies, combined with other modalities for treatment, are underway.

Sedating antihistamines (e.g., diphenhydramine, hydroxyzine) are useful adjunctive therapy, especially during flares. These may have only mild effect on pruritus but can improve the sleeplessness due to scratching during the night. A dose before bedtime is most effective, and additional daytime doses can be added on an individual basis when needed. Nonsedating antihistamines are of little benefit in controlling the pruritus of atopic dermatitis.

Short-term administration of systemic corticosteroids is rarely indicated for cases of severe disease and may be considered when adequate topical therapy failed or is being instituted. Systemic corticosteroid courses should be adequately tapered and used in conjunction with an appropriate atopic skin care regimen. Rebound flare of atopic dermatitis is common following withdrawal of corticosteroids and should be anticipated to avoid misinterpretation of the natural disease severity. Long-term and frequent repeated courses should be avoided to prevent adverse effects.

Ultraviolet light therapy (UVB, narrow band UVB, UVA, or UVA1) can be an option for moderate to severe cases in older children. Typically, light therapy is administered two to three times weekly until improvement is seen, and then is tapered or discontinued once the acute flare has resolved. More frequent use of light therapy in children is hindered by requirements for frequent office visits, ability to cooperate with standing in a light box while wearing protective goggles, and risk of long-term skin damage, including the potential for skin cancer development with excessive UV light exposure. Systemic cyclosporine (up to 5 mg/kg/day) can be effective therapy for atopic dermatitis in severe cases. It is used for periods of up to 1 year to gain control of severe disease and should be tapered once the atopic dermatitis is controlled.

COMPLICATIONS

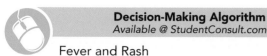

Decision-Making Algorithm
Available @ StudentConsult.com

Fever and Rash

An increased tendency toward bacterial, viral, and fungal skin infections is due to an impaired skin barrier and decrease in innate immune proteins in the skin as well as maladaptive secondary immune responses.

Secondary impetigo with *S. aureus* is the most common secondary skin infection found in atopic dermatitis. Group A streptococcus infection is also common. Infection manifests with pustules, erythema, crusting, scabbing, flare of disease, or lack of response to adequate anti-inflammatory therapy. Localized lesions can be treated with topical mupirocin. Widespread and generalized lesions require oral antibiotic therapy, most commonly with a first-generation cephalosporin, such as cephalexin. Methicillin-resistant *S. aureus* infection is increasingly common, and antibiotic therapy should be tailored based on local resistance rates and patient factors. Diagnosis of superinfection may be made clinically, but a superficial bacterial culture can confirm the diagnosis and provide antimicrobial susceptibilities. Treatment should include a concomitant atopic skin care routine including the continued use of topical corticosteroids. Although secondary skin infection with *S. aureus* is common, progression to cellulitis or septicemia is unusual. Rarely, intravenous antibiotics may nevertheless be required. Children with colonization and frequent infections may benefit from dilute bleach baths two to three times weekly; ¼ to ½ cup of household bleach is added to a half-full or full bathtub.

Eczema herpeticum (Kaposi's varicelliform eruption) is one of the potentially serious infectious complications in atopic dermatitis. After herpes simplex virus (HSV) infection, an eruption of multiple, pruritic, vesiculopustular lesions occurs in a disseminated pattern, both within plaques of atopic dermatitis and on normal-appearing skin. These characteristically rupture and form crusted umbilicated papules and punched-out hemorrhagic erosions (Fig. 190-3). Irritability, anorexia, and fever can also be seen. Systemic and central nervous system disease have been reported. Bacterial superinfection of eroded areas of the skin often occurs. Diagnosis can be made rapidly from a scraping of the skin lesion stained with Giemsa or Wright's stain (**Tzanck test**), though these are not highly sensitive. These stains allow

Figure 190-3 Eczema herpeticum (hand).

microscopic visualization of the presence of multinucleated giant cells indicative of herpes simplex virus or varicella-zoster virus infection. Vesicle fluid can also be sent for polymerase chain reaction (PCR) detection of herpes simplex virus DNA, rapid direct fluorescent antibody testing, or viral culture. Laboratory confirmation of infection is important because similar clinical manifestations can occur with bacterial infections.

The psychosocial impact of atopic dermatitis can be significant. There is often disfigurement, lack of sleep from pruritus resulting in irritability and fatigue, and limitations on participation in sports. Significant time, as well as financial strain, is involved in caring for a child with atopic dermatitis. Thus, management should address these potential issues and provide adequate anticipatory guidance.

PROGNOSIS

Atopic dermatitis frequently remits during childhood and is much less common after puberty. The condition is generally most severe and widespread in infancy and early childhood. Relapse of disease in adults can occur and commonly manifests as face or hand dermatitis. Frequently, adults have generalized dry skin and are aware that their skin is sensitive to many over-the-counter preparations. Patients with atopic dermatitis can also develop asthma and allergic rhinitis. Asthma is more commonly associated with more severe skin disease.

PREVENTION

Individual flares of atopic dermatitis can be prevented by avoiding triggers of inflammation and can be lessened with frequent emollient application. Some evidence suggests that breastfeeding for at least 4 months prevents or delays the occurrence of atopic dermatitis in early childhood. For infants with a parent or sibling with atopic disease and who are not exclusively breastfed for 4 to 6 months, there is modest evidence that the onset of atopic dermatitis may be delayed or prevented by the use of extensively hydrolyzed casein-based formulas. There is insufficient evidence that soy-based formulas, delaying the introduction of complementary foods beyond 4 to 6 months of age, or other dietary intervention prevents the development of atopic disease. There is no convincing evidence that women who avoid peanuts or other foods during pregnancy or while breastfeeding lower their child's risk of allergies.

dermatitis is a cell-mediated immune reaction, also called type IV or delayed-type hypersensitivity. The antigens, or haptens, involved in allergic contact dermatitis readily penetrate the epidermis and are bound by Langerhans cells, the antigen-presenting cells of the skin. The hapten is presented to T lymphocytes, and an immune cascade follows. Contact dermatitis may occur in any age, and girls are more frequently affected than boys.

CLINICAL MANIFESTATIONS

Irritant contact dermatitis is characterized by ill-defined, scaly, pink or red patches and plaques (Fig. 191-1). The eruption is localized to skin surfaces that are exposed to the irritant. Irritant contact dermatitis is observed frequently on the dorsal surfaces of the hands in patients, often from repeated hand washing or exposure to irritating chemicals.

Diaper dermatitis is a common problem in infants and most commonly is a form of irritant contact dermatitis. The dermatitis is caused by irritation from urine and feces, typically affecting the perianal region and the buttocks while sparing the protected groin folds and other occluded areas. Secondary infection by *Candida albicans* or bacterial pathogens may complicate diaper dermatitis as well.

Allergic contact dermatitis may be acute (such as *Rhus* dermatitis) or chronic (such as nickel dermatitis). Acute lesions are bright pink, pruritic patches, often in linear or sharply marginated bizarre configurations. Within the patches are clear vesicles and bullae (Fig. 191-2). Signs and symptoms of the disease may be delayed for 7 to 14 days after exposure if the patient has not been sensitized previously. On reexposure, symptoms begin within hours and are usually more severe. The eruption may persist for weeks. Chronic lesions are pink, scaly, pruritic plaques, often mimicking atopic dermatitis. Even intermittent exposure can result in a persistent dermatitis.

LABORATORY AND IMAGING STUDIES

The diagnosis is established by clinical presentation and history of exposure to a recognized irritant or allergen. Skin-prick testing and serum IgE levels are not helpful in determining the cause of allergic contact dermatitis. Patch testing may be used to determine the allergen causing the reaction in difficult cases.

Chapter 191

CONTACT DERMATITIS

ETIOLOGY AND EPIDEMIOLOGY

Inflammation in the top layers of the skin, caused by direct contact with a substance, is divided into two subtypes: irritant contact dermatitis and allergic contact dermatitis. **Irritant contact dermatitis** is observed after the skin surface is exposed to an irritating chemical or substance. **Allergic contact**

Figure 191-1 Irritant diaper dermatitis.

Figure 191-2 Allergic contact dermatitis to tincture of benzoin.

DIFFERENTIAL DIAGNOSIS

The distribution and appearance of the dermatitis and a detailed exposure history are the most useful diagnostic tools. Involvement of the lower legs and distal arms suggests exposure to plants of the *Rhus* species (poison ivy or poison oak), especially when linear configurations of lesions are present. Dermatitis of the ears (earrings), wrist (bracelet or watch), or periumbilical region (belt buckle or pant buttons) suggests a metal allergy to nickel. Distribution on the dorsal surfaces of the feet indicates a shoe allergy, usually to dyes, rubber, or leather. Topical antibiotics (neomycin) and fragrances (soaps, perfumes, cosmetics) are frequent causes of allergic contact dermatitis.

Diaper rashes caused by *Candida* are quite common. Irritant contact dermatitis primarily affects the prominent, exposed surfaces, whereas *Candida* primarily affects intertriginous areas. The two are frequently present simultaneously, as secondary *Candida* infection may complicate irritant dermatitis.

Psoriasis, seborrheic dermatitis, and Langerhans cell histiocytosis can present with an erythematous rash in the diaper area. Referral to a dermatologist should be considered for any child with severe rash or with diaper rash that does not respond to conventional therapy.

TREATMENT

Topical corticosteroids are effective in treatment of allergic and irritant contact dermatitis. High-potency corticosteroids, and even short courses of oral corticosteroids, may be necessary for severe reactions of allergic contact dermatitis. Oral antihistamines may be required to control itching.

Treatment of candidal diaper dermatitis consists of topical nystatin or topical azole antifungals. Low-potency topical corticosteroids are frequently used in addition to topical antifungal therapy to treat the irritant component of the diaper dermatitis when present concomitantly.

COMPLICATIONS

In addition to superinfection of diaper dermatitis by *C. albicans*, bacterial superinfection may complicate any form of contact dermatitis. This is especially common if the skin barrier is no longer intact because of blistering or scratching.

PREVENTION

Every effort should be made to identify the trigger of allergic or irritant contact dermatitis. With allergic contact dermatitis, reexposure often leads to increasingly severe reactions.

Chapter 192

SEBORRHEIC DERMATITIS

ETIOLOGY

Seborrheic dermatitis is a common, chronic inflammatory disease that has different clinical presentations at different ages. Seborrheic dermatitis classically presents in infants as cradle cap or dermatitis in the intertriginous areas of the axillae, groin, antecubital and popliteal fossae, and umbilicus. It is seen in adolescents as dandruff. The pathogenesis of seborrheic dermatitis is unclear, but it is theorized that there is an abnormal inflammatory response to commensal *Malassezia* species in sebum-rich areas. Areas prone to seborrheic dermatitis include the scalp, eyebrows, eyelids, nasolabial folds, external auditory canals, and posterior auricular folds.

CLINICAL MANIFESTATIONS

Seborrheic dermatitis in infants begins during the first month and persists during the first year of life. It is also called **cradle cap** because of the thick, greasy and waxy, yellow-white scaling and crusting of the scalp (Fig. 192-1). It is usually prominent on the vertex of the scalp, but it may be diffuse. Greasy, scaly, erythematous, nonpruritic patches and plaques may extend to the face and posterior auricular folds, sometimes involving the entire body. Diaper and intertriginous areas can have sharply demarcated, shiny, erythematous patches with yellow, greasy, or waxy-appearing scale. Hypopigmentation may persist after the inflammation has faded. The eruption is usually asymptomatic, which helps differentiate it from infantile atopic dermatitis, which is pruritic.

Classic seborrheic dermatitis during adolescence is typically localized to the scalp. The mild form is commonly known as **dandruff**, a fine, white, dry scaling of the scalp with minor itching. Additional findings of seborrheic dermatitis vary from diffuse, brawny scaling to focal areas of thick, oily, yellow crusts with underlying erythema. The external auditory canals, eyebrows, eyelids, and intertriginous areas may be involved as well. Pruritus may be minimal or severe.

Figure 192-1 Seborrheic dermatitis (cradle cap).

LABORATORY AND IMAGING STUDIES

Laboratory studies and imaging studies are not necessary to diagnose seborrheic dermatitis. Fungal cultures and potassium hydroxide studies may be necessary to help differentiate seborrheic dermatitis of the scalp from tinea capitis (see Chapter 98).

DIFFERENTIAL DIAGNOSIS

Seborrheic dermatitis in an infant may be difficult to differentiate from atopic dermatitis, and in fact, some cases may represent an overlap. In a teenager, seborrheic dermatitis of the scalp and psoriasis of the scalp may have very similar clinical findings; it may be very difficult to differentiate the two disorders, especially if there are no other cutaneous findings to provide additional clues. Intractable, severe, generalized seborrheic dermatitis suggests Langerhans cell histiocytosis. Intractable seborrheic dermatitis, accompanied by chronic diarrhea and failure to thrive, suggests Leiner disease or acquired immunodeficiency syndrome (AIDS).

TREATMENT

Seborrheic dermatitis of the scalp is usually asymptomatic and generally does not require treatment. Minor amounts of scale can be removed easily by frequent shampooing. For infants with cradle cap, oil (such as mineral oil or olive oil) may be gently massaged into the scalp and left on for a few minutes before gently brushing out the scale and shampooing. Daily shampooing with ketoconazole, zinc pyrithione, selenium sulfide, or salicylic acid shampoos can treat scalp scale. Seborrheic dermatitis with inflamed lesions responds rapidly to treatment with low-potency steroids two times daily.

The response to treatment is usually rapid. Secondary bacterial infection can occur but is uncommon. Intractable disease and other complications warrant further evaluation for other etiologies.

PROGNOSIS

Cradle cap is self-limited and resolves during the first year of life. Seborrheic dermatitis does not cause permanent hair loss.

For teenagers, continued use of an antiseborrheic shampoo is often required for control of dandruff.

PREVENTION

Frequent shampooing, especially with early signs of seborrheic dermatitis, may help prevent progression.

OTHER PAPULOSQUAMOUS DERMATOSES
Pityriasis Rosea

Pityriasis rosea is a benign, self-limited eruption that may occur at any age, with peak incidence during adolescence. A solitary, 2- to 5-cm, pink, oval patch with central clearing, the so-called **herald patch**, is the first manifestation of the eruption. The herald patch typically is found on the breast, lower torso, or proximal thigh and is often misdiagnosed as fungal or eczematous in origin. One to 2 weeks later, a generalized eruption occurs on the torso and proximal extremities. Multiple 0.5- to 2-cm, oval to oblong, red or tan macules with a fine, branlike scale are characteristically arranged parallel to skin tension lines (*Christmas tree pattern*). Rarely, the eruption may have an inverse distribution involving the axillae and groin or a papular or papulovesicular appearance. Mild prodromal symptoms may be present with the appearance of the herald patch, and pruritus is present in 25% of cases. The eruption lasts 4 to 14 weeks, with gradual resolution. Residual hyperpigmentation or hypopigmentation can take additional months to clear. Treatment is unnecessary, though pruritus can be managed with oral antihistamines, phototherapy, and low-potency topical corticosteroids.

Psoriasis

Psoriasis is a common papulosquamous condition characterized by well-demarcated, erythematous, scaling papules and plaques. Psoriasis occurs at all ages, including infancy, with onset of 30% of cases during childhood. The disease is characterized by a chronic and relapsing course, although spontaneous remissions can occur. Infections (especially *Streptococcus pyogenes*), stress, trauma, and medications may cause disease exacerbations. Various subtypes of psoriasis exist. The most common variety is **plaque-type psoriasis (psoriasis vulgaris)**, which can be localized or generalized. The lesions consist of round, well-demarcated, red plaques measuring 1 to 7 cm with micaceous scale, which is distinctive in its thick, silvery appearance with pinpoint bleeding points revealed on removal of the scales (**Auspitz sign**). The lesions of psoriasis have a distinctive distribution involving the extensor aspect of the elbows and knees, posterior occipital scalp, periumbilical region, lumbosacral region, and intergluteal cleft. Children often have facial lesions involving the superomedial aspect of the eyelids. Nail plate involvement is common and includes pitting, onycholysis, subungual hyperkeratosis, and oil staining (reddish brown subungual macular discoloration). **Guttate** (numerous small plaques diffusely distributed on the torso), **erythrodermic** (covering large body surface areas), **inverse** (moist red patches affecting body folds), and **pustular** forms may occur.

The foundation of therapy is topical corticosteroids. Treatment of psoriasis with oral corticosteroids can induce pustular psoriasis and should be avoided. Because of the risk of atrophy, striae, and telangiectases, especially when potent fluorinated corticosteroid preparations are administered long-term, the goal is to use the least potent corticosteroid necessary. Topical vitamin D analogs, salicylic acid, and tar preparations are useful adjuvants to topical corticosteroids. Phototherapy with ultraviolet B (UVB) light can be useful as secondary therapy in older children. Extensive plaque or guttate, erythrodermic, and pustular psoriasis may necessitate systemic treatments with immune suppressive medication (methotrexate, cyclosporine, tumor necrosis factor-α antagonists). Disease triggers such as infection or medications should be identified and removed.

Chapter 193

PIGMENTED LESIONS

Birthmark is a term that describes congenital anomalies of the skin. It should not be used as a definitive diagnosis because congenital skin lesions vary greatly in their appearance and prognosis. The differential diagnosis of various birthmarks is listed in Table 193-1.

DERMAL MELANOSIS

The most frequently encountered pigmented lesion is **dermal melanosis**, which occurs in 70% to 90% of African-American, Hispanic, Asian, and Native American infants and in approximately 5% of white infants. This is a congenital lesion caused by entrapment of melanocytes in the dermis during their migration from the neural crest into the epidermis. Although most of these lesions are found in the lumbosacral area (Mongolian spot), they also occur at other sites such as the buttocks, flank, extremities, or, rarely, the face (Fig. 193-1). Single or multiple, poorly demarcated, gray-blue patches up to 10 cm in size may be present. Most lesions gradually disappear during the first few years of life; aberrant lesions in unusual sites are more likely to persist.

CAFÉ AU LAIT MACULES

Café au lait macules are pigmented macules or patches, which may be present in a newborn but tend to develop during childhood (Fig. 193-2). They range in color from very light brown to a chocolate brown. Up to five café au lait macules are found in 1.8% of newborns and 25% to 40% of normal children, and have no significance. Children with six or more café au lait macules (0.5 cm in diameter before puberty or greater than 1.5 cm in diameter after puberty), especially when accompanied by **axillary or inguinal freckling**, should be evaluated carefully

Table 193-1	Common Birthmarks		
COLOR/LESION	**BIRTHMARK**	**LOCATION**	**OTHER FEATURES**
Brown/macule or patch	Cafe au lait macule	Variable	May be associated with genetic syndromes
Brown (<20 cm)/plaque	Congenital melanocytic nevus	Variable	Low risk of melanoma
Brown (>20 cm)/plaque	Giant congenital melanocytic nevus	Trunk most common	Risk of melanoma and neuromelanosis
Brown-"flesh-colored"/plaque	Epidermal nevus	Variable, trunk and neck	May enlarge with time
Red/patch	Port-wine stain (nevus flammeus)	Variable, face most common	May be associated with Sturge-Weber syndrome
Red/patch	Salmon patch (nevus simplex)	Glabella, eyelids, nape of neck	Improves or resolves with time
Red/papule or plaque	Hemangioma	Variable	May be associated with liver hemangiomas, airway hemangiomas, and PHACE syndrome
Gray-blue/patch	Dermal melanosis	Lower trunk (Mongolian spot); face (nevus of Ota); posterior shoulder (nevus of Ito)	Nevus of Ota may be associated with ocular pigmentation
Blue-purple/nodule	Cephalohematoma	Scalp	Resolves with time
Blue-purple/plaque	Venous, lymphatic, or mixed malformation	Variable	Intermittent swelling and pain
Yellow-orange/plaque	Nevus sebaceus	Head and neck	Malignant and benign tumors may arise within
Yellow-orange/nodule	Juvenile xanthogranuloma	Head and neck most common	Spontaneously involutes
Yellow-brown/papule or nodule	Mastocytoma	Variable	Spontaneously involutes
Hypertrichosis/plaque	Smooth muscle hamartoma	Trunk	
Hypertrichosis/tumor	Plexiform neurofibroma	Trunk most common	Associated with neurofibromatosis type 1
White/patch	Nevus anemicus	Variable	
White/patch	Nevus depigmentosus	Variable	

for additional stigmata of neurofibromatosis type 1. Other disorders also associated with café au lait macules include the other forms of neurofibromatosis, Legius syndrome, tuberous sclerosis, McCune-Albright syndrome, multiple lentigines/LEOPARD syndrome, Noonan syndrome, and Russell-Silver syndrome.

Figure 193-1 Dermal hypermelanosis (back).

Figure 193-2 Cafe au lait spots (leg).

CONGENITAL MELANOCYTIC NEVI

Approximately 1% to 2% of newborns have **congenital melanocytic nevi**. Smaller lesions (as opposed to giant pigmented nevi) are brown patches or plaques, often with an oval or lancet configuration. Lesions may resemble café au lait macules initially, but darker pigmentation, variegated speckles, textural changes, and elevation develop with time and help to differentiate these lesions (Fig. 193-3). Thick, dark, coarse hair frequently is associated with congenital melanocytic nevi (Fig. 193-4). These lesions vary in site and size but are most often solitary. Congenital melanocytic nevi pose a very slightly increased risk for the development of malignant melanoma, usually developing during adulthood. Surgical removal may be considered to improve the cosmetic appearance of the patient or to reduce the likelihood of malignant transformation, although some patients and physicians elect for observation. Excisional biopsy is indicated when malignant change is suspected.

CONGENITAL GIANT MELANOCYTIC NEVI

Giant congenital melanocytic nevi are defined as nevi that would be approximately 20 cm in length in adulthood; in a neonate, this translates to 9 cm on the head and neck and 6 cm on the rest of the body. These lesions appear as color variegated, light brown to black patch or plaques, sometimes with smaller macules and papules (**satellite nevi**) in addition. The affected skin may be smooth, nodular, or leathery. Prominent, dark hypertrichosis is often present. **Neuromelanosis**, the presence of melanocytes in the central nervous system, may be associated with giant congenital melanocytic nevi. Affected patients

Figure 193-3 Congenital melanocytic nevus (buttock).

Figure 193-4 Hairy congenital nevus.

may be asymptomatic or have hydrocephalus and seizures; in symptomatic patients, death often results during early childhood. **Malignant melanoma** develops in approximately 2% to 10% of patients with giant congenital melanocytic nevi, in either the cutaneous lesion or the neural melanocytes. In contrast to small and medium congenital melanocytic nevi, melanoma is more likely to develop during childhood. Because of the incidence of malignant degeneration and extensive deformity, surgical excision should be considered for resectable lesions. The use of tissue expansion techniques has greatly improved the capability for surgical removal of large lesions.

ACQUIRED NEVI

Acquired melanocytic nevi are common skin lesions. Melanocytic nevi may occur at any age; however, the lesions develop most rapidly in prepubertal children and teenagers. Melanocytic nevi are well-delineated, round to oval, brown macules and papules. Lesions are most common on the face, upper torso, and arms. Family history, fair skin, and sun exposure are considered major risk factors. Irregular pigmentation, rapid growth, bleeding, and a change in configuration or borders suggest signs of malignant degeneration and biopsy should be performed. Malignant melanoma is rare in childhood; however, there is an alarming increase in incidence in adolescence, especially in those who use indoor tanning. Education of parents and children regarding the risks of sun exposure, appropriate sun protection, and recognition of worrisome lesions is important.

Chapter 194

VASCULAR ANOMALIES

Vascular anomalies can be divided into two major categories: tumors and malformations. Vascular tumors are characterized by hypercellularity, proliferation, and growth. Vascular malformations, however, are developmental defects derived from the capillary, venous, arterial, or lymphatic vessels. In contrast to hemangiomas, vascular malformations remain relatively static over time. Differentiating between these entities is important because they have different prognoses and clinical implications.

VASCULAR TUMORS
Hemangiomas

Decision-Making Algorithms
Available @ StudentConsult.com

Neck Masses
Stridor

Hemangiomas are the most common soft tissue tumors of infancy, occurring in approximately 5% to 10% of 1-year-old infants. In newborns, hemangiomas may originate as a pale

Figure 194-1 Hemangioma (chest).

white macule with threadlike telangiectasia. When the tumor proliferates, it assumes its most recognizable form as a bright red, lobulated plaque or nodule (superficial component, Fig. 194-1). Hemangiomas that lie deeper in the skin are soft, warm masses with a slightly bluish discoloration (deeper component). Frequently, hemangiomas have both a superficial and a deep component. They range from a few millimeters to several centimeters in diameter and are usually solitary; 20% involve multiple lesions. Hemangiomas occur predominantly in females (3:1) and have an increased incidence in premature infants. Approximately 55% are present at birth; the rest develop in the first weeks of life. Superficial hemangiomas reach their maximal size by 6 to 8 months, but deep hemangiomas may grow for 12 to 14 months. They then undergo slow, spontaneous resolution, which takes 3 to 10 years.

Despite the benign nature of most cutaneous hemangiomas, there may be the risk of functional compromise or permanent disfigurement depending on the location and extent. Ulceration, the most frequent complication, can be painful and increases the risk of infection, hemorrhage, and scarring. Areas frequently associated with complications include the periocular region, lip, nasal tip, beard, face (large lesions), groin, and buttocks.

Periorbital hemangiomas pose considerable risk to vision and should be monitored carefully. Amblyopia can result from the hemangioma causing obstruction of the visual axis or pressure on the globe, resulting in astigmatism. If there is any concern, the patient should have urgent evaluation by an ophthalmologist. Treatment may be indicated to prevent blindness. **Subglottic hemangiomas** manifest as hoarseness and stridor; progression to respiratory failure may be rapid. Symptomatic airway hemangiomas develop in more than 50% of infants with extensive facial hemangiomas on the chin and jaw (beard distribution); any infant with a beard hemangioma should be referred for laryngoscopy. Multiple cutaneous (diffuse hemangiomatosis) and large facial hemangiomas may be associated with visceral hemangiomas. Extensive cervicofacial hemangiomas may be associated with multiple anomalies, including posterior fossa malformations, hemangiomas, arterial anomalies of the cerebrovasculature, coarctation of aorta and cardiac defects, and eye abnormalities (**PHACE syndrome**). **Lumbosacral hemangiomas** suggest an occult spinal dysraphism with or without anorectal and urogenital anomalies. Magnetic resonance imaging of the spine is indicated in all patients with midline cutaneous hemangiomas in the lumbosacral area.

Most hemangiomas do not necessitate medical intervention and involute spontaneously; however, if complications arise and treatment is warranted, oral propranolol is the mainstay of therapy.

Pyogenic Granuloma

A pyogenic granuloma is an acquired, benign vascular tumor commonly seen in children. Initially, the lesions appear as pink-red papules that often arise after minor trauma, growing rapidly over a period of weeks into a bright red, vascular, often pedunculated papule measuring 2 to 10 mm. The lesions often have the appearance of granulation tissue and are very friable. They may occur anywhere on the body, but the head, neck, and upper extremities are most commonly affected. When traumatized, these lesions may bleed profusely, often requiring emergent medical attention. Surgical excision is the most definitive treatment option, though pulsed dye laser can be useful for very small lesions.

VASCULAR MALFORMATIONS
Port-Wine Stain

Port-wine stains (nevus flammeus, capillary malformation) are malformations of the superficial capillaries of the skin. These lesions are present at birth and should be considered permanent developmental defects. They do not enlarge after birth; any apparent increase in size is caused by growth of the child. A port-wine stain may be localized to any body surface, but facial lesions are the most common. They are pink-red, sharply demarcated macules and patches in infancy (Fig. 194-2). With time, they darken to a purple or *port-wine* color and may develop a pebbly or slightly thickened surface. Vascular blebs may form within the lesions and become symptomatic or bleed. The most successful treatment modality in use is the pulsed dye laser, which can result in 80% to 90% improvement in these lesions after a series of treatment sessions and can avoid future complications associated with vascular dilation. Treatment is more effective if undertaken in infancy. Overgrowth of underlying bone can occur and is frequently seen with facial lesions. Affected patients often need maxillofacial intervention from malalignment that develops.

Most port-wine stains occur as isolated defects and do not indicate systemic malformations. Rarely, they may suggest ocular defects or specific neurocutaneous syndromes. **Sturge-Weber syndrome** (encephalotrigeminal angiomatosis) may occur with a facial port-wine stain, usually in the cutaneous distribution of the first branch of the trigeminal nerve. Other features include leptomeningeal angiomatosis, mental retardation, seizures, hemiparesis contralateral to the facial lesions, ipsilateral intracortical calcification, and frequent ocular manifestations such as buphthalmos, glaucoma, angioma of the choroid, hemianoptic defects, and optic atrophy. Anticonvulsant therapy and neurosurgical procedures have been of value in some patients. Glaucoma can occur in association with port-wine stains located on the eyelid, even in the absence of Sturge-Weber syndrome, and these patients need lifelong monitoring of ocular pressures. **Klippel-Trénaunay-Weber** syndrome is characterized by the triad of capillary and venous malformations, venous varicosities, and hyperplasia of the soft

Figure 194-2 Port-wine stain (face).

tissues—and often bone—of the involved area. The lower limb is most commonly affected. A port-wine stain overlying the spine may rarely be a marker of spinal dysraphism or an intraspinal vascular malformation.

Salmon Patch (Nevus Simplex)

A salmon patch (nevus simplex, stork bite, angel's kiss) is a variant of nevus flammeus that is present in 70% of normal newborns. They are red, irregular, macular patches resulting from dilation of dermal capillaries and are usually found on the nape of the neck, the eyelids, and the glabella. Most of the facial lesions fade by 1 year of age, but lesions on the neck may persist for life. Surveys of adult populations confirm the persistence of the nuchal lesions in approximately 25% of the population.

Chapter 195

ERYTHEMA MULTIFORME, STEVENS-JOHNSON SYNDROME, AND TOXIC EPIDERMAL NECROLYSIS

Erythema multiforme (EM), Stevens-Johnson syndrome (SJS), and toxic epidermal necrolysis (TEN) are acute hypersensitivity reactions characterized by cutaneous and mucosal necrosis. These syndromes represent a hypersensitivity reaction to a precipitating cause, usually infectious organisms or drugs. These disorders were historically thought to represent a spectrum of the same disease process, and inconsistent use of these disease names led to further confusion. A consensus definition was published in 1993, and current literature favors that EM is distinct from the SJS/TEN spectrum of disease. The differential diagnosis of vesiculobullous eruptions is listed in Table 195-1.

Decision-Making Algorithm
Available @ StudentConsult.com

Vesicles and Bullae

ERYTHEMA MULTIFORME

EM is a common, self-limiting, acute hypersensitivity syndrome characterized by the abrupt onset of round, deep red, well-demarcated macules and papules with a dusky gray or bullous center. The size may range from a few millimeters to a few centimeters, but most lesions are approximately 1 cm in diameter. The classic **target lesion** consists of three concentric rings; the outermost is red, the intermediate is white, and the center is a dusky red or purple. These can progress to edematous plaques or bullae. If blistering occurs, it is circumscribed

Table 195-1	Vesiculobullous Eruptions		
ENTITY	**CLINICAL CLUES**	**ENTITY**	**CLINICAL CLUES**
INFECTIOUS		Stevens-Johnson syndrome and toxic epidermal necrolysis	Prodrome of fever, headache, malaise, sore throat, cough, vomiting, diarrhea Extensive epidermal necrosis with mucosal involvement Frequently related to drugs (e.g., sulfonamides, anticonvulsants) Nikolsky sign
Bacterial			
Staphylococcal scalded skin syndrome	Generalized, tender erythema Nikolsky sign Occasionally associated with underlying infection such as osteomyelitis, septic arthritis, pneumonia Desquamation and moist erosions observed, especially in intertriginous areas More common in children younger than 5 years of age		
		EXTRINSIC	
		Contact dermatitis	Irritant or allergic Distribution dependent on the irritant or allergen Distribution helpful in identifying cause
Bullous impetigo	Localized blisters from staphylococcal infection	Insect bites	Occur occasionally following flea or mosquito bites May be hemorrhagic bullae Often in linear or irregular clusters Very pruritic
Viral			
Herpes simplex	Grouped vesicles on erythematous base May be recurrent at same site—lips, eyes, cheeks, hands Reactivated by fever, sunlight, trauma, stress	Burns	Irregular shapes and configurations May be suggestive of abuse Bullae with second- and third-degree injuries
Varicella	Crops of vesicles on erythematous base ("dewdrops on rose petal") Highly contagious May see multiple stages of lesions simultaneously Associated with fever	Friction	Usually on acral surfaces May be related to footwear Often activity-related
		MISCELLANEOUS	
Herpes zoster	Grouped vesicles on erythematous base limited to one or several adjacent dermatomes Thoracic dermatomes most commonly involved in children Usually unilateral Burning, pruritus	Urticaria pigmentosa	Red-brown macules and papules; bullous lesions are rare Darier sign Lesions appear in infancy and spontaneously resolve in childhood
Hand-foot-mouth syndrome (coxsackievirus infection)	Prodrome of fever, anorexia, sore throat Oval blisters in acral distribution, usually few in number Shallow, oral erosions on erythematous base in oral mucosa Highly infectious Peak incidence in late summer and in fall	Miliaria crystallina	Clean, 1- to 2-mm superficial vesicles occurring in crops Rupture spontaneously Intertriginous areas, especially neck and axillae
		Hereditary: epidermolysis bullosa, incontinentia pigmenti, epidermolytic hyperkeratosis	
HYPERSENSITIVITY		Autoimmune: linear IgA disease, bullous pemphigoid, dermatitis herpetiformis	
Erythema multiforme	Target lesions on acral sites May have involvement of mucosal surfaces Associated with herpes simplex virus infection		

Modified from Nopper AJ, Rabinowotz RG: Rashes and skin lesions. In Kliegman RM, editor: Practical Strategies in Pediatric Diagnosis and Therapy, Philadelphia, 1996, WB Saunders.

and involves less than 10% of the body surface area. Cutaneous lesions are symmetrical and commonly involve acral areas such as the hands, feet, elbows, and knees. Involvement of the ocular, oral, and genital mucosa can be seen in some cases.

Most EM cases in children are precipitated by herpes simplex virus infection, though the infection may no longer be apparent by the time EM develops. *Mycoplasma pneumoniae* and other infectious organisms may also trigger EM. Symptomatic treatment is usually sufficient. Oral antihistamines help suppress pruritus, stinging, and burning. The use of systemic corticosteroids is controversial but may be considered for severe mucosal disease. Antiviral medications targeting herpes simplex virus do not alter the course of the EM, though children with recurrent EM may be candidates for prophylactic antivirals. The prognosis is excellent, with most lesions lasting no more than 2 weeks. Healing occurs without scarring.

STEVENS-JOHNSON SYNDROME AND TOXIC EPIDERMAL NECROLYSIS

SJS, TEN, and SJS/TEN overlap are severe, life-threatening disorders thought to represent the same disease continuum. They are usually preceded by a prodrome of fever, malaise, and upper respiratory symptoms 1 to 14 days before the onset of cutaneous lesions. Red macules appear suddenly and tend to coalesce into large patches, with a predominant distribution over the face and trunk. Atypical targets may be present, causing diagnostic confusion initially with EM, although the atypical targets lack the characteristic three zones. Skin lesions evolve rapidly into bullae and areas of necrosis. SJS is defined as epidermal detachment of less than 10% of the body surface area, whereas SJS/TEN overlap has 10% to 30% and TEN has greater than 30% body surface area involvement. Any mucosal surface may be involved. The upper and lower lips are generally swollen and bright red with erosions and hemorrhagic crusts, and the remainder of the oral mucosa may also be involved. Early in the disease process, there is bilateral conjunctival injection; however, this usually progresses to conjunctival erosions. There may be erosions of the penile, vaginal, or perianal mucosa. Urogenital, esophageal, and tracheal surfaces may be involved in the most severe cases.

Drugs and *Mycoplasma pneumoniae* infections are the most common causes of SJS/TEN in children. The most common drugs implicated are nonsteroidal anti-inflammatory drugs, sulfonamides, anticonvulsants, and antibiotics. Other precipitating factors are viral infections, bacterial infections, syphilis, and deep fungal infections.

SJS/TEN can occur at any age. The diagnosis of SJS/TEN is clinical; there are no diagnostic tests. Confusion with EM, Kawasaki disease, and bacterial toxin-mediated diseases (scarlet fever, toxic shock syndrome, and staphylococcal scalded skin syndrome) may occur. Patients with Kawasaki disease have conjunctival injection and hyperemia of the mucous membranes. Necrosis of the mucosal surfaces does not occur; blistering, erosions, and severe crusting are not observed. The mucosal changes of staphylococcal scalded skin syndrome are minor, and frank erosions are not present. The blistering of the skin is more superficial and favors intertriginous regions.

SJS/TEN is a serious illness with a mortality rate as high as 35% for severe cases of TEN. Prompt discontinuation of the offending agent is key. No controlled clinical trials regarding medical therapy exist, though early initiation of intravenous immunoglobulin has been proposed. Supportive care is another essential component of therapy, and a multidisciplinary care team is often necessary. Sepsis is the major cause of morbidity and mortality, so meticulous wound care is crucial, with stringent surveillance for cutaneous infections and use of antibiotics as warranted. Parenteral or nasogastric feeding should be instituted early to accelerate the healing process. Careful fluid management and monitoring of electrolytes are critical. Ocular complications are a major cause of long-term morbidity, so early involvement of an ophthalmologist is important.

Chapter 196

CUTANEOUS INFESTATIONS

Arthropods are common in the environment. Although many can bite or sting humans, only a few infest humans. Arachnids (mites) are the most common, parasitizing humans and animals by burrowing into the skin and depositing eggs within the skin.

SCABIES

Decision-Making Algorithm
Available @ StudentConsult.com

Vesicles and Bullae

Scabies is caused by the mite *Sarcoptes scabiei*. The female mite burrows into the epidermis and deposits her eggs, which mature in 10 to 14 days. The disease is highly contagious because infested humans do not manifest the typical signs or symptoms for 3 to 4 weeks, facilitating transmission. An immunocompetent person with scabies typically harbors only 10 to 20 mites.

The clinical presentation varies depending on the age of the patient, duration of infestation, and immune status of the patient. Severe and paroxysmal itching is the hallmark, with complaints of itching that is frequently worse than the eruption would suggest. Most children exhibit an eczematous eruption composed of red, excoriated papules and nodules. The classic linear papule or burrow is often difficult to find. Distribution is the most diagnostic finding; the papules are found in the axillae, umbilicus, groin, penis, instep of the foot, and web spaces of the fingers and toes (Fig. 196-1). Infants infested with scabies have diffuse erythema, scaling, and pinpoint papules. Pustules, vesicles, and nodules are much more common in infants and may be more diffusely distributed. The face and scalp usually are spared in adults and older children, but these areas are usually involved in infants. Nodular lesions may represent active infection or prolonged hypersensitivity lesions following resolution of infestation. Immunocompromised or neurologically impaired persons may develop a severe form

Figure 196-1 Scabies (hand).

of the disease known as **Norwegian** or **crusted scabies**, with infestation of 2 million live mites at one time.

The diagnosis of scabies can be confirmed by microscopic visualization of the mite, eggs, larvae, or feces in scrapings of papules or burrows examined under oil immersion. Skin biopsy is rarely necessary but may be useful if lesions have become nodular.

Curative treatment is achieved by a 12-hour (overnight) application of permethrin 5% cream applied to the entire body. Because permethrin is not effective against the eggs, the treatment should be repeated 1 week later to kill any subsequently hatched larvae. All household members and close contacts should be treated simultaneously, even if asymptomatic. Bed linens, towels, and clothes worn for the previous 2 days before treatment should be machine-washed in hot water and machine-dried using high heat; heat is the most effective scabicide. Items that are not washable may be dry-cleaned or placed in a sealed plastic bag for 7 days.

Secondary bacterial infection may occur but is uncommon. In contrast to the pediculoses, scabies is not a vector for infections. Pruritus may persist for 7 to 14 days after successful therapy because of a prolonged hypersensitivity reaction, which does not indicate treatment failure. Inadequate treatment or reinfestation should be suspected if new lesions develop after treatment.

PEDICULOSES

Three species of lice infest humans: *Pediculus humanus capitis*, the **head louse**; *Pthirus pubis*, the **pubic louse** or **crab louse**; and *Pediculus humanus humanus* (also known as *Pediculus humanus corporis*), the **body louse**. Lice are wingless insects 2 to 4 mm in length that cannot fly or jump. Transmission usually occurs by direct contact with another infested individual. Indirect spread through contact with fomites or personal belongings, such as hairbrushes, combs, or caps, is much less frequent.

Pediculosis differs from scabies infestation in that the louse resides on the hair or clothing and intermittently feeds on the host by piercing the skin. The *bite* causes small urticarial papules and itching. Head lice live close to the skin and may live for 30 days, depositing 100 to 400 eggs as **nits** on hair shafts, usually within 6 mm of the scalp.

Head lice are seen most frequently in early school-age children. Head lice infestations are unrelated to hygiene and are not more common among children with long hair or with dirty hair. It is estimated that 6 to 12 million persons in the United States and 1% to 3% of persons in developed countries are infested with head lice each year. In the United States, head lice infestation is rare among African Americans and may be more common in girls, which is attributed to their tendency to play more closely with one another than boys do.

Pubic lice are transmitted by sexual contact. Their presence in children may be a sign of child abuse. Body lice are firm evidence of poor hygiene, such as infrequent washing and clothing changes.

Itching, if present, is the primary symptom. Pediculosis capitis usually causes pruritus behind the ears or on the nape of the neck, or a crawling sensation in the scalp. Pediculosis pubis usually causes pruritus in the groin. Eyelash involvement in children may cause crusting and blepharitis. Pediculosis corporis causes pruritus that, because of repeated scratching, may result in lichenification or secondary bacterial infection. Excoriations and crusting, with or without associated regional lymphadenopathy, may be present.

Infestation with the head louse may be asymptomatic and has little morbidity. The diagnosis can be confirmed by visualizing a live louse. A fine-toothed comb to trap lice is more effective than simply looking at the hair. Wet combing is more time-consuming, but dry combing produces static that may propel the lice away from the comb.

Nits represent the outer casing of the louse ova. Viable nits have an intact operculum (cap) on the nonattached end and a developing louse within the egg. **Brown nits** located on the proximal hair shaft suggest active infestation. **White nits** located on the hair shaft 4 cm or farther from the scalp indicate previous infestation. Because nonviable nits can remain stuck in the hair for weeks to months after an infestation has resolved, many children with nits do not have active lice infestation.

The treatment of head lice is controversial because of resistance to many established options. Over-the-counter permethrin (1%) and pyrethrin-based products (0.17% to 0.33%) are the first choices of therapy. Because 20% to 30% of eggs may survive one treatment, a second treatment should be applied in 7 to 10 days. Drug resistance is on the rise, and malathion (0.5%) lotion may be used as an alternative for resistant cases.

Everyone in the family should be checked for head lice and treated if live lice are found to reduce the risk of reinfestation. Bed linens, towels, and clothes worn for the previous 2 days before treatment should be machine-washed in hot water and machine-dried using high heat. Items that are not washable may be dry-cleaned or placed in a sealed plastic bag for 2 weeks. Brushes and combs should be soaked in dish detergent or rubbing alcohol for 1 hour. Rugs, furniture, mattresses, and car seats should be vacuumed thoroughly.

Manual removal of nits after treatment is not necessary to prevent spread. Children treated for head lice should return to school immediately after completion of the first effective treatment or first wet combing, regardless of the presence of remaining nits. There is no evidence that *no nit* or *nit-free* policies reduce transmission of head lice. If required for return to school, nit removal is best achieved by wetting the hair and combing with a fine-toothed metal comb.

Excoriations can become secondarily infected with skin bacteria, usually *Staphylococcus* and *Streptococcus*. The body louse functions as a vector for potentially serious infectious diseases, including **epidemic typhus**, caused by *Rickettsia prowazekii*; **louse-borne relapsing fever**, caused by *Borrelia recurrentis*; and **trench fever**, caused by *Bartonella quintana*. These louse-borne infections are rare in the United States. In contrast to body lice, head lice and pubic lice are not associated with transmission of other infections.

Suggested Reading

Eichenfield LE, Esterly NB, Frieden IJ: *Textbook of Neonatal Dermatology*, ed 2, Philadelphia, 2008, Saunders.

Holland KE, Drolet BA: Infantile hemangioma, *Pediatr Clin North Am* 57:1069–1083, 2010.

Krakowski AC, Eichenfield LF, Dohil MA: Management of atopic dermatitis in the pediatric population, *Pediatrics* 122:812–814, 2008.

Paller AS, Mancini AJ: *Hurwitz Clinical Pediatric Dermatology*, ed 4, Philadelphia, 2011, Saunders.

Schachner LA, Hansen RC: *Pediatric Dermatology*, ed 4, Philadelphia, 2011, Saunders.

Yan AC, Baldwin HE, Eichenfield LF, et al: Approach to pediatric acne treatment: an update, *Semin Cutan Med Surg* 30:S16–S21, 2011.

Orthopedics

Kevin D. Walter and J. Channing Tassone

Chapter 197

ORTHOPEDICS ASSESSMENT

To care for the pediatric patient, one must understand the growth and development of the musculoskeletal system as well as common orthopedic terms (Table 197-1). Practitioners should recognize common mechanisms for congenital and acquired orthopedic disorders (Table 197-2).

GROWTH AND DEVELOPMENT

The ends of the long bones contain a much higher proportion of cartilage in the skeletally immature child than in an adult (Figs. 197-1 and 197-2). The high cartilage content allows for a unique vulnerability to trauma and infection (particularly in the metaphysis).

The physis is responsible for the longitudinal growth of the long bones. Articular cartilage allows the ends of the bone to enlarge and accounts for growth of smaller bones, such as the tarsals. The periosteum can provide circumferential growth. Trauma, infection, nutritional deficiency (rickets), inborn errors of metabolism (mucopolysaccharidoses), and other metabolic disorders (renal tubular acidosis, hypothyroid) may affect each of the growth processes and produce distinct aberrations.

Table 197-1	Common Orthopedic Terminology
Abduction	Movement away from midline
Adduction	Movement toward or across midline
Apophysis	Bone growth center that has a muscular insertion but is not considered a growth plate (example: tibial tubercle)
Arthroscopy	Surgical exploration of a joint using an arthroscope
Arthroplasty	Surgical reconstruction of a joint
Arthrotomy	Surgical incision into a joint; an "open" procedure
Deformation	Changes in limb, trunk, or head due to mechanical force
Dislocation	Displacement of bones at a joint
Equinus	Plantar flexion of the forefoot, hindfoot, or entire foot
Femoral anteversion	Increased angulation of the femoral head and neck with respect to the frontal plane
Malformation	Defect in development that occurs during fetal life (example: syndactyly)
Osteotomy	Surgical division of a bone
Pes cavus	High medial arch of the foot
Pes planus	Flat foot
Rotation, internal	Inward rotation (toward midline)
Rotation, external	Outward rotation (away from midline)
Subluxation	Incomplete loss of contact between two joint surfaces
Tibial torsion	Rotation of the tibia in an internal or external fashion
Valgus/ valgum	Angulation of a bone or joint in which the apex is toward the midline (example: knock-knee)
Varus/varum	Angulation of a bone or joint in which the apex is away from the midline (example: bowlegs)

Table 197-2	Mechanisms of Common Pediatric Orthopedic Problems	
CATEGORY	**MECHANISM**	**EXAMPLE(S)**
CONGENITAL		
Malformation	Teratogenesis before 12 weeks of gestation	Spina bifida
Disruption	Amniotic band constriction Fetal varicella infection	Extremity amputation Limb scar/atrophy
Deformation	Neck compression	Torticollis
Dysplasia	Abnormal cell growth or metabolism	Osteogenesis imperfecta Skeletal dysplasias
ACQUIRED		
Infection	Pyogenic-hematogenous spread	Septic arthritis, osteomyelitis
Inflammation	Antigen-antibody reaction Immune mediated	Systemic lupus erythematosus Juvenile idiopathic arthritis
Trauma	Mechanical forces, overuse	Child abuse, sports injuries, unintentional injury, fractures, dislocations, tendinitis
Tumor	Primary bone tumor Metastasis to bone from other site Bone marrow tumor	Osteosarcoma Neuroblastoma Leukemia, lymphoma

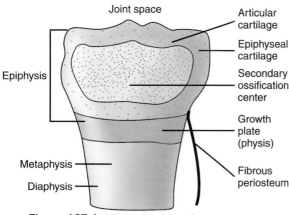

Figure 197-1 Schematic of long bone structure.

Figure 197-2 **The ends of long bones at various ages.** Lightly stippled areas represent cartilage composition, whereas heavily darkened areas are zones of ossification. *(From Tachjidan MO: Congenital Dislocation of the Hip, New York, 1982, Churchill Livingstone, p 105.)*

DEVELOPMENTAL MILESTONES

Neurologic maturation, marked by achievement of developmental motor milestones, is important for normal musculoskeletal development (see Section 2). A neurologic disorder may cause a secondary musculoskeletal abnormality (e.g., extremity contractures in Duchenne muscular dystrophy). Thus, normal motor development must be included in the definition of a normal musculoskeletal system.

Infants

Decision-Making Algorithms
Available @ StudentConsult.com

In-Toeing, Out-Toeing, and Toe-Walking
Bowlegs and Knock-Knees

The in utero position of the fetus can affect the angular and torsional alignment (temporary or permanent) of the skeletal system, especially of the lower extremity (Fig. 197-3). The newborn's hips are externally rotated. Pes planus and genu varum are common. Infants are usually born with a flexed posture. This position usually decreases to neutral within the first 4 to 6 months. The foot is often flat and *tucked under* at birth; the ankle will be inverted and the forefoot is adducted when compared with the hindfoot. The lateral border of the foot must straighten out, even with dorsiflexion, to be considered secondary to in utero positioning.

The head and neck may also be distorted by in utero positioning. The spine and upper extremities are less likely to be affected. By the age of 3 to 4 years, the effects of in utero positioning have usually resolved.

Gait

Normal gait has a stance phase and swing phase; each leg should have symmetrical timing with each phase. The stance phase represents 60% of the gait and begins with foot contact (usually the heel strike) and ends with the toe-off. During the swing phase (40%), the foot is off the ground. The gait cycle is the interval between stance phases on the same limb.

Toddlers will generally walk independently by 18 months of age. Their externally rotated gait is usually inconsistent, is characterized by short, rapid steps, and does not have the reciprocal arm swing. Gait coordination improves over time, with a normal gait usually achieved by the time a child enters elementary school.

Decision-Making Algorithms
Available @ StudentConsult.com

Limp
In-Toeing, Out-Toeing, and Toe-Walking

The Limping Child

The differential diagnosis for a limping child is often categorized by age and presence or absence of a painful limp (Table 197-3). The gluteus medius muscle stabilizes the pelvis during the stance phase, preventing the pelvis from dropping toward the leg in swing phase. An **antalgic gait** is a painful limp; the stance phase and stride of the affected limb are shortened to decrease the discomfort of weight bearing on the affected limb. The **Trendelenburg gait** has a normal stance phase, but excessive swaying of the trunk. **Waddling gait** refers to a bilateral decrease in function of the gluteus muscles.

Toe walking is a common complaint in early walkers. A physician should evaluate any child older than 3 years of age who still toe walks. Although this is most likely habit, a neuromuscular disorder (cerebral palsy, tethered cord), Achilles tendon contracture (heel cord tightness), or a leg-length discrepancy should be considered.

Figure 197-3 Deformation abnormalities resulting from uterine compression.

Table 197-3	Differential Diagnosis of Limping in Children

AGE GROUP	DIAGNOSTIC CONSIDERATIONS	AGE GROUP	DIAGNOSTIC CONSIDERATIONS
Early walker: 1 to 3 years of age	*Painful Limp* Septic arthritis and osteomyelitis Transient monarticular synovitis Occult trauma ("toddler's fracture") Intervertebral diskitis Malignancy *Painless Limp* Developmental dysplasia of the hip Neuromuscular disorder Cerebral palsy Lower extremity length inequality	Adolescent: 11 years of age to maturity	*Painful Limp* Septic arthritis, osteomyelitis, myositis Trauma Rheumatologic disorder Slipped capital femoral epiphysis: acute; unstable Malignancy *Painless Limp* Slipped capital femoral epiphysis: chronic; stable Developmental dysplasia of the hip: acetabular dysplasia Lower extremity length inequality Neuromuscular disorder

Child: 3 to 10 years of age	*Painful Limp*
	Septic arthritis, osteomyelitis, myositis
	Transient monarticular synovitis
	Trauma
	Rheumatologic disorders
	  Juvenile idiopathic arthritis
	Intervertebral diskitis
	Malignancy
	Painless Limp
	Developmental dysplasia of the hip
	Legg-Calve-Perthes disease
	Lower extremity length inequality
	Neuromuscular disorder
	  Cerebral palsy
	Muscular dystrophy (Duchenne)		

Chapter **198**

FRACTURES

Fractures account for 10% to 15% of all childhood injuries. The anatomic, biomechanical, and physiologic differences in children account for unique fracture patterns and management. Fracture terminology helps describe fractures (Table 198-1).

The pediatric skeleton has a higher proportion of cartilage and a thicker, stronger, and more active periosteum, capable of producing a larger callus more rapidly than in an adult. The thick periosteum may decrease the rate of displaced fractures and stabilize fractures after reduction. Because of the higher proportion of cartilage, the skeletally immature patient can withstand more force before deformation or fracture than adult bone. As children mature into adolescence, the rate of healing slows and approaches that of adults.

PEDIATRIC FRACTURE PATTERNS

Buckle or **torus fractures** occur after compression of the bone; the bony cortex does not truly break. These fractures will typically occur in the metaphysis and are stable fractures that heal in approximately 4 weeks with immobilization. A common example is a fall onto an outstretched arm causing a buckle fracture in the distal radius.

Complete fractures occur when both sides of bony cortex are fractured. This is the most common fracture and may be classified as comminuted, oblique, transverse, or spiral, depending on the direction of the fracture line.

Greenstick fractures occur when a bone is angulated beyond the limits of plastic deformation. The bone fails on the tension side and sustains a bend deformity on the compression side. The force is insufficient to cause a complete fracture (Fig. 198-1).

Table 198-1	Useful Fracture Terminology
Complete	The bone fragments separate completely
Incomplete	The bone fragments are still partially joined
Linear	Referring to a fracture line that is parallel to the bone's long axis
Transverse	Referring to a fracture line that is at a right angle to the bone's long axis
Oblique	Referring to a fracture line that is diagonal to the bone's long axis
Spiral	Referring to a twisting fracture
Comminution	A fracture that results in several fragments
Compaction	The bone fragments are driven into each other
Angulation	The fragments have angular malalignment
Rotation	The fragments have rotational malalignment
Shortening	The fractured ends of the bones overlap
Open	A fracture in which the bone has pierced the skin

Bowing fractures demonstrate no fracture line evident on radiographs, but the bone is bent beyond its limit of plastic deformation. This is not a true fracture, but will heal with periosteal reaction.

Physeal Fractures

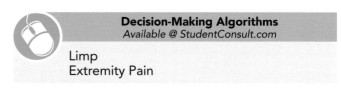

Decision-Making Algorithms
Available @ StudentConsult.com

Limp
Extremity Pain

Fractures involving the growth plate constitute about 20% of all fractures in the skeletally immature patient. These fractures are more common in males (2:1 male-female ratio). The peak incidence is 13 to 14 years in boys and 11 to 12 years in girls. The distal radius, distal tibia, and distal fibula are the most common locations.

Ligaments frequently insert onto epiphyses. Thus, traumatic forces to an extremity may be transmitted to the physis, which is not as biomechanically strong as the metaphysis; it may fracture with mechanisms of injury that may cause sprains in the adult. The growth plate is most susceptible to torsional and angular forces.

Physeal fractures are described using **Salter-Harris classification,** which allows for prognostic information regarding premature closure of the growth plate and poor functional outcomes. The higher the type number, the more likely the patient will have complications. There are five main groups (Fig. 198-2):

Type I: transverse fracture through the physis; growth disturbance is unusual

Type II: fracture through a portion of the physis and metaphysis; most common type of Salter-Harris fracture (75%)

Type III: fracture through a portion of the physis and epiphysis into the joint that may result in complication because of intra-articular component and because of disruption of the growing or hypertrophic zone of the physis

Figure 198-1 The greenstick fracture is an incomplete fracture. *(Modified from White N, Sty R: Radiological evaluation and classification of pediatric fractures, Clin Pediatr Emerg Med 3:94–105, 2002.)*

Type IV: fracture through the metaphysis, physis, and
epiphysis with a high risk of complication
Type V: a crush injury to the physis with a poor functional
prognosis

Types I and II fractures can often be managed by closed
reduction and do not require perfect alignment. A major
exception is the type II fracture of the distal femur, which is
associated with a poor outcome unless proper anatomic alignment is obtained. Types III and IV fractures require anatomic
alignment for successful treatment. Type V fractures are rare
and often result in premature closure of the physis.

MANAGEMENT OF PEDIATRIC FRACTURES

The majority of pediatric fractures can be managed with
closed methods. Some fractures need closed reduction to
improve alignment. Approximately 4% of pediatric fractures
require internal fixation. Patients with open physes are more
likely to require internal fixation if they have one of the following fractures:

Displaced epiphyseal fractures
Displaced intra-articular fractures
Fractures in a child with multiple injuries
Open fractures
Unstable fractures

The goal of internal fixation is to improve and maintain anatomic alignment. This is usually done with Kirschner wires,
Steinmann pins, and cortical screws with subsequent external immobilization in a cast until healing is satisfactory. After
healing, the hardware is frequently removed to prevent incorporation into the callus and prevent physeal damage.

External fixation without casting may be necessary for pelvic fractures causing hemodynamic instability. Fractures associated with soft tissue loss, burns, and neurovascular damage
may benefit from external fixation.

SPECIAL CONCERNS
Remodeling

Fracture remodeling occurs because of a combination of
periosteal resorption and new bone formation. Many pediatric fractures do not need perfect anatomic alignment for
proper healing. Younger patients have greater potential for

fracture remodeling. Fractures that occur in the meta-physis,
near the growth plate, may undergo more remodeling. Fractures angulated in the plane of motion also remodel very well.
Intra-articular fractures, angulated or displaced diaphyseal
fractures, rotated fractures, and fracture deformity not in the
plane of motion tend not to remodel as well.

Overgrowth

Overgrowth occurs in long bones as the result of increased
blood flow associated with fracture healing. Femoral fractures
in children younger than 10 years of age will frequently over-
grow 1 to 3 cm. This is the reason end-to-end alignment for
femur and long-bone fractures may not be indicated. After
10 years of age, overgrowth is less of a problem, so end-to-end
alignment is recommended.

Progressive Deformity

Fractures and injuries to the physis can result in premature
closure. If it is a partial closure, the consequence may be an
angular deformity. If it is a complete closure, limb shortening
may occur. The most commonly affected locations are the distal femur and the distal and proximal tibia.

Neurovascular Injury

Fractures and dislocations may damage adjacent blood vessels
and nerves. The most common location is the distal humerus
(**supracondylar fracture**) and the knee (dislocation and physeal fracture). It is necessary to perform and document a careful neurovascular examination distal to the fracture (pulse,
sensory, and motor function).

Compartment Syndrome

Compartment syndrome is an orthopedic emergency that
results from hemorrhage and soft tissue swelling within the
tight fascial compartments of an extremity. This can result
in muscle ischemia and neurovascular compromise unless it
is surgically decompressed. The most common sites are the
lower leg (tibial fracture) and arm (supracondylar fracture).

Affected patients have severe pain and will eventually have
decreased sensation in the dermatomes supplied by the nerves

Figure 198-2 The types of growth plate injury as classified by Salter and Harris. See text for descriptions of types I to V. (*From Salter RB, Harris WR: Injuries involving the epiphyseal plate, J Bone Joint Surg Am 45:587–622, 1963.*)

located in the compartment. Swollen and tight compartments and pain with passive stretching are present. This can happen underneath a cast and may actually occur when a cast is applied too tightly. It is important to educate all patients with fractures on the signs of compartment syndrome and ensure that they realize it is an emergency.

Toddler's Fracture

This is an oblique fracture of the distal tibia without a fibula fracture. There is often no significant trauma. Patients are usually 1 to 3 years old, but can be as old as 6 and present with limping and pain with weight bearing. There may be minimal swelling and pain. Initial radiographs do not always show the fracture; if symptoms persist, a repeat x-ray in 7 to 10 days may be helpful.

Child Abuse

Decision-Making Algorithm
Available @ StudentConsult.com

Extremity Pain

Child abuse must always be considered in the differential diagnosis of a child with fractures, especially in those younger than 3 years (see Chapter 22). Common fracture patterns that should increase the index of suspicion include multiple fractures in different stages of radiographic healing, metaphyseal corner fractures (shaking), fractures too severe for the history, or fractures in nonambulatory infants. Although spiral fractures of long bones were historically considered pathognomic for abuse, they can be seen in nonabuse situations.

When there is concern for child abuse, the child should have a full evaluation, which may include admission to the hospital. A thorough and well-documented physical examination should focus on soft tissue injuries, the cranium, and a funduscopic examination for retinal hemorrhages or detachment. A skeletal survey or a bone scan may be helpful in identifying other fractures.

Chapter 199

HIP

The hip is a ball (femoral head) and socket (acetabulum) joint that is important for skeletal stability. The femoral head and acetabulum are interdependent for normal growth and development. The femoral neck and head, which contain the capital femoral epiphysis, are intra-articular. The blood supply to this region is unique because the blood vessels are extraosseous and lie on the surface of the femoral neck, entering the epiphysis peripherally. Thus, the blood supply to the femoral head is vulnerable to trauma, infection, and other causes that may increase intra-articular pressure. Damage to the blood supply can lead to **avascular necrosis**.

DEVELOPMENTAL DYSPLASIA OF THE HIP

In developmental dysplasia of the hip (DDH), the hips at birth may be dislocated or dislocatable. The femoral head and acetabulum develop from the same mesenchymal cells; by 11 weeks' gestation, the hip joint is formed. There are two types of DDH: teratologic and typical. **Teratologic dislocations** occur early in utero and are usually associated with neuromuscular disorders (spina bifida, arthrogryposis). **Typical dislocations** occur in the neurologically normal infant and can occur before or after birth. The true incidence of DDH is unknown, but it may be as high as 1.5 cases per 1000 infants.

Etiology

Newborn infants have ligamentous laxity that, if significant enough in the hip, may lead to spontaneous dislocation and reduction of the femoral head. Persistence of this spontaneous pattern can lead to pathologic changes, such as flattening of the acetabulum, muscle contractures that limit motion, and joint capsule tightening. The left hip is affected three times as often as the right hip, possibly because of in utero positioning.

Physiologic risk factors for DDH include a generalized ligamentous laxity, perhaps from maternal hormones that are associated with pelvic ligament relaxation (estrogen and relaxin). Female infants are at higher risk (9:1); family history is positive in 20% of all patients with DDH.

Other risk factors include breech presentation, firstborn child (60%), oligohydramnios, and postnatal infant positioning. In breech presentations, the fetal pelvis is situated in the maternal pelvis. This can increase hip flexion and limit overall fetal hip motion, causing further stretching of the already lax joint capsule and exposing the posterior aspect of the femoral head. The altered relationship between the acetabulum and femoral head causes abnormal acetabular development. Postnatal positioning of the hips in a tight swaddle with the hips adducted and extended can displace the hip joint.

Congenital muscular torticollis, metatarsus adductus, and clubfoot are associated with DDH. An infant with any of these three conditions should receive a careful examination of the hips.

Clinical Manifestations

Every newborn requires a screening physical examination for DDH; further evaluation through at least the first 18 months of life is part of the physical examination for toddlers. DDH evolves over time, so the examination may change as the patient ages. The examination starts with inspection for asymmetrical thigh and gluteal folds with the hips and knees flexed. A relative shortening of the femur with asymmetrical skin folds is a positive **Galeazzi sign** and indicates DDH. Range of motion should be assessed with the pelvis stabilized and the child supine on the examining table, not in the parent's lap (Fig. 199-1). Hip abduction should easily reach or exceed 75°, and hip adduction should reach 30°. Limitations may indicate contractures associated with DDH, especially decreased abduction.

ABDUCTION TEST

1)
90
Normal at birth to 1 month of age

2)
70
Often normal, 1 to 9 months of age

3)
60
Suspected significant limitation

4)
50
Definite limitation

Figure 199-1 Hip abduction test. Place the infant supine, flex the hips 90°, and fully abduct the hips. Although the normal abduction range is broad, hip disease should be suspected in any patient who lacks more than 30° to 45° of abduction. *(From Chung SMK: Hip Disorders in Infants and Children, Philadelphia, 1981, Lea & Febiger, p 69.)*

The **Barlow test** attempts to dislocate an unstable hip (Fig. 199-2). The examiner should stabilize the infant's pelvis with one hand and grasp the abducted and flexed thigh in the other hand. The hip should be flexed to 90°. Next, begin to adduct the hip, while applying a posterior force to the anterior hip. A hip that can be dislocated in this method is readily felt (clunk feeling) and is a positive test. It may reduce spontaneously once the posterior force is removed, or the examiner may need to perform the Ortolani test.

The **Ortolani test** may reduce a dislocated hip (Fig. 199-3). The examiner should stabilize the pelvis and hold the leg in the same method as for the Barlow test. The infant's hip should be in 90° of flexion. Abduct the hip while applying anterior pressure to the posterior thigh. A positive test is the palpable reduction of the dislocation, which may be felt (clunk). After 2 months of age, the hip may develop muscular contractures, preventing positive Ortolani tests.

These tests should be performed with only gentle force and done one hip at a time. The test may need to be repeated multiple times, as they can be difficult to interpret. A click, which is not pathologic, may occur from breaking the surface tension of the hip joint or snapping gluteal tendons.

Bilateral fixed dislocations present a diagnostic dilemma because of the symmetry on exam. The **Klisic test** is useful in this situation; it is done by placing the third finger over the greater trochanter and the index finger over the anterior superior iliac spine, then drawing an imaginary line between the two. The line should point to the umbilicus in a normal child. However, in a dislocated hip, the greater trochanter is elevated, which causes the line to project lower (between the umbilicus and pubis). This test is helpful identifying bilateral DDH, which can otherwise be difficult to diagnose because of the symmetry found on examination.

Older children with unrecognized DDH may present with limping. A patient with increased lumbar lordosis and a waddling gait may have an unrecognized bilateral DDH.

A

B

Figure 199-2 Barlow (dislocation) test. Reverse of Ortolani test. If the femoral head is in the acetabulum at the time of examination, the Barlow test is performed to discover any hip instability. **A,** The infant's thigh is grasped as shown and adducted with gentle downward pressure. **B,** Dislocation is palpable as the femoral head slips out of the acetabulum. Diagnosis is confirmed with the Ortolani test.

Figure 199-3 Ortolani (reduction) test. With the infant relaxed and content on a firm surface, the hips and knees are flexed to 90°. The hips are examined one at a time. The examiner grasps the infant's thigh with the middle finger over the greater trochanter and lifts the thigh to bring the femoral head from its dislocated posterior position to opposite the acetabulum. Simultaneously the thigh is gently abducted, reducing the femoral head in the acetabulum. In a positive finding, the examiner senses reduction by a palpable, nearly audible *clunk.*

Radiographic Evaluation

Ultrasound is used for initial evaluation of infants with DDH. Ultrasonography is necessary for girls with a positive family history or breech presentation in both sexes. This should be obtained after 6 weeks of age to avoid confusion with physiologic laxity. Because the femoral head begins to ossify at 4 to 6 months of age, plain radiographs can be misleading until patients are older.

Treatment

The treatment of DDH is individualized and depends on the child's age at diagnosis. The goal of treatment is a stable reduction that results in normal growth and development of the hip. If DDH is suspected, the child should be sent to a pediatric orthopedic specialist.

The **Pavlik harness** is an effective treatment up to 6 months of age. It provides hip flexion to just over 90° and limits adduction to no more than neutral. This positioning redirects the femoral head toward the acetabulum. The hip must be reduced within 1 to 2 weeks of beginning the Pavlik harness, although the infant will need more time in the device. The Pavlik harness is successful in treating approximately 95% of dysplastic or subluxated hips, and 80% successful for treatment of true dislocations. Persistently dislocated hips should not remain in a Pavlik harness for more than 2 weeks for fear of iatrogenic acetabular damage. Patients failing the Pavlik harness warrant treatment with an abduction orthosis.

Children over 6 months or those who have failed nonoperative treatment should undergo closed reduction using a hip spica cast. This is done under general anesthesia; reduction is evaluated with an intraoperative arthrogram, then confirmed by postoperative computed tomography (CT) or magnetic resonance imaging (MRI). If closed reduction fails, open reduction is indicated. Patients over 18 months of age may require a pelvic and femoral osteotomy.

Complications

The most important and severe complication of DDH is iatrogenic avascular necrosis of the femoral head. This can occur from excessive flexion or abduction during positioning of the Pavlik harness or hip spica cast. Infants under 6 months of age are at highest risk. Pressure ulcers can occur with prolonged casting. Redislocation or subluxation of the femoral head and residual acetabular dysplasia can occur.

TRANSIENT MONOARTICULAR SYNOVITIS

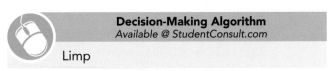

Transient synovitis, also known as **toxic synovitis**, is a common cause of limping in children. It is a diagnosis of exclusion, because **septic arthritis** and **osteomyelitis** of the hip must be excluded (see Chapters 117 and 118).

Etiology and Epidemiology

The etiology of transient synovitis is uncertain, but possible causes are viral illness and hypersensitivity. Approximately 70% of children diagnosed with transient synovitis have an upper respiratory tract viral infection in the preceding 7 to 14 days. Biopsies have revealed nonspecific synovial hypertrophy. Hip joint aspirations, when necessary, are negative for bacterial culture or signs of bacterial infection.

The mean age at onset is 6 years, with a range of 3 to 8 years. It is twice as common in male children.

Clinical Manifestations and Evaluation

The patient or family will describe an acute onset of pain in the groin/hip, anterior thigh, or knee. Irritation of the obturator nerve can cause referred pain in the thigh and knee when the pathology is at the hip. Patients with transient synovitis are often afebrile, walk with a painful limp, and have normal to minimally elevated white blood cell count, C-reactive protein, and erythrocyte sedimentation rate compared with bacterial diseases of the hip (Table 199-1). Table 197-3 lists the differential diagnosis of a limping child.

Anteroposterior and frog-leg radiographs of the hip are usually normal. Ultrasonography may reveal a joint effusion. It is mandatory to rule out septic arthritis in the presence of effusion with a joint aspiration and cell count.

Treatment

The mainstay of treatment is bed rest and minimal weight bearing until the pain resolves. Nonsteroidal anti-inflammatory medication is usually sufficient to decrease pain. Limiting strenuous activity and exercise for 1 to 2 weeks following recovery is helpful. Follow-up will help ensure that there is no deterioration. Lack of improvement necessitates further evaluation for more serious disorders.

LEGG-CALVE-PERTHES DISEASE
Etiology and Epidemiology

Table 199-1	Differences between Bacterial Infection and Transient Synovitis
BACTERIAL INFECTION*	**TRANSIENT SYNOVITIS**
Elevated joint fluid cell count Fever—temperature >38.5° C	Afebrile
Leukocytosis	Normal WBC count
ESR >20 mm/hour	Normal ESR and CRP
Refusal to walk	Painful limp
Hip held in external rotation, abduction, and flexion	Hip held normally
Severe pain and tenderness	Moderate pain and mild tenderness

CRP, C-reactive protein; ESR, erythrocyte sedimentation rate; WBC, white blood cell.
*Examples: Septic arthritis, osteomyelitis of hip.

Legg-Calve-Perthes disease (LCPD) is idiopathic **avascular necrosis (osteonecrosis)** of the capital epiphysis of the femoral head. The etiology is unclear, but it is likely caused by an interruption of the blood supply to the capital femoral epiphysis. There may be an associated hypercoagulability state (factor V Leiden).

LCPD commonly presents in patients 3 to 12 years of age, with a mean age of 7 years. It is four to five times more common in boys.

Clinical Manifestations
Patients may not present for several weeks because of minimal discomfort; the classic presentation is a child with an atraumatic, painless limp. There may be mild or intermittent hip/groin, anterior thigh, or knee pain. Decreased internal rotation and abduction with some discomfort, thigh muscle spasm, and anterior thigh muscular atrophy may be present. Patients have delayed bone age.

Radiologic Evaluation
Anteroposterior and frog-leg radiographs of both hips are usually adequate for diagnosis and management. It is necessary to document the extent of the disease and follow its progression. MRI and bone scan are helpful to diagnose early LCPD.

Treatment and Prognosis
LCPD is usually a self-limited disorder that should be followed by a pediatric orthopedist. Initial treatment focuses on pain control and restoration of hip range of motion. The goal of treatment is prevention of complications, such as femoral head deformity and secondary osteoarthritis.

Containment is important in treating LCPD; the femoral head is contained inside the acetabulum, which acts like a mold for the capital femoral epiphysis as it reossifies. Nonsurgical containment uses abduction casts and orthoses, whereas surgical containment is accomplished with osteotomies of the proximal femur and pelvis.

The short-term prognosis is determined by the magnitude of the femoral head deformity after healing has completed. It is improved by early diagnosis, good follow-up, and compliance with the treatment plan. Older children and children with a residual femoral head deformity are more likely to develop osteoarthritis (OA). The incidence of OA in patients who developed LCPD after 10 years of age is close to 100%; it is negligible in children with onset before 5 years of age. Patients between 6 and 9 years of age have a risk of OA of less than 40%.

SLIPPED CAPITAL FEMORAL EPIPHYSIS

Decision-Making Algorithms
Available @ StudentConsult.com

Limp
Extremity Pain

Etiology and Epidemiology
Slipped capital femoral epiphysis (SCFE) is a common adolescent hip disorder that is an orthopedic emergency. The incidence is 10.8 per 100,000, and it is slightly higher in males. African-American and Hispanic populations are at higher risk. Approximately 20% of patients with SCFE will have bilateral involvement at presentation, and another 20% to 40% may progress to bilateral involvement. The average age is 10 to 16 years, with a mean of 12 years in boys and 11 years in girls. Additional risk factors for SCFE include obesity, trisomy 21, and endocrine disorders (hypothyroid, pituitary tumor, growth hormone deficiency).

Classification
SCFE is classified as stable or unstable. Unstable patients refuse to ambulate even with crutches. Stable patients have an antalgic gait. SCFE can also be characterized as acute (symptoms less than 3 weeks) or chronic (symptoms over 3 weeks). Acute-on-chronic SCFE is seen when more than 3 weeks of symptoms are accompanied by an acute exacerbation of pain and difficulty/inability to bear weight.

Clinical Manifestation
The presentation is variable, based on severity and type of slip. Patients will often report hip or knee pain, limp or inability to ambulate, and decreased hip range of motion. There may or may not be a traumatic event. *Any knee pain mandates an examination of the hip, as hip pathology can cause referred pain to the anterior thigh and knee along the obturator nerve.* The patient usually holds the affected extremity in external rotation. As the hip is flexed, it will progressively externally rotate. There is usually a limitation of internal rotation, but there may also be a loss of flexion and abduction. If the patient can bear weight, it is typically an antalgic gait with the affected leg in external rotation. It is important to examine both hips to determine bilateral involvement.

Radiologic Evaluation
Anteroposterior and frog-leg radiographs are indicated. Patients with known SCFE or with a high index of suspicion should not undergo frog-leg lateral radiographs. Instead, a cross table lateral radiograph reduces the risk of iatrogenic progression. The earliest sign of SCFE is widening of the physis without slippage (**preslip condition**). Klein's line (Fig. 199-4) is helpful in assessing the anteroposterior radiograph for SCFE. The slippage can be classified radiographically as type I (0% to 33% displacement), type II (34% to 50%), or type III (>50%). The likelihood of complications increases with degree of displacement.

Treatment
Patients with SCFE should be immediately made non–weight bearing and referred to a pediatric orthopedist. The goal is to prevent further slippage, enhance physeal closure, and minimize complications, which is usually accomplished with internal fixation in situ with a single cannulated screw. More severe cases may require surgical hip dislocation and reduction to realign the epiphysis. There is controversy surrounding the prophylactic fixation of the nonaffected side. Assessment for endocrine disorders is important, particularly in children outside the range of 10 to 16 years of age.

Figure 199-4 Slipped capital femoral epiphysis (SCFE). **A,** Anteroposterior radiograph reveals a widened physis (*small arrows*) and decreased height of the epiphysis on the left. In addition, there is loss (*large arrow*) of the Capener triangle (*c*) (normal double density of the medial metaphysis superimposed on the posterior acetabular rim on right) and an abnormal lateral femoral neck line (normal on right). **B,** Frog, lateral view confirms the inferomedial position of the SCFE. (*From Blickman H:* Pediatric Radiology, the Requisites, *ed 2, St Louis, 1998, Mosby, p 244.*)

Complications

The two most serious complications of SCFE are **chondrolysis** and **avascular necrosis**. Chondrolysis is destruction of the articular cartilage. It is associated with more severe slips and with intra-articular penetration of operative hardware. This can lead to severe osteoarthritis (OA) and disability. Avascular necrosis occurs when there is a disruption of the blood supply to the capital femoral epiphysis. This usually happens at the time of injury, but may occur during forced manipulation of an unstable slip. Avascular necrosis may occur in up to 50% of unstable SCFEs and may lead to OA.

Table 200-1	Common Causes of In-Toeing and Out-Toeing
IN-TOEING	**OUT-TOEING**
Internal femoral torsion or anteversion	External femoral torsion or retroversion
Internal tibial torsion	External tibial torsion
Metatarsus adductus	Calcaneovalgus feet
Talipes equinovarus (clubfoot)	Hypermobile pes planus (flatfoot)
Developmental dysplasia	Slipped capital femoral epiphysis

In-Toeing

Decision-Making Algorithm
Available @ StudentConsult.com

In-Toeing, Out-Toeing, and Toe-Walking

Femoral Anteversion

Internal femoral torsion or femoral anteversion is the most common cause of in-toeing in children 2 years or older (Table 200-1). It is at its worst between 4 and 6 years of age, and then resolves. It occurs twice as often in girls. Many cases are associated with generalized ligamentous laxity. The etiology of femoral anteversion is likely congenital and is common in individuals with abnormal sitting habits such as *W-sitting*.

Clinical Manifestations. The family may give a history of W-sitting, and there may be a family history of similar concerns when the parents were younger. The child may have *kissing kneecaps* due to increased internal rotation of the femur. While walking, the entire leg will appear internally rotated, and with running the child may appear to have an *egg-beater* gait where the legs flip laterally. The flexed hip will have internal rotation increased to 80° to 90° (normal 60° to 70°) and external rotation limited to about 10°. Radiographic evaluation is usually not indicated.

Chapter 200

LOWER EXTREMITY AND KNEE

Torsional (in-toeing and out-toeing) and angular (physiologic bowlegs and knock knees) variations in the legs are common reasons that parents seek medical attention for their child. Most of these concerns are physiologic and resolve with normal growth. Understanding the natural history allows physicians to reassure the family and to identify nonphysiologic disorders that necessitate further intervention. Physiologic disturbances are referred to as variations; pathologic disturbances are called deformities.

TORSIONAL VARIATIONS

The femur is internally rotated (anteversion) about 30° at birth, decreasing to about 10° at maturity. The tibia begins with up to 30° of internal rotation at birth and can decrease to a mean of 15° at maturity.

Torsional variations should not cause a limp or pain. Unilateral torsion raises the index of suspicion for a neurologic (hemiplegia) or neuromuscular disorder.

Internal Tibial Torsion

Decision-Making Algorithm
Available @ StudentConsult.com

In-Toeing, Out-Toeing, and Toe-Walking

FIGURE 200-1 Thigh-foot angle measurement. The thigh-foot angle is useful for assessment of tibial torsion. The patient lies prone, with knees flexed to 90°. The long axis of the thigh is compared to the long axis of the foot to determine the thigh-foot angle. Negative angles are associated with internal tibial torsion, and positive angles are associated with external tibial torsion.

FIGURE 200-2 Bowleg and knock-knee deformities. A, Bowleg deformity. Bowlegs are referred to as varus angulation (genu varum) because the knees are tilted away from the midline of the body. B, Knock-knee or valgus deformity of the knees. The knee is tilted toward the midline. *(From Scoles P: Pediatric Orthopedics in Clinical Practice, Chicago, 1982, Year Book Medical Publishers, p 84.)*

This is the most common cause of in-toeing in a child *younger* than 2 years old. When it is the result of in utero positioning, it may be associated with metatarsus adductus.

Clinical Manifestations. The child will present with a history of in-toeing. The degree of tibial torsion may be measured using the **thigh-foot angle** (Fig. 200-1). The patient lies prone on a table with the knee flexed to 90°. The long axis of the foot is compared with the long axis of the thigh. An inwardly rotated foot represents a negative angle and internal tibial torsion. If follow-up is warranted, measurements should be done at each visit to document improvement.

Treatment of In-toeing

The mainstay of management is to identify patients who have pathologic reasons for in-toeing and reassurance and follow-up to document improvement for patients with femoral anteversion and internal tibial torsion. It can take until 7 to 8 years of age for correction, so it is important to inform families of the appropriate timeline. Braces (Denis Browne splint) do not improve these conditions. Fewer than 1% of all patients with in-toeing will need surgical intervention because of functional disability or cosmetic appearance.

Out-Toeing

Decision-Making Algorithm
Available @ StudentConsult.com

In-Toeing, Out-Toeing, and Toe-Walking

External Tibial Torsion

External tibial torsion is the most common cause of out-toeing and may be associated with a calcaneovalgus foot (see Chapter 201). This is often related to in utero positioning. It may improve over time, but because the tibia rotates externally with age, external tibial torsion can worsen. It may be an etiologic factor for patellofemoral syndrome, especially when combined with femoral anteversion. Treatment is usually observation and reassurance, but patients with dysfunction and cosmetic concerns may benefit from surgical intervention.

ANGULAR VARIATIONS

Decision-Making Algorithm
Available @ StudentConsult.com

Bowlegs and Knock-Knees

The majority of patients who present with knock-knees (**genu valgum**) or bowlegs (**genu varum**) are normal (Fig. 200-2). Infants are born with maximum genu varum. The lower extremity straightens out around 18 months of age. Children typically progress to maximal genu valgum around 4 years. The legs are usually straight to a slight genu valgum in adulthood.

It is important to inquire about family history and assess overall height. A child who is 2 standard deviations below normal with angular deformities may have skeletal dysplasia. Dietary history should be obtained, as rickets (see Chapter 31) may cause angular deformities. For genu valgum, following the intermalleolar distance (distance between the two tibial medial malleoli with the knees touching) is used. Measurement of the intercondylar distance (the distance between the medial femoral condyles with the medial malleoli touching) is used for genu varum. These measurements track improvement or progression. When obtaining radiographs, it is important to have the patella, not the feet, facing forward. In the child with external tibial torsion, having the feet facing forward gives the false appearance of bowlegs.

Genu Valgum

Decision-Making Algorithm
Available @ StudentConsult.com

Bowlegs and Knock-Knees

Physiologic knock-knees are most common in 3- to 4-year-olds and usually resolve between 5 and 8 years of age. Patients with asymmetrical genu valgum or severe deformity may have underlying disease causing their knock-knees (e.g., renal osteodystrophy, skeletal dysplasia). Treatment is based on reassurance of the family and patient. Surgical intervention may be indicated for severe deformities, gait dysfunction, pain, and cosmesis.

Genu Varum

Decision-Making Algorithm
Available @ StudentConsult.com

Bowlegs and Knock-Knees

Physiologic bowlegs are most common in children older than 18 months with symmetrical genu varum. This will generally improve as the child approaches 2 years of age. The most important consideration for genu varum is differentiating between physiologic genu varum and Blount disease (tibia vara).

Tibia Vara (Blount Disease)

Decision-Making Algorithms
Available @ StudentConsult.com

Extremity Pain
Bowlegs and Knock-Knees

Tibia vara is the most common pathologic disorder associated with genu varum. It is characterized by abnormal growth of the medial aspect of the proximal tibial epiphysis, resulting in a progressive varus deformity. Blount disease is classified according to age of onset:
Infantile (1 to 3 years)
Juvenile (4 to 10 years)
Adolescent (>11 years)

Late-onset Blount disease is less common than infantile disease. The cause is unknown, but it is felt to be secondary to growth suppression from increased compressive forces across the medial knee.

Clinical Manifestations

Infantile tibia vara is more common in African Americans, females, and obese patients. Many patients were early walkers.

Nearly 80% of patients with infantile Blount disease have bilateral involvement. It is usually painless. The patients will often have significant internal tibial torsion and lower extremity leg-length discrepancy. There may also be a palpable medial tibial metaphyseal beak.

Late-onset Blount disease is more common in African Americans, males, and markedly obese patients. Only 50% have bilateral involvement. The initial presentation is usually painful bowlegs. Late-onset Blount disease is usually not associated with palpable metaphyseal beaking, significant internal tibial torsion, or significant leg-length discrepancy.

Radiologic Evaluation

Weight-bearing anteroposterior and lateral radiographs of both legs are necessary for the diagnosis of tibia vara. Fragmentation, wedging, and beak deformities of the proximal medial tibia are the major radiologic features of infantile Blount disease. In late-onset Blount disease, the medial deformity may not be as readily noticeable. It can be very difficult to tell the difference between physiologic genu varum and infantile Blount disease on radiographs in patients younger than 2 years of age.

Treatment

Once the diagnosis of Blount disease is confirmed, treatment should begin immediately. Orthotics to unload the medial compressive forces can be used in children younger than 3 years of age with a mild deformity. Compliance with this regimen can be difficult. Nonoperative management of more severe Blount disease is contraindicated. Any patient older than 4 years should undergo surgical intervention. Patients with moderate to severe deformity and patients who fail orthotic treatment also require surgical intervention. Proximal tibial valgus osteotomy with fibular diaphyseal osteotomy is the usual procedure performed.

LEG-LENGTH DISCREPANCY

Decision-Making Algorithm
Available @ StudentConsult.com

In-Toeing, Out-Toeing, and Toe-Walking

Leg-length discrepancy (LLD) is common and may be due to differences in the femur, tibia, or both bones. The differential diagnosis is extensive, but common causes are listed in Table 200-2. The majority of the lower extremity growth comes from the distal femur (38%) and the proximal tibia (27%).

Measuring Leg-Length Discrepancy

Clinical measurements using bony landmarks (anterior superior iliac spine to medial malleolus) are inaccurate. The **teloradiograph** is a single radiograph of both legs that can be done in very young children. The **orthoradiograph** consists of three slightly overlapping exposures of the hips, knees, and ankles. The **scanogram** consists of three standard radiographs of the hips, knees, and ankles with a ruler next to the extremities. A

Table 200-2	Common Causes of Leg-Length Discrepancy
Congenital	Coxa vara Clubfoot Hypoplasia
Developmental	Developmental dysplasia of the hip (DDH) Legg-Calve-Perthes disease (LCPD)
Neuromuscular	Hemiplegia Disuse secondary to developmental delay
Infectious	Physeal injury secondary to osteomyelitis
Tumors	Fibrous dysplasia Physeal injury secondary to irradiation or neoplastic infiltration Overgrowth
Trauma	Physeal injury with premature closure Malunion (shortening of extremity) Overgrowth of healing fracture
Syndrome	Neurofibromatosis Beckwith-Wiedemann syndrome Klippel-Trenaunay syndrome

FIGURE 200-3 Diagram of the knee extensor mechanism. The major force exerted by the quadriceps muscle tends to pull the patella laterally out of the intercondylar sulcus. The vastus medialis muscle pulls medially to keep the patella centralized. (*Modified from Smith JB: Knee problems in children,* Pediatr Clin North Am 33:1439, 1986.)

computed tomography (CT) scanogram is the most accurate measure of LLD, but also has the highest radiation exposure. Technology such as EOS/slot scanning is an extremely accurate, reduced-radiation alternative to CT scan. The measured discrepancy is followed using Moseley and Green-Anderson graphs.

Treatment

Treating LLD is complex. The physician must take into account the estimated adult height, discrepancy measurements, skeletal maturity, and the psychological aspects of the patient and family. LLD greater than 2 cm usually requires treatment. Shoe lifts can be used, but they will often cause psychosocial problems for the child and may make the shoes heavier and less stable. Surgical options include shortening of the longer extremity, lengthening of the shorter extremity, or a combination of the two procedures. Discrepancies less than 5 cm are treated by epiphysiodesis (surgical physeal closure) of the affected side, whereas discrepancies greater than 5 cm are treated by lengthening. Current use of removable implants, which permit growth modulation without permanent impact on growth plates, has allowed for early and more accurate treatment.

KNEE

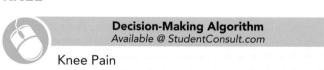

Decision-Making Algorithm
Available @ StudentConsult.com

Knee Pain

The knee joint is constrained by soft tissues rather than the usual geometric fit of articulating bones. The medial and lateral collateral ligaments as well as the anterior and posterior cruciate ligaments maintain knee stability. Weight and force transmission can cross articular cartilage and the meniscus.

The patellofemoral joint is the extensor mechanism of the knee and a common site of injury in the adolescent (Fig. 200-3).

Knee effusion or swelling is a common sign of injury. When the fluid accumulates rapidly after an injury, it is usually a hemarthrosis (blood in the joint) and may indicate a fracture, ligamentous disruption (often of the anterior cruciate ligament [ACL]), or meniscus tear. Unexplained knee effusion may occur with arthritis (septic, Lyme disease, viral, postinfectious, juvenile idiopathic arthritis, systemic lupus erythematosus). It may also occur as a result of overactivity and hypermobile joint syndrome (ligamentous laxity). An aspiration and laboratory evaluation of unexplained effusion can help expedite a diagnosis.

Discoid Lateral Meniscus

Each meniscus is normally semilunar in shape; rarely the lateral meniscus will be disk shaped. A normal meniscus is attached at the periphery and glides anteriorly and posteriorly with knee motion. The discoid meniscus is less mobile and may tear more easily. When there is inadequate posterolateral attachment, the discoid meniscus can displace anteriorly with knee flexion, causing an audible click. Most commonly, patients will present in late childhood or early adolescence after an injury with knee pain and swelling. The anteroposterior radiographs can show increased joint space and a squared-off appearance of the lateral femoral condyle; magnetic resonance imaging (MRI) can confirm the diagnosis. Treatment is usually arthroscopic excision of tears and reshaping of the meniscus.

Popliteal Cyst

A popliteal cyst (**Baker cyst**) is commonly seen in the middle childhood years. The cause is the distension of the gastrocnemius and semimembranous bursa along the posteromedial aspect of the knee by synovial fluid. In adults, Baker cysts are associated with meniscus tears. In childhood, the cysts are usually painless and benign. They often spontaneously resolve, but it may take several years. Knee radiographs are normal. The diagnosis can be confirmed by ultrasound. Treatment is reassurance, because surgical excision is indicated only for progressive cysts or cysts that cause disability.

Osteochondritis Dissecans

Decision-Making Algorithms
Available @ StudentConsult.com

Knee Pain
Extremity Pain

Osteochondritis dissecans (OCD) most commonly involves the knee. It occurs when an area of bone adjacent to the articular cartilage suffers a vascular insult and separates from the adjacent bone. It most commonly affects the lateral aspect of the medial femoral condyle. Patients may complain of knee pain or swelling. The lesions can be seen on anteroposterior, lateral, and tunnel view radiographs. MRI can be helpful in determining the extent of the injury. In young patients with intact articular cartilage, the lesion will often revascularize and heal with rest from activities. The healing process may take several months and requires radiographic follow-up to document healing. With increasing age, the risk for articular cartilage damage and separation of the bony fragment increases. Older patients are more likely to need surgical intervention. Any patient with a fracture of the articular cartilage will not improve without surgical intervention. Patients with OCD should be referred to a specialist.

Osgood-Schlatter Disease

Decision-Making Algorithm
Available @ StudentConsult.com

Knee Pain

Osgood-Schlatter disease is a common cause of knee pain at the insertion of the patellar tendon on the tibial tubercle. The stress from a contracting quadriceps muscle is transmitted through the developing tibial tubercle, which can cause a microfracture or partial avulsion fracture in the ossification center. It usually occurs after a growth spurt and is more common in boys. The age at onset is typically 11 years for girls and 13 to 14 years for boys.

Patients will present with pain during and after activity as well as have tenderness and local swelling over the tibial tubercle. Radiographs may be necessary to rule out infection, tumor, or avulsion fracture.

Rest and activity modification are paramount for treatment. Pain control medications and icing may be helpful. Lower extremity flexibility and strengthening exercise programs are important. Some patients may require immobilization. The course is usually benign, but symptoms frequently last 1 to 2 years. Complications can include bony enlargement of the tibial tubercle and avulsion fracture of the tibial tubercle.

Patellofemoral Disorders

Decision-Making Algorithm
Available @ StudentConsult.com

Knee Pain

The patellofemoral joint is a complex joint that depends on a balance between restraining ligaments of the patella, muscular forces around the knee, and alignment for normal function. The interior surface of the patella has a V-shaped bottom that moves through a matching groove in the femur called the trochlea. When the knee is flexed, the patellar ligaments and the majority of the muscular forces pulling through the quadriceps tendon move the patella in a lateral direction. The vastus medialis muscle counteracts the lateral motion, pulling the patella toward the midline. Problems with function of this joint usually result in anterior knee pain.

Idiopathic anterior knee pain is a common complaint in adolescents. It is particularly prevalent in adolescent female athletes. Previously, this was referred to as chondromalacia of the patella, but this term is incorrect as the joint surfaces of the patella are normal. It is now known as **patellofemoral pain syndrome** (PFPS). The patient will present with anterior knee pain that worsens with activity, going up and down stairs, and soreness after sitting in one position for an extended time. There is usually no associated swelling. The patient may complain of a grinding sensation under the kneecap. Palpating and compressing the patellofemoral joint with the knee extended elicits pain. Patients often have weak hip musculature or poor flexibility in the lower extremities. Radiographs are rarely helpful but may be indicated to rule out other diagnoses such as osteochondritis dissecans.

Treatment is focused on correcting the biomechanical problems that are causing the pain. This is usually done using an exercise program emphasizing hip girdle and vastus medialis strengthening with lower extremity flexibility. Anti-inflammatory medication, ice, and activity modifications may also be helpful. Persistent cases should be referred to an orthopedic or sports medicine specialist.

One must exclude **recurrent patellar subluxation** and **dislocation** when evaluating a patient with PFPS. Acute traumatic dislocation will usually cause significant disability and weight bearing seen in an initial dislocation. Patients with recurrent dislocations often have associated ligamentous laxity, genu valgum, and femoral anteversion. The initial treatment is nonoperative and may involve a brief period of immobilization, followed by an aggressive physical therapy program designed to strengthen the quadriceps and improve function of the patellofemoral joint. Continued subluxation or recurrent dislocation is failure of this treatment plan, and surgical repair is usually necessary.

FOOT

In newborns and non–weight-bearing infants, the difference between posturing and deformity is important. Posturing is the habitual position in which the infant holds the foot; passive range of motion is normal. Deformity produces an appearance similar to posturing, but passive motion is restricted. Most pediatric foot disorders are painless. Foot pain is more common in older children (Table 201-1).

CLUB FOOT (TALIPES EQUINOVARUS)

Decision-Making Algorithm
Available @ StudentConsult.com

In-Toeing, Out-Toeing, and Toe-Walking

A clubfoot deformity involves the entire leg, not just the foot. It affects 1 in 1000 newborns and is bilateral in one half of cases. The tarsals in the affected foot are hypoplastic; the talus is most affected. The muscles of the limb are hypoplastic because of the abnormal tarsal interactions, which leads to a generalized limb hypoplasia, mainly affecting and shortening the foot. There is usually atrophy of the calf musculature.

Etiology
Family history is important. Club foot can be congenital, teratologic, or positional. Although congenital clubfoot (75% of all cases) is usually an isolated abnormality, every infant should be assessed for developmental dysplasia of the hip. Teratologic clubfoot is associated with a neuromuscular disorder, such as myelomeningocele, arthrogryposis, or other syndromes. Positional clubfoot is a normal foot that was held in the deformed position in utero.

Clinical Manifestations
The diagnosis is seldom confused with other disorders (Fig. 201-1). The presence of clubfoot should prompt a careful search for other abnormalities. The infant will have hindfoot equinus and varus, forefoot adduction, and varying degrees of rigidity. All are secondary to the abnormalities of the talonavicular joint. Calf atrophy and foot shortening are more noticeable in older children.

Radiologic Evaluation
In infants, radiographs and advanced imaging are rarely necessary for assessment because their tarsals have incomplete ossification. The navicular ossifies at about 3 years of age for girls and 4 years for boys. As children age, radiographs can be used to follow the tibial calcaneal and lateral talocalcaneal angles and to assess navicular positioning.

Table 201-1	Differential Diagnosis of Foot Pain by Age
AGE GROUP	**DIAGNOSTIC CONSIDERATIONS**
0 to 6 years	Poorly fitting shoes Fracture Puncture wound Foreign body Osteomyelitis Cellulitis Juvenile idiopathic arthritis Hair tourniquet Leukemia
6 to 12 years	Poorly fitting shoes Trauma (fracture, sprain) Juvenile idiopathic arthritis Puncture wound Sever disease Accessory tarsal navicular Hypermobile flatfoot Oncologic (Ewing sarcoma, leukemia)
12 to 18 years	Poorly fitting shoes Stress fracture Trauma (fracture, sprain) Foreign body Ingrown toenail Metatarsalgia Plantar fasciitis Achilles tendinopathy Accessory ossicles (navicular, os trigonum) Tarsal coalition Avascular necrosis of metatarsal (Freiberg infarction) or navicular (Kohler disease) Plantar warts

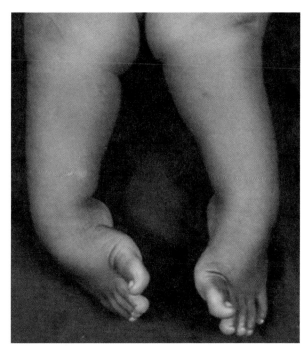

FIGURE 201-1 Clinical picture demonstrating clubfoot deformity. *(From Kliegman RM, Behrman, RE, Jenson HB, et al: Nelson's Textbook of Pediatrics, ed 18, Philadelphia, 2007, Saunders, p 2778.)*

Treatment
The goal of treatment is to correct the deformity and preserve mobility. Nonoperative treatment involves the Ponseti method of serial casting. The Ponseti method also relies on a percutaneous tenotomy of the Achilles tendon to help correct the equinus deformity.

FIGURE 201-2 Clinical picture of metatarsus adductus with a normal foot on opposite side. *(From Kliegman RM, Behrman, RE, Jenson HB, et al: Nelson's Textbook of Pediatrics, ed 18, Philadelphia, 2007, Saunders, p 2777.)*

About 20% of patients will require an anterior tibialis tendon transfer in early childhood. Rarely, more aggressive surgical procedures may need to be done. Complications of untreated clubfoot include severe disability. Complications of treated clubfoot include recurrence and stiffness.

METATARSUS ADDUCTUS

Decision-Making Algorithm
Available @ StudentConsult.com

In-Toeing, Out-Toeing, and Toe-Walking

Metatarsus adductus is the most common foot disorder in infants. It is characterized by a convexity of the lateral foot (Fig. 201-2) and is caused by in utero positioning. It is bilateral in half of cases. Occurring equally in boys and girls, it is more common in first-born children because of the smaller primigravid uterus. Two percent of infants with metatarsus adductus have **developmental dysplasia of the hip**.

Clinical Manifestations

The forefoot is adducted and sometimes supinated, but the midfoot and hindfoot are normal. The lateral border of the foot is convex, while the medial border is concave. Ankle dorsiflexion and plantar flexion are normal. With the midfoot and hindfoot stabilized, the deformity can be pushed beyond a neutral position (into abduction). Older children may present with an in-toeing gait.

Treatment

True metatarsus adductus resolves spontaneously over 90% of the time without treatment, so reassurance is all that is needed. Metatarsus adductus that does not improve within 2 years needs evaluation by a pediatric orthopedist. Persistent cases may benefit from serial casting or bracing, and potentially surgery. The deformity is not associated with a disability.

It is important to differentiate among metatarsus adductus, **metatarsus varus**, and **skewfoot**. Metatarsus varus looks like metatarsus adductus, but it is an uncommon rigid deformity that will need serial casting. Skewfoot is an uncommon deformity that is characterized by hindfoot plantar flexion, midfoot abduction, and forefoot adduction, giving the foot a Z or serpentine appearance. This needs to be managed very carefully with serial casting and surgery to help reduce the risk of disability in adulthood.

CALCANEOVALGUS FOOT

The calcaneovalgus foot is another common foot disorder in newborns that is secondary to in utero positioning. It is characterized by a hyperdorsiflexed foot with forefoot abduction and heel valgus. It is usually unilateral. The appearance may be quite severe dorsiflexion, but it is not a rigid deformity like congenital vertical talus. Simulated weight-bearing radiographs may be necessary for questionable diagnoses. The calcaneovalgus foot will appear normal or have minimal hindfoot valgus.

This disorder requires no treatment beyond reassurance. Parents can be taught passive stretching exercises for their infant's foot. Most affected infants realign by 2 years. A calcaneovalgus foot can be associated with bowing of the tibia, which resolves spontaneously, but a leg length discrepancy may exist.

HYPERMOBILE PES PLANUS (FLEXIBLE FLATFOOT)

Hypermobile or pronated feet are seen in 15% of adults. The child with flatfeet is usually asymptomatic and has no activity limitations. Newborn and toddler flatfoot is the result of ligamentous laxity and fat in the medial longitudinal arch. This is called **developmental flatfoot** and usually improves by 6 years of age. In older children, flatfoot is typically the result of generalized ligamentous laxity, and there is often a positive family history. Hypermobile flatfoot can be thought of as a normal variant.

Clinical Manifestations

In the non–weight-bearing position, the older child with a flexible flatfoot will have a medial longitudinal arch. When weight bearing, the foot pronates (arch collapse) with varying degrees of hindfoot valgus. Subtalar motion (essentially all ankle motion except plantar and dorsiflexion) is normal. Any loss of subtalar motion may indicate a rigid flatfoot, which can be related to tarsal coalition, neuromuscular disorders (cerebral palsy), and heel cord contractures. Radiographs of hypermobile flatfeet are usually not indicated.

Treatment

Hypermobile pes planus cannot be diagnosed until after 6 years of age; before that, it is developmental pes planus. Reassurance that this is a normal variant is very important. Patients who are symptomatic with activity may require education on proper, supportive footwear, orthotics/arch supports, and heel cord stretching.

TARSAL COALITION

Patients with tarsal coalition will usually present with a **rigid flatfoot** (loss of inversion and eversion at the subtalar joint). Coalition is produced by a congenital fusion or failure of segmentation of two or more tarsal bones. The attachment may be fibrous, cartilaginous, or osseous. Tarsal coalition can be unilateral or bilateral and will often become symptomatic in early adolescence. The most common forms of tarsal coalition are **calcaneonavicular** and **talocalcaneal.**

Clinical Manifestations

Decision-Making Algorithms
Available @ StudentConsult.com
Limp
Extremity Pain

The patient will usually present with hindfoot pain, which may radiate laterally because of peroneal muscle spasm. Symptoms are exacerbated by sports, and young athletes can present with frequent *ankle sprains.* There is a familial component. Pes planus is usually present in both weight bearing and non–weight-bearing positions. There is usually a loss of subtalar motion, and passive attempts at joint motion may produce pain.

Radiologic Evaluation

Anteroposterior, lateral, and oblique radiographs should be obtained, but they may not always clearly identify the disorder. The oblique view often identifies the calcaneonavicular coalition. Computed tomography (CT) is the gold standard for diagnosis of tarsal coalition. Even patients with obvious calcaneonavicular coalition on plain radiographs should have a CT scan to rule out a second coalition.

Treatment

Coalitions that are asymptomatic (the majority) do not need treatment. Nonoperative treatment for patients with pain consists of cast immobilization for a few weeks and foot orthotics. The symptoms will often return, necessitating surgery. Surgical excision of the coalition and soft tissue interposition to prevent reossification can be very effective.

CAVUS FOOT

Cavus foot is characterized by increased height of the medial longitudinal arch (**high arch**) and frequently hindfoot varus. It can be classified as physiologic or neuromuscular. Most patients with physiologic cavus foot are asymptomatic. A thorough neurologic examination on all patients with a cavus foot is important. Patients with painful high arches have a high risk of neurologic (tethered cord) and neuromuscular disease, and there is a strong association with **Charcot-Marie-Tooth disease**, a familial neuropathy. The underlying disorder should be treated first. Nonoperative treatment using orthotics is usually not helpful. Progressive, symptomatic cavus foot will likely need surgical reconstruction.

IDIOPATHIC AVASCULAR NECROSIS

Decision-Making Algorithms
Available @ StudentConsult.com
Limp
Extremity Pain

Kohler disease (tarsal navicular) and **Freiberg disease** (head of the second metatarsal) are uncommon and due to avascular necrosis. Patients will present with pain at the affected site with activity and weight bearing. Infection, fracture, and neoplasm should be excluded. Treatment consists of immobilization and activity restriction. The majority of the patients will improve upon subsequent revascularization and re-formation of bone.

SEVER DISEASE (CALCANEAL APOPHYSITIS)

Decision-Making Algorithm
Available @ StudentConsult.com
Extremity Pain

Sever disease is a common cause of heel pain among active young people. The mean age of presentation for girls is about 9 years of age and for boys about 11 to 12 years. Approximately 60% of cases are bilateral. Sever disease is caused by the forces of the calf musculature through the Achilles tendon at the calcaneal apophysis, causing microfracture. As the child ages and the apophysis begins to close, the pain disappears.

Clinical Manifestations

The common presentation is a young athlete who develops heel pain with activity that decreases with rest. Swelling is rare, but limping may be associated with Sever disease. The child will have pain to palpation of the posterior calcaneus and often tight heel cords. Radiographs are rarely indicated, but with persistent pain they should be done to exclude infection or tumor.

Treatment

Activity modification, icing, and anti-inflammatory medications can be helpful. A program designed to improve heel cord flexibility and overall ankle strength may decrease symptoms. Heel elevation using heel wedges or heel cups can be helpful.

TOE DEFORMITIES

Curly toes are the most common deformity of the lesser toes. The fourth and fifth toes are most commonly affected. Curly toes are characterized by flexion at the proximal interphalangeal joint with lateral rotation of the toe. It is caused by contractures of the flexor digitorum brevis and longus tendons. Some curly toes will spontaneously resolve by 3 to 4 years of age. Persistent deformity may be treated by surgical tenotomy.

Polydactyly (extra toes) is usually found on the initial newborn physical examination. When the extra toe is adjacent to the fifth toe and attached by only a stalk of soft tissue or skin, simple ligation or amputation is effective. When the deformity involves the great toe or middle toes, or when the extra digit has cartilage or bone, delayed surgical intervention is indicated. **Syndactyly** (fusion of toes) is more common than polydactyly. It is usually a benign cosmetic problem. Both syndactyly and polydactyly may be associated with malformation syndromes (Table 201-2).

Table 201-2	Disorders Associated with Syndactyly and Polydactyly

POLYDACTYLY	SYNDACTYLY
Ellis-van Creveld syndrome	Apert syndrome
Rubinstein-Taybi syndrome	Carpenter syndrome
Carpenter syndrome	de Lange syndrome
Meckel-Gruber syndrome	Holt-Oram syndrome
Polysyndactyly	Orofaciodigital syndrome
Trisomy 13	Polysyndactyly
Orofaciodigital syndrome	Fetal hydantoin syndrome
	Laurence-Moon-Biedl syndrome
	Fanconi pancytopenia
	Trisomy 21
	Trisomy 13
	Trisomy 18

Chapter 202

SPINE

SPINAL DEFORMITIES

A simplified classification of the common spinal abnormalities, scoliosis and kyphosis, is presented in Table 202-1.

Clinical Manifestations

Decision-Making Algorithm
Available @ StudentConsult.com

Back Pain

Most patients will present for evaluation of an asymmetrical spine, which is usually pain free. A complete physical examination is necessary for any patient with a spinal deformity, because the deformity can indicate an underlying disease. The back is examined from behind (Fig. 202-1). First, the levelness of the pelvis is assessed. Leg-length discrepancy produces pelvic obliquity, which often results in **compensatory scoliosis**. When the pelvis is level, the spine is examined for symmetry and spinal curvature with the patient upright. Cutaneous lesions (hemangioma, skin dimple, or hair tuft) should be noted. The spine should be palpated for areas of tenderness.

The patient is then asked to bend forward with the hands directed between the feet (**Adams forward bend test**). The examiner should inspect for asymmetry in the spine. The presence of the hump in this position is the hallmark for scoliosis. The area opposite the hump is usually depressed because of spinal rotation. Scoliosis is a rotational malalignment of one vertebra on another, resulting in rib elevation in the thoracic spine and paravertebral muscle elevation in the lumbar spine. With the patient still in the forward flexed position, inspection from the side can reveal the degree of roundback. A sharp forward angulation in the thoracolumbar region indicates a **kyphotic deformity**. It is important to examine the skin for café au lait spots (**neurofibromatosis**), hairy patches, and nevi (**spinal dysraphism**). Abnormal extremities may indicate

Table 202-1	Classification of Spinal Deformities

SCOLIOSIS

Idiopathic

Infantile

Juvenile

Adolescent

Congenital

Failure of formation

   Wedge vertebrae

   Hemivertebrae

Failure of segmentation

   Unilateral bar

   Bilateral bar

Mixed

Neuromuscular

Neuropathic diseases

Upper motor neuron disease

   Cerebral palsy

   Spinocerebellar degeneration

   Friedreich ataxia

   Charcot-Marie-Tooth disease

   Syringomyelia

   Spinal cord tumor

   Spinal cord trauma

Lower motor neuron disease

   Myelodysplasia

   Poliomyelitis

   Spinal muscular atrophy

Myopathic diseases

   Duchenne muscular dystrophy

   Arthrogryposis

   Other muscular dystrophies

Syndromes

Neurofibromatosis

Marfan syndrome

Compensatory

Leg-length inequality

KYPHOSIS

Postural roundback

Scheuermann disease

Congenital kyphosis

Adapted from the Terminology Committee of the Scoliosis Research Society, 1975.

skeletal dysplasia, whereas heart murmurs can be associated with Marfan syndrome. It is essential to do a full neurologic examination to determine whether the scoliosis is idiopathic or secondary to an underlying neuromuscular disease, and to assess whether the scoliosis is producing any neurologic sequelae.

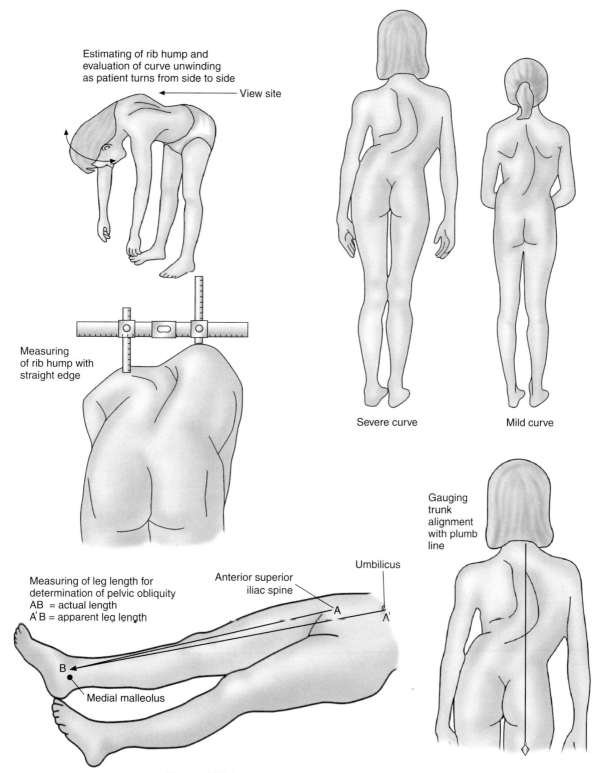

Figure 202-1 Clinical evaluation of a patient with scoliosis.

Radiologic Evaluation

Initial radiographs should include a posteroanterior and lateral standing film of the entire spine. The iliac crests should be visible to help determine skeletal maturity. The degree of curvature is measured from the most tilted or end vertebra of the curve superiorly and inferiorly to determine the Cobb angle (Fig. 202-2). Newer imaging modalities such as slot scanning or EOS provide the ability to obtain accurate measurements with much lower radiation than radiographs.

SCOLIOSIS

Alterations in normal spinal alignment that occur in the antero-posterior plane are termed scoliosis. Most scoliotic deformities

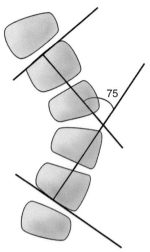

Figure 202-2 Cobb method of scoliotic curve measurement. Determine the end vertebrae of the curve: They are at the upper and lower limits of the curve and tilt most severely toward the concavity of the curve. Draw two perpendicular lines, one from the bottom of the lower body and one from the top of the upper body. Measure the angle formed. This is the accepted method of curve measurement according to the Scoliosis Research Society. Curves of 0° to 20° are mild; 20° to 40°, moderate; and greater than 40°, severe.

are idiopathic. Scoliosis may also be congenital, neuromuscular, or compensatory from a leg-length discrepancy.

Idiopathic Scoliosis
Etiology and Epidemiology
Idiopathic scoliosis is the most common form of scoliosis. It occurs in healthy, neurologically normal children. Approximately 20% of patients have a positive family history. The incidence is slightly higher in girls than boys, and the condition is more likely to progress and require treatment in females. There is some evidence that progressive scoliosis may have a genetic component as well.

Idiopathic scoliosis can be classified in three categories: **infantile** (birth to 3 years), **juvenile** (4 to 10 years), and **adolescent** (>11 years). Idiopathic adolescent scoliosis is the most common cause (80%) of spinal deformity. The right thoracic curve is the most common pattern. Juvenile scoliosis is uncommon, but may be underrepresented because many patients do not seek treatment until they are adolescents. In any patient younger than 11 years of age, there is a greater likelihood that scoliosis is not idiopathic. The prevalence of an intraspinal abnormality in a child with congenital scoliosis is approximately 40%.

Clinical Manifestations
Idiopathic scoliosis is a painless disorder 70% of the time. A patient with pain requires a careful evaluation. Any patient presenting with a left-sided curve has a high incidence of intraspinal pathology (syrinx or tumor). Evaluation of the spine with magnetic resonance imaging (MRI) is indicated in these cases.

Treatment
Treatment of idiopathic scoliosis is based on the skeletal maturity of the patient, the size of the curve, and whether the spinal curvature is progressive or nonprogressive. Initial treatment for scoliosis is likely observation and repeat radiographs to assess for progression. No treatment is indicated for nonprogressive deformities. The risk factors for curve progression include gender, curve location, and curve magnitude. Girls are five times more likely to progress than boys. Younger patients are more likely to progress than older patients.

Typically, curves under 25° are observed. Progressive curves between 20° and 50° in a skeletally immature patient are treated with bracing. A radiograph in the orthotic is important to evaluate correction. Curves greater than 50° usually require surgical intervention.

Congenital Scoliosis
Abnormalities of the vertebral formation during the first trimester may lead to structural deformities of the spine that are evident at birth or early childhood. Congenital scoliosis can be classified as follows (Fig. 202-3):

Partial or complete failure of vertebral formation (wedge vertebra or hemivertebra)
Partial or complete failure of segmentation (unsegmented bars)
Mixed

More than 60% of patients have other associated abnormalities, such as VACTERL association (vertebral defects, imperforate anus, cardiac anomalies, tracheoesophageal fistula, renal anomalies, limb abnormalities such as radial agenesis) or Klippel-Feil syndrome. Renal anomalies occur in 20% of children with congenital scoliosis, with renal agenesis being the most common; 6% of children have a silent, obstructive uropathy suggesting the need for evaluation with ultrasonography. Congenital heart disease occurs in about 12% of patients. **Spinal dysraphism** (tethered cord, intradural lipoma, syringomyelia, diplomyelia, and diastematomyelia) occurs in approximately 20% of children with congenital scoliosis. These disorders are frequently associated with cutaneous lesions on the back and abnormalities of the legs and feet (e.g., cavus foot, neurologic changes, calf atrophy). MRI is indicated in evaluation of spinal dysraphism.

The risk of spinal deformity progression in congenital scoliosis is variable and depends on the growth potential of the malformed vertebrae. A unilateral unsegmented bar typically progresses, but a block vertebra has little growth potential. About 75% of patients with congenital scoliosis will show some progression that continues until skeletal growth is complete, and about 50% will require some type of treatment. Progression can be expected during periods of rapid growth (before 2 years and after 10 years).

Treatment of congenital scoliosis hinges on early diagnosis and identification of progressive curves. Orthotic treatment is not helpful in congenital scoliosis. Early spinal surgery should be performed once progression has been documented. This can help prevent major deformities. Patients with large curves that cause thoracic insufficiency should undergo surgery immediately.

Neuromuscular Scoliosis
Progressive spinal deformity is a common and potentially serious problem associated with many neuromuscular disorders, such as cerebral palsy, Duchenne muscular dystrophy, spinal

Congenital scoliosis

Closed vertebral types
(MacEwen classification)

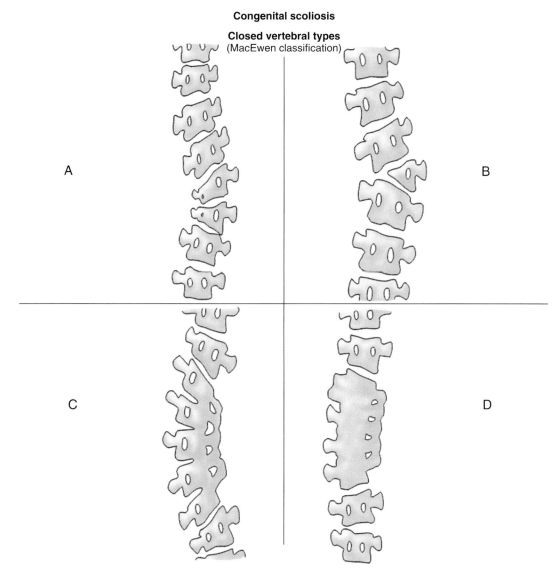

Figure 202-3 Types of closed vertebral and extravertebral spinal anomalies that result in congenital scoliosis. **A,** Partial unilateral failure of formation (wedge vertebra). **B,** Complete unilateral failure of formation (hemivertebra). **C,** Unilateral failure of segmentation (congenital bar). **D,** Bilateral failure of segmentation (block vertebra).

muscular atrophy, and spina bifida. Spinal alignment must be part of the routine examination for a patient with neuromuscular disease. Once scoliosis begins, progression is usually continuous. The magnitude of the deformity depends on the severity and pattern of weakness, whether the underlying disease process is progressive, and the amount of remaining musculoskeletal growth. Nonambulatory patients have a higher incidence of spinal deformity than ambulatory patients. In nonambulatory patients, the curves tend to be long and sweeping, produce pelvic obliquity, involve the cervical spine, and also produce restrictive lung disease. If the child cannot stand, then a supine or seated anteroposterior radiograph of the entire spine, rather than a standing posteroanterior view, is indicated.

The goal of **treatment** is to prevent progression and loss of function. Nonambulatory patients are more comfortable and independent when they can sit in a wheelchair without external support. Progressive curves can impair sitting balance, which affects quality of life. Orthotic treatment is usually ineffective in neuromuscular scoliosis. Surgical intervention may be necessary with frequent fusion to the pelvis.

Compensatory Scoliosis
Adolescents with a leg-length discrepancy (Chapter 200) may have a positive screening examination for scoliosis. Before correction of the pelvic obliquity, the spine curves in the same direction as the obliquity. However, with identification and correction of any pelvic obliquity, the curvature should resolve, and treatment should be directed at the leg-length discrepancy. Thus, it is important to distinguish between a structural and compensatory spinal deformity.

KYPHOSIS

Decision-Making Algorithm
Available @ StudentConsult.com

Back Pain

Kyphosis refers to a roundback deformity or to increased angulation of the thoracic or thoracolumbar spine in the sagittal plane. Kyphosis can be postural, structural (Scheuermann kyphosis), or congenital.

Postural Roundback

Postural kyphosis is secondary to poor posture. It is voluntarily corrected in the standing and prone positions. The patient may also have increased lumbar lordosis. Radiographs are usually unnecessary if the kyphosis fully corrects. If not, radiographs will reveal no vertebral abnormalities. Treatment, if needed, is aimed at improving the child's posture.

Scheuermann Kyphosis

Scheuermann disease is the second most common cause of pediatric spinal deformity. It occurs equally in males and females. The etiology is unknown, but there may be hereditary factors. Scheuermann kyphosis is differentiated from postural roundback on physical examination and by radiographs.

A patient with Scheuermann disease cannot correct the kyphosis with standing or lying prone. When viewed from the side in the forward flexed position, patients with Scheuermann disease will have an abrupt angulation in the mid to lower thoracic region (Fig. 202-4), and patients with postural roundback show a smooth, symmetrical contour. In both conditions, lumbar lordosis is increased. However, half of patients with Scheuermann disease will have atypical back pain, especially with thoracolumbar kyphosis. The **classic radiologic findings** of Scheuermann kyphosis include the following:
Narrowing of disk space
Loss of anterior height of the involved vertebrae producing wedging of 5° or more in at least three consecutive vertebrae
Irregularities of the vertebral endplates
Schmorl nodes
Treatment of Scheuermann kyphosis is similar to idiopathic scoliosis. It is dependent on the degree of deformity, skeletal maturity, and the presence or absence of pain. Nonoperative treatment begins with bracing. Surgical fusion is done for patients who have completed growth, have a severe deformity, or have intractable pain.

Congenital Kyphosis

Congenital kyphosis is a failure of the formation of all or part of the vertebral body (with preservation of posterior elements) or failure of anterior segmentation of the spine, or both. Severe deformities are found at birth and tend to rapidly progress. Progression will not cease until the end of skeletal growth. A progressive spine deformity may result in neurologic deficit. Treatment of congenital kyphosis is often surgical.

Figure 202-4 Note the sharp break in the contour of a child with kyphosis. *(From Behrman RE: Nelson Textbook of Pediatrics, ed 14, Philadelphia, 1992, WB Saunders.)*

TORTICOLLIS
Etiology and Epidemiology

Torticollis is usually first identified in newborns because of a head tilt. Torticollis is usually secondary to a shortened sternocleidomastoid muscle (muscular torticollis). This may result from in utero positioning or birth trauma. Acquired torticollis may be related to upper cervical spine abnormalities or central nervous system pathology (mass lesion). It can also occur in older children during a respiratory infection (potentially secondary to lymphadenitis) or local head or neck infection, and it may herald psychiatric diagnoses.

Clinical Manifestations and Evaluation

Decision-Making Algorithms
Available @ StudentConsult.com

Neck Masses
Stiff or Painful Neck

Infants with muscular torticollis have the ear tilted toward the clavicle on the ipsilateral side. The face will look upward toward the contralateral side. There may be a palpable swelling or fibrosis in the body of the sternocleidomastoid shortly after birth, which is often the precursor of a contracture. Congenital muscular torticollis is associated with skull and facial asymmetry (**plagiocephaly**) and developmental dysplasia of the hip.

After a thorough neurologic examination, anteroposterior and lateral radiographs should be obtained. The goal is to rule out a nonmuscular etiology. A computed tomography (CT) scan or MRI of the head and neck is necessary for persistent neck pain, neurologic symptoms, and persistent deformity.

Treatment

Treatment of muscular torticollis is aimed at increasing the range of motion of the neck and correcting the cosmetic deformity. Stretching exercises of the neck can be very beneficial for infants. Surgical management is indicated if patients do not improve with adequate stretching exercises in physical therapy. Postoperative physical therapy is needed to decrease the risk of recurrence. Treatment in patients with underlying disorders should target the disorder.

BACK PAIN IN CHILDREN
Etiology and Epidemiology

Back pain in the pediatric population should always be approached with concern. In contrast to adults, in whom back pain is frequently mechanical or psychological, back pain in children may be the result of organic causes, especially in preadolescents. Back pain lasting longer than a week requires a detailed investigation. In the pediatric population, approximately 85% of children with back pain for greater than 2 months have a specific lesion: 33% are posttraumatic (spondylolysis, occult fracture), 33% are developmental (kyphosis, scoliosis), and 18% have an infection or tumor. In the remaining 15%, the diagnosis is undetermined.

Clinical Manifestations and Management

Decision-Making Algorithm
Available @ StudentConsult.com

Back Pain

The history must include the onset and duration of symptoms. The location, character, and radiation of pain are important. Neurologic symptoms (muscle weakness, sensory changes, and bowel or bladder dysfunction) must be reviewed. Medical history and family history should be obtained, with a focus on back pain, rheumatologic disorders, and neoplastic processes. The review of systems should include detailed questions on overall health, fever, chills, recent weight loss, and recent illnesses. Physical examination should include a complete musculoskeletal and neurologic evaluation. Spinal alignment, range of motion, areas of tenderness, and muscle spasm should be noted. **Red flags** for childhood back pain include persistent or increasing pain, systemic findings (e.g., fever, weight loss), neurologic deficits, bowel or bladder dysfunction, young age (under 4 is strongly associated with tumor), night waking, pain that restricts activity, and a painful left thoracic spinal curvature.

Anteroposterior and lateral standing films of the entire spine with bilateral oblique views of the affected area should be obtained. Secondary imaging with bone scan, CT scan, or MRI may be necessary for diagnosis. MRI is very useful for suspected intraspinal pathology. Laboratory studies, such as a complete blood count, erythrocyte sedimentation rate (ESR), C-reactive protein (CRP), and specialized testing for juvenile idiopathic arthritis and ankylosing spondylitis, may be indicated.

The differential diagnosis of pediatric back pain is extensive (Table 202-2). Treatment depends on the specific diagnosis. If serious pathology has been ruled out and no definite diagnosis has been established, an initial trial of physical therapy with close follow-up for reevaluation is recommended.

Table 202-2	Differential Diagnosis of Back Pain

INFECTIOUS DISEASES

Diskitis (most common before the age of 6 years)
Vertebral osteomyelitis (pyogenic or tuberculous)
Spinal epidural abscess
Pyelonephritis
Pancreatitis

RHEUMATOLOGIC DISEASES

Juvenile idiopathic arthritis
Reiter syndrome
Ankylosing spondylitis
Psoriatic arthritis
Inflammatory bowel disease

DEVELOPMENTAL DISEASES

Scheuermann kyphosis
Scoliosis (left thoracic)
Spondylolysis
Spondylolisthesis

TRAUMATIC AND MECHANICAL ABNORMALITIES

Hip and pelvic abnormalities (sacroiliac joint dysfunction)
Herniated nucleus pulposus (intervertebral disk)
Overuse injuries (facet syndrome)
Vertebral stress fractures (spondylolysis, spondylolisthesis)
Vertebral compression fracture (steroid, sickle cell anemia)
Upper cervical spine instability (atlantoaxial instability)

NEOPLASTIC DISEASES

Primary vertebral tumors (osteogenic sarcoma)
Metastatic tumor (neuroblastoma)
Primary spinal tumor (astrocytoma)
Bone marrow malignancy (leukemia, lymphoma)
Benign tumors (eosinophilic granuloma, osteoid osteoma)

OTHER

Conversion disorder
Juvenile osteoporosis

SPONDYLOLYSIS AND SPONDYLOLISTHESIS
Etiology and Epidemiology

Spondylolysis is a defect in the pars interarticularis. Spondylolisthesis refers to bilateral defects with anterior slippage of the superior vertebra on the inferior vertebra. The lesions are not present at birth, but about 5% of children will have the lesion by 6 years of age. It is most common in adolescent athletes, especially those involved in sports that involve repetitive back extension. Classically, this was an injury seen in gymnasts and divers. However, with increased intensity and year-round sports, the incidence is increasing. Football interior lineman (extension while blocking), soccer players (extension while shooting), and basketball players (extension while rebounding) are examples of athletes at higher risk. The most common location of spondylolysis is L5, followed by L4.

Spondylolisthesis is classified according to the degree of slippage:
Grade 1: less than 25%
Grade 2: 25% to 50%
Grade 3: 50% to 75%
Grade 4: 75% to 99%
Grade 5: complete displacement or spondyloptosis
The most common location of spondylolisthesis is L5 on S1.

Clinical Manifestations

Decision-Making Algorithm
Available @ StudentConsult.com

Back Pain

Patients will often complain of an insidious onset of low back pain persisting over 2 weeks. The pain tends to worsen with activity and with extension of the back and improves with rest. There may be some radiation of pain to the buttocks. A loss of lumbar lordosis may occur due to muscular spasm. Pain is present with extension of lumbar spine and with palpation over the lesion. Patients with spondylolisthesis may have a palpable *step off* at the lumbosacral area. A detailed neurologic examination should be done, especially because spondylolisthesis can have nerve root involvement.

Radiologic Evaluation

Anteroposterior, lateral, and oblique radiographs of the spine should be obtained. The oblique views may show the classic *Scotty dog* findings associated with spondylolysis. The lateral view will allow measurement of spondylolisthesis. Unfortunately, plain radiographs do not regularly reveal spondylolysis, so advanced imaging may be needed. The most helpful form of advanced imaging among CT, bone scan, single-photon emission CT (SPECT), or MRI continues to be debated. MRI may be required in patients with neurologic deficits.

Treatment
Spondylolysis
Painful spondylolysis requires activity restriction. Bracing is controversial but may help with pain relief. Patients benefit from an aggressive physical therapy plan to improve lower extremity flexibility and increase core strength and spinal stability. It is most beneficial to begin with flexion exercises and progress to extension exercises as tolerated. There is evidence that some patients with an acute spondylolysis can achieve bony union and that these patients have a decreased incidence of low back pain and degenerative change in the low back as they age when compared with spondylolysis patients with nonunion. Rarely, surgery is indicated for intractable pain and disability.

Spondylolisthesis

Decision-Making Algorithm
Available @ StudentConsult.com

Back Pain

Patients with spondylolisthesis require periodic evaluation for progression of their slippage. Treatment of spondylolisthesis is based on grading.

Grade 1: Same treatment as spondylolysis. Failure of nonoperative management may lead to surgical fusion.
Grade 2: Reasonable to try nonoperative management, but if the slippage is progressing, surgical intervention may be needed. Any patient with neurologic symptoms requires surgical intervention.
Grades 3 to 5: Spinal fusion is usually required to prevent further slippage or damage.

DISKITIS

Decision-Making Algorithms
Available @ StudentConsult.com

Back Pain
Stiff or Painful Neck

Diskitis is an intervertebral disk space infection that does not cause associated vertebral osteomyelitis (see Chapter 117). The most common organism is *Staphylococcus aureus*. The infection can occur at any age but is more common in patients under 6 years of age.

Clinical Manifestations
Children may present with back pain, abdominal pain, pelvic pain, irritability, and refusal to walk or sit. Fever is an inconsistent symptom. The child typically holds the spine in a straight or stiff position, generally has a loss of lumbar lordosis due to paravertebral muscular spasm, and refuses to flex the lumbar spine. The white blood cell count is normal or elevated, but the ESR and CRP are usually high.

Radiologic Evaluation
Radiographic findings vary according to the duration of symptoms before diagnosis. Anteroposterior, lateral, and oblique radiographs of the lumbar or thoracic spine will typically show a narrow disk space with irregularity of the adjacent vertebral body end plates. In early cases, bone scan or MRI may be helpful, because they will be positive before findings are noticeable on plain radiographs. MRI can also be used to differentiate between diskitis and the more serious condition of vertebral osteomyelitis.

Treatment
Intravenous antibiotic therapy is the mainstay of treatment. Blood cultures may occasionally be positive and identify the infectious agent. Aspiration and needle biopsy are reserved for children who are not responding to empirical antibiotic treatment. Symptoms should resolve rapidly with antibiotics, but intravenous antibiotics should be continued for 1 to 2 weeks and be followed by 4 weeks of oral antibiotics. Pain control can be obtained with medications and temporary orthotic immobilization of the back.

UPPER EXTREMITY

SHOULDER
The shoulder actually comprises four joints:
Glenohumeral joint (commonly referred to as the shoulder joint)
Acromioclavicular joint
Sternoclavicular joint
Scapulothoracic joint

The glenohumeral joint has minimal geometric stability because the relatively small glenoid fossa articulates with the proportionately larger head of the humerus. The low level of intrinsic stability allows for a large range of motion. The rotator cuff muscles help give the glenohumeral joint more stability, but they need normal contact of the glenohumeral joint to be successful. The scapulothoracic movement also expands the range of motion of the shoulder, but like the glenohumeral joint, it requires strong, coordinated musculature to function efficiently.

Sprengel Deformity
Sprengel deformity is the congenital elevation of the scapula. There are varying degrees of severity; it is usually unilateral. There is restricted scapulothoracic motion (especially with abduction) so most of the shoulder motion is through the glenohumeral joint. There is usually associated hypoplasia of the parascapular muscles. Webbing of the neck and low posterior hairline can be associated problems. There is an association with congenital syndromes, such as Klippel-Feil anomaly, so a thorough history and examination are necessary. Mild forms with a cosmetic deformity and mild loss of shoulder motion do not need surgical correction. Severe forms may have a bony connection (omovertebral) between the scapula and lower cervical spine. Moderate and severe forms may need surgical repositioning of the scapula in early childhood to improve cosmesis and function.

Brachial Plexus Injuries
Obstetric brachial plexus palsy is discussed in Section 11. **Brachial plexopathy** is an athletic injury, commonly referred to as a **stinger** or **burner.** The symptoms are often likened to a *dead arm.* There is pain (often burning), weakness, and numbness in a single upper extremity. There are three mechanisms of injury:
Traction caused by lateral flexion of the neck away from the involved upper extremity
Direct impact to the brachial plexus at Erb's point
Compression caused by neck extension and rotation toward the involved extremity

Symptoms are always unilateral and should resolve within 15 minutes. It is paramount to assess the *cervical spine* for serious injury. Bilateral symptoms, lower extremity symptoms, persistent symptoms, or recurrent injury are all signs of more serious disease and may need a more extensive workup and cervical spine stabilization. Athletes may return to activity if there are no red flags on history or physical examination and the athlete has full pain-free range of motion and strength in the neck and affected extremity.

Glenohumeral Dislocation
Shoulder dislocation is uncommon in childhood but becomes more frequent in adolescence. The younger the patient is at presentation, the more likely it is that the patient will have recurrent dislocation. Anterior dislocation is the most common. If assessment of the neurovascular status of the affected extremity reveals any compromise, urgent reduction is needed to prevent further complications. Patients will need radiographs to assess for fractures of the glenoid (Bankhart lesion) and humeral head (Hill-Sachs lesion). Most patients will require a brief period of protection in a sling or shoulder immobilizer, as well as pain control. As symptoms resolve, a gentle range-of-motion program, followed by an aggressive strengthening program, should be done. Recurrence occurs in nearly 90% of athletes participating in contact sports, so orthopedists consider surgical intervention early rather than awaiting further dislocation.

Overuse Injuries
The incidence of overuse injuries is increasing because of increased opportunities for athletic participation as well as higher levels of intensity during sports. Overuse injuries are inflammatory responses in tendons and bursae that are subjected to repetitive motions and trauma (e.g., rotator cuff tendinopathy in swimmers). These injuries are uncommon in children but may be seen in adolescents. Bony injury, such as physeal fractures and apophysitis, must be ruled out before making the diagnosis of a soft tissue overuse injury. Many overuse injuries in the shoulder, such as rotator cuff tendinopathy, are secondary to joint laxity.

The patient will often present with discomfort over the affected area that worsens with activity. Physical examination usually reveals tenderness to palpation and often weakness of the associated muscles due to pain. It is important to assess for glenohumeral stability. Radiographs may be indicated for acute trauma or when symptoms are not improving. Treatment consists of activity modification, icing, anti-inflammatory medication, and a physical therapy program aimed at strengthening, increasing flexibility, and improving posture.

Proximal Humeral Epiphysiolysis
Proximal humeral epiphysiolysis is commonly referred to as **Little Leaguer's shoulder.** It most commonly occurs in 9- to 14-year-olds who participate in overhead (tennis, volleyball) and throwing sports, particularly baseball pitchers. It is a stress injury that potentially can be a fracture (epiphysiolysis) of the proximal humeral physis. Most patients present with pain during or after throwing. There may be tenderness to palpation over the proximal humerus; if the athlete has been resting for a few days, examination may be normal. Radiographs should include comparison views to assess the physis. There may be widening of the proximal humeral physis in the affected arm, but the films may be normal. Treatment is rest from the offending activity, followed by a rehabilitation program designed to

improve strength in the shoulder muscles. Pitchers should also be encouraged to follow youth pitching guidelines published by Little League baseball.

ELBOW

The elbow consists of three articulations:

Ulnar-humeral joint

Radial-humeral joint

Proximal radioulnar joint

Collectively, these joints produce a hinge-type joint that allows for supination (palm up) and pronation (palm down) positioning of the hand. The elbow has excellent geometric stability, and the musculature around the elbow primarily produces flexion and extension.

Radial Head Subluxation

Decision-Making Algorithm
Available @ StudentConsult.com

Extremity Pain

Radial head subluxation is more commonly known as **nursemaid's elbow**. Because the radial head is not as bulbous in infants and young children, the annular ligament that passes around it can partially slip off the radial head with traction across the elbow (Fig. 203-1). The subluxation is usually caused by a quick pull on the extended elbow when a child is forcefully lifted by the hand or when the child falls while holding hands with an adult. After a subluxation, the child usually holds the hand in a pronated position and will refuse to use the hand or move the elbow. Moving the hand into the supinated position while applying pressure to the radial head will usually reduce the injury. Usually, radiographs are not necessary unless reduction cannot be obtained or there is concern for fracture (swelling and bruising). Once the injury is reduced, the child will begin using the arm again without complaint. Parents should be educated about the mechanism of injury and encouraged to avoid that position. There is a high rate of recurrence for this injury. The problem generally resolves with

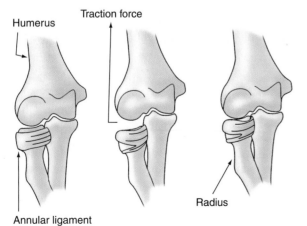

Figure 203-1 Nursemaid's elbow. The annular ligament is torn when the arm is pulled. The radial head moves distally, and when traction is discontinued, the ligament is carried into the joint. *(From Rang M: Children's Fractures, Philadelphia, 1974, JB Lippincott, p 121.)*

maturation, but some children with high recurrence rates may benefit from casting or, rarely, surgical intervention.

Panner Disease

Decision-Making Algorithm
Available @ StudentConsult.com

Extremity Pain

Panner disease is an osteochondritis of the capitellum (lateral portion of distal humeral epiphysis) that occurs spontaneously in late childhood. Clinical features include elbow pain, decreased range of motion, and tenderness to palpation over the capitellum. Radiographs reveal fragmentation of the capitellum. Treatment is activity restriction and follow-up radiographs to demonstrate spontaneous reossification of the capitellum over several months. There is usually no need for further treatment or imaging studies. This is not to be confused with osteochondritis dissecans of the capitellum, which usually will occur in adolescents involved with throwing sports.

Throwing Injuries

The elbow is especially vulnerable to throwing injuries in the skeletally immature athlete. These occur from excessive and repetitive tension forces across the radial aspect of the elbow and compression forces across the lateral aspect of the elbow. These injuries are commonly known as Little Leaguer's elbow.

Decision-Making Algorithm
Available @ StudentConsult.com

Extremity Pain

Although this injury is most common in baseball players who throw frequently (pitcher, catcher, third base, and shortstop), it also occurs in football quarterbacks and tennis players. Patients will usually complain of pain over the medial elbow with throwing that may last for a few days afterward. There may be associated swelling and lateral or posterior elbow pain. Radiation of pain may be secondary to ulnar neuropathy. There is often a flexion contracture of the elbow when compared to the opposite side. Palpation of the medial epicondyle, radial head, capitellum, lateral epicondyle, and olecranon process often reveals tenderness. Ulnar (medial) collateral ligament stability should be assessed. Radiographs should include the contralateral elbow for comparison. Radiographic findings in Little Leaguer's elbow can vary and may include normal anatomy, medial humeral epicondyle apophyseal avulsion fracture, osteochondritis dissecans of the capitellum, radial head abnormalities, and foreign bodies in the elbow. MRI may be helpful.

Treatment depends on the underlying diagnosis but always includes pain control and rest from activity. *Classic Little Leaguer's elbow* refers to medial humeral epicondyle apophysitis. These athletes benefit from rest, ice, anti-inflammatory medication, and a physical therapy program aimed at upper body strengthening. Throwing mechanics and the pitching guidelines published by Little League Baseball/Softball should be reviewed with these players. Switching players to a lower throwing position (e.g., first base) after rehabilitation, to avoid pitching for the remainder of the season, is often recommended.

WRIST AND HAND

Multiple small joints, a delicately balanced intrinsic muscle system, a powerful extrinsic muscle system, dense sensory innervation, and specialized skin combine to make the hand a highly mobile and sensitive yet powerful anatomic part. The extrinsic muscles originate in the forearm and the intrinsic muscles are located in the hand and coordinate small, delicate movements. The movements of opening the hand, extending and spreading the fingers, and then clenching the hand into a fist requires coordinated function of the intrinsic and extrinsic muscles. Tenderness of direct palpation of the bones raises the concern for fracture. **Scaphoid fracture** is the most common carpal bone fracture in the pediatric population. It requires immobilization in a thumb spica cast, whereas displaced fractures require surgical intervention. **Salter-Harris fractures of the distal radius** are also very common. In young gymnasts, there is increased risk for injury at the distal radial physis from repetitive impact and upper extremity weight bearing. This is commonly called **gymnast's wrist** and requires absolute rest from impact and weight bearing to prevent premature closure of the growth plate.

Ganglion cysts are synovial fluid-filled cysts about the wrist. The most common location is the dorsum of the wrist near the radiocarpal joint, followed by the volar radial aspect of the wrist. The defect is in the joint capsule, which allows synovial fluid into the soft tissues with wrist use, where it can become walled off with fibrous tissue. Often, in skeletally immature patients, the process is benign and disappears over time. Large ganglion cysts or cysts that are painful and interfere with function may require more aggressive therapy. Aspiration and steroid injection into the cyst may be helpful, but many will recur. Surgical excision will remove the tract that attaches to the wrist joint, so it is usually curative.

Finger Abnormalities

Polydactyly (extra digits) occurs in simple and complex varieties (see Table 201-2). Skin tags and digit remnants that occur near the metacarpophalangeal joint of the fifth digit and thumb that do not have palpable bones or possess voluntary motion are simple varieties. These may be excised or ligated in the nursery. Complex deformities should be referred to a pediatric orthopedist for amputation. **Syndactyly** (fused digits) are concerning because of the possibility of shared structures and the tethering effects on bone growth (see Table 201-2). All patients with syndactyly should be referred for treatment options.

Trigger thumb and **trigger finger** are secondary to isolated thickening of the flexor tendons. As the thickened nodule enlarges, it may catch in a bent position, then snap or *trigger* straight as it passes through the first pulley that anchors the tendon. Ultimately, as it enlarges, it cannot pass through at all and produces a flexion deformity at the interphalangeal joints. The nodule may be palpable near the metacarpophalangeal joint. These children should be referred for surgical correction.

Chapter **204**

BENIGN BONE TUMORS AND CYSTIC LESIONS

Benign bone tumors and cystic lesions are common in childhood. Some represent fibrous dysplasia. Others are benign bone cysts (unicameral) or benign bone tumors (osteoid osteoma). Subacute osteomyelitis (**Brodie abscess**) and eosinophilic granulomas are lesions not associated with abnormal bone or cartilage growth. Some of these lesions can produce pain, limp, and pathologic fractures. Others can be incidental findings on radiographs. The prognosis is usually excellent. A brief differential diagnosis of bone tumors and their management is listed in Table 204-1. Malignant bone tumors are discussed in Section 21.

Table 204-1	Benign Bone Tumors and Cysts			
DISEASE	**CHARACTERISTICS**	**RADIOGRAPHIC FINDINGS**	**TREATMENT**	**PROGNOSIS**
Osteochondroma (osteocartilaginous exostosis)	Common; distal metaphysis of femur, proximal humerus, proximal tibia; painless, hard, nontender mass	Bony outgrowth, sessile or pedunculated	Excision, if symptomatic	Excellent; malignant transformation rare
Multiple hereditary exostoses	Osteochondroma of long bones; bone growth disturbances	As above	As above	Recurrences
Osteoid osteoma	Pain relieved by aspirin; femur and tibia; found predominantly in boys	Dense sclerosis surrounds small radiolucent nidus, <1cm	As above	Excellent
Osteoblastoma (giant osteoid osteoma)	As above, but more destructive	Osteolytic component; size >1cm	As above	Excellent
Enchondroma	Tubular bones of hands and feet; pathologic fractures, swollen bone; Ollier disease if multiple lesions are present	Radiolucent diaphyseal or metaphyseal lesion; may calcify	Excision or curettage	Excellent; malignant transformation rare

Continued

Table 204-1	Benign Bone Tumors and Cysts—cont'd			
DISEASE	**CHARACTERISTICS**	**RADIOGRAPHIC FINDINGS**	**TREATMENT**	**PROGNOSIS**
Nonossifying fibroma	Silent; rare pathologic fracture; late childhood, adolescence	Incidental radiographic finding; thin sclerotic border, radiolucent lesion	None or curettage with fractures	Excellent; heals spontaneously
Eosinophilic granuloma	Age 5–10 years; skull, jaw, long bones; pathologic fracture; pain	Small, radiolucent without reactive bone; punched-out lytic lesion	Biopsy, excision rare; irradiation	Excellent; may heal spontaneously
Brodie abscess	Insidious local pain; limp; suspected as malignancy	Circumscribed metaphyseal osteomyelitis; lytic lesions with sclerotic rim	Biopsy; antibiotics	Excellent
Unicameral bone cyst (simple bone cyst)	Metaphysis of long bone (femur, humerus); pain, pathologic fracture	Cyst in medullary canal, expands cortex; fluid-filled unilocular or multilocular cavity	Curettage; steroid injection into lesion	Excellent; some heal spontaneously
Aneurysmal bone cyst	As above; contains blood, fibrous tissue	Expands beyond metaphyseal cartilage	Curettage, bone graft	Excellent

Suggested Reading

Herring JA: *Tachdjian's Pediatric Orthopedics*, ed 4, Philadelphia, 2007, Saunders.

Kliegman RM, Stanton BF, St. Geme JW, et al, editors: *Nelson Textbook of Pediatrics*, ed 19, Philadelphia, 2011, Saunders.

Miller MD, Thompson SR: *DeLee & Drez's Orthopaedic Sports Medicine: Principles and Practices*, ed 3, Philadelphia, 2009, Saunders.

Sawyer JR, Kapoor M: The limping child: a systemic approach to diagnosis, *Am Fam Physician* 79:215–224, 2009.

Shipman SA, Helfand M, Moyer VA, et al: Screening for developmental dysplasia of the hip: a systemic literature review for the U.S. Preventive Services Task Force, *Pediatrics* 117:e557–e576, 2006.

Stein CJ, Micheli LJ: Overuse injuries in youth sports, *Phys Sports Med* 38:102–108, 2010.

Wenger DR, Pring ME, Rang M: *Rang's Children's Fractures*, ed 3, Philadelphia, 2005, Lippincott Williams & Wilkins.

Wilson JC, Rodenberg RE: Apophysitis of the lower extremities, *Contemporary Pediatrics* 28:38–46, 2011.

Index

A

AAFP (American Academy of Family Physicians), on immunizations, 318
AAMR (American Association on Mental Retardation) Adaptive Behavioral Scale, 29t
AAP (American Academy of Pediatrics), 64
  on immunizations, 318
ABC (airway, breathing, circulation), for acute illness or injury, 124
ABCDE (airway, breathing, circulation, disability, and exposure) pathway, for trauma patients, 124, 133
Abdomen, of newborn, 200
Abdominal injury, due to child abuse, 71–72
Abdominal mass, due to Wilms tumor, 550
Abdominal muscles, during exhalation, 455
Abdominal pain, 417–422
  acute, 418
    diagnostic approach to, 418, 419t
    differential diagnosis of, 418, 419t–420t
    distinguishing features of, 418, 420t
    onset of, 418
  due to irritable bowel syndrome, 418–422
  functional (recurrent), 418–422
    differential diagnosis of, 420, 421t
    distinguishing features of, 420–421, 422t
    suggested evaluation of, 420–421, 422t
    treatment of, 421–422
    warning signs in, 420–421, 422t
  general considerations with, 418
  referred, 418
  somatic, 418
  somatoparietal, 418
  visceral, 418
Abducens nerve, assessment of, 614
Abduction, 667t
Abnormal uterine bleeding, 243, 243t
ABO blood group incompatibility, 216–217
Abortion(s), adolescent, 2
ABPA (allergic bronchopulmonary aspergillosis)
  vs. asthma, 274
  in cystic fibrosis, 475
ABR (auditory brainstem response), 33
Abscess, 651f
  brain, increased intracranial pressure due to, 640
  breast, 87
  Brodie, 382–383, 693, 693t–694t
  lung, 363
  meningeal, 343t
  peritonsillar, upper airway obstruction, 465t–466t
  renal, 372
  retropharyngeal, upper airway obstruction, 465t–466t

Absence seizures, 620
  atypical, 620
Absolute neutrophil count, in immunocompromised person, 390
Abuse. see Child abuse; Physical abuse
Acanthosis nigricans
  Crouzon syndrome with, 147t
  in type 2 diabetes mellitus, 579
Acapella device, 460
Access, to care, 1, 3
Accessory muscles of exhalation, 455
Accessory muscles of inspiration, 455
Acebutolol, maternal use of, 207t
Acetaminophen
  for analgesia, 145t
  toxicity of, 141t
Acetazolamide, maternal use of, 207t
Acetoacetate, in maple syrup urine disease, 176
Achondroplasia (ACH), genetic basis for, 147t, 148
Acid-base balance, 119
Acid-base disorder, 119–123
  clinical assessment of, 119–120
  metabolic acidosis as, 120–121, 120t
    anion gap in, 120t, 121
    appropriate compensation during, 120t
    clinical manifestations of, 121
    diagnosis of, 121
    etiology of, 120–121
    treatment of, 121
  metabolic alkalosis as, 120t, 121–122
    appropriate compensation during, 120t
    chloride resistant, 122, 122t
    chloride responsive, 122t
    clinical manifestations of, 122
    diagnosis of, 122
    etiology of, 121–122
    treatment of, 122
  mixed, 120
  simple, 119–120
    appropriate compensation during, 120t
Acid-fast mycobacteria, 407
Acid ingestion, due to poisoning, 139
Acid-labile subunit (ALS), 583
Acid lipase deficiency, 181t–182t
Acidemia, 119–120
Acidosis, 119–120
  in acute renal failure, 561
  due to diabetic ketoacidosis, 575
  fetal, 189
  lactic, 121
    due to mitochondrial disorders, 184–185

Acidosis (Continued)
  metabolic, 120–121
  respiratory, 120t
    acute, 120t
    chronic, 120t
    in newborn, 210
ACIP (Advisory Committee on Immunization Practices), 318
Acne, 652–653
  cystic, 652–653
  vulgaris, 652
Acoustic reflectometry, for otitis media, 352
Acquired immunodeficiency syndrome (AIDS), 412–416
  clinical manifestations of, 412–413, 413t
  complications of, 415
  differential diagnosis of, 413
  epidemiology of, 412
  etiology of, 412
  hemophilia and, 529
  laboratory and imaging studies for, 413
  prevention of, 416
  prognosis for, 415–416
  transmission of
    horizontal, 412
    vertical, 412
  treatment of, 413–415
Acquired nevi, 662
Acquired thrombocytopenia, 527
Acrocyanosis, in newborn, 201–202
Acrodermatitis enteropathica, 103t, 105
ACTH. see Adrenocorticotropic hormone (ACTH)
Activated charcoal, for gastrointestinal decontamination, 142–143
Activated partial thromboplastin time (APTT), 524–526, 525f, 526t
  in hemophilia, 529
Acute chest syndrome, in sickle cell anemia, 519, 520t
Acute disseminated encephalomyelitis (ADEM), 345
Acute dystonic reactions, 637
Acute gastrointestinal hypersensitivity, 295t
Acute illness or injury
  common manifestations of, 124
  history of, 124
  initial assessment of, 124
  initial diagnostic evaluation for, 124–125
    diagnostic tests and imaging in, 125
    screening test in, 124–125
  physical examination for, 124, 125t
  resuscitation for, 125–126

Note: Page numbers with "*f*" denote figures; "*t*" tables.

Acute illness or injury (*Continued*)
  cardiopulmonary, 126–127
    airway in, 126
    breathing in, 126
    circulation in, 126
    drugs in, 127
    need for, 124, 125t
    oxygen supplementation for, 125
  warning signs and need for, 124, 125t
Acute labyrinthitis, ataxia due to, 633
Acute life-threatening event (ALTE), 461–462
Acute lung injury (ALI), 128
Acute lymphoid/lymphoblastic leukemia (ALL),
  542
  classification of, 542, 543t
  clinical manifestations of, 542–543
  epidemiology of, 542
  laboratory and imaging studies of, 543
  prognosis for, 544t, 546
  risk factors for, 536t
  T-cell, 542–543
  treatment of, 543–544
Acute myeloid/myelogenous leukemia (AML)
  classification of, 542
  clinical manifestations of, 542–543, 543t
  epidemiology of, 542
  risk factors for, 536t
  treatment of, 546
Acute otitis media (AOM), 351, 352t
Acute phase reactants, in infectious diseases,
  315–316
Acute phase response, in infectious diseases,
  315–316
Acute renal failure (ARF), 561–563
Acute respiratory distress syndrome (ARDS),
  128, 473
Acute retroviral syndrome, 339, 412
Acute stress disorder, 57
Acute tubular necrosis (ATN), acute renal failure
  due to, 561
Acute urethral syndrome, 372
Acute water intoxication, 114
Acyclovir
  for genital herpes, 380–381
  for varicella-zoster virus, 334
Acylcarnitine profile, plasma, 171, 171t
Acylglycine profile, urine, 171, 171t
Adalimumab, for juvenile idiopathic arthritis,
  308
Adams forward bend test, 684
Adapalene, for acne, 652
Adaptive behavior scales, 29t
Adaptive immune system, 252–253
Adderall (Mixed amphetamine salts), for ADHD,
  42t
Addison disease, 611
  clinical manifestations of, 611
  defined, 611
  hypoglycemia due to, 582
  treatment of, 611
Adduction, 667t
ADEM (acute disseminated encephalomyelitis),
  345
Adenoidal hypertrophy, 467
Adenoids, anatomy of, 455
Adenoma(s)
  adrenal, precocious puberty due to, 593–595
  islet cell, hyperinsulinemia due to, 581
  pituitary, 570
  sebaceum, 612, 646
Adenopathy, with anemia, 511
Adenosine
  in cardiopulmonary resuscitation, 127t
  for dysrhythmias, 490
Adenoviruses, conjunctivitis due to, 386

ADH. *see* Antidiuretic hormone (ADH)
ADHD. *see* Attention-deficit/hyperactivity
  disorder (ADHD)
Adjunctive therapy, for meningitis, 346
Adjustment disorder, with depressed mood, 60
Adjuvant chemotherapy, 539–541
Adolescent(s)
  abortions in, 2
  birth rate in, 2
  constitutional delay in, 589, 590t
  defined, 14
  developmental age of, 234, 237t
  eating disorder(s) in, 248–249, 248t
    anorexia nervosa as, 248, 248f
      clinical manifestations and diagnosis of,
        248, 249t
      epidemiology of, 248
      treatment and prognosis for, 248, 249t
    bulimia nervosa as, 248–249, 249t
    issues that can trigger, 248t
    risk factors for, 249f
    slippery slope to, 249f
    treatment and prognosis for, 249t
  genetic assessment of, 155
  interviewing of, 234–237, 237t
    confidentiality in, 234, 237t
    developmental age and, 234, 237t
    on risk-taking behavior, 234
    SCAG tool for, 235f–236f
    STEP guide for, 237f
  leading causes of death in, 234, 234t
  legal rights of, 234, 237t
  medical decision making by, 5
  nutritional issues for, 90
  overview and assessment of, 234–240
  as parents, 77
  physical growth and development of, 13,
    237–240
    for boys, 238–240, 239f
    early, 13
    for girls, 237–238, 238f–239f
    normal variations in, 241–242
      breast asymmetry and masses as, 241,
        241t
      gynecomastia as, 241t, 245–247
      irregular menses as, 241
      physiologic leukorrhea as, 241
  physician-patient relationship with, 20
  prevalence of common chronic illnesses in,
    234, 234t
  psychological growth and development of,
    237t, 241
  psychosocial development of, 14–15
    early, 14–15
    late, 15
    middle, 15
  reaction to divorce by, 83
  sexual maturity rating for, 13
  sexually transmitted infection testing for, 22
  substance use and abuse by, 2
  violence in, 80–81, 81t
  well care of, 240–242
    early, 240
    late, 240
    middle, 240
    pelvic examination in, 240–241
    physical examination in, 240, 240t
Adolescent gynecology, 242–247
  contraception in, 245–247
    abstinence for, 245
    barrier methods of, 247
      condoms and foam as, 247
      sponge, caps, and diaphragm as, 247
    coitus interruptus for, 247
    emergency postcoital, 246, 247t

Adolescent gynecology (*Continued*)
    intrauterine devices for, 246
    oral and anal sex for, 247
    rhythm method (periodic coital abstinence)
      for, 247
    steroidal, 245–247
      combined oral contraceptives for, 245–246,
        245t–246t
      contraceptive patch for, 246
      contraceptive vaginal ring for, 246
      hormonal injections and implants for, 246
      progesterone-only pill or minipill for, 246
  menstrual disorder(s) in, 242–244
    abnormal uterine bleeding as, 243, 243t
    amenorrhea as, 242–243
    dysmenorrhea as, 242, 244
    irregular menses as, 241–242
  pregnancy in, 244–245
    continuation of, 245
    diagnosis of, 244
    termination of, 245
  rape in, 247
Adoption, 78
Adrenal adenoma, precocious puberty due to,
  593–595
Adrenal carcinoma, precocious puberty due to,
  593–595
Adrenal cortex, anatomy of, 607
Adrenal gland
  anatomy of, 607
  physiology of, 607, 608f
Adrenal gland dysfunction, 607–611
  in Addison disease, 611
  in adrenal insufficiency, 608–609, 609t–610t
  in Cushing syndrome, 611
  due to 11-hydroxylase deficiency, 611
  due to 21-hydroxylase deficiency, 609–611
Adrenal hemorrhage, 609
Adrenal hyperplasia
  congenital. *see* Congenital adrenal hyperplasia
  lipoid, 608f
  mild, late-onset, or nonclassic, 608–609
Adrenal insufficiency, 608–609
  clinical and biochemical features of, 608,
    609t–610t
  due to 11-hydroxylase deficiency, 611
  due to 21-hydroxylase deficiency, 609–611
  due to Addison disease, 611
  milder forms of, 608–609
Adrenal steroids
  maternal and fetal, 607
  maternal use of, 207t
  normal variations in, 607
  synthesis and release of, 607, 608f
Adrenal tumor, feminizing, 594t
Adrenarche, 589
  in boys, 238–240, 239f, 589
  in girls, 237–238, 238f–239f, 589
  premature, 596, 593t
Adrenocorticotropic hormone (ACTH)
  in Cushing syndrome, 611
  maternal and fetal, 607
  normal variations in, 607
  physiology of, 607
Adrenoleukodystrophy (ALD), 644
  genetic basis for, 150t
  X-linked, 642t–643t
Adrenomyeloneuropathy, 644
Adriamycin (doxorubicin), for cancer, 540t–541t
Advanced care, 7
Adventitious breath sounds, 458t
Adverse drug reactions, 296–298
  accelerated, 297
  classification of, 296, 297t
  clinical manifestations of, 297

Adverse drug reactions *(Continued)*
   complications of, 298
   defined, 296
   differential diagnosis of, 297
   epidemiology of, 296–297
   etiology of, 296, 297t
   immediate (anaphylactic), 297
   immunologic, 296, 297t
   laboratory and imaging studies for, 297
   late, 297
   nonimmunologic, 296, 297t
   prevention of, 298
   prognosis of, 298
   treatment of, 297–298
   vomiting due to, 423t
Advisory Committee on Immunization Practices
      (ACIP), 318
Advocacy, 5
   with developmental disability, 31t
Aeroallergens, in asthma, 274
Aerosol therapy, 460
Afferent pupillary defect, 614
AFP (alpha-fetoprotein)
   maternal serum screening for, 154
   and myelomeningocele, 647
African tick-bite fever, 398t–400t
African trypanosomiasis, 398t–400t
Afterload, in heart failure, 500, 500t
Afterload reduction
   for cardiomyopathy, 504
   for heart failure, 501t, 502
   for ventricular septal defect, 491–492
Agammaglobulinemia, 256, 258t
   autosomal recessive, 256
   X-linked, 256, 258t
Agoraphobia, 55
AH$_{50}$ test, 268
AIRE (autoimmune regulator) gene, in chronic
      mucocutaneous candidiasis, 261
Airway, breathing
   circulation, disability, and exposure (ABCDE)
         pathway, for trauma patients, 124, 133
   and circulation (ABCs), for acute illness and
         injury, 124, 125t
Airway(s), endoscopic evaluation of, 459
Airway hemorrhage, 474
Airway hyperresponsiveness, in asthma, 273
Airway patency, 126
   in cardiopulmonary resuscitation, 126
   in newborn resuscitation, 194
   in rapid cardiopulmonary assessment, 125t
Airway remodeling, in asthma, 273
Airway resistance, 456, 459
AIS (arterial ischemic stroke), 630–631
Alagille syndrome, 444
Albright hereditary osteodystrophy, 602
Albuterol, for asthma, 276
Alcohol
   acute effects of, 250t–251t
   as teratogen, 206t
Alcohol-induced hypoglycemia, 580t
Alcohol-related birth defects, 79
Alcohol-related neurodevelopmental
      disorder, 79
Alcohol use, during pregnancy, 79
Alcoholism, vitamin and nutrient deficiencies
      with, 97t
ALD (adrenoleukodystrophy), 644
   genetic basis for, 150t
Aldosterone deficiency, clinical manifestations
      of, 609t
Alertness, assessment of, 613
ALI (acute lung injury), 128
Alkalemia, 119–120
Alkali agents, ingestion of, 139

Alkalosis
   hypocalcemia due to, 602
   metabolic, 121–122
   respiratory, 120t
Alkylating agents, for cancer, 540t–541t
ALL. *see* Acute lymphoid/lymphoblastic
      leukemia (ALL)
Allergen, 271
Allergen immunotherapy, for allergic rhinitis,
      284–285
Allergic bronchopulmonary aspergillosis (ABPA)
   vs. asthma, 274
   in cystic fibrosis, 475
Allergic contact dermatitis, 657f, 656
Allergic eosinophilic esophagitis, 295t
Allergic eosinophilic gastroenteritis, 295t
Allergic proctocolitis, 295t
Allergic rhinitis, 282–285
   clinical manifestations of, 282–283
   complications of, 287
   differential diagnosis of, 283–284, 283t
   epidemiology of, 282
   episodic, 282
   etiology of, 282
   laboratory and imaging studies of, 283
   perennial, 282
   prognosis and prevention of, 287–288
   seasonal, 282
   treatment of, 284–285
      immunotherapy for, 284–285
      pharmacotherapy for, 284
Allergic salute, 272, 283
Allergic shiners, 272, 283
Allergy(ies), 653, 657
   allergen in, 271
   assessment of, 271–273
      common manifestations in, 272
      diagnostic imaging in, 275–276
      history in, 272
      initial diagnostic evaluation in, 272–273
      physical examination in, 272
      screening tests in, 272–273, 272t
   atopy in, 271–272
   contact, 657f, 272, 657
   drug, 296–298
      accelerated, 297
      classification of, 296, 297t
      clinical manifestations of, 297
      complications of, 298
      defined, 296
      differential diagnosis of, 297
      epidemiology of, 296–297
      etiology of, 296, 297t
      immediate (anaphylactic), 297
      immunologic, 296, 297t
      laboratory and imaging studies for, 297
      late, 297
      nonimmunologic, 296, 297t
      prevention of, 298
      prognosis of, 298
      treatment of, 297–298
   food, 294
      with atopic dermatitis, 656
      clinical manifestations of, 294, 295t
      complications of, 297–298
      diagnosis of, 206t, 294–296
      etiology and epidemiology of, 294
      laboratory and imaging studies for, 294
      prognosis and prevention of, 298
      treatment of, 297
      vomiting due to, 423t
   hypersensitivity reactions in, 271, 271t
      type I (anaphylactic), 271, 271t, 289
         immediate, 271t
         late-phase, 271

Allergy(ies) *(Continued)*
      type II (antibody cytotoxicity), 271, 271t
      type III (immune complex), 271–272, 271t
         Arthus reaction in, 271–272
         serum sickness in, 271–272
      type IV (cellular immune-mediated, delayed
            type), 271t, 272
   insect, 293–294
      clinical manifestations of, 293, 293t
      complications of, 296
      differential diagnosis of, 293–294
      epidemiology of, 293
      etiology of, 293
      laboratory and imaging studies for, 293
      prevention of, 294
      prognosis of, 296
      treatment of, 296
Allergy skin testing, for asthma, 274
Alper disease, 184
Alpha-antagonists, for ADHD, 42t
Alpha chain hemoglobinopathies, 518
Alpha-fetoprotein (AFP)
   maternal serum screening for, 154
   and myelomeningocele, 647
Alport syndrome, hematuria due to, 558–559
ALS (acid-labile subunit), 583
Alström syndrome, obesity in, 91t
ALTE. *see* Acute life-threatening event (ALTE)
Alternative pathway, of complement activation,
      267–268, 267f
Alternative splicing, 146
Altruism, 5
Alveolar-capillary membrane, gas diffusion
      across, 456
Alveolar cyst disease, 407
Alveolar hemorrhage, 474
Alveolar macrophages, as lung defense
      mechanisms, 456
Alveolar ventilation, 456
Alveoli, 455
Ambiguous genitalia, 606
   approach to infant with, 606–607
   diagnosis of, 607
   due to inadequate masculinization of 46,XY
         male, 605–606, 606t
   due to virilization of 46,XX female, 605, 605t
   normal development and, 604–605, 604f–605f
   treatment of, 177
Amblyomma cajennense, 401
Amblyopia, 31
Amebiasis, 367
Amebic dysentery, 368
Amegakaryocytic thrombocytopenia, 526–527
Amenorrhea, 242–243
   athletic, 591
   in congenital adrenal hyperplasia, 242
   endocrine evaluation for, 242
   history and physical examination for, 242
   in polycystic ovary syndrome, 242
   primary, 592
      defined, 242
      etiology of, 242
   progesterone withdrawal test for, 242
   secondary
      defined, 242
      etiology of, 242
   therapy for, 242–243
   treatment of, 592
   in Turner syndrome, 242
American Academy of Family Physicians
      (AAFP), on immunizations, 318
American Academy of Pediatrics (AAP), 64, 86
   on immunizations, 318
American Association on Mental Retardation
      (AAMR) Adaptive Behavioral Scale, 29t

American dog tick, 401
American trypanosomiasis, 398t–400t
Amino acid(s), in parenteral nutrition, 113
Amino acid disorder(s), 174–177
    of ammonia disposal, 176–177, 176f
        argininosuccinate lyase deficiency as, 177
        ornithine carbamoyltransferase deficiency
            as, 177
        treatment of, 177
    of metabolism, 174
        homocystinuria as, 175, 175f
        maple syrup urine disease as, 176, 176f
        phenylketonuria as, 174–175, 174f
        tyrosinemias as, 174f, 175
    neonatal screening for, 170, 170t
    specialized testing for, 170–171
    that affect specific transport mechanisms in
        kidney and intestine, 177
        cystinuria as, 177
        Hartnup syndrome as, 177
Amino acid profile
    plasma, 171t
    urine, 171, 171t
Aminopterin, as teratogen, 206t
Aminosalicylate drugs, for ulcerative colitis,
    441–442
5-Aminosalicylic acid (5-ASA mesalamine), for
    ulcerative colitis, 441–442
Amiodarone
    in cardiopulmonary resuscitation, 127t
    maternal use of, 207t
Ammonia, in renal function, 553–554
Ammonia disposal, disorders of, 176–177, 176f
Amniocentesis, 155
Amniotic fluid, meconium-stained, 195–196, 214
Amoxicillin
    for endocarditis prophylaxis, 367
    for Lyme disease, 397–400
    for sinusitis, 350
Amoxicillin-clavulanate, for sinusitis, 350
Amphetamines, acute effects of, 250t–251t
Amrinone, for heart failure, 501t
Anabolic steroids, acute effects of, 250t–251t
Anal stenosis, constipation due to, 426t
Analgesia
    epidural, 145
    patient-controlled, 145
Anaphylactic hypersensitivity reactions, 271,
    271t, 289
Anaphylactoid reaction, 288–289
Anaphylatoxins, 288–289
Anaphylaxis, 288–291
    biphasic, 291
    clinical manifestations of, 289–290
    differential diagnosis of, 290–291
    due to insect bites, 293
    epidemiology of, 289
    etiology of, 288–289, 289t
    laboratory and imaging studies for, 290
    prevention of, 291
    protracted, 291
    treatment of, 292f, 291
Anaplasma phagocytophilum, 398t–400t, 401
Anaplasmosis, 398t–400t, 401–402
    clinical manifestations of, 402
    complications and prognosis for, 402
    differential diagnosis of, 402
    epidemiology of, 401
    etiology of, 401
    laboratory and imaging studies for, 402f, 402
    prevention of, 402
    treatment of, 402
Anatomic dead space, 456
Anatomic evaluation, for chronic liver disease,
    449t

Ancylostoma braziliense, 405t
Ancylostoma duodenale, 404, 405t
Ancylostomiasis, infant, 405t
Androgen deficiency, and growth, 584t
Androgen excess, and growth, 584t
Androgen insensitivity, complete syndrome of,
    592, 606
Androgen resistance, complete form of, 606
Androgenic therapy, for Fanconi anemia, 517
Anemia, 104, 509–523
    aplastic, 517–518
        differential diagnosis of, 516t
        etiology and epidemiology of, 517
        Fanconi, 517–518
        idiopathic, 516t
        laboratory studies of, 517
        marrow replacement in, 517
        pancytopenia in, 517–518
        treatment of, 517
    classification of, 509–510, 510f
    clinical manifestations of, 507t, 510–511,
        511t–512t
    congenital hypoplastic, 516t
    Cooley, 518
        clinical manifestations of, 518
        etiology and epidemiology of, 515t, 518
        treatment of, 518
    defined, 509
    diagnosis of
        history in, 511, 511t
        physical examination in, 511, 512t
    differential diagnosis of, 513–523
    drug-induced, 511, 511t
    due to cancer, 539t
    due to chronic kidney disease, 562–563
    etiology of, 509–510, 510f
    Fanconi, 517–518
        clinical manifestations of, 516t, 517
        differential diagnosis of, 516t
        etiology and epidemiology of, 517
        marrow replacement in, 517–518
        treatment of, 517
    hemolytic, 510f, 518–523
        autoimmune
            clinical manifestations of, 522
            etiology of, 510f, 522
            laboratory diagnosis of, 513f, 522–523
            treatment and prognosis of, 523
        due to disorders extrinsic to red blood cells,
            522–523
            clinical manifestations of, 522
            etiology of, 522, 510f
            laboratory diagnosis of, 522–523, 522f
            treatment and prognosis of, 523
        due to enzymopathies, 520–521
            etiology of, 510f
            glucose-6-phosphate dehydrogenase
                deficiency as, 509–510, 513f, 520
            pyruvate kinase deficiency as, 509–510,
                521
        due to major hemoglobinopathies, 518
            etiology of, 510f, 518
            sickle cell disease as, 518–520
            β-thalassemia major (Cooley anemia) as,
                515t, 518
        due to membrane disorders, 521
            clinical manifestations of, 521
            etiology of, 510f, 521
            laboratory diagnosis of, 521
            treatment of, 521
    hypochromic, microcytic, 513–517
        differential diagnosis of, 514t
        due to inflammation, 514t
        due to iron deficiency, 510f, 513–514
            clinical manifestations of, 513

Anemia *(Continued)*
            diagnosis of, 103t, 104, 513f
            differential diagnosis of, 514t
            epidemiology of, 513, 514t
            etiology of, 104, 510f, 513
            pernicious, 101
            prevention of, 514
            treatment of, 104, 513–514
        due to lead poisoning, 514–515
        etiology of, 509–510, 510f
        laboratory studies of, 513f
        thalassemia minor as, 514
            differential diagnosis of, 514t
            etiology and epidemiology of, 514, 515f,
                515t
            laboratory testing for, 514
            treatment of, 514
    of inflammation, 514t, 515
    iron deficiency, 104, 510f, 513–514
        clinical manifestations of, 513
        diagnosis of, 103t, 104, 513f
        differential diagnosis of, 514t
        epidemiology of, 513, 514t
        etiology of, 104, 510f, 513
        prevention of, 514
        treatment of, 104, 513–514
    laboratory studies in, 511, 513f
    macrocytic, 517
        due to marrow failure/pancytopenia, 517
            differential diagnosis of, 517
            etiology of, 517
        etiology of, 509–510, 510f
    microangiopathic, in hemolytic uremic
        syndrome, 560
    in newborn, 216–223
        blood loss, 218
        diagnosis and management of, 218–219
        differential diagnosis of, 216, 217f
        due to blood group incompatibility,
            216–217
        due to decreased red blood cell production,
            216
        due to erythroblastosis fetalis, 216–217
        due to hemolytic disease, 217
        due to increased red blood cell destruction,
            216–218
        etiology, 216
    normocytic, 515–517
        differential diagnosis of, 516t
        etiology of, 509–510, 510f, 515
        treatment of, 515
    pernicious, 101
    physiologic, 216
    screening for, 21
    sickle cell, 518–520
        clinical manifestations of, 519, 520t
        etiology and epidemiology of,
            518–519, 519t
        laboratory diagnosis of, 513f, 520
        treatment of, 520
Anencephalus, 196t
Anencephaly, 647–648
Anergy, in tuberculosis, 408
Anesthetic agents, maternal use of, 207t
Aneuploidy, 157–159
    defined, 157
    monosomies as, 158–159
        defined, 157
        Turner syndrome as, 158–159
    trisomies as, 157–158
        defined, 157
        Down syndrome as, 157
        Klinefelter syndrome as, 158
        trisomy 13 as, 158
        trisomy 18 as, 157–158

Aneurysm(s)
  cerebral, in autosomal dominant polycystic
      kidney disease, 568
  coronary artery, in Kawasaki disease, 303–304
Aneurysmal bone cyst, 693t–694t
Angel dust, acute effects of, 250t–251t
Angelman syndrome (AS), genetic basis for, 153
Angel's kiss, 662
Angina
  Ludwig, 349
  Vincent, 349
Angioedema, 288–291
  acute, 288–289
  chronic, 288–289
  clinical manifestations of, 289–290
  differential diagnosis of, 290–291
  epidemiology of, 289
  etiology of, 288–289
  hereditary, 289, 291t
  laboratory and imaging studies for, 290, 291t
  physical, 288–289
  prevention of, 291
  recurrent, 290, 291t
  treatment of, 291
  upper airway obstruction due to, 465t–466t
Angiography, of pulmonary embolism
  CT, 475
  pulmonary, 475
Angiomas, in Sturge-Weber syndrome,
      662, 646
Angiomatosis, encephalotrigeminal, port-wine
      stain in, 662, 646
Angioneurotic edema, hereditary, genetic basis
      for, 147t
Angiostrongyliasis, abdominal, 405t
Angiostrongylus cantonensis, 405t
Angiostrongylus costaricensis, 405t
Animal dander, and asthma, 275t
Anion gap, in metabolic acidosis, 141t
Anions, in body fluids, 106
Aniridia Wilms tumor association, 159
Ankylosing spondylitis, juvenile, 307t
Anomalous innominate artery, 470
Anorectal malformations, 439–440
  constipation due to, 426t
Anorectal manometry, for Hirschsprung disease,
      440
Anorexia nervosa, 248, 248f
  clinical manifestations and diagnosis of, 248,
      249t
  delayed puberty due to, 591
  epidemiology of, 248
  treatment and prognosis for, 248, 249t
Anovulation, 243
Ant bites, allergic reactions to, 293
Antagonism, of antimicrobial drugs, 325
Antalgic gait, 668
Anterior pituitary gland, 570–571, 571f
Anterior pituitary hormone function testing, 577t
Anterior uveitis, 388t–389t
Anthrax, 398t–400t
Anti-infective therapy, 323–324
  antagonism in, 325
  definitive, 323
  drug-drug interactions in, 325
  drug susceptibilities in, 323
  empirical or presumptive, 323
  oral absorption in, 324
  pharmacokinetic properties of, 324
  site and nature of infection and, 324
  synergism in, 325
Anti-inflammatory medications, for pericarditis,
      505
Anti-Rh-positive immune globulin (RhoGAM),
      218

Anti-*Saccharomyces cerevisiae* antibody, in
      inflammatory bowel disease, 440–441
Antiarrhythmic drugs, 490t
Antibiotic-associated diarrhea, 367
Antibiotic-lock, 395
Antibiotics, 655
  for acne, 652
    oral, 652
    topical, 652
  for cancer, 540t–541t
  for cystic fibrosis, 477–478
  for pneumonia, 364
  topical
    for acne, 652
    for atopic dermatitis, 655
Antibody cytotoxicity hypersensitivity reactions,
      271, 271t
Antibody deficiency disease(s), 256–258
  agammaglobulinemia as, 256, 258t
    autosomal recessive, 256
    X-linked, 256, 258t
  antibody deficiency syndrome as, 257–258,
      258t
  common variable immunodeficiency as, 256,
      258t
    clinical features of, 256
    etiology of, 256, 257f
  IgA deficiency as, 257, 258t
  IgG subclass deficiency as, 257, 258t
  pathogenesis of, 256
  transient hypogammaglobulinemia of infancy
      as, 257, 258t
Antibody deficiency syndrome, 257–258, 258t
Anticholinergics
  for asthma, 276
  toxicity of, 141t
Anticipatory guidance, 23–25, 24t–25t
Anticongestive medications, in truncus
      arteriosus, 498
Antidepressants, for somatoform disorder, 54
Antidiuretic hormone (ADH)
  in regulation of intravascular volume, 106
  in renal function, 553, 555f
  in sodium balance, 112–113
Antiemetic medications, for vomiting, 423
Antihistamines
  for allergic rhinitis, 284
    first-generation, 284
    second-generation, 284
  for atopic dermatitis, 655
  for urticaria and angioedema, 291
Antimetabolites, for cancer, 540t–541t
Antimicrobial therapy, for pneumonia, 360t
Antineutrophil cytoplasmic antibody, in
      inflammatory bowel disease, 440–441
Antinuclear antibody(ies)
  in juvenile idiopathic arthritis, 306
  manifestations of, 303t
  in systemic lupus erythematosus, 309–310
Antioxidant, 101
Antiphospholipid antibodies, and thrombosis,
      531
Antiphospholipid syndrome, maternal, 205
Antiretroviral therapy, for HIV, 415t
Antithrombin deficiency, thrombosis due to, 531
Antithrombin III, in hemostasis, 523
α_1-antitrypsin deficiency, 444
  emphysema due to, 471–472
Anuria, 108
  due to renal disease, 554t
  fluid therapy for, 108, 108t
Anus
  anteriorly displaced, constipation due to, 426t
  imperforate, 439–440
    constipation due to, 426t

Anxiety disorder(s), 55–59
  acute stress disorder as, 57
  common, characteristics of, 55t
  comorbidities, 55t
  diagnosis and differential diagnosis of, 55t
  epidemiology of, 55t
  generalized
    defined, 55–56
    diagnostic criteria for, 56t
  management of, 58
  not otherwise specified, 57
  onset, 55t
  panic disorder, 55
    diagnostic criteria for, 56t
    panic attacks, 55
  post-traumatic stress disorder
    defined, 55–59
    diagnostic criteria for, 57t
  prognosis of, 55t
  treatment of, 58
AOM (acute otitis media), 351, 352t
Aorta
  fetal, Doppler examination of, 189
  overriding, in tetralogy of Fallot, 495
Aortic stenosis, 494
  clinical manifestations of, 494
  etiology and epidemiology of, 494
  imaging studies of, 494
  treatment of, 494
Apgar examination, 194, 194t
Aphasia(s), 613
  acquired epileptic, 621
Apid stings, allergic reactions to, 293
Aplasia cutis congenita, in trisomy 13, 158
Aplastic anemia. *see* Anemia, aplastic
Aplastic crisis(es)
  in chronic hemolytic anemia, 516–517
  in sickle cell anemia, 519, 520t
  transient, due to erythema infectiosum, 333
Apnea, 463–464
  categories of, 463t
  central, 215, 463
  defined, 215, 463
  etiology of, 463, 463t
  mixed, 215
  obstructive, 215, 463
    sleep, 463, 463t
      etiology of, 463
      treatment of, 463–464
  of prematurity, 215–216, 463, 463t
Apnea-hypopnea index (AHI), 463
Apophysis, 667t
Apophysitis, calcaneal, 683
Appearance, of newborn, 196
Appendicitis, 443–444
  abdominal pain due to, 420t
  clinical manifestations of, 443
  etiology and epidemiology of, 443
  laboratory and imaging studies for, 443–444,
      448t
  treatment of, 444
  vomiting due to, 423t
Appendicular ataxia, 631
Appendix testis, torsion of, 569
APTT (activated partial thromboplastin time),
      524–526, 525f, 526t
  in hemophilia, 529
Ara-C (cytosine arabinoside), for cancer,
      540t–541t
Arboviruses, encephalitis due to, 345
Arch, high, 683
ARDS (acute respiratory distress syndrome), 128
ARF. *see* Acute renal failure (ARF)
Argininosuccinate lyase (ASL) deficiency, 177
Ariboflavinosis, 97

Arm recoil, in newborn, 198f
Arm span, 583–584
Arousal, defined, 634
Arrhythmias. *see* Dysrhythmia(s)
Artemis gene, in severe combined immunodeficiency, 260
Arterial blood gas, with respiratory failure, 128
Arterial blood gas analysis, 459
Arterial clots, 524
Arterial ischemic stroke (AIS), 630–631
Arterial partial pressure of carbon dioxide (PaCO$_2$), in newborns, 209–210
Arterial partial pressure of oxygen (PaO$_2$), in newborns, 209–210
Arterial switch, in transposition of the great arteries, 497
Arthralgias, in systemic lupus erythematosus, 309
Arthritis
    due to rheumatic fever, 502
    in Henoch-Schönlein purpura, 302–303
    infectious (suppurative, septic), 384–386
        clinical manifestations of, 384–385
        complications and prognosis for, 389
        differential diagnosis of, 308t, 385–386
        epidemiology of, 384
        etiology of, 384, 384t
        laboratory and imaging studies of, 385
        prevention of, 389
        treatment of, 387–389, 388t–389t
    in juvenile dermatomyositis, 313
    juvenile idiopathic. *see* Juvenile idiopathic arthritis (JIA)
    Lyme, 385t
    poststreptococcal, 307t
    reactive, 308t, 384–385, 384t–385t
    in rheumatic diseases, 299
    in systemic lupus erythematosus, 309
Arthritis-dermatitis syndrome, 384
Arthrocentesis, for juvenile idiopathic arthritis, 307
Arthrogryposis multiplex congenita, 162
Arthroplasty, 667t
Arthroscopy, 667t
Arthrotomy, 667t
Arthus reaction, 271–272
Articular cartilage, 668f
Articulation disorders, 34–35
Artificial airway, 460
Arylsulfatase A deficiency, 181t–182t
Arytenoid cartilages, anatomy of, 455
AS (Angelman syndrome), genetic basis for, 153
5-ASA (5-aminosalicylic acid), for ulcerative colitis, 441–442
Ascariasis, 405
    intestinal, 405t
    pulmonary, 405
Ascaris lumbricoides, 405, 405t
Ascites
    with chronic liver disease, 448, 448t
    urinary, 566
Ascorbic acid deficiency, 96–97, 99t–100t
ASD. *see* Atrial septal defect (ASD)
ASD(s) (autism spectrum disorders), 63
Ash leaf spots, 646
Asparaginase, for cancer, 540t–541t
Aspartylglucosaminidase deficiency, 181t–182t
Aspartylglycosaminuria, 181t–182t
Aspergillosis, allergic bronchopulmonary
    vs. asthma, 274
    in cystic fibrosis, 475
Aspergillus, 475
Asphyxia
    intrauterine, 194
    in newborn
        effects of, 191, 193t

Asphyxia *(Continued)*
    etiology of, 192, 194t
    hypoxic-ischemic injury due to, 191
    metabolic acidosis due to, 191
    pallida, 202
Aspiration, of foreign body, 470–471
    clinical manifestations of, 471
    diagnostic studies for, 471
    epidemiology of, 470–471
    prevention of, 471
Aspirin
    for Kawasaki disease, 304–305
    maternal use of, 207t
Association, in dysmorphology, 161
Asthma, 273–282, 470
    cardiogenic, 359
    clinical manifestations of, 273–274
    complications of, 278, 280f
    diagnosis of, 470
    differential diagnosis of, 274, 274t–275t
        vs. bronchiolitis, 359
    epidemiology of, 273
    etiology of, 273
    factors contributing to severity of, 273–274, 275t
    laboratory and imaging studies of, 274
    monitoring of, 279, 281f
    persistent, 282t, 276, 277f
    prevention of, 279–282, 281f
    prognosis for, 282t, 278–279
    respiratory failure due to, 128
    status asthmaticus in, 278
    treatment of, 274–276
        approach to, 276
            stepwise, 276, 277f–278f
        for exacerbations, 276, 277f
        long-term control medications in, 275–276
            inhaled corticosteroids as, 275–276, 279f
            leukotriene modifiers as, 275–276
            long-acting β$_2$-agonists as, 276
            omalizumab, 276
            theophylline, 276
        minimizing allergen exposure in, 274–275, 275t
        quick-relief medications in, 276
            anticholinergic agents as, 276
            oral corticosteroids as, 276
            short-acting β$_2$-agonists as, 276
        rule of twos for, 276
        self-management guidelines in, 279, 281f
            adherence in, 282
            peak flow monitoring in, 279–282
            written action plan in, 282, 280f
    triad, 284
Astrocytoma
    prognosis for, 549t
    subependymal giant cell, 646
Asymmetric tonic neck reflex, 13
Ataxia, 615
    appendicular, 631
    clinical manifestations of, 631–632
    defined, 631–633
    with developmental disabilities, 28t
    due to acute labyrinthitis, 633
    due to brain tumors, 633
    due to drug intoxication, 632
    due to inborn errors of metabolism, 633
    due to neuroblastoma, 633
    due to paraneoplastic opsoclonus-myoclonus syndrome, 633
    etiology of, 632–633
    Friedreich, 633
        genetic basis for, 150t
    inherited syndromes, 632t
    postinfectious acute cerebellar, 632–633
    truncal, 631

Ataxia-telangiectasia, 260–261, 261t, 633
Atelectasis, 458t
    in respiratory distress syndrome, 211
Atenolol, maternal use of, 207t
Athetosis, 637
Athlete's foot, 337t
Athletic amenorrhea, 591
ATM gene, in ataxia-telangiectasia, 260–261
ATN (acute tubular necrosis), acute renal failure due to, 561
Atomoxetine (Strattera), for ADHD, 42t
Atonic seizures, 620
Atopic dermatitis, 285–288, 653–656
    with bacterial superinfection, 655–656, 655f
    clinical manifestations of, 285–286, 285f, 653–654, 653f–654f
    complications of, 287, 655–656, 655f
    differential diagnosis of, 286–287, 286t, 654
    epidemiology of, 285, 653
    etiology of, 285, 653
    laboratory and imaging studies for, 286, 286t, 654
    lichenified plaques in, 285–286, 286f
    prevention of, 656, 287–288
    prognosis for, 656, 287
    treatment of, 287, 654–655
Atopic march, 653
Atopy, 271–272
Atrial contractions, premature, 489
Atrial dysrhythmias, 489
Atrial fibrillation, 489
Atrial flutter, 489, 490t
Atrial natriuretic peptide, in regulation of sodium balance, 106–107
Atrial pacemaker, wandering, 489
Atrial septal defect (ASD), 492, 492f
Atrioventricular canal defects, 493, 493f
Atrophy, 651t
Atropine, in cardiopulmonary resuscitation, 127t
Attachment, 79
    in infancy, 14
Attention-deficit/hyperactivity disorder (ADHD), 41–42
    clinical manifestations of, 41
    complications of, 42
    defined, 41
    differential diagnosis of, 41
    epidemiology of, 41
    etiology of, 41
    obsessive-compulsive disorder and, 62
    prevention of, 42
    treatment of, 41–42
Atypical depression, 60
Auditory brainstem response (ABR), 33
Aura, migraine, 617
Auscultation, 482
    of clicks, 482
    of heart murmurs, 481
        continuous, 484
        diastolic, 484
        ejection, 482–483
        frequency/pitch, 483
        holosystolic (pansystolic, regurgitation), 482–483
        intensity, 483t
        normal or innocent, 484, 484t
        systolic, 482–483
    of heart sounds, 482
Auspitz sign, in psoriasis, 658
Autism, 63–64
    comorbidities with, 64
    diagnostic criteria for, 65t
    etiology of, 64
    screening for, 18–19, 64

Autism spectrum disorders (ASDs), 63
Autoantibodies
    manifestations of, 303t
    in systemic lupus erythematosus, 309
Autocrine action, of hormones, 570, 570f
Autoimmune hemolytic anemia
    etiology of, 510f
    laboratory diagnosis of, 513f
Autoimmune hepatitis, 450, 449t
Autoimmune polyglandular syndrome, 599
Autoimmune regulator (*AIRE*) gene, in chronic
    mucocutaneous candidiasis, 261
Autoimmune thyroiditis, 599
    with diabetes mellitus, 578
Autologous stem cell rescue, for neuroblastoma,
    549
Autonomic dysfunction, in Guillain-Barré
    syndrome, 625
Autonomy, 5
    in early childhood, 14
    in end-of-life decision making, 9
Autosomal dominant (AD) inheritance, 147–148,
    147t
    achondroplasia due to, 147t
    Crouzon syndrome with acanthosis nigricans
        due to, 147t
    defined, 147
    hereditary angioneurotic edema due to, 147t
    of inborn errors of metabolism, 169
    Marfan syndrome due to, 147t
    myotonic dystrophy due to, 147t
    neurofibromatosis 1 due to, 147t
    neurofibromatosis 2 due to, 147t
    nonsyndromic craniosynostosis due to, 147t
    pedigree drawing of, 148f
    penetrance in, 147, 148f
    rules of, 148t
    thanatophoric dysplasia due to, 147t
    variable expressivity of, 147
Autosomal recessive agammaglobulinemia, 256
Autosomal recessive (AR) inheritance, 148–149
    congenital adrenal hyperplasia due to, 150t
    consanguinity and, 154
    cystic fibrosis due to, 150t
    defined, 148
    Friedreich ataxia due to, 150t
    Gaucher disease due to, 150t
    of inborn errors of metabolism, 169
    pedigree drawing of, 150f
    phenylketonuria due to, 150t
    rules of, 150t
    sickle cell disease due to, 150t
Autosomes, 146
Avascular necrosis, idiopathic, 683
Avian influenza, 359
Azathioprine, for ulcerative colitis, 441–442
Azelaic acid, for acne, 652
Azithromycin
    for *Chlamydia* infection, 380
    for streptococcal pharyngitis, 349t

B
B-cell disorder(s)
    antibody deficiency disease(s) due to,
        256–258
        agammaglobulinemia as, 256, 258t
            autosomal recessive, 256
            X-linked, 256, 258t
        antibody deficiency syndrome as, 257–258,
            258t
        common variable immunodeficiency as,
            256, 258t
            clinical features of, 256
            etiology of, 256, 257f
        IgA deficiency as, 257, 258t

B-cell disorder(s) (*Continued*)
        IgG subclass deficiency as, 257, 258t
        pathogenesis of, 256
        transient hypogammaglobulinemia of
            infancy as, 257, 258t
β₂-agonists, for asthma
    long-acting, 276
    short-acting, 276
β-blockers, for heart failure, 502
Babesia, 396, 398t–400t
Babesiosis, 398t–400t
Babinski reflex, 613t
Babinski response, 615
Babinski sign, 200–201
Baby bottle caries, 429
Bacillary fever, 398t–400t
Bacillus anthracis, 398t–400t
Back pain, 689, 689t
Back to Sleep initiative, 23
Back-to-sleep program, 462–463
Bacteremia, 374
    catheter-associated, 395
    fever and, 324–325
    in nephrotic syndrome, 557–558
    occult, 325
    zoonotic, 398t–400t
Bacterial colonization, of newborn, 191
Bacterial diarrhea, fever due to, 325
Bacterial diseases, zoonotic, 398t–400t
Bacterial enteritis, GI bleeding due to, 427t
Bacterial gastroenteritis, vomiting due to, 423t
Bacterial infection(s)
    in immunocompromised person, 390
    superficial, 335–336
        cellulitis as, 335–336
        folliculitis as, 336
        impetigo as, 335
        perianal dermatitis as, 336
    viral *vs.*, 317, 325
Bacterial meningitis, 641
Bacterial tracheitis, upper airway obstruction due
    to, 465t–466t
Bacterial vaginosis, 374, 375t, 377t–378t
Bag/mask ventilation, for respiratory failure, 126,
    131
Baker cyst, 679–680
Balloon angioplasty, for coarctation of the aorta,
    494
Balloon atrial septostomy, for transposition of the
    great arteries, 497
Balloon valvuloplasty
    for aortic stenosis, 494
    for pulmonary stenosis, 494
Balsalazide, for ulcerative colitis, 441–442
Barbiturates, maternal use of, 207t
Bare lymphocyte syndrome, 259t, 260
Barium enema, for Hirschsprung disease,
    440
Barium esophagram, 458
Barium upper gastrointestinal series, for
    gastroesophageal reflux, 431
Barlow test, 200, 673, 673f
Bart hemoglobin, 518
Bartonella henselae, 339–340, 398t–400t
Bartter syndrome, hypokalemia in, 116
Basilar artery migraines, 637
Basophilic stippling, due to lead poisoning,
    514–515
Batten disease, 181t–182t
Batteries, ingestion of, 139
Battle sign, 638
Bayley Scales of Infant Development (3rd ed),
    29t
Baylisascaris procyonis, 405, 405t
Becker muscular dystrophy, 627

Beckwith-Wiedemann syndrome, 162
    hypoglycemia in, 580–581
    omphalocele in, 439
Beclomethasone HFA, for asthma, 279f
Bed bug bites, anaphylaxis due to, 293
Bee stings, allergic reactions to, 293
Behavioral assessment, issues in, 19–20
Behavioral complications, of hearing impairment,
    33t
Behavioral issues, evaluation of, 20
Behavioral management, of ADHD, 41–42
Behavioral problems
    context of, 19, 19t
    with developmental disability, 31t
    screening for, 16
Behavioral training, for functional constipation,
    45–46
Behaviors, controlling undesirable, 23,
    24t–25t
Bell palsy, 614
Beneficence, 5
    in end-of-life decision making, 9
Benzathine penicillin
    for rheumatic fever, 502
    for streptococcal pharyngitis, 349t
Benzodiazepines, 58–59, 82
    maternal use of, 207t
    for status epilepticus, 621–622, 622t
Benzoyl peroxide, for acne, 652
Bereavement, 8, 82–85
Beriberi, 97, 98t
Bernard-Soulier syndrome, 528
Beta cells, in insulin-dependent diabetes mellitus,
    573
Beta chain hemoglobinopathies, 518
Bi-level positive airway pressure (BiPAP),
    463–464
Bicarbonate, in cardiopulmonary resuscitation,
    127t
Bidirectional cavopulmonary shunt for tricuspid
    atresia, 497
Bidirectional Glenn procedure, for tricuspid
    atresia, 497
Bilharziasis, 406–407
Biliary atresia, 444, 448
Bilirubin
    in breastfed infants, 86–87
    direct conjugated, 219
    in fetus, 219
    indirect unconjugated, 219
    production of, 219
Bilirubin diglucuronide, 219
Bilirubin encephalopathy, 220–221
Biliverdin, 219
Biophysical profile, of fetus, 189
Biopsy
    lung, 460
        transbronchial, 459
    rectal, for Hirschsprung disease, 440
    renal, for acute renal failure, 561
    small bowel, for celiac disease, 442
Biopsychosocial influences, on health and illness,
    3
Biopterin metabolism, disorders in, 174
Biot respiration, 457t
Biotin deficiency, 98t–100t
Biotinidase deficiency, 178–179
    clinical manifestations of, 179
    treatment of, 179
Biotinidase deficiency, neonatal screening for,
    170, 170t
Bipolar disorder (BD), 59–62
    and cyclothymic disorder, 61
    differential diagnosis for, 61
    etiology of, 61

Bipolar disorder (BD) *(Continued)*
  hypomania, 60–61
  mania in, 59t
  not otherwise specified, 61
  with psychotic features, 62, 66
  and suicide, 60
  treatment of, 61
  type II, 61
Bird flu, 359
Birth(s)
  demographics of, 2
  history of, in genetic assessment, 156
Birth injury, 202–203
Birth rate, in adolescents, 2
Birth weight
  low, 188
  very low, 188
Birthmarks, 659, 659t
Births, preterm, 187
bis-chloronitrosourea (BCNU, carmustine, nitrosourea), for cancer, 540t–541t
Bisacodyl, for functional constipation, 47t
Black-legged tick, 396
Blackfly bites, anaphylaxis due to, 293
Blackhead, 652
Blackwater fever, 404
Bladder, neurogenic, vesicoureteral reflux due to, 565
Bladder outlet obstruction, 566
Bladder stones, 567
Blalock-Taussig procedure, for tricuspid atresia, 497
Bleeding
  gastrointestinal, 426–429
  in hematologic disorders, 506
  in hemophilia, 529
  sites of, in hemostatic disorders, 524
Bleeding disorders. *see* Hemostatic disorder(s)
Bleeding time, 524–526, 526t
Bleomycin, for cancer, 540t–541t
Blepharitis, 387, 388t–389t
Blindness, legal, 31
Blister cells, 513f
Blood-brain barrier, chemotherapy and, 541
Blood component therapy, 532–533
  products used in, 532, 532t
  transfusion reactions from, 532–533, 532t
Blood cultures, for infectious diseases, 317
Blood gas analysis, for respiratory distress in newborns, 209–210
Blood glucose testing, for type 1 diabetes, 577–578
Blood group sensitization, maternal, 205t
Blood loss, anemia due to, 511
  in newborn, 218
Blood oxygenation, transition from fetal to newborn, 189–190, 191f
Blood pressure, classification of, 564t
Blood smear, 526t
Blood transfusion, 532–533
  products used in, 532, 532t
  transfusion reactions from, 532–533, 532t
Blood urea nitrogen (BUN), 109, 555
  in acute renal failure, 562
Blood volume, 106
  of newborn, 216
Bloodstream infection, catheter-related, 394
Blount disease, 678
Blue cohosh herbal tea, maternal use of, 207t
BMI. *see* Body mass index (BMI)
BMI age-specific and gender-specific percentile curves, 91
Body composition, fluids and electrolytes in, 106, 107f
Body dysmorphic disorder (BDD), 53–54
  vs. obsessive-compulsive disorder, 64

Body lice, 665
Body mass index (BMI)
  defined, 10
  growth chart for, 11f
  interpretation of, 91t
  and obesity, 91, 91t
Body plethysmography, 459
Body temperature
  instability of, in infants younger than 3 months, 325
  in newborn, 203
  normal, 324
  regulation of, 324
Boil, 336
Bonding, in infancy, 14
Bone(s)
  growth and development of, 667, 668f
  structure of, 668f
Bone cysts, 693–694, 693t–694t
  aneurysmal, 693t–694t
  unicameral (simple), 693t–694t
Bone marrow abnormalities, due to lysosomal storage diseases, 181t–182t
Bone marrow aspiration, for cancer, 542t
Bone marrow examination, for hematologic disorders, 506
Bone marrow failure, 517
  pancytopenia due to, 527
Bone marrow replacement, 517–518
Bone mineral accretion, 103
Bone mineralization, parathyroid hormone and vitamin D in, 602
Bone mineralization diseases, 602–603
  hypocalcemia as, 602–603
  physiologic changes in, 603t
  rickets as, 603
Bone morphogenetic receptor-2 (BMPR2) gene, 473
Bone scan, for cancer, 542t
Bone tumors, 693–694, 693t–694t
Bordetella parapertussis, 356
Bordetella pertussis, 356
Borellia lonestari, 397, 398t–400t
Borrelia, relapsing fever due to, 398t–400t
Bottle mouth, 429
Botulism, infant, 627
Boutonneuse fever, 398t–400t
Bowing fracture, 670
Bowlegs, 677, 677f
Boys, growth and development of, 238–240
BPD (bronchopulmonary dysplasia), 213–214
Brachial plexopathy, 691
Brachial plexus injuries, 691
  in newborn, 202–203
Brachycephaly, 161t
Brachydactyly, 161t
Bradycardia, fetal, 189
Brain, congenital malformations of, 647–649
Brain abscess, increased intracranial pressure due to, 640
Brain cell swelling, in hyponatremia, 114
Brain diseases, and degenerative diseases, 645
Brain hemorrhage, due to hypernatremia, 115
Brain herniations, 636–637, 636t
  bilateral, 636t
  cerebellar, 636t
  subfalcian, 636t
  transtentorial, 636–637, 636t
  uncal, 636–637, 636t
Brain injury, traumatic. *see* Head trauma
Brain swelling, diffuse, 641
Brain tumor(s), 546–548
  ataxia due to, 633
  clinical manifestations of, 546–547
  complications of, 547

Brain tumor(s) *(Continued)*
  differential diagnosis of, 547
  epidemiology of, 546
  etiology of, 546
  increased intracranial pressure due to, 547, 640
  laboratory/imaging studies of, 547, 547f
  primary, 546
  prognosis for, 547–548, 549t
  secondary, 546
  treatment of, 547
  vomiting due to, 423t
Brainstem glioma, prognosis for, 548, 548t
Branched chain amino acids, metabolism of, 176f
Branched chain ketoaciduria, 176
Branching enzyme, 172, 172t, 173f
Breast, of newborn, 197f
Breast abscess, 87
Breast milk, composition of, 88–89, 88t
Breast milk jaundice, 86–87
Breast tenderness, 87
Breastfeeding, 86–88
  adequacy of, 86
  advantages of, 86
  common problems with, 87
  composition of breast milk in, 88–89, 88t
  contraindications and recommendations for, 87t
  demographics of, 87f
  engorgement with, 87
  exclusive, 89
  initiation and maintenance of, 2, 86, 87f
  jaundice with, 86–87
  maternal drug use and, 88
  and micronutrient deficiency, 97t
  for prevention of obesity, 92
  and rickets, 102
  stools with, 86
Breastfeeding jaundice, 86–87
Breath-holding spells, 463t
Breath sounds, 458t
Breathing, 126
  in cardiopulmonary resuscitation, 126
  control of, 461–464, 461f
    disorder(s) of, 461–464, 463t
      acute life-threatening event as, 461–462
      apnea as, 463–464, 463t
      SIDS as, 462–463, 462t
  neonatal onset of, 191
  in newborn resuscitation, 194–195
  work of, 457
Breathing patterns, 457t
Bridging therapy, in juvenile idiopathic arthritis, 308
Brief psychotic disorder, 66
Bright Futures, 20–23
Brill-Zinsser disease, 398t–400t
Broca aphasia, 613
Brodie abscess, 382–383, 693
Bromides, maternal use of, 207t
Bronchial breath sounds, 458t
Bronchiectasis, 363, 469
  in Kartagener syndrome, 472
Bronchiolitis, 357–358, 471
  clinical manifestations of, 357–358
  complications and prognosis for, 363
  defined, 357
  differential diagnosis of, 362
  epidemiology of, 357
  etiology of, 357
  laboratory and imaging studies of, 361–362
  obliterans, 363
  prevention of, 363–364
  treatment of, 362
Bronchoalveolar lavage, 459
Bronchopneumonia, 358–359

Bronchopulmonary dysplasia (BPD), 213–214, 471
Bronchoscopy, 459
Bronchospasm, 458t
Bronchus(i), mainstem, anatomy of, 455
Broviac catheters, infections associated with, 394
Brown dog tick, 401
Brucella, 398t–400t
Brucellosis, 398t–400t
Bruises, due to child abuse, 70–71, 71f, 72t–73t
Buckle fracture, 670
Budesonide DPI, for asthma, 279f
Budesonide inhaled, for asthma, 279f
Bulbar weakness, 625t
Bulimia nervosa, 248–249, 249t
Bulk, muscle, in motor examination, 615
Bulla, 650t, 651f
Bullous impetigo, 335, 663t
Bullous rash, infections with fever and, 329t–330t
Bullying, 80–81
Bumblebee stings, allergic reactions to, 293
BUN (blood urea nitrogen), 109, 555
    in acute renal failure, 562
    in dehydration, 108–111
Burkholderia cepacia, in cystic fibrosis, 475
Burkitt lymphoma
    clinical manifestations of, 545
    endemic (African) form of, 545
    etiology of, 544, 545t
    sporadic (North American) form of, 545
Burn(s), 137–139
    classification of, 137
    clinical manifestations of, 137–138, 137f
    complications of, 138t
    deep partial-thickness, 137
    due to child abuse, 71, 71f, 72t–73t
    epidemiology of, 137
    etiology of, 137
    first-degree, 137
    fluid management, 138
    fourth-degree, 137
    full-thickness, 137
    hypermetabolic response, 138
    inhalation injuries, 137
    laboratory and imaging studies of, 138
    major, 138
    percentage surface area involved in, 137–138, 137f
    prevention of, 141
    prognosis of, 141
    second-degree, 137
    superficial, 137
    systemic capillary leak due to, 138
    third-degree, 137
    treatment of, 138–139
    vesiculobullous eruptions due to, 663t
    wound care, 138–139
Burner, 691
Burrow, 651f
Bursitis, suppurative, 385–386
Button batteries, ingestion of, 139

C
C1-esterase inhibitor deficiency, acquired, 291t
C1-inhibitor, laboratory studies of, 268–269
C1-inhibitor deficiency, 268
    treatment of, 269
C3 deficiency, 268
Café au lait macules, 612, 659–660, 660f
    with developmental disabilities, 28t
    differential diagnosis of, 659t
    in neurofibromatosis type I, 645–646, 645f
CAH. *see* Congenital adrenal hyperplasia (CAH)
Calcaneal apophysitis, 683
Calcaneovalgus foot, 682
Calcidiol, 102

Calcifediol, 99t–100t
Calcineurin inhibitors, topical, for atopic dermatitis, 655
Calcinosis, in juvenile dermatomyositis, 313
Calcinosis universalis, in juvenile dermatomyositis, 313
Calcitriol, 102
    in renal function, 553
Calcium chloride, in cardiopulmonary resuscitation, 127t
Calcium deficiency, 103
Calcium gluconate, for hypocalcemia, 603
Caloric intake, and growth, 10–12
Calories, in parenteral nutrition, 113
CAM (complementary and alternative medicine), 4
Camptodactyly, 161t
Campylobacter jejuni, 398t–400t
    diarrhea due to, 366t, 367
    and Guillain-Barré syndrome, 625
Campylobacteriosis, 398t–400t
Cancer
    assessment for, 534–536, 535f
        common manifestations of, 534, 537t
        differential diagnosis in, 535
        history in, 534, 536t
        initial diagnostic evaluation in, 535–536
            diagnostic imaging in, 536, 542t
            minimum work up in, 542t
            screening tests in, 535–536
        physical examination in, 534
    in children
        epidemiology of, 534, 535f
        risk factors for, 536t
    common manifestations of, 534, 537t
    differential diagnosis of, 535
    emergencies with, 538, 539t
    prevention of, 538
Cancer treatment, 538–541
    adverse effects of, 542t, 541
    chemotherapy as, 539–541
    for oncologic emergencies, 538, 539t
    other forms of, 541
    radiation therapy as, 541
    surgery as, 538
Candida albicans infection, oropharyngeal, 431
Candidal diaper dermatitis, 658
Candidiasis, 337t
    chronic mucocutaneous, 261, 261t
    vulvovaginal, 375t
Canthus, 161t
Capillary hemangiomas, 198
Capillary leak, systemic, due to burns, 138
Capnocytophaga canimorsus, 398t–400t
Captopril
    for heart failure, 501t
    maternal use of, 207t
Caput succedaneum, 202
Carbohydrate disorder(s), 172–174
    fructosuria as, 176
        galactokinase deficiency as, 173–174
        galactosemia as, 173–174, 173f
        glycogen storage diseases as, 172–173, 172t, 173f
    hereditary fructose intolerance as, 176
    neonatal screening for, 170t
Carbohydrate intolerance, formula for, 88t
Carbon dioxide (CO_2), 119, 126
    end-tidal, 459
        in cardiopulmonary resuscitation, 126
    in pulmonary physiology, 455
Carbon dioxide partial pressure (P_{CO_2}), 456t
Carbon monoxide, in bilirubin production, 219
Carbon monoxide, toxicity of, 141t
Carboplatin, for cancer, 540t–541t

Carboxyhemoglobin assessment, for burns, 138
Carbuncle, 336, 651f
Cardiac arrhythmias. *see* Dysrhythmia(s)
Cardiac catheterization, in cardiovascular system assessment, 486f, 486
Cardiac manifestations, of systemic diseases, 481t
Cardiac murmurs. *see* Heart murmurs
Cardiac output
    cardiopulmonary arrest, 126
    oxygen delivery and, 129
Cardiac silhouette, 484–485, 485f
Cardiac syncope, 488t
Cardiomegaly
    in coarctation of the aorta, 494
    due to cardiomyopathy, 503–504
    in hypoplastic left heart syndrome, 499
Cardiomyopathy(ies), 184, 502–504, 503t
Cardiopulmonary arrest, 126–127
    airway management for, 126
    circulatory management for, 126
    drug for, 127
    endotracheal intubation for, 126
    hypoxic-ischemic damage in, 126, 126t
    outcome of, 126
Cardiopulmonary assessment, rapid, 125t
Cardiopulmonary resuscitation (CPR), 126
    airway in, 126
    breathing in, 126
    circulation in, 126
    defibrillation and cardioversion in, 127t
    drugs in, 127, 127t
    need for, 125t
Cardiovascular support, for shock, 132, 132t
Cardiovascular system assessment, 481–486
    history in, 481, 481t–482t
    laboratory and imaging tests in, 484–486
        cardiac catheterization as, 486f, 486
        chest radiography as, 484–485, 485f
        echocardiography as, 486f, 485–486
        electrocardiography as, 484, 485f
        pulse oximetry as, 484
    physical examination in, 481–484
        auscultation, 482
        clicks in, 482
        heart murmurs, 481
            continuous, 484
            diastolic, 484
            ejection, 482–483
            frequency/pitch of, 483
            holosystolic (pansystolic, regurgitant), 482–483
            intensity of, 483t
            normal or innocent, 484
            systolic, 482–483
        heart sounds in, 482
        inspection, 482
        palpation, 482
Cardioversion, 127
    in cardiopulmonary resuscitation, 127, 127t
    synchronized, for dysrhythmias, 490
Carditis, due to rheumatic fever, 502, 503t
Caries, 429–430
    bottle mouth, 429
    epidemiology and treatment of, 429
    etiology of, 429
    prevention of, 429–430
Carnitine(s), plasma, 171t
Carnitine deficiency, 183
Carotid bruit, 484t
Carotid sinus syncope, 488t
Carpenter syndrome, obesity in, 91t
Carriers, for genetic disorders, 147, 147f
Carvedilol, for heart failure, 501t
Caseous lymph node, and skeletal tuberculosis, 409

Cat eye syndrome, 160
Cat-scratch disease, 339–340, 398t–400t
Cataract
  with developmental disabilities, 28t
  in galactosemia, 173
Catarrhal stage, of pertussis, 356
CATCH 22 syndrome, 260
Catch-down growth, 12
Catch-up growth, 10–12, 96
Catecholamines, with neuroblastoma, 548
Cathartic, for poisoning, 143
Catheter-related infections, 394t
  of bloodstream, 394
Catheter-related sepsis, due to parenteral
    nutrition, 114
Catheter-related thrombosis, 394
Cations, in body fluids, 106
Cattell Infant Intelligence Scale, 29t
Caustic esophageal injuries, 434–435
Caustic ingestion, 139
Cavernous hemangiomas, 198
Cavopulmonary shunt, bidirectional, for
    tricuspid atresia, 497
Cavus foot, 683
CBT (cognitive-behavioral therapy)
  for bipolar disorder, 61
  for obsessive-compulsive disorder, 62–63
  for somatoform disorders, 54
CCHS (congenital central hypoventilation
    syndrome), 463
CD. see Crohn's disease (CD)
CD4 cells, for HIV, 412
Cefdinir, for otitis media, 352
Cefixime
  after rape, 247
  for Chlamydia infection, 380
  for gonorrhea, 379
Cefotaxime, for meningitis, 343–344
Ceftriaxone
  after rape, 247
  for gonococcal ophthalmia neonatorum, 389
  for gonorrhea, 379
  for Lyme disease, 397–400
  for meningitis, 343–344
  for otitis media, 352
Cefuroxime axetil, for otitis media, 352
Celiac disease, 295t, 442
  constipation due to, 426t
Cellular immune-mediated hypersensitivity,
    271t, 272
Cellulitis, 335–336
  orbital, 350, 388t–389t
  postseptal, 388t–389t
  preseptal (periorbital), 350, 388t–389t
Central catheters, infections associated
    with, 394
Central chemoreceptors, in control of ventilation,
    461, 461f
Central nervous system (CNS)
  congenital malformations of, 647–649
    of brain, 647–649
    of spinal cord, 647
  embryogenesis of, 647
Central nervous system (CNS) abnormalities
  delayed puberty due to, 590, 590t, 593t
  due to lysosomal storage diseases, 181t–182t
Central nervous system (CNS) depressants,
    maternal use of, 207t
Central nervous system (CNS) depression, in
    newborn, 196
Central nervous system (CNS)-directed therapy,
    for leukemia, 543–544
Central nervous system (CNS) infection,
    depressed consciousness due to, 636
Central nervous system (CNS) lupus, 312

Central nervous system (CNS) reflex(es)
  of child, 615
  of newborn, 13, 613, 613t
Central nervous system (CNS) shunts, infections
    associated with, 397
Central nervous system (CNS) tumor(s),
    546–548
  clinical manifestations of, 546–547
  complications of, 547
  differential diagnosis of, 547
  epidemiology of, 546
  etiology of, 546
  laboratory/imaging studies of, 547, 547f
  primary, 546
  prognosis for, 547–548, 549t
  risk factors for, 536t
  secondary, 546
  treatment of, 547
  vomiting due to, 423t
Central neurogenic hyperventilation, 634–635
Central pontine myelinolysis, 110
  due to overly rapid rehydration, 110
  due to rapid correction of hyponatremia, 114
Central venous catheters
  infections associated with, 394, 395f
  for parenteral nutrition, 113
Central wheal, in allergen-specific IgE in vivo
    skin testing, 272
Cephalexin, for streptococcal pharyngitis, 349t
Cephalhematoma, 659t
  in newborn, 202
Cephalosporins, allergic reaction to, 296–298
Cephalothin, maternal use of, 207t
Cerebellar ataxia, postinfectious acute, 632–633
Cerebellar mutism syndrome, 547
Cerebral aneurysms, in autosomal dominant
    polycystic kidney disease, 568
Cerebral contusion, 638, 638t
Cerebral edema, 110
  due to diabetic ketoacidosis, 575–576
  due to overly rapid rehydration, 110
Cerebral herniation, due to diabetic ketoacidosis,
    575
Cerebral palsy (CP), 35–36
  ataxic, 36t
  choreoathetotic, 36t
  defined, 35
  diagnosis of, 35
  dyskinetic, 36t
  dystonic, 36t
  epidemiology of, 35
  mixed, 36t
  risk factors for, 35t
  by site of involvement, 35t
  spastic, 36t
  treatment of, 35–36
  by type of motor disorder, 36t
Cerebrohepatorenal syndrome, 180–183
Cerebrosidase deficiency, 181t–182t
Cerebrospinal fluid (CSF) analysis, 616t, 615
  for alteration of consciousness, 637
  for cancer, 542t
  for CNS disorders, 343t
  for neonatal meningitis, 228
Cerebrospinal fluid (CSF) leak, 638–639
Cerebrospinal fluid (CSF) rhinorrhea, 283t
Cerebrovascular disease, in sickle cell anemia,
    520t
Cerubidine (daunorubicin), for cancer, 540t–541t
Cervical cap (FemCap), 247
Cervical lymphadenopathy
  clinical manifestations of, 340
  complications and prognosis for, 341–342
  differential diagnosis of, 341
  epidemiology of, 340

Cervical lymphadenopathy (Continued)
  etiology of, 338–340
  in Kawasaki disease, 303
  laboratory and imaging studies for, 340, 341f
  prevention of, 344
  treatment of, 341
Cervical shield (Lea's Shield), 247
Cervical spine injuries, 639
Cervicitis, nongonococcal, 379
Cestodes, 404
Cetirizine, for allergic rhinitis, 284
CFTR (cystic fibrosis transmembrane regulator),
    475
CFTR gene, and pancreatic insufficiency,
    450–451
CGH (comparative genomic hybridization),
    159
CH₅₀ test, 268
Chagas disease, 398t–400t
  congenital infection with, 230t
Chalasia, vs. vomiting, 422
Chalazion, 387
Chancre, 380
Chancroid, 376, 377t
Charcoal, activated, for poisoning, 142–143
Charcot-Marie-Tooth disease, 626
  cavus foot in, 683
CHARGE association, choanal atresia in, 284
Chédiak-Higashi syndrome (CHS), 264t
Chelation therapy, for β-thalassemia major, 518
Chemical(s), as teratogens, 154
Chemoprophylaxis
  for malaria, 404
  for meningitis, 346
Chemoreceptors, in control of ventilation
  central, 461, 461f
  peripheral, 461, 461f
Chemotherapy, 539–541, 540t–541t
  adjuvant, 539–541
  adverse effects of, 542t, 541
  and blood-brain barrier, 541
  high-dose, for neuroblastoma, 549
  for leukemia, induction, 543–544
  neoadjuvant, 539–541
  resistance to, 541
  vomiting due to, 423t
Cherry-red spot, in macula, with developmental
    disabilities, 28t
Chest, of newborn, 199
Chest compression, in cardiopulmonary
    resuscitation, 126
Chest motion, 458t
Chest pain, 487–488, 489t
Chest percussion, 460
Chest physiotherapy, 460
  for cystic fibrosis, 477–478
Chest tubes
  for pleural effusion, 480
  third space losses from, 108
Chest wall disorder(s), 478–480
  pectus carinatum as, 478
  pectus excavatum as, 478
  scoliosis as, 478
Chest x-ray (CXR)
  for asthma, 274
  for cancer, 536, 542t
  in cardiovascular system assessment, 484–485,
    485f
Cheyne-Stokes respiration, 457t, 634–635
Chickenpox, 333–335
  clinical manifestations of, 334
  complications and prognosis for, 335
  defined, 333–334
  differential diagnosis of, 334
  epidemiology of, 334

Chickenpox *(Continued)*
    etiology of, 333–334
    laboratory and imaging studies for, 334
    prevention of, 335
    treatment of, 334–335
Child abuse, 70–74
    defined, 70
    diagnosis of, 70
    domestic violence and, 79–80
    epidemiology of, 70
    management of, 73–74, 74f
    physical, 70–73
        abdominal injury due to, 71–72
        bruises due to, 70–71, 71f, 72t–73t
        burns due to, 71, 71f, 72t–73t
        diagnosis of, 70–73, 70t
        differential diagnosis of, 72–73, 72t–73t
        epidemiology of, 70
        fractures due to, 71, 71f, 72t–73t,
            674–675
        head trauma due to, 72, 72f, 72t–73t
        subdural hemorrhage due to, 226
    prevention of, 74
    reporting of, 70
    risk factors, 70
    sexual, 73
        defined, 73
        diagnosis of
            history in, 73
            laboratory evaluation in, 73
            physical examination in, 73
        epidemiology of, 73
        sexually transmitted infections due to, 73
Child neglect, 70
Child Protective Services (CPS), 70
Childhood
    congenital hemiplegia of, 631
    sleep disorders, 47–50, 49t
Childhood antecedents, of adult health
        conditions, 1
Chinese liver fluke, 406t
Chlamydia trachomatis, 376, 379–380
    clinical features of, 376t
    congenital infection with, 230t, 233
    diagnosis of, 379–380
    epidemiology of, 379
    and gonorrhea, 376t
    pathogenesis of, 379
    pelvic inflammatory disease due to, 379
    pneumonia due to, 359, 363t
    treatment of, 380
Chlamydial conjunctivitis, 233, 387
    clinical manifestations of, 387, 388t
    complications of, 389
    epidemiology of, 387
    treatment of, 388t, 389
Chlamydophila pneumoniae, pneumonia due to,
        359, 363t
Chloral hydrate, for sedation, 145t
Chloroquine, for malaria, 404
Choanal atresia, 283t, 284
Choanal stenosis/atresia, 196t
    upper airway obstruction due to, 467
Cholangiopancreatography, endoscopic
        retrograde, 453
Cholecalciferol, 102
Cholecystitis, abdominal pain due to, 420t
Cholelithiasis, abdominal pain due to, 420t
Cholera-like enterotoxin, 367
Cholestasis, 444–447
    chronic, 449
    clinical manifestations of, 444
    defined, 444
    differential diagnosis of, 445f
    etiology and epidemiology of, 444

Cholestasis *(Continued)*
    laboratory and imaging studies for, 444, 446f,
        446t
    treatment of, 444–447
    vitamin and nutrient deficiencies with, 97t
Cholestatic liver disease, due to parenteral
        nutrition, 114
Cholesterol screening, 22, 22t
Cholesterol side-chain cleavage (CYP11A1)
        enzyme, in congenital adrenal hyperplasia,
        608f
Cholinergics
    maternal use of, 207t
    toxicity of, 141t
Chondritis, *Pseudomonas*, 382
Chondrolysis, 680
"ChooseMyPlate" guidelines, 89–90, 90f
Chordee, 568
Chorea, 633–634
    due to rheumatic fever, 502, 503t
Choreoathetosis, 637
Choriomeningitis, lymphocytic, 398t–400t
Chorionic gonadotropin-secreting tumor,
        precocious puberty due to, 593t
Chorionic villus sampling (CVS), 155
Chorioretinitis, with developmental disabilities,
        28t
Choroid plexus papilloma, prognosis for, 549t
Choroiditis, 388t–389t
Chromatin, 146
Chromium deficiency, 103t
Chromosomal deletion syndrome, 159–160
    aniridia Wilms tumor association as, 159
    of chromosome 22q11.2 deletion syndromes,
        159–160
    cri du chat syndrome as, 159–160
    Williams syndrome as, 159
Chromosomal disorder(s), 156–160
    due to abnormalities in number (aneuploidy),
        157–159
    defined, 157
    monosomies as, 158–159
        defined, 157
        Turner syndrome as, 158–159
    trisomies as, 157–158
        defined, 157
        Down syndrome as, 157
        Klinefelter syndrome as, 158
        trisomy 13 as, 158
        trisomy 18 as, 157–158
    due to chromosomal deletions, 159–160
        aniridia Wilms tumor association as, 159
        of chromosome 22q11.2 deletion
            syndromes, 159–160
        cri du chat syndrome as, 159–160
        Williams syndrome as, 159
    due to chromosome duplication, 160
        cat eye syndrome as, 160
        inverted duplication chromosome 15 as, 160
    epidemiology of, 157
    fetal detection of, 189
Chromosome(s), 146
Chromosome 15, inverted duplication, 160
Chromosome 22q11.2 deletion syndromes,
        159–160
Chromosome analysis, 163
    in genetic assessment, 159
Chromosome duplication syndromes, 160
    cat eye syndrome as, 160
    inverted duplication chromosome 15 as, 160
Chronic carriers, of typhoid fever, 366, 368
Chronic cough, 458
Chronic fatigue syndrome (CFS), 51
Chronic granulomatous disease (CGD), 264–266,
        264t

Chronic illnesses
    in children and adolescents, 234t
    trends in, 1
Chronic kidney disease (CKD), 562–563
Chronic lung disease, 213–214
Chronic lymphocytic thyroiditis, 599
    with diabetes mellitus, 578
Chronic mucocutaneous candidiasis, 261, 261t
Chronic myeloid/myelogenous leukemia (CML),
        542
Chvostek sign, 204, 602
Cigarette smoking, around children, 79
Ciliary dyskinesia, primary, 472
Ciliary elevator system, in pneumonia, 359
Ciliated epithelium, of paranasal sinuses and
        nasal turbinates, as filter, 456
Circadian rhythm disorders, 49
Circulation, transition from fetal to neonatal, 191
Circulatory status, 124
    cardiopulmonary resuscitation, 124
    in newborn resuscitation, 196
    in rapid cardiopulmonary assessment, 125t
Cirrhosis, 448
cis-retinoic acid, for neuroblastoma, 549
Cisplatin, for cancer, 540t–541t
CKD. *see* Chronic kidney disease (CKD)
Classical pathway, of complement activation,
        267–268, 267f
Clavicle fractures, in newborn, 203
Cleft lip and palate, 431–433
Clicks, auscultation of, 482
Clindamycin, for acne, 652
Clinodactyly, 161t
Clitoral enlargement, in newborn, 200
Clonidine (Kapvay), for ADHD, 42t
Clonorchiasis, 406t
Clonorchis sinensis, 406t
C-loop, in midgut malrotation, 437–438
Clostridium difficile-associated diarrhea, 366t,
        367
Clot retraction, 523, 524f
Clotting factors disorders, 528
    disseminated intravascular coagulation (DIC)
        as, 530–531, 530t–531t
    etiology of, 528
    hemophilia as, 528–530
    thrombosis as, 531, 531f
    von Willebrand disease as, 529t, 530
Club drugs, 250
    acute effects of, 250t–251t
Club foot, 681–682, 681f
Clubbing, digital, 457
    in cystic fibrosis, 475
Clue cells, in vulvovaginitis, 374
CMV (cytomegalovirus)
    congenital infection with, 230t, 231
    in immunocompromised person, 391
    pneumonia due to, 359
CO_2 (carbon dioxide)
    in acid-base balance, 119
    end-tidal, 459
        in cardiopulmonary resuscitation, 126
        in pulmonary physiology, 455
Coagulation, 509, 510f
    disseminated intravascular, 528, 530–531
        clinical manifestations of, 531, 531t
        differential diagnosis of, 531t
        due to cancer, 539t
        due to thrombotic microangiopathy, 528
        etiology of, 530, 530t
        in newborn, 222
        treatment of, 531
Coagulation disorder(s), 523–531
    clinical manifestations of, 507t, 524
    differential diagnosis of, 526–531

Coagulation disorder(s) *(Continued)*
  disseminated intravascular coagulation (DIC)
    as, 528, 530–531
  etiology and epidemiology of, 523, 525f, 526t
  with fulminant liver failure, 448t
  GI bleeding due to, 427t
  hemophilia as, 528–530
  laboratory testing for, 524–526, 526t
  in newborn
    clinical manifestations and differential
      diagnoses of, 222–223
    etiology and pathogenesis of, 223
  thrombosis as, 531, 531f
  von Willebrand disease as, 529t, 530
Coagulation factors, 222
  in hemostasis, 523, 525f
Coagulation pathways, 523, 525f
Coagulopathy. *see* Coagulation disorder(s)
Coarctation of the aorta, 494
Cobb angle, 685, 685f
Cocaine, 82, 87t
  acute effects of, 250t–251t
  neonatal addiction to and withdrawal from,
    204
Cocaine use, during pregnancy, 79
Cochlear implants, 34
Cockroach allergens, and asthma, 275t
COCs. *see* Combined oral contraceptives (COCs)
Codeine, for analgesia, 145t
Codon, 146
Cognition, tests of, 29t
Cognitive-behavioral methods, 54
Cognitive-behavioral therapy (CBT), for
  obsessive-compulsive disorder, 62–63
Cognitive development, milestones of, 16t
Cold, common, 283, 346–347
Cold caloric stimulation, 635–636
Cold injury, of infant, 203
Cold sores, 337
Colic, 37–39
  clinical manifestations of, 38, 38f
  differential diagnosis of, 38–39
  epidemiology of, 37
  etiology of, 37
  in normal development, 37
  physical examination, 38
  prevention of, 39
  prognosis for, 39
  treatment of, 39
Colitis
  allergic, GI bleeding due to, 427t
  pseudomembranous, GI bleeding due to, 427t
  Trichuris, 405t
  ulcerative, 440
    clinical manifestations of, 440, 441t
    epidemiology and etiology of, 440
    laboratory and imaging studies for, 440–441,
      441t
    treatment of, 441–442
Collaboration, 5
Collagen vascular diseases, assessment of, 299
  common manifestations in, 299–301, 303t
  diagnostic imaging in, 302
  differential diagnosis in, 299, 300t
  history in, 299
  initial diagnostic evaluation in, 302
  laboratory testing in, 302
  physical examination in, 299
Collecting ducts, 553
Colonic malformations, constipation due to,
  426t
Colonic stricture, constipation due to, 426t
Colonopathy, fibrosing, due to lipase, 478
Colonoscopy, for inflammatory bowel disease,
  441

Colony-stimulating factors, in hematopoiesis,
  509, 510f
Colorado tick fever, 398t–400t
Colorblindness, genetic basis for, 151t
Columella, 161t
Coma
  assessment of, 634–636
  causes of, 142t
  clinical manifestations of, 636–637, 636t
  defined, 634, 635t
  due to inborn errors of metabolism, 167t
  due to poisoning, 139
  etiology of, 636
  laboratory and diagnostic imaging of,
    635t, 637
  prognosis of, 637
  treatment of, 637
Coma scales, 635, 639
Combined immunodeficiency disease(s),
  258–262
  bare lymphocyte syndrome, 259t, 260
  DiGeorge syndrome as, 259t, 260
  hyper-IgM syndrome as, 259t
    autosomal recessive, 258
    clinical features of, 258
    due to defects in NEMO, 258
    pathogenesis of, 258
    X-linked, 258, 259t
  Omenn syndrome as, 259t, 260
  severe, 258–260, 259t
    autosomal recessive, 260
    clinical manifestations of, 260
    due to deficiencies in adenosine deaminase
      and purine nucleoside phosphorylase,
      260
    in Nezelof syndrome, 260
    pathogenesis of, 258–260
    X-linked, 260
Combined oral contraceptives (COCs),
  245–246
Combined ventricular hypertrophy, in truncus
  arteriosus, 497
Comedo(nes), 650t, 651f, 652
Common cold, 283, 346–347
Common variable immunodeficiency (CVID),
  256, 258t
Communication, 5
Communication disorders, 34–35, 34t
Comparative genomic hybridization (CGH),
  159
Compartment syndrome, 671–672
Compassion, 4
Complement assays, 258
Complement component cascade, 267f
Complement evaluation, in angioedema,
  291t
Complement pathways, 263, 267f
Complement proteins, 263
  disorder of, 268
Complement system, 266–269, 267f
  disorders of, 263
  etiology of, 267–268
  laboratory studies for, 268–269
Complementary and alternative medicine
  (CAM), 4
Complementary foods, 89
Complete blood count
  for anemia, 511
  with differential, for immunodeficiency
    disorders, 255
  for gastrointestinal symptoms, 417
  for infectious diseases, 316–317
Complete heart block, 490t
Compound skull fractures, 638
Compulsions, 62, 62t

Computed tomography (CT)
  of brain and spinal cord, 616
  for cancer, 536, 542t
  of chest, 458–459
  contrast enhanced, for infectious diseases, 317
  for head trauma, 637
  for infectious diseases, 317
  for seizures, 622
  of trauma patient, 134
  of urinary system, 557
Computed tomography (CT) angiography, of
  pulmonary embolism, 475
Computed tomography (CT) scanogram, of leg-
  length discrepancy, 678–679
Concerta (Methylphenidate), for ADHD, 42t
Concussion(s), 637–638
Conditioning therapy, for enuresis, 44
Condoms, 247
Conduction, heat loss via, 203
Condylomata acuminata, 338, 376, 383
  clinical features of, 378t
  diagnosis of, 381
  pathogenesis of, 384
  treatment of, 381
Condylomata lata, 380
Confidentiality, 6
  of adolescent interview, 234
  HIPAA on, 5–6
  limited, 5
Confusional arousals, 49t
Confusional migraines, 637
Congenital adrenal hyperplasia (CAH)
  ambiguous genitalia due to, 606, 608
  amenorrhea due to, 242
  genetic basis for, 150t
  pathogenesis of, 608f
  premature adrenarche due to, 596
  salt-losing, 608
Congenital central hypoventilation syndrome
  (CCHS), 463
Congenital complete heart block, 489
Congenital diaphragmatic hernia, 196t,
  215, 471
Congenital giant melanocytic nevi, 660–661
Congenital heart disease, 157
  acyanotic, 491–494, 491t
    aortic stenosis as, 494
    atrial septal defect as, 492, 492f
    coarctation of the aorta as, 494
    endocardial cushion defect as, 493
    etiology and epidemiology of, 491
    patent ductus arteriosus as, 492–493, 492f
    pulmonary stenosis as, 493–494
    ventricular septal defect as, 491–492, 491f
  congenital malformation syndromes associated
    with, 482t
  cyanotic, 495–499
    extracardiac complications of, 500t
    hypoplastic left heart syndrome as,
      498–499, 498f
    with polycythemia, 527
    presenting symptoms in, 495t
    tetralogy of Fallot as, 495–496, 496f
    total anomalous pulmonary venous return,
      498, 498f
    transposition of the great arteries as, 496–
      497, 496f
    tricuspid atresia as, 497, 497f
    truncus arteriosus as, 497–498
  ductal-dependent, 196t
Congenital hemiplegia of childhood, 631
Congenital hip dysplasia. *see* Developmental
  dysplasia of the hip (DDH)
Congenital hypotonia, benign, 629–630
Congenital infection (s), 229–233, 230t

Congenital lobar
  emphysema, 471
  overdistension, 471
Congenital malformations, 146, 160–161
  association in, 161
  of CNS, 647–649
    of brain, 647–649
    of spinal cord, 647
  with congenital heart disease, 482t
  defined, 160–161
  diagnosis of, 163
  due to disruptions of development, 160–161
  due to extrinsic factors, 160–161
  due to inborn errors of metabolism, 168
  due to intrinsic factors, 160–161
  epidemiology of, 161
  history for
    family, 161–162
    pregnancy, 161
  laboratory evaluation of, 163
  life-threatening, 196, 196t
  minor, 161
  multiple, 161
  physical examination, 162–163
    craniofacial, 162
    of extremities, 162–163
    of genitalia, 163
    growth in, 162
    of neck, 162
    of trunk, 162
  sequence in, 160–161
  syndromes in, 160
  terminology used in, 161, 161t
Congenital melanocytic nevi, 198, 660, 660f
  differential diagnosis of, 659t
  giant, 198, 659t, 660–661, 660f
  hairy, 660, 660f
Congenital myasthenic syndrome, 627
Congenital myopathies (CM), 628
Congenital rubella syndrome, 229–231, 230t, 331
Congestive heart failure. see Heart failure
Conjunctival erythema, in Kawasaki disease,
    303, 304f
Conjunctivitis
  acute, 386, 387t
  bacterial, 387, 388t–389t
  chlamydial, 233, 387
  clinical manifestations of, 387, 388t
  complications and prognosis for, 389
  differential diagnosis of, 387–389
  epidemiology of, 387
  etiology of, 386–387
  gonococcal, 387
    complications of, 389
    neonatal, 386–387, 388t–389t
      clinical manifestations of, 387, 388t
      treatment of, 388t
    prophylaxis for, 389
    treatment of, 389
  hyperpurulent, 387
  inclusion, 387, 388t
  laboratory and imaging studies of, 387
  neonatal, 386–387, 388t–389t
    chlamydial, 387
      clinical manifestations of, 387, 388t
      complications of, 389
      epidemiology of, 387
      treatment of, 388t, 389
    clinical manifestations of, 387, 388t
    differential diagnosis of, 387–389
    epidemiology of, 387
    etiology of, 386–387
    gonococcal, 387
    treatment of, 389
  neonatal, chlamydial, 233

Conjunctivitis (Continued)
  prevention of, 389
  treatment of, 388t, 389
  viral, 386, 388t–389t
Connective tissue disease
  assessment of, 299–301
    common manifestations in, 299–301, 303t
    diagnostic imaging in, 302
    history in, 299
    initial diagnostic evaluation in, 302
    laboratory testing in, 302
    physical examination in, 299
  differential diagnosis of, 299, 300t
    vs. juvenile idiopathic arthritis, 308t
Conotruncal anomaly face syndrome, 159–160
Consanguinity, and autosomal recessive
    inheritance, 154
Consciousness
  defined, 634
  depression of, transient, recurrent, 637
  disorders of, 634–637
    acute, 634–637, 635t
      assessment of, 634–636
      clinical manifestations of, 636–637, 636t
      etiology of, 636
      laboratory and diagnostic imaging of,
        635t, 637
      prognosis of, 637
      treatment of, 637
    transient, recurrent, 637
Consolidation, of lung, 458t
Constipation, 425–426
  chronic and soiling, education about, 45t
  defined, 425
  differential diagnosis of, 425, 426t
  distinguishing features of, 425–426
  evaluation and treatment of, 426
  functional, 44–46
    clinical manifestations of, 44–45
    complications of, 46
    defined, 44, 425
    differential diagnosis of, 45, 425, 426t
    epidemiology of, 44
    etiology of, 44
    evaluation of, 426
    prevention of, 46
    treatment of, 45–46, 426
      behavioral training, 45–46
      disimpaction in, 46t
Constitutional delay
  in growth and adolescence, 589, 590t
  short stature due to, 585–586, 586t, 587t
Contact allergies, 657f, 272, 658
Contact dermatitis, 654, 656–657
  allergic, 657f, 656
  atopic vs., 654
  clinical manifestations of, 657f, 656, 656f
  complications of, 658
  differential diagnosis of, 658
  etiology and epidemiology of, 656
  irritant, 656, 658
  laboratory and imaging studies for, 656
  prevention of, 658
  treatment of, 658
  vesiculobullous eruptions due to, 663t
Containment, 675
Continence, 567
Continuous positive airway pressure (CPAP),
    463–464, 470
Contraception, 245–247
  abstinence for, 245
  barrier methods of, 247
    condoms and foam as, 247
    sponge, caps, and diaphragm as, 247
  coitus interruptus for, 247

Contraception (Continued)
  emergency postcoital, 246, 247t
  intrauterine devices for, 246
  oral and anal sex for, 247
  rhythm method (periodic coital abstinence)
    for, 247
  steroidal, 245–247
    combined oral contraceptives for,
      245–246, 245t–246t
    contraceptive patch for, 246
    contraceptive vaginal ring for, 246
    hormonal injections and implants for, 246
    progesterone-only pill or minipill for, 246
Contraceptive patch, 246
Contraceptive vaginal ring (NuvaRing), 246
Contraceptives, oral
  combined, 245–246
    contraindications to, 245t
    missed, 246t
  progesterone-only pill or minipill for, 246
Contrasexual precocity, 593t
Contrast enhanced CT, for infectious diseases,
    317
Contusion, cerebral, 638, 638t
Convalescent stage, of pertussis, 356
Convection, heat loss via, 203
Conversion disorder, 51
  diagnostic criteria for, 53t
  falling out syndrome, 52–53
  nonepileptic seizures in, 53
Convulsion(s). see also Seizure(s)
  benign neonatal, 621
  simple febrile, 620
Cooley anemia, 518
  clinical manifestations of, 518
  etiology and epidemiology of, 515t, 518
  treatment of, 518
Coombs tests, 522f
Coordination, of movement, 615
Copper deficiency, 103t
Copper intrauterine device (ParaGard), 246
Cor pulmonale, 473
Cordocentesis, 189
Corneal cloudiness, with developmental
    disabilities, 28t
Corneal disorders, due to lysosomal storage
    diseases, 181t–182t
Corneal reflex, 614
Coronary artery aneurysms, in Kawasaki disease,
    303–304
Coronary artery disease, syncope due to, 488t
Corporal punishment, 23
Corpus callosum, agenesis of, 648
Corrin ring, 101
Corticospinal tract, 623
Corticospinal tract lesions, 624, 624t
Corticosteroids, 654
  for allergic rhinitis, 284
  for asthma
    inhaled, 275–276, 279f
    oral, 276
  for atopic dermatitis, 654
    systemic, 655
    topical, 287, 654
  for autoimmune hemolytic anemia, 523
  for juvenile dermatomyositis, 313
  for juvenile idiopathic arthritis, 308
  for laryngeal hemangioma, 468
  maternal use of, 207t
  for systemic lupus erythematosus, 311
  topical, 655
    for atopic dermatitis, 287, 654
    complications of, 655
  for urticaria and angioedema, 291
Corticotropin, 607

Corticotropin-releasing hormone (CRH), 607
Cortisol, normal variations in, 607
Cortisol-binding protein, 607
Cortisol deficiency
  clinical manifestations of, 609t
  and growth, 584t
  hypoglycemia due to, 582
Cortisol excess, and growth, 584t
Cortisol insufficiency, 607
Cough
  acute, 458
  chronic, 458
  due to croup, 354
  evaluation of, 458
  as lung defense mechanism, 457–458
Cough assist device, 460
Cough syncope, 488t
Coumarin, as teratogen, 206t
Counseling, on developmental problems, 30, 30t
Counter-regulatory hormones
  hypoglycemia due to defects in, 580t,
    581–582
  in serum glucose regulation, 580, 581f
Cow's milk-based formulas, 88–89, 88t
Coxiella burnetii, 398t–400t
Coxsackievirus infection
  conjunctivitis due to, 386, 388t–389t
  vesiculobullous eruptions due to, 663t
CP. *see* Cerebral palsy (CP)
CPAP. *see* Continuous positive airway pressure
    (CPAP)
CPR. *see* Cardiopulmonary resuscitation (CPR)
CPS (Child Protective Services), 70
Cr. *see* Creatinine
Crab lice, 381, 378t
Cracked lips, in Kawasaki disease, 303, 304f
Crackles, fine, 457
Cradle cap, 657, 658f
Cranial nerve evaluation, 613–614
  of cranial nerve I, 614
  of cranial nerve II, 614
  of cranial nerve(s) III, IV, and VI, 614
  of cranial nerve V, 614
  of cranial nerve VII, 614
  of cranial nerve VIII, 614
  of cranial nerve(s) IX and X, 614
  of cranial nerve XI, 614
  of cranial nerve XII, 614
Cranial nerve palsies, 638–639
Craniofacial dysmorphology, 161t, 162
Craniopharyngioma
  delayed puberty due to, 590
  hypopituitarism due to, 573
  prognosis for, 549t
Craniosynostosis, 612, 648
  genetic basis for, 147t
Craniotabes, 198–199
  in rickets, 102
Creatine biosynthesis, disorders of, 171
Creatinine (Cr)
  in acute renal failure, 562
  plasma, 555
Creatinine clearance, 555
Creatinine concentration, in dehydration, 109
Cretinism, 103t
  endemic, 599
CRH (corticotropin-releasing hormone), 607
Cri du chat syndrome, 159–160
Cricoid portion, of trachea, anatomy of, 455
Cricoid ring, 455
Crigler-Najjar syndrome, hyperbilirubinemia
    due to, 219
Crohn's disease (CD), 440
  clinical manifestations of, 440, 441t
  epidemiology and etiology of, 440

Crohn's disease (CD) *(Continued)*
  laboratory and imaging studies for, 440–441,
    441t
  treatment of, 442
Cross-dressing, 75
Croup, 354–356, 467
  clinical manifestations of, 354, 355t
  complications and prognosis for, 357
  differential diagnosis of, 354
  etiology and epidemiology of, 354
  laboratory and imaging studies of, 354, 355f
  membranous, upper airway obstruction due to,
    465t–466t
  spasmodic
    bacterial, 354
    upper airway obstruction due to,
      465t–466t
  treatment of, 354–356
  upper airway obstruction due to, 465t–466t
Crouzon syndrome, with acanthosis nigricans,
    genetic basis for, 147t
Crust, 651t
Crying
  of colic, 37–39
  duration of, 37
  frequency of, 37
  by infants, 37f
  intensity of, 37
  in normal development, 37, 37f
Cryoprecipitate, 532t
Cryptorchidism, 568
Cryptosporidium parvum, diarrhea due to, 366t,
    367
CT. *see* Computed tomography (CT)
Cullen sign, 451
Cultural concerns, about palliative care and end-
    of-life decisions, 9
Culture(s), 3–4
  for infectious diseases, 317
Cushing syndrome, 611
  obesity in, 91t
Cushing triad, 641
Custody, 82–83
Cutaneous infection(s), 335–338
Cutaneous infestation(s), 664–666
  pediculoses as, 665–666
  scabies as, 664–665, 665f
Cutaneous larva migrans, 405t
Cutaneous manifestations, of systemic diseases,
    651
CVID (common variable immunodeficiency),
    256
CVS (chorionic villus sampling), 155
CXR. *see* Chest x-ray (CXR)
Cyanide, toxicity of, 141t
Cyanosis
  central, 201–202
  due to respiratory failure, 128
  in newborn, 201–202, 201t, 209
  perioral, 482
  peripheral, 482
  with respiratory distress, 495t
  without respiratory distress, 495t
Cyanotic heart disease, maternal, 205t
Cyclic antidepressants, toxicity of, 141t
Cyclic vomiting syndrome (CVS), 437,
    422, 423t
Cyclophosphamide
  for cancer, 540t–541t
  for juvenile dermatomyositis, 313
  for systemic lupus erythematosus, 311
Cyclosporine
  for atopic dermatitis, 655
  for juvenile dermatomyositis, 313
Cyclothymic disorder, 61

CYP11A1 (cholesterol side-chain cleavage
    enzyme, in congenital adrenal hyperplasia),
    608f
Cyst(s), 650t, 651f
  bone, 693–694, 693t–694t
    aneurysmal, 693t–694t
    unicameral (simple), 693t–694t
  duplication
    GI bleeding due to, 427t
    vomiting due to, 423t
  ganglion, 693
  laryngeal, 468
  leptomeningeal, 638
  ovarian, precocious puberty due to, 593t, 595,
    595t
  pancreatic pseudo-, 451–452
  popliteal (Baker), 679–680
Cystathionine ß-synthase deficiency, 175
Cysteinyl leukotriene receptor antagonists, for
    asthma, 275–276
Cystic acne, 652
Cystic fibrosis (CF), 475–478
  clinical manifestations of, 475–476, 476t
  complications of, 476t
  constipation due to, 426t
  diagnostic studies for, 477t
  etiology and epidemiology of, 475
  genetic basis for, 150t
  intestinal atresia in, 439
  pancreatic insufficiency due to, 450–451
  treatment of, 477–478
Cystic fibrosis transmembrane regulator (CFTR),
    475
Cystic lesions, bone, 693–694
Cysticerci, 407, 407t
Cystinosis
  in Fanconi syndrome, 120
  nephropathic, 181t–182t
Cystinuria, 177
Cystitis, 372
Cystogram, radionuclide, for vesicoureteral
    reflux, 565
Cystourethrogram, voiding, 557
  for urinary tract infection, 373
  for vesicoureteral reflux, 565
Cytogenetic analysis, for leukemia, 543
Cytokine synthesis, tests for, 255
Cytokine(s), in hematopoiesis, 510f
Cytomegalovirus (CMV)
  congenital infection with, 230t, 231
  in immunocompromised person, 391
  pneumonia due to, 359
Cytosine arabinoside (Ara-C), for cancer,
    540t–541t
Cytoxan (cyclophosphamide), for cancer,
    540t–541t

D

D-dimers, in pulmonary embolism, 475
Dacryoadenitis, 388t–389t
Dacryocystitis, 387–389, 388t–389t
Dactinomycin, for cancer, 540t–541t
Dactylitis
  in sickle cell anemia, 520t
  in skeletal tuberculosis, 409
Danazol, for C1-inhibitor deficiency, 269
Dander, and asthma, 275t
Dandruff, 657
Dandy-Walker malformation, 648
Danon disease, 181t–182t
Darier sign, 290–291
DAT (direct antiglobulin test), 522f
Date rape, 82
Date-rape drugs, 250
Dating violence, 82

Daunorubicin, for cancer, 540t–541t
DDH. *see* Developmental dysplasia of the hip (DDH)
Death and dying
  cause of, 2, 2t
  explanation to child of, 84
  of parent or family member, 84–85, 84t
  sudden, 7
  understanding, 8
Debranching enzyme, 172t, 173f
Decerebrate posturing, 636
Decongestants, for allergic rhinitis, 284
Decorticate posturing, 636
Deep tendon reflexes, 613, 615
Deep venous thrombi, 524
Deer tick, 396
DEET (N,N-Diethyl-*m*-toluamide), for prevention of zoonoses, 396
Deferoxamine, for iron poisoning, 143t–144t
Defibrillation, in cardiopulmonary resuscitation, 127, 127t
Definitive anti-infective therapy, 323
Deformation, 161
  defined, 667t
  due to uterine compression, 668, 669f
  mechanisms of, 161, 667t
Degenerative disease(s), 642–645
  acquired illnesses mimicking, 645
  with focal manifestations, 644
  gray matter (neuronal), 642–643
  hereditary and metabolic, 642–644
  white matter (leukodystrophies), 642–643
Deglutition syncope, 488t
Degree of effort, 457
Dehydration, 108–111
  approach to, 109–110
  assessing degree of, 108, 109t
  calculation of fluid deficit in, 109
  due to diabetic ketoacidosis, 574
  due to diarrhea, 366
  fluid resuscitation for, 109
  fluid therapy for, 109–110
  hypernatremic, 110
    clinical manifestations of, 115
    monitoring and adjusting, 110
    treatment of, 115
      overly rapid, 115, 110
  hyponatremic, 111f, 110
  laboratory evaluation of, 109
  mild, 108–109
  moderate, 108–109
  oral rehydration for, 110–111
  severe, 108–109, 109t
  signs and symptoms, 109t
Delayed puberty, 589–592
  classification of, 590t
  differential diagnosis of, 591t
  due to constitutional delay, 589, 591t
  due to hypergonadotropic hypogonadism (primary gonadal failure), 590t
    ovarian, 590t, 591–592
    testicular, 590t, 592
  due to hypogonadotropic hypogonadism, 589, 590t–591t
    due to CNS abnormalities, 590, 590t–591t
    due to idiopathic hypopituitarism, 590, 590t
    due to isolated gonadotropin deficiency, 590, 590t–591t
    due to Kallmann syndrome, 590, 591t
    syndromic, 590–591
  primary amenorrhea as, 592
  treatment of, 592
Delayed sleep phase, 49t
Delayed-type hypersensitivity, 255, 271t, 272
Delivery, history of, in genetic assessment, 156

Delivery room care
  resuscitation in, 194
    airway patency in, 194
    algorithm for, 195f
    breathing in, 194–195
    circulation in, 196
    drug administration in, 196
    specific conditions requiring, 201–203
      cyanosis as, 201–202, 201t
      life-threatening congenital malformations as, 202
      shock as, 202
  routine, 191–196
    skin and umbilical cord care in, 191
    silver nitrate instillation in, 191
    vitamin K prophylaxis in, 191
Delta agent, 369, 370t
  complications and prognosis of, 373–374
Dementia(s), 642–645
  acquired illnesses mimicking, 645
  with focal manifestations, 644
  of gray matter (neuronal), 642–643
  hereditary and metabolic, 642–644
  of white matter (leukodystrophies), 642–643
Dengue fever, 398t–400t
Dennie lines, 272
  in atopic dermatitis, 285–286
Dennie-Morgan folds, 272
  in atopic dermatitis, 285–286
Dental care, 23
  with developmental disability, 31t
Dental caries, 429–430
Denver Developmental Screening Test II, 17, 17f–18f
Depo-Provera (medroxyprogesterone acetate)
  for contraception, 246
  for dysmenorrhea, 244
Depressed mood, adjustment disorder with, 60
Depressed skull fractures, 638
Depression, 59–62
  in adjustment disorder with depressed mood, 60
  atypical, 60
  in depressive disorder not otherwise specified, 60
  in dysthymic disorder, 59–60
  major, 59
    comorbid psychiatric disorder with, 61
    diagnostic criteria for, 59t
    etiology of, 61
    with psychotic features, 59, 66
  in seasonal affective disorder, 60
  and suicide, 60
  treatment of, 60
Deprivation dwarfism, 584–585
Dermacentor andersoni, 401
Dermacentor variabilis, 401
Dermal melanosis, 659, 659t, 660f
Dermatitis
  atopic, 285–288, 653
  contact, 654, 656–657
  diaper, 656
    candidal, 658
    irritant contact, 657f, 656, 658
  nickel, 654, 656
  papulosquamous, 658–659
  perianal, 336
  Rhus, 656
  seborrheic, 657
Dermatoglyphics, 163
Dermatographism, 289
Dermatology assessment, 650–651
  common manifestations in, 650–651
    of primary skin lesions, 650–651, 650t, 651f
    of secondary skin lesions, 650–651, 651t

Dermatology assessment *(Continued)*
  history in, 650
  initial diagnostic evaluation and screening tests in, 651
  physical examination in, 650
Dermatomyositis, juvenile, 311–312
Dermatophytosis, 336
DES (diethylstilbestrol), as teratogen, 206t
Desensitization, for penicillin allergy, 297–298
Desloratadine, for allergic rhinitis, 284
Desmopressin
  for enuresis, 44
  for hemophilia, 529
  for von Willebrand disease, 530
Desquamation, in Kawasaki disease, 303–304
Development
  of adolescents
    normal variations in, 241–242
      breast asymmetry and masses as, 241, 241t
      gynecomastia as, 241t, 245–247
      irregular menses as, 241
      physiologic leukorrhea as, 241
    physical, 237–240
      for boys, 238–240, 239f
      for girls, 237–238, 238f–239f
  of bones, 667, 668f
  defined, 10
  disorders of, 15–20
  disruptions of, 160–161
  fostering optimal, 23–25, 24t–25t
  history of, in genetic assessment, 156
  normal, 13–15
    physical, 13
      in adolescence, 13
      in late school-age period/early adolescence, 13
      in later infancy, 13
      in newborn period, 13
    psychosocial, 14–15
      in adolescence, 14–15
      in early childhood, 14
      in infancy, 14
      of school readiness, 14, 14t
Developmental assessment, 26–29
  cognitive, 27, 29t
  educational, 27–29
  history taking in, 26, 27t
  issues in, 19–20
  medical, 26, 27t
  motor, 26
  physical examination in, 26, 28t
  psychological, 27, 29t
  of social environment, 29
Developmental delay, constipation due to, 425, 426t
Developmental disabilities, 26–36
  defined, 26
  due to cerebral palsy, 35–36, 35t–36t
  due to hearing impairment, 32–34, 33t
  due to mental retardation, 31, 31t–32t
  due to speech-language impairment, 34–35
  due to vision impairment, 31–32
  management of, 29–30
    counseling principles for, 30
    goal in, 26
    interdisciplinary team intervention for, 30, 31t
    intervention in primary care setting for, 29–30, 30t
  medical home for, 26
  multifaceted team assessment of, 26–29
    cognitive, 27, 29t
    educational, 27–29
    history taking in, 26, 27t

Developmental assessment *(Continued)*
    medical, 26, 27t
    motor, 26
    physical examination in, 26, 28t
    psychological, 27, 29t
    of social environment, 29
Developmental disorders, pervasive, 63–66, 64t
Developmental dysplasia of the hip (DDH),
        672–674
    Barlow (dislocation) test for, 673, 673f
    clinical manifestations of, 672–673
    complications of, 674
    etiology of, 672
    Galeazzi sign in, 672
    hip abduction test for, 672, 673f
    Klisic test for, 673
    Ortolani (reduction) test for, 673, 673f
    radiographic evaluation of, 674
    risk factors for, 672
    teratologic dislocations in, 672
    treatment of, 674
    typical dislocations in, 672
Developmental hematology, 506–509, 510f
Developmental issues, evaluation of, 20
Developmental milestones, 13–14, 16t
    musculoskeletal, 668
        for infants, 668, 669f
Developmental screening, 15–19
Developmental screening tests, 16
Developmental surveillance, 15–19
Deviated septum, 283t
Dexamethasone
    for CNS tumors, 547
    for croup, 354–355
    for meningitis, 343–344
Dexamethasone suppression test, for Cushing
        syndrome, 611
Dexmethylphenidate (Focalin), for ADHD, 42t
Dextrose
    in maintenance fluids, 107
    in parenteral nutrition, 113
DHT (dihydrotestosterone), in sexual
        differentiation, 604–605, 605f
Diabetes Control and Complications Trial,
        576–577
Diabetes insipidus
    central, 114
    nephrogenic, 114
Diabetes mellitus (DM), 572–579
    classification of, 572, 573t
    constipation due to, 426t
    cystic fibrosis-related, 475
    defined, 572–573
    insulin-dependent (type 1), 573
        chronic lymphocytic thyroiditis with, 578
        classification of, 573t
        clinical manifestations of, 573
        complications of, 578
        diabetic ketoacidosis due to, 573–578
            complications of, 576
            etiology of, 573
            pathophysiology of, 574, 575f
            presentation of, 574
            transition to outpatient management of,
                576
            treatment of, 575–576
        epidemiology of, 573
        etiology of, 573, 574f
        genetic susceptibility to, 573
        honeymoon period in, 574f, 576
        hypoglycemia in, 578
        outpatient management of, 576
            blood glucose testing in, 577–578
            goals of, 576–577
            insulin regimens in, 577

Diabetes mellitus (DM) *(Continued)*
        long-term glycemic control in, 578
        nutrition in, 577
    prognosis for, 578
    maternal, 205t–206t, 206
        gestational, 206, 573t
        as teratogens, 154
    maturity-onset, of youth, 573t, 579
    mitochondrial, 573t
    neonatal, 573t
    non-insulin-dependent (type 2), 572
        classification of, 573t
        clinical manifestations and differential
                diagnosis of, 579
        epidemiology of, 578
        pathophysiology of, 578
        therapy for, 579
Diabetic ketoacidosis (DKA), 573–578
    complications of, 576
    etiology of, 573
    pathophysiology of, 574, 575f
    presentation of, 574
    transition to outpatient management of, 576
    treatment of, 575–576
Diabetic macrovascular disease, 578
Diabetic nephropathy, 578
Diabetic neuropathy, 578
Diabetic retinopathy, 578
Dialysis
    for acute renal failure, 562
    for chronic kidney disease, 563
    for poisoning, 143
Diamond-Blackfan syndrome, 516, 516t
Diaper dermatitis, 656, 658
    candidal, 658
    irritant contact, 657f, 656, 658
Diaphoresis, due to heart failure, 501
Diaphragm
    contraceptive, 247
    during inspiration, 455
Diaphragmatic hernia, congenital, 196t, 215
Diaphysis, 668f
Diarrhea, 104–105, 424–425
    acute, 424–425
    adjusting fluid therapy, 108t, 110
    antibiotic-associated, 367
    bacterial, 366t
        fever due to, 325
    chronic, 424–425
    clinical manifestations of, 367–368
    Clostridium difficile-associated, 367
    common-source, 368
    complications and prognosis of, 372
    defined, 366, 424
    dehydration due to, 366
    differential diagnosis of, 368, 424–425, 424t
    distinguishing features of, 425
    due to decreased motility, 367t
    due to increased motility, 367t
    due to mucosal invasion, 367t
    due to parasites, 366t
    etiology and epidemiology of, 366–367, 366t
    evaluation of, 425
    functional, 424–425
    hypernatremia due to, 114
    hypokalemia due to, 116
    hyponatremia due to, 113
    laboratory and imaging studies of, 368
    mechanisms of, 367t
    metabolic acidosis due to, 120
    osmotic, 367t, 424–425
    prevention of, 372
    secretory, 367t, 424
    toddler's, 424–425
    traveler's, 366t, 367

Diarrhea *(Continued)*
    treatment of, 368–369
    viral, 366–367, 366t
Diastatic skull fractures, 638
Diastematomyelia, 647
Diastolic murmurs, 484
Diazepam
    for neonatal seizures, 226
    for status epilepticus, 621–622, 622t
DIC. *see* Disseminated intravascular coagulation
        (DIC)
Diet
    of the normal child and adolescent, 89–90
    for celiac disease, 442
    and colic, 39
    with developmental disability, 31t
    of the normal infant, 86–89
        breastfeeding in, 86–88
        complementary foods and weaning in, 89
        formula feeding in, 88–89
    for obesity, 92, 92t
    recommendations, 89–90
    of toddlers and older children, 89, 90t
Dietary history, for anemia, 511, 511t
Dietary protein-induced enteropathy, 295t
Diethylstilbestrol (DES), as teratogen, 206t
Differential Abilities Scale, 29t
Difficult child, 17
Diffusion, of gases across alveolar-capillary
        membrane, 456
Diffusion defect, hypoxemia due to, 456t
DiGeorge syndrome, 159–160, 259t, 260
Digestive system assessment, 417–429
    diagnostic imaging in, 417
        endoscopy for, 417, 418f
        radiology for, 417
    history in, 417
    physical examination in, 417
    screening tests in, 417
Digestive system disorders, common
        manifestations of, 417–429
    abdominal pain as, 417–422
    constipation and encopresis as, 425–426, 426t
    diarrhea as, 424–425, 424t
    GI bleeding as, 426–429, 427t–428t, 428f
    vomiting as, 422–423, 423t
Digital clubbing, 457
    in cystic fibrosis, 475
Digitalis, for heart failure, 501t
Digoxin, for ventricular septal defect, 491–492
Dihydrobiopterin reductase, 174
Dihydrotestosterone (DHT), in sexual
        differentiation, 604–605, 605f
1,25-Dihydroxyvitamin D (1,25-[OH]$_2$-D), 102,
        602–603
Dilated cardiomyopathy(ies), 502
    clinical manifestations of, 502
    etiology of, 502
    imaging studies of, 503–504
    treatment of, 504
Dimercaptosuccinic acid (DMSA, succimer), for
        lead poisoning, 143t–144t
DIOS (distal intestinal obstruction syndrome),
        478
Diphenhydramine
    for allergic rhinitis, 284
    for food allergies, 298
Diphtheria, tetanus, pertussis (DTaP) vaccine,
        317–318, 319f–322f, 358
Diplegia, due to cerebral palsy, 35t
Diplopia, 614
Direct antiglobulin test (DAT), 522f
Direct DNA analysis, 160, 163
Directly observed therapy, for tuberculosis, 411
Discipline, 23

Discoid lateral meniscus, 679
Discoid lupus, 309
Disimpaction, 45, 46t
Diskitis, 690
Dislocation, 667t
Disorders of sexual development (DSD), 604–607
    ovotesticular, 606
Disruptions, of development, 160–161, 667t
Disseminated gonococcal infections, 379, 384
Disseminated intravascular coagulation (DIC),
        530–531
    clinical manifestations of, 531, 531t
    differential diagnosis of, 531t
    due to cancer, 539t
    due to thrombotic microangiopathy, 528
    etiology of, 530, 530t
    in newborn, 222
    treatment of, 531
Dissociative states, in post-traumatic stress
        disorder, 56
Distal convoluted tubule, 553
Distal intestinal obstruction syndrome (DIOS),
        478
Distal radius, Salter-Harris fractures of, 693
Distal tubule, 553, 555f
Distributive justice, 6
Diuretics
    for cardiomyopathy, 503t
    for heart failure, 501t
    hypokalemia due to, 116
    for patent ductus arteriosus, 493
Divalproex sodium, for bipolar disorder, 61
Diverticulum, Meckel, 440
    abdominal pain due to, 420t
    GI bleeding due to, 427t
Divorce, 82–85
    outcome of, 83
    reactions of different ages to, 82–83
    role of pediatrician during, 83–84, 84t
Dizziness, etiology of, 488t
DKA. see Diabetic ketoacidosis (DKA)
DM. see Diabetes mellitus (DM); Myotonic
        dystrophy (DM)
DMD. see Duchenne muscular dystrophy (DMD)
DNA (deoxyribonucleic acid), 146
DNA analysis, in genetic assessment, 160
DNA polymerase chain reaction, for HIV, 413
DNA repair, in Fanconi anemia, 517
Do not resuscitate (DNR) orders, 9
Dobutamine
    for heart failure, 501t
    for shock, 132t
Dolichocephalic, 162
Doll's eye maneuver, 614, 635–636
Domestic violence, 79–80, 80t
Donovanosis, 376, 377t
Dopamine
    for heart failure, 501t
    for shock, 132t
Doppler examination, of fetal aorta or umbilical
        arteries, 189
Double-stranded DNA, antibodies to, in systemic
        lupus erythematosus, 309–310
Down syndrome (DS), 157
    newborn assessment for, 196t
Doxorubicin, for cancer, 540t–541t
Doxycycline, 479
    for *Chlamydia* infection, 380
    for Lyme disease, 397–400
    for Rocky Mountain spotted fever, 401
DPIs (dry powder inhalers), 460
Drowning, 136–137
    defined, 136
    near-, 136
Drowsiness, after head injury, 639

Drug(s)
    associated with neutropenia, 265t
    maternal
        small for gestational age due to, 208t
        as teratogens, 206, 206t
        that may adversely affect newborn, 206, 207t
Drug abuse
    by adolescents, 2
    after birth, 79
    during pregnancy, 79, 205t
Drug addiction
    maternal, 79, 205t
    neonatal, 204
        to cocaine, 204
        to opiates, 204
Drug administration, in newborn resuscitation,
        196
Drug-drug interactions, 325
Drug-induced anemia, 511, 511t
Drug-induced hypoglycemia, 580t, 582–583
Drug intoxication, ataxia due to, 632
Drug reactions, adverse, 296–298
Drug susceptibilities, 323
Drug toxicity, therapeutic monitoring for, 143t
Drug withdrawal, neonatal, 204
    from cocaine, 204
    from opiates, 204
Dry powder inhalers (DPIs), 460
DS (Down syndrome), 157
    newborn assessment for, 196t
DTaP (diphtheria, tetanus, pertussis) vaccine,
        317–318, 319f–322f, 358
Duchenne muscular dystrophy (DMD),
        627–628
    clinical manifestations of, 627
    etiology of, 627
    genetic basis for, 151t
    laboratory and diagnostic studies of, 627
    treatment of, 627–628
Ductal-dependent congenital heart disease,
        196t
Ductus arteriosus
    closure of, 190–191
    patent, 190–191, 492–493, 492f
        clinical manifestations of, 213, 492–493
        coarctation of the aorta, 494
        etiology and epidemiology of, 492
        imaging studies of, 493
        respiratory distress syndrome and, 212–213
        treatment of, 493
Ductus venosus, 190–191
Duke Criteria, Modified, for infective
        endocarditis, 365, 365t
Duodenal atresia, 196t, 439
Duodenal hematoma, 135
Duodenal ulcer, abdominal pain due to, 420t
Duplication cysts
    GI bleeding due to, 427t
    vomiting due to, 423t
Dust mites, and asthma, 275t
DV. see Dysfunctional voiding (DV)
Dwarfism
    Laron, 584, 588
    psychosocial or deprivation, 584–585
    zinc deficiency and, 104–105
Dysentery, 368
    amebic, 368
    diarrhea due to, 424
    Trichuris, 405t
Dysfluency, 19
Dysfunctional voiding (DV), 567–568
Dysgerminomas, 611
Dyskeratosis congenita, 516t
Dyskinesia(s), 633
    tardive, 637

Dysmenorrhea
    primary, 244
    secondary, 244
    treatment of, 244, 244t
Dysmetria, 615, 632
Dysmorphology, 160–163
    association in, 161
    defined, 160–161
    diagnosis of, 163
    due to disruptions of development, 160–161
    due to extrinsic factors, 160–161
    due to inborn errors of metabolism, 168
    due to intrinsic factors, 160–161
    epidemiology of, 161
    history for
        family, 161–162
        pregnancy, 161
    laboratory evaluation of, 163
    life-threatening, 196t
    malformation sequence in, 160–161
    physical examination, 162–163
        craniofacial, 162
        of extremities, 162–163
        of genitalia, 163
        growth in, 162
        of neck, 162
        of trunk, 162
    syndromes in, 160
    terminology used in, 161, 161t
Dysostosis multiplex, due to lysosomal storage
        diseases, 181t–182t
Dyspepsia, nonulcer, 436, 436t
Dysphagia, 458, 467
Dysphoric mania, 60–61
Dysplasia, 667t
Dyspnea
    due to pulmonary edema, 473
    exertional, due to pulmonary stenosis, 493
Dysrhythmia(s), 141, 488–490
    atrial, 489
    etiology and differential diagnosis, 488, 489t
    heart block as, 489
    syncope due to, 488t
    treatment of, 490, 490t
    ventricular, 489
Dysthymic disorder, 59–60
Dystonia, 637
    in glutaric acidemia I, 178
Dystrophin, 627
Dystrophy
    Becker, 627
    Duchenne (pseudohypertrophic progressive),
        627–628
        clinical manifestations of, 627
        etiology of, 627
        genetic basis for, 151t
        laboratory and diagnostic studies of, 627
        treatment of, 627–628
    facioscapulohumeral, 628
    limb-girdle muscular, 628
    myotonic, 628

E

EAEC (enteroaggregative *E. coli*), 366t, 367
Ear(s)
    with developmental disabilities, 28t
    of newborn, 197f
    swimmer's. see Otitis externa
Early childhood, developing autonomy in, 14
East African sleeping sickness, 398t–400t
Easy child, 17
Eating disorder(s), 248–249, 248t
    anorexia nervosa as, 248, 248f
        clinical manifestations and diagnosis of,
            248, 249t

Eating disorder(s) (*Continued*)
epidemiology of, 248
treatment and prognosis for, 248, 249t
bulimia nervosa as, 248–249, 249t
issues that can trigger, 248t
risk factors for, 249f
slippery slope to, 249f
Ecchymosis(es), 524, 650t
ECF. *see* Extracellular fluid (ECF)
ECG (electrocardiography), in cardiovascular
system assessment, 484, 485f
ECG (electrocardiographic) changes, 116
Echinococcus, 407, 407t
alveolar, 407t
unilocular (hydatid), 407, 407t
Echinococcus granulosus, 407
Echinococcus multilocularis, 407
Echinococcus vogeli, 407
Echocardiography, in cardiovascular system
assessment, 486f, 485–486
Eclampsia, 187
ECMO (extracorporeal membrane oxygenation)
for heart failure, 501t
for meconium aspiration syndrome, 215
for primary pulmonary hypertension of the
newborn, 215
Economic stresses, 3
Ecstasy, acute effects of, 250t–251t
Ecthyma, 336
gangrenosum, 336
Eczema, 653–654. *see also* Atopic dermatitis
with developmental disabilities, 28t
herpeticum
in atopic dermatitis, 287, 653–654
vs. varicella and zoster, 334
vaccinatum, in atopic dermatitis, 287, 653–654
Edema
cerebral, 110
due to diabetic ketoacidosis, 575–576
due to overly rapid rehydration, 110
due to renal disease, 553, 554t
hereditary angioneurotic, genetic basis for,
147t
in nephrotic syndrome, 556
in newborn, 198
Edetate calcium disodium (EDTA), for lead
poisoning, 143–144t
EDMA (3,4-ethylenedioxy-N-
methylamphetamine), acute effects of,
250t–251t
Edrophonium, maternal use of, 207t
Educational assessment, with developmental
disabilities, 27–29
Educational complications, of hearing
impairment, 33t
Educational intervention, for developmental
disability, 30
EEG (electroencephalogram), for seizures, 622
EEG (electroencephalography), 616, 47
Egg cases, of public lice, 381
Egophony, 458t
EHEC (enterohemorrhagic *E. coli*), 366t, 367
Ehlers-Danlos syndrome
hypermobility in, 313
hypotonia in, 629
Ehrlichia chaffeensis, 398t–400t, 401
Ehrlichia ewingii, 398t–400t, 401
Ehrlichiosis, 396, 398t–400t, 401–402
clinical manifestations of, 402
complications and prognosis for, 402
differential diagnosis of, 402
epidemiology of, 401
etiology of, 401
human granulocytic, 398t–400t
human monocytic, 398t–400t, 401

Ehrlichiosis (*Continued*)
laboratory and imaging studies for, 402f, 402
prevention of, 402
sennetsu, 398t–400t
treatment of, 402
EIEC (enteroinvasive *E. coli*), 366t, 367
Ejection clicks, due to aortic stenosis, 494
Ejection murmurs, 482–483
adolescent, 484t
due to aortic stenosis, 494
due to atrial septal defect, 493
Elbow, 692–693
Little Leaguer's, 692
nursemaid's, 692, 692f
Panner's disease of, 692
radial head subluxation of, 692, 692f
throwing injuries of, 692–693
Electrocardiographic (ECG) changes, in
hypokalemia, 116
Electrocardiography (ECG), in cardiovascular
system assessment, 484, 485f
Electroencephalogram (EEG), for seizures, 622
Electroencephalography (EEG), 616, 47
Electrolyte(s), 107
in body composition, 106
in parenteral nutrition, 113
Electrolyte imbalances, in diabetic ketoacidosis,
575
Electromyography (EMG), 616
Elimination control, 43
and enuresis, 43–44
and functional constipation and soiling, 44–46
normal development of, 41
Elliptocytosis, hereditary
clinical manifestations of, 521
etiology of, 509–510, 521
laboratory diagnosis of, 521
treatment of, 521
EM (erythema multiforme), 290–291, 662–664,
663t
Emancipated minors, 6
Embolism, pulmonary, 474–475
Embolus(i), septic, due to infective endocarditis,
365
Emergencies
hypertensive, 563
oncologic, 538, 539t
Emergency postcoital contraception, 246, 247t
EMG (electromyography), 616
EMLA (eutectic mixture of local anesthetics) for
analgesia, 145
Empathy, 4
Emphysema, 471–472
congenital lobar, 471
interstitial, 471–472
subcutaneous, 471–472
Empirical anti-infective therapy, 323
Empyema, 361, 363, 479
Enalapril
for heart failure, 501t
maternal use of, 207t
Encephalitis, 344–346
causes of, 345t
clinical manifestations of, 345
complications and prognosis for, 347
defined, 344
depressed consciousness due to, 636
differential diagnosis of, 345
epidemiology of, 345
etiology of, 344–345
laboratory and imaging studies for, 345–346
prevention of, 347
treatment of, 347
viral, 344–345
West Nile, 345

Encephaloceles, 647–648
Encephalomyelitis
acute disseminated, 345
due to measles, 331
Encephalomyelopathy, subacute necrotizing,
642t–643t, 644
Encephalopathy
bilirubin, 220–221
due to inborn errors of metabolism,
167, 167t
hepatic, 447–449
stages of, 448t
treatment of, 448t
hypoxic-ischemic
due to near drowning, 136
in newborn, 226–227
clinical manifestations of, 227, 227t
etiology of, 226–227
prognosis for, 227
seizures due to, 225
Encephalotrigeminal angiomatosis, port-wine
stain in, 662, 646
Enchondroma, 693t–694t
Encopresis, 44
clinical manifestations of, 44–45
complications of, 46
defined, 425
differential diagnosis of, 45
epidemiology of, 44
etiology of, 44
prevention of, 46
treatment of, 45–46
End-of-life care, 7–9
access to comprehensive and compassionate, 7
bereavement in, 8
cognitive issues in, 8
commitment to quality improvement of, 8
cultural, religious, and spiritual concerns
about, 9
goals of, 7
interdisciplinary resources in, 8
model of integrated, 7–8
principles of, 7–8
support for caregivers in, 8
End-of-life decision making, ethical issues in, 9
End-of-life issues, 7–9
End-stage renal disease (ESRD), 562
End-tidal carbon dioxide, 459
in cardiopulmonary resuscitation, 126
Endemic cretinism, 599
Endemic goiter, 599
Endobronchial granulomas, 471
Endobronchial mass lesions, 471
Endocardial cushion defect, 493, 493f
Endocardial cushion tissue, 491
Endocarditis, infective, 364–366
acute, 364
clinical manifestations of, 364
complications and prognosis of, 365–366
culture-negative, 364–365
defined, 364
diagnostic criteria for, 365t
differential diagnosis of, 365, 365t
epidemiology of, 364
etiology of, 364, 364t
laboratory studies and imaging of, 364–365
prevention of, 366
subacute, 364
treatment of, 365
Endocervicitis, 376
Endocrine action, of hormones, 570, 570f
Endocrine disorders, manifestations of, 570
Endocrine evaluation, of growth hormone
secretion, 584
Endocrine system, 570

Endocrinology assessment, 570–572
  of hypothalamic-pituitary axis, 570–571, 571f, 571t
Endophthalmitis, 388t–389t, 389
Endoscopic evaluation, of airways, 459
Endoscopic retrograde cholangiopancreatography (ERCP), 453
Endoscopy
  for gastroesophageal reflux, 431
  for gastrointestinal symptoms, 417, 418f
Endotracheal intubation
  in cardiopulmonary resuscitation, 126
  in newborn resuscitation, 194
Energy deficiency, due to inborn errors of metabolism, 168
Energy stores, hypoglycemia due to inadequate, 580t, 582
Engorgement, 87
Entamoeba histolytica, diarrhea due to, 366t, 367
Enteritis. see Gastroenteritis
Enteroaggregative *E. coli* (EAEC), 366t, 367
Enterobiasis, 406
  vulvovaginitis due to, 375t
Enterobius vermicularis, 405t, 406
Enterocolitis
  due to Hirschsprung disease, 440
  food protein-induced, 295t
  GI bleeding due to, 427t
  necrotizing, 223–224
Enterohemorrhagic *E. coli* (EHEC), 366t, 367
Enteroinvasive *E. coli* (EIEC), 366t, 367
Enteropathogenic *E. coli* (EPEC), 366t, 367
Enteropathy, dietary protein-induced, 295t
Enterotoxigenic *E. coli* (ETEC), 366t, 367
Enteroviruses, conjunctivitis due to, 387t
Enteroxigenic disease, 368
Enthesitis, in rheumatic diseases, 299
Enuresis, 43–44
  clinical manifestations of, 43–44
  complications of, 44
  defined, 43
  differential diagnosis of, 44
  epidemiology, 43
    physical examination, 43
  etiology, 43
  nocturnal, 567
  prevention of, 44
  as sleep disorder, 49t
  treatment of, 44
Enuresis alarm, 44
Environmental control
  for allergic rhinitis, 285
  for asthma, 274–275, 275t
Environmental intervention, for developmental disability, 30
Enzootic cycle, 396
Enzymatic disorders, neurodegenerative illnesses due to, 642–643, 642t–643t
Enzymes, for cancer, 540t–541t
Enzymopathy(ies), hemolytic anemia due to, 520–521
  etiology of, 510f
  G6PD deficiency as, 509–510, 513f, 520
  pyruvate kinase deficiency as, 509–510, 521
Eosinophil(s), normal values for, 508t
Eosinophilia
  disorders associated with, 272, 275t
  in infectious diseases, 316–317
  nonallergic rhinitis with, 283–284
Eosinophilic esophagitis (EOE), 431–433
  clinical manifestations of, 431
  etiology and epidemiology of, 431
  laboratory and imaging studies for, 431–432, 432f
  treatment and prognosis of, 432–433

Eosinophilic granuloma, 693t–694t
Eosinophilic meningitis, 405t
Eotaxins, functions of, 253t
EPEC (enteropathogenic *E. coli*), 366t, 367
Ependymoma
  epidemiology of, 546
  prognosis for, 549t
Epidemic typhus, 398t–400t, 666
Epidermal nevus, 659t
Epididymitis, 569
Epidural analgesia, 145
Epidural hemorrhage, 638t
Epiglottitis, 354, 467
  upper airway obstruction due to, 465t–466t
Epilepsy. *see also* Seizure(s)
  benign childhood, with centrotemporal spikes, 621
  defined, 618
  vs. degenerative diseases, 645
  myoclonic, 620–621
    juvenile (of Janz), 621
  rolandic, 621
  status epilepticus in, 621–622
    treatment of, 622t
Epilepsy syndromes, 619t, 621
Epileptic aphasia, acquired, 621
Epileptiform disorders, 621
Epinephrine
  for anaphylaxis, 291
  in cardiopulmonary resuscitation, 127, 127t
  for croup, 354–355
  for food allergies, 298
  in newborn resuscitation, 196
  for shock, 132t
Epiphyseal cartilage, 668f
Epiphyseal fractures, 670–671, 671f
Epiphyseal growth plate, 381
Epiphysiolysis, proximal humeral, 691–692
Epiphysis, 668f
Episcleritis, 388t–389t
Episodic allergic rhinitis, 282
Episodic neurologic disorders, 612
Epstein-Barr virus (EBV)
  anemia due to, 516t
  infectious mononucleosis due to, 339
    clinical manifestations of, 340
    complications and prognosis for, 341
    etiology of, 339
    laboratory studies for, 340
    serologic tests for, 340
  in X-linked lymphoproliferative disease, 261
Equinus, 667t
Erb-Duchenne paralysis, in newborn, 202–203
ERCP (endoscopic retrograde cholangiopancreatography), 453
Ergocalciferol, 102
Erosion, 651t
Erysipelas, 335–336
Erysipeloid, 398t–400t
Erysipelothrix rhusiopathiae, 398t–400t
Erythema infectiosum, 333
Erythema marginatum, due to rheumatic fever, 502, 503t
Erythema migrans, 397
Erythema multiforme (EM), 290–291, 662–664, 663t
  vesiculobullous eruptions due to, 663t
Erythema nodosum, infections with fever and, 329t–330t
Erythema toxicum, 198
Erythematous flare, in allergen-specific IgE in vivo skin testing, 272
Erythroblastopenia, transient, 516t

Erythroblastosis fetalis
  newborn anemia due to, 217
  predicting severity of, 218
  prevention of, 218
Erythrocyte P antigen, in erythema infectiosum, 333
Erythrocytic phase, of *Plasmodium* life cycle, 402
Erythroderma, infections with fever and diffuse, 329t–330t
Erythroid cells, in hematopoiesis, 506
Erythroid colony-forming unit, 506–509
Erythromycin, for acne, 652
Erythromycin estolate, for streptococcal pharyngitis, 349t
Erythromycin ethyl succinate, for streptococcal pharyngitis, 349t
Erythropoiesis, 506–509
  in β-thalassemia major, 518
  embryonic, 216
Erythropoietin, 506–509
  in chronic kidney disease, 562–563
  in renal function, 554
Escherichia coli
  diarrhea due to, 366t, 367
  in peritonitis, 453
  urinary tract infections due to, 372
Esophageal atresia, 433–434, 433f
Esophageal compression, 458
Esophageal disorder(s), 430–437
  caustic esophageal injuries as, 434–435
  due to foreign bodies, 434
  eosinophilic esophagitis as, 431–433
  esophageal atresia as, 433–434, 433f
  gastroesophageal reflux as, 430–431, 432t
  tracheoesophageal fistula as, 433–434, 433f
Esophageal foreign bodies, 434
Esophageal impedance monitoring, for gastroesophageal reflux, 431
Esophageal pH probe monitoring, 24-hour, for gastroesophageal reflux, 431
Esophageal reflux, abdominal pain due to, 420t
Esophageal varices, 448
  GI bleeding due to, 427t
Esophagitis, 436, 436t
  allergic eosinophilic, 295t
Esophagram, barium, 458
Estrogens, 103
  conjugated for delayed puberty, 592
Etanercept, for juvenile idiopathic arthritis, 308
ETEC (enterotoxigenic *E. coli*), 366t, 367
Ethical decision making, 5
Ethical issues
  in end-of-life decision making, 9
  in genetic testing and screening, 6
  in practice, 6–7
Ethical principles, related to infants, children, and adolescents, 5
Ethics, 5–7
  in health care, 5
  religious issues and, 6
Ethinyl estradiol
  for delayed puberty, 592
Ethylene glycol
  metabolic acidosis due to, 121
  toxicity of, 141t
3,4-Ethylenedioxy-N-methylamphetamine (EDMA), acute effects of, 250t–251t
Etonogestrel implant (Implanon), 246
Etoposide (VP-16), for cancer, 540t–541t
Eunuchoid proportions, in hypogonadotropic hypogonadism, 589
Eutectic mixture of local anesthetics (EMLA), for analgesia, 145

Evaluation
of child with special needs, 26–36
due to cerebral palsy, 35–36, 35t–36t
due to hearing impairment, 32–34, 33t
due to mental retardation, 31, 31t–32t
due to speech-language impairment, 34–35, 34t
due to vision impairment, 31–32
management of developmental problems in, 29–30
counseling principles for, 30
interdisciplinary team intervention for, 30, 31t
intervention in primary care setting for, 29–30, 30t
multifaceted team assessment of complex problems in, 26–29
cognitive, 27, 29t
educational, 27–29
history taking in, 26, 27t
medical, 26, 27t
motor, 26
psychological, 27, 29t
of social environment, 29
of well child, 20
Evaporation, heat loss via, 203
Evra (norelgestromin) contraceptive patch, 246
Ewing sarcoma, 552
clinical manifestations of, 551
differential diagnosis of, 552
epidemiology of, 551
laboratory/imaging studies of, 552
prognosis for, 552
risk factors for, 536t
treatment of, 552
Exchange transfusion, for indirect hyperbilirubinemia, 221
Excoriation, 651t
Exercise
hematuria due to, 559
for obesity, 92t
Exertional dyspnea, due to pulmonary stenosis, 493
Exhalation
accessory muscles of, 455
physiology of, 455
Exit site infection, 394
Exocrine pancreatic insufficiency, in cystic fibrosis, 476, 478
Exons, 146
Exostosis(es)
multiple hereditary, 693t–694t
osteocartilaginous, 693t–694t
Expiratory reserve volume, 455f
Expressive language disorders, 35
Extensor plantar reflex, 615
External cardiac massage, in newborn resuscitation, 196
External genitalia
ambiguous, 604
congenital malformations of, 163
with developmental disabilities, 28t
differentiation of, 604f–605f
inadequate masculinization of male, 605–606, 606t
of newborn, 197f
virilization of female, 605, 605t
External intercostal muscles, during inspiration, 455
External tibial torsion, 677
Extinction, 15, 31
Extracellular fluid (ECF), 106, 107f
composition of solutes in, 106
plasma water and interstitial fluid in, 106, 107f
volume of, 106

Extracorporeal membrane oxygenation (ECMO)
for heart failure, 501t
for meconium aspiration syndrome, 215
for primary pulmonary hypertension of the newborn, 215
Extrahepatic biliary atresia, 444
Extrapulmonary shunt, hypoxemia due to, 456t
Extrapulmonary tuberculosis, 410
Extremities
congenital malformations of, 161t, 162–163
with developmental disabilities, 28t
of newborn, 200
Extremity fractures, in newborn, 203
Extrinsic pathway, of coagulation, 523, 525f
Extrinsic tracheal compression, 470
Exudates, 479–480
Eye(s)
with developmental disabilities, 28t
dysmorphology of, 162
foreign body in, 388t–389t
of newborn, 197f
raccoon, 638
Eye movements
assessment of, 614
in coma, 635–636
Eye scrub, for blepharitis, 387

F

FA (Friedreich ataxia), 633
genetic basis for, 150t
Fabry disease, 181t–182t
Face
congenital malformations of, 161t, 162
of newborn, 199
Facial appearance, with developmental disabilities, 28t
Facial nerve, assessment of, 614
Facial nerve injury, in newborn, 203
Facial weakness, 625t
Facioscapulohumeral dystrophy, 628
Factitious disorder, 51–54
Factitious hyperinsulinemia, 581
Factor 5 Leiden, in thrombosis, 531
Factor VIII deficiency, genetic basis for, 151t
Failure to thrive (FTT), 67–69
causes of, 68t
complications of, 69
defined, 67
diagnosis and clinical manifestations of, 67–69
diagnostic criteria for, 67
epidemiology of, 67
etiology of, 67, 68t
treatment of, 69, 69t
Falling out syndrome, 52–53
Famciclovir
for genital herpes, 380–381
for varicella-zoster virus, 334–335
Familial hemophagocytic lymphohistiocytosis, 516t
Familial short stature, 12
Family(ies)
defined, 76
functions of, 76–77, 77t
single-parent, 77
traditional, 77
Family dysfunction, 79
defined, 76
for emotional support, education, and socialization, 79
for physical needs, 79
Family history
for developmental disabilities, 27t
for dysmorphology, 161–162
in genetic assessment, 155
for hemostatic disorders, 523

Family structure
and function, 76–79
adoption as, 78
foster care as, 78–79
homosexual parents as, 77–78
single-parent families as, 77
Family violence, 80, 80t
Fanconi anemia, 517–518
clinical manifestations of, 516t, 517
differential diagnosis of, 516t
etiology and epidemiology of, 517
marrow replacement in, 517–518
treatment of, 517
Fanconi syndrome, 557
proximal renal tubular acidosis in, 120
FAP. see Functional abdominal pain (FAP)
Farber lipogranulomatosis, 181t–182t
Fasciculation, 616, 615
Fasciculations
spinal muscular atrophy, 625
Fasciitis, necrotizing, 336
Fasciola hepatica, 406t
Fascioliasis, 406t
Fasciolopsiasis, 406t
Fasciolopsis buski, 406t
Fat metabolic disorder(s), 179–180
Fat-soluble vitamins, 101–103
Fatigability, due to pulmonary stenosis, 493
Fatigue, 54
chronic, 51
Fatty acid(s), catabolism of, 180f, 179
Fatty acid acyl-coenzyme A (CoA), dehydrogenase deficiencies, hypoglycemia due to, 582
Fatty acid disorder(s), 179–180
carnitine deficiency as, 183
of fatty acid oxidation, 179
glutaric aciduria type II, 179–180
neonatal screening for, 170t
specialized testing for, 170–171
Fatty acid oxidation, disorders of, 180f, 179
and hypoglycemia, 580t, 582
Fatty liver disease, nonalcoholic, 450
FBN1 gene, in Marfan syndrome, 148
Febrile paroxysms, in malaria, 403
Febrile seizures, 620
complex or atypical, 620
simple, 620
Fecalith, in appendicitis, 443
Feeding jejunostomy, for gastroesophageal reflux, 432t
FEF (forced expiratory flow) rates, 459
$FEF_{25-75\%}$ (mean midexpiratory flow rate), 459
FemCap (cervical cap), 247
Femoral anteversion, 667t, 676, 676t
clinical manifestations of, 676
Femoral pulses, in coarctation of the aorta, 494
FE_{Na} (fractional excretion of sodium), in acute renal failure, 561
Fentanyl, for analgesia, 145t
Ferritin levels, in anemia, 515
Ferrous sulfate, for iron deficiency anemia, 104
Fetal acidosis, 189
Fetal alcohol spectrum disorder, 79, 154
Fetal alcohol syndrome, 79
Fetal aorta, Doppler examination of, 189
Fetal growth, 188, 189t
Fetal heart rate monitoring, 189
Fetal hemoglobin, 190, 191f, 216, 509
Fetal hydrops, 187, 211
due to Rh sensitization, 217
respiratory distress in newborn due to, 209
Fetal-maternal hemorrhage, 218

Fetal maturity, 188–189
  pulmonary, 189
Fetal mortality, 187–188, 188t
Fetal physiology, transition to neonatal
    physiology from, 189–190, 191f
Fetal size, 188
Fetal well-being, 189
Fetus
  asphyxia in, 194
  assessment of, 188–189, 189t
  diseases of, 208–209
    hydrops fetalis as, 211
    intrauterine growth restriction and small for
        gestational age as, 208–209, 208t
FEV₁ (forced expiratory volume in 1 second, 459
Fever
  blackwater, 404
  Colorado tick, 398t–400t
  dengue, 398t–400t
  factitious, 326
  in immunocompromised person, 391, 392f
  infections with rash and, 329–335
    differential diagnosis of, 329t–330t
    erythema infectiosum (fifth disease) as, 333
    measles (rubeola) as, 329–331
    roseola infantum (exanthem subitum, sixth
        disease) as, 332–333
    rubella (German or 3-day measles) as,
        331–332
    varicella-zoster virus infection (chickenpox,
        zoster) as, 333–335
  in infectious diseases, 315
  in Kawasaki disease, 303
  normal body temperature and, 324
  Q, 398t–400t
  rat-bite, 398t–400t
  relapsing, 398t–400t
  relapsing, louse-borne, 666
  rheumatic, 501–502
    clinical manifestations of, 501–502, 502t
    etiology and epidemiology of, 501
    treatment and prevention of, 503–504
  in rheumatic diseases, 299
  scarlet, 348
  of short duration, 325
  spotted, 398t–400t
  trench, 666
  typhoid, 366, 368
  without a focus, 324–328
    with bacteremia, 324–325
    in children 3 months to 3 years, 325–326,
        326f
    in infants younger than 3 months, 325
    pattern of, 324
    with sepsis, 324–325
Fever blisters, 337
Fever of unknown origin (FUO), 325–328, 327f
Fexofenadine, for allergic rhinitis, 284
FFA (free fatty acids), in serum glucose
    regulation, 580, 581f
FGFR3 gene, in achondroplasia, 148
Fiber supplements, for irritable bowel syndrome,
    421–422
Fibrillation(s), 616
  atrial, 489
  ventricular, 490t
Fibrillin, in Marfan syndrome, 148
Fibrin, in hemostasis, 524f
Fibrinogen, in hemostasis, 524–526, 524f
Fibrinolysis, in hemostasis, 523, 524f
Fibrinolytic agents, for thrombosis, 531
Fibroma, nonossifying, 693t–694t
Fibromyalgia, 313–314
Fibrosing colonopathy, due to lipase, 478
Fibrous periosteum, 668f

Fine crackles, 457
Fine motor-adaptive development, milestones
    of, 16t
Finger(s)
  abnormalities of, 693
  trigger, 693
FIO₂, low, hypoxemia due to, 456t
Fire ant bites, allergic reactions to, 293
First-degree heart block, 489, 490t
FISH (fluorescent in situ hybridization), 159–160
Fissure, 651t
Fitz-Hugh-Curtis syndrome, 379
Flank mass, due to renal disease, 554t
Flashbacks, in post-traumatic stress disorder, 56
Flatfoot
  developmental, 682
  flexible, 682
  rigid, 682–683
Flatworms
  cestodes as, 407t, 404
  trematodes as, 404, 406t
Flavoprotein metabolism, 179f
Flea bites, anaphylaxis due to, 293
Flexible flatfoot, 682
Floppy infant, 629, 630t
Floppy larynx, 467
Fludrocortisone
  for Addison disease, 611
  for 21-hydroxylase deficiency, 609
Fluency disorders, 34–35
Fluid(s)
  in body composition, 106, 107f
  in cardiopulmonary resuscitation, 127t
Fluid deficit, calculation of, 109
Fluid restriction, for heart failure, 501t
Fluid resuscitation
  for burns, 138
  for dehydration, 109
  for intussusception, 443
Fluid therapy, for dehydration, 110
  monitoring and adjusting, 110
Flukes, 404
Flumazenil, for benzodiazepine intoxication,
    143t–144t
Flunisolide, for asthma, 279f
Flunitrazepam, acute effects of, 250t–251t
Fluorescent in situ hybridization (FISH), 159–160
Fluorescent treponemal antibody-absorption,
    380
Fluoride deficiency, 103t, 105
Fluoride supplementation, 103t, 429–430
Fluorosis, 105, 429–430
Fluoxetine
  maternal use of, 207t
  as teratogen, 206t
Fluticasone HFA/MDI/DPI, for asthma, 279f
Flutter, atrial, 489, 490t
Flutter valve, 460
Fly bites, anaphylaxis due to, 293
Flying squirrel typhus, 398t–400t
FMR-1 gene, in fragile X syndrome, 153
FMRP (fragile X mental retardation protein),
    153
Focal segmental glomerulosclerosis (FSGS),
    nephrotic syndrome due to, 556
Focalin (Dexmethylphenidate), for ADHD, 42t
Focalin XR (Dexmethylphenidate), for ADHD,
    42t
Folate deficiency, 98–100, 98t–100t
  anemia due to, 510f
Folic acid antagonists, as teratogens, 206t
Folie à deux, 66
Follicle-stimulating hormone (FSH), in puberty,
    589
Follicular cyst, precocious puberty due to, 594t

Folliculitis, 336
  hot tub, 336
Fontan procedure, for tricuspid atresia, 497
Fontanelles, 198–199
Food(s), adverse reactions to, 294–296
  clinical manifestations of, 294, 295t
  complications of, 297–298
  diagnosis of, 294–296, 296t
  etiology and epidemiology of, 294
  laboratory and imaging studies for, 294
  prognosis and prevention of, 298
  treatment of, 297
  vomiting as, 423t
Food-borne causes, of diarrhea, 368
Food protein-induced enterocolitis syndrome,
    295t
Foot, 681–683
  calcaneovalgus, 682
  cavus, 683
  club, 681–682, 681f
  hypermobile pes planus (flexible flat-), 682
  idiopathic avascular necrosis of, 683
  metatarsus adductus of, 682
  posturing vs. deformity of, 681
  Sever disease (calcaneal apophysitis) of,
      683
  skew-, 682
  tarsal coalition of, 682–683
  toe deformities of, 683, 689t
Foot pain, differential diagnosis of, 681, 681t
Forbes disease, 172t
Forced expiratory flow (FEF) rates, 459
Forced expiratory volume in 1 second (FEV₁),
    459
Forced vital capacity (FVC), 459
Forchheimer spots, in rubella, 331
Forehead, dysmorphology of, 162
Foreign body(ies), 468
  vs. bronchiolitis, 359
  esophageal, 434
  in eye, 388t–389t
  infections associated with, 324
  in nose, 284
  upper airway obstruction due to, 465t–466t
  vulvovaginitis due to, 375t
Foreign body aspiration, 470–471
Formicid stings, allergic reactions to, 293
Formoterol, for asthma, 276
Formula feeding, 88–89
  with carbohydrate intolerance, 88t
  cow's milk based formulas, 88–89
  hypoallergenic formula, 88t
  premature, 88–89
  soy, 88–89, 88t
  standard, 88t
Formula preparation, for failure to thrive, 69t
Fosphenytoin, for status epilepticus, 621–622,
    622t
Foster care, 2, 78–79
Founder effect, with inborn errors of metabolism,
    169
Fraction of inspired oxygen (FIO₂), low,
    hypoxemia due to, 456t, 460
Fractional excretion of sodium (FE_Na), in acute
    renal failure, 561
Fracture remodeling, 671
Fracture(s), 670–672
  angulation, 670t
  bowing, 670
  buckle (torus), 670
  comminution, 670t
  compaction, 670t
  complete, 670, 670t
  due to child abuse, 71, 71f, 674–675
  epiphyseal, 670–671, 671f

Fracture(s) (*Continued*)
greenstick, 670, 670f
incomplete, 670t
in infants, 38
linear, 670t
management of pediatric, 671
oblique, 670t
open, 670t
patterns of pediatric, 670–671
rotation, 670t
Salter-Harris classification of, 670–671, 671f
shortening, 670t
skull, 638–639
special concern(s) with, 671–672
compartment syndrome as, 671–672
neurovascular injury as, 671
overgrowth as, 671
progressive deformity as, 671
remodeling as, 671
spiral, 670t
terminology for, 670t
toddler's, 674–675
transverse, 670t
Fragile X mental retardation protein (FMRP), 153
Fragile X syndrome (FRAX), genetic basis for, 151t, 153
Frameshift mutation, 146
Francisella tularensis, 398t–400t
FRC (functional residual capacity), 455–456
Free fatty acids (FFAs), in serum glucose regulation, 580, 581f
Freiberg disease, 683
Fremitus, vocal, 458t
Friction, vesiculobullous eruptions due to, 663t
Friedreich ataxia (FA), 633
genetic basis for, 150t
Fröhlich syndrome, obesity in, 91t
Fructose intolerance, hereditary, 176
hypoglycemia due to, 582
Fructose-1,6-diphosphatase deficiency, hypoglycemia due to, 582
Fructosuria, 176
FSGS (focal segmental glomerulosclerosis), nephrotic syndrome due to, 556
FSH (follicle-stimulating hormone), in puberty, 589
α-L-Fucosidase deficiency, 181t–182t
Fucosidosis, 181t–182t
Fulminant liver failure, 447–448. *see also* Liver failure; fulminant
Fumarylacetoacetate hydrolase deficiency, 175
Functional abdominal pain (FAP), 54, 418. *see also* Abdominal pain; functional
Functional residual capacity (FRC), 455–456
Fundoplication procedure, for gastroesophageal reflux, 432t
Funeral, children at, 85
Fungal infection(s)
in immunocompromised person, 390–391
superficial, 336
Fungal meningitis, 343t
Fungemia, catheter-associated, 395
FUO (fever of unknown origin), 325–328, 327f
causes of, in children, 327t–328t
screening tests for, 326–328
Furosemide, for heart failure, 501t
Furuncle, 336, 651f

G

GAD. *see* Generalized anxiety disorder (GAD)
Gadolinium enhanced MRI, in infectious diseases, 317
Gag reflex, 614

Gait
antalgic, 668
assessment of, 613, 615, 668
Trendelenburg, 668
waddling, 668
Galactocerebroside ß-galactosidase deficiency, 181t–182t
Galactokinase deficiency, 173–174
Galactose-1-phosphate uridyltransferase deficiency, 173, 173f
Galactose-6-sulfatase deficiency, 181t–182t
Galactosemia, 173–174
clinical manifestations of, 173
diagnosis of, 173
genetic basis for, 169t
hypoglycemia due to, 582
laboratory manifestations of, 173
neonatal screening for, 170, 170t
treatment of, 173
Galactosialidosis, 181t–182t
α–Galactosidase deficiency, 181t–182t
ß-Galactosidase deficiency, 181t–182t
Galactosyl ceramide lipidosis, 181t–182t
Galeazzi sign, 672
Gallstones, due to anemia, 511
Ganglion cysts, 693
Gangliosidosis
GM$_1$ (generalized, infantile), 181t–182t
GM$_2$, 181t–182t
Gardnerella vaginalis, 374
Gasping, 457t, 634–635
Gastric lavage, for poisoning, 142–143
Gastritis, vomiting due to, 423t
Gastroenteritis
acute, 366–369
clinical manifestations of, 367–368
complications and prognosis of, 372
defined, 366
differential diagnosis of, 368
etiology and epidemiology of, 366–367, 366t
laboratory and imaging studies of, 368
prevention of, 372
treatment of, 368–369
allergic eosinophilic, 295t
bacterial
GI bleeding due to, 427t
vomiting due to, 423t
viral, vomiting due to, 423t
Gastroesophageal reflux (GER), 430–431
clinical manifestations of, 431
etiology and epidemiology of, 430–431
infantile, 422
laboratory and imaging studies of, 431
physiologic, 430–431
treatment of, 431, 432t
vs. vomiting, 422, 423t
Gastrointestinal (GI) bleeding, 426–429
differential diagnosis of, 427, 427t
distinguishing features of, 427
evaluation of, 427, 428t
treatment of, 428–429, 428f
Gastrointestinal (GI) complications, of cystic fibrosis, 476t
Gastrointestinal (GI) decontamination, for poisoning, 142–143
Gastrointestinal (GI) hypersensitivity, acute, 295t
Gastrointestinal (GI) involvement, in Henoch-Schönlein purpura, 302–303
Gastrointestinal (GI) losses, adjusting fluid therapy for, 108, 108t
Gastrointestinal (GI) problems, with developmental disability, 31t
Gastrointestinal (GI) symptoms
abdominal pain as, 417–422
constipation and encopresis as, 425–426, 426t

Gastrointestinal (GI) symptoms (*Continued*)
defined, 425
differential diagnosis of, 425, 426t
diarrhea, 424–425
acute, 424–425
chronic, 424–425
defined, 424
differential diagnosis of, 424–425, 424t
distinguishing features of, 425
evaluation of, 425
functional, 424–425
osmotic, 424–425
secretory, 424
toddler's, 424–425
GI bleeding as, 426–429
of poisoning, 141
vomiting as, 422–423, 423t
Gastrointestinal (GI) system assessment, 417–429
diagnostic imaging in, 417
endoscopy for, 417, 418f
radiology for, 417
history in, 417
physical examination in, 417
screening tests in, 417
Gastrointestinal (GI) system disorders, common manifestations of, 417–429
abdominal pain, 417–422
constipation and encopresis as, 425–426, 426t
diarrhea as, 424–425, 424t
GI bleeding as, 426–429, 427t–428t, 428f
vomiting as, 422–423, 423t
Gastroschisis, 196t, 200, 439
Gaucher disease, 181t–182t, 642t–643t, 643
genetic basis for, 150t
G-CSF (granulocyte colony-stimulating factor)
in hematopoiesis, 509, 510f
for infection in immunocompromised person, 392–394
Gell and Coombs classification, of adverse drug reactions, 296, 297t
Gender identity, 75–76, 75t
Gender identity disorder (GID), 75–76
Gender roles, 75, 75t
Gene(s), 146
General appearance, with developmental disabilities, 28t
Generalized anxiety disorder (GAD), 55–56
defined, 55–56
diagnostic criteria for, 56t
Genetic assessment, 154–156
history in
of delivery and birth, 156
of development, 156
family, 155
laboratory evaluation, 159
chromosome analysis in, 159
direct DNA analysis in, 160
fluorescent in situ hybridization in, 159–160
microarray comparative genomic hybridization in, 160
past medical, 156
physical examination, 159
of pregnancy, 155–156
preconception and prenatal counseling, 154–155
adolescent and adult, 155
familial factors in, 154
maternal factors in, 155
postnatal, 155
screening in, 154–155
Genetic disorder(s)
autosomal dominant, 147t
autosomal recessive, 150t
due to expansion of trinucleotide repeat, 153

Genetic disorder(s) (Continued)
due to genomic imprinting, 153
due to uniparental disomy, 152–153
Angelman syndrome due to, 153
Prader-Willi syndrome as, 153
mitochondrial inheritance, 152
heteroplasmy in, 152
MELAS as, 152
multifactorial disorders (polygenic inheritance)
hypertrophic pyloric stenosis as, 152
neural tube defects as, 152
type of, 146
X-linked recessive, 150
Genetic testing and screening
ethical issues in, 6
for primary immunodeficiency, 258
Genetics, 146–151
Genital ambiguity, 604–607
approach to infant with, 606–607
diagnosis of, 607
due to inadequate masculinization of 46,XY male, 605–606, 606t
due to virilization of 46,XX female, 605, 605t
normal development and, 604–605, 604f–605f
treatment of, 607
Genital herpes, 377t
Genital ulcers, 376, 377t
Genital warts, 338, 376, 383
clinical features of, 378t
diagnosis of, 381
pathogenesis of, 384
treatment of, 381
Genitalia
ambiguous, 604
congenital malformations of, 163
with developmental disabilities, 28t
differentiation of, 604f–605f
inadequate masculinization of male, 605–606, 606t
of newborn, 197f, 200
virilization of female, 605, 605t
Genomic imprinting, 153
Genomics, 146–151
Genu valgum, 677–678, 677f
Genu varum, 677f, 678
Germ cell tumors
malignant, risk factors for, 536t
treatment of, 547
Germinomas, delayed puberty due to, 593
Gesell Developmental Observation-Revised (GDO-R), 29t
Gestation(s). see also Pregnancy
multiple, 187
Gestational age
fetus, 188
large for, 197, 199f
of newborn, 197
and abnormal fetal growth patterns, 197, 199f
cumulative score in, 197, 198f
neurologic criteria in, 197, 198f
physical criteria for, 197, 197f
small for, 208–209
clinical features of, 208
complications of, 189t, 197
defined, 197, 208
etiology of, 208, 208t
management of, 208–209
and mortality rate, 199f
prenatal detection of, 208
Gestational diabetes, 206, 573t
GFR (glomerular filtration rate), 554
GH. see Growth hormone (GH)
GHBP (growth hormone-binding protein), 583
Ghent nosology, 149t

Ghon complex, 408, 410
Ghrelin, in GH secretion, 583
Giant cell pneumonia, due to measles, 331
Giant coronary artery aneurysms, in Kawasaki disease, 303
Giant osteoid osteoma, 693t–694t
Giant pigmented nevi, 198, 660
Giardia lamblia, diarrhea due to, 366t, 367
Giardiasis, vulvovaginitis due to, 375t
Gingivitis, acute necrotizing ulcerative, 349
Gingivostomatitis, 348
herpes, 337
Girls, growth and development of, 237–238
Gitelman syndrome, hypokalemia in, 116
Glabella, 161t
Glands, 570
enlargement of, 570
Glanzmann thrombasthenia, 528
Glasgow Coma Scale, 133, 134t, 635, 639
Glenn procedure, bidirectional, for tricuspid atresia, 497
Glenohumeral dislocation, 691
Glenohumeral joint, 691
Gliomas
precocious puberty due to, 593
prognosis for, 549t
Globin chains, in erythropoiesis, 506–509
Globoid cell leukodystrophy, 642t–643t, 643
Glomerular filtration, 553
Glomerular filtration rate (GFR), 554
Glomerulonephritis (GN), 558–560
acute postinfectious, 558
clinical manifestations of, 558–559
diagnostic studies of, 558t, 559
etiology and epidemiology of, 558
membranoproliferative, nephrotic syndrome due to, 556
poststreptococcal
clinical manifestations of, 558–559
etiology of, 558
prognosis for, 560
treatment of, 559
prognosis and prevention of, 560
rapidly progressive, 558
therapy for, 559
Glomerulosclerosis, focal segmental, nephrotic syndrome due to, 556
Glossitis, 100
Glottis, anatomy of, 455
Glucocerebrosidase deficiency, 181t–182t
genetic basis for, 150t
Glucocorticoids
for 21-hydroxylase deficiency, 609–611
biosynthesis of, 608f
Gluconeogenesis
and hypoglycemia, 580t, 582
in serum glucose regulation, 580, 581f
Glucose
in cardiopulmonary resuscitation, 127t
for hypoglycemia, 582
in maintenance fluids, 107
serum
in hypoglycemia, 572–573
regulation of, 580, 581f
in urine, 555–556
Glucose-6-phosphatase deficiency, 172t
hypoglycemia due to, 582
Glucose-6-phosphate dehydrogenase (G6PD) deficiency
anemia due to, 509–510, 513f, 520
clinical manifestations of, 521
epidemiology of, 520
etiology of, 520
genetic basis for, 151t
laboratory studies of, 521

Glucose-6-phosphate dehydrogenase (G6PD) deficiency (Continued)
Mediterranean variant of, 520–521
phagocytic disorders in, 264t
treatment and prevention of, 521
type A (African) variant of, 520–521
type B variant of, 520–521
Glucose tolerance, 572–573
Glucosylceramide lipidosis, 181t–182t
Glucuronosyltransferase deficiency, 219
Glutaric acidemia type I, 179f, 178
Glutaric aciduria type II, 179–180
Glutaryl-CoA dehydrogenase deficiency, 179f, 178
Gluten, in celiac disease, 442
Glycemic control, for type 1 diabetes mellitus, 578
Glycerin suppository, for functional constipation, 47t, 46t
Glycogen, 172
synthesis and degradation of, 172, 173f
Glycogen storage diseases, 172–173, 172t, 173f
hypoglycemia due to, 582
Glycogen synthetase, 172, 173f
Glycogenolysis,
and hypoglycemia, 580t, 582
in serum glucose regulation, 580, 581f
Glycohemoglobin (HgbA$_{1c}$), 578
Glycolytic enzymes, in erythropoiesis, 506–509
Glycosaminoglycans, 183
Glycosuria, in insulin-dependent diabetes mellitus, 573
GM-CSF (granulocyte-macrophage colony-stimulating factor)
in hematopoiesis, 509, 510f
for infection in immunocompromised person, 392–394
GM$_1$ gangliosidosis, 181t–182t, 642t–643t
GM$_2$ gangliosidosis, 181t–182t, 642t–643t, 643
GN. see Glomerulonephritis (GN)
GnRH (gonadotropin-releasing hormone), in puberty, 589
GnRH (gonadotropin-releasing hormone)-independent sexual precocity, 593–595, 593t, 595t
Goiter, endemic, maternal, 205t
GoLYTELY (polyethylene), for poisoning, 143
Gonadal failure, primary, 590t–591t
ovarian, 590t, 591–592
testicular, 590t, 592
Gonadal steroids, biosynthesis of, 608f
Gonadarche, 589
Gonadoblastomas, 611
Gonadotropin-releasing hormone (GnRH), in puberty, 589
Gonadotropin releasing hormone (GnRH) analogs, 75–76
Gonadotropin-releasing hormone (GnRH)-independent sexual precocity, 593–595, 593t, 595t
Gonococcal conjunctivitis, 387
complications of, 389
neonatal, 388t–389t
clinical manifestations of, 387
treatment of, 388t
prophylaxis for, 389
treatment of, 389
Gonococcal infections, disseminated, 379
Gonococcemia, differential diagnosis of, 300t
Gonorrhea, 379
and Chlamydia trachomatis, 376t
clinical features of, 376t
congenital infection with, 230t, 232–233
disseminated gonococcal infections due to, 379
pathogenesis of, 379

Gonorrhea (Continued)
  pelvic inflammatory disease due to, 379
  recommended treatment for, 233
  treatment of, 379
Gordon syndrome, 118
Gottron papules, in juvenile dermatomyositis, 311
Gower sign, 615, 627
  in juvenile dermatomyositis, 311
G6PD deficiency. see Glucose-6-phosphate dehydrogenase (G6PD) deficiency
Graft-versus-host disease (GVHD)
  acute, 270
  chronic, 270
  due to cancer, 539t
  with hematopoietic stem cell transplantation, 269
  in severe combined immunodeficiency, 262
Gram-negative anaerobic bacilli, pneumonia due to, 363t
Granulation tissue, endobronchial, 471
Granulocyte colony-stimulating factor (G-CSF)
  in hematopoiesis, 509, 510f
  for infection in immunocompromised person, 392–394
Granulocyte-macrophage colony-stimulating factor (GM-CSF)
  in hematopoiesis, 509, 510f
  for infection in immunocompromised person, 392–394
Granuloma(s)
  endobronchial, 471
  eosinophilic, 693t–694t
  inguinale, 376, 377t
  pyogenic, 662
Granulosa cell tumor, precocious puberty due to, 594t
Graphesthesia, 615
Grasp reflex, 13, 613, 613t
Graves disease, 600
  clinical manifestations of, 600, 600t
  maternal, 205t, 206
  treatment of, 600
    drugs for, 600–601
    radioiodine for, 601
    surgical, 601
Great arteries, transposition of, 496–497, 496f
Greenstick fractures, 670, 670f
GRF (growth hormone-releasing factor), 583
Grief, 8
Gross motor development, milestones of, 16t
Ground itch, 405
Group A streptococci, 347, 348t
  osteomyelitis due to, 381–382
  pharyngitis due to
    clinical manifestations of, 347–348
    complications of, 349
    epidemiology of, 347
    etiology of, 347
    laboratory evaluation of, 348
    prevention of, 349
    recurrent, 349
    treatment of, 349, 349t
  pneumonia due to, 363t
Group B streptococci
  osteomyelitis due to, 381–382
  pneumonia due to, 363t
Growing pains, 312–313
Growth abnormalities, 584–588
  short stature as. see Short stature
Growth and development, 583–588
  of adolescents, 237–240
    for boys, 238–240, 239f
    for girls, 237–238, 238f–239f
    normal variations in, 241–242

Growth and development (Continued)
    breast asymmetry and masses as, 241, 241t
    gynecomastia as, 241t, 245–247
    irregular menses as, 241
    physiologic leukorrhea as, 241
  benchmarks for, 10, 10t
  of bones, 667, 668f
  catch-down, 12
  catch-up, 12
  constitutional delay in, 589, 590t
  defined, 10
  disorders of, 10, 12
  hormonal effects on, 584t
  measurement of, 583–584
  normal, 10–15, 583–584
Growth charts
  for body mass index, 11f
  for head circumference, 11f
  for height, 11f
  for weight, 11f
Growth factors, mechanisms of action of, 570f
Growth failure
  with anemia, 511
  in chronic kidney disease, 562–563
  defined, 584, 586f
  screening tests for, 588t
Growth hormone-binding protein (GHBP), 583
Growth hormone (GH) deficiency, 586–588
  classic congenital or idiopathic, 586
  clinical manifestations of, 586–588
  diagnosis of, 588, 588t
  differential diagnosis of, 587t
  etiology and epidemiology of, 585t, 586
  and growth, 584t
  hypoglycemia due to, 580
  treatment of, 587t, 588
Growth hormone (GH) excess, and growth, 584t
Growth hormone (GH) insensitivity, 588
Growth hormone (GH) release inhibitory factor, 583
Growth hormone (GH) resistance, 584, 588
Growth hormone (GH) secretion
  endocrine evaluation of, 584
  physiology of, 583
Growth hormone-releasing factor (GRF), 583
Growth patterns, 583, 586f
  evaluation of, 10, 12t
Growth plate, 668f
Growth plate injury, Salter-Harris classification of, 670–671, 671f
Grunting, 457
Guanfacine (Intuniv), for ADHD, 42t
Guillain-Barré syndrome, 625–626
Gustatory rhinitis, 283–284
Guttate psoriasis, 658
Gymnast's wrist, 693
Gynecologic issue(s), 242–247
  contraception in, 245–247
    abstinence for, 245
    barrier methods of, 247
      condoms and foam as, 247
      sponge, caps, and diaphragm as, 247
    coitus interruptus for, 247
    emergency postcoital, 246, 247t
    intrauterine devices for, 246
    oral and anal sex for, 247
    rhythm method (periodic coital abstinence) for, 247
    steroidal, 245–247
      combined oral contraceptives for, 245–246, 245t–246t
      contraceptive patch for, 246
      contraceptive vaginal ring for, 246

Gynecologic issue(s) (Continued)
    hormonal injections and implants for, 246
    progesterone-only pill or minipill for, 246
  menstrual disorder(s) as, 242–244
    abnormal uterine bleeding as, 243, 243t
    amenorrhea as, 242–243
    dysmenorrhea as, 242, 244
    irregular menses as, 241–242
  pregnancy as, 244–245
    continuation of, 245
    diagnosis of, 244
    termination of, 245
  rape as, 247
Gynecomastia, in adolescent boys, 596, 245–247

H

H₁ antihistamines, for urticaria and angioedema, 291
H₂ receptor antagonist, for gastroesophageal reflux, 432t
H1N1 influenza, 87t
H5N1, 359
HAART (highly active antiretroviral therapy), 413–415
Haddon matrix, 133
Haemophilus ducreyi, 376
Haemophilus influenzae, conjunctivitis due to, 386
Haemophilus influenzae type b (Hib)
  osteomyelitis due to, 381–382
  pneumonia due to, 359, 363t
Haemophilus influenzae type b (Hib) vaccine, 317–318, 319f–322f, 342
Hair, with developmental disabilities, 28t
Hair tourniquets, in infants, 38
Hair tufts, over lumbosacral spine, 197
Hairy congenital nevus, 660, 660f
Hallucinogens, acute effects of, 250t–251t
Haloperidol, maternal use of, 207t
Hamartoma
  precocious puberty due to, 593
  smooth muscle, 659t
  in tuberous sclerosis, 646
Hand, 693
  finger abnormalities of, 693
  fractures of, 693
Hand-foot-mouth syndrome, vesiculobullous eruptions due to, 663t
HANE (hereditary angioneurotic edema), genetic basis for, 147t
Hantavirus pulmonary syndrome, 359, 398t–400t
Haptenation, in adverse drug reactions, 296
Harpeden stadiometer, 583
Hartnup syndrome, 177
Harvester ant bites, allergic reactions to, 293
Hashimoto thyroiditis, 599
Haverhill fever, 398t–400t
Hay fever, 282
HBeAg (hepatitis B early antigen), 371
HBIG (hepatitis B immunoglobulin), 372
HBsAg (hepatitis B surface antigen), 369, 371
HBV. see Hepatitis B virus (HBV)
HD (Huntington disease), genetic basis for, 147t
HDV (hepatitis D virus), 369, 370t
  complications and prognosis of, 373–374
Head, congenital malformations of, 161t, 162
Head circumference (HC)
  benchmarks for, 10, 10t
  with developmental disabilities, 28t
  growth chart for, 11f
  in neurology assessment, 612
Head injuries, 134
Head louse, 665
  clinical manifestations of, 665
  differential diagnosis of, 665

Head louse (*Continued*)
  epidemiology of, 665
  etiology of, 665
  treatment of, 665
Head tilt, 614
Head trauma, 637–640
  disorders of consciousness due to, 634–637
    acute, 634–637, 635t
      assessment of, 634–636
      clinical manifestations of, 636–637, 636t
      etiology of, 636
      laboratory and diagnostic imaging of,
        635t, 637
      prognosis of, 637
      treatment of, 637
      transient, recurrent, 637
  due to child abuse, 72, 72f, 72t–73t
  increased intracranial pressure due to, 640–642
    clinical manifestations of, 641
    etiology of, 636t, 640–641, 640t
    laboratory and diagnostic studies for, 641
    treatment of, 641–642
  with neurologic deficits, 637
    concussion as, 637–638
    drowsiness, headache and vomiting due
      to, 639
    due to cervical spine injuries, 639
    due to cranial nerve palsies, 638–639
    due to CSF leak, 638–639
    due to skull fractures, 638–639
    intracranial hemorrhage in, 638–640, 638t
    seizures as, 639
    transient, 639
Headache, 616–618
  acute, 617t
    recurrent, 617t
  after head injury, 639
  chronic
    daily, 617t
    nonprogressive, 617t
    progressive, 617t
  clinical manifestations of, 617, 617t
  diagnostic studies for, 617–618, 617f
  etiology and epidemiology of, 616
  temporal patterns of, 617, 617t
  treatment of, 620
Health care
  pediatric, 1–4
    changing morbidity and, 3
    culture and, 3–4
    current challenges in, 1
    health disparities in, 3
    landscape of, 1–2
    other health issues affecting, 2–3
Health care-associated infections, 394
Health Care Quality Improvement Act, 4
Health care team, 1
Health insurance coverage, 1–2
Health Insurance Portability and Accountability
  Act (HIPAA), 5–6
Health maintenance and supervision visits, 13,
  15–16
  anticipatory guidance in, 23–25, 24t–25t
  dental care in, 23
  fostering optimal development in, 23–25
  immunizations in, 22
  nutritional assessment in, 23
  safety issues in, 23
  schedule of preventive measures in, 17f, 15–16
  screening tests in, 17f, 21–22
    for anemia, 21
    for cholesterol, 22, 22t
    hearing and vision, 21
    for lead, 21–22, 22t
    newborn, 21

Health maintenance and supervision visits
    (*Continued*)
  for sexually transmitted infections, 22
  for tuberculosis, 22, 22t
  topics for, 15–16, 16t
Hearing, with developmental disabilities, 28t
Hearing assessment, 614
Hearing impairment, 32–34
  etiology of, 32–33, 33t
  interventions for, 34
  levels of, 33t
  neurodevelopmental-behavioral complications
    of, 32–33, 33t
Hearing intervention, for developmental
  disability, 30
Hearing screening, 19, 19t
  of children 3 years of age and older, 21
  of infants and toddlers, 21
  of newborns, 21, 33–34
Heart
  with developmental disabilities, 28t
  of newborn, 200
  normal, 486f
Heart block, 489
  congenital complete, 489
  first-degree, 489
  Mobitz type I (Wenckebach), 489, 490t
  Mobitz type II, 490t
  third-degree, 489
Heart disease, congenital
  acyanotic, 491–494, 491t
    aortic stenosis as, 494
    atrial septal defect as, 492, 492f
    coarctation of the aorta as, 494
    endocardial cushion defect, 493
    etiology and epidemiology, 491
    patent ductus arteriosus as, 492–493, 492f
    pulmonary stenosis as, 493–494
    ventricular septal defect as, 491–492, 491f
  congenital malformation syndromes associated
    with, 482t
  cyanotic, 495–499
    extracardiac complications of, 500t
    hypoplastic left heart syndrome as, 498–499,
      498f
    tetralogy of Fallot as, 495–496, 496f
    total anomalous pulmonary venous return,
      498, 498f
    transposition of the great arteries as, 496–
      497, 496f
    tricuspid atresia as, 497, 497f
    truncus arteriosus as, 497–498
  ductal-dependent, 196t
Heart failure, 499–501
  clinical manifestations of, 501–502
  due to dilated cardiomyopathy, 502
  etiology and epidemiology of, 499–500
    by age presentation, 500t
  imaging studies of, 502
  treatment of, 501
  ventricular function curve in, 499–500, 499f
Heart murmurs, 481, 483f
  continuous, 484
  diastolic, 484
  ejection, 482–483
    due to aortic stenosis, 494
  frequency or pitch, 483
  intensity, 483t
  in newborn, 200
  normal or innocent, 484, 484t
  Still, 484t
  systolic, 482–483
    in total anomalous pulmonary venous
      return, 498
    in truncus arteriosus, 497

Heart murmurs (*Continued*)
  in tetralogy of Fallot, 495–496
  timing, 483f
  vibratory, 484t
Heart rate
  in heart failure, 499–500, 500t
  of newborn, 196
Heart sounds, 482, 483f
  in newborn, 200
  in total anomalous pulmonary venous return,
    498
  with tricuspid atresia, 497
  in truncus arteriosus, 497–498
Heart transplantation, for cardiomyopathy, 504
Heat-labile enterotoxin, 367
Heat loss, mechanisms of, 203
Heat-stable enterotoxin, 367
Heat stress, in newborn, 203
Hecht pneumonia, due to measles, 331
Heel to ear, in newborn, 198f
Height
  benchmarks for, 10, 10t
  midparental, 12
Heinz bodies, in G6PD deficiency, 520
Helicobacter pylori, in peptic ulcer disease, 436
Heliotrope discoloration, in juvenile
  dermatomyositis, 311
Helium dilution, 459
HELLP syndrome, 187
Helminthiasis(es), 404–407
  ascariasis as, 405
  due to cestodes (tapeworms), 407t, 404
  due to nematodes (roundworms), 405t
  due to trematodes (flukes), 404, 406t
  echinococcosis as, 407
  enterobiasis (pinworm) as, 406
  hookworm infections as, 404–405
  neurocysticercosis due to, 407
  schistosomiasis (bilharziasis) as, 406–407
  visceral larva migrans as, 405–406
Helper T cells, in HIV, 412
Hemangioma(s), 661–662
  capillary, 198
  cavernous, 198
  clinical features of, 661, 661f
  complications of, 661
  defined, 661
  with developmental disabilities, 28t
  differential diagnosis of, 659t
  laryngeal, upper airway obstruction due to, 468
  lumbosacral, 661–662
  periorbital, 661–662
  in PHACE syndrome, 661–662
  subglottic, 661–662
  treatment of, 661–662
Hematemesis, evaluation of, 428t
Hematocrit, normal values for, 508t
Hematologic abnormalities, in systemic lupus
  erythematosus, 310
Hematologic disorders
  clinical presentation of, 506, 507t
  vs. juvenile idiopathic arthritis, 308t
Hematologic values, in infancy and childhood,
  506, 508t
Hematology, developmental, 506–509, 510f
Hematology assessment, 506–509
  developmental hematology and, 506–509, 510f
  history in, 506
  initial diagnostic evaluation in, 506, 508t
  physical examination and common
    manifestations in, 506, 507t
Hematoma
  duodenal, 135
  in hemostatic disorders, 524
  subdural, in newborn, 226

Hematopoiesis, 510f
  embryonic, 216
  extramedullary, 506
Hematopoietic stem cell(s), sources of, 269
Hematopoietic stem cell transplantation (HSCT),
      269–270
  for aplastic anemia, 517
  complications of, 270
  for Fanconi anemia, 517
  immunodeficiency diseases curable by, 269,
      269t
  major histocompatibility complex
      compatibility in, 269
  for sickle cell anemia, 520
Hematuria, 558–560
  benign familial, 558–559
  clinical manifestations of, 558–559
  diagnostic studies of, 558t, 559, 559f
  due to renal disease, 554t
  etiology and epidemiology of, 558
  gross, 558
  microscopic, 558
  prognosis and prevention of, 560
  therapy for, 559
Heme, in erythropoiesis, 506–509
Heme iron, 104
Hemiparesis, due to cerebral palsy, 35t
Hemiplegia
  of childhood, congenital, 631
  due to cerebral palsy, 35t
Hemochromatosis, with β-thalassemia major,
      518
Hemodialysis, for chronic kidney disease,
      563
Hemodynamics, for cardiomyopathy(ies), 503t
Hemoglobin
  Bart, 518
  fetal, 190, 191f, 216, 509
  normal values for, 508t
  production of, 509
Hemoglobin A, 509
Hemoglobin C, 518
Hemoglobin D, 518
Hemoglobin E, 518
Hemoglobin electrophoresis
  for hemoglobinopathies, 520
  in newborn screening, 21
Hemoglobin F, 190, 191f, 216, 509
Hemoglobin H, 515t
Hemoglobin level(s)
  after birth, 216
  in anemia, 509
Hemoglobin-oxygen dissociation curve, fetal,
      190, 191f
Hemoglobin S, 518
Hemoglobin S-β-thalassemia, 518–519, 519t
Hemoglobin SC disease, 518–519, 519t
Hemoglobin SS disease, 518–519, 519t. see also
      Sickle cell disease
Hemoglobinopathy(ies)
  alpha chain, 518
  beta chain, 518
  hemolytic anemia due to, 510f, 518
  laboratory diagnosis of, 520
Hemoglobinuria, paroxysmal nocturnal,
      516t
Hemolysis
  isoimmune, 522, 522f
  in newborn
      diagnosis and management of, 218–219
      etiology of, 216
      nonimmune causes of, 218
Hemolytic anemia. see Anemia; hemolytic
Hemolytic crisis, in sickle cell anemia, 520t
Hemolytic disease, of the newborn, 217

Hemolytic uremic syndrome (HUS), 366t, 367,
      560
  clinical manifestations of, 560
  diagnostic studies of, 560, 560t
  due to thrombotic microangiopathy, 528
  etiology and epidemiology of, 560
  GI bleeding due to, 427t
  glomerular injury due to, 558
  schistocytes in, 513f
  treatment and prognosis for, 560
Hemophagocytic syndrome
  due to roseola infantum, 333
  virus-associated, 516t
Hemophilia, 528–530
  clinical manifestations of, 529
  etiology and epidemiology of, 523
  etiology of, 528
  laboratory studies of, 529
  treatment of, 529
Hemophilia A, 528, 529t
  genetic basis for, 151t
Hemophilia B, 528, 529t
Hemoptysis, due to pulmonary hemorrhage,
      474
Hemorrhage
  airway, 474
  alveolar, 474
  brain, due to hypernatremia, 115
  contusion, 638t
  epidural, 638t
  fetal-maternal, 218
  intracranial
      in neonatal alloimmune thrombocytopenic
          purpura (NATP), 527
      in newborn, 226
      post-traumatic, 638t
  intraparenchymal, 638t
  in newborn
      intracranial, 226
      intraventricular. see Intraventricular
          hemorrhage (IVH); in newborn
      periventricular, 226
      retinal, 202
      subarachnoid, 226
      subconjunctival, 202
      subdural, 226
  pulmonary, 473–474
      clinical manifestations of, 473–474
      diagnostic studies for, 474
      differential diagnosis of, 474, 474t
      etiology of, 473
      hemoptysis due to, 474
      treatment of, 474
  subarachnoid
      due to trauma, 638t
      in newborn, 226
  subdural, 638t
      due to child abuse, 72, 72f
      in newborn, 226
Hemorrhagic disease of the newborn, 102–103
  due to vitamin K deficiency, 222
Hemorrhagic disorders. see Hemostatic
      disorder(s)
Hemorrhagic strokes, 630–631
Hemosiderosis, idiopathic pulmonary, 473
Hemostasis
  developmental, 523
  normal, 523, 524f
Hemostatic disorder(s), 523–531
  clinical manifestations of, 524
  clotting factors disorders, 528
      disseminated intravascular coagulation
          (DIC) as, 530–531
      etiology of, 528
      hemophilia as, 528–530

Hemostatic disorder(s) (Continued)
      thrombosis as, 531, 531f
      von Willebrand disease as, 529t, 530
  differential diagnosis of, 526–531
  etiology and epidemiology of, 523, 525f, 526t
  laboratory testing for, 524–526, 526t
  in newborn
      clinical manifestations and differential
          diagnoses of, 222–223
      etiology and pathogenesis of, 223
  of platelet function, 528
  of platelet number, 526, 527f
      idiopathic thrombocytopenic purpura (ITP)
          as, 527–528
      sequestration thrombocytopenia due to
          decreased platelet production as,
          526–527
      thrombocytopenia due to peripheral
          destruction as, 527
      Wiskott-Aldrich syndrome as, 528
Hemostatic plug, 524f, 531f
Hemotympanum, 638
Henoch-Schönlein purpura (HSP), 301–303
  clinical manifestations of, 302, 302f
  complications of, 302–303
  diagnostic criteria for, 302t
  differential diagnosis of, 302, 304t
  epidemiology of, 301
  etiology of, 301
  laboratory and imaging studies of, 302
  prognosis for, 304
  treatment of, 302
Heparin
  for disseminated intravascular coagulation,
      531
  for thrombosis, 531
Hepatic encephalopathy, 447–449
  stages of, 448t
  treatment of, 448t
Hepatic failure, due to inborn errors of
      metabolism, 168t
Hepatic fibrosis, in autosomal recessive polycystic
      kidney disease, 566
Hepatic synthetic function, for gastrointestinal
      symptoms, 417
Hepatitis
  autoimmune, 450, 449t
  fulminant, 373–374
  neonatal, 444
  nonalcoholic fatty, 450
  viral, 369–372
      clinical manifestations of, 370, 371f
      complications and prognosis of, 373–374
      differential diagnosis of, 371
      epidemiology of, 369–370
      etiology of, 369
      laboratory and imaging studies for, 370–371
      prevention of, 374
      treatment of, 371–372
  viral, laboratory and imaging studies for, 449t
  vomiting due to, 423t
Hepatitis A (HepA) vaccine, 372, 317–318,
      319f–322f
Hepatitis A virus (HAV), 370t
  clinical manifestations of, 370, 371f
  complications and prognosis of, 373–374
  epidemiology of, 369–370
  laboratory studies for, 370–371
  prevention of, 374
  treatment of, 371–372
Hepatitis B (HepB) vaccine, 317–318, 319f–322f
Hepatitis B surface antigen (HbsAg), 369, 371
Hepatitis B virus (HBV), 369, 370t
  clinical manifestations of, 370, 371f
  complications and prognosis of, 373–374

Hepatitis B virus (HBV) *(Continued)*
    congenital infection with, 230t
    due to transfusion, 532–533
    epidemiology of, 369–370
    hemophilia and, 529
    laboratory studies for, 370–371
    prevention of, 374
    treatment of, 371–372
Hepatitis C virus (HCV), 369, 370t
    clinical manifestations of, 370, 371f
    complications and prognosis of, 373–374
    due to transfusion, 532–533
    epidemiology of, 369–370
    hemophilia and, 529
    laboratory studies for, 370–371
    treatment of, 371–372
Hepatitis D virus (HDV), 369, 370t
    complications and prognosis of, 373–374
    hemophilia and, 529
Hepatitis E virus (HEV), 370t
    complications and prognosis of, 373–374
    epidemiology of, 369–370
Hepatitis G virus (HGV), 370t
    epidemiology of, 369–370
Hepatoblastoma, risk factors for, 536t
Hepatocellular carcinoma, risk factors for, 536t
Hepatocellular function, impaired, 448–449
Hepatomegaly
    with developmental disabilities, 28t
    due to inborn errors of metabolism, 168t
    in glycogen storage diseases, 172
Hepatorenal syndrome, 447
Hepatosplenomegaly
    with anemia, 511
    in hematologic disorders, 506
HepB (hepatitis B) vaccine, 372, 317–318,
        319f–322f
Herald patch, in pityriasis rosea, 658
Hereditary angioedema (HAE), 268, 289, 291t
    types of, 289, 291t
Hereditary angioneurotic edema (HANE),
        genetic basis for, 147t
Hereditary cancer syndrome, genetic assessment
        of, 155
Hereditary degenerative diseases, 642–644
Hereditary elliptocytosis
    clinical manifestations of, 521
    etiology of, 509–510, 521
    laboratory diagnosis of, 521
    treatment of, 521
Hereditary fructose intolerance, 176
    hypoglycemia due to, 582
Hereditary motor sensory neuropathy (HMSN),
        626
Hereditary pyropoikilocytosis, 521
Hereditary spherocytosis
    clinical manifestations of, 521
    etiology of, 509–510, 521
    laboratory diagnosis of, 521
    treatment of, 521
Hering-Breuer reflex, 461, 461f
Hernia
    congenital diaphragmatic, 196t, 215
    umbilical, 200
Herniation(s), brain, 636–637, 636t
    bilateral, 636t
    cerebellar, 636t
    subfalcian, 636t
    transtentorial, 636–637, 636t
    uncal, 636–637, 636t
Herpangina, 348
Herpes
    genital, 377t
        clinical features of, 377t
        diagnosis of, 380

Herpes *(Continued)*
        pathogenesis of, 380
        primary, 380
        secondary, recurrent, or reactivation
            eruptions in, 380
        treatment of, 380–381
    gingivostomatitis, 337
    gladiatorum, 337–338
    labialis, 337
Herpes simplex, infection of breast, 87t
Herpes simplex virus (HSV)
    congenital infection with, 230t, 231–232
    conjunctivitis due to, 386, 388t
    in immunocompromised person, 391
    pneumonia due to, 363t
    superficial infections due to, 336–338
    superinfection with, in atopic dermatitis, 287,
        653–655, 655f
    vs. varicella and zoster, 334
    vesiculobullous eruptions due to, 663t
Herpesvirus B infection, 398t–400t
Herpetic whitlow, 337–338
Hers disease, 172t
Heterophyes heterophyes, 406t
Heterophyiasis, 406t
Heteroplasmy, 152
Heterosexuality, 75t
Heterotopias, of gray matter, 648–649
Heterozygous, 147
HEV (hepatitis E virus), 370t
    complications and prognosis of, 373–374
    epidemiology of, 369–370
Hexamethonium bromide, maternal use of, 207t
Hexosaminidase A deficiency, 181t–182t
Hexose monophosphate shunt pathway, in G6PD
        deficiency, 520
HgbA$_{1c}$ (glycohemoglobin), 578
HGV (hepatitis G virus), 370t
    epidemiology of, 369–370
HHV-6 (human herpesvirus type 6), roseola
        infantum due to, 332
HHV-7 (human herpesvirus type 7), roseola
        infantum due to, 332
Hib (*Haemophilus influenzae* type b)
    osteomyelitis due to, 381–382
    pneumonia due to, 359, 363t
Hib (*Haemophilus influenzae* type b) vaccine,
        317–318, 319f–322f, 342
Hickman catheters, infections associated with,
        394
High attitude pulmonary edema, 472
High flow nasal cannula (HFNC), 460
High-performance liquid chromatography, for
        hemoglobinopathies, 520
Highly active antiretroviral therapy (HAART),
        413–415
Hip abduction test, 672, 673f
Hip dislocation test, 673, 673f
Hip reduction test, 673, 673f
HIPAA (Health Insurance Portability and
        Accountability Act), 5–6
Hip(s), 672–676
    development dysplasia of, 672–674
    Legg-Calvé-Perthes disease of, 674–675
    slipped capital femoral epiphysis of, 675–676
    transient monoarticular synovitis of, 674, 674t
Hirschsprung disease, 440
    constipation due to, 425, 426t
History
    for cancer, 534, 536t
    for developmental disabilities, 27t
    for dysmorphology
        family, 161–162
        pregnancy, 161
    in genetic assessment

History *(Continued)*
    of delivery and birth, 156
    of development, 156
    family, 155
    laboratory evaluation, 159
    past medical, 156
    physical examination, 159
    of pregnancy, 155–156
    in hematology assessment, 506
    in neurology assessment, 612
    perinatal, 27t, 188–189, 190t
    of skin disorders, 650
HIV. *see* Human immunodeficiency virus (HIV)
Hives, 288, 290f, 650t, 651f
HMSN. *see* Hereditary motor sensory neuropathy
        (HMSN)
Hodgkin disease, 536t
Holocarboxylase deficiency, 178–179
Holoprosencephaly, 574, 648
Homocysteine
    metabolism of, 175f
    plasma total, 171t
Homocysteinemia, and thrombosis, 531
Homocystinuria, 175, 175f
Homosexuality, 75–76, 75t–76t
    supportive health care environments, 76t
Homovanillic acid (HVA), with neuroblastoma,
        548
Homozygous, 147
Honesty, 4
Honeybee stings, allergic reactions to, 293
Hookworm infections, 404–405
Hordeola, 387
Horizontal transmission, of HIV, 412
Hormonal effects, on growth, 584t
Hormone(s)
    abnormal response of end organ to, 570
    for cancer, 540t–541t
    defined, 570
    mechanisms of action of, 570, 570f
    peptide, 570
    steroid, 570
Hormone deficiency, 570
Hormone excess, 570
Horner syndrome, 614
    in newborn, 202–203
Hornet stings, allergic reactions to, 293
Hospice care, 8
Hospital admissions, 2
Hospital ethics committees, 7, 9
Hot spot mutational, 148
Hot tub folliculitis, 336
HPS (hypertrophic pyloric stenosis), genetic basis
        for, 152
HSCT. *see* Hematopoietic stem cell
        transplantation (HSCT)
HSP. *see* Henoch-Schönlein purpura (HSP)
HSV. *see* Herpes simplex virus (HSV)
HTN. *see* Hypertension (HTN)
Human chorionic gonadotropin (HCG),
        maternal serum screening for, 154
Human herpesvirus type 6 (HHV-6), roseola
        infantum due to, 332
Human herpesvirus type 7 (HHV-7), roseola
        infantum due to, 332
Human immunodeficiency virus (HIV), 87t,
        412–416
    clinical manifestations of, 412–413
    complications of, 415
    congenital infection with, 230t
    differential diagnosis of, 413
    due to transfusion, 532–533
    epidemiology of, 412
    etiology of, 412
    hemophilia and, 529

Human immunodeficiency virus (HIV)
  (Continued)
  laboratory and imaging studies for, 413
  maternal infection with, 87
  prevention of, 416
  prognosis for, 415–416
  transmission of
    horizontal, 412
    vertical, 412
  treatment of, 413–415
Human papillomavirus (HPV), 338
  genital warts due to, 338, 376, 383
    clinical features of, 378t
    diagnosis of, 381
    pathogenesis of, 384
    treatment of, 381
  juvenile laryngeal papillomatosis due to,
    465t–466t
Human papillomavirus (HPV) vaccine, 317–318,
    319f–320f
Human parvovirus, anemia due to, 516t
Human parvovirus B19
  congenital infection with, 230t
  erythema infectiosum due to, 333
Humate P (von Willebrand factor-containing
    concentrate), for von Willebrand disease,
    530
Hunter syndrome, 181t–182t, 642t–643t, 644
Huntington disease (HD), genetic basis for, 147t
Hurler syndrome, 181t–182t, 642t–643t, 644
HUS. see Hemolytic uremic syndrome (HUS)
HUS (Hemolytic uremic syndrome), 366t, 367
Hutchinson triad, 232
HVA (homovanillic acid), with neuroblastoma,
    548
Hyaline membrane disease. see Respiratory
    distress syndrome
Hydatid cyst disease, 407
Hydralazine, for heart failure, 501t
Hydranencephaly, 648
Hydrocarbon ingestion, 139
Hydrocephalus, 640–641
  causes of, 640–641, 640t
  communicating, 640–641
  external, 640–641
  increased intracranial pressure due to, 640–641
  macrocephaly due to, 648
  obstructive, 640–641
  treatment of, 642
  vomiting due to, 423t
Hydrocortisone
  for Addison disease, 611
  for 21-hydroxylase deficiency, 609
Hydronephrosis, 196t
Hydrops fetalis, 187, 211
  in anemia, 515t
  due to Rh sensitization, 217
Hydroxychloroquine
  for juvenile dermatomyositis, 313
  for systemic lupus erythematosus, 311
11-Hydroxylase deficiency, 611
21-Hydroxylase deficiency, 118, 609–611
  ambiguous genitalia due to, 609, 611
  biochemical diagnostic studies for, 609
  clinical manifestations of, 609
  genetic basis for, 150t
  incidence of, 609
  treatment of, 609–611
Hydroxymethylglutaryl-CoA lyase deficiency, 179
17-Hydroxyprogesterone (17-OHP), in
    21-hydroxylase deficiency, 609
Hydroxyurea, for sickle cell anemia, 520
25-Hydroxyvitamin D (25-[OH]-D), 102,
    602–603
  for rickets, 603

Hydroxyzine, for allergic rhinitis, 284
Hymenolepis diminuta, 407t
Hymenolepis nana, 407t
Hymenoptera stings, allergic reactions to, 293
Hyper-IgE syndrome, 261t, 262
  disorders of neutrophil migration in,
    264, 264t
Hyper-IgM syndrome, 259t
  autosomal recessive, 258
  clinical features of, 258
  due to defects in NEMO, 258
  pathogenesis of, 258
  X-linked, 258
Hyperactivity, in ADHD, 42t
Hyperammonemia
  depression of consciousness due to, 637
  etiology of, 167, 167t
  in later infancy and childhood, 166f,
    167–168
  neonatal
    moderate, 167
    severe, 167
  treatment of, 177
Hyperbilirubinemia
  conjugated, differential diagnosis of, 445f
  conjugated, in newborn, 220, 220t
  in newborn, 219–222
    conjugated, 220, 220t
    kernicterus (bilirubin encephalopathy) due
      to, 220–221
    unconjugated
      etiology of, 219–220, 220t
      therapy, 221
  unconjugated
    differential diagnosis of, 445f
    in newborn
      etiology of, 219–220, 220t
      therapy of, 221
Hypercalcemia, due to cancer, 539t
Hypercalciuria, hematuria due to, 559
Hypercholesterolemia, in nephrotic syndrome,
    556
Hypercoagulable states, common, 526t
Hyperemia, in otitis media, 351
Hyperextension, 313f
Hyperglycemia
  due to defects in propionate pathway,
    177–178
  due to diabetic ketoacidosis, 574–575
  in insulin-dependent diabetes mellitus, 573
Hyperinflation, 469–470
Hyperinsulinemia
  factitious, 581
  hypoglycemia due to, 580–581, 580t
Hyperinsulinism, obesity in, 91t
Hyperirritable skin, in atopic dermatitis, 285
Hyperkalemia, 117–119
  in acute renal failure, 561
  causes of, 118t
  diagnosis of, 122
  due to cancer, 539t
  etiology of, 117–118
  factitious, 117
  treatment of, 122, 122t
Hyperkeratosis, 175
Hyperkinetic patterns, 633
Hyperleukocytosis, due to cancer, 539t
Hyperlucent lung, unilateral, 363
Hypermetabolic response, to burns, 138
Hypermobile pes planus, 682
Hypermobility, benign, 313, 313f, 313t
Hypernatremia, 114–115, 115f
Hypernatremic dehydration, 110
Hyperosmolality, hyponatremia due to,
    113, 113f

Hyperparathyroidism, 603t
  maternal, 205t
Hyperphenylalaninemia, 174
Hyperphosphatemia
  in acute renal failure, 561
  due to cancer, 539t
  in infant, 204
Hyperpnea, 457
Hypersegmented neutrophils, 100
Hypersensitivity reactions, 271, 271t
  of food, 294
    clinical manifestations of, 294, 295t
    complications of, 297–298
    diagnosis of, 296t, 294–296
    etiology and epidemiology of, 294
    laboratory and imaging studies for, 294
    prognosis and prevention of, 298
    treatment of, 297
  type I (anaphylactic), 271, 271t, 289
    immediate, 271t
    late-phase, 271
  type II (antibody cytotoxicity), 271, 271t
  type III (immune complex), 271–272, 271t
    Arthus reaction in, 271–272
    serum sickness in, 271–272
  type IV (cellular immune-mediated, delayed
    type), 271t, 272
Hypersplenism, in aplastic anemia, 518
Hypertelorism, 161t, 162
Hypertension (HTN), 563–564
  clinical manifestations of, 563–564
  in coarctation of the aorta, 494
  defined, 563
  diagnostic studies of, 564
  due to renal disease, 554t, 563, 564t
  etiology of, 563, 564t
  intracranial. see also Intracranial pressure
    (ICP), increased
  idiopathic, 641
  maternal, 205t
  persistent (primary)
    of newborn, 191
  portal, 448
  primary (essential), 563
  prognosis for, 564
  pulmonary
    arterial
      clinical manifestations and diagnostic
        studies for, 473
      etiology of, 473
      idiopathic, 473
      treatment and prognosis for, 473
    persistent (primary), of newborn, 215
      with meconium aspiration, 215
    syncope due to, 488t
  secondary, 563
  staging of, 564t
  treatment of, 564
Hyperthermia, malignant, 629
Hyperthyroidism, 600–601
  clinical manifestations of, 600, 600t
  congenital, 601
  in Graves disease, 600
  maternal, 205t, 206
  thyroid storm due to, 601
  treatment of, 600
    drugs for, 600–601
    radioiodine for, 601
    surgical, 601
Hypertonia, with developmental disabilities,
    28t
Hypertonic phosphate, for functional
    constipation, 46t
Hypertransfusion program, in β-thalassemia
    major, 518

Hypertrophic cardiomyopathy(ies), 502
 clinical manifestations of, 502
 etiology of, 502
 imaging studies of, 503–504
 treatment of, 504
Hypertrophic pyloric stenosis (HPS), genetic
  basis for, 152
Hyperuricemia, due to cancer, 539t
Hyperventilation
 central neurogenic, 634–635
 in seizures, 620
Hyperviscosity syndrome, in newborn, 221–222
Hypervitaminosis A, 101
Hypoallergenic formula, 88t
Hypocalcemia, 602–603
 in acute renal failure, 561
 clinical manifestations of, 602
 due to hypomagnesemia, 603
 due to neonatal tetany, 602
 due to poisoning, 141t
 due to primary hypoparathyroidism, 602
 due to pseudohypoparathyroidism, 602
 etiology of, 603
 neonatal seizures due to, 225
 in newborn, 204
 transient, 602
 treatment of, 603
Hypochondriasis, 52t, 53
Hypogenitalism, with developmental disabilities,
  28t
Hypoglycemia, 579
 clinical manifestations of, 573, 581t
 definition of, 572–573
 depression of consciousness due to, 637
 diagnosis of, 583
 due to poisoning, 141t
 emergency management of, 583
 etiology of, 580t
 with fulminant liver failure, 448t
 in glycogen storage diseases, 172
 ketotic, due to inborn errors of metabolism,
   168
 ketotic, idiopathic, 582
 neonatal seizures due to, 225
 pathophysiology of, 580–582
  drugs/intoxication in, 580t, 582–583
  energy stores (inadequate substrate) in,
    580t, 582
  hormonal signal in, 580–582, 580t, 581f
   and defects in counter-regulatory
     hormones, 580t, 581–582
   and factitious hyperinsulinemia, 581
   and hyperinsulinemia, 580–581, 580t
  metabolic response pathways in, 580t, 582
   fatty acid oxidation in, 580t, 582
   and gluconeogenesis, 580t, 582
   and glycogenolysis, 580t, 582
  persistent hyperinsulinemic, of newborn,
    580–581
 with type 1 diabetes mellitus, 578
Hypokalemia, 116–117
Hypoketotic hypoglycemia, 179
Hypomagnesemia, 603
 neonatal seizures due to, 225
 in newborn, 204
Hypomania, 60–61
Hyponatremia, 113–114
 clinical manifestations of, 114
 etiology of, 113–114
 euvolemic, 113–114, 113f
 hypervolemic, 113f, 114
 hypovolemic, 113, 113f
 pseudo-, 113, 113f
 symptomatic, 114
 treatment of, 114

Hyponatremic dehydration, 110
Hypoparathyroidism
 primary, 602, 603t
 pseudo-, 602, 603t
  short stature due to, 586
 transient, 602
Hypoperfusion, 495t
Hypophosphatemic rickets, 150–151
Hypopituitarism
 acquired, 573
 congenital, 574
 diagnostic evaluation of, 571t
 due to craniopharyngioma, 573
 hypoglycemia due to, 581–582
 idiopathic, delayed puberty due to, 590, 590t
Hypoplastic left heart syndrome, 498–499, 498f
Hypoplastic nail, 161t
Hypoplastic right ventricle, 497
Hypoproteinemia, in nephrotic syndrome, 556
Hypospadias, 163, 568
Hypothalamic deficiency, 573
Hypothalamic glioma, precocious puberty due
  to, 593
Hypothalamic-pituitary axis, 570–571, 571f
 disorders of, 571–572
Hypothalamic-pituitary-thyroid axis, 597f
Hypothalamic-pituitary tumors, delayed puberty
  due to, 591t
Hypothalamus, 570–571, 571f
 hormonal influences of, 571f
Hypothyroidism, 45, 598–600
 acquired, 599–600
 causes of, 598t
 congenital, 598–599
 and degenerative diseases, 645
 delayed puberty due to, 591
 secondary or tertiary, 598
 symptoms and signs of, 599t
Hypotonia, 615, 623. see also Weakness
 benign congenital, 629–630
 central (without significant weakness),
   629–630, 630t
 with developmental disabilities, 28t
 neonatal and infantile, 629, 629f
 with weakness, 630t
Hypoventilation
 congenital central syndrome, 463
 hypoxemia due to, 456t
Hypoxemia
 causes of, 456, 456t
 in newborn, treatment of, 209–210
Hypoxia
 in cardiopulmonary resuscitation, 126
 with depressed consciousness, 634
 due to pulmonary embolism, 474
Hypoxic-ischemic encephalopathy
 due to near-drowning, 136
 in newborn, 226–227
  clinical manifestations of, 227, 227t
  etiology of, 226–227
  prognosis for, 227
  seizures due to, 225
Hypoxic pulmonary vasoconstriction, 456
Hypoxic spells, in tetralogy of Fallot, 495–496
Hypsarrhythmia, 621

I

I-cell disease, 181t–182t
131I (radioactive iodine)
 for hyperthyroidism, 601
 maternal use of, 207t
 as teratogen, 206t
IBS (irritable bowel syndrome), abdominal pain
  due to, 418–422, 420t
Ibuprofen, maternal use of, 207t

ICF (intracellular fluid), 106, 107f
 solutes in, 106
 volume of, 106
ICP. see Intracranial pressure (ICP)
Icteric phase, of viral hepatitis, 370
Idiogenic osmoles, due to overly rapid
  rehydration, 110
Idiopathic nephrotic syndrome (INS), 556
Idiopathic thrombocytopenia, maternal, 205,
  205t
Idiopathic thrombocytopenic purpura (ITP),
  527–528
 bleeding disorder in newborn due to, 223
 chronic, 528
 clinical manifestations of, 527–528
 diagnosis of, 528
 etiology of, 527
 maternal, 205, 205t
  clinical manifestations of, 527
  etiology of, 527
  neonatal thrombocytopenia due to,
    223
  treatment of, 527
 treatment and prognosis of, 528
Iduronate 2-sulfatase deficiency,
  181t–182t
α-L-Iduronidase deficiency, 181t–182t
IEP (individualized educational plan), 26
Ifosfamide, for cancer, 540t–541t
IGF-1 (insulin-like growth factor-1), 583
IGF-BP3 (insulin-like growth factor-binding
  protein), 583
Ileal atresia, 196t
Illness, as sleep disorder, 49t
Imipramine
 for enuresis, 44
 maternal use of, 207t
Immersion injuries, due to child abuse, 71
Immobilization, physiologic changes due to,
  603t
Immotile cilia syndrome, 472
Immunization, 22, 317–318
 active, 317
 administration of, 317
 adverse events after, 318
 catch-up, 318
 contraindications to, 318
 human papillomavirus, 319f–322f
 informed consent for, 318
 passive, 317
 and prophylaxis, 317–323
 recommended schedule for, 319f–320f
Immunocompromised person, infection in,
  390–394
Immunodeficiency, 101
 common variable, 256, 258t
  clinical features of, 256
  etiology of, 256, 257f
 fever due to, 326
 severe combined, 258–260, 259t
  autosomal recessive, 260
  clinical manifestations of, 260
  due to deficiencies in adenosine deaminase
    and purine nucleoside phosphorylase,
    260
  in Nezelof syndrome, 260
  pathogenesis of, 258–260
  X-linked, 260
Immunodeficiency disease(s)
 antibody-mediated
  agammaglobulinemia as, 256, 258t
   autosomal recessive, 256
   X-linked, 256, 258t
  antibody deficiency syndrome as, 257–258,
    258t

Immunodeficiency disease(s) *(Continued)*
  common variable immunodeficiency as, 256, 258t
    clinical features of, 256
    etiology of, 256, 257f
    IgA deficiency as, 257, 258t
    IgG subclass deficiency as, 257, 258t
    pathogenesis of, 256
    transient hypogammaglobulinemia of infancy as, 257, 258t
  assessment, 252–256
    adaptive immune system and, 252–253
    clinical characteristics of, 254t
    diagnostic evaluation of, 255–256
      imaging in, 256
      laboratory tests in, 255–256, 255t
    differential diagnosis of, 254–255, 254t
    due to defects in anatomic-mucociliary barrier, 252, 252t
    history of, 253–254
    innate immune system and, 252, 253t
    physical examination for, 254
  combined, 258–262
    bare lymphocyte syndrome, 259t, 260
    DiGeorge syndrome as, 259t, 260
    hyper-IgM syndrome as, 259t
      autosomal recessive, 258
      clinical features of, 258
      due to defects in NEMO, 258
      pathogenesis of, 258
      X-linked, 258, 259t
    Omenn syndrome as, 259t, 260
    severe, 258–260, 259t
      autosomal recessive, 260
      clinical manifestations of, 260
      due to deficiencies in adenosine deaminase and purine nucleoside phosphorylase, 260
      in Nezelof syndrome, 260
      pathogenesis of, 258–260
      X-linked, 260
    due to lymphocyte disorders. *see* Lymphocyte disorder(s)
  secondary, 254t
Immunoglobulin A (IgA) deficiency, 257, 258t
Immunoglobulin A (IgA) nephropathy
  hematuria due to, 558
  prognosis for, 560
Immunoglobulin E (IgE)
  disorders associated with elevated, 272, 272t
    screening tests for, 272–273, 282t
  in food allergies, 296
Immunoglobulin G (IgG) subclass deficiency, 257, 258t
Immunomodulating drugs, topical, for atopic dermatitis, 287
Immunophenotype, of leukemia, 543
Immunosuppression, and immunization, 318
Immunotherapy, for allergic rhinitis, 284–285
Impact seizures, 639
Imperforate anus, 439–440
  constipation due to, 426t
Impetigo, 335
  bullous, 335, 663t
  nonbullous (crusted), 335
Implanon (etonogestrel implant), 246
Implanted venous access systems (Port-a-Cath), infections associated with, 394
Impulsivity, in ADHD, 42t
In-toeing, 676–677
  common causes of, 676t
  due to femoral anteversion, 676
  due to internal tibial torsion, 676–677, 677f
  treatment of, 677

In vitro serum testing, for antigen-specific IgE, 272–273, 282t
In vivo skin testing, for allergen-specific IgE, 272, 282t
Inactivated poliovirus (IPV) vaccine, 319f–322f
Inattention, in ADHD, 42t
Inborn errors of metabolism
  assessment of, 164
    clinical, and laboratory findings, 169, 169t
  ataxia due to, 633
  clinical presentation of, 165–168
    congenital malformations or dysmorphic features in, 168
    energy deficiency in, 168
    hyperammonemia in, 167
      etiology of, 167, 167t
      in later infancy and childhood, 166f, 167–168
      moderate neonatal, 167
      severe neonatal, 167
    ketosis and ketotic hypoglycemia in, 168
    metabolic acidosis in, 167–168, 168t
    neurologic signs in, 167, 167t
    specific organ, 168, 168t
    storage disorders, 168
    toxic, 165–167
  genetic aspects of, 169
    identification of molecular pathology as, 169
    mechanisms of inheritance as, 169
  incidence of, 164t
  metabolic acidosis due to, 121
  neonatal screening for, 170–171, 170t
    confirmatory testing principles of, 170
    disorders identified by, 170, 170t
    specialized laboratory and clinical testing after, 170–171, 171t
    strategy of, 170
  overview of treatment for, 171
  pathophysiology of, 165t
  signs and symptoms of, 164–165
Incontinentia pigmenti, 150–151
Individualized educational plan (IEP), 26
Indomethacin, maternal use of, 207t
Induction chemotherapy, for leukemia, 543–544
Infancy
  bonding and attachment in, 14
  physical development in later, 13
  sleep disorders in, 48–50
Infant(s)
  colic in, 37–39
    clinical manifestations of, 38, 38f
    defined, 37
    differential diagnosis of, 38–39
    epidemiology of, 37
    etiology of, 37
    prevention of, 39
    prognosis for, 39
    treatment of, 39
  crying by, 37–39, 37f
  genetic assessment of, 155
  hearing and vision screening of, 21
  low birth weight, 188
  tests of cognition in, 29t
  very low birth weight, 188
Infant botulism, 627
Infant mortality, 2–3, 187–188, 188t
Infantile beriberi, 97
Infantile hypotonia, 629, 629f
Infantile spasms, 621
Infantometer, 583
Infection(s)
  assessment of, 252–256
    adaptive immune system and, 252–253
    clinical characteristics of, 254t
    diagnostic evaluation of, 255–256

Infection(s) *(Continued)*
      imaging in, 256
      laboratory tests in, 255–256, 255t
    differential diagnosis of, 254–255, 254t
    due to defects in anatomic-mucociliary barrier, 252, 252t
    history of, 253–254
    innate immune system and, 252, 253t
    physical examination for, 254
  congenital (TORCH), 229–233, 230t
    with *Chlamydia trachomatis*, 230t, 233
    with cytomegalovirus, 230t, 231
    with hepatitis B virus, 230t
    with herpes simplex virus, 230t, 231–232
    with HIV, 230t
    with *Mycobacterium tuberculosis*, 230t
    with *Neisseria gonorrhoeae*, 230t, 232–233
    with parvovirus B19, 230t
    with rubella, 229–231, 230t
    with syphilis, 230t, 232
    with toxoplasmosis, 229, 230t
    with *Trypanosoma cruzi*, 230t
    with varicella-zoster virus, 230t
  cutaneous (superficial), 335–338
    bacterial, 335–336
      cellulitis as, 335–336
      folliculitis as, 336
      impetigo as, 335
      perianal dermatitis as, 336
    fungal, 336
    viral, 336–338
      due to herpes simplex virus, 336–338
      due to human papillomavirus, 338
      molluscum contagiosum as, 338
  with fever and rash, 329–335
    differential diagnosis of, 329t–330t
    erythema infectiosum (fifth disease) as, 333
    measles (rubeola) as, 329–331
    roseola infantum (exanthem subitum, sixth disease) as, 332–333
    rubella (German or 3-day measles) as, 331–332
    varicella-zoster virus infection (chickenpox, zoster) as, 333–335
  with foreign body, 324
  in immunocompromised person, 390–394
    clinical manifestations of, 391
    differential diagnosis of, 391
    endogenous, 390
    epidemiology of, 391
    etiology of, 390–391, 390t
    exogenous, 390
    laboratory tests and imaging for, 391
    prevention of, 394
    treatment of, 391–394, 392f–393f
  maternal
    effect on fetus or newborn of, 205t
    as teratogens, 154
  medical device-associated, 394–396
    with CNS shunts, 397
    with peritoneal dialysis, 397
    with urinary catheters, 395–396
    with vascular devices, 394–395
    ventilator-associated pneumonia as, 395
  with neutropenia, 265t
  orthopedic problems due to, 667t
  respiratory distress in newborn due to, 209
  in sickle cell disease, 519, 520t
Infectious diseases
  assessment of, 315–317
    diagnostic imaging in, 323
    differential diagnosis in, 315
    history in, 316t
    initial diagnostic evaluation in, 315
    localizing manifestations of, 316t

Infectious diseases (*Continued*)
  physical examination in, 315
  screening tests in, 315–317
    viral *vs.* bacterial, 317t
  with developmental disability, 31t
    viral *vs.* bacterial, 325
Infectious mononucleosis, 339
  clinical manifestations of, 340
  complications and prognosis for, 341
  etiology of, 339
  laboratory studies for, 340
Infectious rhinitis, 283
Infective endocarditis, 364–366
Inflammation
  anemia of, 514t, 515
  orthopedic problems due to, 667t
Inflammatory bowel disease (IBD), 440–442
  clinical manifestations of, 440, 441t
  epidemiology and etiology of, 440
  GI bleeding due to, 427t
  vs. juvenile idiopathic arthritis, 307t, 385t
  laboratory and imaging studies for, 440–441,
    441t
  treatment of, 441–442
Inflammatory diseases, fever due to, 326
Infliximab
  for Crohn's disease, 442
  for juvenile idiopathic arthritis, 308
Influenza, avian, 359
Influenza A, 359
Influenza vaccine, 319f–320f
  for prevention of pneumonia, 363–364
Infuse-a-Port (implanted venous access system),
    infections associated with, 394
Inhalants, acute effects of, 250t–251t
Inhalation challenge test, 459
Inheritance patterns, 146–154
  autosomal dominant disorders, 147–148,
    147t
  autosomal recessive disorders, 148–149, 150t
  expansion of trinucleotide repeat as, 153
  genomic imprinting as, 153
  for inborn errors of metabolism, 169
  mitochondrial, 152
    heteroplasmy in, 152
    for inborn errors of metabolism, 169
    MELAS due to, 152
  multifactorial disorders (polygenic
    inheritance), 151–152
    hypertrophic pyloric stenosis as, 152
    neural tube defects as, 152
  pedigree drawing of, 147, 147f–148f
  uniparental disomy as, 152–153
    Angelman syndrome due to, 153
    Prader-Willi syndrome due to, 153
Inhibin, in puberty, 589
Inhibitors, for hemophilia, 529–530
Injury prevention, 133
  education for, 133–134
Injury(ies), 133
  birth, 202–203
  epidemiology and etiology of, 133
  intestinal, 135
  pancreatic, 135
  prevention of, 24t–25t, 133–134
  renal, 135
  to spleen, 135
Innate immune system, 252, 253t
Innominate artery, tracheal compression due to,
    470
Inotropic drugs
  for cardiomyopathy, 504
  for heart failure, 501t
INS (idiopathic nephrotic syndrome), 556
Insect allergies, 293–294

Insect bites, vesiculobullous eruptions due to,
    663t
Insensible losses, 107, 108t
Insomnia, behavioral, 49t
Inspiration
  accessory muscles of, 455
  physiology of, 455
Inspiratory reserve volume, 455f
Inspiratory stridor, due to laryngomalacia, 467
Insulin
  for diabetic ketoacidosis, 577
    in transition to outpatient management, 576
  intermediate-acting (NPH), 577, 577t
  long-acting, 577, 577t
  multiple daily injections of, 576–578
  in serum glucose regulation, 580, 581f
  short-acting (regular), 577, 577t
  subcutaneous, 576
  for type 1 diabetes mellitus, 573
  very short-acting (lispro, aspart, glulisine),
    577, 577t
Insulin deficiency, in cystic fibrosis, 476
Insulin-like growth factor-1 (IGF-1), 583
Insulin-like growth factor-binding protein (IGF-
    BP3), 583
Insulin pumps, 576–577
Insulin sensitivity, 577
Insulin therapy, hypokalemia due to, 116
Insulin:carbohydrate ratio, 577
Integrity, 4
Intercostal retractions, 457
Interdisciplinary team intervention, for
    developmental problems, 30
Interferon-γ (IFN-γ), functions of, 253t
Interleukin-1 (IL-1), functions of, 253t
Interleukin-2 (IL-2), functions of, 253t
Interleukin-3 (IL-3), functions of, 253t
Interleukin-4 (IL-4), functions of, 253t
Interleukin-5 (IL-5), functions of, 253t
Interleukin-6 (IL-6), functions of, 253t
Interleukin-7 (IL-7), functions of, 253t
Interleukin-8 (IL-8), functions of, 253t
Interleukin-9 (IL-9), functions of, 253t
Interleukin-10 (IL-10), functions of, 253t
Interleukin-12 (IL-12), functions of, 253t
Interleukin-13 (IL-13), functions of, 253t
Interleukin-17 (IL-17), functions of, 253t
Interleukin-18 (IL-18), functions of, 253t
Internal intercostal muscles, during exhalation,
    455
Internal tibial torsion, 676–677, 677f
Intersex, 605
  approach to infant with, 606–607
  diagnosis of, 607
  due to inadequate masculinization of 46,XY
    male, 605–606, 606t
  due to virilization of 46,XX female, 605, 605t
  normal development and, 604–605, 604f–605f
  treatment of, 607
Interstitial edema, 472
Interstitial emphysema, 471–472
Interstitial fluid, 106, 107f
Interstitial process, 458t
Intertriginous areas, dermatitis in, 657
Intestinal atresia, 438–439
  clinical manifestations of, 439
  etiology and epidemiology of, 438
  laboratory and imaging studies for, 439
  treatment of, 439
  types of, 439f
  vomiting due to, 423t
Intestinal injury, 135
Intestinal obstruction
  abdominal pain due to, 420t
  due to congenital anomaly, 196t

Intestinal tract disorder(s), 437–444
  anorectal malformations as, 439–440
  appendicitis as, 443–444
  celiac disease as, 442
  gastroschisis as, 439
  Hirschsprung disease as, 440
  inflammatory bowel disease as, 440–442, 441t
  intestinal atresia as, 438–439, 439f
  intussusception as, 442–443
  Meckel diverticulum as, 440
  midgut malrotation as, 437–438, 438f
  omphalocele as, 439
Intimate partner violence, 79–80, 80t
Intoxication-induced hypoglycemia, 580t, 582–583
Intracellular fluid (ICF), 106, 107f
  solutes in, 106
  volume of, 106
Intracranial hemorrhage
  in newborn, 226
  post-traumatic, 638t
Intracranial hypertension, idiopathic, 641
Intracranial pressure (ICP), increased, 640–642
  clinical manifestations of, 641
  depressed consciousness due to, 636
  due to brain tumors, 547
  due to cancer, 539t
  etiology of, 636t, 640–641, 640t
  laboratory and diagnostic studies for, 641
  treatment of, 641–642
Intrapulmonary shunting, 472
  hypoxemia due to, 456t
Intrauterine growth restriction (IUGR), 208–209
  clinical features of, 208
  complications of, 188, 189t
  defined, 197, 208
  etiology of, 208, 208t
  management of, 208–209
  prenatal detection of, 208
Intravascular volume, regulation of, 106–107
Intravenous (IV) catheters, infections associated
    with, 394
Intravenous (IV) fluids, during labor, 207t
Intravenous (IV) pyelogram, 557
Intraventricular hemorrhage (IVH), in newborn
  clinical manifestations of, 226
  diagnosis of, 226
  pathogenesis of, 226
  seizures due to, 225
  treatment of, 226
Intrinsic factor, 101
Intrinsic pathway, of coagulation, 523, 525f
Introns, 146
Intubation, 460–461
Intuniv (Guanfacine), for ADHD, 42t
Intussusception, 442–443
  abdominal pain due to, 420t
  clinical manifestations of, 442–443
  etiology and epidemiology of, 442
  GI bleeding due to, 427t
  ileocolonic, 442
  laboratory and imaging studies for, 443
  treatment of, 443
  vomiting due to, 423t
Inverse psoriasis, 658
Inverted duplication chromosome 15, 160
Involucrum, in osteomyelitis, 382–383
Iodide(s), maternal use of, 207t
  radioactive, 207t
Iodine, radioactive, as teratogen, 206t
Iodine deficiency, 103t, 104
IP-10, functions of, 253t
Ipecac syrup, for poisoning, 142–143
Ipratropium bromide
  for allergic rhinitis, 284
  for asthma, 276

IPV (inactivated poliovirus) vaccine, 319f–322f
Iridocyclitis, 388t–389t
    in juvenile idiopathic arthritis, 306
Iris coloboma, in cat eye syndrome, 160
Iron, toxicity of, 141t
Iron deficiency, 103t, 104
    hookworm, 405t
Iron deficiency anemia. *see* Anemia; iron
        deficiency
Iron intake
    inadequate, 90
    for toddlers and older children, 90
Irritable bowel syndrome (IBS), abdominal pain
        due to, 418–422, 420t
Irritant contact dermatitis, 657f, 656
Islet cell adenoma, hyperinsulinemia due to,
        581
Islet cells, in insulin-dependent diabetes mellitus,
        573
Isolation effect, with inborn errors of
        metabolism, 169
Isoleucine, metabolism of, 176f
Isotonic fluid, for third space losses, 108
Isotretinoin
    for acne, 652
    for cancer, 540t–541t
    for neuroblastoma, 549
    as teratogen, 206t
Isovaleric acidemia, 178, 178f
    neonatal screening for, 170t
    treatment of, 178
ITP. *see* Idiopathic thrombocytopenic purpura
        (ITP)
IUGR. *see* Intrauterine growth restriction
        (IUGR)
IV (intravenous) catheters, infections associated
        with, 394
IV (intravenous) fluids, during labor, 207t
IV (intravenous) pyelogram, 557
IVIG (intravenous immunoglobulin)
    for autoimmune hemolytic anemia, 523
    for Guillain-Barré syndrome, 626
    for Kawasaki disease, 304–305
Ixodes pacificus, 396
Ixodes scapularis, 396, 401

J
Jacksonian march, 618–619
Jarisch-Herxheimer reaction, 380
JAS (juvenile ankylosing spondylitis), 307t
Jaundice
    breast milk, 86–87, 220
    breastfeeding, 86–87
    differential diagnosis of, 444, 445f
    due to anemia, 511
    due to inborn errors of metabolism, 168t
    on first day of life, 220
    in hematologic disorders, 506
    physiologic, 219
    in pyloric stenosis, 435
JDM. *see* Juvenile dermatomyositis (JDM)
Jejunostomy, feeding, for gastroesophageal reflux,
        432t
Juvenile idiopathic arthritis (JIA), 305–308
    clinical presentation of, 305–307, 306f, 306t
    complications of, 308
    differential diagnosis of, 300t, 307–308,
        307t–308t
    epidemiology of, 305
    etiology of, 305
    laboratory and imaging studies for, 307, 385t
    oligoarticular, 306, 306f, 306t
    polyarticular, 306–307, 306t
    prognosis for, 308
    spondyloarthropathies, 306t, 307

Juvenile idiopathic arthritis (JIA) *(Continued)*
    systemic-onset, 306t, 307
    treatment of, 308
Jock itch, 337t
Joint contractures, with developmental
        disabilities, 28t
Joint custody, 83
Joint hypermobility, 313, 313f, 313t
Joint space, 668f
Jones criteria, for rheumatic fever, 501, 503t
JRA. *see* Juvenile idiopathic arthritis (JIA)
Juice intake, for toddlers and older children, 89
Justice, 5
    distributive, 6
Juvenile ankylosing spondylitis (JAS), 307t
Juvenile dermatomyositis (JDM), 311–312
    clinical manifestations of, 311–312
    diagnostic criteria for, 313t
    differential diagnosis of, 312
    epidemiology of, 311
    etiology of, 311
    laboratory and imaging studies of, 312
    prognosis for, 312
    treatment of, 312
Juvenile laryngeal papillomatosis, upper airway
        obstruction due to, 465t–466t, 468
Juvenile pernicious anemia, 101
Juvenile polyp, GI bleeding due to, 427t
Juvenile rheumatoid arthritis (JRA). *see* Juvenile
        idiopathic arthritis (JIA)

K
Kallman syndrome, delayed puberty in, 590, 590t
Kaposi varicelliform eruption, 337–338
    in atopic dermatitis, 287, 655–656, 655f
    vs. varicella and zoster, 334
Kapvay (Clonidine), for ADHD, 42t
Kartagener syndrome, 472
Karyotype, 158–159
Kasabach-Merritt syndrome, 223
    hemolytic anemia in, 522
Kasai procedure, 444–447
Katayama fever, 407
Kawasaki disease (KD), 303–305, 665
    clinical manifestations of, 303–304
        in acute phase, 303, 304f
        in convalescent phase, 304
        in subacute phase, 303–304
    complications of, 308, 308t
    diagnostic criteria for, 304t
    differential diagnosis of, 300t, 304, 304t
    epidemiology of, 303
    etiology of, 303
    incomplete (atypical), 304
    laboratory and imaging studies for, 304
    prognosis for, 308
    vs. Stevens-Johnson syndrome, 665
    treatment of, 304–305
KCl (potassium chloride), in maintenance fluids,
        107
Kehr sign, 135
Keratitis, 175, 386, 388t–389t
Keratoconjunctivitis, epidemic, 386
Keratolytic agents, for acne, 652
Keratosis pilaris, 272
    in atopic dermatitis, 285–286
Kerion, 337t
Kerley B lines, in pulmonary edema, 473
Kernicterus, 220–221
Ketoacidosis, diabetic, 573–578
Ketoaciduria, branched chain, 176
Ketogenesis
    hypoglycemia due to disorders of, 582
    in insulin-dependent diabetes mellitus, 573
    in serum glucose regulation, 580, 581f

Ketone bodies
    in diabetic ketoacidosis, 573, 575f
    formation of, 180f, 179
    in maple syrup urine disease, 176
Ketosis
    due to defects in propionate pathway, 177–178
    due to inborn errors of metabolism, 168
Ketotic hypoglycemia
    due to inborn errors of metabolism, 168
    idiopathic, 582
Kidney, congenital and developmental anomalies
        of, 565–567
Kidney disease(s)
    chronic, 562–563
        clinical manifestations of, 562–563
        due to vesicoureteral reflux, 565
        etiology and epidemiology of, 563t, 562
        prognosis for, 563
        stages of, 563t
        treatment of, 563
    common manifestations of, 554–555, 554t
    etiology of, 554t
    polycystic, 566
        autosomal dominant, 568
        autosomal recessive, 566
    primary, 554–555, 554t
    risk factors for, 553
    secondary, 554–555, 554t
Kidney function, normal, 553, 555f
Kidney injury, 135
Kidney stones, 567
Kidney transplantation, for end-stage renal
        disease, 563
Kindergarten readiness, 14
Kingella kingae, osteomyelitis due to, 381–382
Kissing bug bites, anaphylaxis due to, 293
Kissing kneecaps, 676
Klinefelter syndrome (KS), 158, 606
    delayed puberty in, 592
Klippel-Trénaunay-Weber syndrome, port-wine
        stain in, 662
Klisic test, 673
Klumpke paralysis, 202–203
Knee(s), 679–680
    discoid lateral meniscus, 679
    effusion or swelling of, 679
    extensor mechanism of, 679, 679f
    knock-, 677, 677f
    Osgood-Schlatter disease of, 680
    osteochondritis dissecans of, 680
    patellofemoral disorders of, 680
    popliteal cyst of, 679–680
Knee pain, idiopathic anterior, 680
Kneecaps, kissing, 676
Knock-knees, 677, 677f
Kohler disease, 683
Koplik spots, 329–330
Kostmann syndrome, neutropenia in, 263
Krabbe disease, 181t–182t, 642t–643t, 643
KS (Klinefelter syndrome), 158
    delayed puberty in, 592
Kugelberg-Welander syndrome, 624–625
Kussmaul respirations, 457t
    in diabetic ketoacidosis, 574
Kwashiorkor, 94–95
Kyphosis, 688
    classification of, 684t
    clinical evaluation of, 684
    congenital, 688
    postural roundback, 688
    Scheuermann, 688, 688f

L
L/S (lecithin to sphingomyelin) ratio, 210–211
La belle indifference, 51–52

Labor and delivery, history of, 190t
Labyrinthitis
    acute, ataxia due to, 633
    vomiting due to, 423t
Lactate, metabolism of, 184–185, 185f
Lactic acidosis, 121
    due to mitochondrial disorders, 184–185
Lactobacillus acidophilus, for prevention of
    diarrhea, 369
Lactose-free cow's milk-based formulas, 88–89
Lactose intolerance, abdominal pain due to, 420t
Lactulose, for functional constipation, 47t
Lacy, reticulated rash, in erythema infectiosum,
    333
LAD-I (leukocyte adhesion deficiency type I),
    264, 264t
LAD-II (leukocyte adhesion deficiency type II),
    264, 264t
Ladd bands, in midgut malrotation, 437, 438f
Lamp-2 deficiency, 181t–182t
Landau-Kleffner syndrome, 621
Landau posture, 629
Langerhans cell histiocytosis, 286–287, 658
Language development, milestones of, 16t
Language function, assessment of, 613
Language intervention, for developmental
    disability, 30
Language screening, 19, 19t
Lanugo, 197f
Large for gestational age, 197
Laron dwarfism, 584
Laron syndrome, 588
Larva migrans, 405t
Laryngeal cysts, 468
Laryngeal hemangioma, upper airway
    obstruction due to, 468
Laryngeal mask airway (LMA), 460–461
Laryngeal papillomatosis, juvenile, upper airway
    obstruction due to, 465t–466t
Laryngeal webs, 468
Laryngitis, upper airway obstruction due to,
    465t–466t
Laryngomalacia, 464, 467
    clinical manifestations of, 467
    diagnostic studies of, 467
    etiology of, 464t, 467
    treatment of, 467
Laryngotracheobronchitis, 354–356
    clinical manifestations of, 354, 355f, 355t
    complications and prognosis for, 357
    differential diagnosis of, 354
    etiology and epidemiology of, 354
    laboratory and imaging studies of, 354
    treatment of, 354–356
    upper airway obstruction due to, 465t–466t
Laser therapy, for laryngeal hemangioma, 468
Lateral meniscus, discoid, 679
Laurence-Moon-Bardet-Biedl syndrome
    obesity in, 91t
    short stature in, 586
Lazy leukocyte syndrome, phagocytic disorders
    due to, 264t
LBW (low birth weight) infants, 188
LCHAD (long-chain hydroxyacyl-CoA
    dehydrogenase), neonatal screening for, 170t
LCHAD (long-chain hydroxyacyl-CoA
    dehydrogenase) deficiency, 179
Lead, maternal ingestion of, 207t
Lead poisoning, anemia due to, 514–515
Lead screening, 21–22, 22t
Lea's Shield (cervical shield), 247
Lecithin to sphingomyelin (L/S) ratio, 210–211
Lectin pathway, of complement activation,
    267–268, 267f
Leflunomide, for juvenile idiopathic arthritis, 308

Left-to-right shunts, 491
Left ventricular diastolic volume, in heart failure,
    500t
Left ventricular hypertrophy
    due to aortic stenosis, 494
    due to tricuspid atresia, 497
Left ventricular outflow tract (LVOT)
    obstruction, syncope due to, 488t
Leg discomfort, in coarctation of the aorta, 494
Leg-length discrepancy (LLD), 678–679
    common causes of, 679t
    measuring, 678–679
    treatment of, 679
Legal issues, 5–6
Legg-Calvé-Perthes disease (LCPD), 674–675
    clinical manifestations of, 675
    etiology and epidemiology of, 674–675
    radiologic evaluation of, 675
    treatment and prognosis for, 675
Legionella pneumophila, 361
Legionnaires' disease, 361
Leigh disease, 184, 644
Leishmania, 398t–400t
Leishmania donovani complex, 398t–400t
Leishmaniasis, 398t–400t
Leiter International Performance Scale, Revised,
    29t
Lemierre syndrome, 349
Length, growth chart for, 11f
Lennox-Gastaut syndrome, 621
Leptomeningeal cyst, 638
Leptospira interrogans, 398t–400t
Leptospirosis, 398t–400t
Lethargy, 634
    due to intussusception, 443
Leucine, metabolism of, 176f
Leukemia, 157, 542–544
    acute lymphoid/lymphoblastic. *see* Acute
        lymphoid/lymphoblastic leukemia (ALL)
    acute myeloid/myelogenous. *see* Acute
        myeloid/myelogenous leukemia (AML)
    chronic myeloid/myelogenous, 542
        epidemiology of, 542
        etiology of, 542
    clinical manifestations of, 542–543
    complications of, 546
    differential diagnosis of, 300t, 543
    epidemiology of, 542
    etiology of, 542
    laboratory and imaging studies of, 543
    prognosis for, 544t, 546
    treatment of, 543–544
Leukocyte(s), normal values for, 508t
Leukocyte adhesion deficiency type I (LAD-I),
    264, 264t
Leukocyte adhesion deficiency type II (LAD-II),
    264, 264t
Leukocyte esterase, in urine, 555–556
Leukocytosis, in infectious diseases, 317t,
    316–317
Leukodystrophy(ies)
    adreno-, 644
        genetic basis for, 151t
    globoid cell, 643
    metachromatic, 181t–182t, 643
Leukokoria, in newborn, 199
Leukomalacia, periventricular, in newborn, 226
Leukorrhea, physiologic, *vs.* sexually transmitted
    infections, 377t–378t
Leukotriene modifiers, for asthma, 275–276
Leukotriene synthesis inhibitors, for asthma,
    275–276
Levalbuterol, for asthma, 276
Levocetirizine, for allergic rhinitis, 284
Levonorgestrel intrauterine device (Mirena), 246

Levonorgestrel (Plan B), for emergency postcoital
    contraception, 246
Leydig cell tumor, precocious puberty due to,
    593t
LH (luteinizing hormone), in puberty, 589
Li-Fraumeni syndrome, 551
Lichenification, 651t
Liddle syndrome, hypokalemia in, 116
Lidocaine, in cardiopulmonary resuscitation,
    127t
Lifestyle modifications, for migraines, 620
Ligament of Treitz, in midgut malrotation, 437
Limb-girdle muscular dystrophy, 628
Limb weakness
    distal, 625t
    ophthalmoplegia and, 625t
Limit(s), knowledge of, 4–5
Limit setting, 25
Limping child, 668, 669t
Linear skull fractures, 638
Lip(s), cracked, in Kawasaki disease, 303, 304f
Lipase, fibrosing colonopathy due to, 478
Lipid emulsion, in parenteral nutrition, 113
Lipidoses, 181t–182t
Lipoid adrenal hyperplasia, 608f
Lipoma, sacral, constipation due to, 426t
Lisch nodules, in neurofibromatosis type I,
    645–646
Lisdexamfetamine (Vyvanse), for ADHD, 42t
Lissencephaly, 648–649
Listeria monocytogenes, 398t–400t
Listeriosis, 398t–400t
Lithium
    for bipolar disorder, 61
    as teratogen, 206t
Little Leaguer's elbow, 692
Little Leaguer's shoulder, 691–692
Liver, with developmental disabilities, 28t
Liver disease, 444–450
    cholestasis as, 444–447
    chronic, 448–449
        autoimmune hepatitis as, 450, 449t
        clinical manifestations of, 448–449
        etiology and epidemiology of, 448
        laboratory and imaging studies for, 449, 449t
        steatohepatitis, 450
        treatment of, 450t, 449
        Wilson disease as, 449–450
    fulminant liver failure as, 447–448
Liver failure
    fulminant, 447–448
        clinical manifestations of, 447, 448t
        defined, 447
        etiology and epidemiology of, 447, 447t
        laboratory and imaging studies for, 447
        treatment of, 447–448, 448t
    in galactosemia, 173
Liver fluke, 406t
Liver function tests
    for chronic liver disease, 449t
    for gastrointestinal symptoms, 417
Liver phosphorylase deficiency, 172t
Liver trauma, 135
LLD. *see* Leg-length discrepancy
Lobar overdistension, congenital, 471
Local anesthetics, for analgesia, 145
Lomustine (CCNU), for cancer, 540t–541t
Long-chain hydroxyl-CoA dehydrogenase
    (LCHAD), neonatal screening for, 170t
Long-chain hydroxyl-CoA dehydrogenase
    (LCHAD) deficiency, 180f, 179
Loop of Henle, 553, 555f
Loratadine, for allergic rhinitis, 284
Lorazepam, for status epilepticus, 621–622, 622t
Loss-of-function mutation, 153

Louse-borne infections, 666
Louse-borne relapsing fever, 666
Low birth weight (LBW) infants, 188
Lower airway disease, 469–475
    acute respiratory distress syndrome, 473
    asthma as. *see* Asthma
    bronchiolitis as. *see* Bronchiolitis
    bronchopulmonary dysplasia as, 213–214, 471
    clinical manifestations of, 469
    cor pulmonale as, 473
    diagnostic studies for, 469–470
    differential diagnosis of, 470–475
    emphysema as, 471–472
    due to endobronchial mass lesions, 471
    etiology of, 469, 469t
    due to extrinsic tracheal compression, 470
    due to foreign body aspiration, 470–471
    pneumonia as. *see* Pneumonia
    primary ciliary dyskinesia as, 472
    pulmonary arterial hypertension as, 473
    pulmonary edema as, 472–473
    pulmonary embolism as, 474–475
    pulmonary hemorrhage as, 473–474, 474t
    tracheoesophageal fistula as. *see*
        Tracheoesophageal fistula
    tracheomalacia as, 470
Lower extremity, 676–680
    angular variations in, 677–678
        genu valgum as, 677–678, 677f
        genu varum as, 677f, 678
        tibia vara (Blount disease) as, 678
    leg-length discrepancy of, 678–679, 679t
    torsional variations in, 676–677
        in-toeing as, 676–677
            common causes of, 676t
            due to femoral anteversion, 676
            due to internal tibial torsion, 676–677, 677f
        out-toeing as, 677
            common causes of, 676t
            due to external tibial torsion, 677
Lower motor neuron disease, 624–630
    of anterior horn cells, 624–625, 624t
    clinical manifestations of, 624t
    due to infant botulism, 627
    due to muscle disease, 627–628. *see also*
        Muscle disease(s)
    due to peripheral neuropathy, 625–626
    laboratory and diagnostic studies for, 629
    malignant hyperthermia with, 629
    myasthenia gravis as, 626–627
    spinal muscular atrophy as, 624–625
    topography of, 624, 625t
Lower motor neurons, 623
Lower motor unit, 623–624
Lower respiratory tract infection, 358–359
LP. *see* Lumbar puncture
LSD (lysergic acid diethylamide), acute effects of, 250t–251t
Lubricant, for functional constipation, 47t
Ludwig angina, 349
Lumbar puncture (LP)
    for increased intracranial pressure, 641
    for infectious diseases, 317
    for leukemia, 543
    traumatic, 615
Lumbosacral hemangioma, 661–662
Lumbosacral spine, hair tufts over, 197
Lung(s)
    anatomy of, 455
    of newborn, 199–200
    physiology of, 455–457
        defense mechanism in, 456–457
        pulmonary mechanics in, 455–456, 455f
        respiratory gas exchange in, 456, 456t
    unilateral hyperlucent, 363

Lung abscess, 363
Lung biopsy, 460
Lung capacities, 455f
Lung compliance, 456
Lung consolidation, 458t
Lung defense mechanisms, 456–457
Lung development, 210–211, 211f
Lung disease
    chronic, 213–214
    obstructive, 459
    restrictive, 456
Lung flukes, 406t
Lung injury, acute, 128
Lung volumes, 455f
Lungworm, rat, 405t
Lupus, discoid, 309
Lupus nephritis, 312
Luteinizing hormone (LH), in puberty, 589
LVOT (left ventricular outflow tract) obstruction, syncope due to, 488t
Lyme disease, 396–400, 398t–400t
    clinical manifestations of, 397
    complications and prognosis for, 400
    differential diagnosis of, 300t, 397
    early disseminated, 397
    early localized, 397
    epidemiology of, 396–397, 397f
    etiology of, 396
    laboratory and imaging studies for, 397
    late, 397
    prevention of, 400
    synovial fluid findings in, 385t
    treatment of, 397–400
Lymphadenitis, 339
    cervical, 339
Lymphadenopathy, 338–342
    cervical, 339
    clinical manifestations of, 340
    complications and prognosis for, 341–342
    defined, 338
    differential diagnosis of, 341
    epidemiology of, 340
    etiology of, 338–340
    generalized, 338, 339t
    in hematologic disorders, 506
    inguinal, 339t
    in Kawasaki disease, 303
    laboratory and imaging studies for, 340, 341f
    prevention of, 344
    regional, 338–340
    treatment of, 341
    in tuberculosis, 408
Lymphangitis, 339
Lymphatic malformation, differential diagnosis of, 659t
Lymphocutaneous syndromes, 339, 339t
Lymphocyte(s)
    atypical
        in infectious diseases, 316–317
        in lymphadenopathy, 340
    normal values for, 508t
Lymphocyte disorder(s), 256–263
    antibody deficiency disease(s) due to, 256–258
        agammaglobulinemia as, 256, 258t
        antibody deficiency syndrome as, 257–258, 258t
        common variable immunodeficiency as, 256, 258t
            clinical features of, 256
            etiology of, 256, 257f
        IgA deficiency as, 257, 258t
        IgG subclass deficiency as, 257, 258t
        pathogenesis of, 256
        transient hypogammaglobulinemia of infancy as, 257, 258t

Lymphocyte disorder(s) (*Continued*)
    combined immunodeficiency disease(s) due to, 258–262
    etiology and clinical manifestations of, 256–262
    other
        ataxia-telangiectasia as, 260–261, 261t
        cartilage-hair hypoplasia (short-limbed dwarf) as, 261t
        chronic mucocutaneous candidiasis as, 261, 261t
        hyper-IgE syndrome as, 261t, 262
        Nijmegen breakage syndrome as, 261t
        Wiskott-Aldrich syndrome as, 260, 261t
        X-linked lymphoproliferative syndrome as, 261, 261t
    pathogenesis of, 256, 257f
    prevention and newborn screening of, 266
    treatment of, 262
Lymphocyte phenotyping, 255
Lymphocytic choriomeningitis, 398t–400t
Lymphocytic thyroiditis, 599
    with diabetes mellitus, 578
Lymphocytosis, due to pertussis, 356
Lymphohistiocytosis, familial hemophagocytic, 516t
Lymphoid hyperplasia, in allergic colitis, 442
Lymphoma, 544–546
    anaplastic, 544
    Burkitt
        clinical manifestations of, 545
        etiology of, 544, 545t
    clinical manifestations of, 545
    complications of, 547
    defined, 544
    diagnosis of, 545
    differential diagnosis of, 545
    epidemiology of, 545
    etiology of, 544–545, 545t
    Hodgkin. *see* Hodgkin disease
    laboratory/imaging studies of, 545, 547f
    large cell, 544, 545t
    lymphoblastic, 544, 545t
    non-Hodgkin. *see* Non-Hodgkin lymphoma (NHL)
    prognosis for, 547–548
    treatment of, 545–546
Lymphoproliferative disease
    with hematopoietic stem cell transplantation, 269
    X-linked, 341
Lysosomal α-glucosidase deficiency, 172t
Lysosomal enzyme activity, 184
Lysosomal membrane, storage diseases caused by defective synthesis of, 181t–182t
Lysosomal proteolysis, storage diseases caused by, 181t–182t
Lysosomal storage disorders, 184
    diagnostic testing for, 184–185
    treatment strategies for, 185
    types of, 181t–182t
Lysosomal transport proteins, storage diseases caused by dysfunction of, 181t–182t
Lysosomes, 183

M

M-CHAT (Modified Checklist for Autism in Toddlers), 18–19
M-CSF (macrophage colony-stimulating factor), in hematopoiesis, 510f
MAC (membrane attack complex), 267–268, 267f
Macro-orchidism, with developmental disabilities, 28t
Macrocephaly, 612, 648, 648t
    with developmental disabilities, 28t
    in glutaric acidemia I, 178

Macrocrania, 648
Macrophage colony-stimulating factor (M-CSF),
    in hematopoiesis, 510f
Macula, cherry-red spot in, with developmental
    disabilities, 28t
Macular rash, infections with fever and,
    329t–330t
Macule, 650t, 651f
Maculopapular rash, infections with fever and,
    329t–330t
Magnesium citrate
    for functional constipation, 46t
    for poisoning, 143
Magnesium hydroxide, for functional
    constipation, 47t
Magnesium sulfate, maternal use of, 207t
Magnetic resonance imaging (MRI), 163
    of autism, 64
    of brain and spinal cord, 616
    for cancer, 536, 542t
    of chest, 458–459
    of CNS tumors, 547
    for infectious diseases, 317
    for seizures, 622
    of urinary system, 557
Mainstem bronchi, anatomy of, 455
Maintenance fluid therapy, 106–107, 107t
    for burns, 138
Maintenance water, adjustments in
    clinical causes of, 108, 108t
    components of, 108t
    due to surgical drains and chest tubes, 108
    due to urine output, 108
        decreased, 108, 108t
        increased, 108, 108t
    gastrointestinal sources of, 108, 108t
    normal sources of, 108
Major depressive disorder (MDD), 59
    diagnostic criteria for, 59t
Major determinant, in skin testing for penicillin
    allergy, 297
Major histocompatibility complex (MHC)
    compatibility, in hematopoietic stem cell
    transplantations, 269
Malabsorption syndromes, vitamin and nutrient
    deficiencies with, 97t
Malar butterfly rash, in systemic lupus
    erythematosus, 309, 310f
Malar region, dysmorphology of, 162
Malaria, 398t–400t, 402–404
    algid, 404
    cerebral, 404
    clinical manifestations of, 403, 403t
    complications and prognosis for, 404
    differential diagnosis of, 403
    epidemiology of, 402
    etiology of, 402
    laboratory and imaging studies for, 403
    prevention of, 404
    relapse of, 403
    treatment of, 404
Malformations, 161
    association in, 161
    congenital, 146
    defined, 160–161, 667t
    diagnosis of, 163
    due to disruptions of development, 160–161
    due to extrinsic factors, 160–161
    due to inborn errors of metabolism, 168
    due to intrinsic factors, 160–161
    epidemiology of, 146, 161
    history for
        family, 161–162
        pregnancy, 161
    laboratory evaluation of, 163

Malformations (Continued)
    life-threatening, 196, 196t, 202
    mechanisms of, 667t
    minor, 161
    multiple, 161
    physical examination for, 162–163
        craniofacial, 162
        of extremities, 162–163
        of genitalia, 163
        growth in, 162
        of neck, 162
        of trunk, 162
    sequence of, 160–161
    syndromes in, 160
    terminology used in, 161, 161t
Malignancies, fever due to, 326
Malignant cells, bone marrow infiltration by,
    anemia due to, 515–516
Malignant hyperthermia, 629
Malignant melanoma, 660–661
    giant congenital nevi and, 660–661
    maternal, 205t
Malingering, 51–54, 52t
Mallory-Weiss syndrome, GI bleeding due to,
    427t
Malnutrition, 93–96
    classification of, 94t
    complications of, 96
    definitions of, 94t
    in failure to thrive, 69, 94. see also Failure to
        thrive
    kwashiorkor as, 94–95
    marasmus as, 94
    mild, 94t
    moderate, 94t
    physical signs of, 95t
    primary, 93–94
    secondary, 93–94, 94f
    severe, 94t
    treatment of, 95–96
Malnutrition-infection cycle, 69
Mandibular region, dysmorphology of, 162
Mania
    dysphoric, 60–61
    symptoms of, 59t
Manic depressive disorder. see Bipolar disorder
    (BD)
Mannitol, for increased intracranial pressure, 641
α-Mannosidase deficiency, 181t–182t
Mannosyl phosphotransferase deficiency,
    181t–182t
Mantoux test, 409
Maple syrup urine disease (MSUD), 176
    clinical manifestations of, 176
    definitive diagnosis of, 176
    laboratory manifestations of, 176
    neonatal screening for, 170t
    treatment of, 176
Marasmus, 94
Marcus Gunn pupil, 614
Marfan syndrome (MS), 148
    diagnostic criteria for, 149t
    genetic basis for, 147t
    hypermobility in, 313
    hypotonia in, 629
Marijuana, acute effects of, 250t–251t
Markers, for cancer, 542t
Maroteaux-Lamy syndrome, 181t–182t
Masculinization, inadequate, of 46,XY male,
    605–606, 606t
Mask ventilation
    in newborn resuscitation, 194
    for respiratory failure, 131
Mass lesions, 640
    upper airway obstruction due to, 468

Mastitis, 87
Mastocytoma, 659t
Mastoiditis, acute, 352
Maternal assessment, 186–187
Maternal deprivation, growth failure due to,
    584–585
Maternal disease(s)
    affecting newborn, 204–206, 205t
        antiphospholipid syndrome as, 205
        diabetes mellitus as, 205t–206t, 206
        hyperthyroidism as, 205t, 206
        idiopathic thrombocytopenia as, 205, 205t
        other, 206
        systemic lupus erythematosus as, 205, 205t
    as teratogens, 154
Maternal health status, effect on fetus of, 1
Maternal hyperphenylalaninemia, 175
Maternal infections, as teratogens, 154
Maternal medications
    small for gestational age due to, 208t
    as teratogen, 206, 206t
    that may adversely affect newborn, 206, 207t
Maternal serum screening, 154
Mature minors, 6
Maturity
    fetal, 188–189
        pulmonary, 189
    of newborn, 197
        and abnormal fetal growth patterns, 197,
            199f
        cumulative score in, 197, 198f
        neurologic criteria in, 197, 198f
        physical criteria for, 197, 197f
Maturity-onset diabetes of youth (MODY), 573t,
    579
MBP. see Munchausen syndrome by proxy (MBP)
MCAD (medium-chain acyl-CoA
    dehydrogenase) deficiency, 179
McArdle disease, 172t
McCarthy Scales of Children's Abilities, 29t
McCune-Albright syndrome, precocious puberty
    in, 593–595, 593t
MCD (multicystic renal dysplasia), 566
MCNS (minimal change nephrotic syndrome),
    556
MCV (meningococcal conjugate vaccine),
    319f–322f
MDIs (metered dose inhalers), 460
MDIs (multiple daily injections), of insulin,
    576–578
Mean midexpiratory flow rate (FEF$_{25-75\%}$), 459
Mean platelet volume (MPV), 526
Measles, 329–331
    black, 329–330
    clinical manifestations of, 329–330
    complications and prognosis for, 331
    differential diagnosis of, 330
    epidemiology of, 329
    etiology of, 329
    laboratory and imaging studies for, 330
    modified, 330
    mumps, and rubella (MMR) vaccine, 317–318,
        319f–322f, 331
    prevention of, 331
    treatment of, 330
Mechanical counterpulsation, for heart failure,
    501t
Mechanical ventilation, 461
    for bronchopulmonary dysplasia, 214
    complications of, 131
    for primary pulmonary hypertension of the
        newborn, 215
    pulmonary air leaks due to, 213
    for respiratory distress syndrome, 212
    for respiratory failure, 131

Meckel diverticulum, 440
  abdominal pain due to, 420t
  GI bleeding due to, 427t
Meconium aspiration pneumonia, 214–215
Meconium aspiration syndrome, 209
Meconium ileus
  in cystic fibrosis, 476, 478
  intestinal atresia due to, 439
Meconium-stained amniotic fluid, 195–196
Mediastinal deviation, 458t
Medical assessment, for developmental
    disabilities, 26, 27t–28t
Medical decision making, 5
Medical device-associated infections, 394–396
Medical history, past, in genetic assessment, 156
Medical home, for child with special needs, 26
Medical intervention, for developmental
    disability, 30, 31t
MedicAlert bracelet
  for adverse drug reactions, 298
  for anaphylaxis, 291
  for food allergies, 298
  for insect allergies, 296
Medications. see Drug(s)
Mediterranean spotted fever, 398t–400t
Medium-chain acyl-CoA dehydrogenase
    (MCAD), neonatal screening for, 170t
Medium-chain acyl-CoA dehydrogenase
    (MCAD) deficiency, 180f, 179
Medroxyprogesterone acetate, for delayed
    puberty, 592
Medullary carcinoma of thyroid, 601
Medulloblastoma
  epidemiology of, 546
  MRI of, 547, 547f
  prognosis for, 547–548, 549t
  treatment of, 547
Mefloquine, for malaria, 404
Megacolon, toxic, 440
Megakaryocytes, production of, 509
Megakaryocytic cells, in hematopoiesis, 506
Megalencephaly, 648
Melanocytic nevi, 659t, 660
  acquired, 662
  congenital, 198, 660, 660f
    differential diagnosis of, 659t
    giant, 198, 659t, 660–661, 660f
    hairy, 660, 660f
Melanoma, malignant, 660–661
  giant congenital nevi and, 660–661
  maternal, 205t
Melanosis
  dermal, 659, 659t, 660f
  pustular, 198
MELAS (mitochondrial encephalomyopathy with
    lactic acidosis and strokelike episodes), 152,
    185, 642t–643t, 644
-melia, 161t
Membrane attack complex (MAC), 267–268, 267f
Membrane disorders, hemolytic anemia due to,
    521
  clinical manifestations of, 521
  etiology of, 510f, 521
  laboratory diagnosis of, 521
  treatment of, 521
Membrane rupture
  premature, 187
  prolonged, 187
Membranoproliferative glomerulonephritis
    (MPGN), nephrotic syndrome due to, 556
Membranous nephropathy, nephrotic syndrome
    due to, 556
Membranous septum, 491
Menaquinone, 102
Menarche, 237–238

Meningeal abscess, 343t
Meningitis, 342–344
  aseptic, 342
  bacterial
    complications and prognosis for, 346
    epidemiology of, 342
    etiology of, 342t
    increased intracranial pressure due to, 641
    laboratory studies for, 343
    partially treated, 343t
    prevention of, 346
    treatment of, 344t, 343–344
  clinical manifestations of, 342–343
  complications and prognosis for, 346
  defined, 342
  depressed consciousness due to, 636
  differential diagnosis of, 343
  eosinophilic, 405t
  epidemiology of, 342
  etiology of, 342
  fever due to, 325
  fungal, 343t
  laboratory and imaging studies for, 343
  in newborn, 227
    clinical manifestations of, 228
    incidence of, 228
    risk factors for, 228
    treatment of, 228
  partially treated, 342
  prevention of, 346
  recurrence of, 346
  relapse of, 346
  treatment of, 343–344
  tuberculous, 343t
  viral, 343t
    epidemiology of, 342
    etiology of, 342
  vomiting due to, 423t
Meningocele, 647
Meningococcal conjugate vaccine (MCV),
    319f–322f
Meningococcus prophylaxis, 318–323
Meningomyelocele, 196t
  constipation due to, 426t
Menstrual disorder(s), 242–244
  abnormal uterine bleeding as, 243, 243t
  amenorrhea as, 242–243
  dysmenorrhea as, 242, 244
  irregular menses as, 241–242
Mental health problems, 3
Mental retardation (MR), 31
  defined, 31
  diagnosis and management of, 31
  etiology of, 31, 32t
  levels of, 31t
  prevalence of, 31
Mental status alteration, due to respiratory
    failure, 128
Mental status examination, 612–613
Mepivacaine, maternal use of, 207t
6-Mercaptopurine
  for cancer, 540t–541t
  for ulcerative colitis, 441–442
MERRF (myoclonus, epilepsy, and ragged red
    fibers), 642t–643t, 644
Merrill-Palmer Scale of Mental Tests, 29t
Mesalamine (5-aminosalicylic acid), for
    ulcerative colitis, 441–442
Mescaline, acute effects of, 250t–251t
Metabolic acidosis, 116, 120–121, 139–141
  anion gap in, 118t, 119, 141t
  appropriate compensation during, 117t
  causes of, 118t
  due to inborn errors of metabolism, 167–168,
    169t

Metabolic acidosis (Continued)
  due to poisoning, 139–141, 141t
  hypokalemia with, 116
  in newborn, 192, 210
Metabolic alkalosis, 116, 121–122
  causes of, 122t
  chloride-resistant, 122, 122t
  chloride responsive, 121–122, 122t
  clinical manifestations of, 122
  diagnosis of, 122
  etiology of, 121–122
  hypochloremic, in pyloric stenosis, 435
  hypokalemia with, 116
  treatment of, 122
Metabolic compensation, appropriate, 120
Metabolic degenerative diseases, 642–644
Metabolic disorder(s)
  assessment of, 164–171
    clinical, and laboratory findings, 169, 169t
  ataxia due to, 633
  clinical presentation of, 165–168
    congenital malformations or dysmorphic
      features in, 168
    energy deficiency in, 168
    hyperammonemia in, 167
      etiology of, 167, 167t
      in later infancy and childhood, 166f,
        167–168
      moderate neonatal, 167
      severe neonatal, 167
    ketosis and ketotic hypoglycemia in, 168
    metabolic acidosis in, 167–168, 168t
    neurologic signs in, 167, 167t
    specific organ, 168, 168t
    toxic, 165–167
  genetic aspects of, 169
    identification of molecular pathology as, 169
    mechanisms of inheritance as, 169
  incidence of, 164t
  neonatal screening for. see Neonatal screening;
    for inborn errors of metabolism
  overview of treatment for, 171
  pathophysiology of, 165t
  signs and symptoms of, 164–165
  storage disorders as, 168
  vomiting due to, 423t
Metabolic response pathways, and hypoglycemia,
    580t, 582
Metabolic syndrome, 579
Metabolic testing, for chronic liver disease, 449t
Metachromatic leukodystrophy, 181t–182t,
    642t–643t, 643
Metadate CD (Methylphenidate), for ADHD, 42t
Metagonimiasis, 406t
Metagonimus yokogawai, 406t
Metaphase analysis, in genetic assessment, 159
Metaphysis, 668f
Metastatic disease, in sarcomas, 552
Metatarsal, head of second, idiopathic vascular
    necrosis of, 683
Metatarsus adductus, 682, 682f
Metatarsus varus, 682
Metered dose inhalers (MDIs), 460
Methadone, for analgesia, 145t
Methanol ingestion, metabolic acidosis due to,
    121
Methimazole
  for hyperthyroidism, 600–601
  maternal use of, 207t
Methionine, metabolism of, 175f
Methotrexate
  for cancer, 540t–541t
  for juvenile dermatomyositis, 313
  for juvenile idiopathic arthritis, 308
Methyl mercury, as teratogen, 206t

Methylmalonic acidemia, 177–178
  clinical manifestations of, 177–178
  neonatal screening for, 170t
  treatment of, 177–178
Methylphenidate (Ritalin, Concerta, Metadate),
    for ADHD, 42t
Methylprednisolone, for systemic lupus
    erythematosus, 311
Methylxanthines, for apnea of prematurity, 220
Metoclopramide, for gastroesophageal reflux,
    432t
Metorchiasis, 406t
Metorchis conjunctus, 406t
Metronidazole
  for peritonitis, 454
  for trichomoniasis, 384
MHC (major histocompatibility complex)
    compatibility, in hematopoietic stem cell
    transplantations, 269
Micaceous scale, in psoriasis, 658
Micro-comedo, 652
Microangiopathy, thrombotic, 522, 528
Microarray comparative genomic hybridization,
    160
Microcephaly, 612, 648, 649t
  with developmental disabilities, 28t
Microhemagglutination assay-*T. pallidum*, 380
Micronutrient deficiencies, 96–105
  etiology of, 97t
  with malnutrition, 95–96
  of minerals, 103–105, 103t
  of vitamins, 96–105
Micronutrients, 96
Microphallus, 606
Micturition, normal, 567
Micturition syncope, 488t
Midazolam, for status epilepticus, 621–622, 622t
Middle ear effusion, persistent, 352
Midface, dysmorphology of, 162
Midgut malrotation, 437–438
  clinical manifestations of, 437
  etiology and epidemiology of, 437, 438f
  laboratory and imaging studies for, 437–438
  with volvulus, 437, 438f
  vomiting due to, 423t
Mifepristone, for emergency postcoital
    contraception, 246
Migraine, 616–618
  basilar artery, 637
  clinical manifestations of, 617, 617t
  confusional, 637
  diagnostic studies for, 617–618, 617f
  etiology and epidemiology of, 616
  treatment of, 620
  vomiting due to, 423t
Milia, 198, 650t, 651f
Miliaria, 198
  crystallina, vesiculobullous eruptions due to,
    663t
Miliary tuberculosis, 408
Military deployment, 3
Milk
  breast, composition of, 88–89, 88t
  cow's, for toddlers and older children, 89
Milk intake
  adequacy of, 86
  for toddlers and older children, 89
Milk intolerance, vomiting due to, 423t
Milk of magnesia, for functional constipation, 47t
Milk of molasses, for functional constipation, 46t
Miller Fisher variant, of Guillain-Barré
    syndrome, 625
Milrinone
  for heart failure, 501t
  for shock, 132t

Mineral deficiencies, 103–105, 103t
  of calcium, 103
  of chromium, 103t
  of copper, 103t
  of fluoride, 103t, 105
  of iodine, 103t
  of iron, 103t, 104
  of selenium, 103t
  of zinc, 103t, 104–105
Mineral oil, for functional constipation, 47t, 46t
Mineralocorticoid deficiency, 608
Mineralocorticoids
  biosynthesis of, 608f
  for 21-hydroxylase deficiency, 609
Minerals, in parenteral nutrition, 113
Minimal change nephrotic syndrome (MCNS),
    556
Minor(s)
  emancipated, 6
  mature, 6
Minor determinant, in skin testing for penicillin
    allergy, 297
Minute dog tapeworm, 407
Minute ventilation, 461
MIP-1α, functions of, 253t
MiraLAX (Polyethylene glycol powder), for
    functional constipation, 47t
Mirena (levonorgestrel intrauterine device), 246
Misoprostol, as teratogen, 206t
Missense mutation, 146
Mitochondrial diabetes, 573t
Mitochondrial disorder(s), 183–185, 644
  biomechanical abnormalities of, 184–185, 185f
  defined, 183
  epidemiology of, 183
  genetics of, 185
  inborn errors of metabolism due to, 169, 169t
  MELAS as, 152, 644
  MERRF as, 644
  NARP as, 644
  pathogenesis of, 183, 184f
  signs and symptoms of, 184
  treatment of, 185
Mitochondrial DNA (mtDNA), 152, 185
Mitochondrial encephalomyopathy with lactic
    acidosis and strokelike episodes (MELAS),
    152, 185, 642t–643t, 644
Mitochondrial genome, 184f, 185
Mitochondrial inheritance, 152
  heteroplasmy in, 152
  of inborn errors of metabolism, 169, 169t
  MELAS as, 152
Mitochondrion(ia), function of, 183, 184f
Mixed amphetamine salts (Adderall), for ADHD,
    42t
Mixed marasmus-kwashiorkor, 95
Mixed venous oxygen saturation, in shock, 131
ML (mucolipidosis[es]), 181t–182t
MMR (measles, mumps, and rubella) vaccine,
    317–318, 319f–322f, 331
Mobitz type I heart block, 490t
Mobitz type II heart block, 490t
Möbius syndrome, in newborn, 203
Modified Checklist for Autism in Toddlers
    (M-CHAT), 18–19
Modified Duke Criteria, for infective
    endocarditis, 365, 365t
MODY (maturity-onset diabetes of youth), 573t,
    579
Mold, and asthma, 275t
Molecular tests, for infectious diseases, 317
Molluscum contagiosum, 338
  vulvovaginitis due to, 375t
Mometasone DPI, for asthma, 279f
Mongolian spots, 197, 659, 659t, 660f

Monocytes, normal values for, 508t
Mononucleosis, infectious
  clinical manifestations of, 340
  complications and prognosis for, 341
  etiology of, 339
  laboratory studies for, 340
Monosomy(ies), 158–159
  defined, 157
  Turner syndrome as, 158–159
Montelukast, for asthma, 275–276
Morbidity, changing, 3
Morbilliform rash, in juvenile idiopathic arthritis,
    307
Moro reflex, 13, 202–203, 613t
Morphine
  for analgesia, 145t
  maternal use of, 207t
Morquio syndrome, 181t–182t
Mosaicism, 157
Mother. *see* Maternal
Motion sickness, vomiting due to, 423t
Motor assessment, with developmental
    disabilities, 26
Motor development, milestones in, 668
Motor examination, 614–615
  of bulk, 615
  of coordination, 615
  of gait, 613, 615
  of power, 614–615
  of reflexes, 615
  of tone, 615
Motor intervention, for developmental disability,
    30
Motor problems, with developmental disability,
    31t
Motor sensory neuropathy, hereditary, 626
Motor vehicle accidents, 2
Mouth. *see also* Oral cavity
  bottle, 429
  of newborn, 199
Mouth sores, in systemic lupus erythematosus,
    309
Movement, in newborn, 613
Movement disorders, 633–634
  causes of, 633t
MPGN (membranoproliferative
    glomerulonephritis), nephrotic syndrome
    due to, 556
MPS (mucopolysaccharidoses), 181t–182t,
    642t–643t, 644
MPV (mean platelet volume), 526
MR. *see* Mental retardation (MR)
MRI. *see* Magnetic resonance imaging (MRI)
MS (Marfan syndrome), hypotonia in, 629
MSUD. *see* Maple syrup urine disease
mtDNA (mitochondrial DNA), 152, 185
MTTL1 gene, in MELAS, 152
Muckle-Wells syndrome, 290–291
Mucolipidosis(es) (ML), 181t–182t
Mucopolysaccharides, 183
Mucopolysaccharidoses (MPS), 181t–182t,
    642t–643t, 644
Mucopurulent cervicitis, 376t
Multicystic renal dysplasia (MCD), 566
Multifactorial disorders, 151–152
  hypertrophic pyloric stenosis due to, 152
  neural tube defects due to, 152
Multiple acyl-CoA dehydrogenase deficiency,
    179–180
Multiple daily injections (MDIs), of insulin,
    576–578
Multiple gestations, 187
Multiple malformation syndrome, 161
Multiple organ dysfunction, due to respiratory
    failure, 131

Multiple sulfatase deficiency, 181t–182t
Mumps vaccine, 319f–322f, 331
Munchausen syndrome, fever due to, 326
Munchausen syndrome by proxy (MBP), 54
    fever due to, 326
    hyperinsulinemia due to, 581
Murine typhus, 398t–400t
Murine typhus-like illness, 398t–400t
Murmurs. *see* Heart murmurs
Muscle bulk, in motor examination, 615
Muscle disease(s), 624t, 627–628
    congenital myopathies as, 628
    Duchenne dystrophy as, 627–628
    Emery-Dreifuss dystrophy as, 628
    facioscapulohumeral dystrophy as, 628
    limb-girdle dystrophy as, 628
    metabolic myopathies as, 629
    myotonic dystrophy as, 628
Muscle fasciculations, 615–616
    spinal muscular atrophy, 625
Muscle fibrillations, 616
Muscle phosphofructokinase deficiency, 172t
Muscle phosphorylase deficiency, 172t
Muscle power, in motor examination, 614–615
Muscle strength, in motor examination, 615
Muscle tone
    in motor examination, 615
    in newborn, 613
Muscular dystrophy (MD)
    Becker, 627
    congenital, 628
    constipation due to, 426t
    Duchenne (pseudohypertrophic progressive),
        627–628
        clinical manifestations of, 627
        etiology of, 627
        genetic basis for, 151t
        laboratory and diagnostic studies of, 627
        treatment of, 627–628
    facioscapulohumeral, 628
    limb-girdle, 628
    obesity in, 91t
Muscular septum, 491
Musculoskeletal pain syndrome(s), 312–314
    benign hypermobility as, 313, 313f, 313t
    defined, 299
    differential diagnosis of, 308t
    growing pain as, 312–313
    myofascial pain syndrome and fibromyalgia
        as, 313–314
Mutations, 146
    frameshift, 146
    hot spot, 148
    loss-of-function, 153
    missense, 146
    nonsense, 146
    point, 146
    single gene, 148
    spontaneous, 147
Myasthenia gravis, 626–627
    congenital, 627
    diagnostic studies of, 627
    juvenile, 626
    maternal, 205t
    transient neonatal, 627
Myasthenic syndrome, congenital, 627
Mycobacteria, 407
    nontuberculous, lymphadenitis due to,
        339–340
Mycobacterial diseases, zoonotic, 398t–400t
Mycobacterium fortuitum, 398t–400t
Mycobacterium kansasii, 398t–400t
Mycobacterium marinum, 398t–400t
Mycobacterium tuberculosis. see Tuberculosis
Mycoplasma catarrhalis, conjunctivitis due to, 386

Mycoplasma hominis, pneumonia due to, 359
Mycoplasma pneumoniae
    pneumonia due to, 359, 363t
    Stevens-Johnson syndrome due to, 664
Myelitis, transverse, 624
Myelodysplasia, obesity in, 91t
Myeloid cells, in hematopoiesis, 506
Myelomeningocele, 647
Myeloperoxidase deficiency, 264t
Myeloproliferative disorder, transient, 543
Myocardial contractility, in heart failure, 500
Myocarditis, syncope due to, 488t
Myoclonic epilepsy, 620–621
    juvenile (of Janz), 621
Myoclonus, 637
    epilepsy, and ragged red fibers (MERRF),
        642t–643t, 644
    in paraneoplastic opsoclonus-myoclonus
        syndrome, 633
Myofascial pain syndromes, 313–314
Myonecrosis, 336
Myopathies
    congenital, 628
    endocrine, 629
    metabolic, 629
    mitochondrial, 629
Myositis, in rheumatic diseases, 299
Myotonia, 628
Myotonic dystrophy (DM), 628
    clinical manifestations of, 628
    diagnosis of, 628
    etiology and epidemiology of, 628
    genetic basis for, 147t
    maternal, 205t
Myxedematous cretinism, 103t

N

N-acetylgalactosamine-4-sulfatase deficiency,
    181t–182t
Na (sodium), fractional excretion of, in acute
    renal failure, 561
Nail, hypoplastic, 161t
Nail-fold capillaries, dilated, in juvenile
    dermatomyositis, 311
Naloxone (Narcan), in newborn resuscitation,
    196
Nanophyetiasis, 406t
Nanophyetus salmincola, 406t
Naphthalene, maternal use of, 207t
Narcotics
    constipation due to, 426t
    maternal use of, 207t
    toxicity of, 141t
NARP (neuropathy, ataxia, and retinitis
    pigmentosa), 642t–643t, 644
Nasal alae, 161t
Nasal cannula, 460
Nasal flaring, 457
Nasal polyposis, in cystic fibrosis, 475
Nasal polyps, 284
Nasal smear, for common cold, 347
Nasal sores, in systemic lupus erythematosus, 309
Nasal turbinates, 455
Nasolabial fold, 161t
Nasopharyngoscopy, 459
National Childhood Vaccine Injury Act, 318
National Practitioner Data Bank, 4
National Vaccine Injury Compensation Program,
    318
NATP (neonatal alloimmune thrombocytopenic
    purpura), 527
NBS (New Ballard Score), 198f
NCL (neuronal ceroid lipofuscinosis), 181t–182t,
    642t–643t, 644
NCVs (nerve conduction velocities), 616

NDT (neurodevelopmental therapy), for
    developmental disabilities, 30
Near-drowning, 136
Nebulizers, 460
Necator americanus, 404, 405t
Neck
    congenital malformations of, 162
    of newborn, 199
Necrotizing enterocolitis (NEC), 223–224
    GI bleeding due to, 427t
Necrotizing fasciitis, 336
Negative-pressure ventilation, for prevention of
    tuberculosis, 416
Negative reinforcement, 15
Neglect, 70–74
Neisseria gonorrhoeae, 376, 379
    and *Chlamydia trachomatis,* 376t
    clinical features of, 376t
    congenital infection with, 230t, 232–233
    conjunctivitis due to, 386
        neonatal, 388t
    disseminated gonococcal infections due to, 379
    pathogenesis of, 379
    pelvic inflammatory disease due to, 379
    treatment of, 379
Neisseria meningitidis, prophylaxis for, 318–323
Nematodes, 405t
NEMO (nuclear factor κB essential modulator),
    in hyper-IgM syndrome, 258
Neoadjuvant chemotherapy, 539–541
Neonatal alloimmune thrombocytopenic
    purpura (NATP), 527
Neonatal drug addiction and withdrawal, 204
    from cocaine, 204
    from opiates, 204
Neonatal hepatitis, 444
Neonatal history, for developmental disabilities,
    27t
Neonatal hypotonia, 629
Neonatal mortality, 187, 188t
Neonatal physiology, transition from fetal to,
    189–190, 190t
Neonatal screening, for inborn errors of
    metabolism, 170–171, 170t
    confirmatory testing principles of, 170
    disorders identified by, 170, 170t
    specialized laboratory and clinical testing after,
        170–171, 171t
    strategy of, 170
Neorickettsia sennetsu, 398t–400t
Nephritis, lupus, 312
Nephrogenic rests, 550
Nephrolithiasis, 567
Nephrology assessment, 553–556
    common manifestations in, 554–555, 554t
    history in, 553
    imaging studies in, 558
    physical examination in, 553
Nephropathic cystinosis, 181t–182t
Nephropathy
    IgA
        hematuria due to, 558
        prognosis for, 560
    reflux, 565
Nephrotic syndrome (NS), 556–558
    clinical manifestations of, 557
    complications of, 557–558
    congenital, 556–557
    diagnostic studies of, 557
    differential diagnosis of, 557
    edema in, 556
    etiology and epidemiology of, 556–557
    hypercholesterolemia in, 556
    hypoproteinemia in, 556
    idiopathic, 556

Nephrotic syndrome (NS) (Continued)
  minimal change, 556
  primary, 556, 556t
  prognosis for, 558
  proteinuria in, 556
  secondary, 556–557, 556t
  treatment of, 557
Nerve conduction velocities (NCVs), 616
Nesidioblastosis, 580–581
Neural crest cells, 548, 647
Neural plate, 647
Neural tube, 647
Neural tube defects (NDTs)
  folate deficiency and, 100
  genetic basis for, 152
  maternal screening for, 154
  newborn assessment for, 196t
Neuralgia, postherpetic, 334
Neuraminidase deficiency, 181t–182t
Neuroblastoma, 548–549
  ataxia due to, 633
  clinical manifestations of, 548
  complications of, 549
  differential diagnosis of, 548–549
  epidemiology of, 548
  etiology of, 548
  laboratory/imaging studies of, 548
  prognosis for, 549
  risk factors for, 536t
  staging of, 549, 549t
  treatment of, 549, 549t
Neuroborreliosis, 397
Neurocardiogenic syncope, 488t
Neurocutaneous disorders, 645–647
  neurofibromatosis as, 645–646, 645f
  Sturge-Weber syndrome as, 662, 646–647
  tuberous sclerosis complex as, 646
Neurocysticercosis, 407, 407t
Neurodegenerative disease(s), 642–645
  acquired illnesses mimicking, 645
  with focal manifestations, 644
  gray matter (neuronal), 642–643
  hereditary and metabolic, 642–644
  white matter (leukodystrophies), 642–643
Neurodevelopmental therapy (NDT), for
    developmental disabilities, 30
Neurofibroma(s), 646
  plexiform, 646, 659t
Neurofibromatosis 1 (NF1), 148, 645–646
  clinical manifestations of, 645–646, 645f
  etiology of, 645
  genetic basis for, 147t, 645
Neurofibromatosis 2 (NF2)
  clinical manifestations of, 646
  genetic basis for, 147t, 646
Neurofibromatosis (NF), 551, 645–646
  clinical manifestations of, 645–646, 645f
  etiology of, 645
  segmental, 645
  with spinal deformities, 684
Neurofibromin, 645
Neurogenic bladder, vesicoureteral reflux due
    to, 565
Neurogenic hyperventilation, central, 634–635
Neuroimaging, 616
Neurologic criteria, for newborn maturity and
    gestational age, 197, 198f
Neurologic deficits, head trauma with, 637
  concussion as, 637–638
  drowsiness, headache and vomiting due to, 639
  due to cervical spine injuries, 639
  due to cranial nerve palsies, 638–639
  due to CSF leak, 638–639
  due to skull fractures, 638–639
  intracranial hemorrhage in, 638–640, 638t

Neurologic deficits, head trauma with (Continued)
  seizures as, 639
  transient, 639
Neurologic signs
  with developmental disabilities, 28t
  of inborn errors of metabolism, 167, 167t
Neurology assessment, 612–616
  of child, 613
    cranial nerve evaluation in, 613–614
      of cranial nerve I, 614
      of cranial nerve II, 614
      of cranial nerve(s) III, IV, and VI, 614
      of cranial nerve V, 614
      of cranial nerve VII, 614
      of cranial nerve VIII, 614
      of cranial nerve(s) IX and X, 614
      of cranial nerve XI, 614
      of cranial nerve XII, 614
    mental status evaluation in, 612–613
    motor evaluation in, 614–615
      of bulk, 615
      of coordination, 615
      of gait, 613, 615
      of power, 614–615
      of reflexes, 615
      of tone, 615
    sensory evaluation in, 613, 615
    special diagnostic procedures in, 615–616
      CSF analysis as, 616t, 615
      electroencephalography, 616
      electromyography and nerve conduction
        studies as, 616
      neuroimaging as, 616
  for coma, 634–636
  history in, 612
  of neonate, 200–203, 612–613
    of movement and tone, 613
    of posture, 613
    reflexes in, 613, 613t
  physical examination in, 612
Neuromuscular criteria, for newborn maturity
    and gestational age, 197, 198f
Neuromuscular disease, 624–630
  of anterior horn cells, 624–625, 624t
  clinical manifestations of, 624t
  infant botulism as, 627
  laboratory and diagnostic studies for, 629
  malignant hyperthermia with, 629
  of muscle, 627–628
  myasthenia gravis as, 626–627
  peripheral neuropathy as, 625–626
  spinal muscular atrophy as, 624–625
  topography of, 624, 625t
Neuronal ceroid lipofuscinosis (NCL), 181t–182t,
    642t–643t, 644
Neuronal migration, disorders of, 648–649
Neuropathy, peripheral, 625–626
Neurosyphilis, 380
Neutropenia, 263
  clinical presentation of, 507t
  congenital, severe, 263
  drugs associated with, 265t
  due to cancer, 539t
  in immunocompromised person, 390–391,
    392f
  infections associated with, 265t
  isoimmune, maternal, 205t
  in Kostmann syndrome, 263
  mechanisms of, 265t
  in reticular dysgenesis, 263–264
  in Schwachman-Diamond syndrome, 263–264,
    264t
Neutrophil(s)
  normal values for, 508t
  production of, 509

Neutrophil chemotactic defects
  in leukocyte adhesion deficiency
    type I, 264, 264t
    type II, 264, 264t
Neutrophil disorder(s), 263–266, 264t
  etiology and clinical manifestations of,
    263–266
  of function, 264–266
  of migration, 264
    laboratory diagnosis of, 266
    in leukocyte adhesion deficiency
      type I, 264, 264t
      type II, 264, 264t
  of number (neutropenia), 263–264
  prognosis and prevention, 266
  treatment, 266
Neutrophil function
  disorders of, 264–266
    in Chediak-Higashi syndrome, 264t, 266
    in chronic granulomatous disease, 264–266,
      264t
  tests for, 258
Neutrophil migration, 264, 266f
  disorders of, 264
    laboratory diagnosis of, 266
    in leukocyte adhesion deficiency
      type I, 264, 264t
      type II, 264, 264t
Neutrophil number, disorders of, 263–264
  autoimmune neutropenia as, 264
  benign congenital neutropenia as, 263–264
  cyclic neutropenia as, 263
  drugs associated with, 265t
  infections associated with, 265t
  isoimmune neutropenia as, 264
  in Kostmann syndrome, 263
  mechanisms of, 265t
  in reticular dysgenesis, 263–264
  in Schwachman-Diamond syndrome,
    263–264, 264t
  severe congenital neutropenia as, 263
Nevus(i), 660
  acquired, 662
  anemicus, 659t
  depigmentosus, 659t
  epidermal, 659t
  flammeus, 662, 197
    differential diagnosis of, 659t
    in Klippel-Trénaunay-Weber syndrome,
      662
    in Sturge-Weber syndrome, 662, 646
  of Ito, 659t
  melanocytic, 659t
    acquired, 662
    congenital, 198, 660
      differential diagnosis of, 659t
      giant, 198, 660–661, 660f
      hairy, 660, 660f
  of Ota, 659t
  satellite, 660–661
  sebaceous, 659t
  simplex, 197
New Ballard Score (NBS), 198f
Newborn(s). see also Neonatal
  anemia in, 216–219. see also Anemia; in
    newborn
  bacterial colonization of, 191
  birth injury, 202–203
  blood volume of, 216
  coagulation disorders in, 222–223
    clinical manifestations and differential
      diagnoses of, 222–223
  congenital infection(s) in, 229–233, 230t
  cyanosis in, 201–202, 201t
  hemolytic disease of, 217

Newborn(s) (Continued)
  hemorrhagic disease of, 102–103
    due to vitamin K deficiency, 222
  hyperbilirubinemia in, 219–222
    direct conjugated, 220, 220t
    indirect unconjugated
      etiology of, 219–220, 220t
      therapy of, 221
      kernicterus (bilirubin encephalopathy) due
        to, 220–221
  hypocalcemia in, 204
  hypoxic-ischemic encephalopathy in,
    226–227
  intracranial hemorrhage in, 226
  life-threatening congenital malformations in,
    196, 196t
  maternal diseases affecting, 204–206, 205t
  maturity of, 197
    and abnormal fetal growth patterns, 197,
      199f
    cumulative score in, 197, 198f
    neurologic criteria in, 197, 198f
    physical criteria for, 197, 197f
  meningitis in, 227
  necrotizing enterocolitis in, 223–224
  neurologic examination of, 612–613
    movement and tone in, 613
    posture in, 613
    reflexes in, 613, 613t
  neutropenia in, 263
  persistent hyperinsulinemic hypoglycemia of,
    580–581
  persistent pulmonary hypertension of, 191,
    215
    with meconium aspiration, 215
  pneumonia in, 233
  polycythemia (hyperviscosity syndrome) in,
    221–222
  respiratory distress in, 209–216
    differential diagnosis of, 209, 210t
    due to apnea of prematurity, 215–216
    due to congenital diaphragmatic hernia, 215
    due to hydrops fetalis, 209
    due to infection, 209
    due to meconium aspiration syndrome, 209,
      214–215
    due to primary pulmonary hypertension,
      215
    due to pulmonary hypoplasia, 209, 215
    due to respiratory distress syndrome,
      210–212
      bronchopulmonary dysplasia due to,
        213–214
      clinical manifestations of, 211, 212f
      complications of, 212–214
      lung development and, 210–211, 211f
      patent ductus arteriosus due to, 212–213
      potential causes of, 212t
      prevention and treatment of, 211–212
      pulmonary air leaks due to, 213
      and retinopathy of prematurity, 214
      risk factors for, 211
    due to transient tachypnea, 214
    etiology of, 210t
    initial laboratory evaluation of, 210t
    treatment of
      for hypoxemia, 209–210
      for metabolic acidosis, 210
      for respiratory acidosis, 210
      supportive care for, 209
  resuscitation of, 194
  routine delivery room care for, 191–196
    silver nitrate instillation in, 191
    skin and umbilical cord care in, 191
    vitamin K prophylaxis in, 191

Newborn(s) (Continued)
  seizures in, 224–226
    benign familial, 225
    clinical characteristics of, 225, 225t
    diagnostic evaluation of, 225–226
    differential diagnosis of, 225, 225t
    focal clonic, 225t
    focal tonic, 225t
    generalized tonic, 225t
    myoclonic, 225t
    treatment of, 226
  sepsis in, 227
    acquired in utero, 227
    bacterial, 228
    early-onset
      clinical manifestations of, 228
      treatment for, 228
    incidence of, 227
    late-onset
      clinical manifestations of, 228
      evaluation of, 231
      treatment of, 231
    preterm, 227
    viral, 227–228
  shock in, 202
  temperature elevation in, 203
  temperature regulation in, 203
  transient myeloproliferative disorder of, 543
  transient tachypnea of, 191, 214
Newborn assessment, 189–200
  Apgar examination in, 194, 194t
  genetic, 155
  of gestational age, 197
    and abnormal fetal growth patterns, 197,
      199f
    cumulative score in, 197, 198f
    neurologic criteria in, 197, 198f
    physical criteria for, 197, 197f
  neurologic, 200–203
  perinatal history in, 189, 190t
  physical examination in, 196–200
    of abdomen, 200
    of appearance, 196
    of extremities, 200
    of face, eyes, and mouth, 199
    of genitalia, 197f, 200
    of heart, 200
    of hips, 200
    of lungs, 199–200
    of neck and chest, 199
    of skin, 197–198, 197f
    of skull, 198–199
    of spine, 200
    of vital signs in, 196
Newborn period, physical development in, 13
Newborn screening, 21
  abnormal results in, 191, 193t
  disorders included in or considered for, 191,
    192t
  for hearing, 21
  hemoglobin electrophoresis in, 21
  metabolic, 21
Nezelof syndrome, 260
NF. see Neurofibromatosis (NF)
NF-κB (nuclear factor κB) essential modulator
  (NEMO), in hyper-IgM syndrome, 258
NF1 gene, 148, 645
NF2 gene, 646
Niacin deficiency, 97, 98t–100t
Nickel dermatitis, 654, 656
Nicotinamide, 97
Nicotine, acute effects of, 250t–251t
Niemann-Pick disease, 181t–182t, 642t–643t, 643
Night blindness, 101
Nighttime fears, 49t

Nikolsky sign, 663t
Nipples, supernumerary, 199
Nissen fundoplication procedure, for
  gastroesophageal reflux, 432t
Nit(s), 665
  of pubic lice, 384
Nitrate test, in urinalysis, 555–556
Nitric oxide analysis, exhaled, for asthma, 274
Nitroblue tetrazolium test, for chronic
  granulomatous disease, 266
Nitrofurantoin, maternal use of, 207t
Nitroprusside, for heart failure, 501t
Nitrosourea (bis-chloronitrosourea), for cancer,
  540t–541t
N,N-Diethyl-m-toluamide (DEET), for
  prevention of zoonoses, 396
NNRTIs (non-nucleoside reverse transcriptase
  inhibitors), for HIV, 413–415
Nocturnal enuresis, 567
Nodular lymphoid hyperplasia, GI bleeding due
  to, 427t
Nodules, 650t, 651f
  subependymal, 646
Non-Hodgkin lymphoma (NHL)
  epidemiology of, 545
  etiology of, 544, 545t
  laboratory/imaging studies for, 545, 547f
  prognosis for, 544
  risk factors for, 536t
  treatment of, 544
Non-nucleoside reverse transcriptase inhibitors
  (NNRTIs), for HIV, 413–415
Non-rapid eye movement (NREM) sleep, 47
Nonadherence, in tuberculosis, 411
Nonalcoholic fatty liver disease, 450
Nonallergic, noninfectious rhinitis, 283–284,
  283t
Nonallergic rhinitis with eosinophilia syndrome,
  283–284, 283t
Noncompliance, in tuberculosis, 411
Nonepileptiform disorders, 620–621
Nongonococcal urethritis and cervicitis, 379
Nonheme iron, 104
Noninvasive ventilation, 131, 461
Nonmaleficence, 5
  in end-of-life decision making, 9
Nonossifying fibroma, 693t–694t
Nonsense mutation, 146
Nonsteroidal anti-inflammatory drugs (NSAIDs)
  GI bleeding due to, 427t
  for juvenile idiopathic arthritis, 308
Nonstress test, of fetal well-being, 189
Nonsyndromic craniosynostosis, genetic basis
  for, 147t
Nontreponemal antibody tests, 380
Nontuberculous mycobacteria, lymphadenitis
  due to, 339–340
Norepinephrine, for shock, 132t
Norepinephrine-reuptake inhibitor, for ADHD,
  42t
Normal saline, for functional constipation, 46t
North American liver fluke, 406t
Nose
  anatomy of, 455
  as filter, 456
  foreign bodies in, 284
  skier's, 283–284
Nosocomial infections, 394
NREM (non-rapid eye movement) sleep, 47
NS. see Nephrotic syndrome (NS)
NSAIDs. see Nonsteroidal anti-inflammatory
  drugs (NSAIDs)
NTDs. see Neural tube defects
Nuclear cystogram (NCG), for vesicoureteral
  reflux, 565

Nuclear factor κB (NF-κB) essential modulator (NEMO), in hyper-IgM syndrome, 258
Nuclear renal scanning, for vesicoureteral reflux, 565
Nucleotides, 146
Nursemaid's elbow, 692, 692f
Nutrition
    of adolescents, 89–90
    and growth, 584–585
    of infant, 86–89
        breastfeeding in, 86–88
        complementary foods and weaning in, 89
        formula feeding, 88–89
        parenteral, 113–114. *see also* Parenteral nutrition
    of toddlers and older children, 89, 90t
    for type 1 diabetes mellitus, 577
Nutritional assessment, 23
Nutritional counseling, 24t–25t
Nutritional deficiency disorder(s), 93–96
    classification of, 94t
    complications of, 96
    in failure to thrive, 94
    kwashiorkor as, 94–95
    marasmus as, 94
    physical signs of, 95t
    primary, 93–94
    secondary, 93–94, 94f
    treatment of, 95–96
Nutritional evaluation, for chronic liver disease, 449t
Nutritional management, for failure to thrive, 69, 69t
Nutritional rehabilitation, 96
Nutritional support, for burns, 138
NuvaRing (contraceptive vaginal ring), 246
Nystagmus, 614

O

O₂. *see* Oxygen
OAE (otoacoustic emissions), 34
Obesity, 2, 90–93
    assessment of, 91–92, 91t–92t
    clinical manifestations of, 91
    complications of, 91, 91t
    defined, 90–91
    diagnosis of, 91
    diseases associated with, 91t
    epidemiology of, 90–91
    prevention of, 92, 93t
    treatment of, 92–93
Obsessions, 62, 62t
Obsessive-compulsive disorder (OCD), 53, 62–63
    diagnosis of, 62t
    diagnostic criteria for, 62t
    differential diagnosis of, 64
    treatment of, 62–63
Obsessive-compulsive personality disorder, 63
Obstructive airway disease, 459
Obstructive sleep apnea (OSA), 49, 49t, 463, 463t
Obstructive stenotic lesions, congenital heart disease due to, 491
Obtunded patients, 634
Occult blood, in stool, with anemia, 511
OCD (osteochondritis dissecans), 680
Ocular examination, in neurology assessment, 612
Ocular hypertelorism, 161t, 162
Ocular infections, 386–389
    clinical manifestations of, 387
    complications and prognosis for, 389
    differential diagnosis of, 387–389, 388t–389t
    epidemiology of, 387

Ocular infections *(Continued)*
    etiology of, 386–387
    laboratory and imaging studies of, 387
    prevention of, 389
    treatment of, 389
Ocular larva migrans, 405, 405t
Oculocephalic response, 635–636
Oculocephalic vestibular reflexes, 614
Oculomotor nerve, assessment of, 614
Oculovestibular response, 635–636
OGTT (oral glucose tolerance test), 572
25-[OH]-D (25-hydroxyvitamin D), 102, 602–603
    for rickets, 603
1,25-[OH]₂-D (1,25-dihydroxyvitamin D), 102, 602–603
OI (oxygenation index), for primary pulmonary hypertension of the newborn, 215
Oligodactyly, 162–163
Oligohydramnios, 186–187
Oligosaccharide chromatography, urine, 171t
Oliguria
    due to renal disease, 554t
    fluid therapy for, 108, 108t
Omalizumab (Xolair), for asthma, 276
Omenn syndrome, 259t, 260
Omphalitis, 200
Omphalocele, 196t, 200, 439
Oncologic disorders, *vs.* juvenile idiopathic arthritis, 308t
Oncology assessment, 534–536, 535f
    common manifestations in, 534, 537t
    differential diagnosis in, 535
    history in, 534, 536t
    initial diagnostic evaluation in, 535–536
        diagnostic imaging in, 536, 542t
        minimum work up in, 542t
        screening tests in, 535–536
    physical examination in, 534
Oncospheres, in echinococcosis, 407
Oncovin (vincristine), for cancer, 540t–541t
Onychomycosis, 336
Ophthalmia neonatorum, 386–387
    chlamydial, 232, 387
    clinical manifestations of, 387
    epidemiology of, 387
    etiology of, 386–387
    gonococcal, 387
Ophthalmoplegia
    and limb weakness, 625t
    progressive external, 184
Opiate(s)
    acute effects of, 250t–251t
    neonatal addiction to and withdrawal from, 204
Opiate use, during pregnancy, 79
Opioids, for analgesia, 145t
Opisthorchiasis, 406t
Opisthorchis viverrini, 406t
Opsoclonus, in paraneoplastic opsoclonus-myoclonus syndrome, 633
Opsomyoclonus, with neuroblastoma, 548
Optic glioma, precocious puberty due to, 593
Optic nerve, assessment of, 614
Optic nerve glioma, prognosis for, 549t
Oral absorption, of antimicrobial drugs, 324
Oral allergy syndrome, 295t
Oral cavity, 429–430
    cleft lip and palate of, 431–433
    deciduous and primary teeth in, 429, 429t
    dental caries in, 429–430
    effects of systemic disease on, 429
    thrush of, 433–434
Oral glucose tolerance test (OGTT), 572

Oral/nasogastric tube: polyethylene glycol electrolyte solution, for functional constipation, 46t
Oral rehydration solution (ORS), 110–111
    for traveler's diarrhea, 407
Oral tolerance, 294
Orbital cellulitis, 350, 388t–389t
Orbivirus, 398t–400t
Orchidopexy, 569
Ordinal Scales of Infant Psychological Development, 29t
Organic acid disorder(s), 177–179
    biotinidase deficiency as, 178–179
    confirmatory testing for, 177
    glutaric acidemia I as, 179f, 178
    holocarboxylase deficiency as, 178–179
    isovaleric acidemia as, 178, 178f
    methylmalonic acidemia as, 177–178, 178f
    neonatal screening for, 170, 170t
    outcome of, 177
    propionic acidemia as, 177–178, 178f
    treatment of, 177
Organic acid profile, urine, 171t
Orientia tsutsugamushi, 398t–400t
Ornithine transcarbamylase (OTC) deficiency, 177
Oropharyngeal *Candida albicans* infection, 431
ORS (oral rehydration solution), 110–111
    for traveler's diarrhea, 369
Orthopedic disorders, 308t
    mechanisms of, 667t
Orthopedics, common terminology in, 667t
Orthopedics assessment, 667–668
    developmental milestones in, 668
        for infants, 668, 669f
    of gait, 668
    growth and development in, 667, 668f
    of limping child, 668, 669t
    of toe walking, 668
Orthoradiograph, of leg-length discrepancy, 678–679
Ortolani test, 200, 673, 673f
OSA. *see* Obstructive sleep apnea (OSA)
Osgood-Schlatter disease, 680
Osmotic fragility test, for hereditary spherocytosis, 521
Osmotic gap, in diarrhea, 425
Osmotics, for functional constipation, 47t
Ossification center, secondary, 668f
Osteoblastoma, 693t–694t
Osteocartilaginous exostosis, 693t–694t
Osteochondritis dissecans (OCD), 680
Osteochondroma, 693t–694t
Osteodystrophy, Albright hereditary, 602
Osteoid osteoma, giant, 693t–694t
Osteoid substance, 551
Osteomalacia, 603
    due to vitamin D deficiency, 102
Osteomyelitis, 381–384
    chronic, 381
    clinical manifestations of, 382
    complications and prognosis for, 386
    differential diagnosis of, 383
    epidemiology of, 382
    etiology of, 381–382, 382f
    vs. Ewing sarcoma, 552
    fever due to, 325
    hematogenous, 381
        complications of, 386
        epidemiology of, 382
        prevention of, 384
        treatment of, 383, 383t
    laboratory and imaging studies of, 382–383, 383f

Osteomyelitis (Continued)
  multifocal
    acute, 383f
    recurrent, 382
  prevention of, 384
  subacute, 381
    focal, 382
  treatment of, 383, 383t
  vertebral, 382
Osteopenia, 90
Osteoporosis, 90
  calcium and, 103
Osteosarcoma, 551
  risk factors for, 536t
Osteotomy, 667t
Ostiomeatal complex, in sinusitis, 350
Otalgia, due to acute otitis media, 351
Otitis externa, 353–354
  clinical manifestations of, 353
  complications of, 353–354
  defined, 353
  differential diagnosis of, 353
  epidemiology of, 353
  etiology of, 353
  laboratory and imaging studies of, 353
  malignant, 353
  prevention of, 354
  treatment of, 353
Otitis media (OM), 351–353
  acute, 351, 352t
  chronic, 352
  clinical manifestations of, 351
  complications and prognosis for, 352
  defined, 351
  differential diagnosis of, 352
  due to common cold, 348
  with effusion, 352
  epidemiology of, 351
  etiology of, 351
  laboratory and imaging studies for, 351–352
  prevention of, 352–353
  recurrent, 351
  treatment of, 352
  with tympanic perforation, 353
  vomiting due to, 423t
Otoacoustic emissions (OAE), 34
Otorrhea
  cerebrospinal fluid, 638
  due to otitis media, 351
  tympanostomy tube, 353
Out-toeing, 677
  common causes of, 676t
  due to external tibial torsion, 677
Ovarian cysts, precocious puberty due to, 593t, 595, 595t
Overgrowth syndrome, 162
Overuse injuries, of shoulder, 691
Overweight children, 2
OxyContin, acute effects of, 250t–251t
Oxygen (O_2)
  administration, 460
  delivery, 124
  for heart failure, 501t
  in pulmonary physiology, 455
  saturation, 459
  supplemental, 460
  supplementation, in resuscitation, 125–126
Oxygen partial pressure (Po_2), 456t
Oxygenation, measurements of, 459
Oxygenation index (OI), for primary pulmonary hypertension of the newborn, 215
Oxytocin, maternal use of, 207t
Oxytocin challenge test, 189

P
P wave, 484
Pachygyria, 648–649
Packed red blood cells, transfusion of, 532
$Paco_2$ (arterial partial pressure of carbon dioxide), in newborns, 209–210
PAH. see Pulmonary arterial hypertension (PAH)
PAH (phenylalanine hydroxylase) deficiency, 150t
Pain
  analgesia for, 145
  back, 689
    clinical manifestations and management of, 689
    differential diagnosis of, 689, 689t
    etiology and epidemiology of, 689
    red flags in, 689
  chest, 487–488
    clinical manifestations of, 489
    diagnostic studies of, 489
    differential diagnosis of, 489t
    etiology of, 487, 489t
Pain crisis, in sickle cell anemia, 519
Pain disorder, 53
  diagnostic criteria for, 53t
Painful crisis, in sickle cell anemia, 520t
Palivizumab, for bronchiolitis, 359
Palliative care, 7–9
  access to comprehensive and compassionate, 7
  bereavement in, 8
  commitment to quality improvement of, 8
  conditions appropriate for, 7
  cultural, religious, and spiritual concerns about, 9
  goals of, 7
  interdisciplinary resources in, 8
  model of integrated, 7–8
  principles of, 7–8
  support for caregivers in, 8
Pallor
  due to anemia, 511
  in hematologic disorders, 506
Palpation, in cardiovascular system assessment, 481
Palpebral fissure, 161t
2-PAM, for organophosphate poisoning, 143t–144t
Pancreatic disease, 450–453
  pancreatic insufficiency as, 450–451
  pancreatitis as
    acute, 451–452
    chronic, 452–453
Pancreatic enzymes, 451
  for pancreatic insufficiency, 451
Pancreatic injury, 135
Pancreatic insufficiency, 450–451
  clinical manifestations of, 451
  etiology and epidemiology of, 450–451
  exocrine, in cystic fibrosis, 476
  laboratory and imaging studies for, 451
  treatment of, 451
Pancreatic pseudocyst, 451–452
Pancreatitis
  abdominal pain due to, 420t
  acute, 451–452
    clinical manifestations of, 451
    etiology and epidemiology of, 451, 452t
    laboratory and imaging studies for, 451–452
    treatment of, 452
  chronic, 452–453
    clinical manifestations of, 453
    etiology and epidemiology of, 452–453
    laboratory and imaging studies for, 453
    treatment of, 453
Pancytopenia
  in aplastic anemia, 517–518
  defined, 517
  differential diagnosis of, 517

Pancytopenia (Continued)
  due to bone marrow failure, 527
  etiology of, 517
PANDAS (pediatric autoimmune neuropsychiatric disorder associated with streptococcal infection), 62
Panencephalitis, subacute sclerosing, due to measles, 331
Panic attacks, 55, 56t
Panic disorder
  diagnostic criteria for, 56t
  panic attacks in, 55
Panner disease, 692
Pansinusitis, in Kartagener syndrome, 472
Pansystolic murmurs, due to ventricular septal defect, 491, 491f
Pantothenic acid deficiency, 98t
Pao_2 (arterial partial pressure of oxygen), in newborns, 209–210
Papilledema, 617, 617f
Papilloma, of CNS, prognosis for, 549t
Papillomatosis, juvenile laryngeal, upper airway obstruction due to, 465t–466t
Papules, 650t, 651f
  in acne, 652
Papulosquamous dermatitis, 658–659
Paracentesis, for peritonitis, 453
Parachute reflex, 613t
Paracrine action, of hormones, 570, 570f
ParaGard (copper intrauterine device), 246
Paragonimiasis, 406t
Paragonimus spp., 406t
Parainfluenza virus, croup due to, 354
Paralysis
  due to hypokalemia, 116
  flaccid, areflexic, 624
  periodic, 629
  tick, 626
Parameningeal infection, 343t
Paraneoplastic opsoclonus-myoclonus syndrome, 631
Paraneoplastic syndromes, with neuroblastoma, 548
Paraphimosis, 568
Parapneumonic effusion, 363, 479
Parasitic disease(s), 402–407
  helminthiasis(es) as, 404–407
    ascariasis as, 405
    due to cestodes (tapeworms), 407t, 404
    due to nematodes (roundworms), 405t
    due to trematodes (flukes), 404, 406t
    echinococcosis as, 407
    enterobiasis (pinworm) as, 406
    hookworm infections as, 404–405
    neurocysticercosis due to, 407
    schistosomiasis (bilharziasis) as, 406–407
    visceral larva migrans as, 405–406
  protozoal, 402–404
    malaria as, 402–404
    toxoplasmosis as, 404
Parasomnias, 48–49, 49t
Parathyroid disorders, 602–603
  hypocalcemia, 602–603
  rickets as, 603
Parathyroid hormone (PTH), and vitamin D, 602
Parenteral nutrition (PN), 111–112
  access for, 113–114
  for burns, 138
  complications of, 114
  indications for, 112t, 111–112
Parinaud syndrome, 340
Paronychia, viral, 337–338
Paroxysmal disorders, 618–623, 618t. see also Seizure(s)
Paroxysmal nocturnal hemoglobinuria, 516t

Paroxysmal stage, of pertussis, 356
Partial FAS, 79
Partial pressure of CO_2 (Pco_2), 119
Partial thromboplastin time (PTT)
    activated, 524–526, 525f, 526t
        in hemophilia, 529
    in newborn, 222–223
Parvovirus
    anemia due to, 516t
    congenital infection with, 230t
Past medical history, in genetic assessment, 156
Pasteurella multocida, 398t–400t
    osteomyelitis due to, 381–382
Patch, 650t, 651f
Patella, 679f
Patellar dislocation, recurrent, 680
Patellar subluxation, recurrent, 680
Patellofemoral disorders, 680
Patellofemoral joint, 680
Patellofemoral pain syndrome (PFPS), 680
Patent ductus arteriosus (PDA), 492–493, 492f
    clinical manifestations of, 213, 492–493
    and coarctation of the aorta, 494
    etiology and epidemiology of, 492
    imaging studies of, 493
    respiratory distress syndrome and, 212–213
    treatment of, 213, 493
Paternalism, 5
Pathogen-associated molecular patterns, 252
Patient-controlled analgesia, 145
Pavlik harness, for developmental dysplasia of
        the hip, 674
PCD. *see* Primary ciliary dyskinesia (PCD)
Pco_2 (carbon dioxide partial pressure), 456t
PCR (polymerase chain reaction), for infectious
        diseases, 317
PCV (pneumococcal conjugate vaccine), 319f–320f
    for otitis media, 353
PDA. *see* Patent ductus arteriosus (PDA)
Peak expiratory flow rate (PEFR), 459
    in asthma, 278
Peak flow monitoring, for asthma, 279–282
Pectoriloquy, 458t
Pectus carinatum, 478
Pectus excavatum, 478
Pediatric autoimmune neuropsychiatric disorder
        associated with streptococcal infection
        (PANDAS), 62
Pediatric health care, 1–4
    changing morbidity and, 3
    culture and, 3–4
    current challenges in, 1
    health disparities in, 3
    landscape of, 1–2
    other health issues affecting, 2–3
Pediatric undernutrition, 94
    classification of, 94t
    complications of, 96
    in failure to thrive, 94
    kwashiorkor as, 94–95
    malnutrition, 94t, 95–96
    marasmus as, 94
    physical signs of, 95t
    primary, 93–94
    secondary, 93–94, 94f
    treatment of, 95–96
Pediculoses, 665–666
    capitis, 665
    clinical manifestations of, 665
    complication of, 665
    corporis, 665
    differential diagnosis of, 665
    epidemiology of, 665
    etiology of, 665
    prognosis and prevention of, 665

Pediculoses *(Continued)*
    pubis, 665
    treatment of, 665
Pediculus humanus capitis, 665
Pediculus humanus corporis, 665
Pediculus humanus humanus, 665
Pedigree, 147, 147f–148f
    for dysmorphology, 161–162
    in genetic assessment, 155
    in hematology assessment, 506
PEFR (peak expiratory flow rate), 459
    in asthma, 278
Pellagra, 97, 98t
Pelvic inflammatory disease, 376t, 379
    dysmenorrhea due to, 244
PEM. *see* Protein-energy malnutrition (PEM)
Penetrance, 147, 148f
Penicillamine, as teratogen, 206t
Penicillin
    allergic reaction to, 296–297
        desensitization for, 297–298
        skin testing for, 297–298
    for rheumatic fever, 502
Penicillin G
    for Lyme disease, 397–400
    for syphilis, 380
        congenital, 232
Penicillin V, for streptococcal pharyngitis, 349t
Penicilloyl polylysine, in skin testing for
        penicillin allergy, 297
Penis, anomalies of, 568
Peptic ulcer disease, 436–437
    clinical manifestations of, 436, 436t
    etiology and epidemiology of, 436, 436t
    GI bleeding due to, 427t
    laboratory and imaging studies for, 436, 436t
    risk factors for, 436, 436t
    treatment of, 436–437
    vomiting due to, 423t
Peptide hormones, 570
Percussion, 458t
Perennial allergic rhinitis, 282
Perianal dermatitis, 336
Pericardiocentesis, for pericarditis, 505
Pericarditis, 504–505, 504t–505t
Perinatal care, 2
Perinatal history, 189, 190t
    for developmental disabilities, 27t
Perinatal mortality, 187, 188t
Periodic fever, aphthous stomatitis, pharyngitis,
        and cervical adenitis (PFAPA), 349
Periodic paralysis, 629
Periorbital cellulitis, 350
Periorbital hemangioma, 661–662
Periosteal destruction, in osteomyelitis, 382–383
Periosteal elevation, in osteomyelitis, 382–383
Periosteal fat line, loss of, in osteomyelitis, 382–383
Peripheral intravenous line, for parenteral
        nutrition, 113
Peripheral neuropathy, 625–626
    in chronic inflammatory demyelinating
            polyneuropathy, 626
    in Guillain-Barré syndrome, 625–626
    in hereditary motor sensory neuropathy
            (Charcot-Marie-Tooth Disease), 626
    in tick paralysis, 626
Peripheral receptors, in control of ventilation,
        461, 461f
Peripheral venous catheters, infections associated
        with, 394
Peripherally inserted central catheters
    infections associated with, 394
    for parenteral nutrition, 113
Peristaltic waves, in pyloric stenosis, 435
Peritoneal dialysis, for chronic kidney disease, 317

Peritoneal dialysis-associated infections, 397
Peritonitis, 453–454
    in nephrotic syndrome, 557–558
Peritonsillar abscess, upper airway obstruction
        due to, 465t–466t
Periventricular hemorrhage, in newborn, 226
Periventricular leukomalacia, in newborn, 226
Permethrin, for prevention of zoonoses, 396
Pernicious anemia, 101
Peroxisomal disorders, 180–183
Peroxisomes, 180–183
Persistent pulmonary hypertension of the
        newborn (PPHN), 191, 215
    with meconium aspiration, 215
Pertussis syndrome, 356–357
Pertussis vaccine, 317–318
Pervasive developmental disorders, 64t
Pes cavus, 667t
    in hereditary motor sensory neuropathy, 626
Pes planus, 667t
    hypermobile, 682
PET (positron emission tomography), for cancer,
        536
Petechiae, 650t
    with anemia, 511
    in hematologic disorders, 506
    in hemostatic disorders, 524
Petechial rash, infections with fever and, 329t–330t
PFA (platelet function analyzer), 524–526, 526t
PFAPA (periodic fever, aphthous stomatitis,
        pharyngitis, and cervical adenitis), 349
PFPS (patellofemoral pain syndrome), 680
pH, in newborns, 209–210
PHACE syndrome, 661–662
Phagocytic disorders, 264t
Phagocytosis, 255t
Pharmacokinetic properties, of antimicrobial
        drugs, 324
Pharmacotherapy, for enuresis, 44
Pharyngitis, 347–349
    bacterial, 348t
    clinical manifestations of, 347–348
    complications and prognosis for, 349
    differential diagnosis of, 348–349
    epidemiology of, 347
    etiology of, 347
    laboratory evaluation of, 348
    prevention of, 349
    treatment of, 349, 349t
    viral, 348t
Pharynx, anatomy of, 455
Phencyclidine (PCP), acute effects of, 250t–251t
Phenobarbital
    maternal use of, 207t
    for neonatal seizures, 226
    for status epilepticus, 621–622, 622t
Phenylalanine, metabolism of, 174f
Phenylalanine hydroxylase (PAH) deficiency, 150t
Phenylephrine, for allergic rhinitis, 284
Phenylketonuria (PKU), 174–175, 174f
    due to tetrahydrobiopterin deficiency, 174–175
    genetic basis for, 150t, 169t
    laboratory diagnosis of, 174
    maternal, 205t
    outcome of, 174–175
    screening for, 170t, 174
    sustained control of, 174–175
    as teratogens, 154
    treatment of, 174
Phenytoin, 226
    for status epilepticus, 621–622, 622t
    as teratogen, 206t
Philtrum, 161t
Phimosis, 568
Phlebitis, due to parenteral nutrition, 113

Phobia(s), 55–59
agora-, 55
school, 57
social, 57
specific, 57
defined, 57
diagnostic criteria for, 58t
treatment of, 58
Phosphoenolpyruvate carboxykinase deficiency, hypoglycemia due to, 582
Phosphorylase kinase deficiency, 172t
Photosensitivity, in systemic lupus erythematosus, 309
Phototherapy, for indirect hyperbilirubinemia, 221
PHOX2B gene, in congenital central alveolar hypoventilation, 463
Phrenic nerve palsy, 202–203
Phthirus pubis, vulvovaginitis due to, 375t
Phylloquinone, 102
Physical abuse
abdominal injury due to, 71–72
bruises due to, 70–71, 71f, 72t–73t
burns due to, 71, 71f, 72t–73t
diagnosis of, 70–73, 70t
differential diagnosis of, 72–73, 72t–73t
epidemiology of, 70
fractures due to, 71, 71f, 72t–73t
head trauma due to, 72, 72f, 72t–73t
reporting of, 70
risk factors for, 70
subdural hemorrhage due to, 226
Physical activity, 2
for obesity, 92, 92t
Physical criteria, for newborn maturity and gestational age, 197, 197f
Physical examination
for cancer, 534
in cardiovascular system assessment, 481–484
of colic, 38
for developmental disabilities, 26, 28t
in hematology assessment, 506, 507t
of hemostatic disorders, 524
in neurology assessment, 612
of newborn, 196–200
of skin disorders, 650
Physical growth and development. *see* Growth and development
Physical punishment, 23
Physician-patient relationship, with adolescents, 20
Physiologic nadir, in erythropoiesis, 509
Physis, 668f
Pica, due to lead poisoning, 514–515
Pierre Robin sequence, 160–161, 196t
Pigmented lesions, 659–661
acquired nevi as, 662
café au lait macules as, 659–660, 660f
congenital melanocytic nevi as, 660, 660f
giant, 660–661
hairy, 660, 660f
dermal melanosis as, 659, 659t, 660f
differential diagnosis of, 659, 659t
Pigmented nevi, giant, 660
Pill ulcers, 434–435
Pimecrolimus, for atopic dermatitis, 287
Pineal germinoma, prognosis for, 549t
Pinworms, vulvovaginitis due to, 375t
Pirbuterol, for asthma, 276
Pituitary adenoma, 570
Pituitary function, assessment of, 571, 577t
Pituitary gland, hormonal influences of, 570–571, 571f
Pituitary hormone(s), 570–571, 571f
Pituitary hormone deficiencies, idiopathic multiple, delayed puberty due to, 591t

Pituitary tumors, delayed puberty due to, 591t
Pityriasis rosea, 658
PKD (polycystic kidney disease), 566
autosomal dominant, 568
autosomal recessive, 566
PKU. *see* Phenylketonuria (PKU)
Placenta previa, 186
Placental abnormalities, intrauterine growth restriction and small for gestational age due to, 208t
Placental abruption, 186
Placing reflex, 613t
Plagiocephaly, 161t
and torticollis, 688
Plague, 398t–400t
Plain radiographs, for infectious diseases, 317
Plan B (levonorgestrel), for emergency postcoital contraception, 246
Plantar surface, of newborn, 197f
Plantar warts, 338
Plaque, 650t, 651f
Plasma, fresh frozen, 532t
Plasma creatinine, 555
Plasma osmolality, regulation of, 106
Plasma volume, and sodium excretion, 113
Plasma water, 106, 107f
Plasmin, in hemostasis, 524f
Plasminogen, in hemostasis, 524f
Plasmodium, 398t–400t, 402
Plasmodium falciparum, 403t
Plasmodium knowlesi, 403t
Plasmodium malariae, 403t
Plasmodium ovale, 403t
Plasmodium vivax, 403t
Platelet(s), activated, 523
Platelet concentrate, 532t
Platelet count, 524–526, 526t
Platelet function, disorders, 528
Platelet function analyzer (PFA), 524–526, 526t
Platelet number, disorders of, 526, 527f
idiopathic thrombocytopenic purpura (ITP) as, 527–528
sequestration thrombocytopenia due to decreased platelet production as, 526–527
thrombocytopenia due to peripheral destruction as, 527
thrombotic microangiopathy as, 528
Wiskott-Aldrich syndrome as, 528
Platelet plug, 523, 524f
Platelet production, sequestration thrombocytopenia due to decreased, 526–527
Platelet volume, mean, 526
Pleiotropy, 148
Pleural disorder(s), 478–480
pleural effusion as, 479–480
pneumomediastinum as, 479
pneumothorax as, 478–479
Pleural effusion, 458t, 479–480, 480t
Plexiform neurofibroma, 646, 659t
Pluripotential progenitor stem cells, in hematopoiesis, 506
Pneumatic otoscopy, for otitis media, 351
Pneumatic vests, 460
Pneumatocele, 363
Pneumatosis intestinalis, due to necrotizing enterocolitis, 225
Pneumococcal conjugate vaccine (PCV), 319f–322f
for otitis media, 353
Pneumococcal polysaccharide vaccine (PPSV), 319f–322f
Pneumocystis jirovecii, 412–413
in immunocompromised person, 390
Pneumomediastinum, 479

Pneumonia, 104–105, 358–364, 472
afebrile, 359, 360t
atypical
clinical manifestations of, 359
defined, 358–359
etiology of, 358–359
imaging of, 361–362, 362f
bacterial
clinical manifestations of, 359
imaging of, 361–362, 361f
laboratory studies of, 361–362
broncho-, 358–359, 361f
clinical manifestations of, 359
complications and prognosis for, 363
defined, 358–359
differential diagnosis of, 362, 362t
epidemiology of, 359
etiology of, 358–359, 360t
fever due to, 325
giant cell (Hecht), due to measles, 331
in immunocompromised persons, 362
laboratory and imaging studies of, 361–362, 361f–362f
lobar, 358–359, 361f
meconium aspiration, 214–215
in neonates, 228, 233, 359, 360t
prevention of, 363–364
recurrent, differential diagnosis of, 362t
treatment of, 362, 363t
ventilator-associated, 395
viral
clinical manifestations of, 359
imaging of, 361–362, 361f
laboratory studies of, 361–362
vomiting due to, 423t
Pneumonitis, 358–359
Pneumothorax, 458t, 478–479
clinical manifestations of, 478–479
defined, 478
diagnostic studies for, 479
due to assisted ventilation in newborn, 213, 213f
etiology of, 478
in newborn, 196
secondary, 478
spontaneous primary, 478
tension, 478–479
treatment of, 479
Po$_2$ (oxygen partial pressure), 456t
Point mutation, 146
Poisoning, 139–143
clinical manifestations of, 139, 140t–141t
complications of, 139–141
coma as, 139
direct toxicity as, 139
dysrhythmias as, 141
gastrointestinal symptoms as, 141
metabolic acidosis as, 139–141, 141t
seizures as, 141, 142t
systemic and pulmonary toxicity as, 139
epidemiology of, 139
etiology of, 139
laboratory and imaging studies of, 141–142, 143t
therapeutic monitoring for, 143t
treatment of, 142–143
gastrointestinal decontamination of, 142–143
specific antidotes of, 143, 143t–144t
supportive care of, 142
Poliovirus vaccine, 317–318
Pollen-food allergy syndrome, 295t
Polyarthritis, due to rheumatic fever, 503t
Polycystic kidney disease (PKD), 566
autosomal dominant, 568
autosomal recessive, 566

Polycystic ovary syndrome, amenorrhea due to, 242
Polycythemia
    clinical presentation of, 507t
    cyanotic congenital heart disease with, 527
    in newborn, 221–222
Polydactyly, 161t, 162–163
    of fingers, 693
    of toes, 683, 689t
Polydipsia, in insulin-dependent diabetes
        mellitus, 573
Polyethylene glycol (GoLYTELY), for poisoning,
        143
Polyethylene glycol powder (MiraLAX), for
        functional constipation, 47t
Polygenic inheritance, 151–152
    hypertrophic pyloric stenosis due to, 152
    neural tube defects due to, 152
Polyhydramnios, 187
Polymerase chain reaction (PCR)
    for HIV, 413
    for infectious diseases, 317
Polymicrogyria, 648–649
Polymorphonuclear cells, as lung defense
        mechanism, 456
Polyp, juvenile, GI bleeding due to, 427t
Polysomnogram, 48, 463
Polyuria, 108
    due to renal disease, 554t
    fluid therapy for, 108t
Pompe disease, 172t, 629
Popliteal angle, in newborn, 198f
Popliteal cyst, 679–680
Pork tapeworm, 407
Port-a-Cath (implanted venous access system),
        infections associated with, 394
Portal hypertension, 448
Portion sizes, for prevention of obesity, 92
Portosystemic shunt, 449
Port-wine stain, 662f, 662, 197
    clinical manifestations of, 662f, 662
    differential diagnosis of, 659t
    in Klippel-Trénaunay-Weber syndrome, 662
    in Sturge-Weber syndrome, 662, 646
Positive-pressure ventilation, 461
Positive reinforcement, 15
Positron emission tomography (PET), for cancer,
        536
Postcoital urethritis, 372
Postconcussive syndrome, 632t
Posterior fossa syndrome, 547
Posterior fossa tumors, ataxia due to, 633
Posterior urethral valves, 566
Posterior uveitis, 388t–389t
Postexposure prophylaxis, for measles, 331
Postherpetic neuralgia, 334
Postinfectious acute cerebellar ataxia, 632–633
Postmitotic maturing cells, in hematopoiesis, 506
Postnatal genetic assessment, 155
Postpericardiotomy syndrome, 504
Poststreptococcal arthritis (PsA), 307t
Poststreptococcal glomerulonephritis (PSGN)
    clinical manifestations of, 558–559
    etiology of, 558
    prognosis for, 560
    treatment of, 559
Posttraumatic stress disorder (PTSD)
    defined, 56
    diagnostic criteria for, 57t
    due to domestic violence, 80
    treatment of, 58
Postural roundback, 688
Posture
    assessment of, 614
    with depressed consciousness, 636
    of newborn, 198f, 613

Posturing vs. foot deformity, 681
Potassium, 116–119
    for diabetic ketoacidosis, 575
    transcellular shifts
        hyperkalemia due to, 118t
        hypokalemia due to, 116
Potassium balance, 116
Potassium chloride (KCl)
    in gastrointestinal losses, 108t
    in maintenance fluids, 107
Potassium disorders, 116–119
    hyperkalemia as, 117–119
    hypokalemia as, 116–117
Potter syndrome, 186–187, 196t
    renal agenesis in, 565–566
Pott disease, 409
Pott puffy tumor, 350
Poverty, and health disparities, 3
Power, in motor examination, 614–615
PPD-S (purified protein derivative standard), in
        Mantoux test, 409
PPHN (persistent pulmonary hypertension of the
        newborn), 191, 215
    with meconium aspiration, 215
PPSV (pneumococcal polysaccharide vaccine),
        319f–320f
PR interval, 484
Prader-Willi syndrome (PWS)
    genetic basis for, 153, 160
    hypotonia in, 629
    obesity in, 91t
    short stature in, 586
Pralidoxime (2-PAM, Protopam), for
        organophosphate poisoning, 143t–144t
Preadoption visit, 78
Precocious puberty, 592–596
    central (constitutional, familial), 592–593, 595t
    classification of, 592–593, 593t
    contrasexual, 593t
    defined, 592
    differential diagnosis of, 594t
    evaluation of, 595
    incomplete (GnRH-independent), 593t, 595t
    peripheral, 592–593
    premature adrenarche (pubarche) as, 596, 593t
    premature thelarche as, 596, 593t
    treatment of, 595–596, 595t
    true or complete, 593t, 595t
Preconception genetic assessment, 154–155
    adolescent and adult, 155
    familial factors in, 154
    maternal factors in, 155
    postnatal, 155
    screening in, 154–155
Precordium, hyperdynamic, with patent ductus
        arteriosus, 492–493
Prednisolone, for croup, 354–355
Prednisone, 475
    for asthma, 276
    for cancer, 540t–541t
    for Henoch-Schönlein purpura, 302
    for nephrotic syndrome, 557
    for serum sickness, 294
Preeclampsia, 187
Pregnancy
    adolescent, 244–245
        continuation of, 245
        diagnosis of, 244
        termination of, 245
    assessment during, 186–204
        genetic, 154–155
            familial factors in, 154
            maternal factors in, 155
            postnatal, 155
            screening in, 154–155

Pregnancy (Continued)
    complication(s) of, 186
        hydrops fetalis as, 187
        maternal medical, 186
        with multiple gestations, 187
        obstetric, 186
        oligohydramnios as, 186–187
        placenta previa as, 186
        placental abruption as, 186
        polyhydramnios as, 187
        preeclampsia/eclampsia as, 187
        premature rupture of membranes as, 187
        prolonged rupture of membranes as, 187
        vaginal bleeding as, 186
    high-risk, 186
    maternal diseases during, 204, 205t
        antiphospholipid syndrome as, 205
        diabetes mellitus as, 205t–206t, 206
        hyperthyroidism as, 205t, 206
        idiopathic thrombocytopenia as, 205, 205t
        other, 206
        systemic lupus erythematosus as, 205, 205t
    substance abuse during, 79, 205t
    toxemia of, 187
    vomiting due to, 423t
Pregnancy history
    for dysmorphology, 161
    in genetic assessment, 155–156
    present, 190t
    prior, 190t
Preicteric phase, of viral hepatitis, 370
Preload, in heart failure, 500, 500t
Premature atrial contractions, 489
Premature formula, 88–89
Premature rupture of the membranes, 187
Premature ventricular contractions (PVCs), 489,
        490t
Prematurity
    apnea of, 215–216, 463, 463t
    retinopathy of, 214
Premutation carriers, in fragile X syndrome, 153
Prenatal care, 2
Prenatal genetic assessment, 154–155
    adolescent and adult, 155
    familial factors in, 154
    maternal factors in, 155
    postnatal, 155
    screening in, 154–155
Prenatal history
    in cardiovascular system assessment, 481
    for developmental disabilities, 27t
Prerenal azotemia, due to shock, 132
Preschool children
    reaction to divorce by, 82–83
    tests of cognition in, 29t
Preschool readiness, 14
Preseptal cellulitis, 350
Preslip condition, 675
Presumptive anti-infective therapy, 323
Preterm births, 187
    demographics of, 2
Preterm infants, sepsis in, 227
Preventive measures, schedule for, 17f, 15–16
Priapism, in sickle cell anemia, 519–520, 520t
Primaquine, maternal use of, 207t
Primary care counseling, on developmental
        problems, 29–30, 30t
Primary ciliary dyskinesia (PCD), 472
    clinical manifestations of, 472
    diagnostic studies for, 472
    etiology of, 472
    treatment of, 472
Primary pulmonary hypertension, 473
Primary pulmonary tuberculosis, 408
Primary survey, of trauma patient, 133

Primitive neuroectodermal tumors, treatment of, 547
Probiotic, for prevention of diarrhea, 369
Proctocolitis, allergic, 295t
Professionalism, 4–5
Progestational agent, for delayed puberty, 592
Progesterone withdrawal test, for amenorrhea, 242
Progressive symptoms, of neurologic disorder, 612
Prolonged rupture of the membranes, 187
Promoter sequence, 146
Pronator drift, 615
Properdin, 267–268
    deficiency, 268
Prophase analysis, in genetic assessment, 158–159
Prophylaxis, 318–323
    immunization and, 317–323
    meningococcus, 318–323
    postexposure, for measles, 331
    primary, 318
    rabies, 323
    secondary, 318
    tetanus, 323, 323
Propionate pathway, 177–178, 178f
Propionibacterium acnes, 652
Propionic acidemia, 178
    clinical manifestations of, 178
    neonatal screening for, 170t
    treatment of, 178
Propofol, for sedation, 145t
Propranolol, maternal use of, 207t
Propylthiouracil
    for hyperthyroidism, 600–601
    maternal use of, 207t
Prostaglandin E$_1$
    for coarctation of the aorta, 494
    for hypoplastic left heart syndrome, 499
    for transposition of the aorta, 497
Protectaid (vaginal sponge), 247
Protein C, in hemostasis, 523
Protein C deficiency, thrombosis due to, 531
Protein S, in hemostasis, 523
Protein S deficiency, thrombosis due to, 531
Protein-energy malnutrition (PEM), 93–94
    classification of, 94t
    complications of, 96
    in failure to thrive, 94
    kwashiorkor as, 94–95
    marasmus as, 94
    mild, 94t
    moderate, 94t
    physical signs of, 95t
    primary, 93–94
    secondary, 93–94, 94f
    severe, 94t
    treatment of, 95–96
Proteinuria, 556
    asymptomatic, 556
    clinical manifestations of, 557
    complications of, 557–558
    diagnostic studies of, 557
    differential diagnosis of, 557
    etiology and epidemiology of, 556–557
    fixed, 556
    glomerular, 556–557
    nephrotic, 556
    persistent, 556
    postural (orthostatic), 557
    prognosis for, 558
    symptomatic, 556
    transient, 556–557
    treatment of, 557
    tubular, 556–557

Prothrombin time (PT), 524–526, 525f, 526t
    in newborn, 222–223
Proton-pump inhibitor, for gastroesophageal reflux, 432t
Protozoal disease(s), 402–404
    malaria as, 402–404
    toxoplasmosis as, 404
    zoonotic, 398t–400t
Proximal humeral epiphysiolysis, 691–692
Proximal tubule, 553, 555f
Pruritus ani, 406
PsA (poststreptococcal arthritis), 307t
Pseudocyst, pancreatic, 451–452
Pseudoephedrine, for allergic rhinitis, 284
Pseudo-Hurler polydystrophy, 181t–182t
Pseudohypertrophic progressive muscular dystrophy, genetic basis for, 151t
Pseudohypertrophy, 615
Pseudohypoaldosteronism type 1, hyperkalemia in, 118, 118t
Pseudohypoaldosteronism type 2, hyperkalemia in, 118, 118t
Pseudohyponatremia, 113, 113f
Pseudohypoparathyroidism, 602, 603t
    obesity in, 91t
    short stature due to, 586
Pseudomembranous colitis, GI bleeding due to, 427t
Pseudomonas aeruginosa
    conjunctivitis due to, 386, 388t
    in cystic fibrosis, 477–478
    folliculitis due to, 336
    osteomyelitis due to, 382
    otitis externa due to, 353
Pseudoparalysis, due to osteomyelitis, 382
Pseudoseizures, 53, 620–621
Pseudotumor cerebri, 641
PSGN. *see* Poststreptococcal glomerulonephritis (PSGN)
Psilocybin, acute effects of, 250t–251t
Psoriasis, 658–659
    vs. atopic dermatitis, 654, 658
    differential diagnosis of, 658
    plaque-type, 658
    treatment of, 658
    vulgaris, 658
Psychological assessment, with developmental disabilities, 27, 29t
Psychological development, of adolescent, 237t
Psychological intervention, for developmental disability, 30
Psychological problems, in sickle cell anemia, 520t
Psychophysiologic disorder, 52t
Psychosocial assessment, 14–15
    of adolescence, 14–15
    of bonding and attachment in infancy, 14
    of developing autonomy in early childhood, 14
    of school readiness, 14, 14t
Psychosocial behaviors, modification of, 15
Psychosocial dwarfism, 584–585
Psychosocial problems, 3
Psychosocial short stature, 69
Psychostimulants, 64
Psychotic disorder
    brief, 66
    not otherwise specified, 66
    schizophrenia as. *see* Schizophrenia
    shared, 66
    substance-induced, 66
Psychotic features
    for bipolar disorder, 62
    bipolar disorder with, 66
    major depression, 66
    major depression with, 59

Psychotropics, constipation due to, 426t
PT (prothrombin time), 524–526, 525f, 526t
    in newborn, 222–223
PTH (parathyroid hormone), and vitamin D, 602
PTSD. *see* Posttraumatic stress disorder (PTSD)
PTT (partial thromboplastin time)
    activated, 524–526, 525f, 526t
        in hemophilia, 529
    in newborn, 222–223
Pubarche, 589
    in boys, 238–240, 239f, 589
    in girls, 237–238, 238f–239f, 589
    premature, 596, 593t
Pubertal development, 237–240
    in boys, 238–240, 239f
    in girls, 237–238, 238f–239f
    variations in, 593t
        breast asymmetry and masses as, 241, 241t
        gynecomastia, 596
        gynecomastia as, 241t, 245–247
        irregular menses as, 241
        physiologic leukorrhea as, 241
        premature adrenarche (pubarche) as, 596, 593t
        premature thelarche as, 596, 593t
Puberty, 589–596
    delayed, 589–592
        classification of, 590t
        differential diagnosis of, 591t
        due to constitutional delay, 589, 590t
        due to hypergonadotropic hypogonadism (primary gonadal failure), 590t
            ovarian, 590t, 591–592
            testicular, 590t, 592
        due to hypogonadotrophic hypogonadism, 589, 590t–591t
            due to CNS abnormalities, 590, 590t
            due to idiopathic hypopituitarism, 590, 590t
            due to isolated gonadotropin deficiency, 590, 590t–591t
            due to Kallmann syndrome, 590, 591t
            syndromic, 590–591
        primary amenorrhea as, 592
        treatment of, 592
    precocious, 592–596
        central (constitutional, familial), 592–593, 595t
        classification of, 592–593, 593t
        contrasexual, 593t
        defined, 592
        differential diagnosis of, 594t
        evaluation of, 595
        incomplete (GnRH-independent), 593t, 595t
        peripheral, 592–593
        premature adrenarche (pubarche) as, 596, 593t
        premature thelarche as, 596, 593t
        treatment of, 595–596, 595t
        true or complete, 593t, 595t
Pubic hair growth
    in boys, 238–240, 239f
    in girls, 237–238, 238f–239f
Pubic lice, 378t, 384, 665
    clinical manifestations of, 665
    epidemiology of, 665
    etiology of, 665
Public health, in medical decision making, 6
Pulmonary air leaks, due to assisted ventilation in newborn, 213
Pulmonary angiography, of pulmonary embolism, 475
Pulmonary arterial hypertension (PAH), 473

Pulmonary blood flow, in cardiovascular system assessment, 484–485
Pulmonary capillary blood flow, 456
Pulmonary edema, 472–473
    clinical manifestations of, 472–473
    in coarctation of the aorta, 494
    defined, 472
    diagnostic studies for, 473
    etiology of, 472
    high altitude, 472
    interstitial, 472
    neurogenic, 472
    postobstructive, 472
    treatment and prognosis for, 473
Pulmonary embolism, 474–475
Pulmonary function testing, 459
Pulmonary hemorrhage, 473–474, 474t
Pulmonary hemosiderosis, idiopathic, 473
Pulmonary hypertension, syncope due to, 488t
Pulmonary hypoplasia, 209, 215, 471
Pulmonary maturity of fetus, 189
Pulmonary mechanics, 455–456, 455f
Pulmonary physiology, 455–457
    defense mechanism in, 456–457
    pulmonary mechanics in, 455–456, 455f
    respiratory gas exchange in, 456, 456t
Pulmonary stenosis, 493–494
    clinical manifestations of, 493
    etiology of, 493
    imaging tests for, 493
    peripheral, 493
    subvalvular, 493
    supravalvular, 493
    in tetralogy of Fallot, 495
    treatment of, 494
    valvular, 493
Pulmonary surfactant, 189
    in lung development, 210–211, 211f
Pulmonary toxicity, due to poisoning, 139
Pulse oximetry, 459
    for bronchiolitis, 359
    in cardiovascular system assessment, 484
    with respiratory failure, 128
Pulse pressure
    in cardiovascular system assessment, 481–482
    in dilated cardiomyopathy, 502
    with patent ductus arteriosus, 492–493
Pulsed Doppler studies, of urinary system, 557
Puncture wounds, osteomyelitis due to, 382
Punishment, 15
    physical (corporal), 23
Pupil, Marcus Gunn, 614
Pupillary defect, afferent, 614
Pupillary light reaction, 614
Pupillary responses, in coma, 636–637, 636t
Purified protein derivative standard (PPD-S), in Mantoux test, 409
Purine nucleotides, 146
Purpura, 650t
    with anemia, 511
    in hematologic disorders, 506
    in hemostatic disorders, 524
    idiopathic thrombocytopenic, 527–528
        bleeding disorder in newborn due to, 223
        chronic, 528
        clinical manifestations of, 527–528
        diagnosis of, 528
        etiology of, 527
        maternal, 205, 205t
            clinical manifestations of, 527
            etiology of, 527
            neonatal thrombocytopenia due to, 223
            treatment of, 527
        treatment and prognosis of, 528

Purpura (Continued)
    neonatal alloimmune thrombocytopenic
        clinical manifestations of, 527
        etiology of, 527
        treatment of, 527
    palpable, 302
    thrombotic thrombocytopenic, 528, 560
Purpural rash, infections with fever and, 329t–330t
Pustular melanosis, 198
Pustular rash, infections with fever and, 329t–330t
Pustules, 650t, 651f
    in acne, 652
PVCs (premature ventricular contractions), 489, 490t
PWS. see Prader-Willi syndrome (PWS)
Pyelogram, intravenous, 557
Pyelonephritis, 372
    abdominal pain due to, 420t
Pyloric stenosis, 422, 435–436
    clinical manifestations of, 435
    etiology and epidemiology of, 435
    genetic basis for, 152
    laboratory and imaging studies for, 435, 435f
    vs. salt-losing congenital adrenal hyperplasia, 608
    treatment of, 436
    vomiting due to, 423t, 435
Pyogenic granuloma, 662
Pyrazinamide, for tuberculosis, 410–411, 411t
Pyridostigmine, maternal use of, 207t
Pyridoxal phosphate, 98
Pyridoxine, 98
    deficiency, 98, 98t–100t
Pyrimidine nucleotides, 146
Pyrogens, 324
Pyropoikilocytosis, hereditary, 521
Pyruvate, metabolism of, 184–185, 185f
Pyruvate kinase deficiency, anemia due to, 509–510, 521
Pyuria, 373

Q
Q fever, 398t–400t
QRS complex, 484
QT interval, 484
Quad screen, 154
Quadriplegia, due to cerebral palsy, 35t
Quartan periodicity, of *P. malariae*, 403

R
Rabies, 398t–400t
Rabies immune globulin (RIG), 323
Rabies prophylaxis, 323
Raccoon eyes, 638
Rachitic rosary, in rickets, 102
Radiation
    heat loss via, 203
    as teratogen, 154, 206t
Radiation therapy, 541
    adverse effects of, 542t, 541
    and sarcomas, 551
Radioactive iodine (^{131}I)
    for hyperthyroidism, 601
    maternal use of, 207t
    as teratogen, 206t
Radioallergosorbent test (RAST)
    for antigen-specific IgE, 272–273
    for asthma, 274
Radiofrequency ablation, 490
Radionuclide cystogram, for vesicoureteral reflux, 565
Radionuclide renography, of renal anomalies, 568

Radionuclide scans, for infectious diseases, 317
Radioulnar synostosis, 162
RAG1 (recombinase activating gene 1), in severe combined immunodeficiency, 260
RAG2 (recombinase activating gene 2), in severe combined immunodeficiency, 260
Rales, 457
Ramsay Hunt syndrome, due to zoster, 334
RANTES, functions of, 253t
Rape, 247
    date, 82
    defined, 247
    forensic material from, 247
    therapy after, 247
Rapid eye movement (REM) sleep, 47
Rapid plasma reagin (RPR) test, 380
Rapid tests, for infectious diseases, 317
Rapidly progressive glomerulonephritis (RPGN), 558
Rapport building, 19–20
Rash
    infections with fever and, 329–335
        differential diagnosis of, 329t–330t
        erythema infectiosum (fifth disease) as, 333
        measles (rubeola) as, 329–331
        roseola infantum (exanthem subitum, sixth disease) as, 332–333
        rubella (German or 3-day measles) as, 331–332
        varicella-zoster virus infection (chickenpox, zoster) as, 333–335
    in juvenile dermatomyositis, 311
    in juvenile idiopathic arthritis, 307
    in systemic lupus erythematosus, 309
RAST (radioallergosorbent test)
    for antigen-specific IgE, 272–273
    for asthma, 274
Rat-bite fever, 398t–400t
Rat lungworm, 405t
Rebuck skin window, 266
Receptive language disorders, 35
Recoil, in newborn, 613
Recombinase activating gene 1 (*RAG1*), in severe combined immunodeficiency, 260
Recombinase activating gene 2 (*RAG2*), in severe combined immunodeficiency, 260
Recrudescent typhus, 398t–400t
Rectal biopsy, for Hirschsprung disease, 440
Recurrent laryngeal nerve injury, vocal cord paralysis due to, 468
Red blood cell(s) (RBCs)
    decreased production of, newborn anemia due to, 216
    increased destruction of, newborn anemia due to, 216–218
Red blood cell (RBC) aplasia, congenital pure, 516, 516t
Red blood cell (RBC) morphology, in anemia, 511, 513f
Red blood cell (RBC) production, 506–509
Red reflex, in newborn, 199
Red strawberry tongue, 348
5α-Reductase deficiency, ambiguous genitalia due to, 606
Reed-Sternberg cells, 545
Refeeding syndrome, 69, 96
Reflex(es)
    of child, 615
    of newborn, 13, 613, 613t
    primitive, 613
Reflex rhinitis, 283–284
Reflux, vesicoureteral. see Vesicoureteral reflux (VUR)
Reflux nephropathy, 565

Regurgitation, 430–431
  vs. vomiting, 422
Rehydration, 108
  for dehydration, 108
  oral, 110–111
  overly rapid
    central pontine myelinolysis due to, 110
    cerebral edema due to, 110
Reinforcement
  negative, 15
  positive, 15
Reiter syndrome, 385t
Relapsing fever, 398t–400t
  louse-borne, 666
Reliability, 4
Religious concerns, about palliative care and end-of-life decisions, 9
Religious issues, and ethics, 6
REM (rapid eye movement) sleep, 47
Renal abscess, 372
Renal agenesis, 196t
  bilateral, 566
  unilateral, 565–566
Renal anomalies, 565–567
Renal biopsy, for acute renal failure, 561
Renal disease
  common manifestations of, 554–555, 554t
  end-stage, 562
  etiology of, 554t
  primary, 554–555, 554t
  risk factors for, 553
  secondary, 554–555, 554t
Renal dysplasia, 566
  multicystic, 566
Renal failure
  acute, 561–563
    clinical manifestations of, 561, 562t
    defined, 561
    diagnostic studies of, 561, 562t
    due to shock, 132
    etiology and pathophysiology of, 561, 561t
    intrinsic, 561, 561t–562t
    nonoliguric, 561
    oliguric, 561
    postrenal (obstructive), 561, 561t–562t
    prerenal, 561, 561t–562t
    prognosis for, 562
    treatment of, 561–562
  chronic, 562–563
    clinical manifestations of, 562–563
    due to vesicoureteral reflux, 565
    etiology and epidemiology of, 563t, 562
    prognosis for, 563
    stages of, 563t
    treatment of, 563, 563t
  with fulminant liver failure, 448t
Renal hypoplasia, 566
Renal injury, 135
  in hemolytic uremic syndrome, 560
Renal involvement
  in Henoch-Schönlein purpura, 302
  in systemic lupus erythematosus, 309
Renal medullary carcinoma, risk factors for, 536t
Renal osteodystrophy (ROD), 562–563
Renal output
  decreased, 108, 108t
  increased, 108, 108t
Renal physiology, 553–554, 555f
Renal replacement therapies, for acute renal failure, 562, 562t
Renal salvage, for shock, 132
Renal scarring, due to vesicoureteral reflux, 565
Renal transplantation, for end-stage renal disease, 563

Renal tubular acidosis (RTA), 120
  distal, 120
  hyperkalemic, 120–121
  proximal, 120
Renal tubular function, disordered, in galactosemia, 173
Renal ultrasound (RUS), of renal anomalies, 568
Renin, in renal function, 553
Renin-angiotensin system, in regulation of sodium balance, 106–107
Renography, radionuclide, of renal anomalies, 568
Replacement fluids, 107
Replacement solution, for gastrointestinal losses, 108, 108t
Replacement therapy, 106
  for hemophilia, 529
Research, children as human subject in, 6–7
Reserpine, maternal use of, 207t
Residual volume (RV), 455–456, 455f
Resonance disorders, 34–35
Respect, in palliative care, 7
Respect for others
  and autonomy, 5
  in professionalism, 4
Respiration(s)
  Biot, 457t
  Cheyne-Stokes, 457t, 634–635
  Kussmaul, 457t
    in diabetic ketoacidosis, 574
Respiratory acidosis, 122, 122t
  in newborn, 210
Respiratory alkalosis, 122, 122t
Respiratory compensation, appropriate, 119–120
Respiratory complications, of cystic fibrosis, 476t
Respiratory control, 461–464, 461f
  disorder(s) of, 461–464, 463t
    acute life-threatening event as, 461–462
    apnea as, 463–464, 463t
    SIDS as, 462–463, 462t
Respiratory disease
  assessment for
    breathing patterns in, 457t
    endoscopic evaluation of airways in, 459
    examination of sputum in, 459–460
    history in, 457
    imaging techniques in, 458–459
    lung biopsy in, 460
    measures of respiratory gas exchange in, 459
    physical examination in, 457–458, 457t–458t
    pulmonary function testing in, 459
  obstructive, 459
  physical signs of, 458t
  restrictive, 456
  therapeutic measures for, 460–461
    aerosol therapy as, 460
    chest physiotherapy and clearance techniques as, 460
    intubation as, 460–461
    mechanical ventilation as, 461
    oxygen administration as, 460
    tracheostomy as, 461
Respiratory distress
  with desaturation, 495t
  in newborn, 209–216
  with normal saturation, 495t
Respiratory distress syndrome (RDS), 210–212
  acute, 128
  bronchopulmonary dysplasia due to, 213–214
  clinical manifestations of, 211, 212f
  lung development and, 210–211, 211f
  patent ductus arteriosus due to, 212–213
  potential causes of, 212t
  prevention and treatment of, 211–212
  pulmonary air leaks due to, 213

Respiratory distress syndrome (RDS) *(Continued)*
  and retinopathy of prematurity, 214
  risk factors for, 211
Respiratory failure, 124, 128–129
  chronic, 128
  clinical manifestations of, 128
  complications for, 130–131
  differential diagnosis of, 128–129
  epidemiology of, 128
  etiology of, 128
  hypercarbic, 128
  hypoxemic, 128
  laboratory and imaging studies of, 128
  mixed forms of, 128–129
  prevention of, 131
  prognosis for, 131
  treatment for, 130
Respiratory gas exchange, 456, 456t
  measures of, 459
Respiratory patterns, 457t
Respiratory rate
  assessment of, 457
  of newborn, 196
Respiratory support, for shock, 125–126, 132
Respiratory syncytial virus (RSV)
  bronchiolitis due to, 357
  croup due to, 354
Respiratory system
  anatomy of, 455
  assessment of, 455–461
    breathing patterns in, 457t
    history in, 457
    physical examination in, 457–458, 457t–458t
  physiology of, 455–457
    lung defense mechanism in, 456–457
    pulmonary mechanics in, 455–456, 455f
    respiratory gas exchange in, 456, 456t
Responsibility, 4
Rest, for heart failure, 501t
Restrictive airway disease, 456
Restrictive cardiomyopathy(ies)
  clinical manifestations of, 502
  etiology of, 502
  imaging studies of, 503–504
  treatment of, 504
Restrictive defect, 459
Resuscitation, 109, 125–126
  fluid
    for dehydration, 109
    for shock, 131–132
  isotonic crystalloids in, 125
  for near-drowning, 136
  of newborn, 194
    airway patency in, 194
    algorithm for, 195f
    breathing in, 194–195
    circulation in, 196
    drug administration in, 196
    specific conditions requiring, 201–203
      cyanosis as, 201–202
      life-threatening congenital malformations as, 202
      shock as, 202
  oxygen supplementation in, 125
  vasoactive substance in, 125
Reticular dysgenesis, neutropenia in, 263–264
Reticulate bodies, in *Chlamydia* infection, 379
Reticulocyte(s)
  in erythropoiesis, 506–509
  normal values for, 508t
Reticulocyte count, in anemia, 511
Retinal disorders, due to lysosomal storage diseases, 181t–182t
Retinal hemorrhage, in newborn, 202
Retinoblastoma, risk factors for, 536t

Retinoids, topical, for acne, 652
Retinol, 101
Retinopathy of prematurity (ROP), 214
Retrolental fibroplasia, 214
Retropharyngeal abscess, upper airway
    obstruction due to, 465t–466t
Retroviral syndrome, acute, 339
Rett syndrome, 63–64, 150–151, 642t–643t, 644
    genetic basis for, 151t, 160
Reverse transcriptase, in HIV, 412
Reye syndrome, *vs.* hyperammonemia, 167–168
Rh antigen system, 217
Rh blood group incompatibility, erythroblastosis
    fetalis due to, 217
Rh isoimmunization, hydrops fetalis due to, 210
Rh sensitization
    management of, 217
    maternal, 205t
    prevention of, 218
Rhabdomyolysis, 184
    due to hypokalemia, 116
Rhabdomyosarcoma, 551
    alveolar, 551–552
    clinical manifestations of, 551
    differential diagnosis of, 552
    embryonal, 551–552
    epidemiology of, 551
    laboratory/imaging studies of, 551–552
    prognosis for, 552
    risk factors for, 536t
    treatment of, 552
Rheumatic diseases, assessment of, 299–301
    common manifestations in, 299–301, 303t
    diagnostic imaging in, 302
    differential diagnosis in, 299, 300t
    history in, 299
    initial diagnostic evaluation in, 302
    laboratory testing in, 302
    physical examination in, 299
Rheumatic fever, 501–502
    clinical manifestations of, 501–502, 502t
    etiology and epidemiology of, 501
    treatment and manifestations of, 503–504
Rheumatoid factor, in juvenile idiopathic
    arthritis, 306–307
Rhinitis, 346
    allergic, 282–285
    defined, 282
    differential diagnosis of, 283–284, 283t
    gustatory, 283–284
    infectious, 283
    medicamentosa, 284
    nonallergic, 283–284, 283t
        noninfectious, 283–284
    reflex, 283–284
    vasomotor, 283–284
Rhinorrhea, 638
Rhinosinusitis, 346
    chronic infectious, 283
Rhinoviruses, 348t
Rhipicephalus sanguineus, 401
Rhodopsin, 101
RhoGAM, (anti-Rh-positive immune globulin),
    218
Rhonchi, 457
Rib notching, in coarctation of the aorta, 494
Riboflavin deficiency, 97, 98t–100t
Rickets, 98t, 102, 120, 603
    clinical manifestations of, 102
    diagnosis of, 102
    etiology of, 102, 603
    familial hypophosphatemic, 603, 603t
    in Fanconi syndrome, 120
    pathophysiology of, 102
    treatment of, 99t–100t, 603

Rickets *(Continued)*
    vitamin D-dependent, 603
    vitamin D-resistant, 150
Rickettsia africae, 398t–400t
Rickettsia akari, 398t–400t
Rickettsia conorii, 398t–400t
Rickettsia felis, 398t–400t
Rickettsia prowazekii, 398t–400t
Rickettsia rickettsii, 396, 398t–400t, 401
Rickettsia typhi, 398t–400t
Rickettsial diseases, zoonotic, 398t–400t
Rickettsialpox, 398t–400t
Rifampin, for tuberculosis, 410–411, 411t
RIG (rabies immune globulin), 323
Right-to-left shunts, 491
Right ventricular hypertrophy, 493
    in hypoplastic left heart syndrome, 499
    in tetralogy of Fallot, 495
Right ventricular impulse
    in tetralogy of Fallot, 495
    in total anomalous pulmonary venous return,
        498
Rigidity, 615
Ring form, in *Plasmodium* life cycle, 402
Ringworm, 337t
Ristocetin cofactor assay, for von Willebrand
    disease, 530
Ritalin (Methylphenidate), for ADHD, 42t
RNA polymerase chain reaction, for HIV, 413
Rocky Mountain spotted fever, 398t–400t, 401
ROD (renal osteodystrophy), 562–563
Rohypnol (flunitrazepam), 82
Rolandic epilepsy, 621
Rome III Criteria, for Pediatric Functional
    Gastrointestinal Syndromes, 421t
Rooting reflex, 13, 202–203, 613–614, 613t
ROP (retinopathy of prematurity), 214
Roseola infantum, 332–333
Rotation
    external, 667t
    internal, 667t
Rotavirus (RV), diarrhea due to, 366, 366t
Rotavirus (RV) vaccine, 317–318, 319f–322f
Round worms, 405, 405t
RPGN (rapidly progressive glomerulonephritis),
    558
RPR (rapid plasma reagin) test, 380
RSV (respiratory syncytial virus)
    bronchiolitis due to, 357
    croup due to, 354
Rubella, 331–332
    clinical manifestations of, 331
    complications and prognosis for, 332
    congenital, 229–231, 230t, 331
    contraindications to, 332
    differential diagnosis of, 332
    epidemiology of, 331
    etiology of, 331
    laboratory and imaging studies for, 331–332
    prevention of, 332
    as teratogens, 154
    treatment of, 332
Rubella vaccine, 317–318, 319f–322f, 331
Rule of twos, for asthma, 276
Rupture of the membranes
    premature, 187
    prolonged, 187
RUS (renal ultrasound), of renal anomalies, 568
RV (residual volume), 455–456, 455f
RV (rotavirus), diarrhea due to, 366, 366t
RV (rotavirus) vaccine, 317–318, 319f–322f

S
S_1 (First heart sound), 482
S_2 (Second heart sound), 482

S_3 (Third heart sound), 482
S_4 (Fourth heart sound), 482
Saccharomyces cerevisiae, in inflammatory bowel
    disease, 440–441
Sacral lipoma, constipation due to, 426t
Sacral teratoma, constipation due to, 426t
SAD. *see* Separation anxiety disorder (SAD)
Safety issues, 23
Salicylate(s), for rheumatic fever, 502
Salicylate intoxication, 141t
    metabolic acidosis due to, 121
Salicylic acid, for acne, 652
Salla disease, 181t–182t
Salmeterol, for asthma, 276
Salmon-colored rash, in juvenile idiopathic
    arthritis, 307
Salmon fluke, 406t
Salmon patch, 662, 659t
Salmon patches, 197
Salmonella
    nontyphoidal, 366–367, 398t–400t
    osteomyelitis due to, 383
Salmonella paratyphi, 366
Salmonella typhi, 366
Salmonellosis, 398t–400t
Salter-Harris classification, 670–671, 671f
Salter-Harris fractures, of distal radius, 693
Sandhoff disease, 642t–643t
Sanfilippo syndrome, 181t–182t, 642t–643t, 644
Sarcoma(s), 551–552
    bone, 551
    clinical manifestations of, 551
    complications of, 552
    differential diagnosis of, 552
    epidemiology of, 551
    etiology of, 551
    Ewing. *see* Ewing sarcoma
    laboratory/imaging studies of, 551–552
    prognosis for, 552
    soft tissue, 551
    treatment of, 552
Sarcoptes scabiei, 664
    vulvovaginitis due to, 375t
SARS (severe acute respiratory syndrome), 359
Satellite nevi, 660–661
SC (subcutaneous) emphysema, 471–472
SC (subcutaneous) insulin, 576
SC (subcutaneous) nodules, due to rheumatic
    fever, 503t
Scabies, 664–665
    vs. atopic dermatitis, 286–287
    clinical manifestations of, 664–665, 665f
    complications and prognosis of, 664–665
    etiology and epidemiology of, 664
    laboratory and imaging studies of, 665
    Norwegian or crusted, 664–665
    prevention of, 665
    treatment of, 665
    vulvovaginitis due to, 375t
SCAD (short-chain acyl-CoA dehydrogenase)
    deficiency, 180f, 179
SCAG (Structured Communication Adolescent
    Guide), 235f–236f
Scalding injuries, due to child abuse, 71, 71f
Scale, 651t
Scalene muscles, during inspiration, 455
Scanogram, of leg-length discrepancy, 678–679
Scaphocephaly, 161t
Scaphoid fracture, 693
Scar, 651t
Scarf sign, in newborn, 198f
Scarlet fever, 348
Scheuermann kyphosis, 688, 688f
    classic radiologic findings of, 688
    treatment of, 688

Schistocytes, 513f
Schistosoma haematobium, 406–407, 406t
Schistosoma intercalatum, 406–407
Schistosoma japonicum, 406–407, 406t
Schistosoma mansoni, 406–407, 406t
Schistosoma mekongi, 406–407, 406t
Schistosomiasis, 406–407, 406t
    intestinal or hepatic, 406t
Schizencephaly, 648
Schizoaffective disorder, 66
Schizogony, in *Plasmodium* life cycle, 402
Schizophrenia, 64–66
    diagnostic criteria for, 65t
    etiology of, 64
    subtypes of
        catatonic, 66
        disorganized, 65
        paranoid, 65
        residual, 66
        undifferentiated, 66
    symptoms of
        negative, 65
        positive, 64–65
    treatment of, 66
Schizophreniform disorder, 66
Schnitzler syndrome, 290–291
School-age children
    reaction to divorce by, 83
    tests of cognition in, 29t
School-age period, late, physical development
    in, 13
School phobia, 57
School readiness, 14, 14t
Schwachman-Diamond syndrome, neutropenia
    in, 263–264, 264t
SCID. *see* Severe combined immunodeficiency
    (SCID)
SCIWORA (spinal cord injury without radiologic
    abnormality), 134
Scleritis, 388t–389t
Sclerosis, 651t
Scolding, 23
Scoliosis, 478, 685–687
    adolescent, 686
    classification of, 684t
    clinical evaluation of, 684, 685f
    compensatory, 684, 687
    congenital, 686, 687f
        treatment of, 686
    idiopathic, 686
        clinical manifestations of, 686
        etiology and epidemiology of, 686
        treatment of, 686
    infantile, 686
    juvenile, 686
    neuromuscular, 686–687
        treatment of, 687
    radiologic evaluation of, 685, 686f
Screening
    anemia, 21
    autism, 18–19
    cholesterol, 22, 22t
    developmental, 15–19
    hearing, 19, 19t
        of children 3 years of age and older, 21
        of infants and toddlers, 21
        of newborn, 21
    language (speech), 19, 19t
    lead, 21–22, 22t
    newborn, 21
        hearing, 21
        hemoglobin electrophoresis in, 21
        metabolic, 21
    for sexually transmitted infections, 22
    tuberculosis, 22, 22t

Screening (*Continued*)
    vision, 21
        of children 3 years of age and older, 21
        of infants and toddlers, 21
Screening tests
    for cancer, 535–536
    during well child visits, 17f, 21–22
        for anemia, 21
        for cholesterol, 22, 22t
        hearing and vision, 21
        for lead, 21–22, 22t
        newborn, 21
        for sexually transmitted infections, 22
        for tuberculosis, 22, 22t
Screening tools, 54
Scrofula, 408
Scrotum, disorders and abnormalities of,
    568–569
    clinical manifestations of, 568
    complications of, 569
    etiology of, 568
    treatment of, 569
Scrub typhus, 398t–400t
Scurvy, 96–97, 98t
Seasonal affective disorder, 60
Seasonal allergic rhinitis, 282
Seborrheic dermatitis, 657–659
    atopic *vs.*, 654, 658
    clinical manifestations of, 657, 658f
    differential diagnosis of, 658
    etiology of, 657
    laboratory and imaging studies of, 658
    prevention of, 658
    prognosis for, 658
    treatment of, 658
Second-degree heart block, 489, 490t
Second-hand cigarette smoke, 79
Second heart sound (S_2), 482
    abnormal, 483t
    in tetralogy of Fallot, 495
    in total anomalous pulmonary venous return,
        498
    with tricuspid atresia, 497
    in truncus arteriosus, 497
Second impact syndrome, 638
Secondary ossification center, 668f
Secondary pneumothorax, 478
Sedation, 144–145
    nonprocedural, 144
    procedural, 144
Sedation and analgesia, 144–145, 145t
Sedatives, acute effects of, 250t–251t
Sedentary behavior, and obesity, 92
Sedentary lifestyle, 2
Seizure(s), 662, 141, 618–623
    absence, 620
        atypical, 620
        due to inborn errors of metabolism, 167t
    atonic, 620
    classification of, 618, 619t
    clonic, 619–620
    depression of consciousness due to, 637
    with developmental disability, 31t
    differential diagnosis of, 618, 620t
    in epilepsy syndromes, 619t, 621
    etiology and epidemiology of, 618, 618t–619t
    febrile, 620
        complex or atypical, 620
        simple, 620
    focal, 618–619
        complex partial, 618–619
        simple, 618
    generalized, 619–621
    immediate treatment of, 621–622, 629f
    impact, 639

Seizure(s) (*Continued*)
    jacksonian, 618–619
    laboratory and diagnostic evaluation of, 622
    long-term therapy for, 622–623, 622t
    myoclonic, 620
    neonatal, 224–227
        benign familial, 225
        clinical characteristics of, 225, 225t
        diagnostic evaluation of, 225–226
        differential diagnosis of, 225, 225t
        focal clonic, 225t
        focal tonic, 225t
        generalized tonic, 225t
        myoclonic, 225t
        treatment of, 226
    nonepileptic, 53
    post-traumatic, 639
    pseudo-, 620–621
    psychogenic nonepilepsy, 620–621
    status epilepticus with, 621–622
        treatment of, 622t
    in Sturge-Weber syndrome, 662, 646–647
    tonic, 619–620
    tonic-clonic, 619–620
Selective serotonin reuptake inhibitors (SSRIs),
    58–59
    for obsessive-compulsive disorder, 64
Selenium deficiency, 103t
Self-awareness, 4–5
Self-improvement, 4
Seminiferous tubular dysgenesis, delayed puberty
    due to, 592
SEN-V virus, 370t
Senna, for functional constipation, 47t
Sensory and motor neuropathy, 101
Sensory examination, 613, 615
Sensory impairments, with developmental
    disability, 31t
Sensory integration therapy, for developmental
    disabilities, 30
Sensory receptors, peripheral, in control of
    ventilation, 461f
Separation, 82–85
    from parents, 84, 84t
Separation anxiety disorder (SAD), 57
Sepsis
    bacterial, 228
    early-onset
        clinical manifestations of, 228
        treatment for, 228
    fever and, 324–325
    incidence of, 227
    late-onset
        clinical manifestations of, 228
        evaluation of, 231
        treatment of, 231
    in newborn, 227–229
        acquired in utero, 227
        preterm, 227
        viral, 227–228
Septic emboli, due to infective endocarditis,
    365
Septic thrombophlebitis, 394
Septo-optic dysplasia, 574
Sequence, of malformations, 160–161
Sequestration thrombocytopenia, due to
    decreased platelet production, 526–527
Sequestrum(a), in osteomyelitis, 382–383
Serologic tests, for infectious diseases, 317
Serositis, in rheumatic diseases, 299
Serum glucose
    in hypoglycemia, 572–573
    regulation of, 580, 581f
Serum immunoglobulin levels, for
    immunodeficiency disorders, 255

Serum sickness, 271–272, 292–293
    clinical manifestations of, 292
    epidemiology of, 292
    etiology of, 292
    laboratory and imaging studies for, 292–293
    treatment and prevention of, 294
Sever disease, 683
    clinical manifestations of, 683
    treatment of, 683
Severe acute respiratory syndrome (SARS), 359
Severe combined immunodeficiency (SCID),
        258–260, 259t
    autosomal recessive, 260
    clinical manifestations of, 260
    due to deficiencies in adenosine deaminase
            and purine nucleoside phosphorylase, 260
    hematopoietic stem cell transplantation for,
            269
    in Nezelof syndrome, 260
    pathogenesis of, 258–260
    X-linked, 260
Sex assignment, with ambiguous genitalia, 606
Sex chromosomes, 146
Sex-determining region (SRY) gene, 604–605,
        605f
Sex steroids
    for delayed puberty, 592
    in puberty, 589
Sexual abuse, 73
    defined, 73
    diagnosis of
        history in, 73
        laboratory evaluation in, 73
        physical examination in, 73
    epidemiology of, 73
    management of, 73–74, 74f
    prevention of, 74
    reporting of, 70
    risk factors for, 70
    sexually transmitted infections due to, 73
Sexual development
    abnormal, 605–606
        approach to infant with, 606–607
        diagnosis of, 607
        due to inadequate masculinization of 46,XY
                male, 605–606, 606t
        due to virilization of 46,XX female, 605, 605t
        treatment of, 607
    disorders of, 604–607
    normal, 604–605, 604f–605f
Sexual differentiation disorders, 604–607
    approach to infant with, 606–607
    diagnosis of, 607
    due to inadequate masculinization of 46,XY
            male, 605–606, 606t
    due to virilization of 46,XX female, 605, 605t
    normal development and, 604–605, 604f–605f
    treatment of, 607
Sexual identity, development of, 75
Sexual infantilism, 589–592
    classification of, 590t
    differential diagnosis of, 591t
    due to constitutional delay, 589, 591t
    due to hypergonadotropic hypogonadism
            (primary gonadal failure), 590t
        ovarian, 590t, 591–592
        testicular, 590t, 592
    due to hypogonadotropic hypogonadism, 589,
            590t–591t
        due to CNS abnormalities, 590, 590t–591t
        due to idiopathic hypopituitarism, 590, 590t
        due to isolated gonadotropin deficiency,
                590, 590t–591t
        due to Kallmann syndrome, 590, 591t
        syndromic, 590–591

Sexual infantilism (Continued)
    primary amenorrhea as, 592
    treatment of, 592
Sexual maturity rating, 13
Sexual phase, of Plasmodium life cycle, 402
Sexual precocity, 592–596
    central (constitutional, familial), 592–593, 595t
    classification of, 592–593, 593t
    contrasexual, 593t
    defined, 592
    differential diagnosis of, 594t
    evaluation of, 595
    incomplete (GnRH-independent), 593t, 595t
    peripheral, 592–593
    premature adrenarche (pubarche) as, 596, 593t
    premature thelarche as, 596, 593t
    treatment of, 595–596, 595t
    true or complete, 593t, 595t
Sexuality, with developmental disability, 31t
Sexually transmitted infections (STIs), 243,
        376–381
    abnormal uterine bleeding due to, 243, 243t
    bacterial vaginosis (Gardnerella vaginalis-
            associated vaginitis), 377t–378t
    chancroid (Haemophilus ducreyi) as, 376, 377t
    Chlamydia trachomatis as, 376, 379–380
        clinical features of, 376
        diagnosis of, 379–380
        epidemiology of, 379
        and gonorrhea, 376t
        pathogenesis of, 379
        pelvic inflammatory disease due to, 379
        treatment of, 380
    genital ulcers due to, 376, 377t
    genital warts (condylomata acuminata, human
            papillomavirus) as
        clinical features of, 378t
        diagnosis of, 381
        pathogenesis of, 384
        treatment of, 381
    gonorrhea (Neisseria gonorrhoeae) as, 376, 379
        and Chlamydia trachomatis, 376t
        clinical features of, 376t
        disseminated gonococcal infections due
                to, 379
        pathogenesis of, 379
        pelvic inflammatory disease due to, 379
        treatment of, 379
    granuloma inguinale (donovanosis,
            Calymmatobacterium granulomatis) as,
            376, 377t
    herpes simplex virus (genital herpes) as, 376,
            380–381
    lymphadenopathy due to, 339t
    mucopurulent cervicitis (endocervicitis) due
            to, 376
    pediculosis pubis (pubic lice, crab lice, Phthirus
            pubis) as, 378t, 384
    pelvic inflammatory disease due to, 376t, 379
    syphilis (Treponema pallidum) as, 376, 377t,
            380
    testing for, 22
    trichomoniasis (Trichomonas vaginalis) as, 376,
            377t–378t, 383
    urethritis due to, 376, 376t
    vaginal discharge due to, 376, 377t–378t
    vulvovaginal candidiasis (Candida albicans)
            as, 378t
SGA. see Small for gestational age (SGA)
SH2D1A gene, in X-linked lymphoproliferative
        disease, 261
Shagreen patches, 646
Shared psychotic disorder, 66
Shawl sign, in juvenile dermatomyositis, 311
Sheep liver fluke, 406t

Shift-to-the-left, in infectious diseases, 317t,
        316–317
Shiga toxin, 367
Shiga-like toxin, 367
Shigella, vulvovaginitis due to, 375t
Shigella dysenteriae, 366t, 367
Shock, 125–126, 129–133
    cardiogenic, 125–126, 130
        clinical manifestations of, 130–131
        etiology of, 129–130, 130t
    classification of, 130t
    clinical manifestations of, 130–131
    complications of, 132
    dissociative, 130
        clinical manifestations of, 130–131
        etiology of, 129–130, 130t
    distributive, 130
        clinical manifestations of, 130–131
        etiology of, 129–130, 130t
    etiology and epidemiology of, 129
    hypovolemic, 125–126, 129–130
        clinical manifestations of, 130–131
        etiology of, 129–130, 130t
    laboratory and imaging studies of, 131
    obstructive, 130
        clinical manifestations of, 130–131
        etiology of, 129–130, 130t
    prevention of, 133
    prognosis of, 132
    treatment of, 131–132
        cardiovascular support of, 132
        fluid resuscitation in, 131–132
        general principles of, 131
        organ-directed therapeutics in, 131–132
        renal salvage of, 132
        respiratory support of, 132
    warm, 131
Shock, in newborn, 202
Short bowel syndrome, parenteral nutrition for,
        111–112
Short-chain acyl-CoA dehydrogenase (SCAD)
        deficiency, 180f, 179
Short stature
    causes of, 585t
        endocrine, 584, 585t
        nonendocrine, 584–586, 585t
    constitutional, 12
    defined, 584
    differential diagnosis of, 587t
    due to chronic disease, 585t, 587t
    due to constitutional delay, 585–586, 586f, 587t
    due to deprivational dwarfism, 587t
    due to endocrine disorders, 585t
    due to GH deficiency, 586–588
        classic congenital or idiopathic, 586
        clinical manifestations of, 586–588
        diagnosis of, 588, 588t
        differential diagnosis of, 587t
        etiology and epidemiology of, 585t, 586
        treatment of, 587t, 588
    due to hypothyroidism, 585t, 587t
    due to lysosomal storage diseases, 585t
    due to skeletal dysplasias, 585t
    due to Turner syndrome, 586, 587t
    familial, 12
    genetic or familial, 585–586, 586f, 587t
    psychosocial, 69
    syndromes of, 585t
    therapy for, 587t
Shortness of breath, due to heart failure, 481, 501
Shoulder, 691–692
    brachial plexus injuries of, 691
    glenohumeral dislocation of, 691
    Little Leaguer's, 691–692
    overuse injuries of, 691

Shoulder (*Continued*)
  proximal humeral epiphysiolysis of, 691–692
  Sprengel deformity of, 691
Shoulder drooping, 614
Shprintzen syndrome, 159–160
Shunt infections, 400
SIADH (syndrome of inappropriate antidiuretic
    hormone), hyponatremia in, 113–114
Sialidosis type I, 181t–182t
Sialidosis type II, 181t–182t
Sickle cell(s), 513f
Sickle cell disease, 518–520
  clinical manifestations of, 519, 520t
  etiology and epidemiology of, 518–519,
    519t
  fever due to, 326
  genetic basis for, 150t
  hematuria due to, 559
  laboratory diagnosis of, 513f, 520
  treatment of, 520
SIDS. *see* Sudden infant death syndrome (SIDS)
Silent stroke, in sickle cell anemia, 520
Silver nitrate instillation, in newborn, 191
Silver sulfadiazine, for burns, 138–139
Single gene mutation, 148
Single-parent families, 77
Sinus arrhythmia, 488
Sinus rhythm, 488
Sinus tachycardia, 490t
Sinus venosus defect, 492
Sinusitis, 283, 350–351
  clinical manifestations of, 350
  complications and prognosis for, 350–351
  defined, 350
  differential diagnosis of, 350
  epidemiology of, 350
  etiology of, 350
  laboratory and imaging studies of, 350
  prevention of, 352–353
  treatment of, 350
SIRS (systemic inflammatory response
    syndrome), 130
Situs inversus, in Kartagener syndrome, 472
SJS (Stevens-Johnson syndrome), 662–666, 663t
Skeletal infections, in infants, 38
Skeletal radiographs, 163
Skeletal tuberculosis, 409
Skewfoot, 682
Skier's nose, 283–284
Skin
  with developmental disabilities, 28t
  of newborn, 197–198, 197f
Skin color, in cardiovascular system assessment,
    482
Skin disorder(s), 650
  assessment of, 650–651
    history in, 650
    initial diagnostic evaluation and screening
      tests in, 651
    physical examination in, 650
  common manifestations of, 650–651
    with primary lesions, 650–651, 650t, 651f
    with secondary lesions, 650–651, 651t
  with developmental disability, 31t
Skin grafting, for burns, 137
Skin lesions
  primary, 650–651, 650t, 651f
  secondary, 650–651, 651t
Skull, of newborn, 198–199
Skull fractures, 638–639
  in newborn, 203
"Slapped cheek" rash, in erythema infectiosum,
    333
SLE. *see* Systemic lupus erythematosus (SLE)
Sleep, normal, 47–50

Sleep disorders, 48–50
  clinical manifestations of, 48
    physical examination, 48
  complications of, 50
  differential diagnosis of, 48–49
  epidemiology of, 48
  evaluation of, 48
  prevention of, 49–50, 50t
  treatment of, 49–50
Sleep-onset association disorders, 49t
Sleep phase, delayed, 49t
Sleep position, 24t–25t
Sleep terrors, 49t
Sleep-wake pattern, irregular, 49t
Sleepwalking, 49t
Slipped capital femoral epiphysis (SCFE),
    675–676
  classification of, 675
  clinical manifestations of, 675
  complications of, 680
  etiology and epidemiology of, 675
  radiologic evaluation of, 676f, 675
  treatment of, 675
Slow to warm up child, 17
Sly syndrome, 181t–182t, 642t–643t, 644
Small, round, blue cell tumors, 551
Small bowel biopsy, for celiac disease, 442
Small for gestational age (SGA), 90–91,
    208–209
  clinical features of, 208
  complications of, 189t, 197
  defined, 197, 208
  etiology of, 208, 208t
  management of, 208–209
  prenatal detection of, 208
SMART goals, 92–93
Smell, assessment of sense of, 614
Smooth muscle hamartoma, 659t
Sniffing position, in epiglottitis, 354
Social and environmental intervention, for
    developmental disability, 30
Social development, milestones of, 16t
Social disruptions, as sleep disorders, 49t
Social environment, with developmental
    disabilities, 29
Social history, for developmental disabilities, 27t
Social phobia, 57, 58t
Societal stresses, 3
Sodium (Na), fractional excretion of, in acute
    renal failure, 561
Sodium balance, 112–113
  regulation of, 106–107
Sodium benzoate, for hyperammonemia, 177
Sodium bicarbonate, 127
Sodium chloride, for 21-hydroxylase deficiency,
    609–611
Sodium disorder(s), 112–115
  hypernatremia as, 114–115
  hyponatremia as, 113–114
Sodium excretion, plasma volume and, 112–113
Sodium intoxication, 114, 115f
Sodium phenylacetate, for hyperammonemia,
    177
Sodium restriction, for heart failure, 501t
Soiling. *see* Encopresis
Solid foods, complementary feeding of, 89
Somatic pain, in appendicitis, 443
Somatization disorder, 51, 52t
  diagnostic criteria for, 52t
Somatoform disorder(s)
  body dysmorphic disorder as, 51, 53–54
  chronic fatigue syndrome as, 51
  cognitive-behavioral methods, 54
  conversion disorder as, 51
  defined, 51

Somatoform disorder(s) (*Continued*)
  factitious disorder (Munchausen syndrome),
    52t, 54
  falling out syndrome, 52–53
  features of, 52t
  hypochondriasis as, 52t, 53
  malingering as, 51–54, 52t
  Munchausen syndrome by proxy as, 54
  pain disorder as, 53
  psychophysiologic disorder, 52t
  somatization disorder as. *see* Somatization
    disorder
  treatment of, 54
  undifferentiated, 51, 52t
Somatostatin, for pancreatitis, 453
Somatostatin release inhibitory factor (SRIF), 583
Somnolence syndrome, 50, 547
Sorbitol
  for functional constipation, 47t
  for poisoning, 143
Sotos syndrome, 162
Southeast Asian liver fluke, 406t
Southern tick-associated rash illness, 397,
    398t–400t
Soy formulas, 88–89, 88t
Soy protein intolerance, vomiting due to, 423t
Spasms, infantile, 621
Spasticity, 615
Special needs, children with, 26–36
  defined, 26
  due to cerebral palsy, 35–36, 35t–36t
  due to hearing impairment, 32–34, 33t
  due to mental retardation, 31, 31t–32t
  due to speech-language impairment, 34–35,
    34t
  due to vision impairment, 31–32
  goal in management, 26
  management of developmental problems in,
    29–30
    counseling principles for, 30
    interdisciplinary team intervention for, 30,
      31t
    intervention in primary care setting for,
      29–30, 30t
  medical home for, 26
  multifaceted team assessment of complex
    problems in, 26–29
    cognitive, 27, 29t
    educational, 27–29
    history taking in, 26, 27t
    medical, 26, 27t
    motor, 26
    physical examination in, 26, 28t
    psychological, 27, 29t
    of social environment, 29
Speculum examination, for adolescents, 241
Speech-language complications, of hearing
    impairment, 33t
Speech-language impairment, 34–35, 34t
Speech-language pathologists, 35
Speech-language therapy, 35
  for developmental disability, 30
Speech screening, 19, 19t
Spherocytes, 513f
Spherocytosis, hereditary
  clinical manifestations of, 521
  etiology of, 509–510, 521
  laboratory diagnosis of, 521
  treatment of, 521
Sphingolipidoses, 643
Sphingomyelin lipidosis A, 181t–182t
Sphingomyelin lipidosis B, 181t–182t
Sphingomyelinase deficiency, 181t–182t
Spina bifida, 647
  occulta, 647

Spinal cord, congenital anomalies of, 647
  diagnostic studies of, 647
  diastematomyelia, 647
  etiology and clinical manifestations of, 647
  treatment and prevention of, 647
Spinal cord compression, due to cancer, 539t
Spinal cord injuries, 134, 639
  in newborn, 202
Spinal cord injury without radiologic
    abnormality (SCIWORA), 134
Spinal cord lesions, weakness due to, 624
Spinal deformities, 684–685
  classification of, 684t
  clinical manifestations of, 684
  kyphosis as, 688
    classification of, 684t
    clinical evaluation of, 684
    congenital, 688
    postural roundback, 688
    Scheuermann, 688, 688f
  radiologic evaluation of, 685, 686f
  scoliosis as, 685–687. *see also* Scoliosis
Spinal dysraphism, 684, 686
Spinal muscular atrophy (SMA), 614, 624–625
  clinical manifestations of, 625
  etiology of, 624–625
  laboratory and diagnostic studies for, 625
  treatment of, 625
Spine, 684–690
  back pain of, 689, 689t
  deformities of, 684–685
    classification of, 684t
    clinical manifestations of, 684
    kyphosis as, 688
      classification of, 684t
      clinical evaluation of, 684
      congenital, 688
      postural roundback, 688
      Scheuermann, 688, 688f
    radiologic evaluation of, 685
    scoliosis as, 685–687. *see also* Scoliosis
  diskitis as, 690
  of newborn, 200
  spondylolysis and spondylolisthesis of,
    689–690
  torticollis of, 688–689
Spirillum minus, 398t–400t
Spiritual concerns, about palliative care and end-
    of-life decisions, 9
Spirochetal diseases, zoonotic, 398t–400t
Spirometry, 459
  for asthma, 274
Spitting up, 430–431
  vs. vomiting, 422
Spleen injuries, 135
Splenectomy
  for β-thalassemia major, 518
  for hereditary spherocytosis, 521
Splenic infarction, in sickle cell disease, 519
Splenic sequestration crisis, in sickle cell anemia,
  519, 520t
Splenomegaly, due to anemia, 511
Spondylitis, juvenile ankylosing, 307t
Spondyloarthropathies, 306t–307t, 307
Spondylolisthesis, 689–690
  classification of, 689
  clinical manifestations of, 690
  defined, 689
  etiology and epidemiology of, 689
  radiologic evaluation of, 690
  treatment of, 690
Spondylolysis, 689–690
  clinical manifestations of, 690
  defined, 689
  etiology and epidemiology of, 689

Spondylolysis *(Continued)*
  radiologic evaluation of, 690
  treatment of, 690
Spontaneous mutation, 147
Spontaneous primary pneumothorax, 478
Sporogony, in *Plasmodium* life cycle, 402
Spot urine protein/creatinine, 557
Spotted fever, 398t–400t
Sprengel deformity, 691
Spur cells, in hemolytic anemia, 522
Sputum examination, 459–460
Square window wrist, in newborn, 198f
SRIF (somatostatin release inhibitory factor), 583
SRY (sex-determining region) gene, 604–605,
  605f
SSRIs (selective serotonin reuptake inhibitors)
  for anxiety disorders, 58–59
  for obsessive-compulsive disorder, 64
St. Vitus dance, due to rheumatic fever, 502
Standard formula, 88t
Stanford-Binet Intelligence Scale (4th ed.), 29t
Stanozolol, for C1-inhibitor deficiency, 269
Staphylococcal scalded skin syndrome, 663t, 665
Staphylococcus, vulvovaginitis due to, 375t
Staphylococcus *aureus*
  in cystic fibrosis, 477–478
  osteomyelitis due to, 381–382
    prevention of, 384
    subacute focal, 382
    treatment of, 383
  pneumonia due to, 363t
StAR (steroidogenic acute regulatory protein), in
  lipoid adrenal hyperplasia, 608f
Start codons, 146
Starvation, 69
Static neurologic abnormalities, 612
Stature
  with developmental disabilities, 28t
  growth charts for, 11f
Status asthmaticus, 278
Status epilepticus, 621–622
  treatment of, 622t
Steatohepatitis, 450
Steatorrhea
  in cystic fibrosis, 475
  due to pancreatic insufficiency, 451
Steeple sign, in croup, 354
Steinert disease, genetic basis for, 147t
STEP guide, for adolescent interviewing, 234,
  237f
Stepped down therapy, for asthma, 276,
  277f–278f
Stepped up therapy, for asthma, 276, 277f–278f
Stepwise approach, to asthma management, 276,
  277f–278f
Stereognosis, 615
Sternocleidomastoid muscles, during inspiration,
  455
Steroid hormones, 570
  adrenal
    maternal and fetal, 607
    maternal use of, 207t
    normal variations in, 607
    synthesis and release of, 607, 608f
Steroidal contraception, 245–247
  combined oral contraceptives for, 245–246,
    245t–246t
  contraceptive patch for, 246
  contraceptive vaginal ring for, 246
  hormonal injections and implants for, 246
  progesterone-only pill or minipill for, 246
Steroidogenic acute regulatory protein (StAR), in
  lipoid adrenal hyperplasia, 608f
Stevens-Johnson syndrome (SJS), 662–666, 663t
Stilbestrol, as teratogen, 206t

Stillbirth, 187
Still's murmur, 484t
Stimson line, in measles, 329–330
Stimulants
  acute effects of, 250t–251t
  for ADHD, 42, 42t
  for functional constipation, 47t
Stimulation, appropriate, 79
Stinger, 691
STI(s). *see* Sexually transmitted infections (STIs)
Stocking glove anesthesia, 52–53
Stomach disorder(s), 430–437
  peptic disease as, 436–437, 436t
  pyloric stenosis as, 435–436, 435f
Stomatitis, vesicular, 398t–400t
Stool(s), of breastfed infants, 86
Stool impaction, 45
Stool softener, for functional constipation, 426
Stop codons, 146
Storage diseases, 168
  caused by defective synthesis of lysosomal
    membrane, 181t–182t
  caused by defects in lysosomal proteolysis,
    181t–182t
  caused by dysfunction of lysosomal transport
    proteins, 181t–182t
  metabolic testing for, 170–171
Stork bite, 662
Stranger anxiety, 14
Strattera (Atomoxetine), for ADHD, 42t
Strawberry tongue
  in Kawasaki disease, 303
  red, 348
  white, 348
Strength, in motor examination, 615
Streptobacillus moniliformis, 398t–400t
Streptococcal carriers, 348
Streptococcal infection, 62
  in rheumatic fever, 501
Streptococcal pharyngitis
  clinical manifestations of, 347–348
  complications of, 349
  epidemiology of, 347
  etiology of, 347
  laboratory evaluation of, 348
  prevention of, 349
  recurrent, 349
  treatment of, 349, 349t
Streptococcus(i)
  group A
    osteomyelitis due to, 381–382
    pneumonia due to, 363t
  group B
    osteomyelitis due to, 381–382
    pneumonia due to, 363t
Streptococcus, vulvovaginitis due to, 375t
Streptococcus pneumoniae, 479
  conjunctivitis due to, 386, 388t
  immunization against, 346
  osteomyelitis due to, 381–382
  pneumonia due to, 359, 363t
Streptococcus pyogenes
  osteomyelitis due to, 383t
  pharyngitis due to, 347
Streptomycin, as teratogen, 206t
Stress, increased energy needs with, 94f
Stress-diathesis model, of depression, 59
Stressful states, glucocorticoid doses during,
  609–611
Stressors
  and adult health challenges, 3
  social and economic, 3
Stridor, 457, 464
  due to croup, 354
  due to laryngomalacia, 467

Stridor (*Continued*)
due to subglottic stenosis, 468
due to upper airway obstruction, 467
String sign, in pyloric stenosis, 435
Stroke, 630–631
clinical manifestations of, 631
diagnostic tests and imaging for, 631
differential diagnosis of, 631
etiology of, 630–631, 630t
hemorrhagic, 630–631
in sickle cell anemia, 520, 520t
treatment of, 631
Stroke volume, and oxygen delivery, 129
Strongyloides fuelleborni, 405t
Strongyloides stercoralis, 405t
Structured Communication Adolescent Guide
(SCAG), 235f–236f
Structured weight management, for obesity,
92–93
Stunting, 67, 94, 94t, 104–105
moderate, 94t
severe, 94t
Stupor, 634
Sturge-Weber syndrome, 662, 646–647
port-wine stain in, 662, 646
Stuttering, 19, 34–35
Styes, 387
Subacute bacterial endocarditis prophylaxis, 496
Subacute necrotizing encephalomyelopathy,
642t–643t, 644
Subacute sclerosing panencephalitis, due to
measles, 331
Subarachnoid hemorrhage
aneurysmal, 617t
due to trauma, 638t
in newborn, 226
Subconjunctival hemorrhage, in newborn, 202
Subcutaneous (SC) emphysema, 471–472
Subcutaneous (SC) insulin, 576
Subcutaneous (SC) nodules, due to rheumatic
fever, 502, 503t
Subdural hematoma, in newborn, 226
Subdural hemorrhage, 638t
due to child abuse, 72, 72f
in newborn, 226
Subependymal giant cell astrocytomas, 646
Subependymal nodules, 646
Subgaleal bleed, in newborn, 202
Subglottic hemangioma, 661–662
Subglottic obstruction, 466t
Subglottic space, 455
Subglottic stenosis, 468
Subluxation, 667t
Substance abuse
by adolescents, 2, 250–251
acute illness due to, 251
acute overdose due to, 250, 250t–251t
chronic, 251
screening for, 250, 250t
treatment for, 251
maternal
after birth, 79
during pregnancy, 79, 207t
Substance-induced psychotic disorders, 66
Substernal retractions, 457
Substrate, hypoglycemia due to inadequate, 580t
Succinylacetone, urine or blood, 171t
Sucking reflex, 13
Sudden infant death syndrome (SIDS), 462–463
defined, 462
differential diagnosis of, 462t
etiology and epidemiology of, 462
with medium-chain acyl-CoA dehydrogenase
deficiency, 179
prevention of, 23, 462–463

Suicide
bipolar disorder and, 60
depression and, 60
Sulfasalazine, for ulcerative colitis, 441–442
Sulfisoxazole, for otitis media, 352–353
Sulfonamides, maternal use of, 207t
Sulfonylurea, maternal use of, 207t
Sunsetting, 641
Superficial infection(s)
bacterial, 335–336
cellulitis as, 335–336
folliculitis as, 336
impetigo as, 335
perianal dermatitis as, 336
fungal, 336
viral, 336–338
due to herpes simplex virus, 336–338
due to human papillomavirus, 338
molluscum contagiosum as, 338
Superior vena cava syndrome, due to cancer,
539t
Supplemental oxygen, 460
Supportive care
for cancer, 541
for poisoning, 142
for Stevens-Johnson syndrome and toxic
epidermal necrolysis, 665
Supraclavicular retractions, 457
Supracondylar fracture, 671
Supracristal septum, 491
Supraglottic obstruction, 466t
Suprasternal retractions, 464
Supraventricular tachycardia (SVT), 489, 490t
Surfactant, 189
in lung development, 210–211, 211f
Surgical drains, third space losses from, 108
Susceptibilities, to anti-infective drugs, 323
Sutures, of newborn, 198–199
SVT (supraventricular tachycardia), 489, 490t
Swallowing study, videofluoroscopic,
469–470
Sweat test, for cystic fibrosis, 476, 477t
Swimmer's ear. *see* Otitis externa
Swinging flashlight test, 614
Swollen belly syndrome, 405t
Swyer-James syndrome, 363
Sydenham disease, due to rheumatic fever, 502,
503t
Sylvatic typhus, 398t–400t
Sympathomimetic agents
maternal use of, 207t
toxicity of, 141t
Symptomatic hyponatremia, 114
Synchronized cardioversion, for dysrhythmias,
490
Syncope, 486–487
cardiac, 488t
carotid sinus, 488t
clinical manifestations of, 486–487
cough (deglutition), 488t
defined, 486
diagnostic studies of, 488
etiology of, 486
loss of consciousness due to, 637
micturition, 488t
neurocardiogenic (vasopressor), 488t
Syndactyly, 161t, 162–163
of fingers, 693
of toes, 683, 689t
Syndrome of inappropriate antidiuretic hormone
(SIADH), hyponatremia in, 113–114
Synergism, of antimicrobial drugs, 325
Synophrys, 161t
Synovial fluid findings, in various joint diseases,
385t

Synovitis
in juvenile idiopathic arthritis, 305
in rheumatic diseases, 299
transient (toxic), 384, 674
clinical manifestations and evaluation of,
674, 674t
etiology and epidemiology of, 674
treatment of, 674
Syphilis, 376, 380
clinical features of, 377t
congenital, 230t, 232
diagnosis of, 380
latent, 380
neuro-, 380
pathogenesis of, 380
primary, 380
secondary, 380
tertiary, 380
treatment of, 380
Syrup of ipecac, for poisoning, 142–143
Systemic capillary leak, due to burns, 138
Systemic diseases, cardiac manifestations of,
481t
Systemic inflammatory response syndrome
(SIRS), 130
Systemic lupus erythematosus (SLE), 309–311
clinical manifestations of, 309, 310f, 310t
complications of, 312
diagnostic criteria for, 309t
differential diagnosis of, 300t, 309t, 312
epidemiology of, 309
etiology of, 309
laboratory and imaging studies for, 309–311,
385t
maternal, 205, 205t
prognosis for, 312
treatment of, 312
Systolic murmurs, 482–483
ejection, 482–483
due to aortic stenosis, 494
in total anomalous pulmonary venous
return, 498
in truncus arteriosus, 497

T

T-cell disorder(s), combined immunodeficiency
disease(s) due to, 258–262
T-cell proliferation, 255
T_3 (triiodothyronine)
in embryogenesis, 596–597
in thyroid function, 596–597, 597f
T_4. *see* Thyroxine (T_4)
Tachycardia
due to respiratory failure, 128
fetal, 189
sinus, 490t
supraventricular, 489, 490t
ventricular, 489, 490t
Tachypnea, 457
due to heart failure, 501
due to respiratory failure, 128
transient, of newborn, 191
Tacrolimus, for atopic dermatitis, 287
Taenia solium, 407, 407t
Talipes equinovarus, 681–682, 681f
Tanner stages
in boys, 238–240, 239f
in girls, 237–238, 238f–239f
Tantrums. *see* Temper tantrums
Tapeworms, 407t, 404
echinococcosis due to, 407
neurocysticercosis due to, 407
Tardive dyskinesia, 637
Target lesions, in erythema multiforme, 663–664
Targeted therapies, for cancer, 541

Tarsal coalition, 682–683
    calcaneonavicular, 682–683
    clinical manifestations of, 683
    radiologic evaluation of, 683
    talocalcaneal, 682–683
    treatment of, 683
Tarsal navicular, idiopathic avascular necrosis
        of, 683
Tarui disease, 172t
Tay-Sachs disease, 181t–182t, 642t–643t, 643
Tazarotene, for acne, 652
TBG (thyroxine-binding globulin)
    serum, 598t
    in thyroid function, 596–597
TBG (thyroxine-binding globulin) deficiency,
        congenital, 598
TBSA (total body surface area), 138
TBW (total body water), 106
    compartments of, 106, 107f
TCAs (tricyclic antidepressants), for somatoform
        disorder, 54
Td (tetanus-diphtheria toxoid), 321f–322f
Tdap (tetanus and diphtheria toxoids and
        acellular pertussis) vaccine, 319f–322f
TEE (transesophageal echocardiography), in
        cardiovascular system assessment, 486
Teeth
    deciduous (primary), 429, 429t
    eruption of, 429, 429t
        delayed, 429
    natal, 429
    permanent, 429, 429t
TEF. see Tracheoesophageal fistula (TEF)
Telangiectasia, 650t
    with developmental disabilities, 28t
Telecanthus, 161t
Teloradiograph, of leg-length discrepancy,
        678–679
Temper tantrums, 39–40, 40f
Temperament, 15
Temperature elevation, in newborn, 203
Temperature instability, in infants younger than 3
        months, 325
Temperature regulation, in newborn, 203
TEN (toxic epidermal necrolysis), 662–666, 663t
Tender points, in myofascial pain syndromes, 313
Tension pneumothorax, 478–479
Tension-type headache, 617
Teratogen(s), 153–154
    drugs used to treat maternal illnesses as, 206,
        206t
    isotretinoin as, 652
Teratoma, sacral, constipation due to, 426t
Tertian periodicity, of P. vivax and P. ovale, 403
Tertiary care intervention, for obesity, 93
Testicular pain, differential diagnosis of, 569
Testicular torsion, 569
Testis(es)
    detorsion and fixation of, 569
    differentiation of, 604–605, 605f
    disorders and abnormalities of, 568–569
        clinical manifestations of, 568
        complications of, 569
        etiology of, 568
        treatment of, 569
    retractile, 568
    torsion of, 569
    undescended, 568
Testosterone, in sexual differentiation, 604–605,
        604f–605f
Testosterone cypionate, for delayed puberty, 592
Testosterone enanthate, for delayed puberty, 592
Testosterone-like drugs, as teratogens, 206t
Testotoxicosis, familial, precocious puberty due
        to, 593t–594t

Tet spells, 495–496
Tetanus and diphtheria toxoids and acellular
        pertussis (Tdap) vaccine, 319f–322f
Tetanus-diphtheria toxoid (Td), 321f–322f
Tetanus immunoglobulin (TIG), 323
Tetanus prophylaxis, 323, 323t
Tetany, 602
    neonatal, 204, 602
Tethered cord, constipation due to, 426t
Tetracycline
    for acne, 652
    as teratogen, 206t
Tetrahydrobiopterin deficiency, 174–175
Tetralogy of Fallot, 495–496, 496f
TGF-β (transforming growth factor-β)
    functions of, 253t
    in Marfan syndrome, 148
α-Thalassemia, 514, 515f, 515t
β-Thalassemia intermedia, 515t
β-Thalassemia major, 518
    etiology and epidemiology of, 515t
Thalassemia minor, 514
    differential diagnosis of, 514t
    etiology and epidemiology of, 514, 515f, 515t
    laboratory testing for, 514
    treatment of, 514
β-Thalassemia minor, 514, 515t
α-Thalassemia trait, 515t
Thalidomide, as teratogen, 206t
Thanatophoric dysplasia, 147t
Thelarche, 237–238, 589
    premature, 596, 593t
Theophylline, for asthma, 276
Therapeutic monitoring, for drug toxicity, 143t
Thermal environment, of newborn, 203
Thermogenesis, in newborn, 203
Thiamine deficiency, 97, 98t–100t
Thiazides, maternal use of, 207t
Thigh-foot angle, 677, 677f
Thin basement membrane disease, 558–559
Third-degree heart block, 489
Third heart sound (S₃), 482
Third space losses, 108
Thoracic injury, 134–135
Thoracic scoliosis, 478
Thoracoscopic procedure, 460
Thoracotomy, 460
Threats, 23
Threshold, in hypertrophic pyloric stenosis,
        152
Throat culture, for streptococcal pharyngitis,
        348
Thrombasthenia, Glanzmann, 528
Thrombin, in hemostasis, 523, 524f
Thrombin time, 526t
Thrombocytopenia, 525f
    acquired, 526–527
    amegakaryocytic, 526–527
    bleeding disorder in newborn due to, 223
    clinical presentation of, 507t
    differential diagnosis of, 526–531, 527f
    due to cancer, 539t
    due to peripheral destruction, 527
    due to viral infections, 527
    in hemolytic uremic syndrome, 560
    isoimmune
        maternal, 205t
        in newborn, 223
    maternal
        idiopathic, 205, 205t
        isoimmune, 205t
    sequestration, due to decreased platelet
        production, 526–527
Thrombocytopenia with absent radii syndrome,
        526–527

Thrombocytopenic purpura
    idiopathic. see Idiopathic thrombocytopenic
        purpura (ITP)
    neonatal alloimmune, 527
    thrombotic, 528, 560
Thromboembolism, in nephrotic syndrome,
        557–558
Thrombophlebitis, 394
    septic, 394
Thromboplastin time, partial
    activated, 524–526, 525f, 526t
        in hemophilia, 529
    in newborn, 222
Thrombopoietin, 509
Thrombosis, 531
    catheter-related, 394
    clinical manifestations of, 507t, 531
    diagnostic and imaging studies of, 531
    etiology of, 531, 531f
    treatment of, 531
Thrombotic microangiopathy, 522, 528
Thrombotic thrombocytopenic purpura (TTP),
        528, 560
Thrush, 433
Thumb, trigger, 693
Thumb sign, in epiglottitis, 354
Thyroid carcinoma, 601
Thyroid disorders, 596–601
    hyperthyroidism as, 600–601
    hypothyroidism as, 598–600
    laboratory test results for, 598t
    tumors as, 601
Thyroid function, 596, 597f
Thyroid function tests, 597, 598t
Thyroid gland, physiology and development of,
        596–598, 597f
Thyroid hormone, and GH secretion, 584
Thyroid scan, 597–598
Thyroid-stimulating hormone (TSH), 596
    in embryogenesis, 596
    serum, 596, 598t
    in thyroid function, 596–597
Thyroid stimulating immunoglobulins (TSIs),
        600
Thyroid storm, 601
Thyroid tumors, 601
Thyroidectomy, for hyperthyroidism, 601
Thyroiditis, Hashimoto (autoimmune, chronic
        lymphocytic), 599
    with diabetes mellitus, 578
Thyrotropin-releasing hormone (TRH), 596, 597f
Thyroxine (T₄)
    in embryogenesis, 596
    free, 597, 598t
    in thyroid function, 596–597, 597f
    total, 598t
Thyroxine (T₄) deficiency, and growth, 584t
Thyroxine (T₄) excess, and growth, 584t
Thyroxine-binding globulin (TBG)
    serum, 598t
    in thyroid function, 596–597
Thyroxine-binding globulin (TBG) deficiency,
        congenital, 598
Tibia vara, 678
Tibial torsion, 667t
    external, 677
    internal, 676–677, 677f
Tibial tubercle, 679f
Tic(s), 637
Tick-borne infections, 396
Tick paralysis, 626
Tidal volume (TV), 455–456, 455f
TIG (tetanus immunoglobulin), 323
Timeout, 31
Tinea capitis, 336, 337t, 658

Tinea corporis, 336, 337t
Tinea cruris, 336, 337t
Tinea pedis, 336, 337t
Tinea unguium, 337t
Tinea versicolor, 337t
Tissue factor, in hemostasis, 523, 524f–525f
Tissue factor pathway inhibitor, in hemostasis, 523, 524f–525f
TLC (total lung capacity), 455–456, 455f
Tobacco smoke, and asthma, 275t
α-tocopherol, 101
Toddlers
    hearing and vision screening of, 21
    nutritional issues for, 89, 90t
Toddler's fracture, 674–675
Toe(s)
    curly, 683
    extra, 683, 689t
    fusion of, 683, 689t
Toe deformities, 683, 689t
Toe walking, 668
Tofranil (imipramine), maternal use of, 207t
Toilet training, 43
Tolerance, oral, 294
Toluene, as teratogen, 206t
Tone, in motor examination, 615
Tongue, strawberry
    in Kawasaki disease, 303
    red, 348
    white, 348
Tonic neck reflex, 613t
Tonsillar hypertrophy, 467
Tonsillitis, 347
Tonsillopharyngitis, 347
TORCH infection(s), 229–233, 230t
Torticollis, 688–689
Torus fracture, 670
Total anomalous pulmonary venous return, 498, 498f
Total body surface area (TBSA), 138
Total body water (TBW), 106
    compartments of, 106, 107f
Total lung capacity (TLC), 455–456, 455f
Tourette syndrome, 637
Toxemia, of pregnancy, 187
Toxic epidermal necrolysis (TEN), 662–666, 663t
Toxic ingestions, metabolic acidosis due to, 121
Toxic megacolon, 440
Toxic synovitis, 674, 674t
Toxocara canis, 405, 405t
Toxocara cati, 405, 405t
Toxocariasis, 405
Toxoids, for immunization, 317
Toxoplasma gondii, 398t–400t, 404
    congenital infection with, 229, 230t
    in immunocompromised person, 390
Toxoplasmosis, 398t–400t, 404
    congenital infection with, 229, 230t
Trachea, anatomy of, 455
Tracheal compression
    due to cancer, 539t
    extrinsic, 470
Tracheitis, bacterial, 354
    upper airway obstruction due to, 465t–466t
Tracheoesophageal fistula (TEF), 433–434, 470
    clinical manifestations of, 196t, 433, 433f
    complications of, 433–434
    etiology and epidemiology of, 433
    H-type, 433, 433f
    laboratory and imaging studies for, 433
    treatment and prognosis of, 433
Tracheomalacia, 470
Tracheostomy, 461
Tranquilizers, acute effects of, 250t–251t
Transbronchial lung biopsy, 459

Transcellular shifts, of potassium, 116
    hyperkalemia due to, 118t, 121
    hypokalemia due to, 116, 117t
Transcortin, 607
Transcription, 146
Transcutaneous electrodes, for respiratory gas exchange measurements, 459
Transesophageal echocardiography (TEE), in cardiovascular system assessment, 486
Transforming growth factor-β (TGF-β)
    functions of, 253t
    in Marfan syndrome, 148
Transfusion, 532
    products used in, 532, 532t
    transfusion reactions from, 532–533, 532t
Transfusion reactions, 532–533, 532t
Transfusion-transmitted virus (TTV), 370t
Transient erythroblastopenia of childhood, 516, 516t
Transient hypogammaglobulinemia of infancy, 257, 258t
Transient monoarticular synovitis, 674, 674t
Transient myeloproliferative disorder, 543
Transient tachypnea of the newborn, 191, 214
Translation, 146
Transplantation, for heart failure, 501t
Transposition of the great arteries, 496–497, 496f
Transtentorial (central) herniation, 636–637, 636t
Transudates, 479
Transverse myelitis, 624
Trauma, 133–136. *see also* Injury(ies)
    abdominal, 135
    assessment and resuscitation for, 133–134, 134t
    clinical manifestations and treatment of, 134–135
    complications of, 135
    degree of, in hemostatic disorders, 524
    Glasgow Coma Scale for, 133, 134t
    intestinal, 135
    laboratory and imaging studies for, 134, 134t
    liver, 135
    orthopedic problems due to, 667t
    pancreatic, 135
    prehospital care for, 133
    primary survey for, 133
    prognosis of, 136
    renal, 135
    secondary survey for, 134
    spinal cord, 134
    to spleen, 135
    tertiary survey for, 134
    thoracic, 134–135
Traumatic brain injury, 637–640
    disorders of consciousness due to, 634–637
        acute, 634–637, 635t
            assessment of, 634–636
            clinical manifestations of, 636–637, 636t
            etiology of, 636
            laboratory and diagnostic imaging of, 635t, 637
            prognosis of, 637
            treatment of, 637
            transient, recurrent, 637
    increased intracranial pressure due to, 640–642
        clinical manifestations of, 641
        etiology of, 636t, 640–641, 640t
        laboratory and diagnostic studies for, 641
        treatment of, 641–642
    with neurologic deficits, 637
        concussion as, 637–638
        drowsiness, headache and vomiting due to, 639
        due to cervical spine injuries, 639
        due to cranial nerve palsies, 638–639
        due to CSF leak, 638–639
        due to skull fractures, 638–639

Traumatic brain injury *(Continued)*
        intracranial hemorrhage in, 638–640, 638t
        seizures as, 639
        transient, 639
Traveler's diarrhea, 366t, 367
Trematodes, 404, 406t
Tremor, 637
Trench fever, 666
Trench mouth, 349
Trendelenburg gait, 668
Treponema pallidum, 376, 380
    congenital infection with, 230t, 232
Treponemal antibody tests, 380
Tretinoin (vitamin A analog)
    for acne, 652
    for cancer, 540t–541t
TRH (thyrotropin-releasing hormone), 596, 597f
Triad asthma, 284
Triamcinolone acetonide, for asthma, 279f
Triatoma bites, anaphylaxis due to, 293
Trichinella spiralis, 405t
Trichinellosis, 405t
Trichomonas vaginalis, 376, 383
Trichomoniasis, 376, 377t–378t, 383
Trichotillomania, 64
Trichuris trichiura, 405t
Tricuspid atresia, 497, 497f
Tricyclic antidepressants (TCAs), 58–59
Trifunctional protein
    in fatty acid catabolism, 180f, 179
    neonatal screening for, 170t
Trigeminal nerve, assessment of, 614
Trigger finger, 693
Trigger thumb, 693
Triiodothyronine (T_3)
    in embryogenesis, 596–597
    in thyroid function, 596–597, 597f
Trimethadione, as teratogen, 206t
Trimethadione, as teratogen, 206t
Triptans, for migraines, 620
Trisomic rescue, 157
Trisomy(ies), 157–158
    defined, 157
    Down syndrome as, 157
    Klinefelter syndrome as, 158
    trisomy 13 as, 158
    trisomy 18 as, 157–158
Trisomy 13, 158, 158t
Trisomy 18, 157–158, 158t
Trisomy 21, 157
    newborn assessment for, 196t
Trochlear nerve, assessment of, 614
Trophozoite, in *Plasmodium* life cycle, 402
Trousseau sign, 204, 602
Truncal ataxia, 631
Truncus arteriosus, 497–498, 497f
Trunk, congenital malformations of, 162
Trunk incurvation reflex, 613t
Trypanosoma brucei gambiense, 398t–400t
Trypanosoma brucei rhodesiense, 398t–400t
Trypanosoma cruzi, 398t–400t
    congenital infection with, 230t
Trypanosomiasis
    African, 398t–400t
    American, 398t–400t
Trypsin, 451
Tryptophan, 97
TSC1 gene, 646
TSC2 gene, 646
TSH. *see* Thyroid-stimulating hormone (TSH)
TSIs (thyroid stimulating immunoglobulins), 600
TTP (thrombotic thrombocytopenic purpura), 528, 560
TTV (transfusion-transmitted virus), 370t
Tubercle bacilli, 408
Tuberculin skin test (TST), 409, 409t–410t

Tuberculosis, 407–412
  clinical manifestations of, 408–409
  complications and prognosis of, 411
  congenital infection with, 230t
  differential diagnosis of, 410
  epidemiology of, 408
  etiology of, 407
  extrapulmonary, 410
  groups at high risk for, 22t
  laboratory and imaging studies of, 409–410
  latent, 408
  miliary, 408
  prevention of, 411–412
  primary
    progressive, 408
    pulmonary, 408
  pulmonary, 408
    primary, 408
    reactivation, 408
  screening and diagnosis of
    culture for, 409–410
    imaging for, 410
    tuberculin skin test for, 22, 409
  skeletal, 409
  synovial fluid findings in, 385t
  transmission of, 408
  treatment of, 410–411, 411t
  urogenital, 409
Tuberculous meningitis, 343t, 408–409
Tuberculous peritonitis, 409
Tuberculous pleural effusion, 408
Tuberous sclerosis, 646
  infantile spasms due to, 621
Tubers, 646
Tubular function, 553
Tularemia, 398t–400t
Tumor(s), 650
  bone, 693–694, 693t–694t
  CNS, 546–548
  orthopedic problems due to, 667t
  of skin, 650t, 651f
  syncope due to, 488t
Tumor lysis syndrome, 538, 539t
Tumor necrosis, degree of, 552
Tunnel infection, 394–395
Turner syndrome (TS), 158–159, 606
  amenorrhea due to, 242
  delayed puberty in, 592
  obesity in, 91t
  short stature in, 588, 588t
Twin-to-twin transfusion syndrome, 187
Twinning, 187
Two-point discrimination, 615
TYK2 gene, in hyper-IgE syndrome, 262
Tympanic membranes, of newborn, 199
Tympanic perforation, otitis media with, 353
Tympanocentesis, for otitis media, 352
Tympanometry, for otitis media, 351–352
Tympanostomy tube otorrhea, 353
Tympanostomy tubes, and otitis externa, 353
Typhoid fever, 366, 368
Typhus, 398t–400t
  epidemic, 398t–400t, 666
Tyrosine, metabolism of, 174f
Tyrosinemia(s), 175
  neonatal screening for, 170t
  type I, 175
  type II, 175
  type III, 175
Tzanck test, 655–656

U
UBE3A gene, in Angelman syndrome, 153
UC. see Ulcerative colitis

Ulcer(s), 651t
  duodenal, abdominal pain due to, 420t
  genital, 376, 377t
  peptic, 436
  pill, 434–435
Ulcerative colitis (UC), 440, 441t
Ultrasonography, 459
  for infectious diseases, 317
  of renal anomalies, 568
  of urinary system, 557
    for urinary tract infection, 373
Ultraviolet light therapy, for atopic dermatitis, 655
Umbilical arteries, Doppler examination of, 189
Umbilical cord
  care of, 191
  clamping or milking (stripping) of, 216
Umbilical hernias, 200
Uncal herniation, 636–637, 636t
Undescended testes, 568
Unilateral hyperlucent lung, 363
Unilocular cyst disease, 407
Uniparental disomy (UPD), 152–153
  Angelman syndrome due to, 153
  Prader-Willi syndrome as, 153
Upper airway obstruction, 464–468
  clinical manifestations of, 464
  defined, 464
  diagnostic studies for, 464
  differential diagnosis of, 467–468
    for acute disease, 465t–466t
    age-related, 464t
  due to adenoidal and tonsillar hypertrophy, 467
  due to angioedema, 465t–466t
  due to choanal stenosis/atresia, 467
  due to epiglottitis, 465t–466t
  etiology of, 464
  due to foreign body, 465t–466t
  due to laryngeal papillomatosis, 465t–466t
  due to laryngitis, 465t–466t
  due to laryngomalacia (floppy larynx), 467
  due to laryngotracheobronchitis (croup), 465t–466t
  due to mass lesions, 468
  due to membranous croup (bacterial tracheitis), 465t–466t
  due to peritonsillar abscess, 465t–466t
  due to retropharyngeal abscess, 465t–466t
  due to spasmodic croup, 465t–466t
  due to subglottic stenosis, 468
  supraglottic vs. subglottic, 466t
  due to vocal cord paralysis, 468
Upper extremity, 691–693
  elbow in, 692–693
    Panner disease of, 692
    radial head subluxation of, 692, 692f
    throwing injuries of, 692–693
  shoulder in, 691–692
    brachial plexus injuries of, 691
    glenohumeral dislocation of, 691
    overuse injuries of, 691
    proximal humeral epiphysiolysis of, 691–692
    Sprengel deformity of, 691
  wrist and hand in, 693
    finger abnormalities of, 693
    fractures of, 693
    ganglion cysts of, 693
Upper gastrointestinal (GI) series
  for gastroesophageal reflux, 431
  for inflammatory bowel disease, 441
Upper motor neuron disease, 624, 624t

Upper motor neurons, 623
Upper-to-lower segment ratio, 583–584
Urea cycle, 176f
Urea cycle disorders, neonatal screening for, 170t
Ureaplasma urealyticum, pneumonia due to, 359
Ureteropelvic junction obstruction, 566t, 568
Ureterovesical (UV) junction, in vesicoureteral reflux, 564–565
Ureters, vesicoureteral reflux due to duplication of, 565
Urethral syndrome, acute, 372
Urethral valves, posterior, 566
Urethritis
  nongonococcal, 379
  postcoital, 372
Urgency, due to renal disease, 554t
Urinalysis, 555–556
  in acute renal failure, 561
  for infectious diseases, 317
  macroscopic, 555–556
  microscopic, 555–556
  for urinary tract infection, 373
Urinary anion gap, 553–554
Urinary ascites, 566
Urinary calculi, 567
Urinary catheters, infections associated with, 395–396
Urinary concentrating capacity, 554
Urinary continence, 567
Urinary tract anomalies, 565–567
Urinary tract infections (UTIs), 372–374
  clinical manifestations of, 373, 554–555
  complications and prognosis for, 375
  differential diagnosis of, 373
  epidemiology of, 373
  etiology of, 372
  fever due to, 325
  hematuria due to, 559
  laboratory and imaging studies of, 373
  prevention of, 374
  relapse rate for, 374
  treatment of, 373–374
  urinary catheters and, 395
  vomiting due to, 423t
Urinary tract obstruction, 566, 566t
Urinary tract stones, 567–569
Urine amino acid profile, 171, 171t
Urine culture, for urinary tract infection, 373
Urine dipstick, 555–556
Urine formation, 553, 555f
Urine output, 108, 108t
Urine specific gravity, in dehydration, 109
Urine specimen, for urinary tract infection, 373–374
Urolithiasis, 567
  abdominal pain due to, 420t
  clinical manifestations of, 567
  diagnostic studies of, 567
  etiology of, 567
  hematuria due to, 559
  treatment of, 567
Urology assessment, 553–556
  common manifestations in, 554–555, 554t
  history in, 553
  imaging studies in, 558
  laboratory studies in, 555–556
  physical examination in, 553
Urticaria, 288–291
  acute, 288–289, 288t
  cholinergic, 289
  chronic, 288–289, 288t
  clinical manifestations of, 289–290, 290f
  cold, 289

Urticaria (Continued)
differential diagnosis of, 290–291
epidemiology of, 289
etiology of, 288–289
acute, 288–289, 288t
chronic, 288–289, 288t
laboratory and imaging studies for, 290, 290t
physical, 288–289
pigmentosa, vesiculobullous eruptions due to, 663t
prevention of, 291
treatment of, 291
Urticarial rash, infections with fever and, 329t–330t
Urticarial vasculitis, 290–291
Uterine abnormalities, intrauterine growth restriction and small for gestational age due to, 208t
Uterine compression, deformation, abnormalities due to, 668, 669f
UTIs. see Urinary tract infections
UV (ureterovesical) junction, in vesicoureteral reflux, 564–565
Uveitis
anterior, 388t–389t
in juvenile idiopathic arthritis, 306
posterior, 388t–389t

V

V/Q (ventilation-perfusion) matching, 456
V/Q (ventilation-perfusion) mismatching, 456, 456t
Vaccine Adverse Event Reporting System (VAERS), 318
Vaccine Information Statements, 318
Vaccines and vaccination
administration of, 317
catch-up, 321f–322f
contraindications to, 318
human papillomavirus, 319f–322f
informed consent for, 318
recommended schedule for, 319f–320f
VACTERL association, 161
and tracheoesophageal fistula, 433
VAERS (Vaccine Adverse Event Reporting System), 318
Vagal maneuvers, 490
Vaginal bleeding, during pregnancy, 186
Vaginal discharge
physiologic, 374, 375t
vs. sexually transmitted infections, 377t–378t
Vaginal sponge (Protectaid), 247
Vaginitis
Gardnerella vaginalis-associated, 374
nonspecific, 374, 375t
vulvo-. see Vulvovaginitis
Vaginosis, bacterial, 374, 375t, 377t–378t
Valacyclovir
for genital herpes, 380–381
for varicella-zoster virus, 334–335
Valgum, 667t
Valgus, 667t
Valine, metabolism of, 176f
Valproate, as teratogen, 206t
Valproic acid, for status epilepticus, 621–622, 622t
Value differences, ethical issues due to, 5
Vanillylmandelic acid (VMA), with neuroblastoma, 548
Variable expressivity, 147
Varicella, 333–334
vesiculobullous eruptions due to, 663t
Varicella vaccine, 335, 317–318, 319f–322f
Varicella-zoster immunoglobulin (VZIG), 335
in immunocompromised person, 394

Varicella-zoster virus (VZV), 333–335
clinical manifestations of, 334
complications and prognosis for, 662
congenital infection with, 230t
differential diagnosis of, 334
epidemiology of, 334
etiology of, 333–334
in HIV, 415
in immunocompromised person, 391
laboratory and imaging studies for, 334
prevention of, 335
treatment of, 334–335
vesiculobullous eruptions due to, 663t
Varix(ices), esophageal, 448
GI bleeding due to, 427t
Varum, 667t
Varus, 667t
Vascular anomalies, 661–662
Vascular catheters, infections associated with, 394
Vascular device infections, 394–395
Vascular malformation(s), 662
defined, 661
port-wine stain (nevus flammeus) as, 662f, 662
pyogenic granuloma as, 662
salmon patch stain (nevus simplex) as, 662
tracheal compression due to, 470
Vascular rings, tracheal compression due to, 470
Vasculitis(ides)
vs. angioedema, 291t
differential diagnosis of, 302, 304t
in rheumatic diseases, 299
urticarial, 290–291
Vasoconstriction, hypoxic pulmonary, 456
Vasodepressor syncope, 488t
Vasomotor rhinitis, 283–284
Vasoocclusive painful events, in sickle cell anemia, 519
Vasopressin, in renal function, 553, 555f
VATS (video-assisted thoracoscopic surgery), for pleural effusion, 480
VC (vital capacity), 455–456, 455f
VCUG (voiding cystourethrogram), 557
for urinary tract infection, 373
for vesicoureteral reflux, 565
Vegans, vitamin and nutrient deficiencies in, 97t
Vegetations, in infective endocarditis, 364
Velban (vinblastine), for cancer, 540t–541t
Velocardiofacial syndrome, 159–160, 260
Venereal Disease Research Laboratory (VDRL) test, 232, 380
Venom immunotherapy, for insect allergies, 296
Venous hum, 484, 484t
Venous malformation, 659t
Ventilation, 126
control of, 461–464, 461f
disorder(s) of, 461–464, 463t
acute life-threatening event as, 461–462
apnea as, 463–464, 463t
SIDS as, 462–463, 462t
minute, 461
noninvasive, for respiratory failure, 131
Ventilation-perfusion (V/Q) matching, 456
Ventilation-perfusion (V/Q) mismatching, 456, 456t
Ventilator-associated pneumonia, 395
Ventricular contractions, premature, 489, 490t
Ventricular dysrhythmias, 489
Ventricular fibrillation, 490t
Ventricular function curve, 499–500, 499f
Ventricular septal defect (VSD), 491–492, 491f
clinical manifestations of, 491
etiology and epidemiology of, 491
imaging studies of, 491
perimembranous, 491

Ventricular septal defect (VSD) (Continued)
in tetralogy of Fallot, 495–496
treatment of, 491–492
tricuspid atresia with, 497f
Ventricular tachycardia, 489, 490t
Ventriculoperitoneal shunts
for hydrocephalus, 642
infections associated with, 400
VER (visual evoked response), 32
Vernix caseosa, 197
Verotoxins (VTs), in hemolytic uremic syndrome, 560
Verruca
plana, 338
vulgaris, 338
Vertebral osteomyelitis, 382
Vertical transmission, of HIV, 412
Very long chain acyl-CoA dehydrogenase (VLCAD), neonatal screening for, 170t
Very long chain acyl-CoA dehydrogenase (VLCAD) deficiency, 180f, 179
Very low birth weight (VLBW) infants, 188
Vesicle, 650t, 651f
Vesicoureteral reflux (VUR), 564–565
classification of, 565f
clinical manifestations of, 565
defined, 564–565
diagnostic studies of, 565, 565f
etiology and epidemiology of, 564–565
treatment of, 565
urinary tract infection due to, 373, 565
Vesicular rash, infections with fever and, 329t–330t
Vesicular stomatitis, 398t–400t
Vesiculobullous eruptions, 663t
Vespid stings, allergic reactions to, 293
Vibratory murmurs, 484t
Video-assisted thoracoscopic surgery (VATS), for pleural effusion, 480
Video endoscopy, for gastrointestinal symptoms, 417
Videofluoroscopic swallowing study, 469–470
Vinblastine (Velban), for cancer, 540t–541t
Vinca alkaloids, for cancer, 540t–541t
Vincent angina, 349
Vincent infection, 349
Vincristine (Oncovin), for cancer, 540t–541t
Vineland Adaptive Behavior Scale-II (2nd ed), 29t
Violence, 79–82
dating, 82
domestic, 79–80, 80t
prevention of, 24t–25t, 81–82
youth, 80–82, 81t
Violent crime, 3
Viral diseases, zoonotic, 398t–400t
Viral encephalitis, 344–345
Viral gastroenteritis, vomiting due to, 423t
Viral hepatitis, 369–372
Viral infection(s)
and asthma, 275t
bacterial vs., 317t, 325
in immunocompromised person, 391
superficial, 336–338
due to herpes simplex virus, 336–338
due to human papillomavirus, 338
molluscum contagiosum as, 338
thrombocytopenia due to, 527
Viral meningitis, 343t
Virilization, of 46,XX female, 605, 605t
Virus-associated hemophagocytic syndrome, 516t
Visceral larva migrans, 405–406, 405t
Visceral pain, in appendicitis, 443
Visceral trauma, in newborn, 203
Vision, partial, 31

Vision impairment, 31–32
    developmental implications of, 32
    diagnosis of, 32
    epidemiology of, 31
    etiology of, 31
    interventions for, 32
    mild to moderate, 32
    severe, 31
Vision screening
    of children 3 years of age and older, 21
    of infants and toddlers, 21
    of newborns, 32
Visual acuity, assessment of, 614
Visual evoked response (VER), 32
Vital capacity (VC), 455–456, 455f
Vital signs, of newborn, 196
Vitamin A, as teratogen, 206t
Vitamin A analog (tretinoin)
    for acne, 652
    for cancer, 540t–541t
Vitamin A deficiency, 96, 98t–100t, 101
Vitamin B$_1$ deficiency, 97, 98t–100t
Vitamin B$_2$ deficiency, 97, 98t–100t
Vitamin B$_3$ deficiency, 97, 98t–100t
Vitamin B$_6$ deficiency, 98, 98t–100t
Vitamin B$_{12}$ deficiency, 98t–100t, 100–101
    anemia due to, 510f
Vitamin C deficiency, 96–97, 99t–100t
Vitamin D
    parathyroid hormone and, 602
    for rickets, 603
    as teratogen, 206t
Vitamin D deficiency, 98t–100t, 102, 603,
    603t
Vitamin D-dependent rickets, 603
Vitamin D$_2$, 102
Vitamin D$_3$, 102
Vitamin deficiencies, 96–105
    of ascorbic acid (Vitamin C), 96–97, 99t–100t
    of biotin, 98t–100t
    fat soluble, 98t, 101–103
    of folate, 98–100, 98t–100t
    of niacin (vitamin B$_3$), 97, 98t–100t
    of pantothenic acid, 98t
    of pyridoxine (vitamin B$_6$), 98, 98t–100t
    of riboflavin (vitamin B$_2$), 97, 98t–100t
    of thiamine (vitamin B$_1$), 97, 98t–100t
    of vitamin A, 98t–100t, 101
    of vitamin B$_{12}$, 98t–100t, 100–101
    of vitamin D, 98t–100t, 102
    of vitamin E, 98t–100t, 101
    of vitamin K, 98t–100t, 102–103
    treatment of, 99t
    water-soluble, 96–101, 98t
Vitamin E deficiency, 98t–100t, 101
    hemolytic anemia due to, 522
Vitamin K deficiency, 98t–100t, 102–103
    coagulation disorders due to, 222
Vitamin K prophylaxis, for newborn, 191
Vitamin K$_1$, 102
Vitamin K$_2$, 102
Vitamins, in parenteral nutrition, 113
VLBW (very low birth weight) infants, 188
VLCAD (very long chain acyl-CoA
    dehydrogenase), neonatal screening for,
    170t
VLCAD (very long chain acyl-CoA
    dehydrogenase) deficiency, 180f, 179
VMA (vanillylmandelic acid), with
    neuroblastoma, 548
Vocal cord(s), anatomy of, 455–456
Vocal cord paralysis, 468
    clinical manifestations of, 468
    etiology of, 468
    treatment and prognosis for, 468

Vocal fremitus, 458t
Voice disorders, 34–35
Voice signs, 458t
Voiding cystourethrogram (VCUG), 557
    for urinary tract infection, 373
    for vesicoureteral reflux, 565
Voiding dysfunction, 567–568
    clinical manifestations of, 567–568
    diagnostic studies of, 568
    etiology of, 567
    treatment of, 568
Volume depletion, 106–107
Volume expansion, 106–107
Volume overload, 106–107
Volume status, regulation of, 106
Volvulus, 196t
    GI bleeding due to, 427t
    midgut malrotation with, 437, 438f
Vomiting, 422–423
    after head injury, 639
    assessment of, 422
    cyclic, 422, 423t
    defined, 422
    differential diagnosis of, 422, 423t
        vs. regurgitation, 422
    distinguishing features of, 422–423, 423t
    treatment of, 423
von Recklinghausen disease
    clinical manifestations of, 645–646
    genetic basis for, 645
von Willebrand disease
    clinical manifestations of, 530
    differential diagnosis of, 529t
    epidemiology of, 523
    etiology of, 523, 530
    laboratory testing for, 530
    treatment of, 530
von Willebrand factor (vWF)
    in hemostasis, 523, 524f
    in von Willebrand disease, 530
von Willebrand factor (vWF) antigen,
    530
VP-16 (etoposide), for cancer, 540t–541t
VTs (verotoxins), in hemolytic uremic syndrome,
    560
Vulnerable child syndrome, 79
Vulvovaginal candidiasis, 378t
Vulvovaginitis, 374–375
    characteristics of, 375t
    clinical manifestations of, 374
    complications and prognosis for, 375
    defined, 374
    diagnosis of, 375t
    differential diagnosis of, 374
    epidemiology of, 374
    etiology of, 374
    laboratory and imaging studies for, 374
    prevention of, 375
    treatment of, 374–375
VUR. see Vesicoureteral reflux (VUR)
vWF. see von Willebrand factor (vWF)
Vyvanse (Lisdexamfetamine), for ADHD,
    42t
VZIG (varicella-zoster immunoglobulin),
    325
    in immunocompromised person, 394
VZV. see Varicella-zoster virus (VZV)

W

Waddling gait, 668
WAGR (Wilms tumor, aniridia, genitourinary
    anomalies, and mental retardation)
    syndrome, 159, 550
WAIS-III (Wechsler Adult Intelligence
    Scale-Revised), 29t

Wandering atrial pacemaker, 489
Warfarin, for thrombosis, 531
Warts, 338
    common, 338
    filiform, 338
    flat, 338
    genital, 338, 376, 383
        clinical features of, 378t
        diagnosis of, 381
        pathogenesis of, 384
        treatment of, 381
    plantar, 338
Wasp stings, allergic reactions to, 293
Wasting, 94t
    severe, 94t
Water
    in body composition, 106, 107f
    plasma, 106, 107f
    total body, 106
    compartments of, 106, 107f
Water balance, and sodium balance,
    112–113
Water losses
    clinical causes of, 108t
    due to increased urine output, 108, 108t
    gastrointestinal sources, 108
    hypernatremia due to, 114, 115f
    insensible, 107
    normal causes of, 108
WBC (white blood cell) abnormalities, due to
    lysosomal storage diseases, 181t–182t
Weakness, 623–631
    clinical manifestations of, 623–624, 624t
    disorders causing, 624t
    due to lower motor neuron, 624–630
        infant botulism as, 627
        of muscle, 627–628
        myasthenia gravis as, 626–627
        peripheral neuropathy as, 625–626
        spinal muscular atrophy as, 624–625
    due to spinal cord disease, 624
    due to stroke, 630–631, 630t
    due to upper motor neuron disease,
        624
        clinical manifestations of, 624, 624t
        etiology and epidemiology of, 624
    etiology of, 623
    facial and bulbar, 625t
    hypotonia without significant, 629–630,
        630t
    limb
        distal, 625t
        ophthalmoplegia and, 625t
    malignant hyperthermia, 629
    in neonatal and infantile hypotonia, 629, 629f,
        630t
    proximal muscle, 625t
Wechsler Adult Intelligence Scale-Revised
    (WAIS-III), 29t
Wechsler Intelligence Scale for Children (4th ed)
    (WISC IV), 29t
Wechsler Primary and Preschool Test of
    Intelligence-Revised (WPPSI-R), 29t
Weight
    benchmarks for, 10, 10t
    growth charts for, 11f
Well child visits, 15–16
    anticipatory guidance in, 23–25, 24t–25t
    dental care in, 23
    fostering optimal development in, 23–25
    immunizations in, 22
    nutritional assessment in, 23
    safety issues in, 23
    schedule of preventive measures in,
        15–16, 17f

Well child visits *(Continued)*
screening tests in, 17f, 21–22
for anemia, 21
for cholesterol, 22, 22t
hearing and vision, 21
for lead, 21–22
newborn, 21
for sexually transmitted infections, 22
for tuberculosis, 22, 22t
topics for, 15–16, 16t
Wenckebach heart block, 489, 490t
Werdnig-Hoffman disease, 624–625
Wernicke aphasia, 613
Wessel's rule of threes, 37
West African sleeping sickness, 398t–400t
West Nile encephalitis, 345
West syndrome, 621
Western black-legged tick, 396
Wet beriberi, 97
Wheal, 650t, 651f
Wheezing, 457
defined, 469
differential diagnosis of, 359, 469t
due to lower airway disease, 469
White blood cell (WBC) abnormalities, due to
lysosomal storage diseases, 181t–182t
White reflex, in newborn, 199
White strawberry tongue, 348
Whitehead, 652
Whitlow, herpetic, 337–338
Whole blood, transfusion of, 532
Whole-bowel irrigation, for drug toxicity, 143
Whooping cough syndrome, 356
Williams syndrome, 159
Wilms tumor, 550–551
aniridia, genitourinary anomalies, and mental
retardation (WAGR) syndrome, 159, 550
bilateral, 550
clinical manifestations of, 550
complications of, 550
differential diagnosis of, 550
epidemiology of, 550
etiology of, 550
laboratory/imaging studies of, 550
prognosis for, 550–551
risk factors for, 536t
treatment of, 550

Wilson disease, 449–450, 642t–643t, 644
Window period, for hepatitis B virus, 371
Wireless capsule endoscopy, for gastrointestinal
symptoms, 417
WISC IV (Wechsler Intelligence Scale for
Children (4th ed)), 29t
Wiskott-Aldrich syndrome, 260, 261t, 286–287,
528
Wolman disease, 181t–182t
Wood smoke, and asthma, 275t
Wood tick, 401
Wound care, for burns, 138–139
Wound infection, zoonotic, 398t–400t
WPPSI-R (Wechsler Primary and Preschool Test
of Intelligence-Revised), 29t
Wrist, 693
finger abnormalities of, 693
fractures of, 693
ganglion cysts of, 693
square window, in newborn, 197f
WT genes, 550

X
X chromosome, 146
X-linked agammaglobulinemia, 256, 258t
X-linked dominant inheritance, 150–151
incontinentia pigmenti due to, 150–151
Rett syndrome due to, 150–151
vitamin D-resistant rickets due to,
150–151
X-linked hyper-IgM syndrome, 258, 259f,
259t
X-linked lymphoproliferative disease, 261, 261t,
341
X-linked recessive inheritance, 150, 151t
adrenoleukodystrophy due to, 151t
colorblindness due to, 151t
defined, 150
Duchenne muscular dystrophy due to,
151t
fragile X syndrome due to, 151t
G6PD deficiency due to, 151t
hemophilia A due to, 151t
Rett syndrome due to, 151t
X-linked thrombocytopenia, isolated,
260
Xanthines, for apnea of prematurity, 220

Xanthogranuloma, juvenile, 659t
Xerophthalmia, 101
Xerosis
of conjunctiva and cornea, 101
due to allergy, 272
Xolair (omalizumab), for asthma, 276

Y
Y chromosome, 146
Yale-Brown obsessive-compulsive scale
(Y-BOCS), 62
Yeast infections, superficial, 337t
Yellow jacket stings, allergic reactions to,
293
Yersinia enterocolitica, 398t–400t
diarrhea due to, 366t, 367
Yersinia pestis, 398t–400t
Yersinia pseudotuberculosis, 398t–400t
Yersiniosis, 398t–400t
Youth violence, 80–82, 81t

Z
Zafirlukast, for asthma, 275–276
Zellweger syndrome, 180–183
Zileuton, for asthma, 275–276
Zinc deficiency, 96, 103t, 104–105
Zinc deficiency dwarfism, 104–105
Zoonosis(es), 396–402
defined, 396
ehrlichiosis and anaplasmosis as, 401–402
epidemiology of, 396
Lyme disease as, 396–400
prevention of, 402
Rocky Mountain spotted fever as, 401
spread of, 396
Zoster, 333–335
clinical manifestations of, 334
complications and prognosis for, 335
defined, 333–334
differential diagnosis of, 334
epidemiology of, 334
etiology of, 333–334
in immunocompromised person, 391
laboratory and imaging studies for, 334
prevention of, 335
treatment of, 334–335
vesiculobullous eruptions due to, 663t